HOWKINS & BOURNE

SHAW'S TEXTBOOK OF GYNAECOLOGY

17th Edition

HOWKINS & BOURNE
SHAW'S TEXTBOOK OF GYNAECOLOGY

Edited by

Sunesh Kumar, MD (AIIMS)
Professor and Chief Gynae Oncology Services,
Department of Obstetrics and Gynaecology,
All India Institute of Medical Sciences,
New Delhi

Emeritus Editors

VG Padubidri, MS, FRCOG (LOND)
Formerly Director Professor and Head,
Department of Obstetrics and Gynaecology
Lady Hardinge Medical College, New Delhi

Shirish N Daftary, MD, DGO, FICS, FIC, FICOG
Emeritus Professor, Formerly Dean and Medical Advisor,
Nowrosjee Wadia Maternity Hospital, Mumbai
Past President, FOGSI

ELSEVIER

ELSEVIER

RELX India Pvt. Ltd.
Registered Office: 818, Indraprakash Building, 8th Floor, 21, Barakhamba Road, New Delhi-110001
Corporate Office: 14th Floor, Building No. 10B, DLF Cyber City, Phase II, Gurgaon-122002, Haryana, India

Shaw's Textbook of Gynecology, 17e, Sunesh Kumar, VG Padubidri, and Shirish N Daftary

ISBN: 978-81-312-5411-0
e-Book ISBN: 978-81-312-5412-7

First printed in India 2018, Reprinted 2019 (twice)

Content Strategist: Sheenam Aggarwal
Content Project Manager: Shivani Pal
Sr Cover Designer: Milind Majgaonkar
Sr Production Executive: Ravinder Sharma

Typeset by GW Tech India
Printed in India by Replika Press Pvt. Ltd.

Dedicated to my teachers, especially Late Prof. Vera Hingorani

Preface to the 17th Edition

Seventeenth Edition of this popular book *"Shaw's Textbook of Gynaecology"* is in your hands. Writing preface to this new edition brings me the nostalgic memory of my student days when all the students read this book and when each word written in the book was like a statement from experts. Last sixty years since first edition of the book has seen lot of advancement in the speciality of gynaecology. IVF and Endoscopic surgery are two very important advances which has made speciality of gynaecology challenging with a bright future.

I have made best efforts to update most of the topics. Such an endeavour was possible only with active support of my colleagues, residents and other staff. My special thanks are due to Dr. Anshu Yadav, Dr. Aarthi S Jayraj, Dr. Rohitha C and other Residents in my department for helping me reviewing the text, video recording and collecting photographs. Professor Sandeep Mathur of Pathology at AIIMS, New Delhi provided excellent coloured photomicrographs.

I do not have enough words to express my thanks to my secretary, Ms. Sapna Gulati for doing writing, editing and correction work in the textbook in a professional manner. Special thanks are due to Ms. Shivani Pal and Ms. Sheenam Agarwal of Elsevier India for their patience and persistence.

Realizing extreme hardship faced by students before final examinations a new section of Audio-visual presentation on important topics has been added.

Do send your comments for improving future publications.

Sunesh Kumar

Preface to the 16th Edition

We, the editors of *Howkins and Bourne Shaw's Textbook of Gynaecology*, are pleased to acknowledge that this book has continued to provide basic foundation of this speciality since 1936. Keeping in view of the popularity of the book, the first Indian edition (10th edition) was published in 1989. Since then, the book has been updated from time to time in the light of the advances made in this speciality. The 15th edition was revised in 2010. Our commitment to the students to improve and update the quality of the book, and provide them with the advanced knowledge prompted us to bring out the 16th edition.

In this edition, not only we have added the latest knowledge on the subject, but also inserted more illustrations, flowcharts and tables to make the reading easier and understandable. We have added more MRI, CT, and many other illustrations wherever required.

Considering the high associated morbidity and mortality of gynaecological malignancies, we have approached the topic of genital tract cancers more exhaustively in this edition. Emphasis has also been laid on the gynaecological problems amongst adolescents and menopausal women. Minimal invasive surgery for the benign conditions is now being replaced by non-surgical therapy such as MRI-guided ablative therapy without the need for hospitalization. Hopefully these procedures will turn safe and effective in near future.

A website of the book has been created for more information on the subject in the form of video clips, online testing and MCQs for entrance tests and the latest updates on the subject.

We owe our special thanks to the entire staff of Elsevier for their wholehearted support and encouragement. We will fail in our duty if we did not make a special reference to Shabina Nasim with whom we interact on a daily basis and also Renu Rawat. We appreciate their professional attitude and their knowledge towards the project, their efficiency and enormous patience to bring out the best for this project.

Our very special thanks and gratitude go to Mr YR Chadha, Publishing Consultant, BI Churchill Livingstone, New Delhi, who initiated and guided us in the First Indian Edition in 1989, without whose persuasion and encouragement this book would not have seen the day. There are many others who have worked behind the scene, we acknowledge our thanks to them.

Last, but not the least, we thank our readers and the student community for their unstinted support over the last 25 years.

VG Padubidri
Shirish N Daftary

Preface to the 10th Edition

Ever since *Shaw's Textbook of Gynaecology* appeared in the United Kingdom in 1936, it has maintained its popularity with teachers, examiners and the student community. It has gone through several editions. The ninth edition, edited by Dr John Howkins and Dr Gordon Bourne, was brought out in 1971, and its popularity in India has remained undiminished. It is therefore timely and opportune that this standard textbook should be revised by Indian teachers of gynaecology to meet the requirements of our undergraduate students. We consider ourselves fortunate for having been assigned this challenging task by the publishers.

In revising the book we have endeavoured to update the contents to include new methods of investigations and treatment. In particular, recent advances in the physiology of menstruation and its hormonal control, carcinoma of the cervix and related preventive measures, endometriosis, and the management of tuberculosis of the genital tract have been incorporated. In addition, the latest methods of birth control and a separate chapter on Medical Termination of Pregnancy have been added to equip our students with the knowledge required to promote India's family welfare programme.

We have also tried to make the text more concise by deleting information that we felt was unnecessary for the Indian undergraduate student, without substantially changing the original style.

We are indebted to Mr YR Chadha, Publishing Director of BI Churchill Livingstone, New Delhi for his constant encouragement and invaluable suggestions in the preparation of this edition. Sincere thanks are extended to Churchill Livingstone, Edinburgh, for their assistance in making this edition possible.

VG Padubidri
Shirish N Daftary

Table of Content

To access the videos and lecture PPTs, scan the symbols and provided in the chapters.

Approach to a Gynaecological Patient

1

CHAPTER OUTLINE

The term *gynaecology* (from the Greek, *gynae* meaning woman and *logos* means discourse) pertains to the diseases of women and is generally used for diseases related to the female genital organs.

The interaction of a patient with a physician can often be an anxiety-producing event, particularly so in the practice of gynaecology because of the sensitive nature of the problems that need to be discussed; hence, the observance of the highest standards of ethical and professional behaviour is required to establish rapport, while not creating a hostile environment in which the patient feels embarrassed or uncomfortable to allow a meaningful assessment of her underlying medical problem.

The following four ethical principles must be integrated into the care and nature of services offered to every patient.

1. **Privacy and respect:** Nowadays, counselling forms an important aspect of consultation. The nature of the gynaecological ailment, reason for a particular investigation and its predictive value should be discussed. The discussion on treatment options with their demerits and merits will enable a woman to choose the treatment she considers best for her. The gynaecologist should, however, guide her in making the right decision. The clinician must respect the patient as an individual. Remember that the patient has the right to make decisions about her health care. It is not ethically or morally right to enforce the physician's opinion on the patient. This will safeguard against any charge of negligence, if a medicolegal problem arises at a later date. The records should be properly maintained and the documents should be preserved. The patient should feel assured at all times about 'privacy and confidentiality'. Talking softly and patiently listening are of a great help.
2. **Beneficence:** The medical attendant must be vigilant to ensure that the therapeutic advice rendered to the patient should be in 'good faith'. It should be aimed at benefiting her. All medical measures adopted during the course of medical treatment should be guided and evaluated on the basis of the principle of the cost/benefit ratio accruing out of the medical advice given.
3. **Justice:** This is rendered when the physician makes access to care, the type of care, the attention provided and the cost of care equitable to the needs of the patient.
4. **Avoiding litigations**: In modern times, it is important to avoid investigations and treatment which may lead to possible litigations in future. For a detailed description it is advised to consult descriptions given by Ley P, Lipkin M Jr, Simpson M, Buckman R, Stewart M, Todd AD, Fisher S.

History and physical examination constitute the fundamental tools on which rest the tentative diagnosis, the tests to be undertaken and the treatment to be recommended (Table 1.1).

HISTORY

Careful history and physical examination form the basis of patient evaluation, clinical diagnosis and management. Investigations are made to confirm the diagnosis and for the follow-up of treatment.

It is advisable to ask the patient to describe her main complaint in her own words and take her own time narrating the evolution of the problem, the aggravating and relieving factors and the investigations and treatment she has already undergone. Good and patient listening is essential to obtain maximum cooperation during the subsequent pelvic examination.

History begins with the recording of the basic information about the patient as shown in the sample pro forma in Table 1.1.

PRESENT ILLNESS

The clinician must record the patient's complaints in the sequence in which they occurred, noting their duration, their aggravating and relieving factors and their relation to menstruation, micturition and defecation. The investigations performed and the response to treatment given so far should be noted.

PAST AND PERSONAL HISTORY

Past medical and surgical problems may have a bearing on the present complaints. For example, a history of diabetes

Table 1.1 1 History: Gynaecological Case Record Form

Name	Age	Marital Status Married/Single/ Unmarried
Presenting complaints:		
Menstrual History: Last menstrual period (LMP) Present menstrual cycles Previous menstrual cycles Age at menarchae Age at Menopause		
Previous Obstetric History: Full term deliveries Preterm deliveries Abortions (Spontaneous/ Induced) Ectopic pregnancy Living issues		
Contraception used:		
Past Medical History: Diabetes Hypertension Thyroid disorders Tuberculosis Any surgery		
Family History: History of cancers in family members History of DM/hypertension		
Personal History: Smoking Addictions Drugs		

may suggest that pruritus vulva may be due to genital candidiasis, and history of sexually transmitted disease (STD) may have a direct bearing on future infertility.

History of pelvic inflammatory disease (PID) or puerperal sepsis may be associated with menstrual disturbances, lower abdominal pain, congestive dysmenorrhoea and infertility. Tuberculosis may lead to oligomenorrhoea and infertility. History of endocrinopathy may affect her sexual functions. Medical diseases such as hypertension, cardiac disease, anaemia, diabetes, asthma and the like will require to be controlled before a planned surgery. Previous blood transfusion and drug allergy should be noted. This has special reference to HIV and hepatitis B infection.

Previous abdominal surgery such as caesarean section, removal of the appendix and excision for ovarian cyst may lead to pelvic adhesions, which may be the cause of abdominal pain, backache, retroverted fixed uterus, infertility and menstrual disturbances. Dyspareunia is often the result of pelvic adhesions.

Allergies to any drug, current medication, use of alcohol, smoking, drug abuse and lifestyle have relevance in the management.

FAMILY HISTORY

Certain problems run in families, e.g. menstrual patterns tend to be similar amongst members of the family. Premature menopause, menorrhagia and dysmenorrhoea may occur in more than one member in a family. Similarly, female members of some families are more prone to cancer of the ovary, uterus and breast. Diabetes, hypertension, thyroid disorders, allergic diathesis and functional disorders are often familial in nature. Genetic and hereditary disorders affect more than one member in the family, e.g. thalassaemia. Tuberculosis may affect many members in the family.

MARITAL AND SEXUAL HISTORY

Note the details of her marital life such as the frequency of coitus, dyspareunia, frigidity, achievement of orgasm, libido, use of contraceptives and the method used. The relevance of dyspareunia to infertility should be noted.

MENSTRUAL HISTORY

Normal menarche and menstrual cycle have been described in Chapter 4.

The term *menorrhagia* denotes excessive blood loss (increase in duration of bleeding/heavier blood flow) without any change in the cycle length. The term menorrhagia is now replaced by 'abnormal uterine bleeding' (AUB) and will be addressed in this chapter. The term *polymenorrhoea* or *epimenorrhoea* refers to frequent menstrual cycles as a result of shortening of the cycle length. Sometimes women suffer from a menstrual disorder characterized by a shorter duration of the cycles coupled with a heavier flow or prolongation in the duration of the flow; this condition is termed as *polymenorrhagia*. The severity of AUB can be assessed by taking into account the number of sanitary pads required per day, history of passing blood clots, the presence of anaemia and evaluating the presence of accompanying symptoms such as fatigue, palpitation, dizziness, breathlessness on exertion and the presence of pallor. Menorrhagia and polymenorrhagia are frequently present in women with myomas, adenomyosis and PID in women wearing intrauterine contraceptive devices (IUCDs) and also due to hormonal imbalance causing dysfunctional uterine bleeding (DUB) in perimenopausal women. AUB now replaces the word DUB.

Oligomenorrhoea is the term used to describe infrequent menses. In this condition, the cycle length is prolonged without affecting the duration and amount of flow. *Hypomenorrhoea* refers to the condition in which the cycle length remains unaltered; however, the duration of bleeding or the amount of blood loss, or both are substantially reduced. When the complete cessation of menstruation occurs, the condition is described as amenorrhoea. The problems of *oligomenorrhoea* and *hypomenorrhoea* are encountered in conditions such as *polycystic ovarian disease (PCOD)*, *hyperprolactinaemia* and *genital tuberculosis,* in women on oral contraceptive pills, in association with certain neoplasms of the pituitary or ovary, in functional hypothalamic disorders and in psychiatric disorders. Drugs may occasionally be implicated. Oligomenorrhoea and hypomenorrhoea may occasionally progress to amenorrhoea. Amenorrhoea is physiological during pregnancy, lactation, before puberty and after menopause. *Metrorrhagia* (now addressed as intermenstrual bleeding) means the occurrence of intermenstrual bleeding, and it may occur in association with ovulation (mittelschmerz); however, it is commonly associated with the presence of neoplasms such as uterine polyps, carcinoma cervix and uterine and lower genital tract malignancy. It may occur with conditions such as vascular erosions, using intrauterine devices or breakthrough bleeding in oral pill users. However, this symptom calls for thorough investigation because of a possible malignant cause. Sometimes the patient may present with the complaint of *continuous bleeding*, so that the normal pattern can no longer be distinguished. Such episodes may be of functional origin due to hormonal disturbances often witnessed as puberty bleeding and perimenopausal bleeding disorders (DUB). However, during the childbearing years, conditions due to complications of early pregnancy such as ectopic pregnancy and abortion often present in this manner. Genital tract neoplasms such as submucous polyps and genital malignancies may present with continuous bleeding. *Postmenopausal bleeding* is often related to genital malignancy in 30%–40%; hence, this symptom should not be treated lightly, it should be evaluated carefully and all efforts made to exclude such a possibility. Postcoital bleeding often suggests cervical lesion, i.e. erosion, polyp and cancer.

The presence of dysmenorrhoea and dyspareunia may have organic cause in the pelvis, i.e. endometriosis, fibroid and PID.

Vaginal discharge is common in lower genital tract infections.

OBSTETRIC HISTORY

Record the details of every conception and its ultimate outcome, the number of living children, the age of the youngest child and the details of any obstetric complications encountered, e.g. puerperal or postabortal sepsis, postpartum haemorrhage (PPH), obstetrical interventions, soft tissue injuries such as cervical tear, an incompetent cervical os and repeated abortions, genital fistulae, complete perineal tear and genital prolapse, stress urinary incontinence and chronic backache. Severe PPH and obstetric shock may lead to pituitary necrosis and 'Sheehan syndrome'. Thus, many a gynaecological problem has its beginnings rooted in earlier inadequate obstetric care.

Medical termination of pregnancy and spontaneous abortions should also be enquired.

Abdominal pain: Abdominal pain is a complaint in pelvic tuberculosis, PID and endometriosis. Acute lower abdominal pain occurs in ectopic pregnancy, torsion or rupture of an ovarian cyst and chocolate cyst.

PHYSICAL EXAMINATION

Physical examination (Table 1.2) includes general examination, systemic examination and gynaecological examination with a female attendant present to assist the patient and reassure her, particularly so when the attending clinician is a male doctor.

Table 1.2 Physical Examination

General Physical Examination	
Height	**Weight**
Pulse	**BP**
Pallor	**Lymphadenopathy**
Thyroid	**Breast**
Systemic Examination	
Cardiovascular System	
Respiratory System	
Abdominal Examination	
Inspection	
Palpation	
Percussion	
Pelvic Examination	
External Genitalia	
Per Speculum Examination	
Per Vaginal Examination	
Per-rectal Examination	
Provisional Diagnosis	

GENERAL EXAMINATION

General examination includes data mentioned in the pro forma (Table 1.2). Pallor of the mucous membranes, the tongue and conjunctivae together with pale appearance of the skin and nails is highly suggestive of anaemia, fullness of the neck is suggestive of a thyroid enlargement and enlarged lymph nodes are indicative of chronic infection, tuberculosis or metastasis following malignancy. Bilateral oedema of the feet may be found in women with large abdominal tumours, and unilateral non pitting oedema is highly suggestive of malignant growth involving the lymphatics. Breast examination should be included in general examination. Hirsutism is a feature of PCOD. Breast secretion is noted in hyperprolactinaemia, an important feature in amenorrhoea.

SYSTEMIC EXAMINATION

All gynae patients must be examined as a whole. This includes the examination of the cardiovascular and respiratory systems. The presence of any neurological symptoms calls for a detailed neurological evaluation, otherwise testing of the reflexes should generally suffice. Liver should be palpated in suspected malignancy for metastasis.

ABDOMINAL EXAMINATION

INSPECTION

Many gynaecological tumours arising out of the pelvis grow upwards into the abdominal cavity. They cause enlargement of the abdomen, particularly the lower abdomen below the umbilicus, and their upper and lateral margins are often apparent on inspection. However, very large tumours can give rise to a diffuse enlargement of the entire abdomen. *Pseudomucinous cystadenomas* of the ovary can enlarge to mammoth proportions, sometimes to an extent of causing cardiorespiratory distress. Eversion of the umbilicus can occur as a result of raised intraabdominal pressure and is observed with large tumours, ascites and pregnancy. The mobility of the abdominal wall with breathing should be observed carefully. In case of an intraabdominal tumour, the abdominal wall moves over the tumour during breathing so that its upper margin is apparently altered. In case of pelvic peritonitis, the movements of the lower abdomen below the umbilicus are often restricted. The presence of striae is seen in parous women, pregnant women, in obese subjects and in women harbouring large tumours.

PALPATION

With the clinician standing on the right side of the patient, it is desirable to palpate the liver, spleen and kidneys with the right hand, and to use the sensitive ulnar border of the left hand from above downwards to palpate swellings arising from the pelvis. The upper and lateral margins of such swellings can be felt, but the lower border cannot be reached.

Myomas feel firm and have a smooth surface, unless they are multiple, when they present a bossed surface. Ovarian neoplasms often feel cystic, and may be fluctuant. The upper margin of these swellings is often well felt, unless the swelling is too large. The pregnant uterus feels soft and is known to harden intermittently during the Braxton Hicks contractions; this is characteristic of pregnancy. The full bladder bulges in the lower abdomen and feels tense and tender. Extreme tenderness on palpation below the umbilicus is suggestive of peritoneal irritation, seen in women with ectopic pregnancy, PID, twisted ovarian cyst, a ruptured corpus luteum haematoma or red degeneration in a fibroid often associated with pregnancy. In women with an acute surgical condition, guarding in the lower abdomen and rigidity on attempting deep palpation are noted.

PERCUSSION

Uterine myomas and ovarian cysts are dull to percussion, but the flanks are resonant. Dullness in the flanks and shifting dullness indicate the presence of a free fluid in the peritoneal cavity. Ascites may be associated with tuberculous peritonitis, malignancy or pseudo-Meig syndrome.

AUSCULTATION

This reveals peristaltic bowel sounds, fetal heart sounds in pregnancy, souffle in vascular neoplasms and pregnant uterus. Hyperperistalsis may indicate bowel obstruction; feeble or absent peristalsis indicates ileus, calling for aggressive attention. Return of peristaltic sounds following pelvic surgery is a welcome sign of recovery and an indication to start oral feeds.

GYNAECOLOGICAL EXAMINATION

Most prefer dorsal position, so that bimanual examination of the pelvic organs can be conducted following abdominal examination without changing the position. Some may prefer left lateral (Sims' position). Verbal consent should be obtained for bimanual examination.

EXAMINATION OF EXTERNAL GENITALIA

It is a good practice to inspect the external genitalia under a good light. Notice the distribution of pubic hair. Normal pubic hair is distributed in an inverted triangle, with the base centred over the mons pubis. The extension of the hair line upwards in the midline along the linea nigra up to the umbilicus is seen in about 25% of women, especially in women who are hirsute or mildly androgenic as in PCOD. With the patient in lithotomy and her thighs well parted, note the various structures of the vulva. Look for the presence of any discharge or blood. Ask the patient to bear down and observe for any protrusion due to polyp or genital descent such as cystocele, rectocele, uterine descent or procidentia. Separate the labia wide apart and examine the fourchette to see whether it is intact or reveals an old healed tear.

SPECULUM EXAMINATION

Speculum examination should ideally precede bimanual vaginal examination especially when the Papanicolaou (Pap) smear and vaginal smear need to be taken.

A bivalve self-retaining speculum such as Cusco's speculum is ideal for an office examination (Figs 1.1 and 1.2). It allows satisfactory inspection of the cervix, taking of a Pap smear, collection of the vaginal discharge from the posterior fornix for hanging drop/KOH smear and colposcopic examination.

Sims' vaginal speculum (Fig. 1.3) with an anterior vaginal wall retractor can be used for the above examination. It permits an assessment of the vaginal wall for cystocele and rectocele. However, an assistant is required to help the clinician during this examination and the woman needs to be brought to the edge of the table. Stress-incontinence should be looked for especially in the presence of vaginal prolapse. In this case, the patient is examined with a full bladder.

BIMANUAL EXAMINATION

After separating the labia with the thumb and index fingers of the left hand, two fingers of the right hand (index and forefinger), after lubrication, are gradually introduced beyond the introitus to reach the fornices. If the fingers encounter the anterior lip of the cervix first, it denotes the cervix is pointing downwards and back towards the posterior vaginal wall, and that the uterus is in the anteverted position, conversely when the posterior lip of the cervix is encountered first, it is indicative of a retroverted uterus.

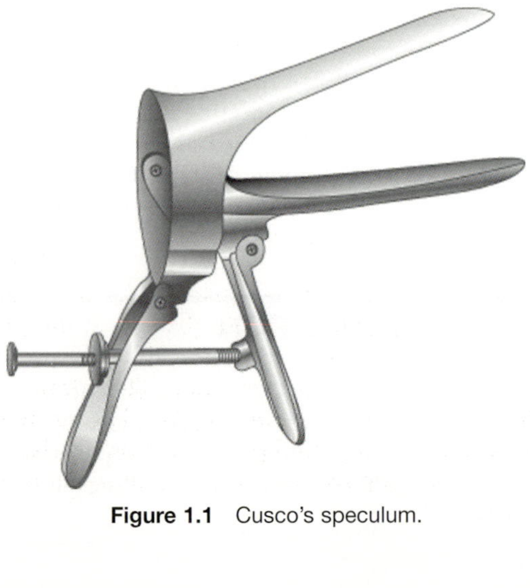

Figure 1.1 Cusco's speculum.

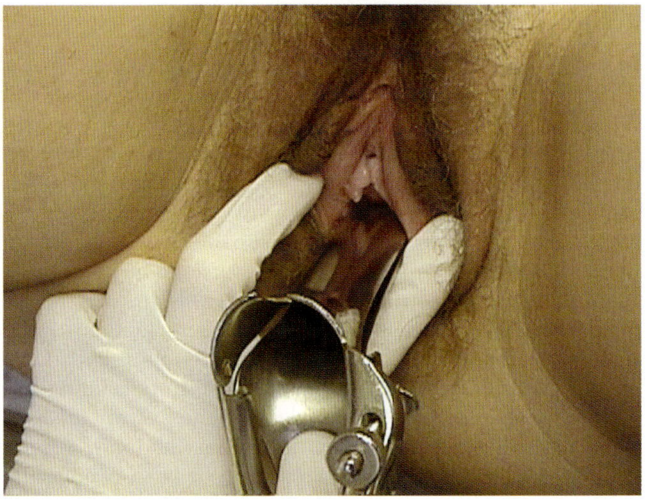

Figure 1.2 Speculum examination of the cervix. The patient is lying in the dorsal position and a Cusco's speculum has been inserted into the vagina. (*Source*: Mike Hughey, MD, President, Brookside Associates, Ltd.)

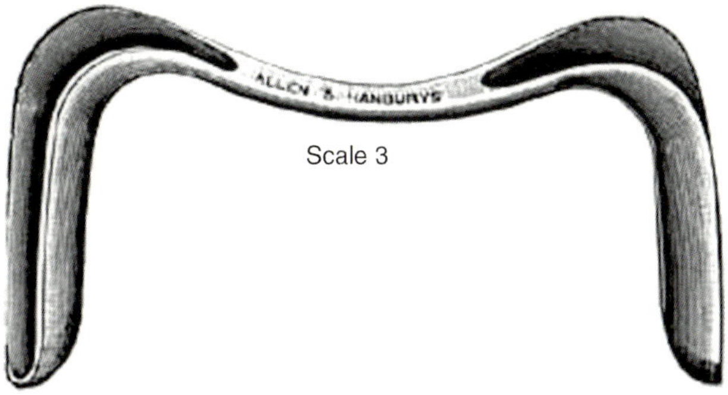

Figure 1.3 Sims' speculum.

The clinician next observes the consistency of the cervix: it is soft during pregnancy and firm in the nonpregnant state. Observe whether the movements of the cervix during the examination cause pain; this is seen in an ectopic pregnancy, as also in women with acute salpingo-oophoritis. The examining fingers now lift up the cervix and thereby elevate the uterus towards the left hand, which is placed over the lower abdomen and brought behind it (Fig. 1.4). The uterus can thus be brought within reach of the abdominal hand and palpated for position, size, shape, mobility, tenderness and the presence of any uterine pathology, e.g. fibroids (Fig. 1.5).

In case of the retroverted uterus, it will be felt through the posterior fornix.

Thereafter, the clinician directs the tips of the examining fingers in the vagina into each of the lateral fornices and, by lifting it up towards the abdominal hand, attempts to feel for masses in the lateral part of the pelvis between the two examining hands. Should this reveal the presence of a swelling separate from the uterus, then the presence of some adnexal pathology is confirmed. The common swellings identified include ovarian cyst (Fig. 1.6) or neoplasm, a paraovarian cyst, e.g. fimbrial cyst, tubo-ovarian masses (Fig. 1.7), hydrosalpinx, and swelling in chronic ectopic pregnancy.

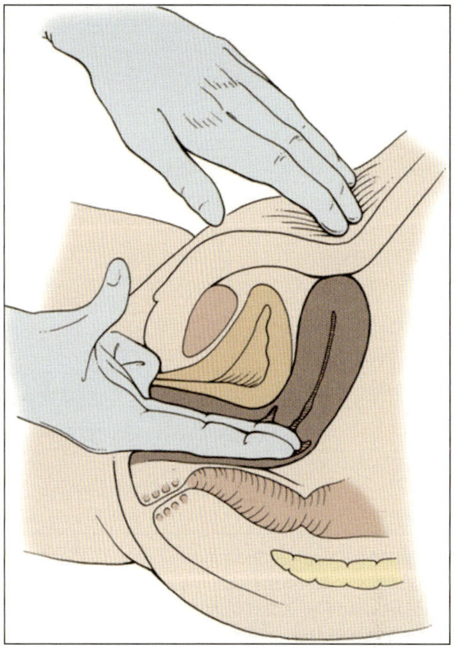

Figure 1.4 Bimanual examination of the pelvis in the female. Two fingers of the right hand are introduced into the vagina and the left hand is placed well above the symphysis pubis. (*Source*: Swartz MH: Textbook of Physical Diagnosis. Philadelphia, WB Saunders, 1989, p 405, Copyright © 2007 Saunders, An Imprint of Elsevier.)

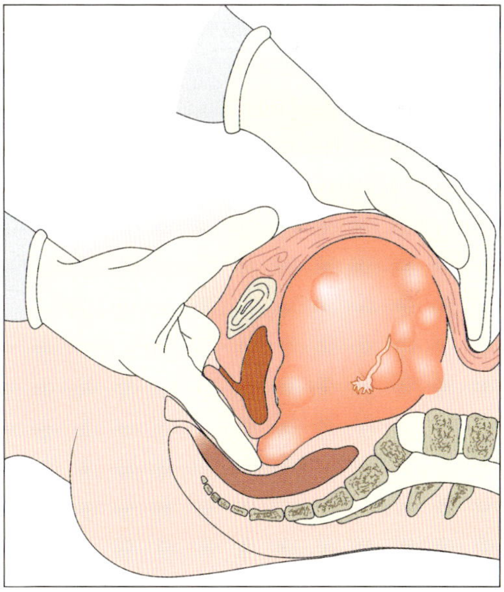

Figure 1.5 Bimanual examination in the case of multiple uterine myomas. Note how the external hand is placed high in the abdomen, well above the level of the tumour. Movements are transmitted between the two hands directly through the tumour.

The appendages are normally not palpable unless they are swollen and enlarged. The ovary is not easily palpable; however, when palpated, it evinces a peculiar painful sensation that makes the patient to wince. Next in turn is the palpation of the posterior fornix. This enables the palpation of the contents of the pouch of Douglas. The most common swelling is the loaded rectum, particularly if she is constipated. Others in order of diminishing frequency

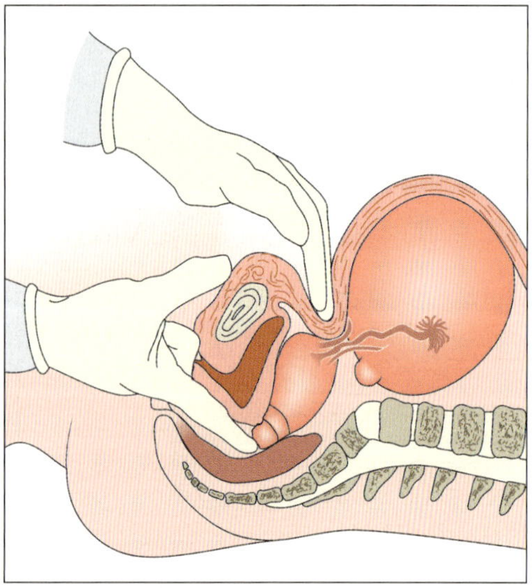

Figure 1.6 Bimanual examination in the case of an ovarian cyst. The nature of the tumour is determined on bimanual examination because the uterus can be identified apart from the abdominal tumour. Compare Fig. 1.5. In some cases the pedicle can be distinguished if the fingers in the vagina are placed high up in the posterior fornix. Movements of the abdominal tumour are clearly not transmitted to the cervix.

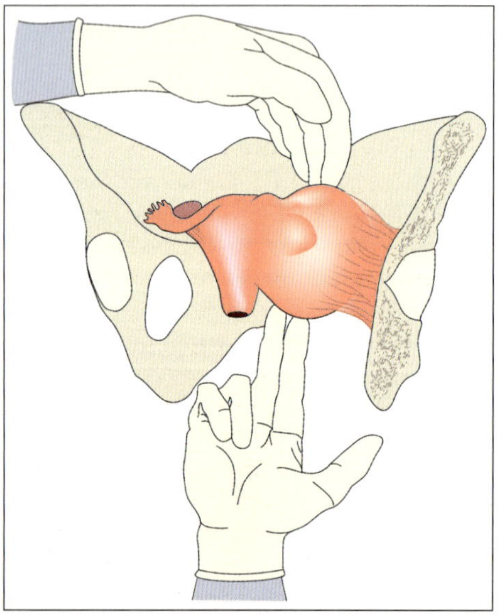

Figure 1.7 Bimanual examination in the case of a pyosalpinx. Note that the uterus is displaced to the opposite side. The fingers in the vagina are moved to one side of the cervix, and they feel the lower pole of the swelling.

include a retroverted uterus, ovaries prolapsed into the pouch of Douglas, uterine fibroid, ovarian neoplasm, chocolate cyst of the ovary, endometriotic nodules, pelvic inflammatory masses resulting from the adhesions of tubo-ovarian masses to the posterior surface of the uterus and the floor of the pouch of Douglas, pelvic abscess pointing in the posterior pouch and pelvic haematocele commonly associated with a ruptured ectopic pregnancy. To recognize the uterus from the adnexal mass, push the cervix upwards, and if this is transmitted to the swelling it is the uterus. Alternately, pushing down the uterus causes the cervix to move down. Adnexal mass does not move with cervical or uterine movement.

RECTAL EXAMINATION

In virgins, a vaginal examination is avoided. Instead a well-lubricated finger inserted into the rectum can be used for a bimanual assessment of the pelvic structures. Nowadays, practically all gynaecologists prefer ultrasonic scanning to rectal examination, which, apart from being unpleasant, is not that accurate. A rectal examination is a very useful additional examination whenever there is any palpable pathology in the pouch of Douglas. It often allows the ovaries to be more easily identified. In parametritis and endometriosis, the uterosacral ligaments are often thickened, nodular and tender. It confirms the swelling to be anterior to the rectum, and if the rectum is adherent to that swelling. This is important in case of carcinoma of the cervix to determine the extent of its posterior spread. A rectal examination is mandatory in women having rectal symptoms. This should begin by inspecting the anus in a good light, when lesions such as fissures, fistula-in-ano, polyps and piles may come to light. Introduction of a well-lubricated proctoscope to inspect the rectum and anal canal helps to complete the examination. Ultrasound nowadays has reduced the importance of rectal examination except in cancer of the cervix and pelvic endometriosis.

INVESTIGATIONS

Detailed history and clinical examination often clinch the diagnosis or reduce the differential diagnosis to a few possibilities. However, investigations may be necessary to confirm the diagnosis, to assess the extent of the disease, to establish a baseline for future comparison regarding the response to a therapy and finally to determine the patient's fitness to undergo surgery.

Common disorders: Age related (see table 1.3)

Table 1.3 Common Gynaecological Disorders – Age Related

I. Adolescent and Prepubertal Girls
- Vaginal discharge
- Disorders of growth
- Precocious puberty
- Delayed puberty
- Sexually transmitted diseases
- Tumors of ovary, vagina and vulva

II. Reproductive Age
- Disorder of menstruation
- Ectopic pregnancy
- Abnormal uterine bleeding
- Contraception related issues
- Infertility
- Pelvic inflammatory diseases
- Malignancies: GTN, Carcinoma Cervix, Ovarian Tumors

III. Menopause and Post Menopausal Age
- Menopause related problems
- Prolapse of uterus
- Post menopausal bleeding
- Malignancies: Cancer Cervix, Carcinoma Endometrium, Carcinoma Ovary and Vulval Cancer

Preoperative investigations are described in the chapter on preoperative and postoperative care. Special investigations are discussed as follows.

Special investigations:

- **Special tests** such as tumour markers: CA-125 in suspected adenocarcinoma of the ovary; carcinoembryonic antigen (CEA), α-fetoproteins and β-hCG in suspected ovarian teratoma and other germ cell tumours of ovary.
- **Bacterial examinations of the genital tract**. These include the following: (a) examination of the vaginal discharge for trichomoniasis; (b) 10% KOH-treated smear for detecting candida; (c) 1% brilliant cresyl violet for staining trichomonad, but not the other bacteria and leucocytes; (d) platinum loop for collection of discharge (in suspected gonorrhoea) from the urethra, ducts of Bartholin and the endocervical secretion for culture on chocolate agar; (e) immunofluorescent examination of the discharge of endocervical cells for suspected chlamydial infection; and (f) microscopic examination of the clue cells for diagnosis of bacterial vaginosis (Chapter 9).

Feinberg–Whittington medium is used for trichomonad and Nickerson–Sabouraud for candiasis. The presence of clue cells indicates bacterial vaginosis.

Polymerase chain reaction (PCR) staining has been extensively utilized in the diagnosis of various infections.

SPECIAL TESTS

HANGING DROP PREPARATION

In women complaining leucorrhoea, the discharge collected from the posterior fornix on the blade of the speculum should be suspended in saline and submitted to microscopic examination. Normal vaginal discharge shows the presence of exfoliated vaginal epithelial cells and the presence of large rod-like lactobacilli known as Döderlein's bacilli. A fresh suspension of the discharge may reveal the motile flagellated organisms known as *Trichomonas vaginalis*. Another common cause of vaginal infection is fungal infection or *vaginal candidiasis*; this can also be detected from a microscopic examination of the vaginal discharge. To the suspension of the vaginal discharge, add an equal amount of 10% KOH solution. Place a drop of the mixture on a slide, cover it with a cover slip, warm the slide and examine it under the low power of the microscope. The KOH dissolves all cellular debris, leaving behind the more resistant yeast-like organisms. Typical hyphae or mycelia and budding spores can be easily detected. Many cases of vaginitis are attributed to *bacterial vaginosis* (nonspecific vaginitis); also known as *Gardnerella vaginalis*. The visualization of 'clue cells' seen preferably in a stained smear of the vaginal discharge is highly suggestive of the infection. Vaginal infections have been discussed later in detail in Chapter 9.

PAPANICOLAOU TEST

Screening for Cancer

First described by Papanicolaou and Traut in 1943, this screening test is often referred to as the 'Pap test' or a surface biopsy or exfoliative cytology (cytology is a Greek word, meaning study of cells). It forms a part of the routine gynaecological examination in women. All sexually active women older than 21 years should undergo an annual check-up with three yearly Pap test. Aside from premalignant and malignant changes, other local conditions can often be recognized by the cytologist. The Pap smear is only a screening test. Positive test (abnormal cells) requires further investigations such as colposcopy, cervical biopsy and fractional curettage. Unfortunately, the Pap test can detect only about 60%–70% of precancer and cancer of the cervix and less than 70% of endometrial cancer. Reliability of the report depends on the slide preparation and the skill of the cytologist. Although a single test yields as much as 10%–15% false-negative reading, it is reduced to only 1% with repeated tests. A false-positive finding is reported in the presence of infection. A yearly negative Pap smear for 3 years is assuring, and thereafter 5-yearly test is adequate.

The Pap smear should be obtained before vaginal examination, because the fingers may remove the desquamated cervical cells and give a false-negative report, lubricant may prevent detection of organisms and any vaginal bleeding during examination may preclude a proper visualization of the cervix. The patient should not have intercourse or touch for 24 hours before the Pap test. The best time to do Pap smear is around ovulation, but any other time can also do. The patient is placed in the dorsal position, with the labia parted, and Cusco's self-retaining speculum is gently introduced without the use of lubricant or jelly. The cervix is exposed; the squamocolumnar junction is now scraped with Ayre's spatula by rotating the spatula all around (Fig. 1.8). The scrapings are evenly spread onto a glass slide and immediately fixed by dipping the slide in the jar containing equal parts of 95% ethyl alcohol and ether. After fixing it for 30 minutes, the slide is air-dried and stained with Pap or short stain. The slide is considered satisfactory, if endocervical cells are seen. To improve the predictive valve, endocervix is also scraped with a brush and added to the slide. Nowadays, a fixative spray (cytospray) is available and can be used conveniently in an office set-up. For hormonal cytological evaluation, the scrapings are taken from the upper lateral part of the vaginal walls; three types of cells are found in the normal smear: (i) the basal and parabasal cells are small, rounded and basophilic with large nuclei; (ii) the cells from the middle layer are squamous cells, transparent and basophilic with vesicular nuclei; and (iii) the cells from the superficial layer are acidophilic with characteristic pyknotic nuclei. In addition, endometrial cells, histiocytes, blood cells and bacteria can be seen. Malignant cells are hyperchromatic with a great increase in chromatin content. The nuclei vary in size and there is usually only a small amount of cytoplasm in the undifferentiated malignant cell (Figs 1.9 and 1.10). The nucleus/cytoplasmic ratio is increased in malignant cells.

Papanicolaou classification:

Grade I	Normal cells (Fig. 1.9)
Grade II	Slightly abnormal, suggestive of inflammatory change; repeat smear after treating the infection
Grade III	A more serious type of abnormality, usually indicative of the need for biopsy
Grade IV	Distinctly abnormal, possibly malignant and definitely requiring biopsy
Grade V	Malignant cells seen (Fig. 1.10)

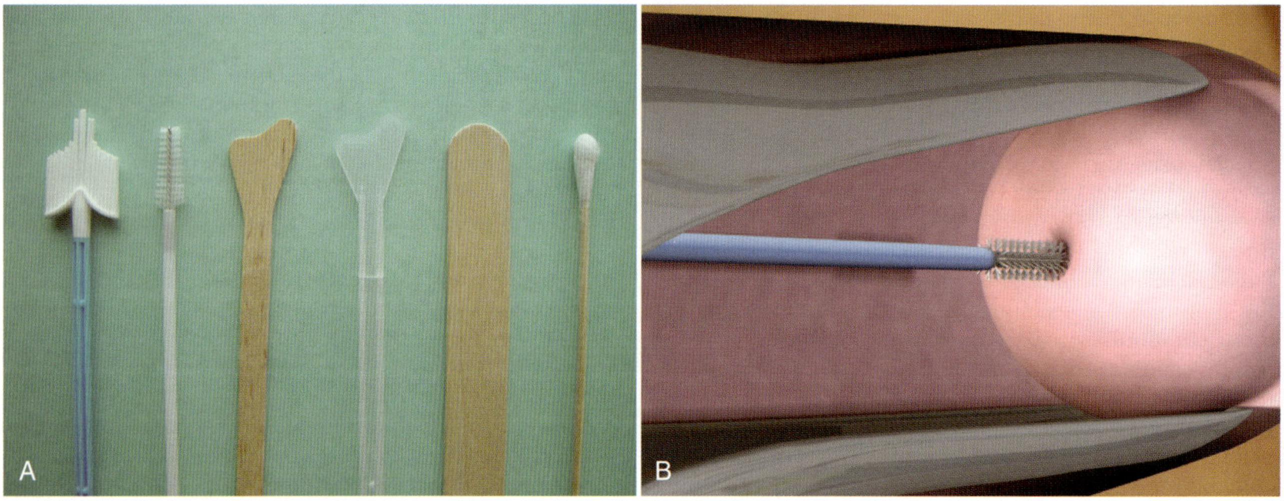

Figure 1.8 **(A)** Papanicolaou sampling devices. Left to right: Cervix-Brush, Cytobrush, wooden spatula, plastic spatula, tongue blade and cotton swab applicator. **(B)** Pap smear with a brush. (*Source* for **(A)**: From Figure 16, Pre-procedure. Procedure Consult. Pap Smear. Editors: Michael L Tuggy and Jorge Garcia; *Source* for **(B)**: From Figure 1, Pre-procedure. Procedure Consult. Papanicolaou Testing. Editors: Todd W Thomsen and Gary S Setnik.)

Scan to play How to take pap smear

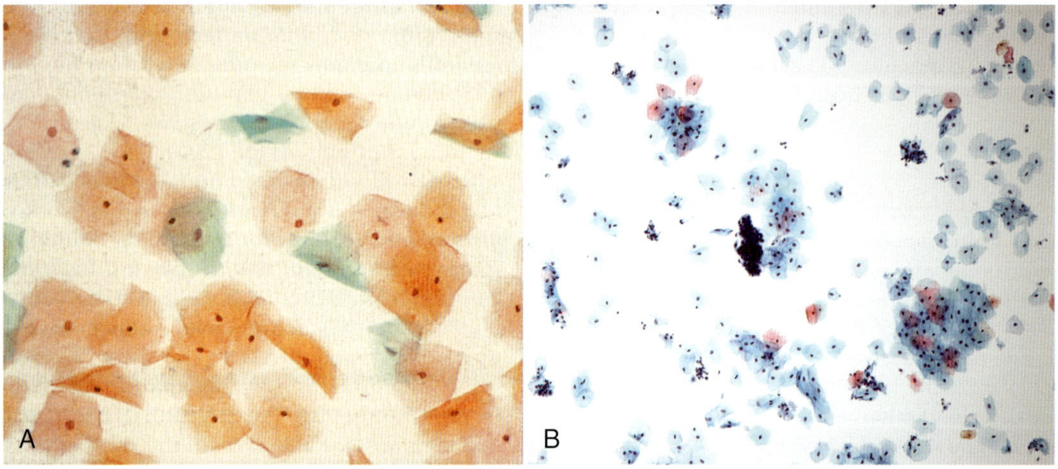

Figure 1.9 Normal cervical smear showing superficial (pink) and intermediate (blue/green) exfoliated cervical cells (low power magnification). (*Source*: From Figure 20-5, Ian Symonds and Sabaratnam Arulkumaran: Essential Obstetrics and Gynaecology, 5th Ed. Elsevier, 2013.)

A newer classification (Table 1.4) describes the cytology smears as follows:

1. Normal cytology
2. Inflammatory smear
3. Cervical intraepithelial neoplasia (CIN I) or mild dysplasia
4. CIN II, III and carcinoma in situ nuclear abnormalities
5. Malignant cells and tadpole cells with nuclear abnormalities

It is reasonable to enquire about the percentage of unsuspected cancers, including carcinoma in situ, that are likely to be diagnosed on routine cytology. The Indian Council of Medical Research (ICMR), New Delhi, screened the population of women older than 30 years and found 5–15 smears to be abnormal per 1000 women examined. The incidence of dysplasia reported at the All India Institute of Medical Sciences, New Delhi, was 16/1000 patients screened. In a postmenopausal woman, if the squamocolumnar junction is indrawn due to oestrogen deficiency, a 10-day course of oestrogen cream exposes the squamocolumnar junction better and yields an accurate result. Postradiation cytology is difficult to sample because of scarring and atrophy of the vagina. The cells are often enlarged, vacuolated with multiple nucleation and nuclear wrinkling. Inflammatory cells may be present (Table 1.5).

Liquid-based cytology using a thin preparation is superior to Pap smear (Fig. 1.11). The liquid is used to screen for papilloma virus. Cervical cancer screening is described in Fig. 1.12. This is described in detail in Chapter 33. Other methods of cervical screening are also described in Chapter 33.

VISUAL INSPECTION AFTER ACETIC ACID APPLICATION (VIA)

Gross inspection of cervix after application of 3% or 5% acetic acid for 1 minute helps in detecting acetowhite area which may harbour CIN/neoplasia.

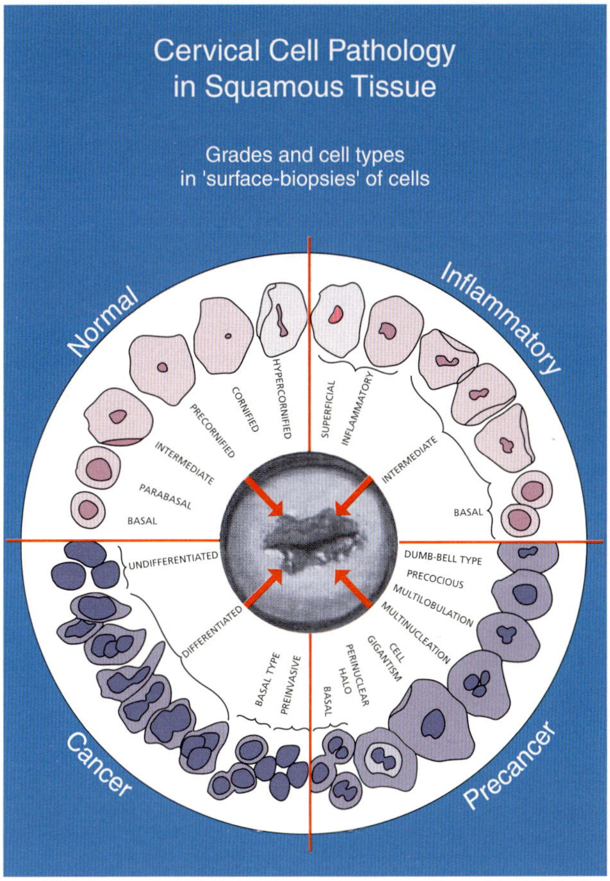

Figure 1.10 Illustration of pathological grades of epidermoid cells in the squamocolumnar junction of the cervix. Cells arising in this location were produced by a uniform cell-scraping technique. Classification of cell types is based upon thorough study, evaluation of cell characteristics and pathological features and is finally correlated with corresponding histological studies of the tissue. No attempt is made to classify cells exfoliated from other tissue areas, such as the endometrium. The squamocolumnar junction is a vital zone to the female, because this is the focal point where cancer arises. Grading of cells depends upon knowledge of origin of cell sample, on securing a rich concentration of cells, and of greatest importance, correct correlation with histological findings.

Table 1.4 Comparison of Different Classification System for Pre-invasive Lesion

Papsmear	Dysplasia	CIN	Bethesda
I			
II			
III	Mild	I	LSIL
IV	Moderate	II	HSIL
V	Severe	III	HSIL

L, low; H, high; SIL, squamous intraepithelial lesion.

Table 1.5 Bethesda Classification

- Sample—adequate, unsatisfactory
- Squamous cell abnormalities
- Atypical squamous cells (ASC)
- Atypical squamous cells of undetermined significance ASCUS
- ASC—cannot exclude high grade lesion ASC-H
- Low-grade squamous intraepithelial lesion (LSIL)
- High-grade squamous intraepithelial lesion (HSIL)
- Squamous cell carcinoma
- Adenocarcinoma

Source: Bethesda Guidelines.

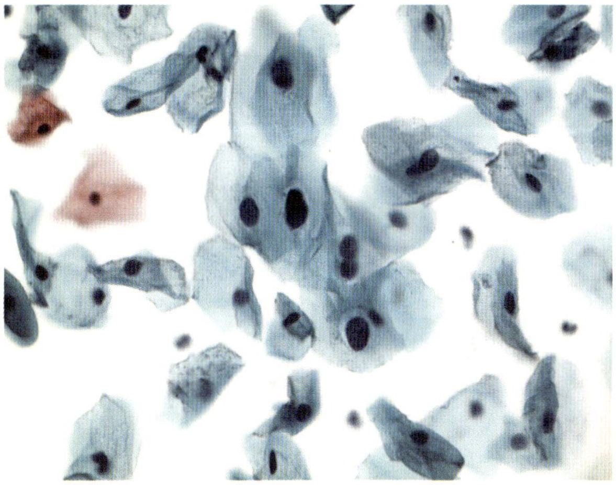

Figure 1.11 Liquid-based cytology classified as epithelial cell abnormality, low-grade squamous intraepithelial lesion (LSIL). Note particularly the cells in the centre. They have enlarged nuclei compared with those in the cells to the left and below. This feature is required for a diagnosis of LSIL. The nuclear contours are irregular. One cell to the right of centre is binucleated, a common feature in LSIL. (*Source*: From Figure 12-1, Barbara S Apgar, Gregory L Brotzman and Mark Spitzer: Colposcopy: Principles and Practice, 2nd Ed. Saunders: Elsevier, 2008.)

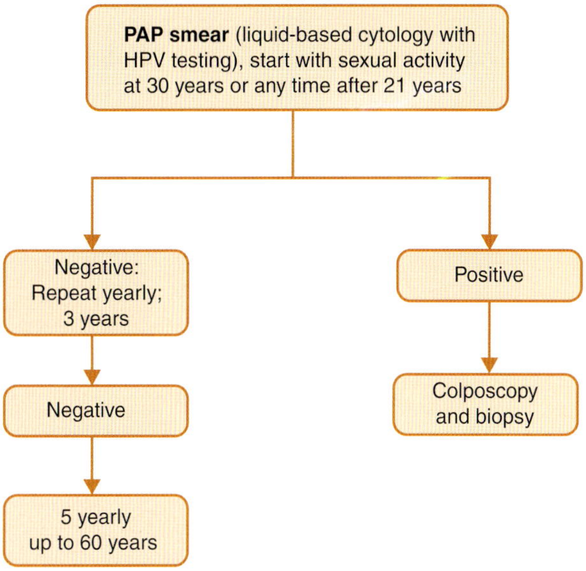

Figure 1.12 Cervical cancer screening.

SCHILLER TEST (VISUAL INSPECTION AFTER LUGOL'S IODINE APPLICATION – VILI)

▶ Scan to play VIA and VILI

This test detects the presence of glycogen in the superficial cells of the vaginal epithelium. The vaginal wall is stained with Lugol's iodine (Lugol's iodine contains 5% iodine and 10% potassium iodide in water [1g iodine + 2g KI]). The vaginal epithelium takes mahogany brown colour in the presence of glycogen. Unstained areas (negative test) are abnormal and require biopsy for histological examination.

CYTOHORMONAL EVALUATION

The ovarian hormones oestrogen and progesterone influence the vaginal mucosa; thus, the epithelial cells exfoliated in the vagina reflect the influence of the prevailing dominant hormone in the system at that time. The oestrogen-dominated smear appears clean and shows the presence of discrete cornified polygonal squames. The progesterone-dominated smear appears dirty and reveals the predominance of intermediate cells. During pregnancy, the cytology smear shows intermediate cells and navicular cells. After the menopause due to the deficiency of the ovarian hormones, the vaginal *mucosa* thins down and the exfoliated cells are predominantly parabasal and basal types. In human papilloma virus (HPV) infection, one can recognize koilocytes with perinuclear halo and peripheral condensation of cytoplasm. The nucleus is irregular and hyperchromatic (Fig. 1.10).

Karyopyknotic Index or KPI (Maturation Index)

It is the ratio of mature squamous cells over the intermediate and basal cells. It is more than 25% in proliferative (oestrogenic) phase (Fig. 1.13) and low in secretory (progestational) phase (Fig. 1.14) and during pregnancy. During pregnancy, a ratio of more than 10% indicates progesterone deficiency. Normally, a peak value of KPI is reached on the day of ovulation (2 days after serum E_2 peak).

UTERINE ASPIRATION CYTOLOGY

Perimenopausal and postmenopausal women on a hormone therapy are now being screened for endometrial cancer. The uterine aspiration syringe or brush is found to be satisfactory for obtaining adequate samples. It can be utilized as an office procedure; about 90% accuracy with no false-positive findings is claimed with this procedure.

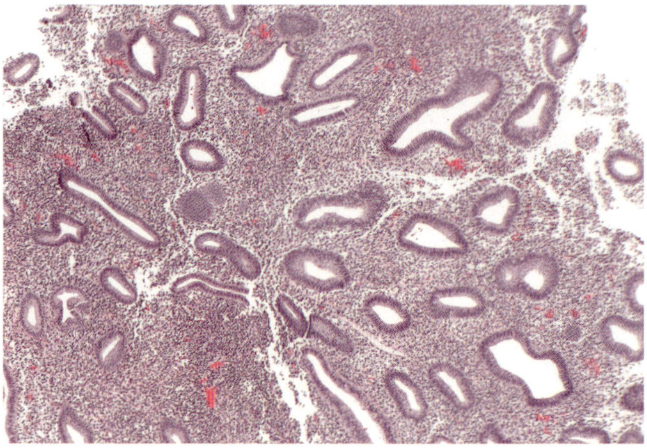

Figure 1.13 Histology of proliferative phase. (*Courtesy:* Dr Sandeep Mathur, AIIMS.)

COLPOSCOPY

The colposcope is a binocular microscope giving a 10–20 times magnification. It is useful in locating abnormal areas and accurately obtaining directed biopsy from the suspicious areas on the cervix and vagina in women with positive Pap smears. This way the frequency of false-negative biopsy is reduced, so also the need for conization, a procedure that is accompanied with considerable amount of bleeding and morbidity (Chapter 18).

ENDOMETRIAL BIOPSY (Fig. 1.14A and B)

An office or outpatient procedure was at one time very popular in the investigations of the female partner for infertility. It is performed in the premenstrual phase. A fine curette is introduced into the uterine cavity to obtain a small strip of the endometrial lining for histopathological examination, secretory endometrium denotes ovulatory cycle. With the availability of ultrasound, a noninvasive method for the detection of ovulation, this procedure is now generally not employed.

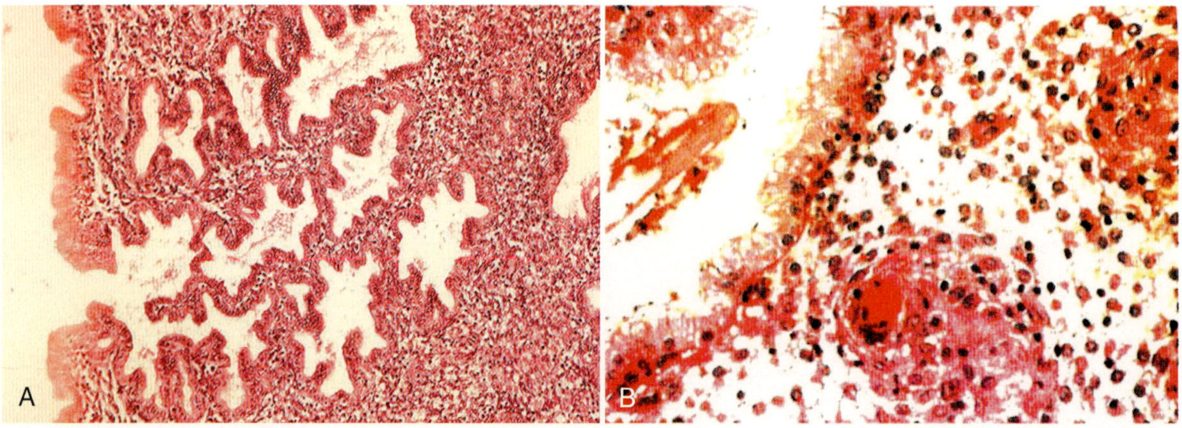

Figure 1.14 **(A)** Histology of secretory phase. **(B)** Midsecretory endometrium. (*Source* for **(A)**: Copyright 2009 by the University of Florida.)

It is still used if tubercular endometritis is suspected. It is useful in the diagnosis of corpus luteal phase defect.

HORMONAL ASSAYS

In present-day practice, it is possible to study the levels of several hormones using radioimmunoassays and/or the ELISA tests. The commonly assayed hormones include FSH, LH, PRL, ACTH, T_3, T_4, TSH, progesterone, oestradiol, testosterone, cortisol, aldosterone, hCG, dehydroepiandrosterone and androstenedione. These assays are used in the diagnosis of menopause, PCOD and prolactinomas, and for monitoring treatment regimes in induction of ovulation and in assisted reproduction.

ULTRASONOGRAPHY

Ultrasonography is a simple noninvasive and painless diagnostic procedure that has the advantage of being devoid of any radiation hazard. The pelvis and the lower abdomen are scanned in both the longitudinal and transverse planes. Generally, this scan is done when the patient's bladder is full as it helps to elevate the uterus out of the pelvis, and displaces the gas-filled bowel loops away, thus providing the sonologist with a window to image the pelvic organs. In most cases, a transvaginal probe can be usefully employed to obtain finer details of the pelvic organs. The bladder need not be full, if the vaginal probe is used. The scan can collaborate the clinical impression or uncover a hitherto unsuspected pathology. Lately, rectal and perineal routes are also available. D3 ultrasound is now capable of providing three-dimensional images of the pelvic organs and is recently available especially to detect genital tract malformations and is less costly than MRI. Ultrasound is also used in certain therapeutic procedures such as in vitro fertilization and aspiration of a cyst or pelvic abscess.

OTHER IMAGING MODALITIES

Radiological investigation such as hysterosalpingography is utilized for studying the patency of the fallopian tubes in an infertile patient. CT scan and MRI are advanced investigations that determine the extent of tumours and their spread. For details, refer to Chapter 40. Sonosalpingography is employed in women with infertility and when uterine polyp is suspected.

GYNAECOLOGICAL ENDOSCOPY

Both diagnostic laparoscopy and hysteroscopy are established useful tools in the armamentarium of the gynaecologist. For details, refer to Chapter 41 (Endoscopy in Gynaecology).

PREGNANCY TEST

The first morning sample of urine is used in a rapid immunological test to confirm pregnancy, by detecting the presence of human chorionic hormone. The pregnancy test becomes positive by the beginning of 6th week, from the last menstrual period. With modern kits, any sample of urine can be used, and it may become positive within 1-2 days after missing the periods.

KEY POINTS

- Most gynaecological diseases can be diagnosed by a proper and detailed history and pelvic examination.
- While approaching a female patient, utmost care should be taken to respect her feelings, ensure privacy and using simple words to know details of her sexual history, contraceptive used, abortions and surgical treatment.
- A wide range of investigations are now available with the gynaecologists which finally confirm the diagnosis, detect the extent of the disease and help in planning the management.
- Pap smear is now an established screening procedure in carcinoma cervix.
- Ultrasound examinations have simplified gynaecological diagnosis.
- Selective gynaecological endoscopy helps definitive diagnosis.
- Hormonal assays are necessary in infertility work up, in vitro fertilization and various hormonal disturbances.
- CT and MRI have added to the imaging modalities and are useful when diagnosis is in doubt on the basis of physical examination.

SELF-ASSESSMENT

1. List the simple steps in history taking of a gynaecological patient.
2. Describe the importance of Pap smears in clinical practice.
3. What is the role of imaging and endoscopy in the clinical practice of gynaecology?

SUGGESTED READING

Ley P. Communications with Patients. London, Croom Helm, 1988.

Lipkin M Jr. The medical interview and related skills. In Branch WT (ed). Office Practice of Medicine. Philadelphia, WB Saunders, 1987; 1287–306.

Simpson M, Buckman R, Stewart M, et al. Doctor patient communication. The Toronto consensus statement. BMJ 1991; 303: 1386–7.

Todd AD, Fisher S. The Social Organization of Doctor-Patient Communication, 2nd ed. Norwood, NJ, Ablex Publishing, 1993; 243–65.

SECTION 1

ANATOMY, PHYSIOLOGY AND DEVELOPMENT OF FEMALE REPRODUCTIVE ORGANS

SECTION OUTLINE

Anatomy of Female Genital Tract

2

CHAPTER OUTLINE

The anatomical knowledge of the female genital organs (Fig. 2.1) and their relation to the neighbouring structures help in the diagnosis of various gynaecological diseases and in interpreting the findings of ultrasound, computed tomography (CT) and magnetic resonance imaging (MRI) scanning. During gynaecological surgery, distortions of the pelvic organs are better appreciated and dealt with and a grave injury to the structures such as bladder, ureter and rectum is avoided. The understanding of the lymphatic drainage of the pelvic organs is necessary in staging various genital tract malignancies and in their surgical dissection.

THE VULVA

The vulva is an ill-defined area which in gynaecological practice comprises the whole of the external genitalia and conveniently includes the perineum. It is, therefore, bounded anteriorly by the mons veneris (pubis), laterally by the labia majora and posteriorly by the perineum.

LABIA MAJORA

The labia majora pass from the mons veneris to end posteriorly in the skin over the perineal body. They consist of folds of skin which enclose a variable amount of fat and are best developed in the childbearing period of life. In children before the age of puberty and in postmenopausal women, the amount of subcutaneous fat in the labia majora is relatively scanty, and the cleft between the labia is therefore conspicuous. At puberty, pudendal hair appear on the mons veneris, the outer surface of the labia majora and in some cases on the skin of the perineum as well. The inner surfaces of the labia majora are hairless and the skin of this area is softer, moister and pinker than over the outer surfaces (Fig. 2.2). The labia majora are covered with squamous epithelium and contain sebaceous glands, sweat glands and hair follicles. There are also certain specialized sweat glands called apocrine glands, which produce a characteristic aroma and from which the rare tumour of hidradenoma of the vulva is derived. The secretion increases during sexual excitement.

The presence of all these structures in the labia majora renders them liable to common skin lesions such as folliculitis, boils and sebaceous cysts (Fig. 2.3). Its masculine counterpart is the scrotum.

LABIA MINORA

The labia minora are thin folds of skin which enclose veins and elastic tissue and lie on the inner aspect of the labia majora. The vascular labia minora are erectile during sexual activity; they do not contain any sebaceous glands or hair follicles (Fig. 2.4). Anteriorly, they enclose the clitoris to form the prepuce on the upper surface and the frenulum on its undersurface. Posteriorly, they join to form the fourchette. The fourchette is a thin fold of skin, identified when the labia are separated, and it is often torn during parturition. The fossa navicularis is the small hollow between the hymen and the fourchette. Labia minora is homologous with the ventral aspect of the penis.

The *clitoris* is an erectile organ and consists of a glans, covered by the frenulum and prepuce, and a body which is subcutaneous; it corresponds to the penis and is attached to the undersurface of the symphysis pubis by the suspensory ligament. Normally, the clitoris is 1–1½ cm long and 5 mm

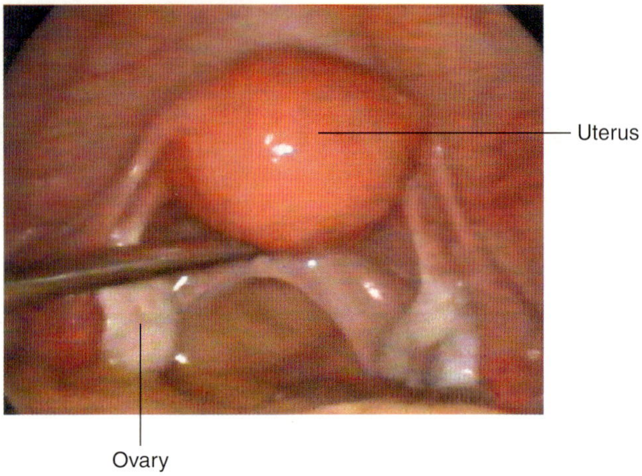

Figure 2.1 General view of internal genital organs showing the normal uterus and ovaries.

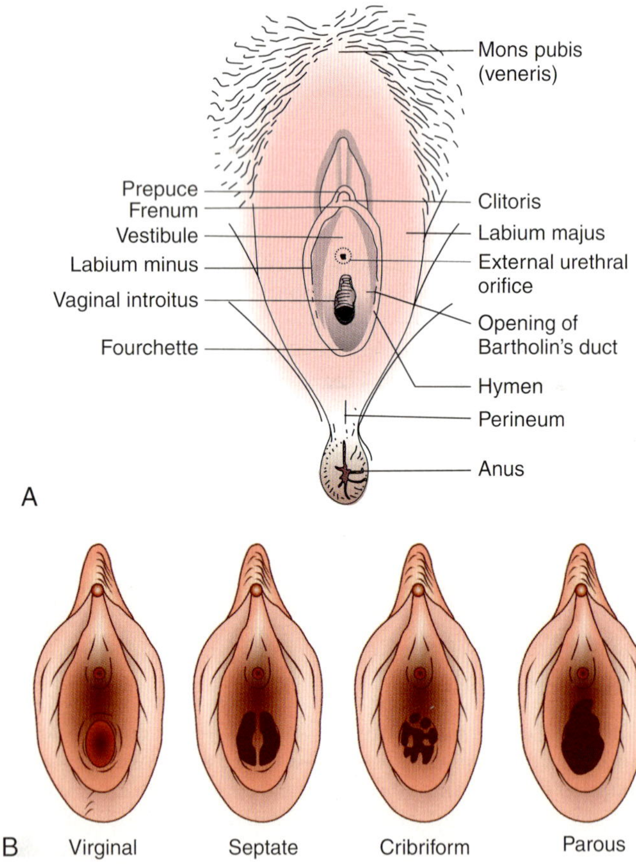

Figure 2.2 **(A)** Anatomy of the vulva. **(B)** Variations of the hymen.

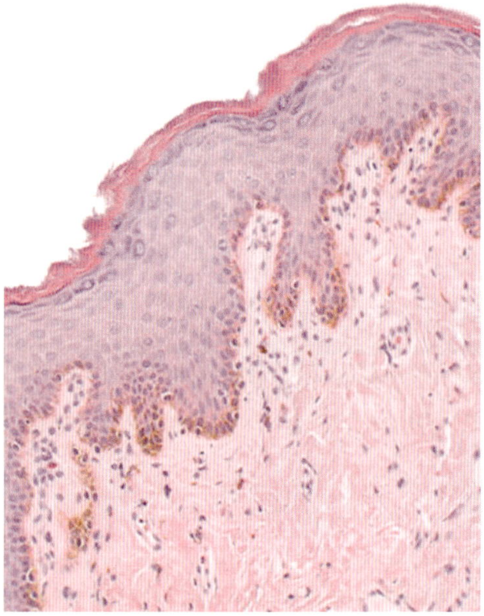

Figure 2.3 Histological section of the labium majus showing squamous epithelium with hair follicle and sebaceous gland (×55).

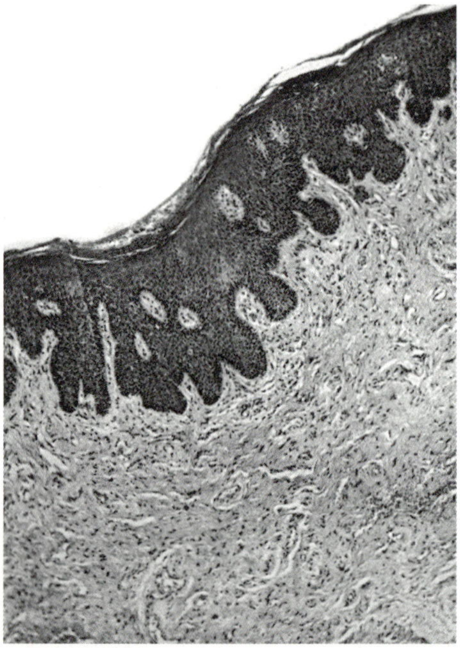

Figure 2.4 Histological section of the labium minus showing squamous epithelium. Note complete absence of hair follicles and sebaceous and sweat glands.

in width. Clitoris of more than 3.5 cm in length and 1 cm in width is called clitoromegaly, and occurs in virilism due to excess of androgen hormone. The clitoris is well supplied with nerve endings and is extremely sensitive. During coitus, it becomes erect and plays a considerable part in inducing orgasm in the female. The clitoris is highly vascular. An injury to the clitoris causes profuse bleeding and can be very painful.

The *vestibule* is the space lying between the anterior and the inner aspects of the labia minora and is bounded posteriorly by the vaginal introitus. The *external urinary meatus* lies immediately posterior to the clitoris. The vaginal orifice lies posterior to the meatus and is surrounded by the hymen. In virgins, the hymen is represented by a thin membrane covered on each surface by squamous epithelium. It generally has a small eccentric opening, which is usually not wide enough to admit the fingertip. Coitus results in the rupture of the hymen; the resulting lacerations are radially arranged and are multiple. Occasionally, coital rupture can cause a brisk haemorrhage. During childbirth, further lacerations occur: the hymen is widely stretched and subsequently is represented by the tags of skin known as the carunculae myrtiformes. With the popularity of the use of internal sanitary tampons, the loss of integrity of the hymen is no longer an evidence of loss of virginity.

The vulval tissues respond to hormones, especially oestrogen, during the childbearing years. After menopause, atrophy due to oestrogen deficiency makes the vulval skin thinner and drier, and this may lead to atrophic vulvitis and itching. *Mons pubis* is an area which overlaps the symphysis pubis and contains fat. At puberty, abundant hair grow over it.

BARTHOLIN'S GLAND

Bartholin's gland lies posterolaterally in relation to the vaginal orifice, deep to the bulbospongiosus muscle and superficial to the outer layer of the triangular ligament. It is embedded in the erectile tissue of the vestibular bulb at its posterior extremity. It is normally impalpable when healthy, but can be readily palpated between the finger and the thumb when enlarged by inflammation. Its vascular bed accounts for the brisk bleeding, which always accompanies its removal. Its duct passes forwards and inwards to open, external to the hymen, on the inner side of the labium minus. The gland measures about 10 mm in diameter and lies near the junction of the middle and posterior thirds of the labium majus. The duct of the gland is about 25 mm long and a thin mucous secretion can be expressed from it by pressure upon the gland. Bartholin's gland and its duct are infected in acute gonorrhoea, when the reddened mouth of the duct can easily be distinguished on the inner surface of the labium minus to one side of the vaginal orifice below the level of the hymen. Bartholin's gland is a compound racemose gland and its acini are lined by low columnar epithelium (Fig. 2.5). The epithelium of the duct is cubical near the acini, but becomes transitional and finally squamous near the mouth of the duct. The function of the gland is to secrete lubricating mucous during coitus. The labia majora join at the posterior commissure and merge imperceptibly into the perineum.

THE VAGINA

The vagina is a fibromuscular passage that connects the uterus to the introitus. The lower end of the vagina lies at the level of the hymen and of the introitus vaginae. It is surrounded at this point by the erectile tissue of the *bulb*, which corresponds to the corpus spongiosum of the male. The direction of the vagina is approximately parallel to the plane of the brim of the true pelvis; the vagina is slightly curved forwards from above downwards, and its anterior and posterior walls lie in a close contact. It is not of uniform calibre, being nearly twice as capacious in its upper part and somewhat flask shaped. The vaginal portion of the cervix projects into its upper end and leads to the formation of the anterior, posterior and lateral fornices. The depth of the fornices depends upon the development of the portio vaginalis of the cervix. In girls before puberty and in elderly women in whom the uterus has undergone postmenopausal atrophy, the fornices are shallow whereas in women with congenital elongation of the portio vaginalis of the cervix, the fornices are deep. The vagina is attached to the cervix at a higher level posteriorly than elsewhere, and this makes the posterior fornix the deepest of the fornices and the posterior vaginal wall longer than the anterior. The posterior wall is 4.5 inch (11.5 cm) long, whereas the anterior wall measures 3.5 inch (9 cm). Transverse folds which are present in the vaginal walls of nulliparae allow the vagina to stretch and dilate during coitus and parturition. These folds are partly obliterated in women who have borne many children. In the anterior vaginal wall, three sulci can be distinguished. One lies immediately above the meatus and is called *submeatal sulcus* (Fig. 2.6). About 35 mm above this

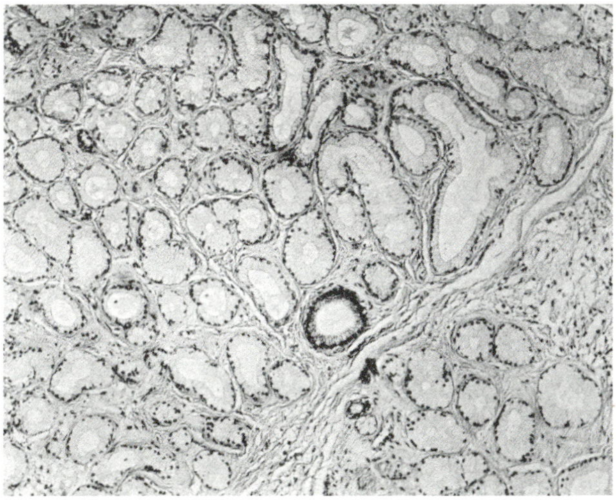

Figure 2.5 Bartholin's gland. Low-power view showing the structure of a compound racemose gland with acini lined by low columnar epithelium (×92).

Scan to play Bartholin's abscess

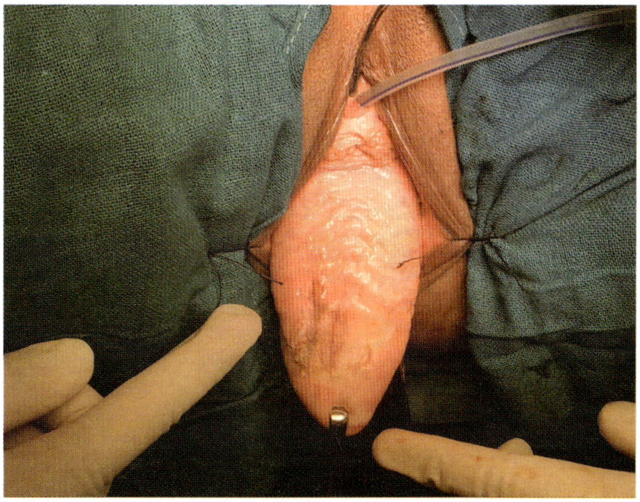

Figure 2.6 A case of prolapse in which the cervix has been drawn down. Parameatal recess, hymen, submeatal sulcus, paraurethral recess, oblique vaginal fold, transverse sulcus of the anterior vaginal wall, arched rugae of the vaginal wall and bladder sulcus.

sulcus in the anterior vaginal wall is a second sulcus, known as the *transverse vaginal sulcus,* which corresponds approximately to the junction of the urethra and the bladder. Further upwards is the *bladder sulcus,* indicating the junction of the bladder to the anterior vaginal wall.

The vaginal mucosa is lined by nonkeratized squamous epithelium which consists of a basal layer of cuboidal cells, a middle layer of prickle cells and a superficial layer of cornified cells (Fig. 2.7). In the newborn, the epithelium is almost transitional in type and cornified cells are scanty until puberty is reached. No glands open into the vagina, and the vaginal secretion is derived partly from the mucous discharge of the cervix and partly from transudation through the vaginal epithelium. The subepithelial layer is vascular and contains much erectile tissue. A muscle layer consisting of a complex interlacing lattice of plain muscle lies external to the subepithelial layer, whereas the large vessels lie in the connective tissues surrounding the vagina. If the female fetus is exposed to diethylstilboestrol (DES) taken by the mother during pregnancy, columnar epithelium appears in the upper two-thirds of vaginal mucosa, which can develop vaginal adenosis and vaginal cancer during adolescence. The keratinization of vaginal mucosa occurs in prolapse due to the exposure of vagina to the outside and ulcer may form over the vaginal mucosa (decubitus ulcer). The keratized mucosa appears skin-like and brown. Menopause causes atrophy of the vagina.

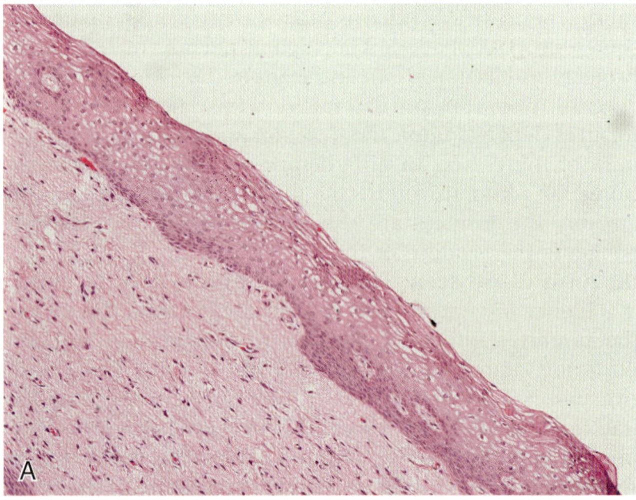

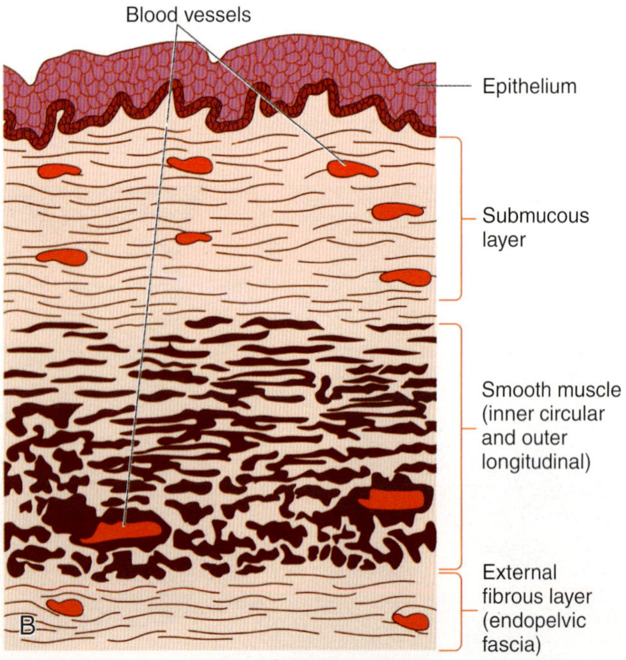

Figure 2.7 **(A)** Low-power (×36) microscopic appearance of the vaginal wall showing the corrugated squamous epithelium and bundles of plain muscle cells subjacent to the vascular subepithelial layer. **(B)** Structure of the vaginal wall. (*Courtesy* for **(A):** Dr Sandeep Mathur, AIIMS.)

The *vaginal secretion* is small in amount in healthy women and consists of white coagulated material. When it is examined under a microscope, squamous cells shed from the vaginal epithelium and Döderlein's bacilli alone are found. *Döderlein's bacillus* is a large Gram-positive rod-shaped organism, which grows anaerobically on acid media. The vaginal secretion is acidic due to the presence of lactic acid, and this acidity inhibits the growth of pathogenic organisms. The pH of the vagina averages about 4.5 during reproductive life. The acidity, which is undoubtedly oestrogen dependent, falls after menopause to neutral or even alkaline. Before puberty, the pH is about 7. This high pH before puberty and after menopause explains the tendency for the development of mixed organism infections in these age groups.

The synthesis of lactic acid is probably influenced by either enzyme or bacterial activity (Döderlein's) on the glycogen of the epithelial cells, which itself is dependent on the presence of oestrogen, so that its deficient activity can be boosted by the administration of oral or local oestrogen. During the puerperium and also in cases of leucorrhoea, the acidity of the vagina is reduced and pathogenic organisms are then able to survive. The squamous cells of the vagina and cervix stain a deep brown colour after being painted with iodine solution, owing to the presence of glycogen in healthy cells (positive Schiller's test). In a postmenopausal woman, because of the absence of or low glycogen-containing superficial cells, Schiller's test becomes negative.

The vaginal epithelium is under the ovarian hormonal influences of oestrogen and progesterone. Oestrogen proliferates the glycogen-containing superficial cells and progesterone causes proliferation of intermediate cells. Lack of these hormones in a menopausal woman leaves only the basal cells with a thin vaginal mucosa.

The abnormal and malignant cells also do not contain glycogen and do not take up the stain. Similarly, these abnormal cells turn white with acetic acid due to coagulation of protein. These areas are selected for biopsy in the detection of cancer.

RELATIONS OF VAGINA

ANTERIOR RELATION

In its lower half, the vagina is closely related to the urethra and the paraurethral glands (Skene's tubules), so closely in fact that the urethrovaginal fascia is a fused structure and only separable by a sharp dissection. In its upper half, the vagina is related to the bladder in the region of the trigone, and here the vesical and vaginal fasciae are easily separable by a blunt dissection via the vesicovaginal space. There is a considerable vascular and lymphatic intercommunication between the vesical and the vaginal vessels, a sinister relationship having a bearing on the surgery of a malignant disease of this area.

POSTERIOR RELATIONS

The lower third of the vagina is related to the perineal body, the middle third to the ampulla of the rectum and the upper third to the anterior wall of the pouch of Douglas, which contains large and small bowel loops. This partition dividing the vagina from the peritoneal cavity is the thinnest area in the whole peritoneal surface and, therefore, a site of election for pointing and opening of pelvic abscess or the production of a hernia or enterocele. This is also an ideal site for colpocentesis in the diagnosis of ectopic pregnancy.

Pouch of Douglas (Fig. 2.8) is a peritoneal cul-de-sac in the rectovaginal space in the pelvis. It is bounded anteriorly by the peritoneum covering the posterior vaginal wall and posteriorly by the peritoneum covering the sigmoid colon and the rectum. Laterally, the uterosacral ligaments limit its boundary whereas the floor is the reflection of the peritoneum of the peritoneal cavity.

The endometriotic nodules and metastatic growth of an ovarian cancer are felt in the pouch of Douglas, so also pelvic inflammatory mass. The uterosacral ligaments are thickened and become nodular in advanced cancer cervix.

LATERAL RELATIONS

The lateral relations from below upwards are the cavernous tissue of the vestibule; the superficial muscles of the perineum; the triangular ligament and at about 2.5 cm from the introitus the levator ani, lateral to which is the ischiorectal fossa. Above the levator lies the endopelvic cellular tissue, and its condensation, called Mackenrodt's ligament, on the either side. The ureter traverses this tissue in the ureteric canal and is about 12 mm anterolateral to the lateral fornix.

SUPERIOR RELATIONS

The cervix with its four fornices – anterior, posterior and two lateral – are related to the uterine vessels, Mackenrodt's ligament and the ureter. Posteriorly, surrounding the pouch of Douglas lie the uterosacral ligaments which can be identified on vaginal examination, especially if thickened by disease such as endometriosis and cancer cervix.

Squamocolumnar junction, also known as transitional zone, is clinically a very important junction where the squamous epithelium lining the vagina merges with the columnar epithelium of the endocervix and is 1–10 mm (Fig. 2.9). Here, the constant cellular activity of the cells takes place, and the cells are highly sensitive to irritants, mutagens and viral agents such as papilloma virus 16, 18. These agents cause nuclear changes that can eventually lead to dysplasia and carcinoma cervix, which is the most common malignancy of the female genital tract in India. Squamocolumnar junction is of two types: first one is embryonic when columnar epithelium spreads over the external os. After puberty, metaplasia of columnar epithelium under the influence of oestrogen brings squamous epithelium close to the external os, thus creating a transitional zone between the two junctions. In women exposed to DES in utero, this zone is well outside the os, spreading over the vaginal vault. In a menopausal woman, it gets indrawn inside the os. During pregnancy and with oral contraceptives, it pouts out of os.

The squamocolumnar junction is well outside the external os during the reproductive period, and in Pap smear this area is scraped and the cytology of its cells studied for the nuclear changes, in the screening programme for cancer cervix.

During pregnancy, the external os becomes patulous and the squamocolumnar junction is well exposed all round. Pap smear yields the most accurate cytological findings.

In menopausal women, the cervix shrinks and the squamocolumnar junction gets indrawn into the cervical canal.

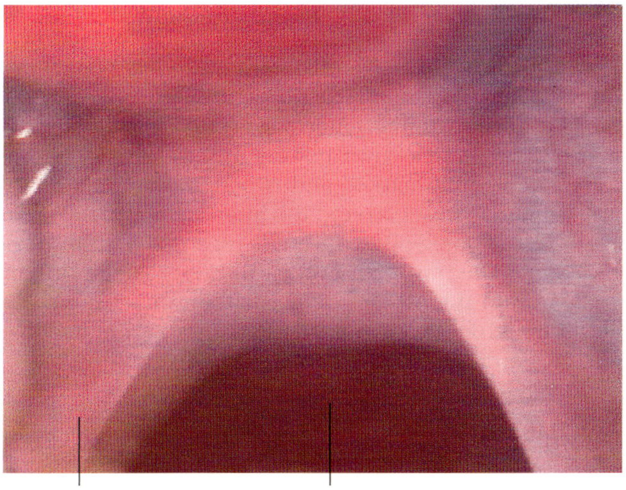

Figure 2.8 Pouch of Douglas showing uterosacral ligaments as upper border.

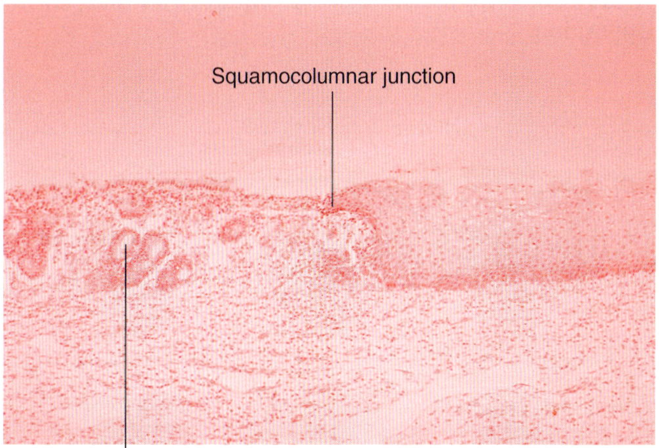

Figure 2.9 Squamocolumnar junction. In the 'ideal' cervix, the original squamous epithelium abuts the columnar epithelium. (*Source*: Hacker NF, Gambone JC, Hobel CJ, Hacker and Moore's Essentials of Obstetrics and Gynecology, 5th ed. Philadelphia: Elsevier, 2010.)

It is therefore not easily accessible, and ill exposed to the vagina, for visual inspection. This explains high false-negative findings in Pap smear in older women. Giving oestrogen locally or orally or prostaglandin E (misoprostol) pessary allows this junction to pout out and improves the efficacy of the Pap smear cytology.

The squamocolumnar junction is studied colposcopically when the Pap smear shows abnormal cells, and the abnormal areas are biopsied for cancer detection.

THE UTERUS

The uterus is pyriform in shape and measures approximately 9 cm in length, 6.5 cm in width and 3.5 cm in thickness. It is divided anatomically and functionally into body and cervix. It weighs 1 ounce (60 g). The line of division corresponds to the level of the internal os, and here the mucous membrane lining the cavity of the uterus becomes continuous with that of the cervical canal (Fig. 2.10). At this level, the peritoneum of the front of the uterus is reflected on to the bladder, and the uterine artery, after passing almost transversely across the pelvis, reaches the uterus, turns at right angle and passes vertically upwards along the lateral wall of the uterus. The cervix is divided into vaginal and supravaginal portions. The fundus of the uterus is that part of the corpus uteri which lies above the insertion of the fallopian tubes. The cavity of the uterus communicates above with the openings of the fallopian tubes, and by way of their abdominal ostia is in direct continuity with the peritoneal cavity. The uterine cavity is triangular in shape with a capacity of 3 mL. The lower angle is formed by the internal os. The lateral angle connecting to the fallopian tube is called the cornual end. The wall of the uterus consists of three layers, the peritoneal covering called perimetrium, the muscle layer or myometrium and the mucous membrane or endometrium.

The uterus is capable of distension during pregnancy, haematometra as well as with distended media during hysteroscopic examination. Otherwise the two walls are in opposition.

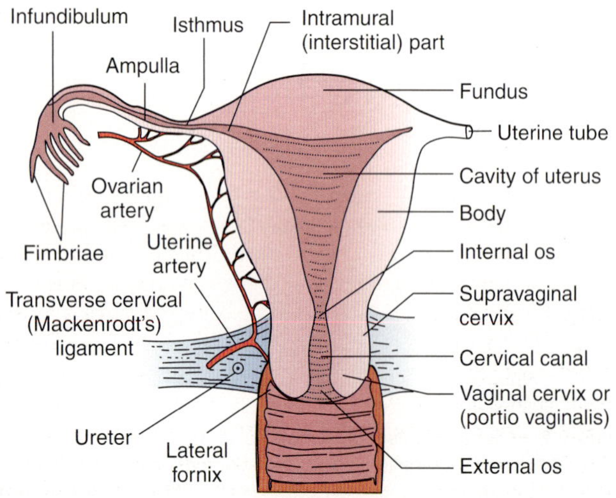

Figure 2.10 A nulliparous uterus showing the anatomical structures.

PERITONEAL COVERING

The peritoneal covering of the uterus is incomplete. Anteriorly, the whole body of the uterus is covered with peritoneum. The peritoneum is reflected on to the bladder at the level of the internal os. The cervix of the uterus has therefore no peritoneal covering anteriorly. Posteriorly, the whole body of the uterus is covered by peritoneum, as is the supravaginal portion of the cervix. The peritoneum is reflected from the supravaginal portion of the cervix on to the posterior vaginal wall in the region of the posterior fornix. The peritoneal layer is incomplete laterally because of the insertion of the fallopian tubes, the round and ovarian ligaments into the uterus, and below this level the two sheets of peritoneum, which constitute the broad ligament, leave a thin bare area laterally on each side.

MYOMETRIUM

The myometrium is the thickest of the three layers of the wall of the uterus. In the cervix, the myometrium consists of plain muscle tissue together with a large amount of fibrous tissue, which gives it a hard consistency. The muscle fibres and fibrous tissues are mixed together without an orderly arrangement. In the body of the uterus, the myometrium measures about 10–20 mm in thickness, and three layers can be distinguished which are best marked in the pregnant and puerperal uterus. The external layer lies immediately beneath the peritoneum and is longitudinal, the fibres passing from the cervix anteriorly over the fundus to reach the posterior surface of the cervix. This layer is thin and cannot easily be identified in the nulliparous uterus. The main function of this layer is a detrusor action during the expulsion of the fetus. The middle layer is the thickest of the three and consists of bundles of muscle separated by a connective tissue, the exact amount of which varies with age; plain muscle tissue is best marked in the childbearing period, especially during pregnancy whereas before puberty and after menopause it is much less plentiful. There is a tendency for the muscle bundles to interlace, and as the blood vessels supplying blood to the uterus are distributed in the connective tissues, the calibre of the vessels is in part controlled by the contraction of the muscle cells. The purpose of this layer is therefore in part haemostatic, though its expulsive role is equally important. This layer is described as *living ligatures of the uterus*, and is responsible for control of bleeding in the third stage of labour. Inefficient contraction and retraction of these muscle fibres cause prolonged labour and atonic postpartum haemorrhage (PPH).

The inner muscle layer consists of circular fibres. The layer is never well marked and is best represented by the circular muscle fibres around the internal os and the openings of the fallopian tubes. It can be regarded as sphincteric in action. The myometrium is thickest at the fundus (1–2 cm) and thinnest at the cornual end (3–4 mm), one should therefore be careful during curettage and endometrial ablation not to perforate the cornual end.

ENDOMETRIUM

The endometrium or mucous membrane lining the cavity of the uterus has a different structure from that of the endocervix. It is described in Chapter 3, 'Normal histology of Ovary and Endometrium'.

The **cervix** is spindle shaped and measures 2.5 cm or a little more. It is bounded above by the internal os and below by the external os (Fig. 2.10). The mucosal lining of the cervix differs from that of the body of the uterus by the absence of a submucosa. The endocervix is lined by a single layer of high columnar ciliated epithelium with spindle-shaped nuclei lying adjacent to the basement membrane with abundant cytoplasm and mucin. The direction of the cilia is downwards towards the external os. The glands are racemose in type (Fig. 2.11A and B) and secrete mucus with a high content of fructose glycoprotein, mucopolysaccharide and sodium chloride. The secretion is alkaline and has a pH of 7.8 and its fructose content renders it attractive to ascending spermatozoa. This secretion collects as a plug in the cervical canal and possibly hinders ascending infections. In gonococcal and chlamydial infections of the cervix, the organisms collect amongst the crypts of the cervical glands. In nulliparous women, the external os is circular but vaginal delivery results in the transverse slit which characterizes the parous cervix. The cervix contains more of fibrous tissue and collagen than the muscle fibres, which are dispersed scarcely amongst the fibrous tissue. Cervix contains mainly collagen and only 10% of muscle fibres. Light microscopic examination reveals 29% muscle fibres in its upper one-third, 18% in the middle one-third and only 6% in the lower one-third, whereas the body of the uterus contains 70% muscle fibres. The change from fibrous tissue of cervix to the muscle tissue of the body is quite abrupt. In late pregnancy and at term, under the influence of prostaglandin, collagenase dissolves collagen into fluid form and renders the cervix soft and stretchable during labour.

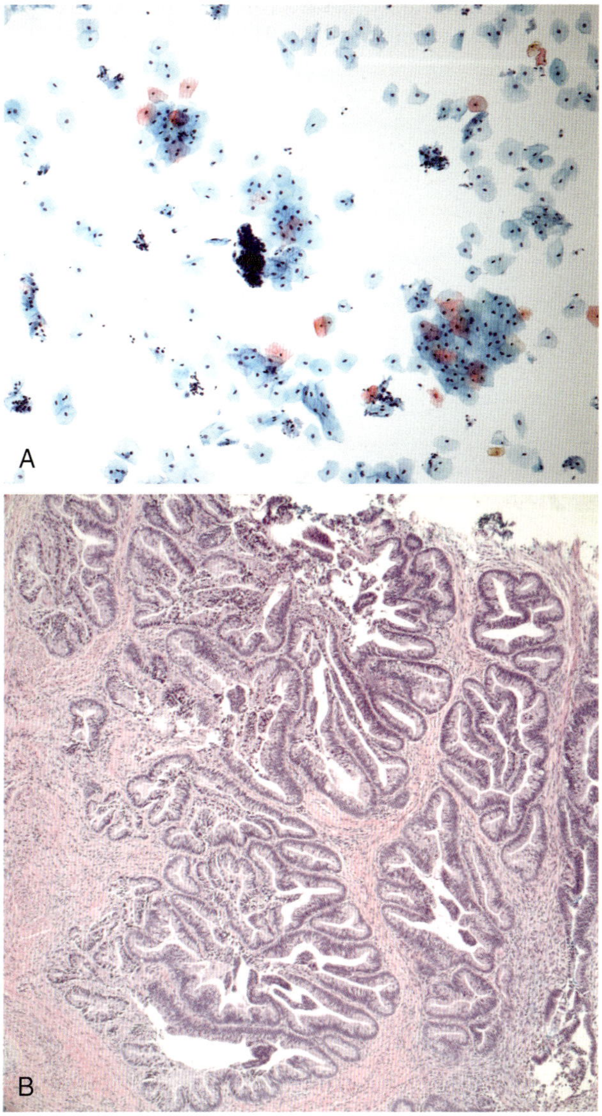

Figure 2.11 **(A)** Normal endocervical cells. **(B)** Normal cervical glands. These are of the racemose type and are lined by high columnar epithelium which secretes mucous (×250). (*Source* for (B): Seema Khutti, Cervix.Premalignant/preinvasive lesions. 2003–2017, PathologyOutlines.com, Inc.)

Functions of the endocervical cell lining are as follows:

- The cilia are directed downwards and prevent ascending infection.
- The cells sieve out abnormal sperms and allow healthy sperms to enter the uterus.
- It provides nutrition to the sperms.
- It allows capacitation of sperms.

Structurally and functionally, the body of the uterus and that of the cervix are in marked contrast. The cervical epithelium shows no periodic alteration during the menstrual cycle, and the decidual reaction of pregnancy is seen only rarely in the cervix. Similarly, the malignant disease of the uterus is an adenocarcinoma of the endometrium, whereas carcinoma of the cervix is usually a squamous cell growth of high malignancy.

An intermediate zone, *the isthmus,* 6 mm in length, lies between the endometrium of the body and the mucous membrane of the cervical canal. Its epithelial lining resembles and behaves like the endometrium of the body. The isthmic portion stretches during pregnancy and forms the lower uterine segment in late pregnancy. This isthmic portion is less contractile during pregnancy and labour but further stretches under uterine contractions. It is identified during caesarean delivery by the loose fold of peritoneal lining covering its anterior surface.

The relationship between the length of the cervix and that of the body of the uterus varies with age. Before puberty, the cervix to corpus ratio is 2:1. At puberty, this ratio is reversed to 1:2, and during the reproductive years, cervix to corpus ratio may be 1:3 or even 1:4. After menopause, the whole organ atrophies and the portio vaginalis may eventually disappear.

Although the endometrial secretion is scanty and fluid in nature, the cervical secretion is abundant and its quality and quantity change in the different phases of the menstrual cycle, under different hormonal effects. The cervical mucous is rich in fructose, glycoprotein and mucopolysaccharides. Fructose is nutritive to sperms during their passage in the cervical canal. Under oestrogenic influence in the preovulatory phase, the glycoprotein network is arranged parallel to each other and facilitates sperm penetration, whereas under the progesterone secretion, the network forms interlacing bridges and prevents their entry into the cervical canal. This property of progesterone is used in a contraceptive pill and progesterone-impregnated intrauterine contraceptive device. Sodium chloride content in the mucous increases at ovulation and forms a fern-like pattern when a drop of mucous is dried on a slide and studied under a microscope.

POSITION OF THE UTERUS

The uterus normally lies in a position of anteversion and anteflexion. The body of the uterus is bent forwards on the cervix approximately at the level of the internal os, and this forward inclination of the body of the uterus on the cervix constitutes anteflexion. The direction of the axis of the cervix depends upon the position of the uterus. In anteversion (Fig. 2.12B), the external os is directed downwards and backwards so that on vaginal examination the examining fingers find that the lowest part of the cervix is the anterior lip. When the uterus is retroverted the cervix is directed downwards and forwards, and the lowest part of the cervix is either the external os or the posterior lip. As a result of its normal position of anteflexion, the body of the uterus lies against the bladder. The pouch of peritoneum that separates the bladder from the uterus is the uterovesical pouch. The peritoneum is reflected from the front of the uterus on to the bladder at the level of the internal os.

Posteriorly, a large peritoneal pouch lies between the uterus and the rectosigmoid colon. If the uterus is pulled forwards, two folds of peritoneum can be seen to pass backwards from the uterus to reach the parietal peritoneum lateral to the rectum. These folds, the uterosacral folds, lie at the level of the internal os and pass backwards and upwards. The uterosacral ligaments are condensation of the pelvic cellular tissues and lie at a lower level and within the uterosacral folds. The pouch of peritoneum below the level of the uterosacral folds, which is bounded in front by the peritoneum covering the upper part of the posterior vaginal wall and posteriorly by the peritoneum covering the sigmoid colon and the upper end of the rectum, is the pouch of Douglas. The posterior fornix of the vagina is in close relation to the peritoneal cavity, as only the posterior vaginal wall and a single layer of peritoneum separate the vagina from the peritoneal cavity. Collection of pus in the pouch of Douglas can therefore be evacuated without difficulty by incising the vagina in the region of the posterior fornix. On the contrary, the uterovesical pouch is approached with difficulty from the vagina; first the vagina must be incised and then the bladder separated from the cervix and the vesicocervical space traversed before the uterovesical fold of the peritoneum is reached (Fig. 2.12A).

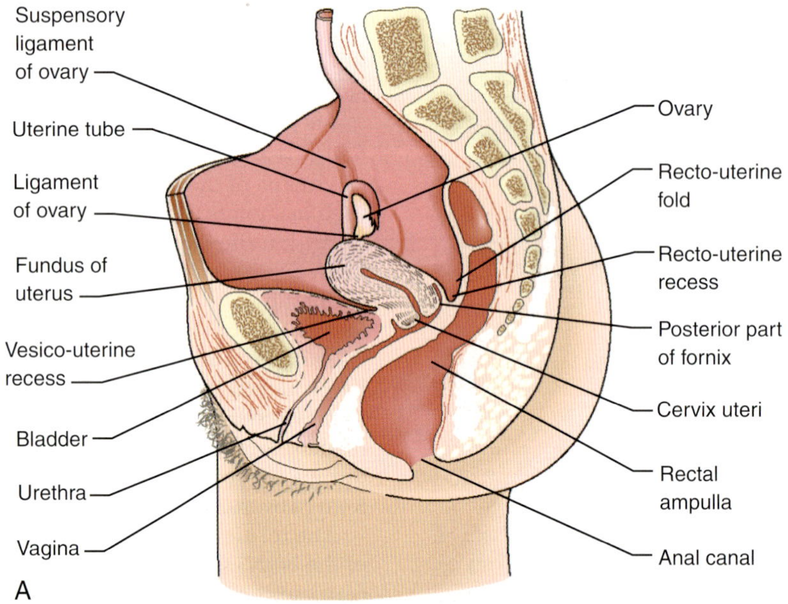

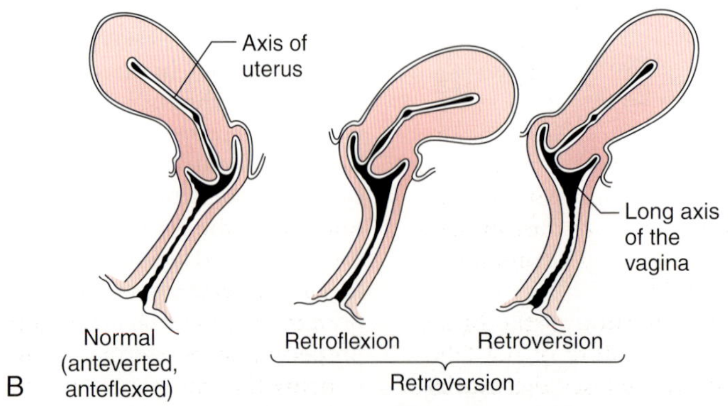

Figure 2.12 (A) The relationship of the female reproductive organs: sagittal section. **(B)** Anteverted, anteflexed and retroverted uterus. (*Source* for **(A)**: From Fig. 7.1. Chris Brooker: Alexander's Nursing Practice, 4th Ed. Churchill Livingstone: Elsevier, 2011.)

THE UTERINE APPENDAGES

The uterus projects upwards from the pelvic floor into the peritoneal cavity and carries on each side of it two folds of peritoneum, which pass laterally to the pelvic wall and form the *broad ligaments*. The fallopian tubes pass outwards from the uterine cornua and lie in the upper border of the broad ligaments. The ovarian ligaments posteriorly, and the round ligaments anteriorly, also pass into the uterine cornua, but at a slightly lower level than the fallopian tubes. Both these ligaments and the fallopian tubes are covered with peritoneum.

The *round ligament* passes from the uterine cornua beneath the anterior peritoneal fold of the broad ligament to reach the internal abdominal ring. In this part of its course it is curved and lies immediately beneath the peritoneum, and is easily distinguished. The round ligament passes down the inguinal canal and finally ends by becoming adherent to the skin of the labia majora. The ligaments consist of plain muscle and connective tissue and vary considerably in thickness. They hypertrophy during pregnancy. The round ligaments are much better developed in multiparae than in nulliparae. They are most remarkably hypertrophied in the presence of large fibroids when they may attain a diameter of 1 cm. They correspond developmentally to the gubernaculum testis and are morphologically continuous with the ovarian ligaments, as during intrauterine life the ovarian and round ligaments are continuous and connect the lower pole of the primitive ovary to the inguinal canal. The round ligaments are lax and, except during labour, are free of tension. There is no evidence that the normal position of anteflexion and anteversion of the uterus is produced by contraction of the round ligaments. The ligaments, however, may be shortened by operation or they may be attached to the anterior abdominal wall, both procedures being used to cause anteversion in a uterus which is pathologically retroverted. The round ligaments are supplied by a branch of the ovarian artery derived from its anastomosis with the uterine artery, hence there is the necessity for ligation of the round ligament during hysterectomy. Along it lymphatic vessels pass from the fundus, which connect with those draining the labium majus into the inguinal glands. This explains the possibility of metastases in these glands in late cases of cancer of the endometrium of the fundus.

The *ovarian ligaments* pass upwards and inwards from the inner poles of the ovaries to reach the cornua of the uterus (Fig. 2.13) below the level of the attachment of the fallopian tubes. They lie beneath the posterior peritoneal fold of the broad ligament and measure about 2.5 cm in length. Like the round ligaments, they consist of plain muscle fibres and connective tissue, but they are not so prominent because they contain less plain muscle tissue. They are morphologically a continuation of the round ligament (contents of broad ligaments are listed in Table 2.1).

Infundibulopelvic ligament is that portion of the broad ligament that extends from the infundibulum of the fallopian tube to the lateral pelvic wall. It encloses the ovarian vessels, lymphatics and nerves of the ovary. The ureter is also in a close contact and can be damaged during clamping of this ligament.

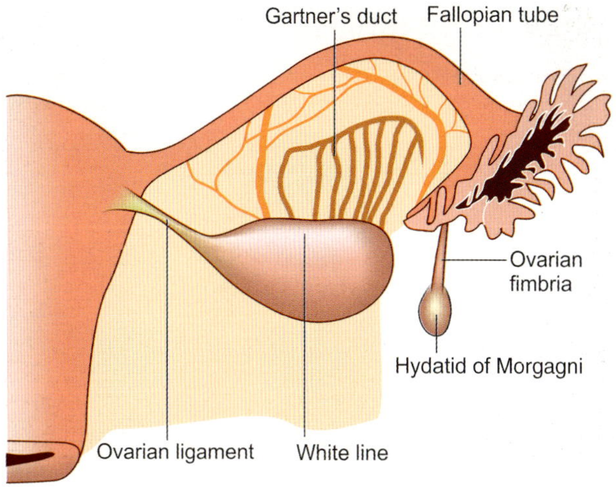

Figure 2.13 The right uterine appendages viewed from behind.

Table 2.1 Contents of Broad Ligament

- Fallopian tube – upper portion
- Round ligament – anteriorly
- Ovarian ligament – posterior fold
- Vestigial structures of Wolffian body – epoophoron and paroophoron
- Vestigial structure of Wolffian duct – Gartner's duct
- Ureter
- Uterine vessels
- Pelvic nerves
- Parametrial lymph node
- Pelvic cellular tissue condensed to form Mackenrodt's ligament
- Infundibulopelvic ligament

Mesovarium attaches the ovary to the posterior fold of peritoneum of the broad ligament and contains vessels, lymphatics and nerves of the ovary. Mesosalpinx lies between the fallopian tube and the ovary and contains the anastomotic vessels between the ovary and uterus and the vestigial structures of the Wolffian body and the duct (see section on The Ovaries).

FALLOPIAN TUBES

Each fallopian tube (Figs 2.13 and 2.14) is attached to the uterine cornu and passes outwards and backwards in the upper part of the broad ligament. The fallopian tube measures 4 inch (10 cm) or more in length and approximately 8 mm in diameter, but the diameter diminishes near the cornu of the uterus to 1 mm. The fallopian tube is divided anatomically into four parts:

1. *The interstitial portion* is the innermost part of the tube which traverses the myometrium to open into the endometrial cavity. It is the shortest part of the tube, its length being the thickness of the uterine muscle, about 18 mm. It is also the narrowest part, its internal diameter being 1 mm or less so that only the finest cannula can be passed into it during falloscopy examination. There are no

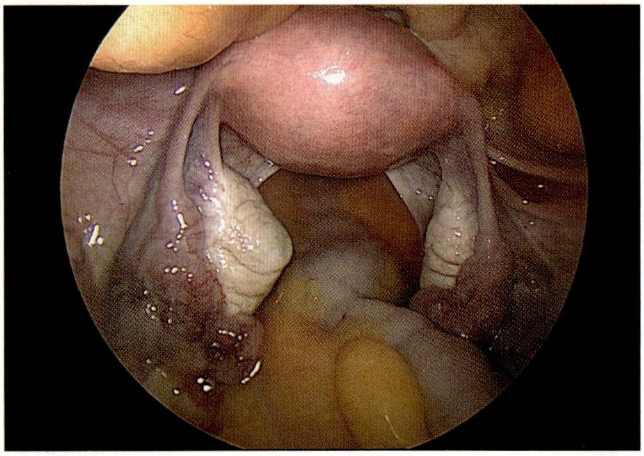

Figure 2.14 Laparoscopic view of the pelvis showing normal uterus and bilateral adnexa. (*Courtesy*: Dr Marwah.)

longitudinal muscle fibres here but the circular fibres are well developed.

2. *The isthmus* comprises the next and inner part of the tube and represents about one-third of the total length, i.e. 35 mm. It is narrow but a little wider than the interstitial part and its lumen has a diameter of 2 mm. Its muscle wall contains both longitudinal and circular fibres, and it is covered by peritoneum except for a small inferior bare area related to the broad ligament. It is relatively straight.
3. *The ampulla* is the lateral, widest and longest part of the tube and comprises roughly two-thirds of the tube, measuring 2.5–3 inch (60–75 mm) in length. Here the mucosa is arborescent with many complex folds (Fig. 2.15). Fertilization occurs in the ampullary portion of the fallopian tube.
4. *The fimbriated extremity or infundibulum* is where the abdominal ostium opens into the peritoneal cavity. The fimbriae are motile and almost prehensile, and enjoy a considerable range of movement and action. One fimbria – the ovarian fimbria – is larger and longer than the others and is attached to the region of the ovary. This fimbria embraces the ovary at ovulation, picks up the ovum and carries it to the ampullary portion.

The fallopian tube represents the cranial end of the Müllerian duct, and its lumen is continuous with the cavity of the uterus. Consequently, spermatozoa and the fertilized ovum can pass along the tube. Fluids such as dyes and gases such as carbon dioxide may be injected through the uterus and by the way of the fallopian tubes into the peritoneal cavity, and by these means the patency of the fallopian tubes can be investigated clinically by a dye test (Fig. 2.16). The fallopian tubes lie in the upper part of the broad ligaments and are covered with peritoneum except along a thin area inferiorly, which is left bare by the reflection of the peritoneum to form the two layers of the broad ligament. The blood supply of the fallopian tube is mainly derived from the tubal branches of the ovarian artery, but the anastomosing branch of the uterine artery supplies its inner part. Unlike the vermiform appendix, the fallopian tube does not become gangrenous when acutely inflamed, as it has two sources of blood supply which reach it at opposite ends. The lymphatics of the fallopian tube communicate with the lymphatics of the fundus of the uterus and with those of the ovary, and they drain along the infundibulopelvic ligament to the para-aortic glands near the origin of the ovarian artery from the aorta. Some drain into the pelvic glands.

The fallopian tubes have three layers: serous, muscular and mucous. The serous layer consists of the mesothelium of the peritoneum. Intervening between the mesothelium and the muscle layer is a well-defined subserous layer in which numerous small blood vessels and lymphatics can be demonstrated. The muscular layer consists of outer longitudinal and inner circular fibres. The circular fibres are best developed in the isthmus and are thinned out near the fimbriated extremity. The mucous membrane is thrown into folds or plicae. Near the isthmus three folds can be recognized, but when traced laterally they divide and subdivide so that in the ampullary region they become highly complex. Each plica consists of stroma which is covered by epithelium. The stroma is cellular and its cells are in some ways

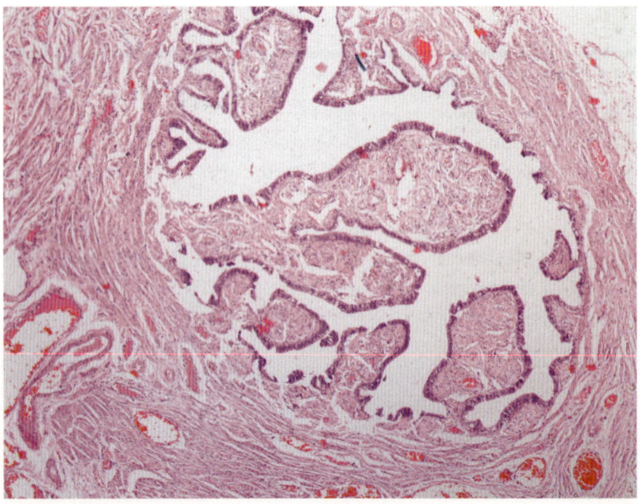

Figure 2.15 Ampullary portion of fallopian tube to show arrangement of plicae (×18) (*Courtesy*: Dr Sandeep Mathur, AIIMS.)

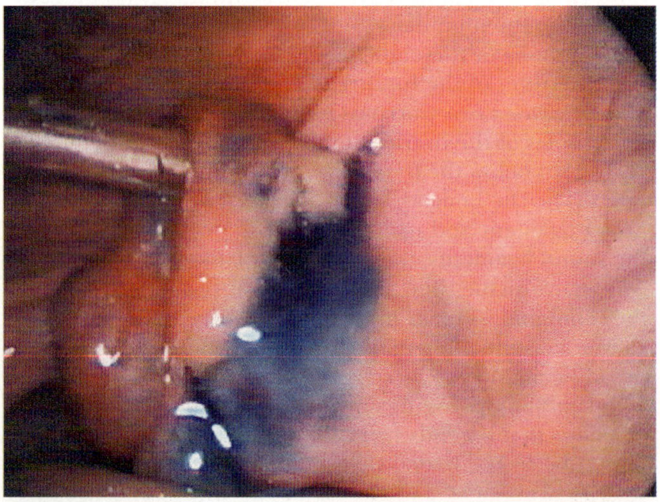

Figure 2.16 Fimbrial end of a patent fallopian tube. Dye test shows spill.

similar to those of the endometrium. The blood vessels of the stroma are plentiful and are particularly well marked in the ampullary region. The epithelium of the mucous membrane consists of three types of cells: the most common is ciliated, and is either columnar or cubical in type. Its function is to propel a fluid current towards the uterus and plays some part in the transport of the inert ovum which, unlike the sperm, has no motile power of its own. Next in order of frequency is a goblet-shaped cell, not ciliated, which does not give the histochemical reactions for mucin. Its function is lubricant and possibly nutritive to the ovum. A cell intermediate in type to the two already mentioned can be distinguished, and small rod-shaped cells are also present. These are the so-called peg cells whose purpose is not known. It has been possible to demonstrate differences in the histological appearances of the epithelium of the fallopian tubes during the menstrual cycle. The *hysterosalpingogram, sonosalpingogram* and *laparoscopic chromotubation* are the clinical methods of testing the patency of the fallopian tubes. Laparoscopy also identifies external tubal adhesions.

THE OVARIES

Each ovary weighs 4–8 g and measures about 35 mm in length, 25 mm in width and 18 mm in thickness. The ovary (Figs 2.14 and 2.17) is almond shaped, pearly grey due to a compact tunica albuginea, and the surface is slightly corrugated. Before puberty, the ovaries are small and located near the pelvic brim. After menopause they atrophy and become shrunken and the grooves and furrows on the surface become well marked. The menopausal ovary measures 20 mm × 10 mm × 15 mm with a volume of 8 mL or less. An ovary larger than this as measured ultrasonically is of great concern in menopausal women. The ovary is attached to the back of the broad ligament by a thin mesentery, the *mesovarium.* Laterally, the ovary is related to the fossa below the bifurcation of the common iliac artery and the ureter. Medially, it is close to the fimbria of the fallopian tube, which stretches over it around ovulation. It is attached to the cornu of the uterus by the ovarian ligament. The infundibulopelvic ligament is the outer border of the broad ligament and contains the ovarian vessels, nerves and lymphatics. The ovaries are not normally palpable during bimanual examination, but cause pain on touch. The *epoophoron,* also known as the organ of Rosenmüller, represents the cranial end of the Wolffian body. It consists of a series of vertical tubules in the mesovarium and mesosalpinx between the fallopian tube above and the ovary below. Each tubule is surrounded by plain muscle and is lined by cubical cells.

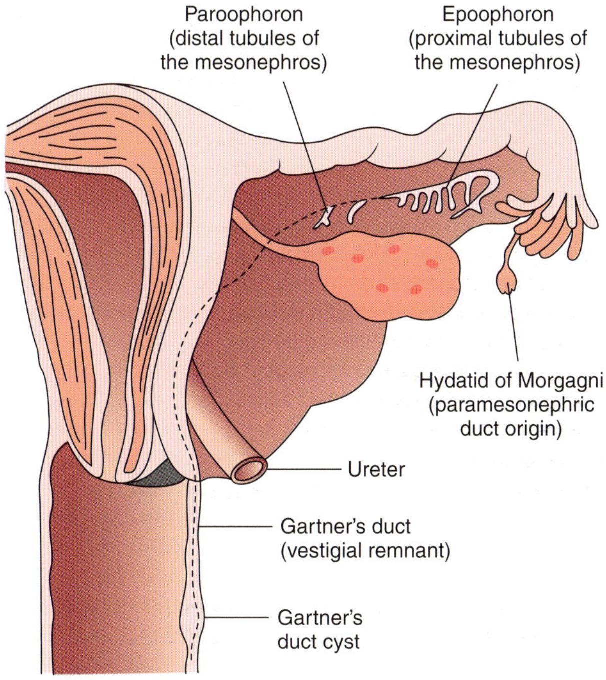

Figure 2.17 Remnants of the mesonephric (Wolffian) ducts that may persist in the anterolateral vagina or adjacent to the uterus within the broad ligament or mesosalpinx.

The paroophoron represents the caudal end of the Wolffian body and similarly contains vertical tubules. It sometimes forms paraovarian cyst.

The Wolffian duct (Gartner's duct) is an imperfect duct which runs parallel to, but below, the fallopian tube in the mesosalpinx. The duct passes downwards by the side of the uterus to the level of the internal os where it passes into the tissues of the cervix. It then runs forwards to reach the anterolateral aspect of the vaginal wall and may reach as far down as the hymen. The duct sometimes forms a cyst, called Gartner cyst, in the broad ligament or in the vagina, and may need surgical enucleation (Fig. 2.17). Histology of the ovary is described in Chapter 3.

THE URETHRA

The urethra measures 35 mm in length and 5–6 mm in diameter. It passes downwards and forwards from the base of the bladder behind the symphysis pubis to end in the external meatus. Its epithelial lining consists of squamous epithelium at the external meatus, but becomes transitional in the canal. Deep to the epithelium is a layer rich in small vessels and connective tissue. The urethral wall comprises inner longitudinal and outer circular involuntary muscle fibres, which are arranged as crisscross spirals. The longitudinal fibres contract and shorten the urethra during micturition. The outer circular fibres keep the internal sphincter closed.

The neck of the bladder (internal urethral sphincter) lies above the levator ani muscles and thus maintains the continence of urine by receiving the same abdominal pressure as the bladder. The bladder base forms an angle of 100° with the posterior urethral wall (posterior urethrovesical angle), which is also responsible for maintaining urinary continence.

RELATIONS

Posteriorly, upper portion of the urethra is loosely connected to the vagina by vesicovaginal fascia and can be dissected easily. In its lower one-third, it is firmly attached to the vagina by pubourethral ligament and requires a sharp dissection. Laterally, it is surrounded by the areolar tissue, the compressor urethra and the superficial perineal muscles. Pubourethral ligament fixes the mid-urethra to the pubic bone and the lateral pelvic wall and maintains continence of urine. Anteriorly, the urethra is separated from the pubic bone by the areolar tissue.

The external urinary meatus lies in the vestibule, 2 cm below the clitoris and is partly concealed by the upper end of the labia minora. Numerous periurethral glands surround the urethra and open by tiny ducts into its lumen. These are analogues of the prostate in males. The paraurethral glands of Skene are important paired glands which lie alongside the floor of the urethra and open by tiny ducts close to the external meatus. The glands when infected form periurethral abscess and cysts.

The proximal urethra derives blood supply from the inferior vesical artery and distal urethra from internal pudendal artery. The veins drain into the vesical plexus and internal pudendal vein. The urethra is innervated by the internal pudendal nerve. The urethra is developed from the cloaca.

The proximity of the urethra to the vagina makes it susceptible to infection spreading from the lower genital tract. The commonest infective organisms are *N.* gonorrhoea, Chlamydia trachomatis and trichomonads. The urethral swab, culture and urine culture can identify the organisms.

THE BLADDER

The bladder is a smooth muscle organ with a body and a trigone. It lies between the symphysis pubis in front and the uterus behind, being separated from the uterus by the uterovesical peritoneum. It is a pelvic organ with a capacity to hold 500–600 mL of urine. The bladder distends upwards with a fixed base at the trigone, and then becomes palpable abdominally.

The bladder has an apex, a base, a superior and two inferolateral surfaces. The neck of the bladder (internal urinary sphincter) lies above the levator ani muscles, so that the raised abdominal pressure transmits the pressure equally to the bladder and its neck, hence maintaining urinary continence during coughing and sneezing. Anteriorly, lies the cave of Retzius (retropubic space). Posteriorly, it is in proximity to the uterus and supravaginal portion of the cervix, separated from them by the uterovesical pouch of peritoneum.

The ureters enter the bladder obliquely, and the area between the ureteric openings and the internal urinary sphincter forms a fixed triangular area called trigone. The apex is continuous with the urachus.

The bladder receives blood supply from the superior and inferior vesical arteries, and the pubic branch of the inferior epigastric artery. The venous plexus drains into internal iliac vein. The lymphatics drain into internal and external iliac glands.

NERVE SUPPLY

The sympathetic outflow is from first and second lumbar segments of the spinal cord which inhibits contractions of the detrusor (bladder) muscle and maintains internal sphincteric contraction. The parasympathetic outflow from S2, S3 and S4 stimulates the detrusor muscle and relaxes the internal sphincter, thus initiating micturition. The sensory nerve fibres reach the central nervous system via the splanchnic nerves (parasympathetic S2–S4). The somatic afferent fibres travel with sympathetic nerves via hypogastric plexus and enter the first and second lumbar segments of the spinal cord. The bladder wall is lined by transitional epithelium, which gets folded when empty but allows bladder distension. The lining membrane of the trigone is fixed to the muscle wall. The muscular coat of the bladder is composed of smooth muscle known as detrusor. The neck of the bladder (internal urinary sphincter) is surrounded by circular muscle fibres.

THE URETERS

Every gynaecologist should be familiar with the anatomy of the pelvic portion of the ureter, as injury can occur during pelvic surgery. The ureter needs to be dissected during Wertheim's hysterectomy for cancer of the cervix. The ureter may run in a close relation to the broad ligament cyst and myoma.

The pelvic portion of the ureter is 13 cm long and 5 mm in diameter. It passes over the bifurcation of the common iliac artery and runs downwards and forwards in the ovarian fossa deep to the peritoneum, where it enters the true pelvis at the brim, it is crossed by the ovarian vessels, and on the left side the mesosigmoid is an anterior relation. In this situation, the obturator vessels and nerve lie laterally, and the hypogastric lymph nodes are closely related. The course of the ureter is then downwards and forwards immediately beneath the peritoneum to which it is always closely attached.

On the pelvic floor, the ureter pierces Mackenrodt's ligament where a canal, the ureteric canal, is developed. It is necessary that the ureter must have room for normal peristalsis without any pressure from the surrounding structures, and the ureteric canal protects the ureter from the outside pressure. In its passage through the ureteric canal, the ureter is crossed by the uterine artery above and the uterine plexus of veins below, thus being forked between the uterine vessels. After leaving the ureteric canal, the ureter passes forwards and medially to reach the bladder, being separated from the cervix by a distance of 1–2 cm (Fig. 2.18). The course of the ureter through the pelvis is not always constant. At operation, the ureter is recognized by its pale glistening appearance and by a fine longitudinal plexus of vessels on its surface, but more particularly by its peristaltic movements. It can also be recognized by palpation between the finger and the thumb as a firm cord, which, as it escapes, gives a characteristic snap. The ureter is rarely duplicated. In advanced stage of cancer of the cervix with extensive involvement of the parametrium, stricture of the ureter causes hydronephrosis and uraemia.

The ureter derives its blood supply from the common, external and internal iliac arteries in addition to a constant vessel from the uterine and inferior vesical artery. The vessels form a longitudinal anastomosis up and down the ureter which protects the ureter from ischaemia if one vessel is ligated or injured. However, damage of several small vessels can cause avascular necrosis and ureteric fistula. The small branches of the renal artery also supply blood to the ureter above the pelvic brim.

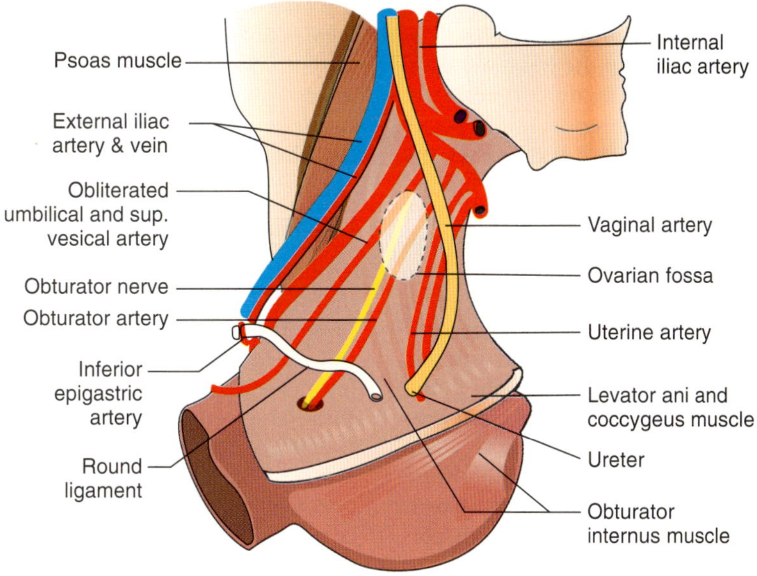

Figure 2.18 Relation of the ureter to the pelvic vessels in the ovarian fossa.

The blood supply to the pelvic ureter is principally from the lateral side, and the ureteric dissection should be done along its medial side.

The injury to the ureter occurs at the infundibulopelvic ligament on the lateral pelvic wall, in the ureteric canal when the uterine vessels are ligated, near the internal cervical os and near the uterosacral ligament. It is important to identify the ureter during Wertheim hysterectomy, broad ligament tumour dissection and while ligating the internal iliac artery.

The lymphatics drain into internal and external iliac glands. The sympathetic nerve supply comes from hypogastric and pelvic plexus; para sympathetic from sacral plexus.

THE RECTUM AND ANAL CANAL

The rectum is the continuation of the pelvic colon and lies in the pelvis at the level of third sacral vertebrae. It measures 12–15 cm and continues as anal canal. It is covered anteriorly and laterally by pelvic peritoneum which forms the posterior surface of the pouch of Douglas. Lower down, it is in a close contact with the posterior vaginal wall, separated by rectovaginal septum. The anal canal is separated from the lower one-third of posterior vaginal wall by the perineal body. Posteriorly, it lies close to the sacrum and coccyx with loose articular tissue, middle sacral artery and pelvic nerve plexus. Laterally lie the two uterosacral ligaments above and levator ani muscles below and ischiorectal fossa. The rectum is surrounded by rectal fascia. The anal canal measures 2.5 cm. Anteriorly, it is related to the perineal body and posteriorly to the anococcygeal body. It has two sphincters: (i) involuntary internal sphincter in the upper two-thirds and (ii) voluntary external sphincter surrounded by puborectalis muscle of the levator ani muscle below.

The rectum and anal canal receive the blood supply from (i) superior rectal branch of interior mesenteric artery and (ii) middle and inferior rectal branches of internal iliac artery. The rectum and upper one-third of anal canal drain via superior rectal veins into portal circulation. Lower one-third portion of anal canal drains into inferior rectal vein (systemic circulation).

THE LYMPHATICS

The rectum and upper one-third of anus drain into internal iliac and preaortic lymphatic nodes. Lower one-third drains into superficial inguinal lymph nodes.

Autonomic pelvic plexus innervates the rectum and upper portion of the anal canal. The lower portion of the anal canal is innervated by the inferior haemorrhoidal nerve. The rectum and upper two-thirds of the anal canal develop from the dorsal portion of the cloaca. The lower anal canal is derived from ectoderm.

THE PELVIC MUSCULATURE

The pelvic muscles of importance in gynaecology are those of the pelvic floor. These muscles are grouped into three layers: (i) those of the pelvic diaphragm, (ii) those of the urogenital diaphragm and (iii) the superficial muscles of the pelvic floor.

PELVIC DIAPHRAGM

The pelvic diaphragm consists of two levator ani muscles. Each levator ani muscle consists of three main divisions: the pubococcygeus, the iliococcygeus and the ischiococcygeus. The pubococcygeus muscle arises from the posterior surface of the body of the pubic bone and passes backwards, lateral to the vagina and the rectum, to be inserted into the anococcygeal raphe and into the coccyx. The inner fibres which come together posterior to the rectum are known as the puborectalis portion of the muscle: they sling up and support the rectum. Some of the inner fibres of the puborectalis fuse with the outer wall of the vagina as they pass lateral to it. Other fibres decussate between the vagina and the rectum in the situation of the perineal body. These decussating fibres divide the space between the two levator ani muscles into an anterior portion, the hiatus urogenitalis, through which passes the urethra and vagina, and a posterior portion, the hiatus rectalis, through which passes the rectum. The dimensions of the hiatus urogenitalis depend upon two main factors: the tone of the levator muscles and the existence of the decussating fibres of the puborectalis muscle.

Perineal tears occurring during parturition divide these decussating fibres, causing the hiatus urogenitalis to become patulous and lead to prolapse. In visceroptosis and asthenic states, the levator muscles become lax, the dimensions of the hiatus urogenitalis are increased and there is a tendency for the pelvic viscera to prolapse. The iliococcygeus is a fan-shaped muscle arising from a broad origin along the white line of the pelvic fascia and passing backwards and inwards to be inserted into the coccyx. The ischiococcygeus or coccygeus muscle has a narrow origin from the ischial spine and spreads out posteriorly to be inserted into the front of the coccyx (Figs 2.19 and 2.20).

The levator muscles together constitute the pelvic diaphragm and support the pelvic viscera: contraction of the levator muscle pulls the rectum and vagina towards the symphysis pubis; the rectum is thereby kinked and closed, and the vagina narrowed anteroposteriorly. The origin of the levator muscle is fixed because the muscle arises anteriorly either from bone or from fascia which is attached to the bone; posteriorly the insertion is either into the anococcygeal raphe or into the coccyx, both of which are moveable. It follows that the contraction of the levator muscles leads to the posterior attachments being pulled towards the symphysis pubis. The movement of the internal rotation of the presenting part during parturition is assisted by this property of the levator muscles. Uterine contractions push the presenting part down upon the levator ani (pelvic floor) and cause the muscles to contract as a result of the direct pressure of the presenting part. The lowest part of the fetus is carried forwards during the contractions of the levator muscles, and as the anterior fibres of the muscles are directed inwards as well as forwards, the presenting part rotates forwards and inwards.

The superior and inferior surfaces of the levator muscles are covered by the pelvic fascia, which separates the muscles from the cellular tissues of the parametrium above and from the fibrous and fatty tissues of the ischiorectal fossa below.

UROGENITAL DIAPHRAGM

The urogenital diaphragm is also called the triangular ligament. It is not so well developed in the female as in the male. It extends from the pubic arch anteriorly to the central point of the perineum posteriorly and consists of two layers of fascia through which pass the vagina and the urethra. The central point of the female perineum lies between the vagina and the rectum. Within the two fascial layers of the urogenital diaphragm lies the deep transverse perineal muscle, which extends laterally on each side to reach the ramus of the pubic bone. This muscle is so poorly developed that it is difficult to dissect in anatomical specimens and needs a special histological technique for its demonstration. Its functional significance is dubious. The striped muscle or voluntary sphincter of the urethra also lies between the two layers of the triangular ligament.

SUPERFICIAL MUSCLES

Four muscles are identified in this layer. The external sphincter muscle of the anus is attached anteriorly to the central point of the perineum and surrounds the anus. The bulbospongiosus muscle, or as it is sometimes called the sphincter vaginae, extends from the central point of the perineum along each side of the vagina to be attached anteriorly to the symphysis pubis. It lies around and lateral to the urethral bulb. The ischiocavernosus muscle extends on each side of the ischial tuberosity in relation to the crura of the clitoris to reach it in the midline. The superficial transverse muscle of the perineum passes laterally on each side from the central point of the perineum to the pubic ramus (Fig. 2.21). Deep to these superficial muscles and between them and the inferior layer of the triangular ligament lie the vestibular bulb and the greater vestibular glands of *Bartholin*.

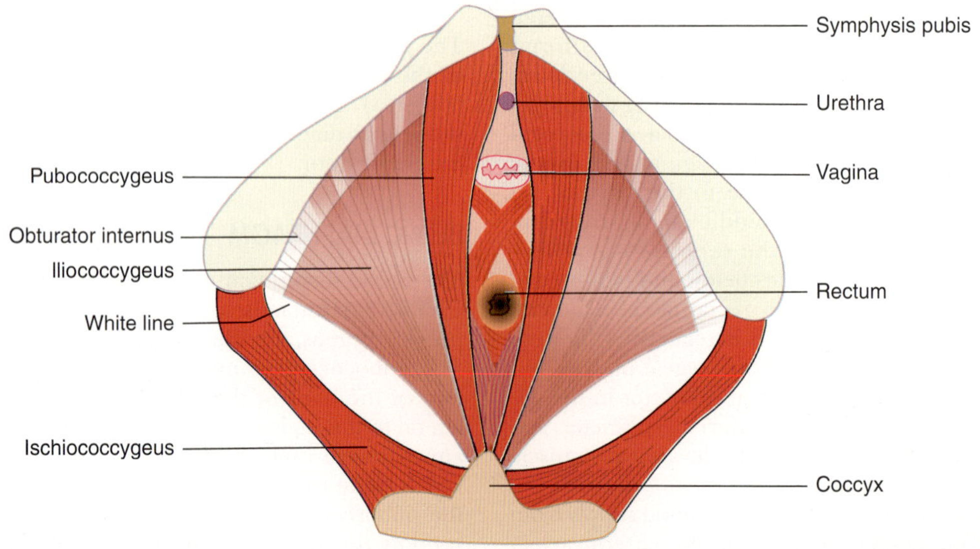

Figure 2.19 The muscular pelvic floor seen from above after the removal of the pelvic viscera and pelvic fascia.

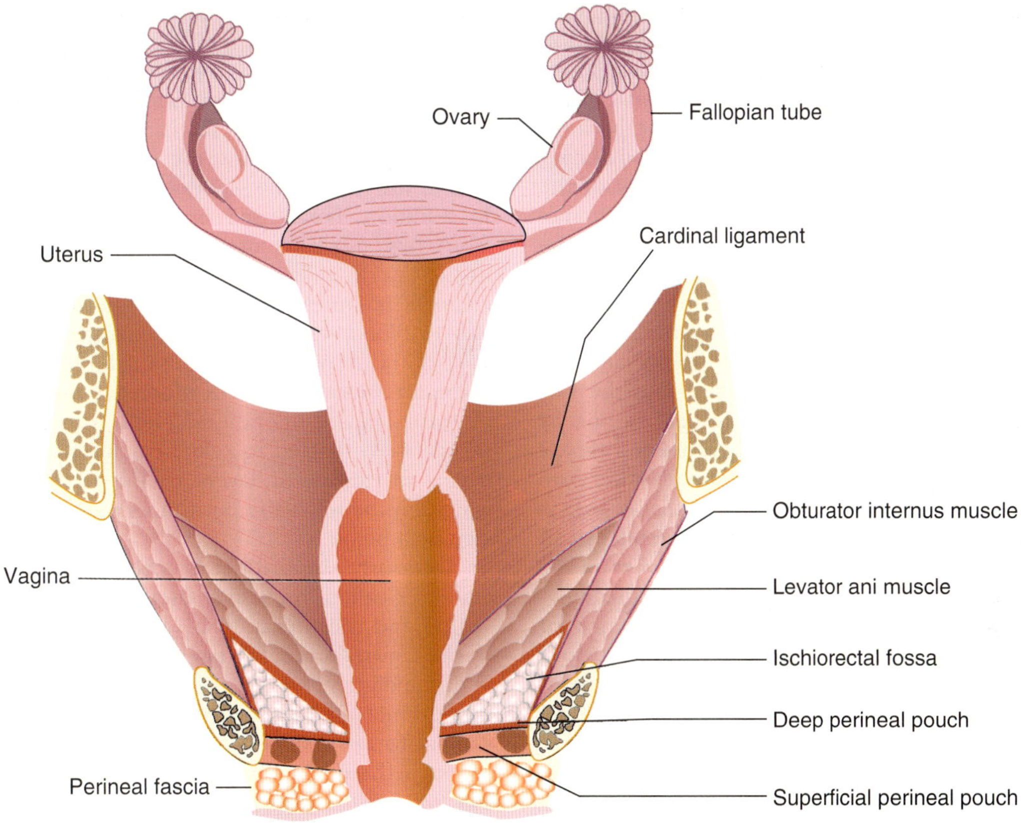

Figure 2.20 Anatomy of the pelvic floor in coronal section.

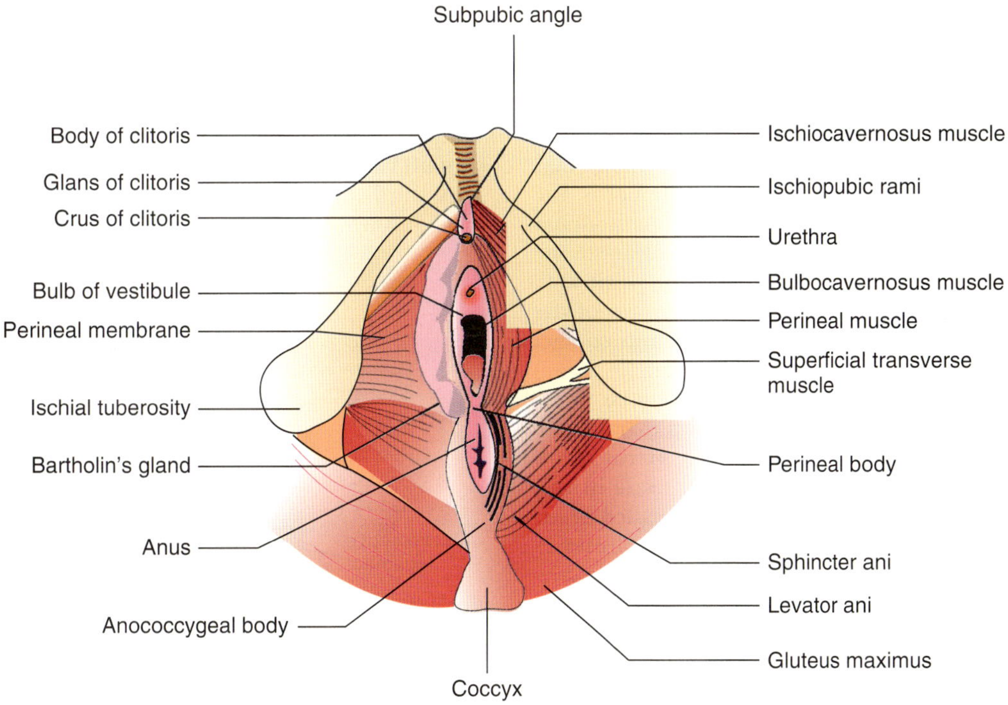

Figure 2.21 The perineum.

The *perineal body* intervenes between the posterior vaginal wall and the anal canal. It is pyramidal in shape with its apex on a level with the junction of the middle and lower thirds of the posterior vaginal wall. The three layers of the muscles of the pelvic floor are represented in the perineal body, and the intervening tissue consisting of fat and fibrous tissue. Superficially, passing from the central point of the perineum are the external sphincter of the anus, the bulbospongiosus and the superficial transverse muscle of the perineum. Deep to this layer lies the fascial layer of the urogenital diaphragm (triangular ligament) enclosing the deep transverse muscle of the perineum. Deeper still, the pelvic diaphragm is represented by the fibres of the levator ani muscles which decussate between the vagina and the rectum. The perineal body is examined by inspection and by palpation. Two fingers are placed in the vagina and flexed laterally; the thumb being applied externally over the labium majus, the levator muscles can be palpated with a remarkable ease and the size of the hiatus urogenitalis can be assessed. On asking the patient to contract her pelvic floor muscles, the tone of these muscles can be estimated.

Prolapse of the genital tract, stress incontinence of urine and faecal incontinence are all related to laxity and atonicity of the muscles of the pelvic floor as well as denervation of pelvic nerves during childbirth. Lately, perineal ultrasound and MRI have greatly improved our knowledge of these supportive structures in maintaining the uterine position and continence of urine and faeces.

THE PELVIC CELLULAR TISSUE

The pelvic cellular tissue consists of loose areolar tissue which intervenes between the pelvic peritoneum above and the pelvic fascia below. It is continuous with the subperitoneal connective tissue and with the loose tissue of the perinephric region. The areolar tissue is loose, and when inflamed in the condition of pelvic cellulitis it may lead to the formation of a palpable swelling. As there is a direct continuation between the perinephric and pelvic cellular tissues, effusions arising in either of these situations may track to point as an abscess in the other. In the pelvis, the pelvic cellular tissue is bounded above by the peritoneum and below by the fascia which covers the upper surface of the levator ani muscles. Laterally it is bounded by the pelvic wall, mainly by the fascia which covers the inner surface of the obturator internus whereas medially it comes into contact with the uterus and the upper part of the vagina.

The *parametrium* is that part of the pelvic cellular tissue which surrounds the uterus. It is by definition extraperitoneal and is most plentiful on each side of the uterus below the level of the internal os. The endopelvic fascia in this region thickens to form ligamentous supports called *Mackenrodt's* or *cardinal ligaments*. Above this level, the presence of the broad ligaments reduces the amount of parametrium to a minimum. It should be remembered that the level of the levator ani muscle is well below the level of the cervix, being more than halfway down the vagina. The pelvic cellular tissue is usually very plentiful on each side of the vagina, where it is called paravaginal cellular tissue or paracolpos.

A distinction is drawn between the pelvic fascia and the endopelvic fascia. The pelvic fascia consists of the dense connective tissue which covers the surfaces above and below the levator ani and the obturator internus muscles. On the contrary, the endopelvic fascia forms the connective tissue coverings for the vagina, the supravaginal portion of the cervix, the uterus, the bladder, the urethra and the rectum. In addition, condensed bands of endopelvic fascia pass from these moveable organs to the back of the pubic bones, to the lateral walls of the pelvis and to the front of the sacrum. The function of the endopelvic fascia is partly to convey blood vessels to the pelvic organs and partly to support them. Between the different layers of the endopelvic fascia are bloodless spaces which are important to identify in vaginal plastic operations. The term pelvic cellular tissue should be restricted to cellular tissue which intervenes between the different layers of the endopelvic fascia and which lies between the peritoneum above and the true pelvic fascia below.

Anteriorly, the bladder is covered by an endopelvic fascial layer called the vesical fascia, whereas behind it lie the vagina and the supravaginal portion of the cervix covered by their own endopelvic fascial layers.

Immediately behind the uterus and vagina, the peritoneum which covers the back of the uterus and the posterior vaginal fornix reduces the pelvic cellular tissue to a minimum in these situations. Deep to the uterosacral folds of peritoneum the endopelvic fascia is plentiful, and here it is condensed to form the uterosacral ligaments which pass backwards and upwards from the uterus in the front to reach the sacrum lateral to the rectosigmoid. The uterosacral ligaments help to support the uterus and prevent it from being forced down by intraabdominal pressure. By their tone they also tend to pull back the cervix and thereby antevert the uterus. Plain muscle fibres can be demonstrated in them. They contain sympathetic and parasympathetic nerves. Mackenrodt's ligaments, similar to uterosacral ligaments, help to support the uterus and prevent it from being forced down when the intraabdominal pressure is raised. They are composed almost entirely of connective tissue and contain very little plain muscle (Fig. 2.22).

A third and equally important part of the supporting mechanism of the pelvic viscera is the pubovesicocervical

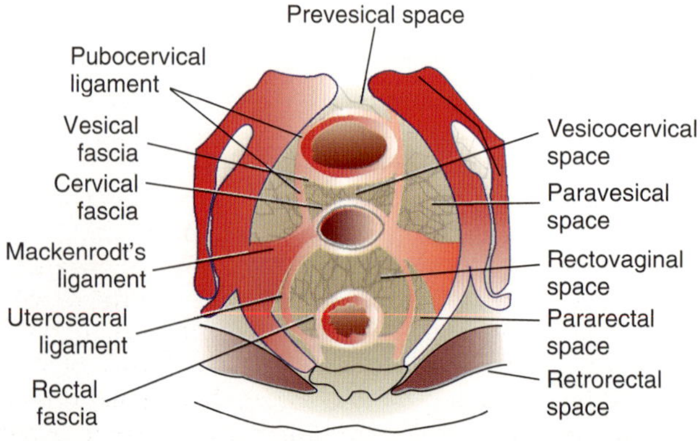

Figure 2.22 The pelvic cellular tissue shown in the cross-section of the pelvis.

fascia or the pubocervical fascia. This is a condensation of the endopelvic fascia which passes from the anterolateral aspect of the cervix to be attached to the back of the pubic bone lateral to the symphysis. Some of its cervical attachment fans out laterally and imperceptibly into the transverse cervical or Mackenrodt's ligament. It can, therefore, be regarded morphologically and functionally as a part of this structure.

If Fig. 2.22 is studied, the supports of the uterus and the bladder are seen to be triradiate condensation of endopelvic fascia:

1. The anterior spoke is the pubocervical fascia or so-called pubocervical ligament.
2. The lateral spoke is Mackenrodt's ligament.
3. The posterior spoke is the uterosacral ligament.

All these three embrace and insert into the cervix and, when intact, operate on it such as the strings of a hammock, preventing descent. If one or two strings are torn, the contents of the hammock prolapse with resulting descent of the bladder and the uterus.

The endopelvic fascial tissue contains the uterine arteries and veins, together with the venous plexus around the cervix and the lateral fornices of the vagina. The lymphatics from the upper two-thirds of the vagina and from the uterus, the ovaries and the fallopian tubes also pass through the pelvic cellular tissue. On each side of the uterus there is sometimes a small inconstant lymphatic gland known as the gland of the parametrium, about the size of the pin's head, near the ureteric canal. The ureter passes through the parametrium via the ureteric canal in an anteroposterior direction, about 1 cm lateral to the cervix to reach the bladder. It passes below the level of the uterine vessels, which cross it as they run transversely through the pelvis to reach the uterus. Sympathetic nerve ganglia and nerve fibres are plentiful in the parametrium (Frankenhauser's plexus).

In the condition of parametritis, the parametrium is inflamed and thickened. Rarely a large swelling forms which extends as far down as the fascia covering the levator ani muscles, and medially it comes directly into contact with the uterus and the upper part of the vagina. Laterally it extends as far out as the pelvic wall. Posteriorly it extends along the uterosacral ligaments in a close relation to the rectosigmoid. Such a swelling may track upwards out of the pelvis to reach the subperitoneal tissues of the iliac region when the effusions may point above Poupart's ligament lateral to the great vessels. In other cases, the swelling may track upwards to the perinephric region. In advanced cases of carcinoma of the cervix, the cancer cells infiltrate the parametrium when they spread either laterally along Mackenrodt's ligaments or posteriorly along the uterosacral ligaments. Clinically, infiltration of the parametrium is detected by determining the mobility of the cervix and the body of the uterus, by palpating in the situation of Mackenrodt's ligament through the lateral fornix of the vagina and by examining the uterosacral ligaments by rectal examination. The fibrosis resulting from chronic parametritis causes chronic pelvic pain and ureteric obstruction (Table 2.2).

Table 2.2 Supports of the Genital Organs

Level	Supports
Level I	Uterosacral ligaments and cardinal ligaments support the uterus and vaginal vault
Level II	Pelvic fascia and paracolpos which connect the vagina to the white line on the lateral pelvic wall through arcus tendinous
Level III	Levator ani muscles support the lower one-third of vagina

THE PELVIC BLOOD VESSELS

The ovarian arteries arise from the aorta, just below the level of the renal arteries. They pass downwards to cross first the ureter and then the external iliac artery, and then they pass into the infundibulopelvic fold. The ovarian artery sends branches to the ovaries and to the outer part of the fallopian tubes; it ends by anastomosing with the terminal part of the uterine artery after giving off a branch to the cornu and one to the round ligament.

Internal iliac artery is one of the bifurcations of the common iliac artery. It is 2 cm in length. The ureter lies anterior and the internal iliac vein posterior to it. It divides into an anterior and a posterior branch. The anterior branch supplies the pelvic organs. In obstetric and gynaecological surgery, profuse haemorrhage is controlled by ligating the internal iliac artery on the either side. During this procedure, the anterior relation of the ureter to the artery should be remembered and injury to the ureter avoided.

The *uterine artery* arises from the anterior trunk of the internal iliac (or hypogastric artery). Its course is at first downwards and forwards until it reaches the parametrium when it turns medially towards the uterus. It reaches the uterus at the level of the internal os, where it turns upwards, at right angles, and follows a spiral course along the lateral border of the uterus to the region of the uterine cornu; here it sends a branch to supply the fallopian tube and ends by anastomosing with the ovarian artery. The tortuosity is lost when the uterus enlarges during pregnancy. During the vertical part of its course, it sends branches which run transversely and pass into the myometrium (Fig. 2.23). These are called the arcuate arteries and from them arises a series of radial arteries almost at right angles. These radial arteries reach the basal layers of the endometrium where they are termed as the basal arteries. From these the terminal spiral and straight arterioles of the endometrium are derived. The least vascular part of the uterus is in the midline. The vaginal branch of the uterine artery arises before the uterine artery passes vertically upwards at the level of the internal os. It passes downwards through the parametrium to reach the vagina in the region of the lateral fornix. This descending vaginal artery is of great importance during the operation of total hysterectomy because, if not separately clamped and tied, it may lead to dangerous operative haemorrhage. The arcuate arteries that supply the cervix are sometimes called the circular artery of the cervix. From these or the descending vaginal branches the anterior and posterior azygos arteries of the vagina are derived (Fig. 2.24).

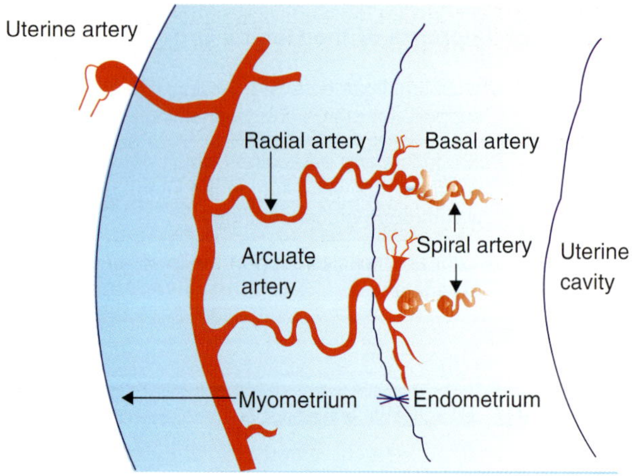

Figure 2.23 The uterine artery and its branches in the uterus.

The following are the branches of the uterine artery:

- Ureteric
- Descending vaginal – these unite to form the anterior and posterior azygos artery of the vagina
- Circular cervical
- Arcuate → radial → basal → spiral and straight arterioles of the functional layer of the endometrium
- Anastomotic with the ovarian artery

The relation of the uterine artery to the ureter is of great importance. The uterine artery crosses above the ureter in the parametrium where it gives off an important ureteric branch to that structure. The artery runs transversely whereas the ureter runs approximately anteroposteriorly through the ureteric canal of the parametrium.

Middle sacral artery is a single artery which arises from the terminal aorta. It descends in the middle of the lumbar vertebra and the sacrum to the tip of the coccyx.

There is an extensive network of collateral connections in the pelvic arterial vasculature that provides a rich anastomotic communication between major vessel systems. This degree of communication is important to ensure adequate supply of oxygen and nutrients in the event of major trauma or other vascular compromise. Hypogastric (internal iliac) artery ligation continues to be used as a strategy for the management of massive pelvic haemorrhage when other measures have failed. Bilateral hypogastric artery ligation effectively reduces pulse pressure in the pelvis, converting flow characteristics from that of an arterial to a venous system and allowing collateral channels of circulation to provide with adequate blood supply to the pelvic structures. This function is best illustrated by the example of preservation of reproductive functions, followed by successful pregnancies occurring after undertaking the lifesaving operation of bilateral ligation, of both hypogastric and ovarian arteries for uncontrolled atonic PPH after delivery. Details of collateral circulation are given in Table 2.3.

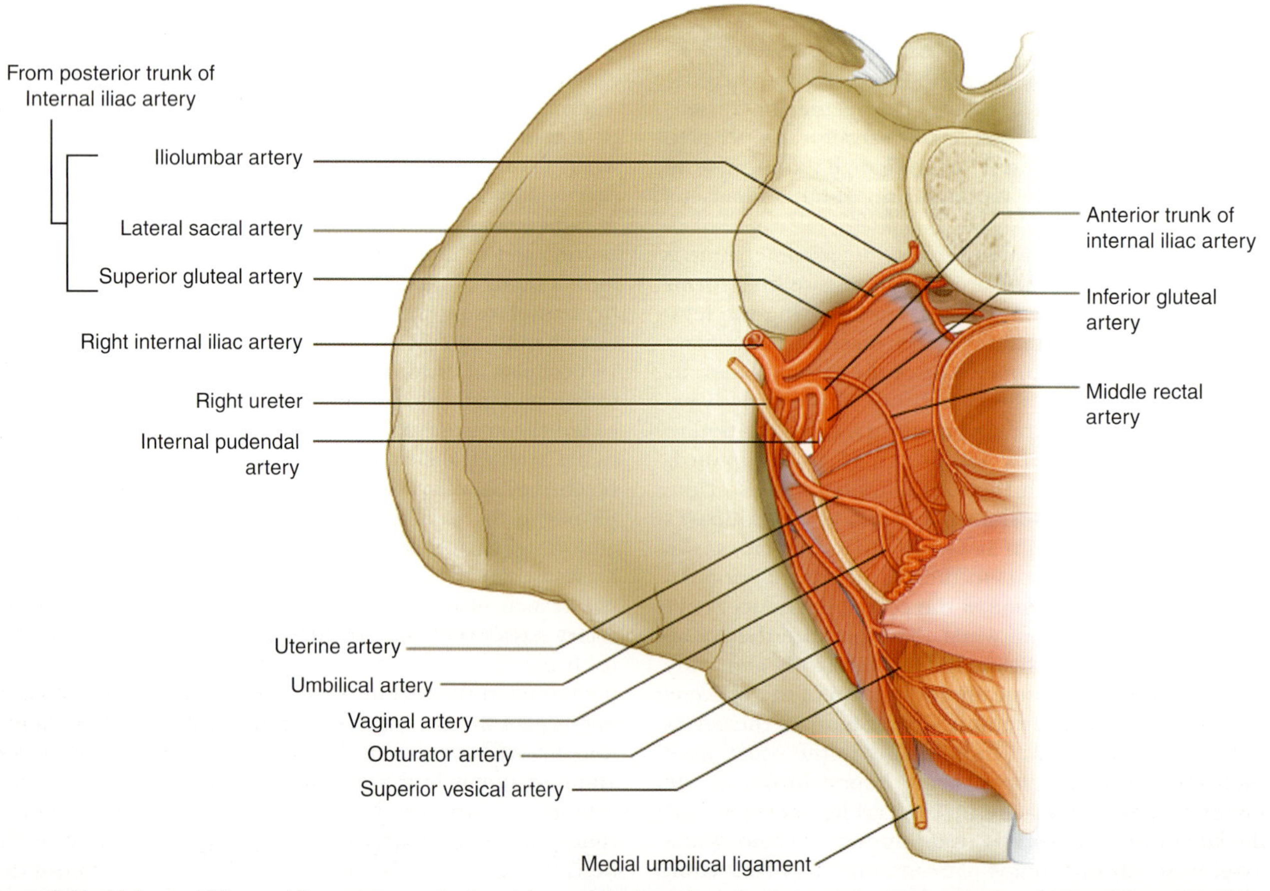

Figure 2.24 Major and Minor pelvis vessels seen in the picture are the branches of anterior and posterior division of internal iliac artery. (*Source*: Raveendranath Veeramani, Sunil Jonathan Holla, Parkash Chand, Sunil Chumber: Gray's Anatomy for Students, First South Asia Ed. Elsevier, 2017.)

Table 2.3 Collateral Arterial Airculation of the Pelvis

Primary Arteries	Collateral Arteries
Aorta	
Ovarian artery	Uterine artery
Superior rectal artery (inferior mesenteric artery)	Middle rectal artery Inferior rectal artery (internal pudendal)
Lumbar arteries	Iliolumbar artery
Vertebral arteries	Iliolumbar artery
Middle sacral artery	Lateral sacral artery
External iliac	
Deep iliac circumflex artery	Iliolumbar artery; superior gluteal artery
Inferior epigastric artery	Obturator artery
Femoral	
Medial femoral circumflex artery	Obturator artery; inferior gluteal artery
Lateral femoral circumflex artery	Superior gluteal; iliolumbar artery

THE VAGINAL ARTERIES

Usually the blood supply of the upper part of the vagina is derived from the vaginal branch of the uterine artery. This vessel reaches the lateral fornix of the vagina and then passes downwards along the lateral vaginal wall. It sends branches transversely across the vagina, which anastomoses with branches on the opposite side to form the azygos arteries of the vagina, which run down longitudinally, one in front of the vagina and one behind. These small vessels are encountered in the operations of anterior and posterior colporrhaphy. In some cases, the vaginal artery does not arise direct from the uterine artery but arises from the anterior division of the hypogastric artery, when it corresponds to the inferior vesical artery in the male.

THE ARTERIES OF THE VULVA AND PERINEUM

The blood vessels of the perineum and external genitalia are derived from the internal pudendal artery, a terminal branch of the anterior division of the internal iliac artery. The artery leaves the pelvis through greater sciatic foramen, winds round the ischial spine and enters the ischiorectal fossa. The main vessel passes forwards in the ischiorectal fossa adjacent to the obturator internus muscle in Alcock's canal. It gives off the inferior haemorrhoidal artery and the transverse perineal artery which supplies the perineum and the region of the external sphincter. It then pierces the urogenital diaphragm and sends another transverse branch to supply the posterior part of the labia and to supply the erectile tissue which surrounds the vaginal orifice. The internal pudendal artery ends as the dorsal artery of the clitoris, supplying the clitoris and vestibule. The tissues around the vaginal orifice, the clitoris and the crura of the clitoris contain a large amount of erectile tissue. Lacerations of the anterior part of the vulva during childbirth may be accompanied by severe bleeding. The terminal branches of the internal pudendal artery anastomose with superficial and deep pudendal arteries which are branches of the femoral artery. This anastomosis is important as it provides an alternative blood supply to the bladder in extended pelvic surgery when the vesical branches of the hypogastric are tied off or even the main trunk of the hypogastric itself may have been ligated at its source.

THE PELVIC VEINS

The left ovarian vein ends by passing into the left renal vein. The right ovarian vein terminates in the inferior vena cava. The most important feature of the pelvic veins is that they form plexuses. These are well marked in the case of the ovarian veins in the infundibulopelvic fold where they form a pampiniform plexus and cause chronic pelvic pain. Occasionally, this plexus becomes varicose and the large dilated veins form a varicocele similar to the condition seen in the male. The uterine plexus is found around the uterine artery near the uterus and the vaginal plexus around the lateral fornix of the vagina. These venous plexuses are well developed in the presence of large myomas and also during pregnancy when a venous plexus can be distinguished between the base of the bladder and the uterus. The uterine plexus of vein drains into the internal iliac vein. There are two additional channels of venous drainage which are of interest in explaining unexpected sites of metastases in malignant disease of the genital tract:

- A portal systemic anastomosis exists between the hypogastric vein and the portal system via the middle and inferior haemorrhoidal veins of the systemic and the superior haemorrhoidal veins of the portal system. This accounts for some liver metastases of the genital tract malignancies.
- A combination between the middle and lateral sacral and lateral lumbar venous system and the vertebral plexus, which may explain some vertebral and even intracranial metastases, is rarely seen in genital tract cancers. In such patients, the lungs may escape metastases as they are bypassed by the malignant emboli.
- Uterine veins communicate with the vaginal veins. This explains vaginal metastasis in uterine cancer and endometriosis. The middle sacral veins are two in number on the either side of the artery and drain into the left common iliac vein. These veins are encountered during presacral neurectomy, vaginal vault sacropexy and exenteration operation.

THE LYMPHATIC SYSTEM

The lymphatics and lymphatic glands which drain the female genital organs are of special importance in malignant disease. The surgical removal or radiation should include all the regional glands for curative effect.

THE LYMPHATIC GLANDS OR NODES

The lymphatic glands which drain the female genital organs are as follows (Fig. 2.25).

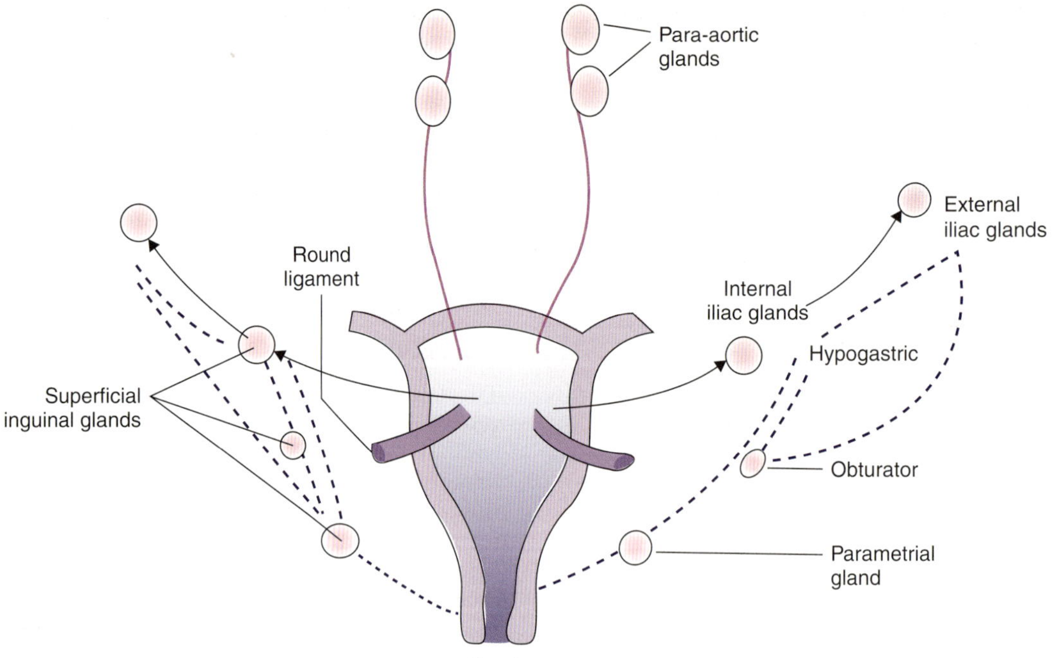

Figure 2.25 Pelvic lymphatic drainage of the cervix.

THE INGUINAL GLANDS

This group of glands consists of a horizontal and a vertical group. The horizontal group lies superficially, parallel to Poupart's ligament whereas the vertical group, otherwise known as the deep femoral glands, follows the saphenous and femoral veins. The uppermost of the deep femoral glands, called the gland of Cloquet or the gland of Rosenmüller, lies beneath Poupart's ligament in the femoral canal between Gimbernat's ligament and the femoral vein. Inconstant deep inguinal nodes are found in the inguinal canal, along the course of the round ligament, and in the tissues of the mons veneris. In such conditions, as primary sore and Bartholin's abscess, the horizontal inguinal group becomes inflamed. There is some evidence that lymphatics from the fundus of the uterus pass along the round ligament and drain into the horizontal inguinal group. It is more likely that these glands will become involved after the appearance of the late suburethral metastasis seen in advanced carcinoma corporis uteri, where the growth has spread down the vagina by a retrograde lymphatic spread. The inguinal glands drain the vulva and lower third of the vagina, the lymphatics of the medial portion of the vulva communicate with lymphatics of the opposite side. It is therefore necessary to perform bilateral inguinal lymphadenectomy when cancer occurs in the medial portion of the vulva.

THE GLANDS OF THE PARAMETRIUM

The hypogastric group (internal iliac glands) contains all the regional glands for the cervix, the bladder, the upper third of the vagina and also the greater part of the body of the uterus. This group of glands may be extensively involved in carcinoma of the uterus, cervix and vagina. The glands are most numerous immediately below the bifurcation of the common iliac group. A further group of these glands situated in the obturator fossa is often called the obturator glands and is frequently the most obviously involved in carcinoma of the cervix. These drain into external and common iliac glands.

EXTERNAL ILIAC GLANDS

This group of glands, several in number, is situated in relation to the external iliac artery and vein. A clean dissection of the external iliac glands can only be made if both vessels are completely mobilized as some of the glands lie lateral to the vessels between them and the lateral pelvic wall. These glands receive drainage from the obturator and hypogastric glands and are involved in late cervical cancer.

COMMON ILIAC GLANDS

This group is the upward continuation of the external and hypogastric group and, therefore, involved next in genital tract cancer.

THE SACRAL GROUP

These glands lie on each side of the rectum and receive lymphatics from the cervix of the uterus and from the upper third of the vagina which have passed backwards along the uterosacral ligaments. Two groups of glands can be recognized, a lateral group lying lateral to the rectum and a medial group lying in front of the promontory of the sacrum. The lymphatics from these glands pass directly either to the inferior lumbar group or to the common iliac group.

THE LUMBAR GROUP OF GLANDS

These lymphatic glands are divided into an inferior group that lies in front of the aorta below the origin of the inferior mesenteric artery and a superior lumbar group which lies near the origin of the ovarian arteries. The superior group of lumbar glands receives lymphatics from the ovaries and fallopian tubes as well as from the inferior lumbar glands. The lymphatics from the fundus of the uterus join the ovarian lymphatics to pass to the same group.

The lymphatic glands already mentioned, namely, the glands of the parametrium, the superficial inguinal, the hypogastric, external and common iliac, the sacral and the lumbar receive lymphatics 'direct' from the female generative organs and are known as the 'regional lymphatic glands' of the female genitalia.

These regional lymph nodes are not palpable clinically, but can be identified on CT and MRI scan if they are enlarged to 1 cm or more. At surgery, these glands should be palpated, removed or biopsied. This helps in staging the cancer and in the postoperative radiotherapy.

THE NERVE SUPPLY

Both sympathetic and parasympathetic systems supply the female genital organs as well as the bladder (Fig. 2.26).

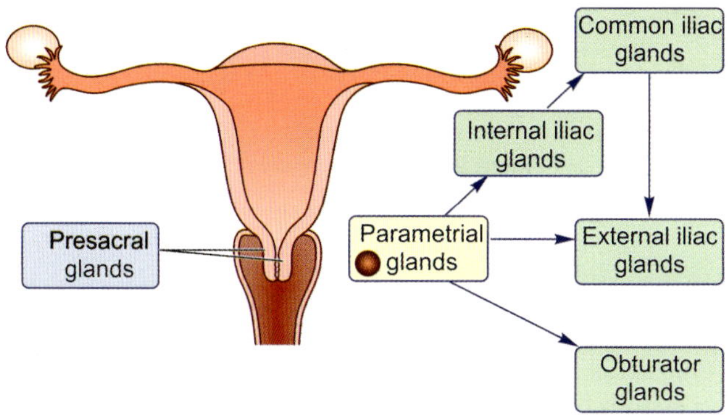

Figure 2.26 Lymphatic drainage of the pelvic lymph nodes.

The sympathetic system consists of the presacral nerve which lies in front of the sacral promontory. This nerve plexus divides into two hypogastric nerves which pass downwards and laterally along the pelvic wall to terminate in the inferior hypogastric plexus. This plexus is diffuse and lies in the situation of the uterosacral ligaments. It also receives fibres from the parasympathetic system consisting of sacral fibres 2, 3 and 4. From here, the nerve fibres pass to all the pelvic organs.

The cervix is well surrounded by a rich plexus of nerves called Frankenhauser's plexus. The lower vagina is innervated by pudendal nerve.

The ovaries derive their nerve supply from the coeliac and renal ganglia which follow the course of the ovarian vessels.

The ilioinguinal nerve, derived from L1, and the genital branch of the genitofemoral nerve (L1 and L2) supply the mons, the upper and outer aspect of the labia majora and the perineum.

The pudendal nerve derived from sacral second, third and fourth segments supplies the lower vagina, clitoris, posterior part of the labia majora and the perineum. Presacral neurectomy is rarely performed to relieve chronic pelvic pain, and pain due to endometriosis. Pudendal block is needed in operative vaginal deliveries (Table 2.4).

APPLIED ANATOMY AND ITS CLINICAL SIGNIFICANCE

1. **Vulva.** The skin of the external genitalia is prone to local and general dermatitis. The moist intertriginous parts of the vulva are susceptible to chronic infection. Mucous glands in the vestibular location may become cystic. A cyst of the canal of Nuck may be mistaken for an indirect inguinal hernia. The loose areolar tissue of the vulva and its rich vascularity account for the large haematomas that

Table 2.4 Nerve Supply in the Pelvis

Organ	Spinal Segments	Nerves
Perineum, vulva, lower vagina	S2–4	Pudendal, inguinal, genitofemoral, posterofemoral cutaneous
Upper vagina, cervix, lower uterine segment, posterior urethra, bladder trigone, uterosacral and cardinal ligaments, rectosigmoid, lower ureter	S2–4	Pelvic parasympathetics
Uterine fundus, proximal fallopian tubes, broad ligament, upper bladder, caecum, appendix, terminal large bowel	T11–12, L1	Sympathetics via hypogastric plexus
Outer two-thirds of fallopian tubes, upper ureter	T9–10	Sympathetics via aortic and superior mesenteric plexus
Ovaries	T9–10	Sympathetics via renal and aortic plexus and celiac and mesenteric ganglia
Abdominal wall	T12–L1	Iliohypogastric
	T12–L1	Ilioinguinal
	L1–2	Genitofemoral

are formed as a consequence of vascular injury during childbirth or accidental injuries. Vulval cancer is rare and occurs in old age. Lymphatic drainage of vulva is relevant in radical vulvectomy for cancer. Pudendal nerve block is required in episiotomy and forceps delivery. The internal pudendal block is performed by injecting local anaesthetic drug into the nerve at the level of ischial spine, as the nerve winds round this spine.

2. **Vagina.** The posterior vaginal fornix lies in proximity to the peritoneal pouch of Douglas. It is a convenient site for access to the peritoneal cavity, colpopuncture, colpocentesis and diagnostic culdoscopy in the diagnosis of pelvic abscess, ectopic pregnancy and pelvic endometriosis. The ureters have a close relation to the lateral vaginal fornices, particularly in patients with uterine prolapse. Ureteric injury should be guarded against during vaginal surgery on the uterus, as also when attempting to suture vaginal lacerations (colporrhexis) high in the vaginal vault. The anatomic proximity of the bladder base, urethra and vagina and the interrelationship between their vascular and lymphatic networks result in inflammation of the vagina (vaginitis) causing urinary tract symptoms such as frequency and dysuria. Gartner's duct cysts represent a cystic dilatation of the remnants of the embryonic mesonephros. They are present in the lateral walls of the vagina. These are generally asymptomatic, but they may cause dyspareunia or vaginal discomfort. In the lower third of the vagina, Gartner's duct cysts are located anteriorly and may mimic a large urethral diverticulum. Squamous cell carcinoma of vagina is very rare and occurs usually over the decubitus ulcer in a woman with vaginal prolapse. Adenocarcinoma of vagina has been reported in young girls who were exposed to DES in utero and can occur in the upper part of the vagina. Lymphatic drainage of vulva is relevant in radical vulvectomy for cancer. Pudendal nerve block is required in episiotomy and forceps delivery. The internal pudendal block is performed by injecting local anaesthetist drug into the nerve at the level of ischial spine as the nerve winds round this spine.
3. **Cervix.** The major vascular supply of the cervix is located laterally. Deep lateral sutures placed laterally to include the vaginal mucosa and the substance of the cervix would help to control bleeding during surgical procedures on the cervix such as conization or the surgical evacuation of the cervical canal in cervical ectopic pregnancy. The stroma of the endocervix unlike the ectocervix is rich in nerve endings; hence, manipulation of the cervical canal can cause an unexpected vasovagal attack and severe bradycardia or even cardiac arrest. The lymphatics of the cervix are very complex involving multiple chains of nodes. The principal regional nodes are the obturator, common iliac, internal iliac and visceral nodes of the parametria; others may also be occasionally involved, hence the need for a wide nodal dissection during the treatment of cancer cervix employing radical surgery. Squamocolumnar junction is the site of cancer of the cervix. Precancerous lesion of the cervix needs ablation or excision depending upon the age of the woman and its grade (Fig. 2.27).

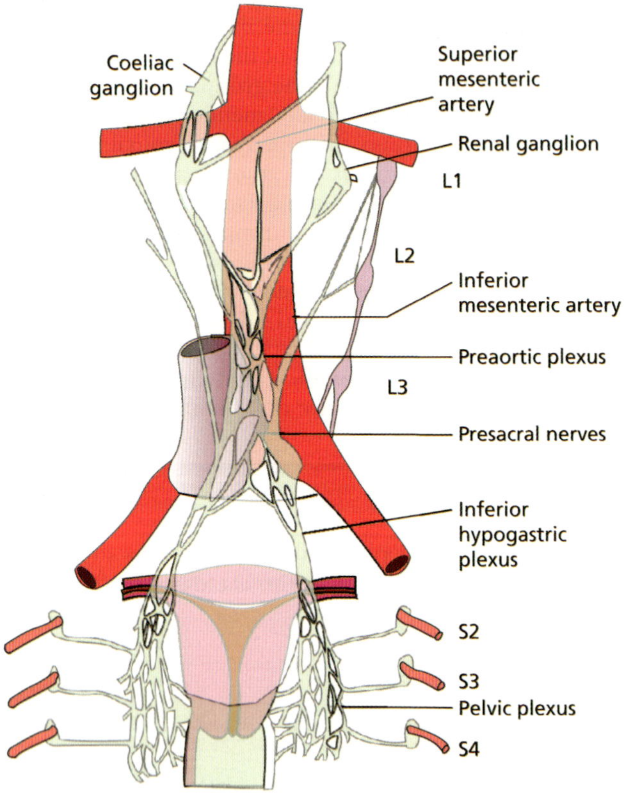

Figure 2.27 Pelvic innervation.

4. **Uterus.** Dysmenorrhoea is not an uncommon symptom, necessitating treatment in day-to-day practice. Although most cases of primary dysmenorrhoea are treated successfully by prostaglandin synthetase inhibitors, there are occasional cases where oral medications may not suffice. In these women, the division of the sensory nerves that accompany the sympathetic nerves can lead to relief. The operations of presacral neurectomy and the endoscopic division of the uterosacral ligaments near the uterine attachment (laparoscopic uterosacral nerve ablation) have been designed to meet this end. The surgeon must be careful to avoid injury to the ureters. The uterus receives its main blood supply from the laterally placed uterine arteries, so the operation of myomectomy of anterior wall uterine fibroids through a midline incision is attended with the least amount of blood loss. Earlier, it has been discussed that the uterus has a rich blood supply from the branches of the vascular anastomotic arcade between the uterine arteries and the ovarian arteries. There is also presence of an extensive pelvic collateral circulation to ensure enough blood supply in emergency situations wherein bilateral surgical ligation of the hypogastric vessels becomes necessary as a life-saving procedure, such as postpartum haemorrhage.
5. **Fallopian tubes.** The right fallopian tube lies in proximity to the appendix. Therefore, it is often difficult to differentiate between acute appendicitis and acute salpingitis. The wide mesosalpinx of the ampullary portion of

the tube permits this part to undergo torsion. Mesonephric remnants in the broad ligament may be the cause of formation of paraovarian cysts. These often mimic ovarian neoplasms. They have been reported to undergo torsion. Falloscopy visualizes the tubal mucosa and patency of the medial end and salpingoscopy studies the mucosa and patency of the ampullary end of the fallopian tube, and enables us to decide between tubal surgery and in vitro fertilization in tubal infertility.

6. **Ovaries.** There is a wide variation in the size of the ovaries during the childbearing years and after menopause. Atrophic menopausal ovaries are not palpable on vaginal examination. Therefore, any palpable adnexal mass in a postmenopausal woman should be viewed with suspicion and investigated thoroughly to exclude a neoplasm. The location of the ovary in the ovarian fossa lies in proximity to the ureters. Hence, during pelvic surgical procedures for severe endometriosis or pelvic inflammatory disease that involve the ovaries, great caution must be exercised to avoid ureteric injury. Ultrasound scanning for any adnexal mass, polycystic ovarian disease and ovulation monitoring is possible and is easy, cost effective, accurate and noninvasive. Additional hormonal monitoring is, however, required in in vitro fertilization programme.
7. **Surgical precautions during gynaecological operations.** The anatomic proximity of female reproductive organs with the ureters, urinary bladder and rectum in the pelvis is a major consideration during gynaecologic surgery. Surgical compromise of the ureter may occur during clamping or ligation of the infundibulopelvic folds, clamping and ligation of the cardinal ligaments, reperitonealization of the lateral wall following hysterectomy or during wide approximation of endopelvic fascia during anterior colporrhaphy repair.

At the base of the broad ligaments, the uterine artery crosses the ureter. During Wertheim's operation, when in doubt whether the structure under view is a blood vessel or the ureter, the feel of the structure is helpful; also, mild stroking lengthwise invokes a wave of peristalsis in the ureter. During abdominal hysterectomy for benign uterine disease, the practice of intrafascial clamping of the parametrium also helps to prevent ureteric injury. Subtotal hysterectomy in younger women in whom the cervix is healthy (Pap test normal) has the advantage of retaining the cervix for sexual reasons and for reducing the risk of future vault prolapse. The urinary bladder if well drained during pelvic surgery will be less vulnerable to inadvertent trauma. During colposuspension operations for stress urinary incontinence, there may be significant venous bleeding in the cave of Retzius. If proper drainage is not provided, there is a possibility of occurrence of a large subfascial haematoma that may extend up to the umbilicus. Rectal injuries occur most frequently during vaginal hysterectomy associated with high posterior colporrhaphy and enterocele repair. The rectum is also vulnerable to injury in the presence of wide adhesions, obliterating the pouch of Douglas in cases of extensive pelvic endometriosis, chronic pelvic inflammatory disease or advanced pelvic malignancy.

The genital prolapse is caused by atonicity, relaxation or damage to the nerve of the pelvic floor muscles and the supporting ligaments. The knowledge of these anatomical structures is necessary in the repair of various types of prolapse and in enhancement and buttressing these structures.

Stress incontinence of urine can be cured by elevating the neck of the bladder and mid-urethral ligamentary suspension.

KEY POINTS

- Anatomical knowledge of the pelvic organs is essential to interpret the clinical findings as well as those of ultrasound, CT and MRI to make an accurate gynaecological diagnosis.
- Normal vaginal secretions are small in amount and varies with the phase of the menstrual cycle. Döderlein's bacilli are Gram-positive microorganisms which grow anaerobically in an acid medium of 4.5 pH. Low acidity of vagina does not allow other organisms to grow and cause vaginitis.
- Normal cervix has several physiological functions. The alkaline secretion attracts sperms at ovulation and sieves out the abnormal sperms in their ascent. The plug of cervical mucous prevents entry of sperms as well as bacteria, and prevents pregnancy and pelvic inflammatory disease. Capacitation of sperms occurs in the cervical canal. The internal os remains closed during pregnancy, but effaces as its collagen dissolves near term.
- Fallopian tube. The secretions of endosalpinx, peristaltic movements of the tube and ovarian fimbria play important role in fertility.
- Knowledge of lymphatic drainage of the pelvic organs is important in staging of cancers, radiation planning and complete surgical removal of tumour. Remnants of the Wolffian duct can cause paraovarian cyst and Gartner's duct cyst.
- The pelvic portion of the ureter lies close to the genital organs. It is recognized by its pale glistening appearance and peristalsis. It needs to be dissected and protected against injury during gynaecological surgery.
- Pelvic floor muscles and fasciae hold the pelvic organs in place. Prolapse of uterus, stress incontinence of urine are related to the laxity and atonicity of these structures. Denervation of the pelvic nerves during childbirth can predisposed to urinary and faecal incontinence.
- The bladder, rectum and anal canal share the same muscular and ligamentary supports. Laxity of these supportive structures causes genital prolapse as well as urinary, faecal incontinence.

SELF-ASSESSMENT

1. Describe the anatomy of Bartholin's gland and its clinical significance.

2. Describe the anatomy of pelvic diaphragm and its importance in genital organ prolapse.
3. Describe the pelvic cellular tissue supports of the uterus.
4. Describe the course of the ureter in the pelvis. What are the sites where ureter is vulnerable to injury during pelvic surgery?

SUGGESTED READING

Cunningham FG, Leveno KL, Bloom SL et al. (eds). William's Obstetrics. 23rd Ed. New York, McGraw Hill, 2010; 14–35.

Schorge JO, Schaffer JI, Halvorson LM et al. (eds). William's Gynaecology. 1st Ed. New York, McGraw Hill, 2008; 798.

Normal Histology of Ovary and Endometrium

3

CHAPTER OUTLINE

Histological study of the endometrium is needed to detect the hormonal causes of infertility and abnormal menstrual patterns. However, lately, studying ovulation pattern in infertility by endometrial examination has lost considerable importance and is superseeded by ultrasonic scanning, which is noninvasive and accurate in detecting the timing of ovulation and the result is available on the spot. Endometrial study is needed in suspected genital tract tuberculosis and cancer. The morphological study of the ovary and adnexal mass is also possible with ultrasound scanning.

THE OVARY

At term, the fetal ovary measures 10–16 mm in length and is situated at the level of the brim of the pelvis. If a section is taken through the ovary and examined histologically, the following can be recognized:

The surface epithelium. This is a single layer of cuboidal cells, which later gives rise to the surface epithelium of the adult ovary. It is morphologically continuous with the mesothelium of the peritoneum.

The subepithelial connective tissue layer. This layer gives rise to the tunica albuginea of the adult ovary and to the basement membrane beneath the surface epithelium.

The parenchymatous zone. This area is the cortex and also the most important area, as it contains the sex cells. It can be divided into the following zones:

- Immediately beneath the surface epithelium, the sex cells are still grouped together in bunches to form egg nests.
- Below this area, the sex cells take the form of primordial follicles and are packed together without orderly arrangement (Fig. 3.1).
- Developing follicles are seen in the deeper parts (Fig. 3.2). The rete ovary in the medulla represents primary sex cords. Leydig cells, analogues of testis, are also seen in the medulla.

Zona vasculosa. This contains the blood vessels. It constitutes the medulla of the ovary (Fig. 3.3). A few hilar cells homologues to interstitial cells of the testes are present in the medulla and rarely cause hilar cell tumour of the ovary.

THE PRIMORDIAL FOLLICLE

As early as in the 3rd week of gestation, primordial germ cells appear in the endoderm of the yolk sac, and these migrate along the dorsal mesentery to the urogenital ridge by the 8th week. The first evidence of primordial follicle appears at about 20 weeks of fetal life. The fetal ovary contains 7 million primordial follicles but most degenerate, and the newborn contains only 2 million follicles. The primordial follicle consists of a large cell, the primordial ovum (oogonia), which is surrounded by flattened cells, best termed as the *follicle epithelial cells.* The follicle epithelial cells give rise to the granulosa cells of the Graafian follicle.

The primitive ovum (primary oocyte) is roughly spherical in shape and measures 18–24 microns in diameter, the nucleus 12 microns and nucleolus 6 microns. It has a well-defined nuclear membrane and its chromatin stains clearly. The primary oocytes remain in the prophase of the first meiotic division until puberty.

The ovary of the newborn is packed with primordial follicles, approximately 2 million, dropping to a few hundreds at puberty. One of the most curious features of the ovary is the tendency of the sex cells to undergo degeneration. An enormous number disappears during intrauterine life (IUL), and this process of degeneration continues throughout childhood and the childbearing period, with the result that no ovum can be detected in the ovaries of a woman who has passed the menopause. At birth, about 2 million follicles seen are reduced to 400,000 at puberty; only 400 follicles are available during the childbearing period for fertilization. The oogonia enter the prophase of the first meiotic division and remain so until puberty.

THE GRAAFIAN FOLLICLE (Fig. 3.2)

The Graafian follicle, described by Regnier de Graaf in 1672, is a vesicle whose size measures on an average between 12 and 16 mm in diameter after puberty. Before puberty, it seldom reaches more than 5 mm in diameter.

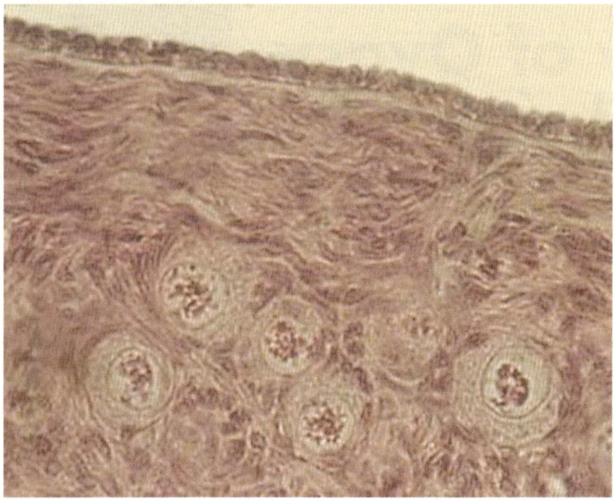

Figure 3.1 Ovary of a newborn child showing germinal epithelium and the stroma packed with primordial follicles. (*Source*: Andrei Gunin, MD, PhD, Dr Sci, Professor, Department of Obstetrics and Gynecology, Medical School Chuvash State University.)

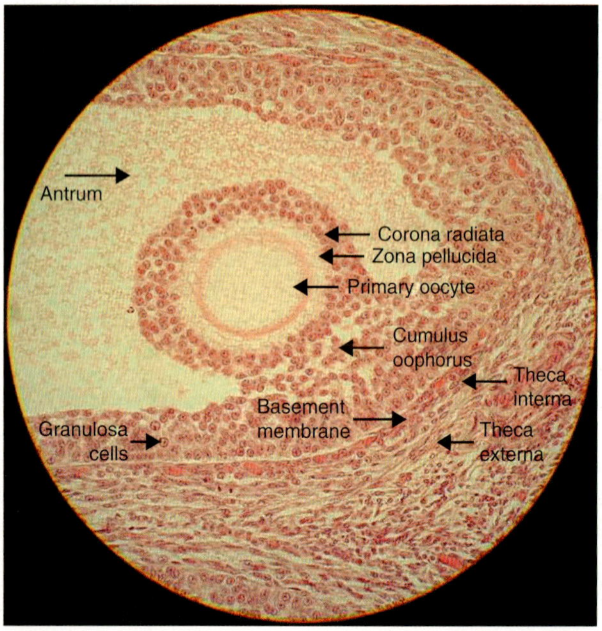

Figure 3.2 Graafian follicle. Discus proligerus showing granulosa cells, the ovum and the membrana limitans externa. Theca interna cells are few. (*Source*: David B Fankhauser, PhD.)

The mature Graafian follicle is spheroidal or ovoid in shape and contains pent-up secretion, the liquor folliculi. The lining consists of two layers: (i) theca interna and (ii) granulosa layer. The outer or *theca interna* layer consists of cells that are derived from the stroma cells of the cortex. The theca cell is responsible for the production of ovarian hormones, oestrogen and progesterone, sometimes extended to the production of androgens. Within the theca interna layer lies the *granulosa cell layer,* which consists of cells that have a characteristic appearance. The cells are 8–10 microns in diameter. The nuclei always stain deeply and the cells contain relatively little cytoplasm. In one area, the granulosa cells are collected together to form a projection into the cavity of the Graafian follicle. This projection is referred to as the *discus proligerus or cumulus oophorus.* The ovum itself lies within the discus proligerus. With the exception of the area around the discus proligerus, the peripheral granulosa cells form a layer only a few cells in thickness, whereas at the discus, the cells are between 12 and 20 layers thick. The granulosa layer itself is nonvascular and capillaries cannot be identified in it. Scattered amongst the granulosa cells, particularly in the vicinity of the discus proligerus, are small spherical globules around which the granulosa cells are arranged radially. These structures form *Call-Exner* bodies. The formation of *Call-Exner bodies* is a distinct feature of granulosa cells and can be readily recognized in certain types of granulosa cell tumours. Between the granulosa layer and the theca interna is a basement membrane called the *membrana limitans externa,* upon which lies the basal layer of granulosa cells (Fig. 3.4).

The mature ovum measures 120–140 microns in diameter and its nucleus measures 20–25 microns. At the periphery of the deutoplasm is a vitelline membrane outside which a clear translucent capsular acellular layer of glycoprotein, known as the zona pellucida, envelops the ovum. The granulosa cells surround the entire periphery of the ovum (Fig. 3.5). The ovum remains in the meiotic arrest until about 36 hours before ovulation when first meiotic division is completed and first polar body is extruded. Second meiotic division occurs only if the sperm penetrates the zona.

Those granulosa cells, which are immediately adjacent to the ovum, have a radial arrangement and form the corona radiata. The corona radiata remains attached to the ovum after its discharge into the peritoneal cavity at ovulation. The theca interna cells enlarge during the maturation of the follicle, and shortly before ovulation, they are larger

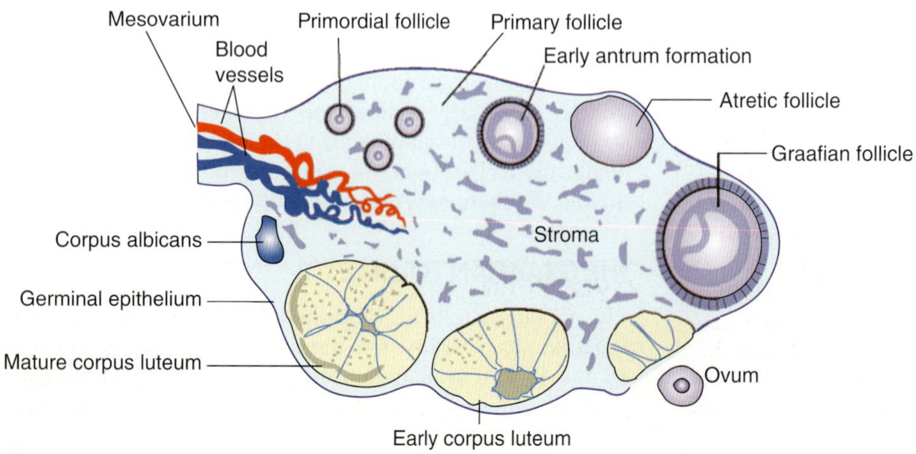

Figure 3.3 Structure of the adult ovary.

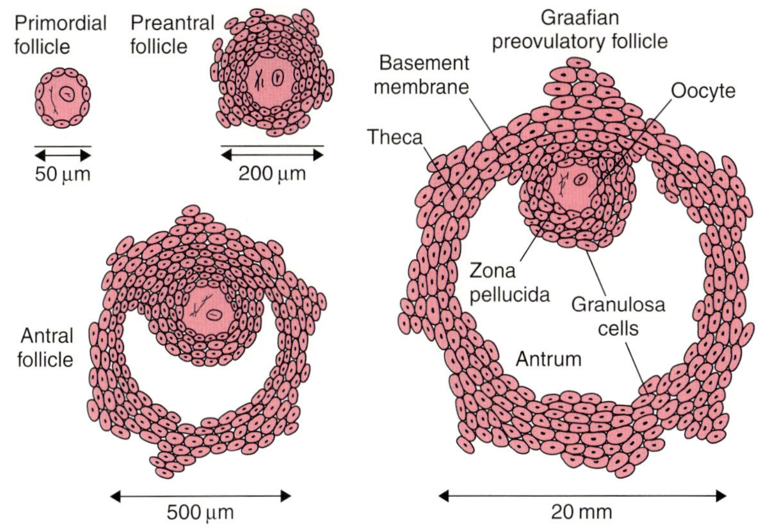

Figure 3.4 Follicular development: Graafian follicle showing granulosa cells, the ovum and theca interna cells. Graafian follicle measures 20 mm at ovulation.

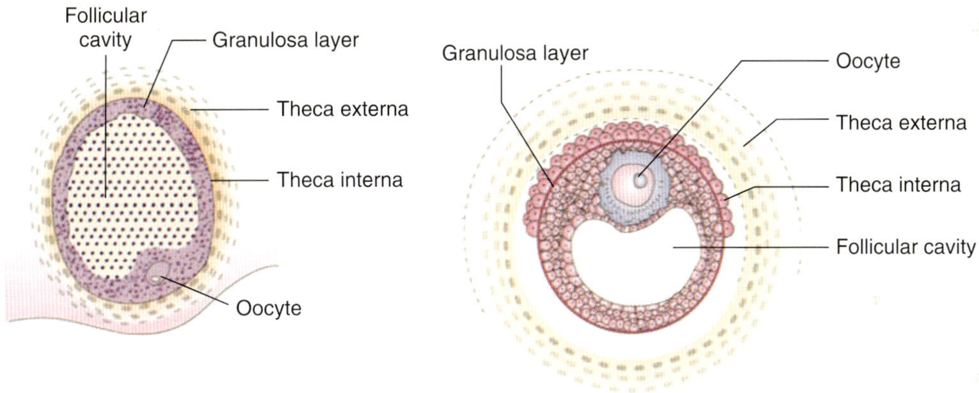

Figure 3.5 Oocyte.

than the granulosa cells. The third layer, the theca externa, is ill-defined in the ovary.

The liquor folliculi is a clear fluid-containing protein which coagulates after formalin fixation. It is secreted by the granulosa cells and contains the ovarian hormone oestrogen.

THE FATE OF THE GRAAFIAN FOLLICLE

The process whereby a primordial follicle is converted into a Graafian follicle, follicularization, can be recognized as early as the 32nd week of IUL. Until puberty, most primordial follicles in the ovary undergo retrogression by a process which is termed as follicle atresia. Ovulation, whereby the follicle discharges its ovum into the peritoneal cavity, is first seen at puberty and is restricted to the childbearing period of life. The development of a primordial follicle into a Graafian follicle is under the control of the follicle-stimulating hormone (FSH) secreted by the anterior pituitary gland. Several follicles commence to develop in each menstrual cycle. In response to FSH, small gap junctions develop between the granulosa cells and the oocyte, and these gap junctions provide a pathway for nutrition and metabolic interchange between them. Of the several follicles developing in both ovaries, one follicle grows faster than the rest and produces more FSH receptors and oestrogen. The rising oestrogen level stimulates luteinizing hormone (LH) receptors in the theca cells but causes a negative feedback to the anterior pituitary gland, leading to a progressive fall in the level of FSH and gonadotropic support to the other lesser developed follicles which atrophy. The number of follicles that develop in any one cycle depends upon the levels of FSH and LH as well as the sensitivity of the follicles. Induction of multiple ovulations in in vitro fertilization is based on this observation. In a spontaneous normal menstrual cycle, only one dominant follicle develops into a Graafian follicle resulting in a single ovulation. Follicular atresia begins first in the ovum and later in the granulosa cells. Hyaline degeneration occurs and hyaline tissue is deposited as a glass membrane. Gradual absorption of liquor folliculi causes collapse of the follicle. The theca interna cells persist longer as dark-stained interstitial cells at the periphery of the follicle.

OVULATION

Ovulation occurs when the ovum surrounded by the corona radiata escapes out of the Graafian follicle. It is quickly picked up by the tubal fimbria, which hugs the ovary at ovulation

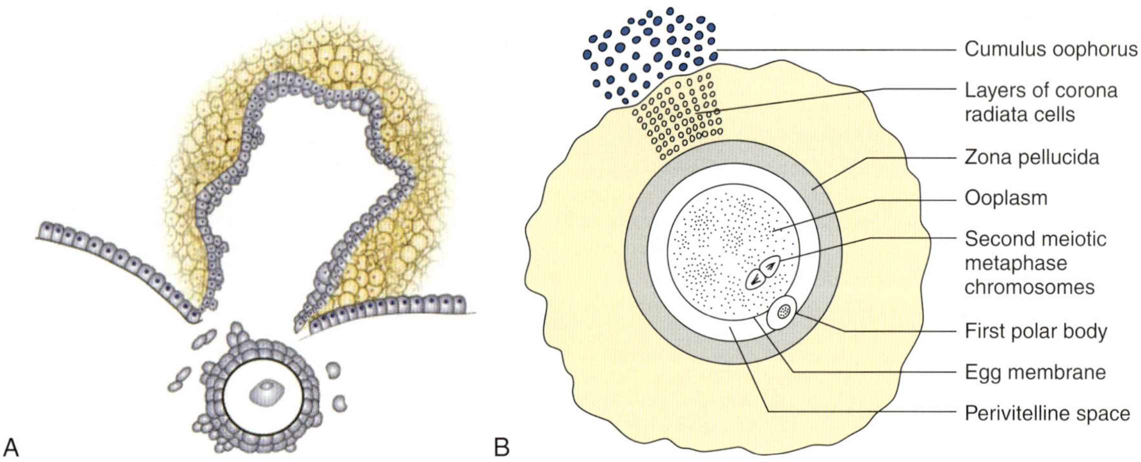

Figure 3.6 **(A)** Ovulation. **(B)** Freshly ovulated ovum.

(Fig. 3.6). The peak level of 75 ng/mL of LH is required for ovulation. LH peak lasts for 24 hours.

The rupture of the Graafian follicle occurs because of the contraction of micromuscle present over the theca externa. The contractions are brought about by prostaglandin secreted under the influence of LH. The process of maturation and ovulation can be minutely studied by serial ultrasonography. The Graafian follicle grows at the rate of 1–2 mm daily and attains the size of 20 mm or more at ovulation. The sudden shrinkage in the size of a follicle, appearance of free fluid in the pouch of Douglas and regrowth of the collapsed cyst thereafter suggest that ovulation has occurred. Knowledge of the timing of ovulation is needed in in vitro fertilization, in artificial insemination and in the control of fertility. Ovulation is estimated to occur 14 days before the 1st day of the succeeding cycle, and this interval is more or less fixed. In case of irregular cycles, it is the follicular phase which varies, but the luteal phase remains more or less constant at 14 days. However, we do encounter cases of infertility with a short luteal phase, when menstruation begins in less than 14 days after ovulation.

Normally, *one single ovum* is discharged from the Graafian follicle. However, multiple ovulations can occur and result in a multiple dizygotic pregnancy. Multiple ovulations can also be therapeutically induced with hormones during in vitro fertilization.

The aperture through which an egg escapes from the ovary is called the stigma, appearing on laparoscopy as a red spot that heals in 3–4 days' time. The indirect methods of detecting ovulation are based on serial vaginal cytology, serial cervical mucus study, premenstrual endometrial biopsy, observing daily basal body temperature (BBT) and estimation of blood progesterone levels (or urinary pregnanediol levels) in the postovulatory or immediate premenstrual phase. Rarely, rupture of the Graafian follicle fails, but the follicle grows into a corpus luteum. This is termed as luteinized unruptured follicle, which causes infertility.

The most important physiological marker of imminent ovulation is LH surge and not E_2 peak, as the latter may not always culminate into ovulation. LH surge causes the following:

1. Completion of meiosis of ovum
2. Ovulation
3. Development of corpus luteum

Anovulation occurs in about 10% cases of infertility, and sporadically during the childbearing years, but its occurrence is not uncommon for a few cycles after the menarche and just prior to the onset of menopause.

Unless fertilized, the ovum does not survive for more than 24 hours. Thereafter, it degenerates in the fallopian tube without leaving behind any trace.

CORPUS LUTEUM (Fig. 3.7A and B)

Soon after ovulation, the Graafian follicle cyst collapses and luteinization of the theca cells and the granulosa cells takes place. The cells bloat up and increase in size, with

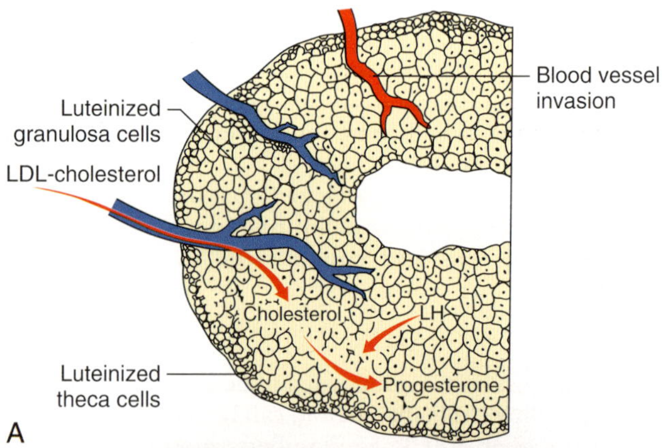

A

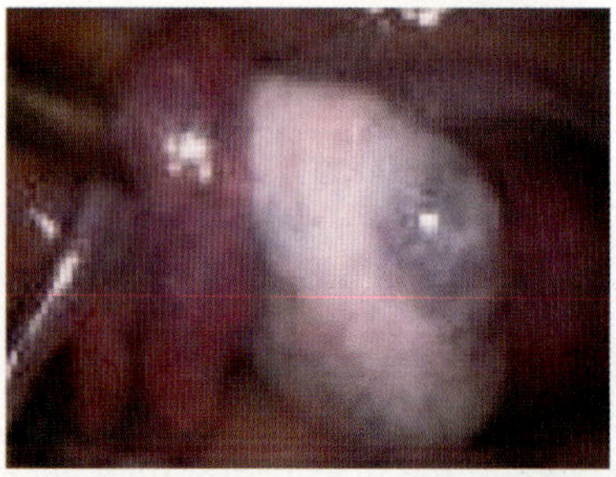

B

Figure 3.7 **(A)** Formation of corpus luteum. **(B)** Laparoscopic appearance of Graafian follicle at the time of ovulation. (*Courtesy* for **(B)**: Dr Shyam Desai, Mumbai.)

pale staining cytoplasm. The nuclei therefore appear small. The cells proliferate and become 8- to 10-fold in size due to which the cyst wall becomes crenated. At the same time, the corpus luteum becomes vascularized from the vessels in the theca interna layer. Some bleeding may occur in the cavity of the cyst. The corpus luteum reaches maximum maturity by the 22nd day of the normal cycle, when it attains the size of 2 cm or more. If pregnancy fails to occur, by the 8th postovulatory day, the corpus luteum starts degenerating and hyalinization sets in. The corpus luteal fluid contains phospholipid, cholesterol and carotene. Although it appears initially grey, later the corpus luteum acquires a yellow colour due to carotene, also known as lutein. During the last premenstrual week, vascularity of the corpus luteum diminishes when atrophy and degeneration of granulosa cells can be demonstrated in the form of vacuolated cells. Later hyaline tissue is deposited, and this hyaline body is known as the corpus albicans. Retrogression of the corpus luteum is a slow process and it is calculated that 9 months may elapse before it is completely replaced by hyaline tissue (Fig. 3.8). The regression is attributed to fall in the LH level and rise in the level of oestrogen and $PGF_2\alpha$.

MENSTRUATION

Menstruation is brought about by fall in the levels of oestrogen and progesterone following the degeneration of the corpus luteum. In anovulatory cycles, fall in the level of oestrogen alone can bring about withdrawal bleeding in the form of menstruation. However, the oestrogen withdrawal bleeding is far heavier than the progesterone withdrawal bleeding.

CORPUS LUTEUM OF PREGNANCY

Following fertilization, the corpus luteum continues to grow and forms the corpus luteum of pregnancy. This corpus luteum is larger and more cystic than the corpus luteum of menstruation and may attain the size of 2.5 cm. The convolutions are larger and more intricate. The individual granulosa cell is also large and measures as much as 40–50 microns. The secretion also increases. The theca cells are seen up to the 20th week, but thereafter they cannot be identified.

The corpus luteum of pregnancy is functionally active up to the 10th to 12th week in human beings. Thereafter, the placenta takes over the secretory function and carries pregnancy to term. Extirpation of the corpus luteum after the 14th week in humans will not therefore induce abortion.

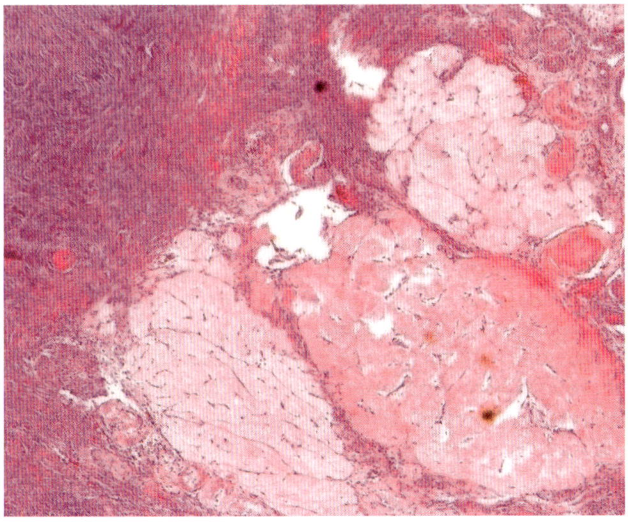

Figure 3.8 Corpus atreticum. The end result of atresia of a Graafian follicle. The granulosa cells have disappeared and a hyaline lamina has been deposited. The follicle is in the process of collapse.

THE ENDOMETRIUM

The endometrium is the special epithelial lining of that part of the cavity of the uterus which lies above the level of the internal os. It consists of a surface epithelium, glands and stroma. It was not until 1907 that the variations in the histological structure of the endometrium during the menstrual cycle were established by Hitschmann and Adler. This formed the basis upon which much of the modern work on the sex hormones rests.

The endometrium of the body of the uterus can be divided into two zones: a superficial termed the functional layer, and a deeper one termed the basal layer, which lies adjacent to the myometrium. The stroma cells of the basal layer stain deeply and are packed closely together. Islands of lymphoid tissue are found in the basal layer. This layer is not shed during mensuration, and regeneration starts before the end of mensuration.

The vascular system of the endometrium is of great importance. Two types of arteries supply the endometrium. One of these is restricted to the basal third and consists of small, straight and short arteries. The superficial two-thirds of the endometrium is supplied by coiled arteries.

THE PROLIFERATIVE PHASE

The phase of the menstrual cycle which starts when regeneration of menstruating endometrium is complete and lasts until the 14th day of a 28-day cycle is referred to as the proliferative or oestrogenic phase. At the end of menstruation, which may occupy from 3 to 5 days, the necrotic superficial layers have been exfoliated and the endometrium is represented by only the deep or basal layer. The coiled arteries have been lost and the terminal ends of the straight arteries are sealed off by fibrin. The stroma is heavily infiltrated with leucocytes and red cells. Regeneration is remarkably rapid and all elements of the endometrium, including glands and new sprouting vessels, are present at the end of 48 hours. The proliferative phase therefore starts and proceeds rapidly for about 3–5 days, and not later than 7 days after the start of the menstrual cycle. During proliferation the functional and the basal layers are well defined. The basal layer measures 1 mm in thickness, whereas the functional layer, commencing with an average of 2.5 mm, reaches about 3.5 mm by the 14th day, and during the secretory phase it hypertrophies still further so that immediately before menstruation its average thickness is about 8–10 mm. During the proliferative phase, the glands of the functional layer are simple tubules with regular epithelium (Fig. 3.9). About the 10th day of the cycle, the glands become slightly sinuous and their columnar epithelium becomes taller than before. The glands sometimes show a characteristic appearance in

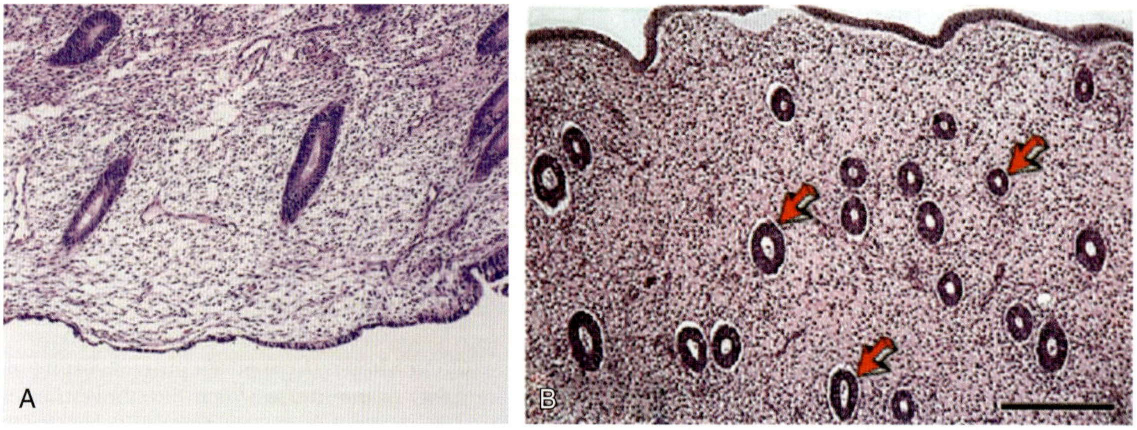

Figure 3.9 **(A)** Normal endometrium in the proliferative phase. **(B)** The glands are simple tubules and are shown in longitudinal and transverse sections (×66). (*Source*: The image belongs to Rex Bentley, MD, Department of Pathology, Duke University Medical Center, taken from link: http://www.pathologypics.com/PictView.aspx?ID=1149. © University of Kansas Medical Center, Department of Anatomy and Cell Biology.)

the later proliferative phase as if the glandular epithelium has been telescoped into the lumen, rather like an intussusception. This appearance is false and this telescoping is in reality due to the tuft of epithelium which has budded off from the gland wall. It is, therefore, merely an evidence of oestrogenic activity in the glandular epithelium. The stroma becomes extremely oedematous with wide separation of individual cells. During the 1st postmenstrual week, the coiled arteries extend only half way through the endometrium. Afterwards they grow more rapidly than the endometrium so that they become more coiled and spiralled. In some cases, the vascularity is so intense that blood oozes into the cavity of the uterus at the time of ovulation to be discharged from the vagina. Regular intermenstrual bleeding of this kind is a well-known clinical symptom and is due to the intense hyperaemia at the end of the proliferative phase. It almost certainly indicates that ovulation has occurred.

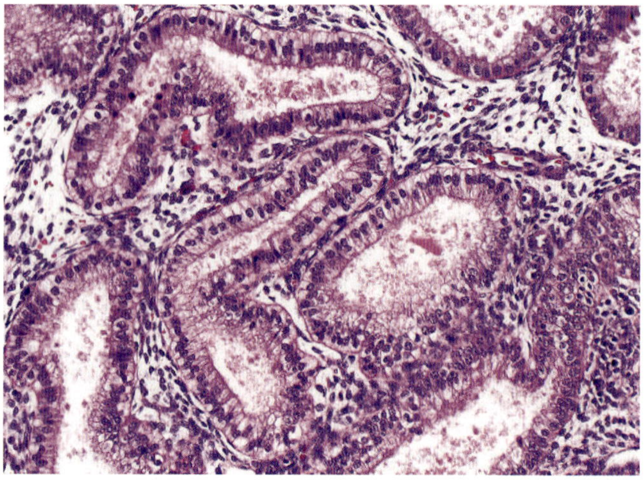

Figure 3.10 Endometrium – secretory hypertrophy (early stage).The gland is crenated, the lumen contains mucous secretion and the inner border of the cells is irregular. Subnuclear vacuolation is well seen. The surrounding stroma is oedematous and the hypertrophied stroma cells are widely separated from each other (×200). (*Source*: The image belongs to Rex Bentley, MD, Department of Pathology, Duke University Medical Center, taken from link: http://www.pathologypics.com/PictView.aspx?ID=1149.)

THE SECRETORY PHASE

Progesterone induces secretory changes only if the endometrium is primed by oestrogen, which produces progesterone receptors in the endometrial cells. The secretory phase of the endometrium begins on the 15th day and persists until the onset of menstruation. The most characteristic signs of this phase are found in the glands. Their epithelial cells develop spherical translucent areas between the nuclei and the basement membrane which contain the precursors of the glandular secretion and which persist until about the 21st day of the cycle. This characteristic appearance is called subnuclear vacuolation and is a presumptive evidence of progesterone activity and, therefore, of ovulation. The fluid in these subnuclear vacuoles consists of mucin and glycogen (Fig. 3.10), the function of which is presumably to provide nutrition to the fertilized ovum. The phase of subnuclear vacuolation is rapidly followed by an increase in intracellular secretion which pushes the nuclei to the basement membrane and fills the cell. The subnuclear vacuole later migrates past the nucleus to the surface of the cell. In the latter part of the secretory phase, the inner border of the epithelial cells become irregular through the discharge of the secretion into the lumina of the glands, which shortly before menstruation are full of coagulated secretion that stains deeply with eosin. The glands become crenated and assume a characteristic corkscrew-shaped form (Fig. 3.11A and B). The stroma of the functional layer remains oedematous, but further interstitial haemorrhage is rare except immediately prior to the onset of menstruation. The coiled arteries become more spiral and form closely wound perpendicular columns through the mucosa. The stroma cells become swollen, and after the 21st day of the cycle they tend to be collected immediately beneath the surface epithelium where they surround the ducts of the glands in such a way that the functional layer can be subdivided into two zones: the superficial or compact zone and a deeper spongy layer. The swollen stroma cells of the compact part of the functional layer represent young decidual cells, and in every respect the reaction of the compact zone corresponds to

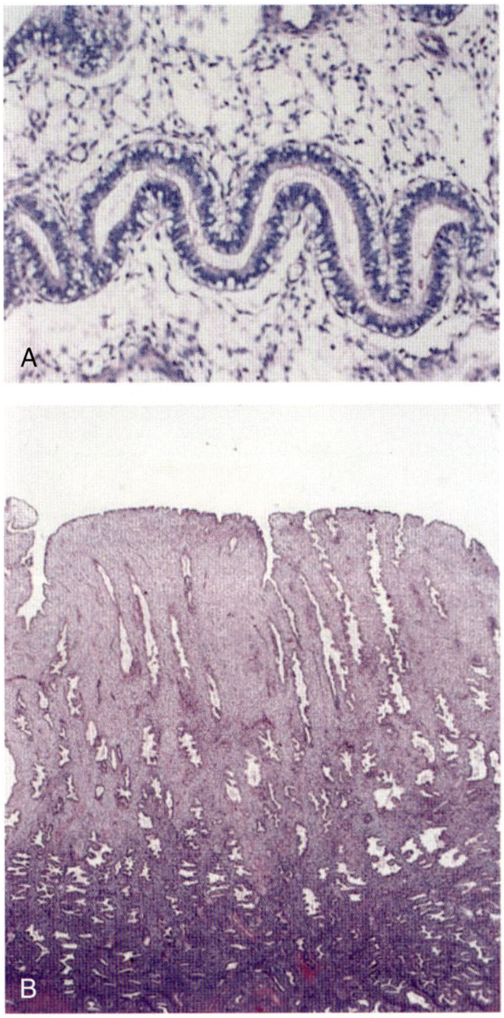

Figure 3.11 **(A)** Endometrium – secretory hypertrophy – at a slightly later stage than Fig. 3.10. The secretory vacuoles are now near the apex of the cell (×124). **(B)** Endometrium showing compacta, spongiosa and basalis layers. (*Source*: The image belongs to Rex Bentley, MD, Department of Pathology, Duke University Medical Center, taken from link: http://www.pathologypics.com/PictView.aspx?ID=1149.)

what is found in this part of the endometrium during pregnancy. The islands of lymphoid tissue in the basal layer of the endometrium scatter lymphocytes into the functional layer so that at this stage, there is a well-marked lymphocytic infiltration of the whole of the endometrium. The endometrium measures 8–10 mm in thickness in the secretory phase. The endometrial thickness can be studied ultrasonically. This study is useful in indicating the optimal time for embryo transfer in in vitro fertilization (Fig. 3.12). In spite of the intense secretory activity of the functional layer, the basal layer glands are not similarly affected and retain non-secretory pattern and mitosis is rare in this phase.

The secretory phase reaches its peak by the 22nd day of the cycle, after which no further growth ensues. About the 24th day of the cycle some shrinkage of the glands is apparent, partly due to the dehydration of the stroma. The corkscrew pattern now becomes saw-toothed. No superficial necrosis has yet occurred but the superficial layers are noticeably less vascular. Just before menstruation, there is a well-marked local leucocytic infiltration.

Dating of the endometrium and the diagnosis of luteal phase defect (LPD) are recognized by correlating the post-ovulatory endometrial picture with the menstrual date. A lag of 2 or more days is confirmative of corpus LPD. The estimation of progesterone level in the mid-secretory phase also indicates progesterone deficiency.

THE MENSTRUATING ENDOMETRIUM

The menstrual changes in the endometrium are essentially degenerative. The spiral-coiled arteries undergo vasoconstriction a few hours before the onset of menstrual bleeding under the influence of prostaglandin $F_2\alpha$. It is believed that the ischaemia thereby produced leads to the necrosis of zones in the walls of the small arteries in the superficial part of the endometrium. In addition, the buckling of the coiled arteries produces blood stasis, which may also cause necrosis. This buckling results from the decrease in the depth of the endometrium as a whole and causes further tightening of the arterial coils. Several additional coils may be detected in a single vessel. Bleeding from the endometrium is restricted only to the times when the coiled arteries relax and when the blood is discharged from the artery through the damaged necrotic areas in its wall. The straight arteries immediately beneath the coiled arteries undergo vasospasm at the time of the menstrual bleeding and thereby provide a simple safety mechanism for haemostasis. This vasospasm limits the menstrual loss. Deficiency of the mechanism may account for some forms of menorrhagia. The vasospasm is selective as it only affects the superficial layers and does not extend to the basal layer, which is thereby assured of an adequate blood supply necessary for regeneration. The compact zone of the functional layer becomes infiltrated with a large number of cells, and the surface epithelium may be pushed away from the sub-adjacent stroma. A little later the glands of the spongy zone of the functional layer disintegrate so that the epithelial cells separate from each other and become scattered amongst the red blood cells, leucocytes and the cells of the stroma (Fig. 3.11B). The degenerative process is rapid so that by the 2nd day of the period of bleeding, the compact zone and the superficial part of the spongy zone have degenerated and a large part of it has been discharged into the cavity of the uterus. It is certain that the whole of the compact zone of the functional layer is shed, and probably most of the spongy zone of the endometrium is also shed. The basal layer is not shed during menstruation. On the 3rd day of the period of bleeding, the surface of the endometrium is raw and the patulous glands of the functional layer open directly into the cavity of the uterus. Active degeneration seems to be restricted to the first 2 days of menstruation. The subsequent bleeding is the result of oozing from the capillaries of the denuded stroma. It is common to find relics of the glands and stroma of the endometrium in the shreds and clots passed on the 5th day of the period of bleeding, which affords conclusive proof that a large part of the endometrium is shed in normal menstruation. There is reason to believe, however, that in some cases of abnormal uterine haemorrhage, the disintegration process is not spread uniformly over the entire endometrium but may be localized to limited areas.

The menstrual blood loss is controlled by interaction between PGE_2, $PGF_2\alpha$ and PGI_2 (prostacyclin) secreted by the

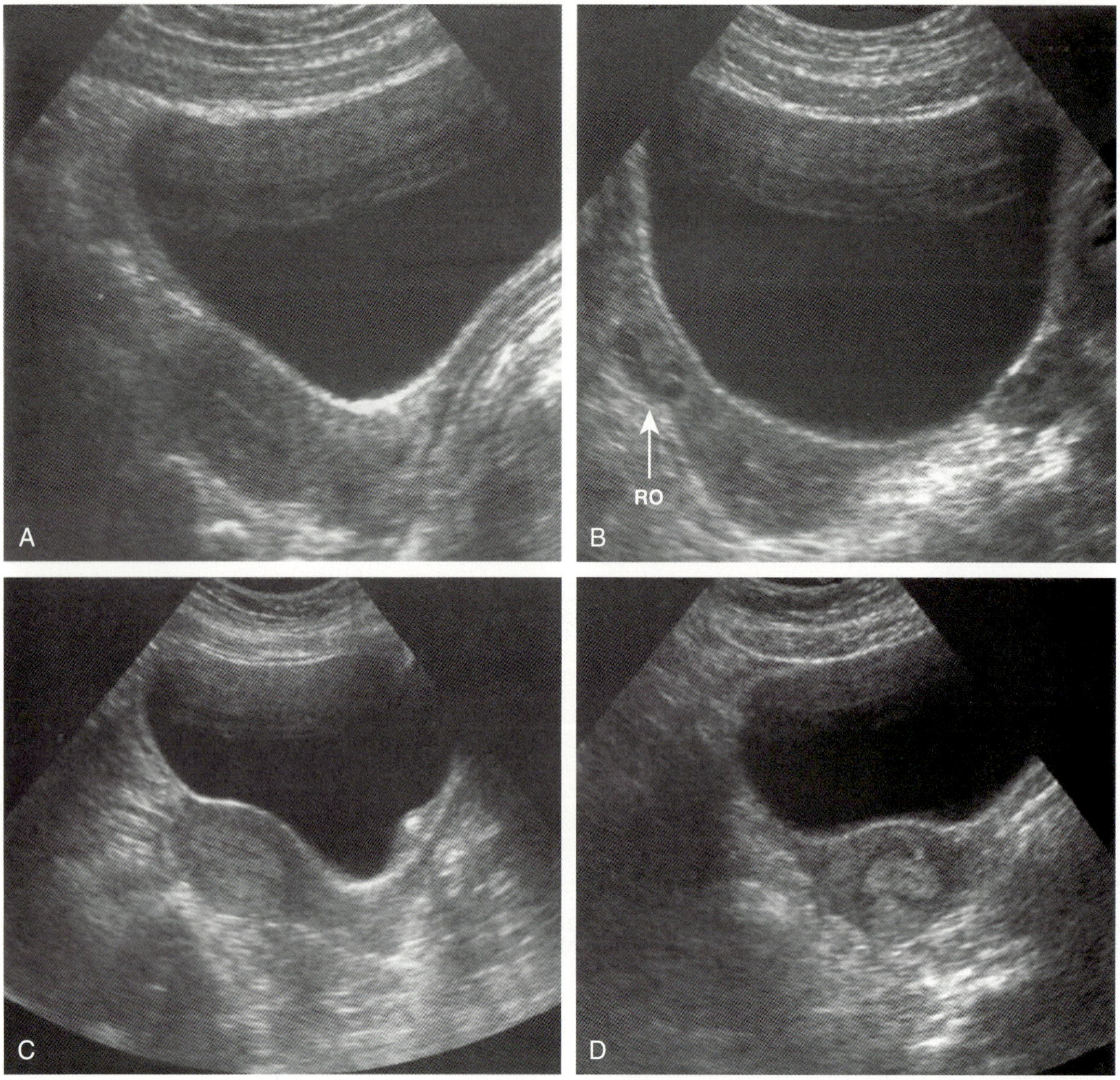

Figure 3.12 Pelvic sonography showing normal anteverted position of the uterus in sagittal views **(A** and **C)** of two separate patients. Note the polycystic (right) ovary adjacent to the uterus in the sagittal view **(B)** and the thickened endometrial linings in the views **(C** and **D)**. (*Courtesy*: Dr Ketan Gundavda, Mumbai.)

endometrium. Whereas PGE_2, $PGF_2\alpha$ and thromboxane cause vasoconstriction of the vessels, prostacyclin causes vasodilation and menorrhagia. The combined oral contraceptive pills (OCPs) cause atrophic endometrium. PGE_2 predominates in the proliferative phase and $PGF_2\alpha$ in the luteal phase.

ENDOMETRIAL REGENERATION

Regeneration of the denuded epithelium is already in progress before the menstrual bleeding has stopped and is completed 48 hours after the end of menstruation. Repair is brought about by the glandular epithelium growing over the bare stroma (Fig. 3.13). This is brought about by vascular endothelial growth factor (VEGF) produced by oestriol stimulation. It is not uncommon for relics of crenated glands to be found in the endometrium during the first 2 days following menstruation, and one of the great characteristics of the endometrium at this time is the presence of a large number of lymphocytes in the stroma. The relation

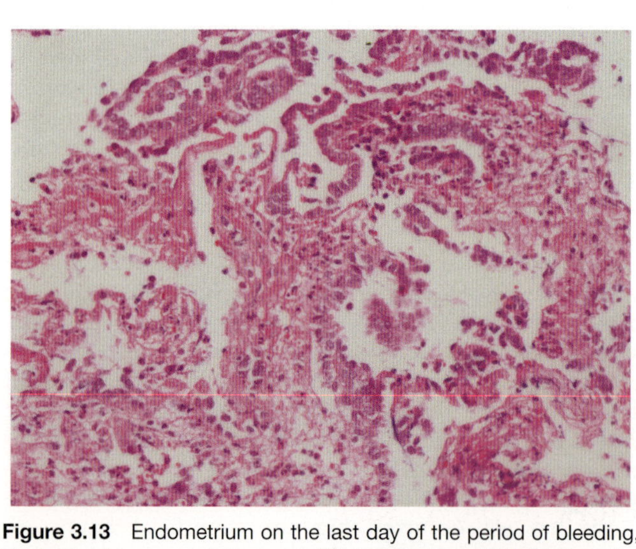

Figure 3.13 Endometrium on the last day of the period of bleeding, illustrating the compact stroma and the method by which the denuded area is covered by the epithelium which grows over it from the glands.

of the cyclical changes between the ovaries and the endometrium is discussed in Chapter 4.

FUNCTIONAL LAYERS OF ENDOMETRIUM

Using magnetic resonance imaging (MRI) technique, Haicak described three layers of endometrium: (1) high-intensity endometrial strip; (2) medium signal intensity over the myometrium; and (3) in between these two layers, a 'junctional zone' or 'subendometrial halo'. Ultrasound shows peristaltic movements in this subendometrial halo zone. These movements are under hormonal influence. This zone is thin before puberty and after the menopause, and also in those on oral combined pills. It increases in size during pregnancy and becomes vascular under oestrogen influence. This zone is maximum at the time of ovulation. At this time, the increased peristaltic movement helps in the transport of sperms into the fallopian tubes. The peristaltic movements diminish during the luteal phase under the effect of progesterone and help in the implantation of fertilized egg.

The contractions or these movements in the subendometrial zone have important bearing on reproductive process. They help in the rapid transport of sperms to the fallopian tubes within a few minutes during ovulation, and also help in implantation during the luteal phase.

Abnormal function of this zone is one of the factors responsible for failure of conception in IVF programme, or occurrence of a tubal pregnancy.

THE DECIDUA OF PREGNANCY

In the early weeks of pregnancy, the structure of the endometrium is very similar to that found in the late secretory phase. The division into compact and spongy zones of the functional layer is more clearly defined. The basal layer can still be identified, but its glands, although staining more deeply than the hypertrophied glands of the spongy layer, show some degree of crenation and contain secretion. The lymphoid islands of the basal layer are not easily identified, for in the early weeks of pregnancy lymphocytes are disseminated extensively into the stroma of the spongy layer. The glands of the spongy layer retain the general form found in the late secretory phase, but they are much more crenated, so much that the impression is given that they have increased in number. The cells lining the glands are irregular in shape and tend to be elongated with irregular processes projecting into the lumina of the glands and discharging secretion. It is not uncommon for small papillae to be formed which project into the glands, but in spite of the activity of the epithelium, the basement membrane remains well defined. Activity is not restricted to the immediate vicinity of the implanted ovum but is distributed uniformly throughout the endometrium of the body of the uterus. The compact layer shows the typical decidual reaction of pregnancy. The decidual cells are derived from stroma cells: they are stellate in shape, contain glycogen and are surrounded by an intercellular fibrillary ground substance and lymphocytes (Fig. 3.14).

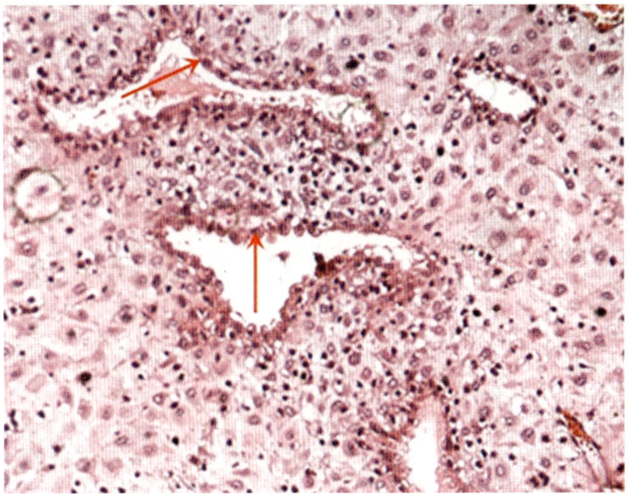

Figure 3.14 Decidua of early pregnancy. The large decidual cells have a faintly staining cytoplasm which is eosinophilic. They are always surrounded by lymphocytes and the cells fuse with an intercellular matrix. (*Source*: Taha M. M. Hassan, Ahmad M. S. Hegazy, Mohammed M. Mosaed, Anatomical and Histopathologic Analysis of Placenta in Dilation and Evacuation Specimens, 2(2):2014.)

ECTOPIC DECIDUAL CELLS

Decidual cells are not restricted to the endometrium of the body of the uterus. Decidual reaction has been demonstrated in various ectopic situations in the pelvis. The best example of ectopic decidual reaction is found on the surface of the ovaries during pregnancy, when small irregular reddish areas are easily recognized with the naked eye and show typical decidual reaction on histological examination. In the ovaries, the decidual reaction is limited to the surface with very little invasion of the cortex. Ectopic decidual reaction is always very well marked beneath the peritoneum of the back of the uterus in the pouch of Douglas. It has been demonstrated in adenomyomas, in the walls of chocolate cysts, on the uterovesical fold of peritoneum and in the omentum. Decidual reaction can invariably be demonstrated in the isthmical region of the endometrium during pregnancy, but only rarely is the typical reaction found in the glands of the cervical canal. Decidual reaction occurs in the fallopian tube in an ectopic pregnancy, but it is incomplete and deficient. A thick decidua develops in hydatidiform mole under the influence of hormones. The significance of ectopic decidual cells is unknown. The decidual reaction is controlled by the corpus luteum, but it is unknown why only cells with this curious distribution respond to the stimulus.

VAGINAL EPITHELIUM

The upper portion of the lateral vaginal epithelium displays cyclic changes in response to the ovarian hormones. These changes can be studied cytologically by scraping this portion of the vaginal epithelium and staining it with Shorr stain. Details of vaginal cytology are discussed in Chapter 9.

OVARIAN FUNCTIONS

Apart from producing an ovum monthly, ovaries produce hormones responsible for maturation of the Graafian follicle, ovulation, menstruation and maintenance of pregnancy in the early weeks of gestation. The steroidal hormones are oestrogen and progesterone. Oestrogen is mainly secreted by the Graafian follicle in the follicular phase (preovulatory phase). A small amount is also secreted by the corpus luteum in the premenstrual phase. Progesterone is secreted by the corpus luteum, and the absence of progesterone in the premenstrual phase denotes anovulation. The control of these hormones is described in Chapter 4. Inhibin is a nonsteroidal hormone present in the Graafian follicle. It is a protein that inhibits FSH and stimulates LH secretion by the anterior pituitary. Excess of inhibin seen in polycystic ovarian disease (PCOD) is responsible for the high level of LH.

The other hormones which the ovary produces in small amounts are testosterone and androstenedione, mainly secreted by the stromal cells and stimulated by LH. Androstenedione gets converted peripherally into oestrone through aromatization in the fat tissue. After menopause, ovarian oestrogen level falls as Graafian follicles disappear, and progesterone fails to be produced. The increased stromal cells of the menopausal ovary continue to produce some androstenedione which gets converted into oestrone. Although a weak oestrogen, oestrone is capable of exerting oestrogenic effect on the target tissues. Obese women have, therefore, more oestrone than a lean woman, and hence a greater tendency to endometrial hyperplasia and malignancy.

PREGNANCY

In some cases of uterine and ectopic pregnancies, the endometrium shows intense adenomatous and hypersecretive activity within the glandular epithelium. The cells are enlarged; epithelial nuclei show mitosis, hyperchromasia, polyploidy and atypical cell types. The cells are hypersecretive without glycogen content. This condition is called the *Arias—Stella reaction.* These changes are focal and often associated with decidual reaction in the stroma. Besides pregnancy, this endometrial reaction is seen in endometriosis, reaction to oestrogen and to gonadotropins as well as in gestational trophoblastic disease (GTD).

MENOPAUSAL ENDOMETRIUM

In the majority of women, oestrogen withdrawal at menopause causes endometrial atrophy, and the endometrium is only 1–3 mm in thickness. The atrophic endometrium is susceptible to infection, resulting in senile endometritis and postmenopausal bleeding. In rare cases, the endometrium becomes hyperplastic under the influence of extragenital oestrogen (oestrone) produced in the peripheral fat from epiandrostenedione. The postmenopausal endometrium measuring more than 4 mm is considered abnormal. Endometrial hyperplasia and polyp also occur when tamoxifen is administered to a woman with breast cancer.

CERVICAL MUCUS

In 1948, Papanicolaou described the fern test and the cyclical changes in the cervical mucus under the influence of various hormones. A drop of cervical mucus spread and dried on a glass slide in the preovulatory phase (oestrogenic phase) presents a palm leaf or fern type of reaction, due to the presence of sodium chloride in it (Fig. 3.15). This reaction disappears after ovulation under progesterone influence. Under the influence of progesterone, the cervical mucus becomes thick and tenacious and impenetrable to sperms and bacteria. The details of cervical mucus are described in Chapter 16.

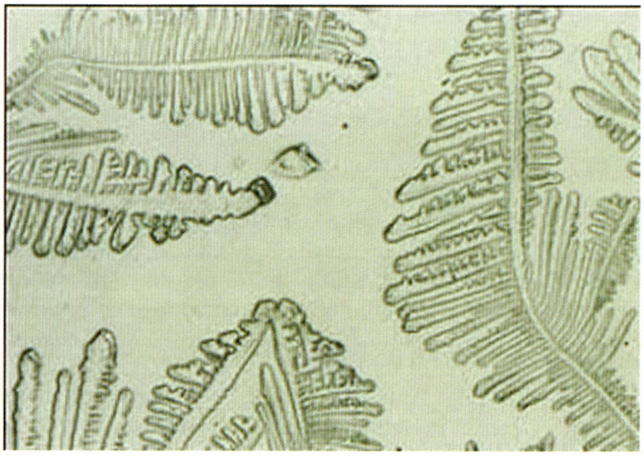

Figure 3.15 Microscopic appearance of dried cervical mucus showing the 'fern appearance'. (*Source*: http://gynaeonline.com/cervical_cycle.htm.)

Endocervical lining does not exhibit cyclical changes like the endometrium. In pregnancy, however, adenomatous hyperplasia may occur, and decidual changes are seen in 10% of the patients.

Oral combined hormonal pills over the years also cause hyperplasia of endocervical epithelium and an abnormal 'Pap smear'. Lately, an increased incidence of endocervical carcinoma has been observed in young women who have been on hormonal contraception use. Contrary to this, the pills cause atrophic endometrium in the body uterus.

PROCESS OF FERTILIZATION

Certain changes are necessary before the primary oocyte can mature for fertilization. Oogonia that enter the prophase of the first meiotic division are known as primary oocytes, whereas those oogonia which do not begin the first meiotic division and not surrounded by granulosa layer undergo atrophy. At puberty, under the LH surge, primary oocyte completes the first meiotic division and gives rise to secondary oocyte, containing most of the cytoplasm, 23X chromosomes and a small polar body. This secondary oocyte completes its second meiotic division only after fertilization, and gives out second polar body.

Thus, the first stage of maturation of the oocyte occurs within the Graafian follicle, but the second division occurs only after the fertilization in the fallopian tube.

KEY POINTS

- The ovary of the newborn has about 2 million primordial follicles. These are reduced to about 400,000 at puberty, and of these around 400 are available during the reproductive lifespan.
- Cyclic changes in the Graafian follicle – leading to ovulation, corpus luteum formation and menstruation – are under the control of the hypothalamus, which controls the release of gonadotropins from the anterior pituitary.

- Oestrogen causes regeneration of the endometrium and leads to proliferative phase. Progesterone is responsible for secretory transformation of the endometrium, rendering it favourable for implantation of fertilized ovum.
- Peak level of 40–75 ng/mL of LH is noted just before ovulation.
- In the present-day practice, serial ultrasound monitoring of the Graafian follicle is the most preferred method to detect ovulation in patients undergoing treatment for infertility.
- Endometrial histology is useful to diagnose endometrial tuberculosis, endometrial cancer and hormonal dysfunction.
- Endometrial thickness of 8–12 mm is considered normal in the premenstrual phase. In postmenopausal women, endometrial thickness should not exceed 4 mm.
- LH surge is an important indicator of imminent ovulation.

SELF-ASSESSMENT

1. Describe the microscopic appearance of the endometrium during the proliferative phase.
2. Describe the histological appearance of the endometrium in the secretory phase.
3. Describe the endometrial changes during pregnancy.
4. What is the significance of cervical mucus changes in fertility practice?

SUGGESTED READING

Berek and Novak's Textbook of Gynaecology, Adashi EY, Hillard PA (eds). Novak's Gynecology. 15th ed. Philadelphia, PA, Williams & Wilkins, 2014.

Mishell DR Jr, Davajan V (eds). Infertility, Contraception and Reproductive Endocrinology. 2nd Ed. Oradell, NJ, Medical Economics Books Oradell, 1986.

Novak E, Novak ER (eds). Textbook of Gynecology. 4th Ed. Baltimore, Philadelphia, PA, Williams & Wilkins, 1952.

4 Physiology of Ovulation and Menstruation

CHAPTER OUTLINE

Cyclical menstruation and reproductive functions in a woman occur as a result of fine interaction between hypothalamus and anterior pituitary. Hormone production (follicle-stimulating hormone [FSH] and luteinizing hormone [LH]) from anterior pituitary in turn is responsible for follicular maturation, ovulation, corpus luteum formation and production of oestrogen and progesterone hormones from ovary. Therefore, an understanding of hypothalamic–pituitary–ovarian (H–P–O) axis is important for knowing physiology of reproduction and management of various diseases associated with their malfunction.

Neuroendocrinology with vast hormonal interactions is responsible for menstrual cycle and reproductive functions in a woman.

HYPOTHALAMIC-PITUITARY-OVARIAN AXIS

It is now well established that a normal menstrual cycle depends on cyclical ovarian steroid secretions, which in turn are controlled by the pituitary and the hypothalamus and, to some extent, are influenced by the thyroid and adrenal glands. It is therefore essential to understand the H–P–O axis in normal women and apply this knowledge in therapeutic management in infertility, family planning and various gynaecological disorders.

HYPOTHALAMUS

Hypothalamus with its several nuclei and extrinsic connections is now considered the main neuroendocrine gland and the regulatory factor in the chain of hypothalamic–pituitary–ovarian–uterine axis. Hypothalamus regulates the functions of the anterior pituitary gland through portal vessels by releasing both stimulatory and inhibitory hormones that in turn influence the functions of the target tissues through the systemic circulation (Fig. 4.1A and B). These hormones in turn are controlled by positive and negative feedback loops from ovarian hormones. External and internal stimuli further modify or influence hypothalamic functions.

Hypothalamus is located at the base of the brain behind optic chiasma and below the thalamus above the pituitary and forms the base of the third ventricle. The base of the hypothalamus forms tuber cinereum, which merges to form the pituitary stalk. The origin of this stalk is known as median eminence, which is rich in capillary loops as well as nerve endings. Median eminence is an important site of storage of chemical signals, which get transferred into portal circulation to reach the anterior pituitary gland. Schally and Guillemin were the first to discover a decapeptide called gonadotropin-releasing hormone (GnRH) in 1971. GnRH is secreted by the median eminence and the arcuate nucleus, which modulates the neural control of FSH and LH by the anterior pituitary gland. It (arcuate nucleus) also secretes prolactin-inhibiting factor (PIF), which is dopamine that inhibits the release of prolactin. During late pregnancy and lactation, a low or absent inhibitory factor leads to a high secretion of prolactin that initiates and maintains lactation.

Hypothalamus is also responsible for secretion of thyrotropin-releasing factor, corticotropin-releasing factor, insulin-like growth factor and melanocyte-releasing factor.

Hypothalamus is connected to the anterior pituitary gland through special hypophysis pituitary portal system of vessels but connected directly to the posterior pituitary gland (neurohypophysis) by the supraoptic and paraventricular nuclei (Fig. 4.2).

GnRH (decapeptide) is synthesized in arcuate nucleus and is released at the nerve endings near tuber cinereum. GnRH has a half-life of 2–4 minutes and is therefore difficult to assay. Its level is assessed through the LH level. It is released in a pulsatile manner into the portal vessels and reaches the anterior pituitary gland. *The pulsatility and amplitude of its release vary with the various phases of the menstrual cycle.* In the preovulatory phase (the follicular phase), it pulses once in every 60 minutes, but it slows down to once in 3 hours in the luteal phase, with increased amplitude of each pulse.

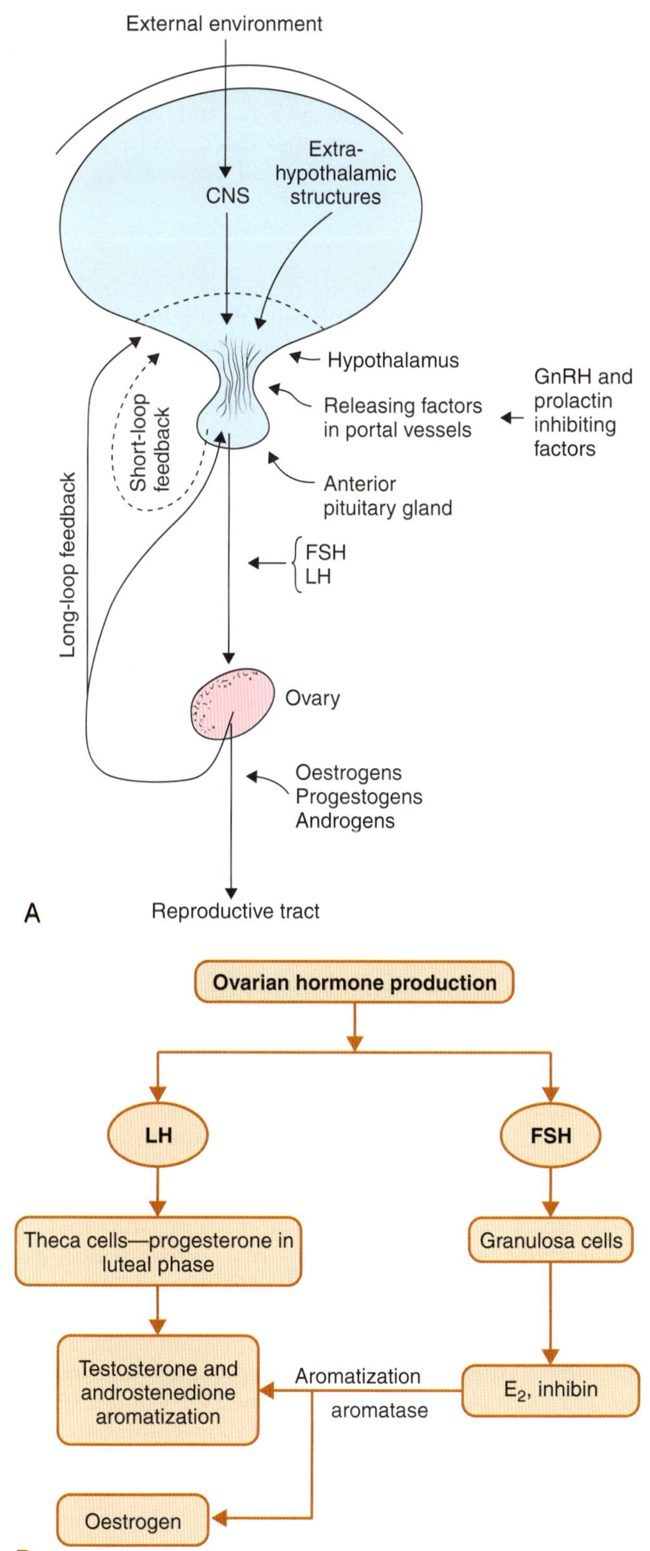

Figure 4.1 **(A)** Hypothalamic–pituitary–ovarian axis. **(B)** Ovarian hormone production.

GnRH exhibits different actions depending on the manner in which it is released. Its continuous release causes suppression of gonadotropins and thereby the ovarian functions through the process of 'downregulation' or desensitization of pituitary hormones. This mode of administration is now employed in therapy using synthetic analogues of GnRH in regulating ovulation in in vitro fertilization and suppressing menstruation in precocious puberty, in reducing the size of the uterine fibroids and in causing shrinkage of endometriosis. Its suppressive effect on ovulation is also being tried as a contraceptive, but the drug has proved expensive as of today. The pulsatile administration, on the other hand, causes cyclical release of gonadotropins – FSH first and later LH which induces ovulation and the possibility of a pregnancy. This therapy is applied in women with anovulatory infertility.

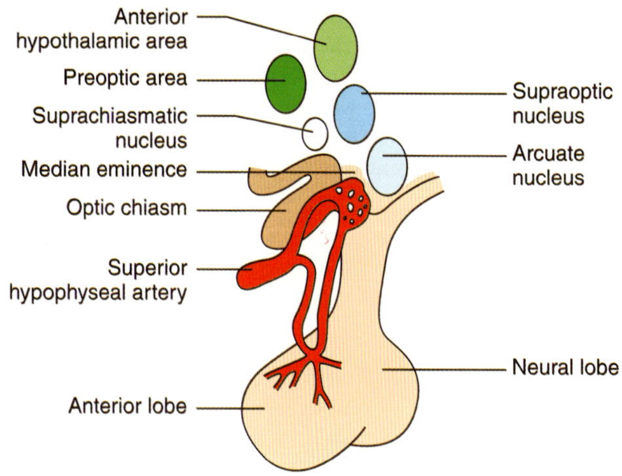

Figure 4.2 Hypothalamic nuclei.

Hypothalamus can be influenced by the higher cortical centres, especially the temporal lobe. Emotional upsets are known to stimulate or depress the H–P–O axis and disturb the menstrual cycles. Neuroendocrine system works through several loops, both positive and negative.

- Long loops through oestrogen and progesterone
- Short loop through anterior pituitary gland
- Ultrashort loop within the hypothalamus

Epinephrine and oestrogen stimulate whereas dopamine, serotonin and opioids inhibit the release of GnRH by the hypothalamus. Gonadotropins also inhibit GnRH secretion.

Until puberty, the hypothalamus is in a dormant state under the inhibitory influence of adrenal cortex, and the higher cortical centres, or it may be insensitive and nonresponsive to these stimuli. It becomes gradually sensitive around 8–12 years and starts its hormonal functions, fully establishing the H–P–O axis by the age of 13–14 years. What triggers GnRH to start functioning is not clear, but perhaps leptin produced by the adipose tissue that initiates the response. Initially, GnRH is released in a pulsatile manner during sleep, but later throughout 24 hours. In the follicular phase, with low oestrogen (E_2) level, pulsatility is every 90 minutes, and with rise in E_2 level, the frequency rises to every 60 minutes. In the luteal phase, the frequency slows down to 1 pulse in 3 hours. Hypothalamus is sexually differentiated at birth. GnRH secretion is continuous in males but pulsatile in females. Administration of testosterone to a female rat at birth is shown to cause a continuous secretion of GnRH in later life and alter the hormonal function to a male type.

Synthetic analogues of GnRH are nonapeptides and are now available and used in the following:

- Preoperative shrinkage of uterine fibroids
- Shrinkage of endometriosis
- Shrinkage of the endometrium prior to endometrial ablation
- Hirsutism
- Precocious puberty
- In vitro fertilization
- Prostatic cancer

Prolonged administration over 6 months can cause oestrogen deficiency and osteoporosis, and therefore the therapy should be used on a short-term basis. This peptide is degraded in the gastrointestinal tract and is therefore given intravenously, subcutaneously or intranasally. Its short life mandates repeated administration at short intervals. However, depot monthly injections are available.

Side effects of GnRH are as follows:

- Insomnia
- Nausea
- Osteoporosis caused by oestrogen deficiency, but reverts to normal after stoppage of the drug
- Decrease in breast size – reversible
- Myalgia, oedema
- Dizziness
- Decreased libido
- Decrease in high-density lipoprotein (HDL) and increase in cholesterol by 10% each

The drugs and their administration are as follows:

- Nafarelin 200 mcg intranasally daily for 6 months.
- Buserelin 300 mcg t.i.d. subcutaneously daily × 5 days.
- Depot injection of goserelin i.m. or implant 3.6 mg monthly.
- Leuprolide 3.75 mg i.m. monthly × 5 months.
- Triptorelin 3.7 mg i.m. 4 weekly.
- Antagon is GnRH antagonist used in downregulation in in vitro fertilization.
- Hypothalamus also secretes insulin-like growth factor, thyroxin and corticotrophin releasing factors.

PITUITARY GLAND

Pituitary gland lies in the sella turcica. It measures 1.2 × 1 × 0.6 cm and weighs 500–900 mg. It comprises the anterior pituitary gland (adenohypophysis) and the posterior pituitary gland (neurohypophysis). The anterior pituitary gland originates at the roof of the embryonic pharynx called Rathke's pouch and contains chromophil and chromophobe cells. The posterior lobe develops from the floor of the brain. The two lobes of the pituitary gland develop independently of each other. The anterior lobe is ectodermal in origin.

ANTERIOR PITUITARY GLAND (ADENOHYPOPHYSIS)

The anterior pituitary gland, measuring 30 × 6 × 9 mm in size, is located at the base of the brain in a bony cavity called sella turcica below the hypothalamus. It consists of three histologically distinguishable cells: (i) the chromophobe or parent cell, (ii) the chromophil cells described as eosinophil or alpha (α) cells and (iii) basophil or beta (β) cells. The β-cells secrete the gonadotropins that control the ovarian function and menstrual cycles. These gonadotropins are FSH, LH, thyroid-stimulating hormone (TSH) and corticosteroid hormone. Each of these hormones has α- and β-fractions. Although α-fraction is identical in all (contains 92 amino acids), β-fraction is specific in its action.

Follicle-Stimulating Hormone

FSH is a water-soluble glycoprotein of high molecular weight and is secreted by the β-cells; it contains 115 amino acids in β-fraction. The carbohydrate fraction is mannose. FSH controls the ripening of the primordial follicles, and in conjunction with the LH, it activates the secretion of oestrogen. Its activity builds up as the bleeding starts to cease, reaches a peak around the 7th day of the cycle (40 ng/mL) and then declines to disappear around the 18th day. Another small peak occurs after ovulation, perhaps as a result of a fall in the level of oestrogen in the premenstrual phase. The half-life of FSH is 4 hours. Low FSH causes defective folliculogenesis and short or defective corpus luteal phase. Oestrogen suppresses FSH secretion through negative feedback mechanism. It develops LH receptors in the granulosa cells.

Gemzell initially isolated FSH from the pituitary of human cadavers at autopsy, but it required 10 pituitaries to produce enough FSH for one ovulation. FSH is now commercially obtained from the urine of menopausal women. The preparation contains both FSH and LH. Pure FSH is now available on the market but is very expensive. FSH is stimulated by GnRH, but suppressed by oestrogen and inhibin B.

Luteinizing Hormone

LH is a water-soluble glycoprotein of high molecular weight secreted by β-cells; it also contains 115 amino acids. The carbohydrate fraction is mannose. Initially, LH pulse occurs only during sleep, but later extends throughout the day. LH surge initiated by oestrogen lasts for 48 hours and is preceded by a small amount of progesterone 2 hours earlier. LH level doubles in 2 hours and the peak plateaus for 14 hours before declining. Progesterone secretion begins 34 hours after LH peak. In conjunction with FSH, it activates the secretion of oestrogen, brings about the maturation of the ovum and causes ovulation. LH stimulates the completion of the reduction division of the oocyte. Following ovulation, it produces luteinization of the granulosa and the theca cells and initiates progesterone secretion. The LH surge precedes ovulation by 24–36 hours (mean 30 hours) and a minimum of 75 ng/mL is required for ovulation. This time relationship of LH peak to ovulation is helpful in predicting the exact time of ovulation in infertile women on gonadotropin therapy, making it possible to retrieve ova in in vitro fertilization and to arrange for timely artificial insemination to enhance chances of conception. LH stimulates the secretion of testosterone and androstenedione in the ovarian stroma (theca cells), which diffuse into the follicular fluid and are aromatized into oestradiol. Low level causes unruptured follicle, non-ovulation and corpus luteal phase defect.

Nowadays, for diagnostic and therapeutic purposes, a rapid, visual, semi-quantitative enzyme immunoassay dipstick test, called OvuSTICK, is available for testing urine to

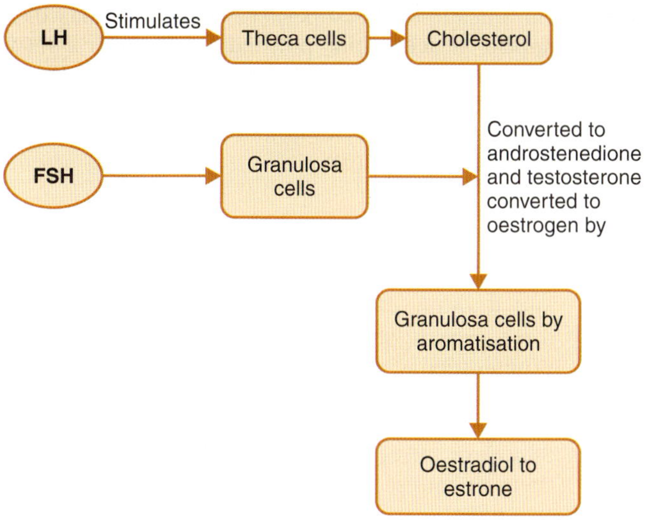

Figure 4.3 Two-cell two-gonadotropin theory of ovarian steroidogenesis.

detect LH surge by undertaking daily LH estimations around the period of ovulation. These kits are expensive. The half-life of LH is 30 minutes (Fig. 4.3). Inadequate LH peak causes unruptured corpus luteum, anovulation and corpus luteal phase defect.

Human Chorionic Gonadotropin

Secreted by the trophoblastic tissue in pregnancy, human chorionic gonadotropin (hCG) has a luteinizing action and is available in injectable form for use in cases of anovulatory infertility, in vitro fertilization, corpus luteal insufficiency and habitual abortions. hCG contains α- and β-fractions. The α-fraction resembles LH and TSH, but the β-fraction is exclusively specific to chorionic tissue. It is commercially obtained from the urine of pregnant women. The level is increased in trophoblastic tumours and some ovarian tumours. Recombinant hCG is now available, which has fewer side effects at the site of injection. 250 μg recombinant hCG is equivalent to 5000Gu of hCG.

Prolactin

Prolactin is an alcohol-soluble protein (polypeptide) (198 amino acids) without a carbohydrate fraction and with a half-life of 30 minutes. It is secreted by α-cells. Its main action is on lactation. It has a suppressive effect on the pituitary–ovarian axis, and therefore the patient who suffers from hyperprolactinaemia may develop amenorrhoea or oligomenorrhoea due to anovulatory cycles, with or without galactorrhoea. Normal prolactin level is 25 ng/mL. Up to 100 ng/mL occurs in hyperprolactinaemia but over 100 ng/mL is seen in pituitary tumours. The prepubertal level of 7 ng/mL rises to 13 ng/mL at puberty and 25 ng/mL in an adult woman. Active prolactin is present in the form of monomer or 'little prolactin' (50%), whereas dimeric and multimetric (big prolactin) forms have negligible biological activity. Normally, the prolactin release is under inhibitor control by hypothalamic release of prolactin inhibiting factor probably dopamine and is released in to the portal system (Hypophysio pituitary portal system). The level of prolactin is raised during sleep, nipple stimulation and the secretion of thyroid-releasing hormone, β-endorphin, serotonin and oestrogen.

Prolactin level does not fluctuate much during the menstrual cycle. It suppresses LH but not FSH, so hyperprolactinaemia decreases the LH/FSH ratio.

Growth hormone, insulin-like growth factor, epidermal growth factor, adrenal cortex and *TSH* also participate in the endocrinological functions in a woman, through their action on the hypothalamus and anterior pituitary gland. A high level of TSH stimulates prolactin secretion and causes ovulatory and menstrual dysfunction. Interleukin-1 is a cytokine with antigonadotropic activity and it prevents luteinization of granulose cells.

POSTERIOR PITUITARY GLAND (NEUROHYPOPHYSIS)

Oxytocin and vasopressin are nonapeptides formed in the hypothalamus and released directly into the posterior pituitary gland. Oxytocin is produced by the paraventricular nucleus and vasopressin by the supraoptic nucleus of the hypothalamus.

Oxytocin

Oxytocin acts mainly on the smooth muscle of the uterus, causing contraction of the muscles and controlling the bleeding in the third stage of labour. By intermittent uterine contractions and relaxation, it induces and enhances the labour pains in the first and second stage of labour. It causes contraction of the myoepithelial cells lining the mammary ducts and ejects milk during suckling.

Vasopressin

Vasopressin maintains the blood volume and blood pressure. Both have antidiuretic action when given in large quantities (over 20 units of oxytocin in 24 hours). The therapeutic applications of these hormones are described in chapter on Hormone Therapy.

OVARIAN STEROIDOGENESIS

The active hormones of the ovary are the steroids derived from cholesterol. These include oestrogens, progesterone, testosterone and androstenedione (Fig. 4.1A). Relaxin and inhibin are other nonsteriod secretions. Oestrogen is produced during follicular phase and progesterone is luteal phase.

OESTROGEN

Natural oestrogens are C18 steroids, the main source of which are the theca and granulosa cells of the Graafian follicles and corpus luteum, while the adrenal cortex is the secondary source of supply. Oestrogen is secreted as oestradiol. It is bound to albumin (30%) and sex hormone–binding globulin (SHBG, 69%), and only 1% is biologically active. It acts by binding to cytoplasmic receptors in the cells. It is inactivated by the liver and excreted as conjugates of oestrone, oestradiol and oestriol in urine and bile (85% in urine, 10% in faeces). The plasma oestradiol level rises approximately 6–7 days before ovulation from 50 mcg daily to the peak level of 300–600 mcg about 2 days before ovulation and approximately 24 hours before the LH peak (level up to 350 pg/mL). Thereafter, the oestradiol concentration falls to 150–200 mcg daily, but a small rise is seen again in the mid-luteal phase. The urinary excretory level follows the pattern seen in the plasma. The oestradiol peak seen before ovulation is not a good marker for indicating ovulation as LH, because follicular maturation does not always end in ovulation. A serum level of oestrogen with ultrasonic monitoring is used to monitor the optimal time to administer hCG for the therapeutic induction of ovulation. Although oestradiol, which is 10 times as potent as oestrone, is present during reproductive period, it is oestrone derived from peripheral aromatization of androstenedione that is predominant in menopausal women. The placenta is the main source of oestriol. Each cycle produces 10 mg of oestradiol.

Synthetic oestrogens are readily available in the market and are used in various gynaecological disorders. They are absorbed orally and through vagina and skin.

ACTIONS OF OESTROGENS (Fig. 4.4)

1. **Feminization and secondary sex characteristics**. The texture of female skin and hair and the shape of female form are considerably influenced by oestrogen.
2. **Specific action on the genital tract**

   Vulva and vagina
   - Development of vulva
   - Vascular stimulation of vulva and vagina
   - Epithelial stimulation of vulva and vagina
   - Cornification of the superficial layers of vagina which appear as acidophilic polyhedral cells with a small pyknotic nucleus. Oestrogen raises the karyopyknotic index in vaginal cytology (Chapter 1)
   - Deposition and metabolism of intracellular glycogen in vaginal epithelium

   Uterus
   - Causes myohyperplasia of myometrium and cervix
   - Increases uterine vascularity
   - Regenerates the endometrium after menstruation and is responsible for the proliferative (preovulatory) growth of endometrium. Oestrogen causes proliferation of epithelial lining, glandular cells and stroma and mitosis. Spiral vessels elongate and stretch the entire length of endometrium, and dilate
   - Stimulant effect on the glands of endocervix and their mucous secretion

   Fallopian tubes

   Oestrogen stimulates the tubal musculature, which is, in fact, morphologically specialized myometrium

   Ovary

   No action
3. **Breast**. Hypertrophy of the ductal and parenchymal tissue of breast, increased vascularity, areolar pigmentation, but no galactogenic effect. Large doses suppress lactation.
4. **Action on other endocrine glands**. Oestrogen suppresses FSH and thyrotropic hormones. It can be used to inhibit

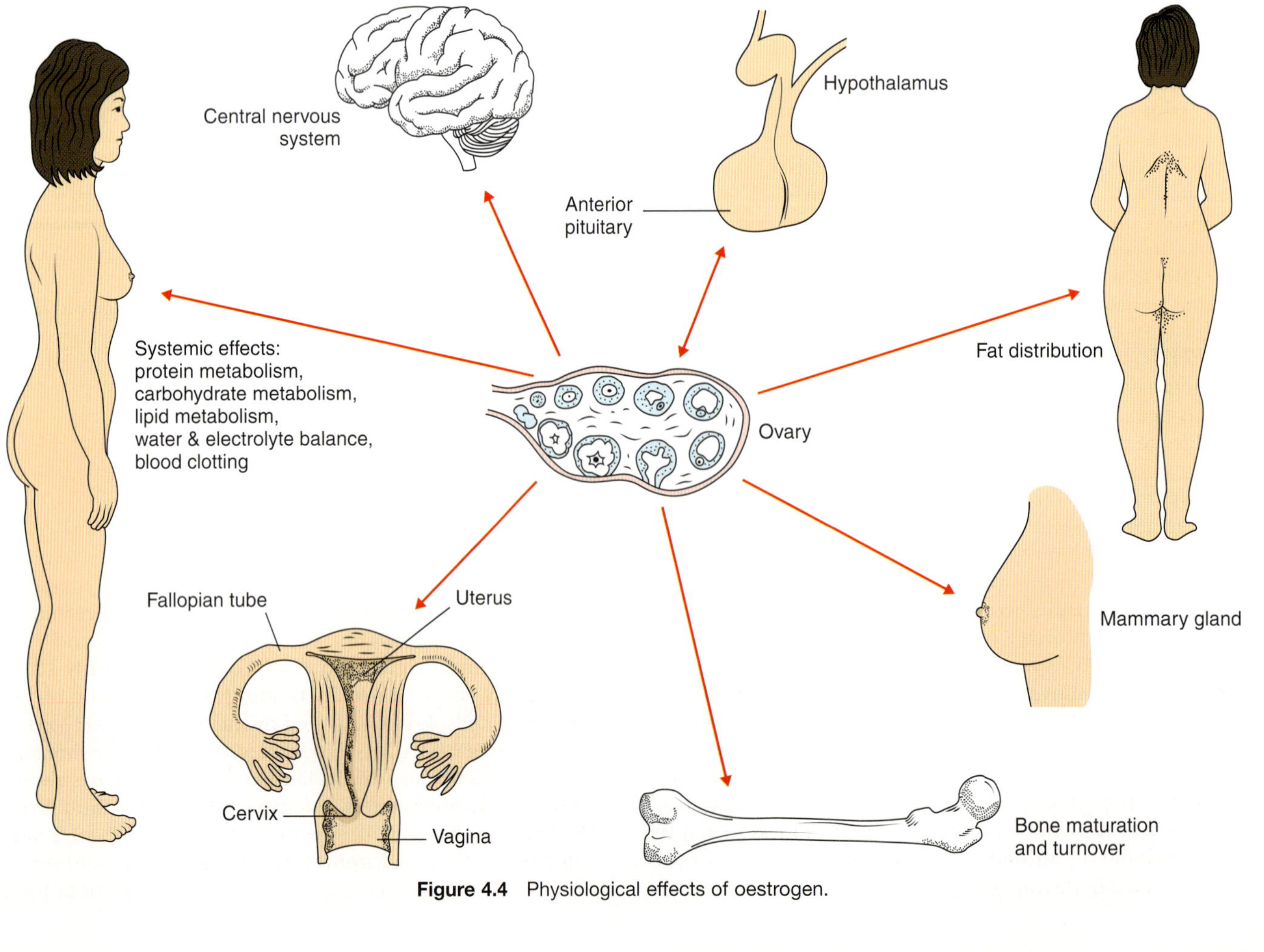

Figure 4.4 Physiological effects of oestrogen.

ovulation as also production of milk in puerperal patient. It is a stimulant for LH and thereby corpus luteum formation, and, to a lesser extent, for ACTH.

5. **Skeletal system**. It increases calcification of bone and the closure of epiphyses in adolescent and is antagonistic to somatotropin. In postmenopausal women, decalcification of bone (osteoporosis leading to kyphosis) is, in fact, due to oestrogen deficiency.
6. **Water and sodium metabolism**. Oestrogen tends to cause water and sodium retention. An example is premenstrual tension, which is caused by congestion and water retention. It also causes calcium and nitrogen retention.
7. **Blood cholesterol**. Blood cholesterol levels are to a small extent controlled by oestrogen, hence the importance of ovarian conservation when performing hysterectomy in a young woman. HDL increases under oestrogen influence and is cardioprotective.
   - Oestrogen improves skin by producing collagen
   - By raising fibrinogen level, it can cause thromboembolism, and is a major side effect of oestrogen
   - It increases SHBG by the liver

PROGESTERONE

The corpus luteum is the main source of progesterone, and a small amount is derived from adrenal gland (2–3 mg) seen in the proliferative phase. Although progesterone is an important intermediary product in the synthesis of adrenal corticosteroids, it has little, if any, biological action from this extraovarian source. The plasma level of progesterone rises after ovulation and reaches a peak level of 15 ng/mL at mid-luteal phase. With the degeneration of the corpus luteum, its level falls and this brings about menstruation. In an anovulatory cycle, progesterone is absent or is in negligible amount (from extraovarian sources). Menstruation is then brought about by a fall in the level of oestrogen. If pregnancy occurs, the corpus luteum persists, even enlarges and continues to secrete progesterone. This high level of hormone prevents menstruation and leads to amenorrhoea of pregnancy. It is excreted in urine as sodium pregnanediol 3-glucuronide and recovered as such for assay in the secretory phase of menstrual cycle. Progesterone is bound to albumin (80%) and corticosteroid-binding globulin (20%). Daily production in the luteal phase is 20–40 mg and daily urine excretion is 3–6 mg. Mid-luteal phase level of less than 15 ng/mL suggests corpus luteal phase defect (LPD) and ovulatory dysfunction.

Radioimmunoassay is currently used to estimate the plasma progesterone levels in mid-luteal phase in cases of infertility. However, with development of enzyme immunoassay, a home 'dipstick' test can estimate urinary pregnanediol to determine occurrence of ovulation. Salivary progesterone level is estimated by direct use of solid-phase enzyme immunoassay (Dooley). Several synthetic progesterones (progestogens) are now available for commercial use (Fig. 4.1A and B).

ACTIONS OF PROGESTERONES

Endometrium. Progesterones cause secretory hypertrophy and decidual formation if the endometrium has been previously primed with oestrogen. Glycogen and mucus collect in tortuous glands.

Pregnancy. Progesterone initially from the corpus luteum and later from the placenta is essential for the continuation of pregnancy.

Uterus. Progestogens cause myohyperplasia of the uterus. They increase the strength but diminish the frequency of uterine contractions.

Fallopian tube. Progestogens cause hyperplasia of the muscular lining of the fallopian tube and make peristaltic contractions more powerful as well as increase the secretion by tubal mucous membrane.

Cervix. Progestogen causes hypertrophy of the cervix and makes cervical mucus more tenacious. It renders internal os competent and holds the pregnancy to term.

Vagina. During early pregnancy, the vagina becomes violet in colour due to venous congestion. The epithelial cells fail to mature and cornify. They are classically basophilic with fairly large nuclei and folded edges. Karyopyknotic index falls to below 10%.

Breasts. Progestogens, with oestrogen, cause breast hypertrophy. They increase acinar epithelial growth.

Pituitary. The exact action of progestogens on the pituitary is not known. Progestogens may inhibit the production of FSH and suppress ovulation. A certain percentage of progestogens is metabolized to oestrogen, and it may well be that the oestrogen so produced is responsible for inhibiting pituitary activity.

Fluid retention. Progestogens cause water and sodium retention and are a contributory factor in premenstrual tension and weight gain.

Smooth muscles. Progestogens relax smooth muscles. The uterine muscles therefore relax in pregnancy. Ureter dilates under its effect.

Thermogenic. Progestogens raise the body temperature by 0.5°C. Basal body temperature (BBT) chart is based on its thermogenic effect during the menstrual cycle.

Anabolic effect. Progestogens exert anabolic effect and this partly accounts for some of the weight gain which may follow their administration.

Libido. Diminution of libido infrequently occurs.

Virilization. Although part of the administered progestogen is metabolized to oestrogen, it is also partly metabolized to testosterone. If administered to a patient during pregnancy, some progestogens have virilizing effect on female fetus.

- Lipid metabolism decreases HDL but increases low-density lipoprotein. Thus, it is harmful for heart.
- It improves immune response.

SIDE EFFECTS

If given in large doses, progestogen can cause gastrointestinal symptoms, nausea and vomiting. Headache and mild elevation of temperature are also seen. In fact, all symptoms of pseudopregnancy state may be observed – water retention, breast enlargement and tenderness, and moderate uterine enlargement. Virilism has been reported with some synthetic progestogens, especially 19-nortestosterones. Some exhibit adverse effects on lipid metabolism and increase the risk of breast cancer. Thrombosis of deep veins, pulmonary embolism and arterial thrombosis are rare but are reported with third generation of synthetic progestogens (gestodene and desogestrel) (Table 4.1).

Table 4.1 Effects of Oestrogen and Progesterone on the Female Genital Tract

Organ	Oestrogen	Progesterone
Breasts	Ductal/stromal growth	Alveolar growth
Vagina	Superficial cells with glycogen	Intermediate cells
Cervix	Abundant mucus thin, viscous, penetrable to sperms	Thick tenacious mucus, impenetrable to sperms
Uterus	Myohyperplasia	Myohyperplasia
Endometrium	Proliferative endometrium	Secretory endometrium
Fallopian tube	Secretion	Increased peristaltic movements
Ovary	No action	No action

RELAXIN

This hormone relaxes the connective tissue and is probably secreted by the ovary. Relaxin is a water-soluble protein and nonsteroid. It may have a role in pregnancy and may be responsible for relaxation of pelvic joints and pelvic floor muscles.

INHIBIN

Inhibin is a nonsteroidal water-soluble protein (peptide) secreted by the Graafian follicle. McCullagh identified this protein and named it inhibin because it is known to suppress pituitary FSH. Inhibin consists of two peptides, namely inhibin A (α-fraction) and inhibin B (β-fraction). In normal ovarian folliculogenesis, FSH and LH initiate secretion of oestrogen by the Graafian follicle. Oestrogen is responsible for secretion of inhibin in the Graafian follicle, which in turn suppresses FSH but stimulates LH secretion. Administration of inhibin in the early follicular phase can delay folliculogenesis and inhibit ovulation and luteinization. Inhibin may have an important role in the control of fertility in both males and females. It causes agglutination of sperms, prevents cervical mucus penetration and interferes with egg interaction. In polycystic ovarian disease (PCOD), there is an increased secretion of inhibin. This causes a low FSH but a high LH secretion by the anterior pituitary gland and is responsible for anovulation. Although the extraction of purified inhibin is not yet successful, there is a possible hope of its availability in the near future. Normal level of 50 pg/mL (>45 pg) drops to less than 15 pg/mL after menopause due to oestrogen deficiency. It is studied by ELISA test.

ACTIVIN

Activin is secreted by the anterior pituitary gland and granulosa cells, stimulates FSH release and enhances action in the ovary.

Follistatin suppresses FSH activity by acting against activin.

ANTI-MÜLLERIAN HORMONE

Anti-Müllerian hormone (AMH) is a peptide secreted by Sertoli cells in the testis and granulosa cells in the ovary. In males, AMH starts to be secreted by the 7th week of intrauterine life and it continues until puberty. It inhibits the development of *Müllerian* system. Absence of AMH results in hermaphrodite.

In females, AMH is secreted by granulosa cells after puberty. It helps in follicular development and oocyte maturation.

Normal value is 2–6.8 ng/mL; level < 1 ng/mL shows poor ovarian reserve, level > 10 ng/mL is seen in PCOD and hyperstimulation syndrome. Its level is related to precocious and delayed puberty, infertility and premature menopause. Its level is related and reflects the number of growing follicles.

Estimation of serum AMH is used in the study of ovarian reserve in an infertile woman and a woman with secondary amenorrhoea. In in vitro fertilization programme, it carries a prognostic value and helps to decide on donor egg.

SEX HORMONE–BINDING PROTEINS

Most of oestrogens and androgens are bound to sex hormone–binding proteins (SHBP) secreted by the liver, and remain inactive. Only free hormones are biologically active and influence their target organs (1%–2%). Oestrogen and thyroid hormones increase the secretion of these proteins, but androgens lower their levels.

TESTOSTERONE

Fifty per cent testosterone comes from ovaries and the rest from adrenal gland. The ovarian stromal tissue secretes androgenic products, namely testosterone, dehydroepiandrosterone (DHEA) and androstenedione. Androstenedione gets converted in the peripheral fat to oestrone. The normal increase in stromal tissue at ovulation causes a slight increase in the secretion of these hormones. After menopause, the increased ovarian stroma is responsible for the rise in these hormones and development of hirsutism in some postmenopausal women. Total daily production of testosterone is 0.2–0.3 mg and plasma level is 0.2–0.8 ng/mL. The daily production of androstenedione is 3 mg and plasma level is 1.3–1.5 ng/mL. Normal 17-ketosteroid level is 5–15 mg in 24 hours. More than 25 mg indicates adrenal hyperplasia. Plasma level of DHEA sulphate over 5 mcg/mL is seen in adrenal hyperplasia.

Eighty to eighty-five per cent androgens are bound to SHBP and 10%–15% to albumin. One to two per cent free testosterone remains biologically active and acts at peripheral targets, i.e. hair growth and acne by conversion to dihydrotestosterone by hydroxylase enzyme. Clinically, administration of androgen causes follicular atresia and anovulation.

PHYSIOLOGY OF MENSTRUATION

The proliferative phase of the endometrium represents the oestrogenic part of menstrual cycle. It is initiated and controlled by oestrogen. The secretory phase of the endometrium is controlled by progesterone, although the effect of progesterone is obtained only after the endometrium has been sensitized with oestrogen. This is because oestrogen produces progesterone receptors on which progesterone acts.

Although the activity of endometrium is directly controlled by the ovarian function and by the two hormones secreted by the ovary, the ovary itself is activated by the pituitary gland, the secretion of which is under the nerve control of the hypothalamus.

At birth, the ovaries are populated with lifetime complement of eggs located in the primordial follicles, but most of these follicles undergo atresia throughout childhood and only about 400 of these primordial follicles are present during reproductive age. At puberty, the hypothalamus starts a pulsatile secretion of GnRH, resulting in the activation of H–P–O uterine axis and in the establishment of menstrual cycles.

Pulsatile GnRH initiates secretion of FSH and LH. FSH released by the anterior pituitary gland stimulates the growth of a few primordial follicles into the Graafian follicles. Multiple follicles start growing in both the ovaries, but only one dominant Graafian follicle is selected which ripens to full maturity and ovulates whereas other follicles become atretic. The Graafian follicles under the influence of FSH together with only a minimal amount of the LH secrete 17-β-oestradiol (Fig. 4.5A and B). 17-β-Oestradiol has several functions: in the first place, it produces proliferative changes in the endometrium, secretes inhibin and inhibits further secretion of FSH by the anterior pituitary and stimulates LH receptors in the theca cells and stimulates the anterior pituitary to secrete LH. Inhibin produced by the Graafian follicle under oestrogenic effect is also responsible for a fall in the FSH level and stimulation of LH secretion. The maximum peak of oestrogen secretion is seen about 48 hours before ovulation, whereas the LH peak occurs about 24–36 hours before ovulation. LH has the following functions: In the first place, it stimulates a Graafian follicle to secrete 17-β-oestradiol, and secondly, it causes the follicle to rupture at ovulation and to form a corpus luteum (Fig. 4.6). It also stimulates the secretion of testosterone and androstenedione by theca cells.

The corpus luteum secretes progesterone, the level of which starts rising. The hormone progesterone has two functions. In the first place, it stimulates the endometrium to undergo secretory hypertrophy, and secondly, it inhibits further production of LH by the anterior pituitary. *The gonadotropins seem to have no direct effect upon the endometrium of the uterus* (Fig. 4.6).

In the absence of pregnancy, both oestrogen and progesterone levels decline gradually and fall in the level of these hormones brings about menstruation. A fall in the level of these hormones also starts off a fresh positive feedback mechanism and triggers the hypothalamus to release gonadotropin. This is how a menstrual cycle is regulated. The luteal phase, i.e. time between ovulation and menstruation, is fairly constant at 14 days in a menstrual cycle. The growth of ovarian follicles and endometrial thickness can be studied by serial ultrasound. Oestrogen, LH and mid-luteal progesterone levels can be conveniently and speedily measured by radio-immunoassays (Fig. 4.7; Table 4.2).

As mentioned earlier, thyroid hormones and adrenal hormones react with sex hormones and alter the H–P–O

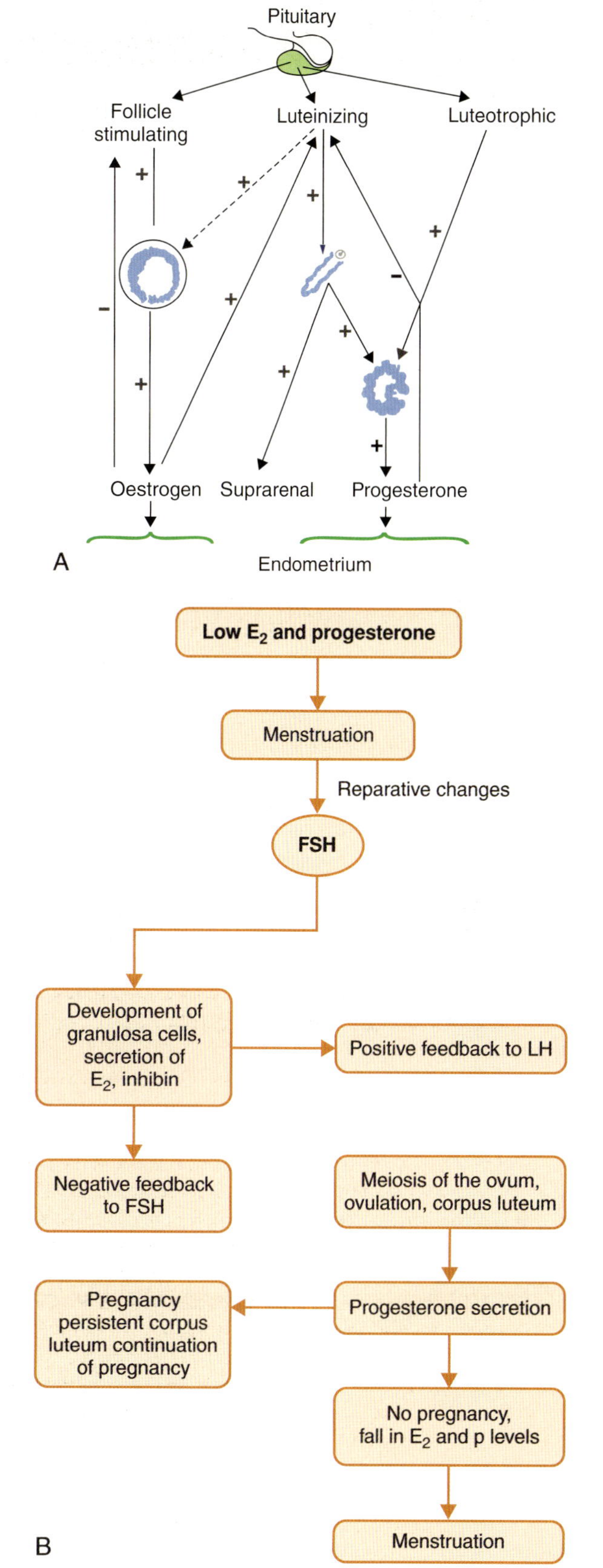

Figure 4.5 **(A)** A scheme illustrating interrelation of pituitary gonadotropic hormones. '+' indicates stimulation and '–' indicates inhibition. **(B)** Flowchart of menstruation.

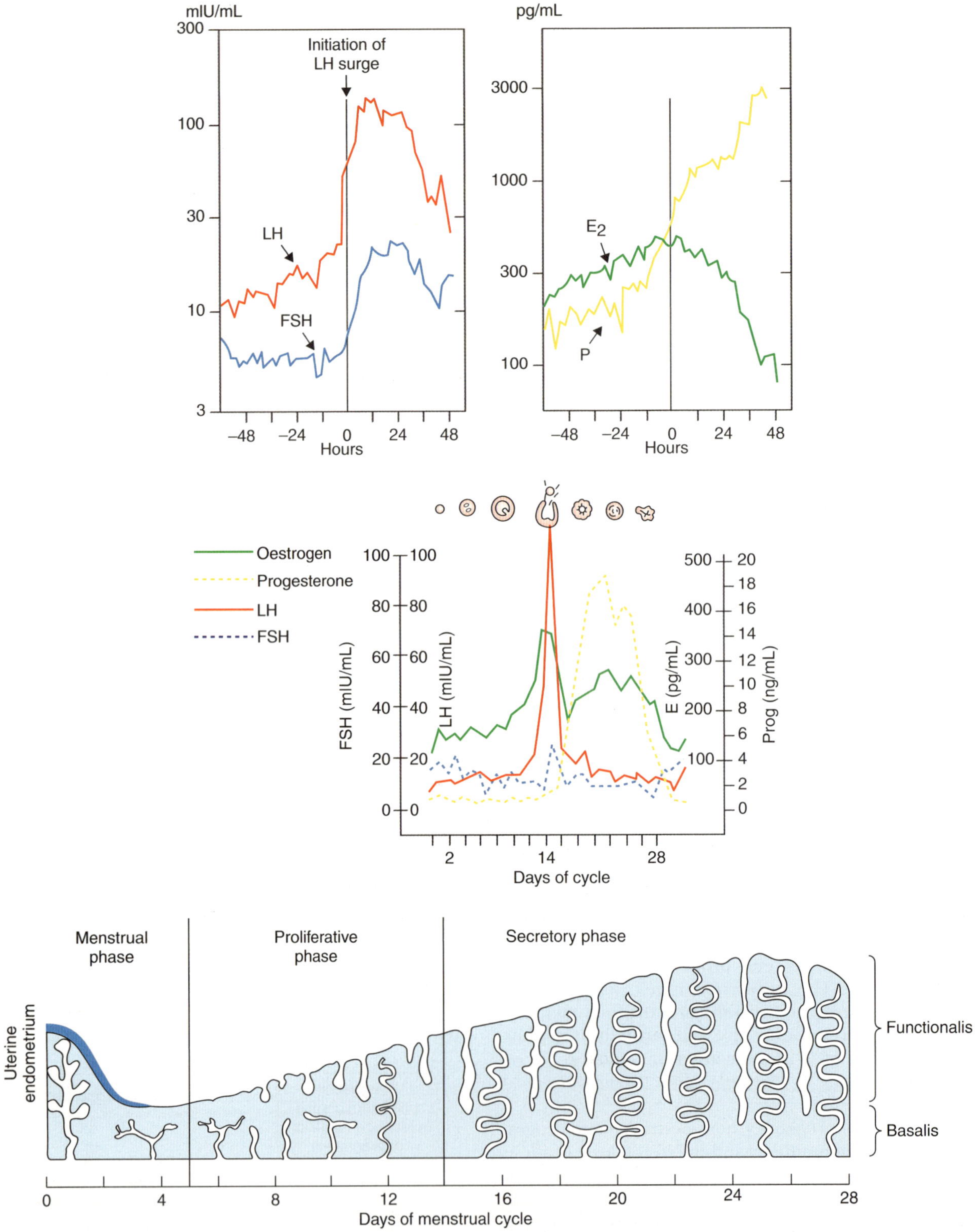

Figure 4.6 Plasma hormone levels in normal menstrual cycles.

pathway by inhibiting GnRH secretion. Oral combined pills, by virtue of inhibiting GnRH and preventing ovulation, cause atropic endometrium. Continuous oestrogen stimulation leads to endometrial hyperplasia (Fig. 4.8).

FEEDBACK MECHANISM IN THE H–P–O AXIS

As mentioned in the beginning, the various hormones liberated by the hypothalamus, the anterior pituitary gland and the ovaries are dependent upon each other, each

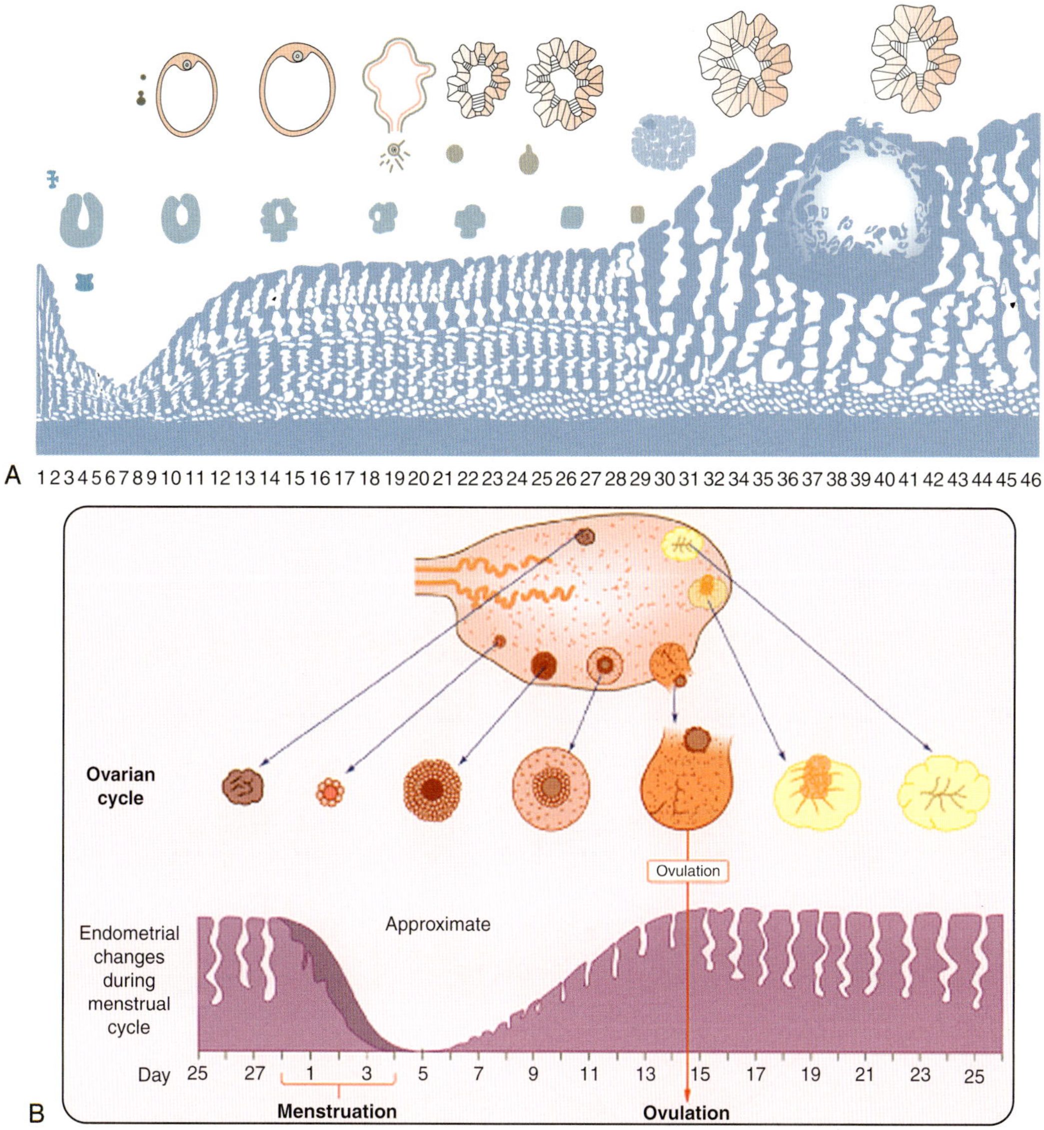

Figure 4.7 **(A)** Schroder's illustration of the relation between ovarian function and the changes in the endometrium during early pregnancy. **(B)** Ovarian cycle with corresponding endometrial thickness.

Table 4.2 Normal Hormonal Levels in Different Phases of Menstrual Cycle

Hormone	Follicular Phase	Ovulation	Luteal Phase	Menstrual Phase
FSH	4–14 mIU/mL	12–30	2–9	3–15 mIU/mL
LH	6–14 mIU/mL	14–40	2–13	3–12 mIU/mL
E_2	50–250 pg/mL	300–500 pg/mL	100–200	–
P	1 ng/mL	–	3-15 ng/mL	–
17 OH steroids	Normal	5–10 mg/daily	–	>25 mg in adrenal hyperplasia
Testosterone	Normal	0.2–0.8 ng/mL	–	>2 ng/mL in androgen-producing ovarian tumours
Androstenedione	Normal	1.3–1.5 ng/mL	–	–
DHEA	Normal	<5 mcg/mL	–	>5 mcg in adrenal hyperplasia
Cortisol	–	<5 mcg/dL	–	–
DHEA-S	800 ng/mL	–	–	>800ng/ml (Adrenal hyperplasia, adrenal tumours)

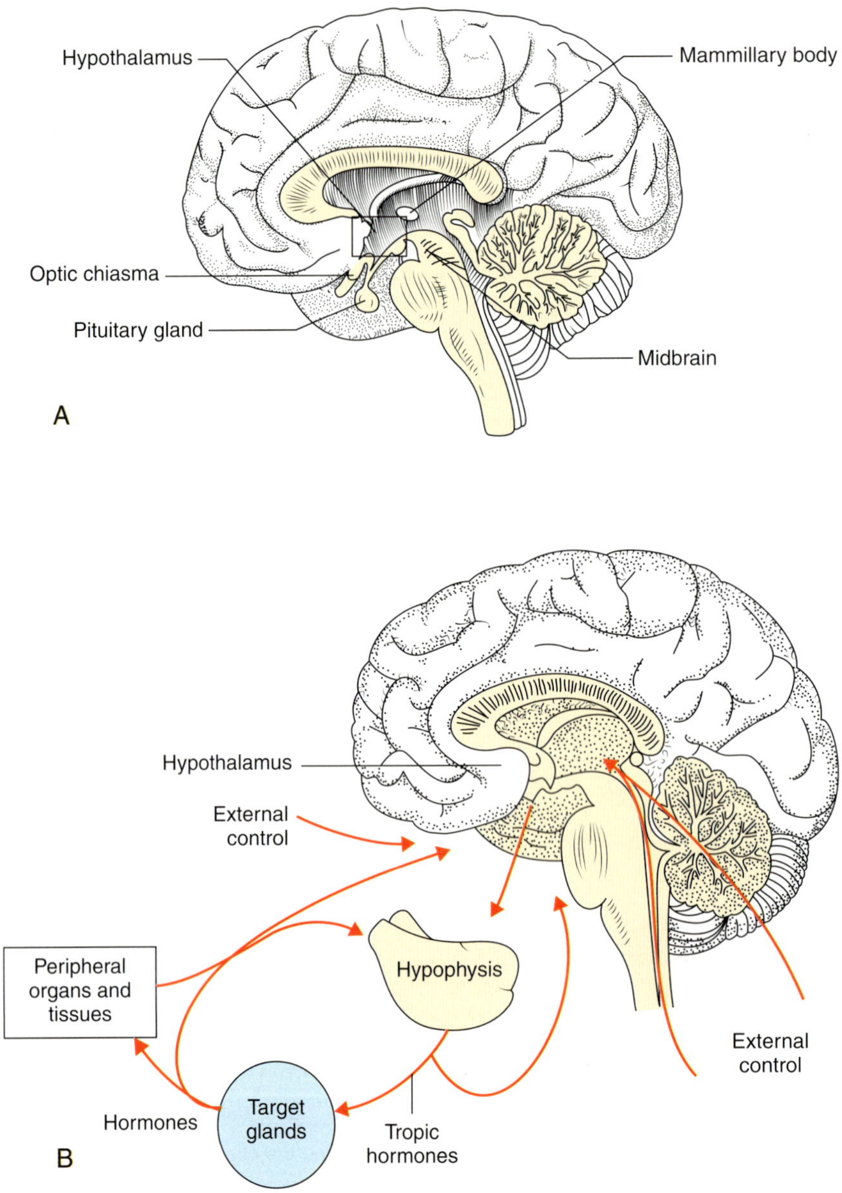

Figure 4.8 Neuroendocrine control of menstruation.

reaching positive as well as negative feedback at different levels.

The following are the feedback:

1. Long feedback mechanism from the ovaries to the pituitary and the hypothalamus.
2. Short feedback mechanism between the anterior pituitary gland and the hypothalamus.
3. Ultrashort feedback mechanism.

Autoregulation of release of GnRH by the hypothalamus. Increased secretion of GnRH suppresses its own synthesis and vice versa.

LEPTIN

Since its discovery in 1994, leptin (adipocyte protein hormone) is linked to nutrition and may bear an important role in the control of H–P–O axis. A diet restriction has a negative impact on the hypothalamus and decreases LH secretion causing amenorrhoea as seen in anorexia nervosa. Leptin is found in follicular fluid in the ovaries and presumably stimulates pulsatile secretion of GnRH around puberty. Hence, an obese adolescent reaches menarche earlier than a lean girl. Lean girls have a delayed puberty. More research is required in this field.

MENSTRUATION

Menstruation is the end point in the cascade of events starting at the hypothalamus and ending in the uterus. Menstrual cycle is usually of 28 days, measured by the time between the first day of one period and the first day of the next. The duration of bleeding is about 3–5 days and the estimated blood loss is between 50 and 200 mL. The regular cycle of 28 days is seen only in a small proportion of women. A deviation of 2 or 3 days from the 28-day rhythm is quite

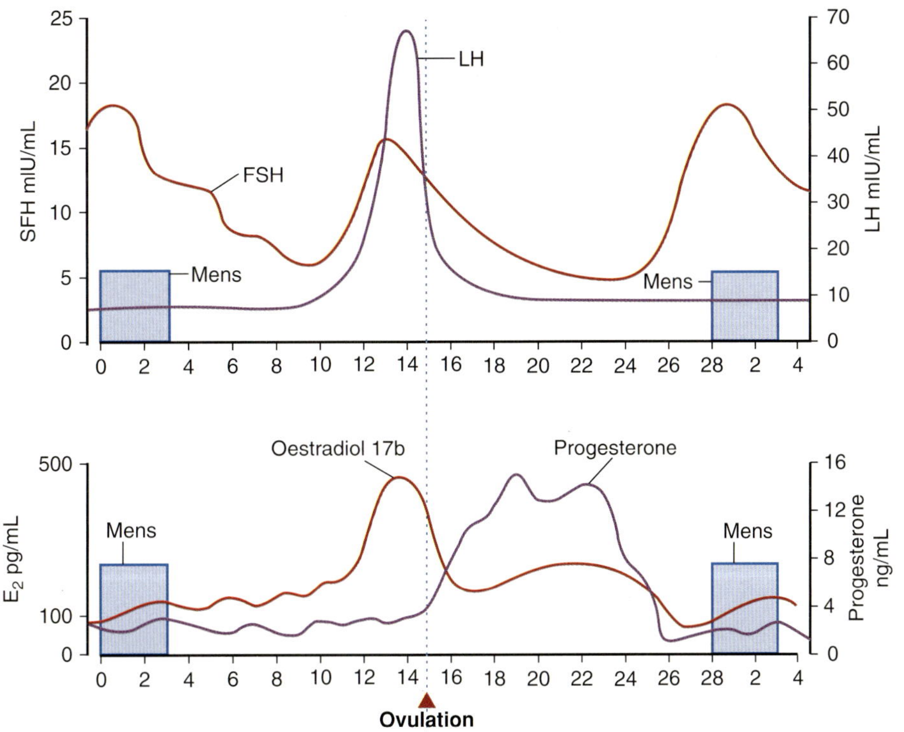

Figure 4.9 Hormonal level during menstrual cycle.

common. The menstrual rhythm depends on the H–P–O function whereas the amount of blood loss depends upon uterine condition.

A study of the coiled arteries of the endometrium shows that there is a slight regression of endometrium shortly after ovulation and that a rapid decrease in thickness can be demonstrated even before menstruation starts. In the regression that starts a few days prior to the onset of menstruation, there is a decreased blood flow which may cause shrinkage of the endometrium from dehydration. During menstruation itself, reduction in the thickness of the endometrium is determined by both desquamation and resorption. The coiled arteries become buckled with subsequent stasis of blood flow. Necrosis of the superficial layers of the endometrium is produced either by local stasis or by the clearly demonstrated vasoconstriction of coiled arteries. Menstrual bleeding occurs when the open arteries damaged by necrosis relax and discharge blood in the uterine cavity. Some degree of venous haemorrhage also occurs. Fragments become detached from the superficial layer of the endometrium by the end of the first day (Figs 4.7–4.10).

An important feature of menstrual changes is the contraction and constriction of coiled arteries. Ischaemia causes necrosis and disintegration of the superficial zone. The regeneration of vascular system is probably brought about by the development of anastomosing arteries. The re-epithelialization is brought about by the cells growing from the mouth of the base of the glands that remain in the unshed basal layer of the endometrium.

In anovulatory menstruation, there is the same shedding of a thin necrotic superficial layer of the endometrium, and it is to be presumed that exactly the same factor is at work to cause vascular changes with resultant ischaemia.

Vascular changes in the endometrium and the amount and duration of menstrual bleeding are controlled by the interaction of different prostaglandins secreted by the endometrium.

Prostaglandin E_2 (PGE_2) causes myometrial contractions but vasodilatation of vessels. Prostaglandin $F_2\alpha$ ($PGF_2\alpha$) causes vasoconstriction as well as myocontraction. Prostacyclin (PGI_2) is responsible for muscle relaxation and vasodilatation. According to this, PGE_2 and $PGF_2\alpha$ are responsible for dysmenorrhoea, and PGI_2 can cause menorrhagia.

Improved ultrasonic imaging and colour Doppler study of the endometrium have improved our knowledge related to menstrual disorders.

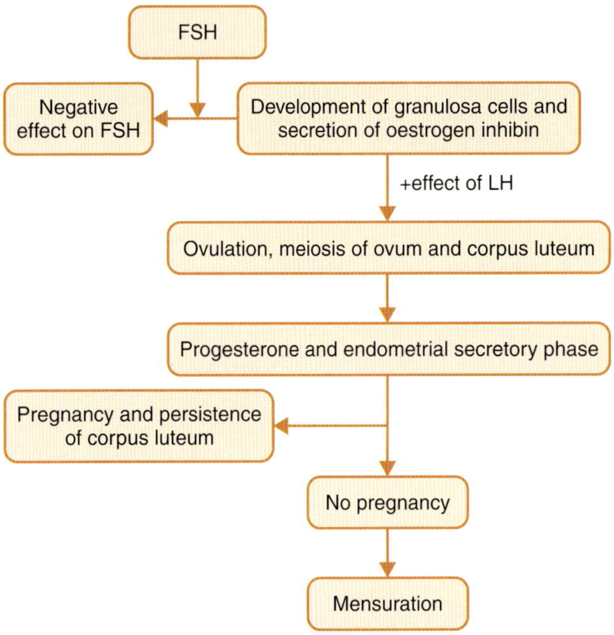

Figure 4.10 Mensuration and pregnancy.

MENSTRUAL FLUID IN 'STEM CELL' THERAPY

The stem cells are the basic building blocks of every other cell in the body. Whereas organ cells have specific functions, the stem cells are 'blank' but have the potential to take up any function. Under suitable environment and surrounded by specific organ cells, the stem cells divide into either stem cells or another type of cells with their attached functions. Thus, the stem cells have a vital role in 'regenerative medicine' in degenerative and life-threatening diseases such as Alzheimer disease, atherosclerosis, diabetes, heart disease, bowel disease, Parkinson disease and rheumatoid arthritis.

The sources of stem cells were until recently seen in bone marrow, embryo, amniotic fluid and umbilical cord blood but now in menstrual fluid as well. The menstrual fluid contains mesenchymal cells such as mononuclear cells and fibroblasts. These cells, however, deteriorate with advancing age. Therefore, cells from young women are suitable for donation, and for self-use at a later age if needed. The kit contains antibiotics to prevent infection, and the menstrual fluid is cryopreserved and harvested. The procedure is simple, noninvasive and painless as well as possible.

KEY POINTS

- Neuroendocrinology with its vast hormonal network is key to normal menstrual cycles and reproductive function in a woman.
- Hypothalamus, with its pulsatile secretion of GnRH (decapeptide), is the main neuroendocrine gland and regulatory factor in the chain of H–P–O axis. The higher cortical centres can modify or influence hypothalamic secretion.
- Pulsatile secretion of GnRH results in secretion of FSH and LH from anterior pituitary gland.
- FSH and LH secreted from anterior pituitary in turn results in follicular maturation and ovulation, which in turn are responsible for secretion of oestrogen and progesterone from ovary.
- Proliferative phase of endometrium represents oestrogenic action of ovary.
- Progesterone causes secretory endometrium only if the latter is primed with oestrogen.
- Therapeutic management in infertility, family planning and gynaecological disorders is based on a sound knowledge of neuroendocrinology and the interaction of various hormones.
- Synthetic analogues of GnRH, FSH and LH are used in infertility and amenorrhoea.
- Oestrogen and progesterone have specific roles in menstrual cycle and in the development of genital organs.
- Other hormones participate in the maintenance of normal menstruation.
- LH surge is the key marker of imminent ovulation.
- LH causes maturation of Graafian follicle, meiosis of ovum before ovulation, ovulation and development of corpus luteum.
- Leptin appears to have a role in the development and onset of puberty.
- Menstrual fluid is recently discovered to contain stem cells and may prove useful in stem cell therapy. Only young women are suitable for donation.

SELF-ASSESSMENT

1. Describe the neuroendocrine control of menstrual cycle.
2. Describe the formation and processes that lead to the formation of Graafian follicles.
3. Describe the mechanism of ovulation.
4. Describe the microscopic appearance of endometrium during the various phases of menstrual cycle.

SUGGESTED READING

Bloom FE. Neuroendocrine mechanisms: cells and systems. In Yen SCC, Jaffe RB (eds). Reproductive Endocrinology. Philadelphia, WB Saunders Co, 1991; 2–24.

Plant TM, Krey LC, Moossy J et al. The arcuate nucleus and the control of the gonadotropin and prolactin secretion in the female rhesus monkey. Endocrinology 1978; 102: 52–62.

Rabin D, McNeil LW. Pituitary and gonadal desensitization after continuous luteinizing hormone releasing hormone infusion in normal females. J Clin Endocrinol Metab 1980; 51: 873–6.

Schwanzel-Fukuda M, Pfaff DW. Origin of Luteinizing hormone releasing hormone neurons. Nature 1989; 338: 161–4.

Soules MR, Steiner RA, Cohen M et al. Nocturnal slowing of pulsatile luteinizing hormone secretion in women during the follicular phase of the menstrual cycle. J Clin Endocrinol Metab 1985; 61: 43–9.

Development of Female Reproductive Organs and Related Disorders

5

CHAPTER OUTLINE

Anomalies of Müllerian ducts are seen in 1%–2% of females. Most anomalies do not have any effect on menstrual or reproductive function and remain undiagnosed. However, some of the anomalies can cause recurrent abortions, preterm delivery, malpresentations or other obstetric complications. Menstrual irregularities are uncommon with these anomalies but at times can cause haematocolpos, cyclical pain in abdomen, etc. Knowledge of anatomical development of genital organs is helpful in understanding these conditions.

DEVELOPMENT OF THE FEMALE GENITAL ORGANS

Urogenital differentiation is a complex process involving genetic, hormonal and environmental influences. The genital and urinary systems develop in close relationship, so developmental errors in both these systems often coexist. If a transverse section is cut through the upper part of the coelomic cavity of an embryo of 8 weeks, the primitive mesentery is seen to project into the coelomic cavity posteriorly near the midline. On each side of the primitive mesentery, another projection, the intermediate cell mass, can be distinguished. On the inner side of the *intermediate cell mass,* by the end of the 8th week, a ridge has appeared – the genital ridge. The *Wolffian body* with primitive tubules and primitive glomeruli occupies the rest of the intermediate mass (Figs 5.1 and 5.2).

DEVELOPMENT OF URINARY SYSTEM

The *primitive urinary system* consists of the pronephros, the mesonephros or Wolffian body and the metanephros, which gives rise to the permanent kidney. Each of these systems is derived from the urogenital plates of the primitive somites. In the human female, the pronephros disappears, and the Wolffian body is represented by the straight tubules of the epoophoron, or organ of Rosenmüller, found in the mesosalpinx of an adult whereas the tubules of the paroophoron represent the relics of the renal tubules of the Wolffian system, and the Gartner's duct represents the Wolffian duct (Fig. 5.3). The metanephros gives rise to the tubules of the permanent kidney whereas the ureter and renal pelvis are formed from a diverticulum from the lower end of the Wolffian duct. In an embryo, two ridges appear between fifth and eighth week, mesonephric (Wolffian) and paramesonephric ducts. The former disappears in females, and the latter, paramesonephric duct (Müllerian), develops into female genital organs. The Müllerian duct is formed as a result of invagination of the mesothelium of the coelomic cavity on the ventral part of the intermediate cell mass. The invagination extends from the pronephros region above to the sacral region below, and both ducts terminate in the primitive cloaca. The position of the Müllerian duct is of importance, for it lies ventral to the Wolffian duct on the outer surface of the intermediate cell mass. In human embryo, the caudal parts of the two Müllerian ducts fuse to form the uterus, whereas the upper parts remain as the fallopian tubes (Fig. 5.3).

DEVELOPMENT OF THE UTERUS, CERVIX AND VAGINA

The uterus can be identified as early as by the end of the 3rd month. Uterus, fallopian tubes and most of the vagina are derived from the Müllerian duct in the absence of Y chromosome. The upper end of the Müllerian duct becomes the abdominal ostium of the fallopian tube, and it is not uncommon for small accessory ostia to be found (Fig. 5.4). In the 7th week of intrauterine life (IUL) of the embryo, an invagination of coelomic mesothelium occurs

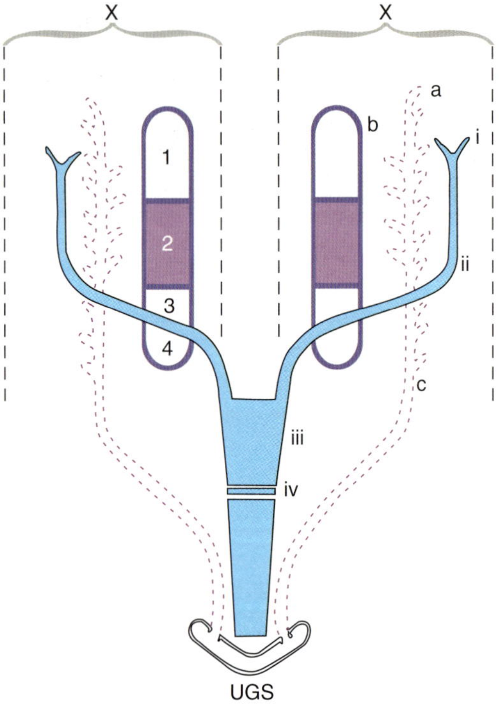

Figure 5.1 Diagram of urogenital system: X – intermediate cell mass, shaded area is the genital ridge. (1) Infundibulopelvic ligament, (2) ovary, (3) ovarian ligament and (4) round ligament. Dotted outline is Wolffian duct (Gartner's duct). (a) Pronephros, (b) epoophoron and (c) mesonephros. Solid block is Müllerian ducts. (i) Fimbria, (ii) fallopian tube, (iii) uterus, (iv) upper three-fourths of the vagina. UGS – urogenital sinus.

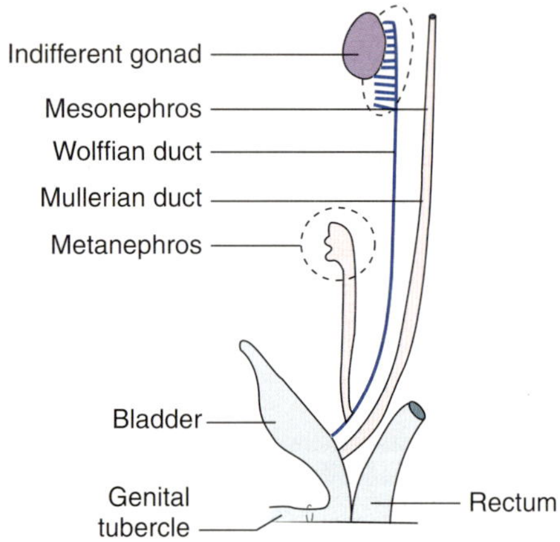

Figure 5.3 Development of genital tract – undifferentiated stage.

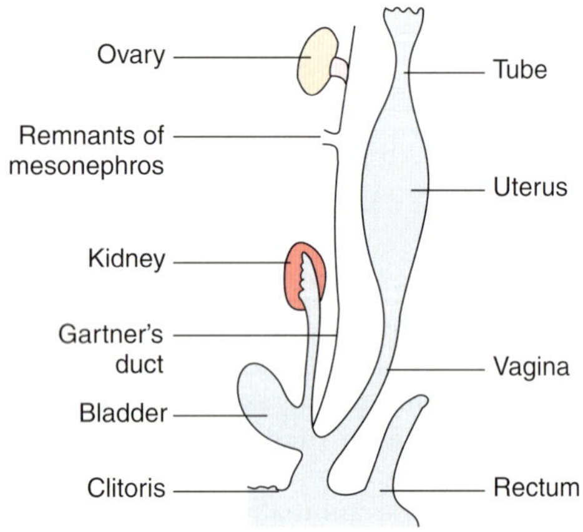

Figure 5.4 Female genital tract development.

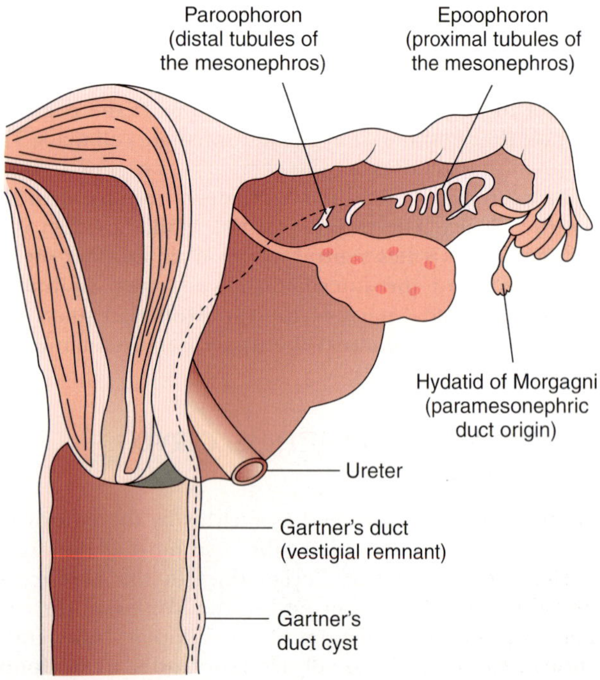

Figure 5.2 Remnants of the mesonephric (Wolffian) ducts that may persist in the anterolateral vagina or adjacent to the uterus within the broad ligament or mesosalpinx.

close to the primitive gonad in the upper lateral portion of the intermediate cell mass; this is called the Müllerian duct (paramesonephric duct). As the two Müllerian ducts, one on either side, develop and grow caudally, they approach each other in the midline after crossing the Wolffian duct (mesonephric duct) and fuse (Figs 5.1 and 5.2). The cranial-free part of the Müllerian ducts develops into fallopian tubes. The middle fused portion forms the uterus and cervix, and the caudal fused portion forms the upper one-third of vagina. Initially, the intervening septa are present but later disappear as a single continuous passage. *Thus, the normal development of the Müllerian system comprises organogenesis, fusion and later septal resorption.*

The muscle wall of the uterus is differentiated from mesoblastic tissues, and during the 5th month, a circular layer of muscle can be distinguished. The longitudinal muscles of uterus can be recognized during the 7th month, and this muscle layer is continuous morphologically with the plain muscle tissue of the ovarian ligament, the round ligament and the muscle fibres found in the uterosacral ligaments (Fig. 5.5).

In the early stage of the development, the cervix of the uterus is longer and thicker than the body, and this proportion persists until puberty. The proportion may persist in adult life, when the uterus is described as infantile in type.

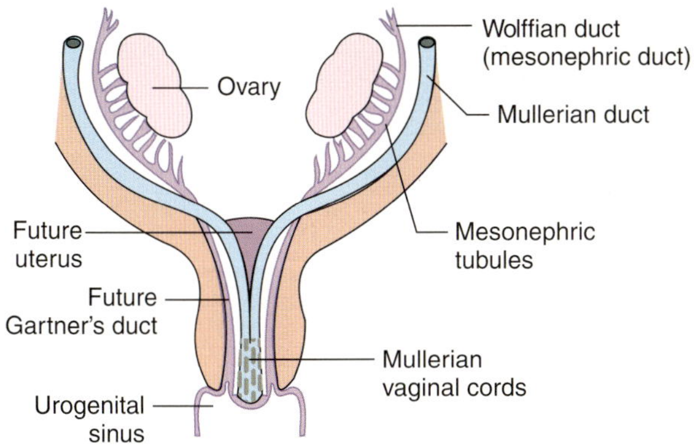

Figure 5.5 Müllerian and Wolffian systems.

The cervical glands can be recognized in the 6th month, whereas the glands of the body of the uterus develop only during the last month of IUL, although primitive glands are present at the 4th month.

The *primitive cloaca* is divided by the formation of the urorectal septum into a ventral part, the urogenital sinus (UGS) and a dorsal part, the rectum. The urorectal septum ultimately develops into the perineal body.

DEVELOPMENT OF VAGINA

The lower ends of the Müllerian ducts terminate in the urogenital sinus, into the posterior part of which they project as a solid Müllerian tubercle. A solid vaginal cord results from proliferation of cells at the caudal tip of fused Müllerian ducts, the cord elongates to meet the bilateral endodermal evaginations (sinovaginal bulbs) from the posterior aspect of urogenital sinus below, and both fuse to form vaginal plate. Vagina is formed by the subsequent canalization of the vaginal cord followed by epithelialization with cells derived from urogenital sinus. Recent proposals hold that only the upper one-third of vagina is formed from Müllerian ducts and the lower vagina develops from the vaginal plate of urogenital sinus. The hymen is the embryologic septum between the sinovaginal bulbs above and the urogenital sinus below.

DEVELOPMENT OF THE EXTERNAL GENITAL ORGANS (Figs 5.6 and 5.7)

The cloaca becomes divided into two parts by the development of the urorectal septum, which originally consists of two folds which project on each side and then fuse caudally to divide the cloaca into a dorsal part, the rectum, and a

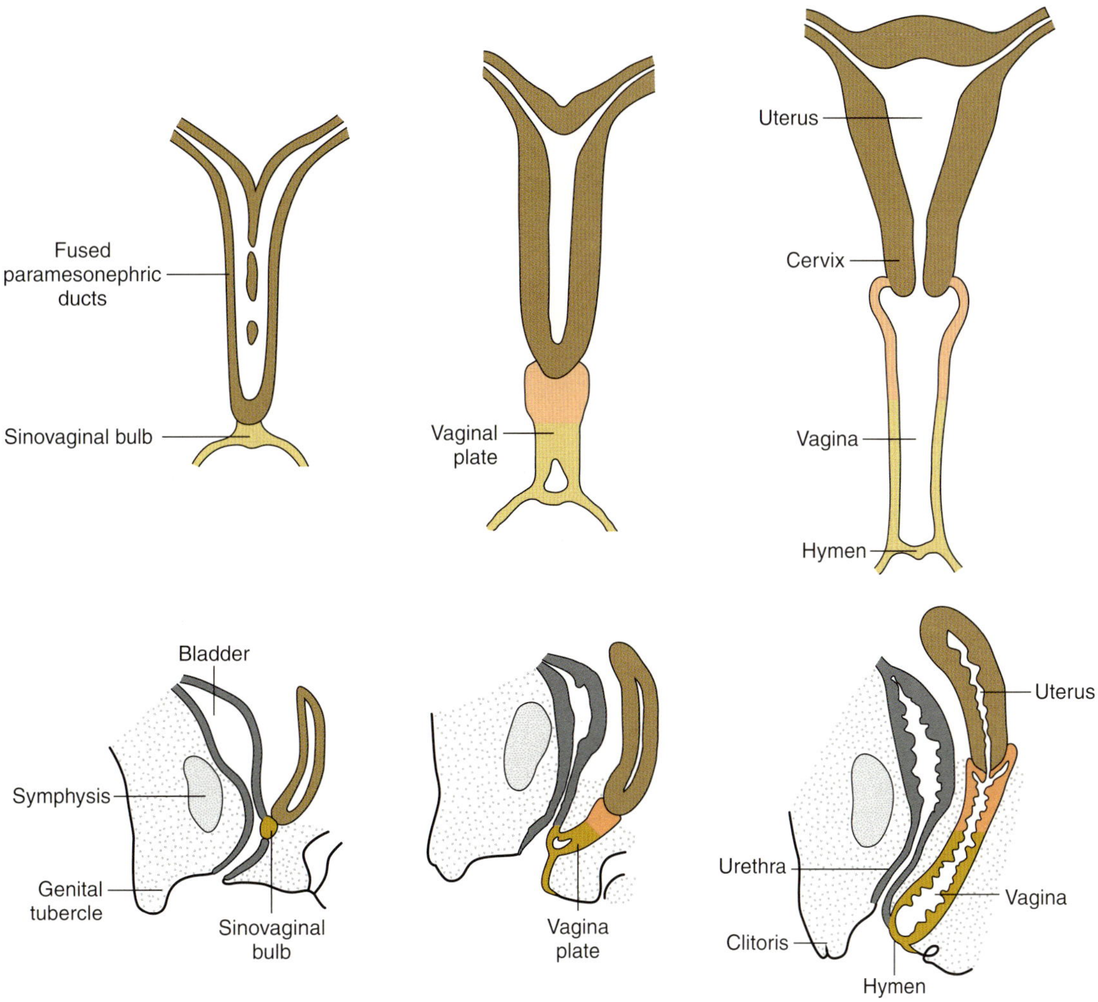

Figure 5.6 Development of the lower genital organs.

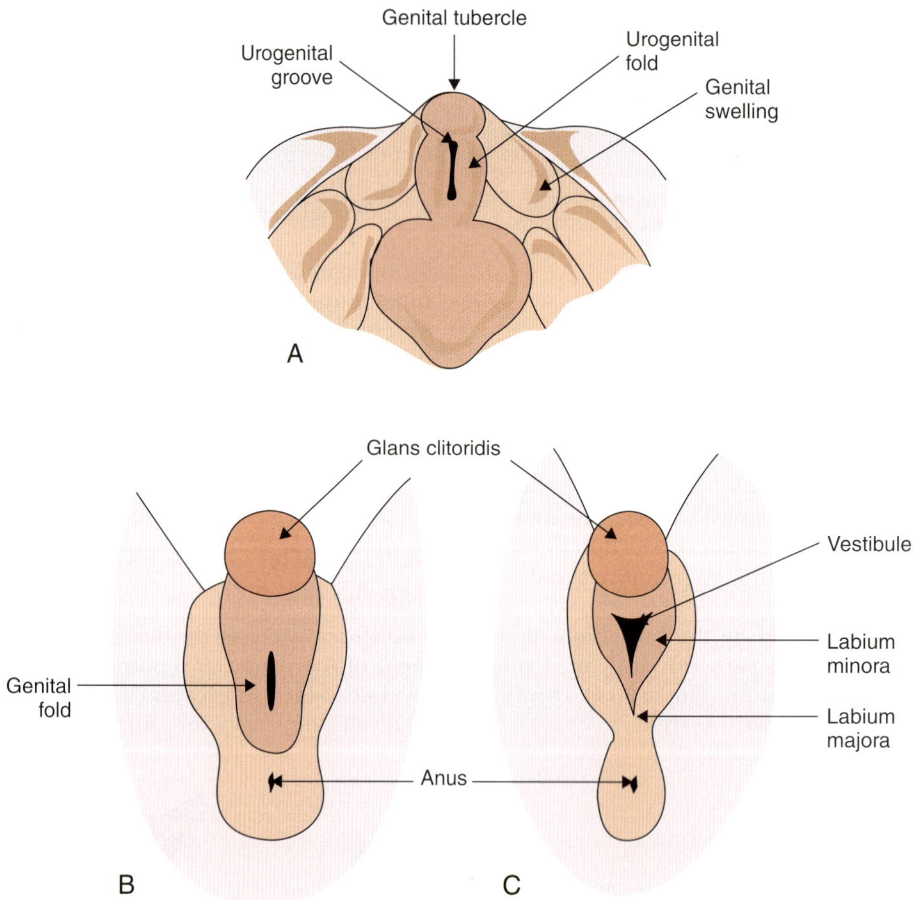

Figure 5.7 Development of the external genitalia.

ventral portion, the urogenital sinus. The primitive cloaca is closed by the cloacal membrane, which can be recognized very early in the development of the embryo and from which the vessels of the allantois are developed. The primitive intestines enter the dorsal part of the cloaca. Both Wolffian ducts, both Müllerian ducts and the allantois, from which the bladder and the urethra are differentiated, enter the urogenital sinus. Originally, the ureter arises from the lower end of the Wolffian duct near the opening of the duct into the urogenital sinus. Subsequently, as a result of the growth of the surrounding mesoblastic tissues, the ureter is displaced cranially so that it enters the urogenital sinus independently of the Wolffian duct. This displacement of the ureter explains the aberrant type of ureter which is sometimes encountered in gynaecological surgery. The part of the urogenital sinus which lies ventral to the mouths of the Wolffian ducts becomes differentiated into the bladder, whereas the allantois is represented by the urachus passing upwards from the apex of the bladder to the umbilicus. Before the 9th week, it is not possible to recognize the fetal sex by external genitalia.

The clitoris develops from the genital tubercle, which appears about the 5th week and is originally a bilateral structure derived from mesoderm. From the region of the genital tubercle, a genital fold passes backwards lateral to the urogenital sinus to form the labium majus (scrotum in the male). Between the genital folds lies the urogenital or anterior part of the cloacal membrane, which breaks down to form the labia minora (6th week). The vestibule and urethra are thus derived from the anterior part of the urogenital sinus, and Bartholin's glands and Skene's paraurethral glands are developed from downgrowths of the urogenital sinus. The female urethra represents the upper part of the male urethra, and the para- and periurethral glands are homologous to the male prostate. The external genitalia are recognizable by the 12th week of IUL. In females, urethral groove remains open to form the vestibule.

DEVELOPMENT OF THE OVARIES

Ovaries begin to develop by the 5th week. The ovarian differentiation is determined by the presence of a determinant located on the gene of the short arm of X-chromosome, although the autosomes are also involved in the ovarian development. Two intact sex chromosomes (XX) are necessary for the development of the ovaries.

The genital ridge extends from the pronephric region above to the sacral region below, and, in its earliest form, is represented by an elongated vertical prominence. Very soon it develops a mesentery of its own, the mesovarium, by which it is attached to intermediate cell mass. The infundibulopelvic fold passes upwards from the upper pole of the ovary and contains the ovarian vessels. The ovarian vessels of an adult, arising from the abdominal aorta, illustrate the original lumbar position of the upper part of the genital ridge. The genital fold of peritoneum passes downwards from the lower pole of the ovary to the region of the internal abdominal ring. The Müllerian duct originally lies on the outer aspect of the genital ridge but crosses the genital fold below. As the Müllerian duct crosses the genital fold, the two structures fuse, and after muscle tissue has formed around the Müllerian duct, it passes into the tissues of the genital fold. The part of the genital fold lying proximal to its point of intersection with the Müllerian duct becomes the ovarian ligament, whereas the distal portion becomes the round ligament (Fig. 5.1). This corresponds to the gubernaculum of the male. The ovaries are developed by the 12th week.

Undescended ovaries. At birth, the ovaries are located at the pelvic brim. They gradually descend to the pelvis by puberty. Undescended ovaries (rare) are associated with absent Müllerian system in as much as 40% cases and unicornuate uterus in 20% cases, and can confuse the ultrasound scanning. The undescended ovaries are at risk of malignancy as with undescended testes. It is a rare condition.

The ovaries can be located by ultrasound scanning, computed tomography (CT) and magnetic resonance imaging (MRI).

The significance of undescended ovaries is as follows:

- They are associated with the Müllerian duct anomalies and may adversely influence the menstrual and reproductive functions.
- Ovulation monitoring may be difficult.
- Ovarian pain may be misinterpreted as appendicitis or intestinal pain.
- Ovarian tumour may be misinterpreted as other abdominal tumour.
- Risk of malignancy.

These abnormally located ovaries may develop malignancy, so it may be advisable to remove them and put the woman on hormonal replacement therapy. In vitro fertilization with donor egg may be possible if the uterus is present.

The ovary descends from its original lumbar position so that at term it lies at the level of the pelvic brim with its long axis directed vertically.

The sex germ cells first appear in the genital ridge. Presently, it is accepted that the germ cells originate in the endodermal cells of the yolk sac by the 4th week from the hind gut of the embryo and migrate along the dorsal mesentry to the genital ridge. At first, the sex cells are arranged in columns perpendicular to the surface by the 6th week. These columns are called primary sex cords and they lie deeply in the substance of the genital ridge. At a later date, secondary cords develop nearer to the surface epithelium. Both primary and secondary cords consist of cells derived from the local stroma of the genital ridge. The egg cells or primordial ova are distinguished by their large size and peculiar mitochondria. It is believed that the sex cells act as organizers to the adjacent stroma cells, which then are converted into granulosa cells. In the male, the cells of the primary cords predominate whereas in the ovary the secondary cords are marked most.

Urogenital differentiation in the embryo is a rather complex process involving genetic, hormonal and environmental influences. The genital and urinary systems develop in close relationship, so developmental errors in both of these systems often coexist. Some anomalies are obvious at birth, but most come to light only at puberty, when the girl fails to menstruate.

GONADS

The chromosomal sex of the fertilized ovum determines the development of the embryonic gonad into the ovaries or the testes, and this in turn directs the further differentiation and development of the internal and external genital organs. The gonads remain undifferentiated until 6th week.

About the 6th week of IUL, a genital ridge appears (crown-rump length of 5 mm) (Figs 5.1–5.5) on the dorsal aspect of the embryo on either side of the midline. It consists of proliferation and thickening of the coelomic epithelium overlying some mesenchymal tissue near the developing kidney. In the female embryos, germ cells originate in the endoderm of the yolk sac near the developing hindgut; they migrate along the root of the dorsal mesentery to enter the developing gonad. Columns of coelomic epithelial cells designated as sex cords invade the cortex of the developing gonad and surround the germ cells, thus forming the primitive primordial follicles. The primordial follicles are recognizable by 20th week of IUL. These proliferate to reach about 7 million in the 7th month of fetal life. However, as the gonadal stroma proliferates, many of these follicles degenerate so that the ovaries at birth contain about 2 million follicles. Of these, only 300–400 will ever ovulate.

The first meiotic division begins in the oocyte by the 20th week in the embryo, but remains dormant in the prophase until ovulation occurs at puberty. The second meiotic division occurs only at fertilization when the sperm penetrates the zona pellucida. The ovary plays no role in the development of internal genital organs.

By the 10th week of IUL, the female gonad assumes histological characteristics of the ovary. The basic sexual pattern is female in all embryos. It is the androgen of testicular origin in the male embryo which causes the male elements to grow. Its absence in embryo develops along the female line. In the male embryo, the fetal testis elaborates two substances: (i) a Müllerian suppression substance which inhibits the development of the Müllerian ducts, Müllerian-inhibiting factor (MIF) glycoprotein secreted by the Sertoli cells of the testes, and (ii) testosterone derived from Leydig cells which is responsible for completing the development of the Wolffian structures, and fusion of the labioscrotal folds and development of the phallus so that the external genitalia develop along the male line. In the absence of androgen, the genital organs develop along the female line. The male external genitalia develop in response to dihydrotestosterone derived by conversion of testosterone by enzyme 5 α-reductase.

However, if the early embryonic state of bisexuality persists into adult life, it results in a state of true hermaphrodism wherein masculine and feminine elements are observed in the gonad as well as in the external and internal genitalia. The ovary plays no role in the development of internal genital organs.

In a female pseudohermaphrodite, the gonad and the Müllerian system are normal, though perhaps underdeveloped as far as the level of the urogenital sinus. The Wolffian vestigial persist as usual, but the phallus (clitoris) is hypertrophic, the labia appear fused in the midline and the urogenital sinus opens at the base of the phallus. Such females may be regarded as males with a hypospadias. The source of the androgen responsible for the altered development of the external genitalia is commonly of adrenal origin such as in congenital adrenal hyperplasia. Knowledge of the nuclear sex at birth is essential to decide the proper sex of rearing.

If the female embryo in utero is exposed to androgen secreted by maternal ovarian or adrenal neoplasms (arrhenoblastoma or hilar cell tumour), or to progestogens, which are mildly androgenic, then such altered hormonal environment can lead to varying degrees of masculinization of the female fetus.

Complete aplasia of ovary is rare, agenesis may appears as streak ovary as in Turner syndrome. The streak ovary contains undifferentiated stroma devoid of germ cells. This happens if the chromosome pattern is 45/XO, when the germ cells fail to migrate along the dorsal mesentery into the gonad.

MÜLLERIAN DUCTS

It is desirable to recapitulate the development of the Müllerian ducts described in the beginning of the chapter.

Arrest in the normal development of the Müllerian ducts can cause several anomalies as listed below (Jones' classification).

1. *Aplasia*, in which the organs fail to develop.
2. *Hypoplasia*, in which the organs are rudimentary.
3. *Atresia*, in which there is partial or complete failure of canalization of these ducts, leading to varying degrees of gynatresia.
4. *Müllerian duct anomalies*, such as asymmetric development, may lead to a unicornuate uterus, with or without a rudimentary horn. Failure of fusion in part or its entirety may lead to duplication of the genital tract, and failure of disappearance of the intervening septum may lead to a septate or subseptate uterus, which may coexist with a septate vagina.
5. *Hermaphroditism* and *pseudohermaphroditism* may be the result of abnormalities of development of the gonads, sex ducts and external genitalia.
6. *Developmental defects* of the urogenital sinus may manifest in the form of defective development of the urinary bladder, hymen and the perineum.

Structural homologues in males and females are discussed in Table 5.1.

Müllerian duct anomalies: Some anomalies are detected at birth, i.e. external genital organs. Some may be detected at puberty while investigating for primary amenorrhoea. Some are revealed during investigations of infertility and repeated pregnancy losses. Although a great number of anomalies of the uterus have been described, these can be broadly grouped as follows:

1. ***Agenesis***
2. ***Anomalies arising out of defects in vertical fusion* (Fig. 5.8; see also Fig. 5.16)** between the downgrowing fused Müllerian ducts and the upgrowing derivative from the

Table 5.1 Structural Homologues in Males and Females

	Male	Female	Determining Factors
Gonadal			
Germ cells	Spermatozoa	Oogonia	Sex chromosomes
Coelomic epithelium	Sertoli cells	Granulosa cells	
Mesenchyme	Leydig cells	Theca cells rete ovarii	
Ductal			
Paramesonephric duct (Müllerian)	Hydatid testis	Fallopian tubes, uterus and upper three-fourths of vagina	Absence of Y-chromosome
Mesonephric duct (Wolffian)	Vas deferens seminal vesicles epididymis	Epoophoron Paroophoron Gartner's duct	Testosterone MIF
External genitalia			
Urogenital sinus	Prostrate Cowper's glands	Lower vagina Skene's tubercles Bartholin's gland	Presence or absence of testosterone and dihydrotestosterone
Genital tubercle	Penis	Clitoris	
Urogenital folds	Corpora spongiosa	Labia minora	
Genital folds	Scrotum	Labia majora	
Urogenital sinus	Bladder, urethra prostrate, bulbo-urethral glands	Lower portion of vagina, Bartholin's gland, paraurethral gland, urinary bladder, urethra	

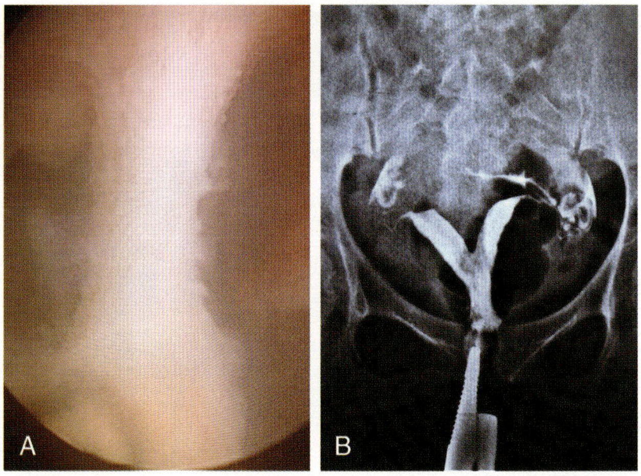

Figure 5.8 **(A)** Hysteroscopy showing septum in the uterus dividing the uterine cavity. **(B)** Hysterosalpingography film of the same patient. (*Courtesy* **(A):** Dr Shyam Desai, Mumbai.)

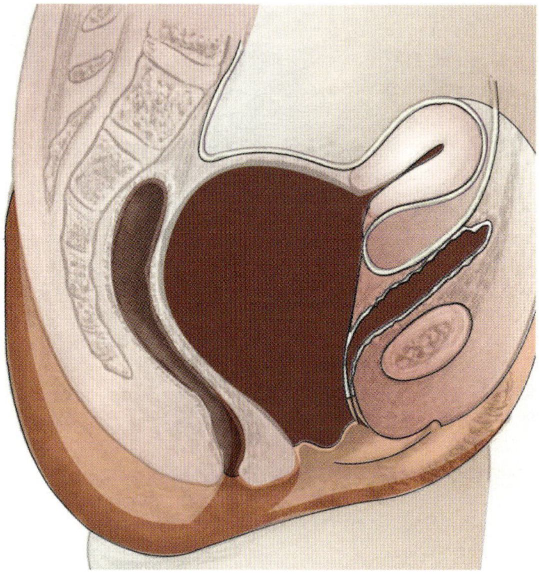

Figure 5.9 Haematocolpos. The illustration shows the distended vagina filled with blood.

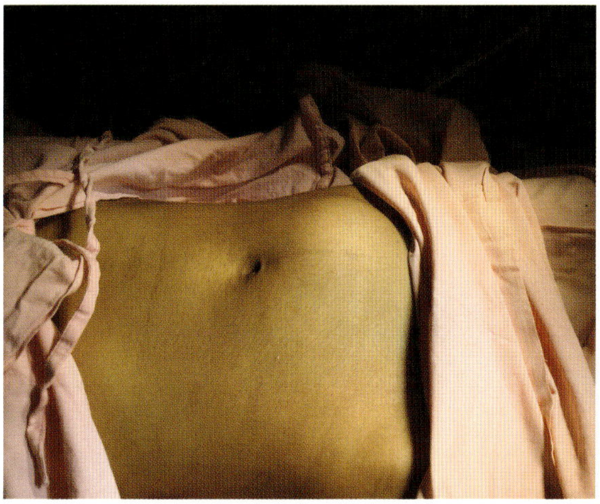

Figure 5.10 Suprapubic bulge caused by haematocolpos.

urogenital sinus. These may manifest as (a) obstructive lesions or (b) nonobstructive lesions.

3. ***Anomalies arising out of defects of lateral fusion or resorption*** resulting in duplication defects. These may manifest as (a) obstructive lesions or (b) nonobstructive lesions.

Congenital defects can occur because of the following:

(a) Failure of initial descent – agenesis.
(b) Failure of vertical fusion – transverse vaginal septum, imperforate hymen.
(c) Failure of lateral fusion – this may result in complete or partial duplication, which may be either symmetrical or asymmetrical. Symmetrical fusion defects would lead to bicornuate uterus or uterus didelphys whereas the asymmetrical fusion defects would result in one well-developed uterine horn with the other being rudimentary. Noncommunicating horn of the uterus is an example of obstructive defect.
(d) Defects in the resorption of the septum – example, septate uterus.

DETAILED CONSIDERATION OF MÜLLERIAN DEFECTS

(a) ***Vertical fusion defects***

1. *Vaginal atresia:* Simpson (1976) stated that vaginal atresia is a condition in which the lower portion of the vagina is represented merely by fibrous tissue, whereas the contiguous superior structures (uterus) are well differentiated.
2. *Transverse vaginal septum:* It occurs in the upper portion of vagina in 50%, middle portion in 30%–40% and lower portion in 10% cases.
   (a) *Imperforate hymen* – this is entirely of urogenital origin. Failure of canalization may lead to formation of a mucocolpos; this may be recognized in early infancy and get treated. However, the anomaly often continues unrecognized until puberty, when amenorrhoea in the presence of secondary sexual characters, cyclic abdominal discomfort, urinary symptoms (retention of urine) and often the palpation of a midline hypogastric lump leads to the examination of the external genitalis, parting of the labia reveals the presence of a tell tale bluish bulging membrane in the region of the hymen that points to the diagnosis of haematocolpos. A simple cruciate incision followed by excision of the tags of hymen allows drainage of the retained menstrual blood. The operation should be performed under aseptic conditions and under an adequate antibiotic cover to avoid any ascending infection. The vagina regains its tone very quickly (Figs 5.9–5.14).
   (b) *Congenital absence of vagina* – Müllerian agenesis (absent vagina)

INTRODUCTION

The common synonyms in clinical usage include Müllerian agenesis (MA), Mayer–Rokitansky–Kuster–Hauser (MRKH)

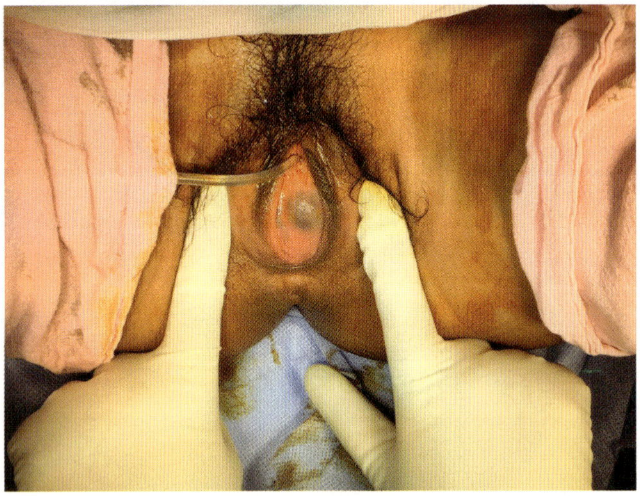

Figure 5.11 Vaginal introitus showing the bulging membrane caused by haematocolpos.

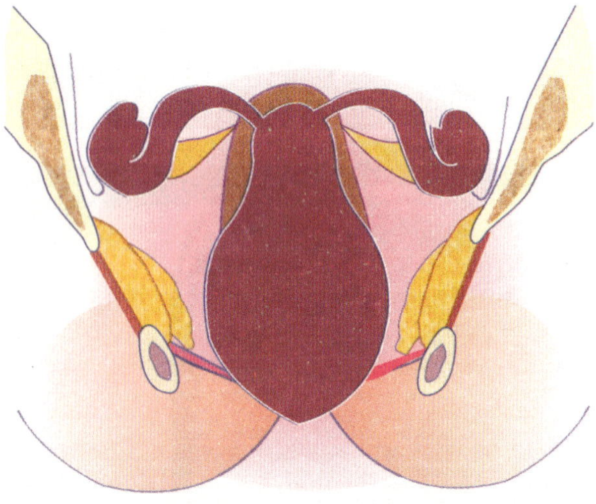

Figure 5.12 Imperforate hymen causing haematocolpos, haematometra and haematosalpinx.

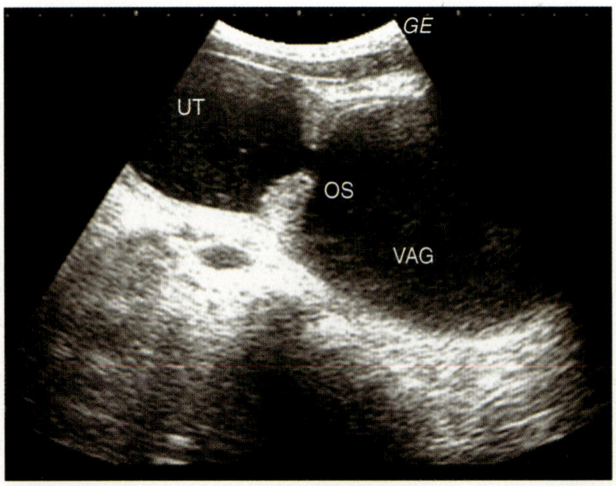

Figure 5.13 Imperforate hymen – ultrasonography showing haematocolpos (distended vagina) and haematometra (distended uterus). (*Courtesy*: Dr Rajeev H Kothari, Mumbai.)

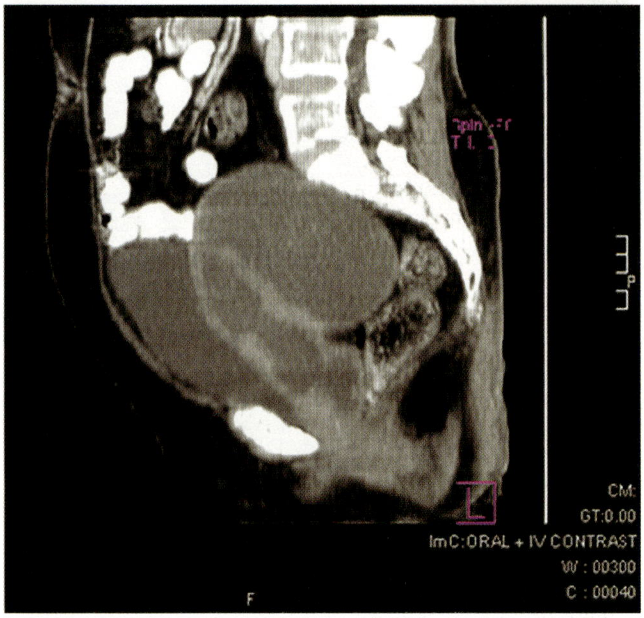

Figure 5.14 CT showing haematometra and haematocolpos. (*Courtesy:* Dr Parveen Gulati, New Delhi.)

syndrome and vaginal agenesis. This condition, though commonly referred to as *congenital absence of the vagina* – a misnomer, is truly a developmental defect of the Müllerian ducts resulting in the condition described as the *MRKH syndrome.* The MRKH syndrome occurs in 1:5000–1:20,000 women at birth, and is diagnosed in approximately 1:1500 gynaecologic admissions.

DEFINING FEATURES

Clinically identified by the absence of structures derived from Müllerian ducts, namely the uterus, cervix and upper vagina, 25% patients may have a short vaginal pouch. Rudimentary tubes are often present. The gonads are ovaries. The karyotype is XX; the disorder seems to be an accident of development. In clinical practice, the working diagnosis for any individual presenting with primary amenorrhoea, feminine secondary sexual characteristics and an absent vagina is MRKH syndrome (Griffin et al., 1976), with a familial tendency in uterus is present in only 7%–8% cases.

CHARACTERISTIC FEATURES

- Congenital absence of uterus and vagina (small rudimentary uterine bulbs are usually present).
- Normal ovarian function, including ovulation.
- Sex of rearing – female.
- Phenotypic sex – female (normal development of breasts, body proportions, hair distribution and external genitalia).
- Genetic sex – female (46, XX – karyotype).
- Frequent association with other congenital anomalies, skeletal and spine abnormalities (20%–30%) urologic abnormalities such as malrotation of kidney, ectopic kidney (horseshoe kidney, pelvic kidney) and anomalies of urinary-collecting system need to be investigated for – by intravenous pyelogram or ultrasound (40%).

DIFFERENTIAL DIAGNOSIS

- Imperforate hymen
- Transverse vaginal septum
- Complete androgen insensitivity syndrome (testicular feminization syndrome)

Imperforate hymen can be detected by observing the vaginal outlet. On performing the Valsalva manoeuvre, the membrane bulges. Pelvic sonography reveals presence of haematocolpos and internal genitalia. Transverse septum reveals presence of a short vagina, absence of bulging on Valsalva manoeuvre. Testicular feminization or androgen insensitivity syndrome closely mimics one another, and efforts to differentiate between these two have therapeutic bearings.

INVESTIGATIONS

- Pelvis and abdomen ultrasound – pelvic organs and kidneys.
- 3-D ultrasound is very precise in detecting these malformations (100% sensitive and specific), less costly than MRI. One should move on to MRI only if any doubt prevails.
- MRI gives more precise definition of pelvic viscera.
- Karyotype.
- Laparoscopy (invasive procedure) may be avoided, extirpation of the Müllerian remnants is not necessary unless it is causing problems such as fibroids, haematometra, endometriosis or symptomatic herniation into the inguinal canal.
- Radiology – descending pyelography to delineate urinary tract anomalies, X-ray L-S spine.

MANAGEMENT

- Nonsurgical methods – act by intermittent pressure on the perineum.
- Frank's nonsurgical method of active dilatation using graduated vaginal dilators of 0.5–1.0 inch diameter and 4–5 inches in length is used to apply constant pressure to the vaginal dimple for 20 minutes t.i.d. for 6–8 weeks to achieve clinically acceptable results. Normal sexual function is possible in over 75% individuals. To maintain patency, vaginal dilator use should be continued until regular sexual intercourse begins. Other modifications of Frank's artificial vagina include Ingram's bicycle seat stool used for 2 hours daily to maintain constant perineal pressure. Jaffe successfully modified Frank's dilation technique by using increasing sizes of syringe containers. Oestrogen creams help in vaginal epithelial transformation.
- Surgical method of vaginoplasty – to be delayed till the marriage or until the patient becomes sexually active. The McIndoe operation of vaginoplasty using split-thickness skin graft spread over a mould and held in place in an artificial space created between the bladder in front and the rectum behind has been successfully performed and has served functional use. Surgeons have also successfully used fresh amniotic membrane graft to line the vaginal space. HIV testing of the donor is required. Another surgical procedure which is simple to perform has been devised by Williams using labial skin. However, the axis of the artificial vagina points directly backwards.
- Tissue expansion vaginoplasty using tissue expander has also been tried with success. Water balloon is employed.
- Shirodkar used a section of the Sigmoid colon to prepare an artificial vagina, but this method was technically difficult to perform, and the mucus secretion caused discomfort; hence, this method is not currently practiced.

Transverse vaginal septum can be very easily mistaken for congenital absence of the vagina. It is a rare condition having an incidence of 1:84,000 gynaecologic visits. The clinical symptoms will depend entirely on whether the septum is imperforate or otherwise. In case of a perforated septum, menstruation occurs and no difficulty is suspected until the time of marriage when apareunia may lead the patient to seek consultation, or at the time of pregnancy. If the septum is imperforate, the symptoms of amenorrhoea and those resulting from mucocolpometra may call for attention. Ultrasonography helps to arrive at the diagnosis. The commonest site for the occurrence of a transverse septum is the junction of the upper and middle third of the vagina. Treatment consists of either manual dilatation from the microperforation or surgical excision of the septum. If the septum is thick and wide, reanastomosis of the upper and lower vagina may be difficult; it may require skin grafting to cover the intervening raw area.

Androgenic insensitivity syndrome – originally described as testicular feminization syndrome – needs to be differentiated from the Müllerian duct anomaly causing MRKH syndrome, which also presents with amenorrhoea and absent uterus. Androgen insensitivity syndrome is a genetically transmitted androgen receptor defect in a 46 XY individual with testes and normal testosterone levels. These individuals present with amenorrhoea, they have no internal male or female genitalia (absent uterus), normal female external genitalia, an absent or shallow vagina, a normal female phenotype with well-developed breasts, and scanty body hair. Ultrasound/MRI examination coupled with a karyotype XY helps to settle the diagnosis. The abnormal gonads are prone to malignancy, so these should be removed surgically at an early date, soon after sexual maturity has been achieved.

(b) ***Lateral fusion defects*** – these include partial or complete duplication.

1. *Double or septate vagina* – this may occur with an entirely normal fallopian tubes, uterus and cervix, or with duplication of the uterus. The longitudinal antero-posterior septum may be partial or complete, extending right down to the vaginal outlet. Generally, both sides are patent, but in rare instances the septum may deviate from the centre and fuse with one lateral vaginal wall so that one side of the vagina and uterus are obstructed and there is unilateral haematocolpos. The asymptomatic longitudinal septum may only come to light when the patient complains of soiling her clothes in spite of using a tampon during menses. Examination may reveal a septum with Müllerian

duplication, wherein her placement of the tampon in one vagina cannot prevent egress from the other side, or it may be detected after marriage when it may be a cause of dyspareunia, or become apparent only at the time of labour. Symptomatic septum requires excision. A thick septum can be very vascular.

Complete Nonfusion of the Müllerian Ducts Results in Duplication of the Genital Tract

2. *Duplication of the uterus* –defects in lateral fusion of the Müllerian ducts may result in partial or complete duplication, the two halves may be symmetrically developed or asymmetrically formed. These may result in obstructive or nonobstructive malformations. Symmetrical malformations include uterus didelphys, bicornuate uterus with double or single cervix, or an arcuate uterus depending on the extent of nonfusion. Asymmetric malformations include uterine duplication in which one uterine horn is fully developed and represented by a hemi uterus, and the other exhibits varying degrees of rudimentary development or may even be totally absent, clinically presenting as a rudimentary uterine horn communicating with the main well-developed horn, a noncommunicating rudimentary functional horn, a nonfunctioning rudimentary horn with considerable disproportion between the two horns or a unicornuate uterus. Wolffian duct anomalies often coexist with Müllerian duct anomalies, hence the importance in clinical practice to undertake an intravenous pyelography or ultrasound in all cases of Müllerian duct anomalies to detect presence of any coexisting urinary tract anomalies.

DETAILED CONSIDERATION OF RELEVANT ANOMALIES OF THE MÜLLERIAN DUCTS

Classification

Recently, a newer classification for Müllerian duct anomalies has been introduced by the European Society of Human Reproduction and Embryology (ESHRE) (Table 5.2).

A new classification of the Müllerian duct anomalies was given by ESHRE/European Society of Gastrointestinal Endoscopy (ESGE) in 2013.

It has the following general characteristics:

1. Anatomy is the basis for the systematic categorization of anomalies.
2. Deviations of uterine anatomy deriving from the same embryological origin are the basis for the design of the main classes.
3. Anatomical variations of the main classes expressing different degrees of uterine deformity and being clinically significant are the basis for the design of the main subclasses.
4. Cervical and vaginal anomalies are classified in independent supplementary subclasses.

- Class U0 incorporates all cases with normal uterus.
- Class U1 or dysmorphic uterus incorporates all cases with normal uterine outline but with an abnormal shape of the uterine cavity excluding septa.
- Class I is further subdivided into three categories:
- Class U1a or T-shaped uterus characterized by a narrow uterine cavity due to thickened lateral walls with a correlation of two-third uterine corpus and one-third cervix.
- Class U1b or uterus infantilis also characterized by a narrow uterine cavity without lateral wall thickening and an inverse correlation of one-third uterine body and two-third cervix.
- Class U1c or others which is added to include all minor deformities of the uterine cavity, including those with an inner indentation at the fundal midline level of 50% of the uterine wall thickness.
- Class U2 or septate uterus incorporates all cases with normal fusion and abnormal absorption of the midline septum. Septate is defined as the uterus with normal outline and an internal indentation at the fundal midline exceeding 50% of the uterine wall thickness. This indentation is characterized as septum and it could divide partly or completely the uterine cavity, including, in some cases, cervix and/or vagina. Class U2 is further divided into two subclasses according to the degree of the uterine corpus deformity.
- Class U2a or partial septate uterus characterized by the existence of a septum dividing partly the uterine cavity above the level of the internal cervical os.
- Class U2b or complete septate uterus characterized by the existence of a septum fully dividing the uterine cavity up to the level of the internal cervical os.
- Class U3 or bicorporeal uterus incorporates all cases of fusion defects. Bicorporeal uterus is defined as the uterus with an abnormal fundal outline; it is characterized by the presence of an external indentation at the fundal midline exceeding 50% of the uterine wall thickness.
- Class U3a or partial bicorporeal uterus characterized by an external fundal indentation partly dividing the uterine corpus above the level of the cervix.
- Class U3b or complete bicorporeal uterus characterized by an external fundal indentation completely dividing the uterine corpus up to the level of the cervix.
- Class U3c or bicorporeal septate uterus characterized by the presence of an absorption defect in addition to the main fusion defect. In patients with bicorporeal septate uterus (Class U3c), the width of the midline fundal indentation exceeds by 150% of the uterine wall thickness.

  U3b and U3c defects are associated with reproductive failure in about 25% of affected women. These women often suffer from miscarriages, preterm births, intrauterine growth restriction (IUGR) and abnormal fetal presentations such as breech and oblique presentations. Incidence of dystocia during labour is high, and the 3rd stage complications, such as adherent placenta and postpartum haemorrhage, are more frequent. Unification surgical procedures undertaken at laparotomy (Strassman operation, Tompkins operation or Jones' wedge metroplasty operation) or hysteroscopic resection of uterine septum help to improve obstetric performance in 60%–85% cases.
- Class U4 or hemi-uterus incorporates all cases of unilateral formed uterus. Hemi-uterus is defined as the unilateral

Table 5.2 ESHRE/ESGE Classification for Female Genital Tract Anomalies

	Uterine Anomaly		Cervical/Vaginal Anomaly
	Main Class	**Sub-Class**	**Co-Existent Class**
U0	Normal uterus	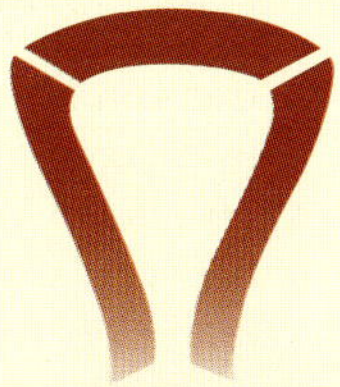	
U1	Dysmorphic uterus	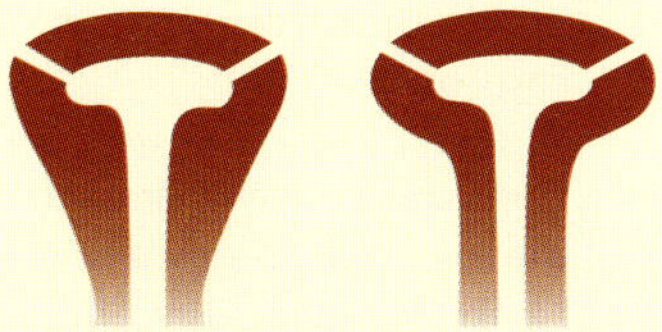 a. T-shaped; b. Infantilis; c. Others	
U2	Septate uterus	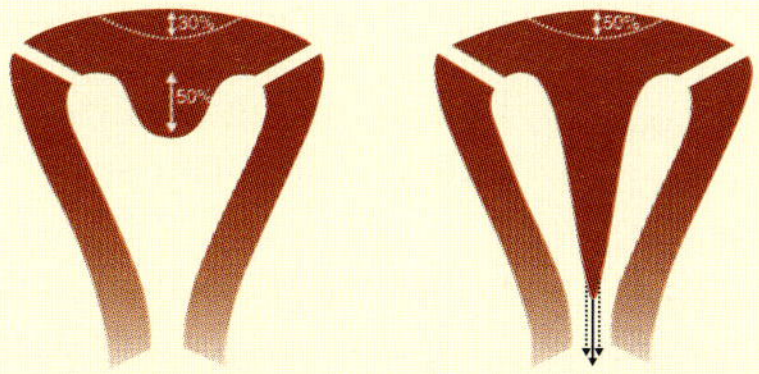 a. Partial; b. Complete	
U3	Bicorporeal uterus	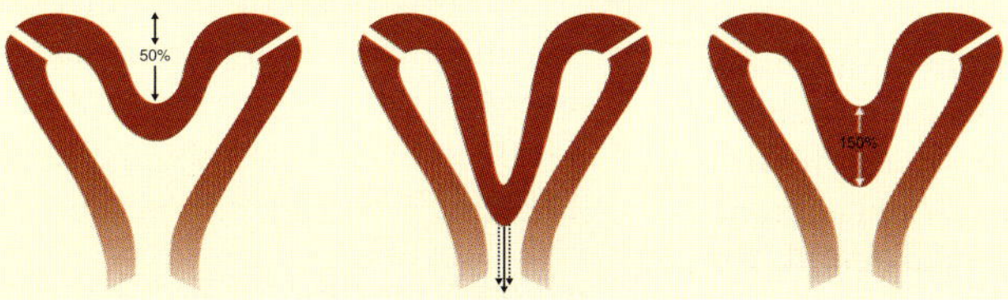 a. Partial; b. Complete; c. Bicorporeal septate	
U4	Hemi-uterus	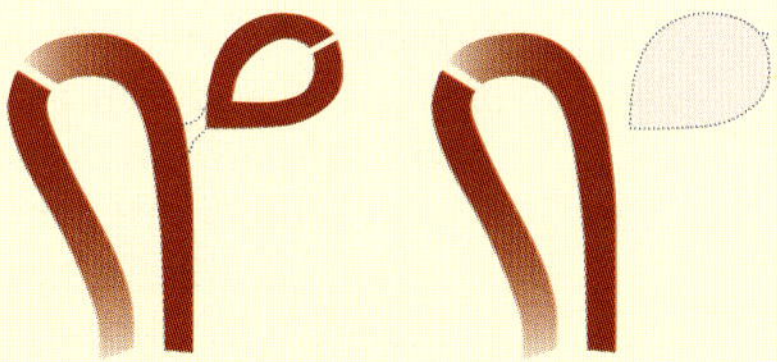 a. With rudimentary cavity; b. Without rudimentary cavity	
U5	Aplastic	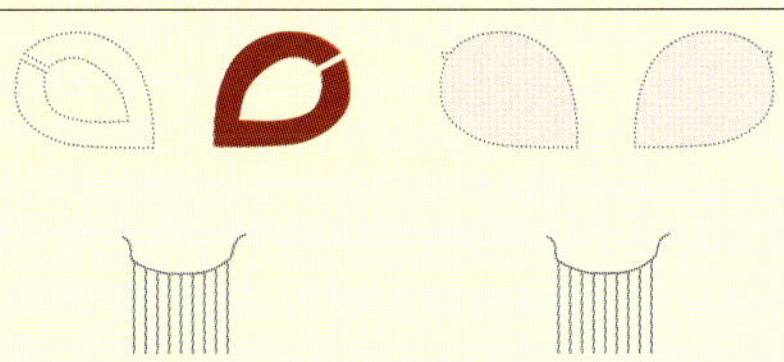 a. With rudimentary cavity; b. Without rudimentary cavity	
U6	Unclassified malformations		
U			*C* *V*
Associated anomalies of non-Müllerian origin:			

Class	Co-Existent Class
C0	*Normal cervix*
C1	*Septate cervix*
C2	*Double "normal" cervix*
C3	*Unilateral cervical aplasia*
C4	*Cervical aplasia*
V0	*Normal vagina*
V1	*Longitudinal non-obstructing vaginal septum*
V2	*Longitudinal obstructing vaginal septum*
V3	*Transverse vaginal septum and/or imperforate hymen*
V4	*Vaginal aplasia*

Development of uterus and vagina: during the 10th week, the paramesonephric ducts fuse at their caudal ends to establish a common channel and come in contact with a thickened portion of posterior urogenital sinus called sinovaginal bulb. This is followed by development of vaginal plate, which elongates between the 3rd and 5th month, and become canalized to form the inferior vaginal lumen. (*Source*: Modified from Sadler TW. Langman's Medical Embryology. Baltimore: William and Wilkins, 1985.)

uterine development; the contralateral part could be either incompletely formed or absent. It is a formation defect; the necessity to classify it in a different class than that of aplastic uterus (formation defect) is due to the existence of a fully developed functional uterine hemi-cavity.

- Class U4a or hemi-uterus with a rudimentary (functional) cavity, characterized by the presence of a communicating or noncommunicating functional contralateral horn.
- Class U4b or hemi-uterus without rudimentary (functional) cavity, characterized either by the presence of a nonfunctional contralateral uterine horn or by aplasia of the contralateral part. Presence of a functional cavity in the contralateral part is the only clinically important factor for complications, such as haemato-cavity or ectopic pregnancy in the rudimentary horn, or haemato-cavity and treatment (laparoscopic removal) are always recommended even if the horn is communicating.

  It accounts for 1%–2% of all uterovaginal anomalies and is often associated with a poor reproductive performance. Spontaneous abortion rates are high, as also the incidence of prematurity. A third of these patients have breech presentations, and a high incidence of severe IUGR has been recorded. It is worth noting that fetal survival has been recorded in only 40% of women with unicornuate uteri. The incidence of caesarean sections is high in this subgroup of women.

  U4a and b defects need to be investigated by intravenous pyelography (IVP) to detect urinary tract anomalies. These are generally present on the side where the Müllerian abnormality is most pronounced. Renal agenesis may be present or the kidney may be malrotated, low lying or pelvic in location.
- Class U5 or aplastic uterus incorporates all cases of uterine aplasia characterized by the absence of any fully or unilaterally developed uterine cavity.
- Class U5a or aplastic uterus with rudimentary (functional) cavity characterized by the presence of bi- or unilateral functional horn.
- Class U5b or aplastic uterus without rudimentary (functional) cavity characterized either by the presence of uterine remnants or by full uterine aplasia.
- Class U6 unclassified includes under anomalies.

Prevalence

- About 1.0% in normal fertile and subfertile women
- About 3.3% in cases of recurrent pregnancy loss

Background

- Congenital uterine anomalies resulting from the Müllerian duct fusion defects are the commonest malformations encountered in clinical practice.
- Septate uterus is most common. About 25% incidence of spontaneous first trimester abortions, and 6% second trimester abortions.
- Implantation into a poorly vascularized fibrous septum might be a contributory factor (Fedele et al. 1996).
- Bicornuate uterus is not generally associated with recurrent pregnancy losses (Proctor et al. 2003).

Diagnosis

- *Combined hysteroscopy and laparoscopy* help to differentiate between bicornuate uterus and septate uterus. The presence of the uterine fundus suggests a septate uterus.
- *Ultrasonography* – septate uterus appears as two cavities without sagittal notching, and the intercornual distance < 4.0 cm. Diagnosis of bicornuate uterus is favoured if the fundal midpoint indentation is >5 mm above the interostial line.
- *Hysterosalpingography (HSG)* – cannot reliably differentiate between septate and a bicornuate/arcuate uterus. If the angle of divergence between the two uterine cavities is $\leq 75°$, the defect is most likely to be septate uterus. If the angle of divergence is $>75°$ but $<105°$, a diagnosis cannot be made.
- *Magnetic resonance imaging (MRI)* – it is an accurate and noninvasive investigation to make a diagnosis of septate uterus. If the septum extends to $\geq 30\%$ of the septal cavity, surgical resection is indicated.

Adverse Obstetric Outcomes

The following adverse obstetric events have been associated with septate uterus:

- First and second trimester pregnancy losses: (between 8- and 16-week gestation) spontaneous abortions – 25%, preterm delivery – 14.5% and live births – 62%.
- About two-thirds of abortions occur in the first trimester.
- It constitutes an important cause of repeated pregnancy losses.
- Other adverse obstetric outcomes include abnormal presentation and IUGR.

Surgical Resection of the Intrauterine Septum (Metroplasty)

Nowadays hysteroscopic resection is considered best as it avoids uterine scar and need for elective caesarean section. The septum is resected with resectoscope or scissors.

Indication: Presence of uterine septum in association of adverse reproductive outcome.

Postoperative management: Oral oestrogen for 3 months after completion of surgery has been the accepted practice. Insertion of a Foley catheter with its bulb distended with 4–8 mL of sterile water has been used for 5–7 days to keep the uterine cavity open and prevent intrauterine adhesions. This is coupled with the administration of antibiotics (doxycycline 100 mg b.i.d. for 5–7 days) and nonsteroidal anti-inflammatory drugs (NSAID) to control pain and prevent adhesions. Asherman syndrome with uterine adhesions and adherent placenta are the late complications.

Amongst the uterine anomalies, bicornuate uterus is seen in 35%–40%, arcuate uterus in 15%, uterus didelphys in 10% and uterine septum in 5%–10% cases.

Diagnosis of Müllerian anomalies: This is based on the following information.

1. Clinical data – family history, menstrual history, past obstetric history and detailed pelvic examination.
2. Imaging sciences – hysterosalpingography, ultrasonography, MRI imaging.

3. Endoscopic examination – laparoscopy and hysteroscopy.

Arterio-venous anastomosis causing menorrhagia not responding to medical therapy and occasional rupture with internal haemorrhage is known. It responds to embolization of uterine arteries. The diagnosis is made by Doppler ultrasound.

MALFORMATIONS OF THE RECTUM AND ANAL CANAL

IMPERFORATE ANUS

Imperforate anus results from the failure or breakdown of the cloacal membrane between the anal depression and the terminal intestine (Fig. 5.15). The diagnosis is made at birth when corrective surgery is required forthwith.

ATRESIA RECTI

Atresia recti is a condition in which the lower part of the rectum fails to develop. This is a much more serious situation than an imperforate anus. Major surgical intervention is called for, and the prognosis is guarded.

CONGENITAL RECTOVAGINAL FISTULA

Various types have been described; these result from the imperfect separation of the rectum from the urogenital sinus. In some cases the anus is represented by a depression in the expected normal position but the rectum opens on to the exterior somewhere else on the perineum. It is called a perineal anus, or it opens partly by way of an anal canal and partly as a fistula in the location of the perineal body, or it opens through the lower part of the posterior vaginal wall into the navicular fossa just within the fourchette. This is often termed as vaginal anus. It is surprising how many women with an ectopic anus suffer little inconvenience and acquire satisfactory bowel control. During childbirth, however, there is a danger of severe and complicated third-degree perineal tear; hence, these patients are best delivered by caesarean section. It should be remembered that if surgical correction of an ectopic anus is undertaken, the sphincteric control of the transplanted anal canal may not be as satisfactory as in the previous situation.

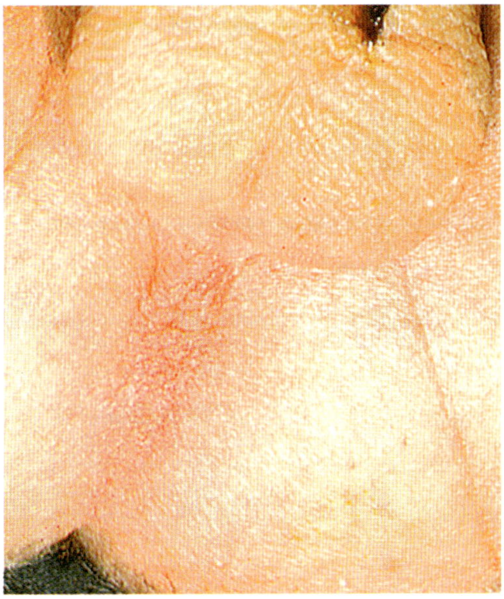

Figure 5.15 Imperforate anus. (*Source*: Jane C. Rothrock, Alexander's Care of the Patient in Surgery, Pediatric Surgery. Mosby, 2011.)

WOLFFIAN DUCT ANOMALIES

The upper portion of the Wolffian duct may at times dilate to form a paraovarian cyst, and the lower portion forms a Gartner cyst (Fig. 5.16). The paraovarian cyst may appear like an ovarian cyst. Its true nature is revealed at laparotomy when the ovary is normal, and the cyst lies in the broad ligament. During its removal, one should look for the ureter, and not injure it. A small Gartner cyst can be left alone but will require marsupialization or excision if it causes dyspareunia.

RENAL TRACT ABNORMALITIES

A double ureter is rarely encountered. Its recognition at laparotomy is necessary if injury to it is to be avoided.

An ectopic ureter sometimes communicates with the vagina, and the diagnosis is made by pyridium test and IVP. It is performed by a urosurgeon.

In a fetus, the kidneys initially develop in the pelvis. They migrate upwards as the ureter starts growing cranially. In a rare instance, the kidneys remain in the pelvis and are mistaken for a retroperitoneal tumour. IVP should be done before surgery is planned for the removal of retroperitoneal tumour.

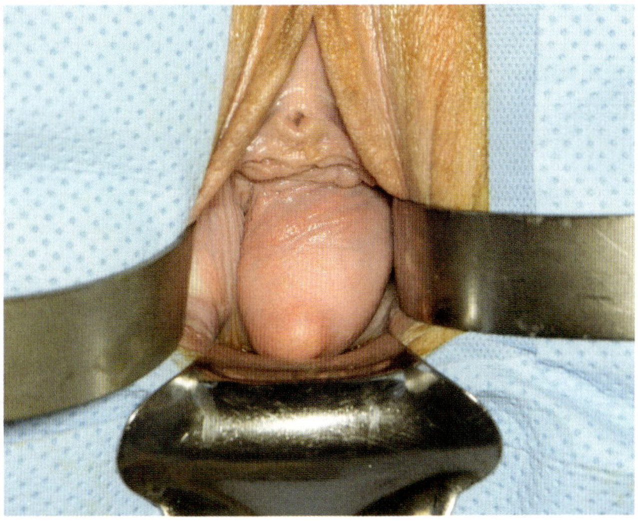

Figure 5.16 Gartner's duct cyst.

KEY POINTS

- There is a close and parallel development of Müllerian duct and Wollfian ducts during IUL. Therefore, anomaly of one system may coexist with the anomaly of other system.
- Although genital tract abnormalities are encountered in only 1% of gynaecological patients, a variety of anomalies starting from aplasia, hypoplasia, atresia and nonfusion have been described. A new classification system given by the European Society of Obstetrics and Gynaecology is useful for describing various types of anomalies.
- A great majority of anomalies go undiagnosed, as they do not cause any interference in menstruation or reproduction.
- For symptomatic patients, investigations, such as hysterosalpingography, hysteroscopy and laparoscopy, are required to confirm and assess the degree of uterine malformation.
- Ultrasound, besides diagnosing genital tract malformation, can detect associated renal anomalies.
- Some abnormalities do not require correction if the woman is asymptomatic. Some are not amenable to correction. Some need plastic surgery to improve fertility, avoid pregnancy loss and solve gynaecological problems such as haematocolpos and haematometra.
- Vaginoplasty to create an artificial vagina requires surgical expertise. It restores sexual function.
- A rare condition of arterio-venous anastomosis causing menorrhagia. it is diagnosed by Doppler ultrasound and responds well to embolization of uterine arteries if excessive bleeding does not respond to medical treatment.

SELF-ASSESSMENT

1. Describe anomalies arising from the fusion defects of the Müllerian ducts.
2. What are the various complications which can occur during pregnancy associated with Müllerian anomalies?
3. How would you differentiate between Müllerian agenesis and testicular feminization syndrome (androgen insensitivity) as the cause of absent vagina?
4. Describe the various types of vaginoplasty.
5. Describe the investigations that assist in establishing the diagnosis of Müllerian anomalies, their limitations and comparative usefulness.

SUGGESTED READING

Bariar LM, Mohsin S, Hakim S, et al. McIndoe vaginoplasty. J Obstet Gynecol India 2002;52:145–6.

Bhadra D, Goswami S, Pradhan M, et al. Two unusual cases of hematometra in adolecent girls with simultaneous menstruation. J Obstet Gynecol India 2002;52:146.

Carrington BM, Hricak H, et al. Müllerian duct anomalies: MR imaging evaluation. Radiology 1990;176:715.

Chakravarty BN. Reconstructive Surgery in Infertility. In: Saraiya UB, Rao KA, chatterjee A (eds). Principles and Practice of Obstetrics and Gynecoogy for Postgraduates, 2nd ed. FOGGI Publication, New Delhi: Jaypee, 2003, p.452.

Dabirashrafi H, Bahadori M, et al. Septate uterus: New idea on the histologic features of the septum in this abnormal uterus. Am J Obstet Gynecol 1995;172:105.

Daly DC, Walters CA, Soto-Albors C. Hysteroscopic metroplasty: Surgical technique and obstetric outcome. Fertil Steril 1983;39:623.

Eli Reshef, Sanfilippo JS. Hysteroscopic evaluation and therapy of Müllerian anomalies. In: Quilligan EJ, Zuspan FP (eds). Current Therapy in Obstetrics and Gynecology. 5th ed. Philadelphia: W. B. Saunders Company; 2000. p. 77.

Evans TN, Poland M, Boving RL. Vaginal malformations. Am J Obstet Gynecol 1981;141:910.

Fedele L, Bianchi S, Marchini M, et al. Ultrastructural aspects of endometrium in infertile women with septate uterus. Fertil Steril 1996;65:750–2.

Frank RT. Formation of artificial vagina without operation. Am J Obstet Gynecol 1938;35:1053.

Green LK, Harris RE. Uterine anomalies. Frequency of diagnosis and associated obstetric complications. Obstet Gynecol 1976; 47:427.

Griffin JE, Edwards C, Madden JE, et al. Congenital absence of the vagina. The Mayer–Rokitansky–Kuster–Hauser syndrome. Ann Int Med 1976;85:224.

Grimbizis GF, Gordts S, Di Spiezio Sardo A, et al. The ESHRE/ESGE consensus on the classification of female genital tract congenital anomalies. Hum Reprod Oxf Engl. 2013;28(8):2032–2044. doi:10.1093/ humrep/det098.

Homer HA, Li TC, Cooke ID, et al. The septate uterus: A review of management and reproductive outcome. Fertil Steril 2000;73:1.

Ingram JN. The bicycle seat stool in the treatment of vaginal agenesis and stenosis: A preliminary report. Am J Obstet Gynecol 1982; 140:867–73.

Israel R, March CM. Hysteroscopic incision of the septate uterus. Am J Obstet Gynecol 1984;149:66.

Jones HW Jr. Reproductive impairment and the malformed uterus. Fertil Steril 1981;36:137.

Jophy R, Padmashi V, Jairaj P. Testicular feminization syndrome. J Obstet Gynecol India 2002;52:165.

Jotwani MJ, Godbole SV, Bhute SB, et al. Pregnancy in a rare case of unicornuate uterus after vaginoplasty. J Obstet Gynecol India 2003;53:84.

Kaur V, Dhar A. Double Uterus with obstructed hemivagina and Ipsilateral renal agenesis. J Obstet Gynecol India 2001;51:46.

Li S, Qayyum A, Coakley FV, et al. Association of renal agenesis and Müllerian duct anomalies. J Comput Assist Tomogr 2000;24:829.

McIndoe A. The treatment of congenital absence and obliterative condition of the vagina. Br J Plast Surg 1950;2:254–67.

Muller P, Musset R, Netter A, et al. State of upper urinary tract in patients with uterine malformations. Study of 133 cases. Presse Med 1967;75:1331.

Parikh MN. Congenital absence of vagina in MRHK syndrome. J Obstet Gynecol India 2000;50:128–30.

Proctor JA, Haney AF. Recurrent first trimester pregnancy loss is associated with uterine septum but not with bicornuate uterus. Fertil Steril 2003;80:1212.

Raga F, Bauser C, Remohi J, et al. Reproductive impact of congenital Müllerian anomalies. Hum Reprod 1997;12:2277.

Richardson DA, Evans MI, Talerman A, et al. Segmental absence of the mid-portion of the fallopian tube. Fertil Steril 1982;37:577.

Rock JA, Murphy AA, Jones HW. Surgery of the cervix. Am J Obstet Gynecol 1992;94:12.

Rock JA, Schlaff WD. The obstetric consequences of uterovaginal anomalies. Fertil Steril 1985;43:681.

Rock JA. Surgery for anomalies of the Müllerian ducts. In: Thompson JD, Rock JA (eds). TeLinde's Operative Gynecology. 7th ed. Philadelphia PA, J.B: Lippincott; 1992. p. 603–46.

Romer T, Lober R. Hysteroscopic correction of a complete septate uterus using a balloon technique. Hum Reprod 1997;12:478.

Puberty, Adolescence and Related Gynaecological Problems

6

CHAPTER OUTLINE

INTRODUCTION

It is being increasingly recognized as a fact that gynaecologic disorders can have their origin in childhood disorders such as congenital defects, neglected infections acquired in childhood, failure to diagnose and treat endocrinopathies in childhood, tumours overlooked and a general tendency to belittle physical and psychological trauma of sexual abuse. All these can cast their shadow on future reproductive health of the individual during adult life.

REPRODUCTIVE ENDOCRINOLOGY OF THE GROWING GIRL CHILD

During childhood, the endocrine changes in the growing female child are directed towards preparing her for the maturation of the hypothalamus–pituitary–ovarian–uterine axis to achieve full reproductive potential. The fetal hypothalamus (arcuate nucleus) begins to produce gonadotropin-releasing hormone (GnRH) by the 10th week of intrauterine life, gonadotropin secretion follows, levels of circulating follicle-stimulating hormone (FSH) and luteinizing hormone (LH) steadily rise up to the 20th week of gestation when the fetal hypothalamus becomes increasingly sensitive to the negative feedback inhibition of the placental steroids resulting in a rapid decline in levels of the circulating gonadotropins. With the birth and expulsion of the placenta, its inhibitory effect ceases and there is once again a transient rise in circulating levels of gonadotropins and a gradual decline to nadir by the age of 2–3 years. Throughout early childhood the levels of circulating gonadotropins continues to remain low, there is a minimal pituitary response to administered GnRH and the hypothalamic secretion of GnRH is profoundly suppressed.

The transition to puberty is characterized by episodic LH secretion associated with the circadian sleep–wake cycle. The rise in LH values becomes two to four times higher during sleep compared to the waking hours. This change is noted during the early phase of onset of puberty. Gradually, the levels of FSH begin to rise and reach a plateau at mid-puberty, and the LH levels continue to rise even thereafter until late puberty. Such changes are observed even in girls suffering from Turner syndrome indicating that these are not dependent on the ovarian steroid hormones but represent the effects of the rapidly maturing hypothalamic–pituitary relationship.

The sequential changes occurring in the growing girl child indicate that the initial development begins with progressively increasing GnRH secretion, which leads to increased pituitary sensitivity and responsiveness to GnRH stimulation. This results in rise in levels of circulating gonadotropins, which promote follicular development in the ovaries. The ovaries in response to the above stimulus produce oestrogens that act on the uterine endometrium to initiate proliferation and endometrial growth, a prelude to menarche. In time, the pulsatile secretion of GnRH is established followed by a cyclic ovarian function and regular menstrual cycles.

Once the hypothalamus becomes active, GnRH may prime the pituitary gonadotrops and increase its sensitivity to subsequent GnRH stimulation. A pulsatile pattern of GnRH secretion slowly evolves. The fact that earlier in the course of development, the GnRH manifests as low-frequency pulses favours FSH secretion, explaining why this is the first gonadotropin to register a rise. Later as the GnRH

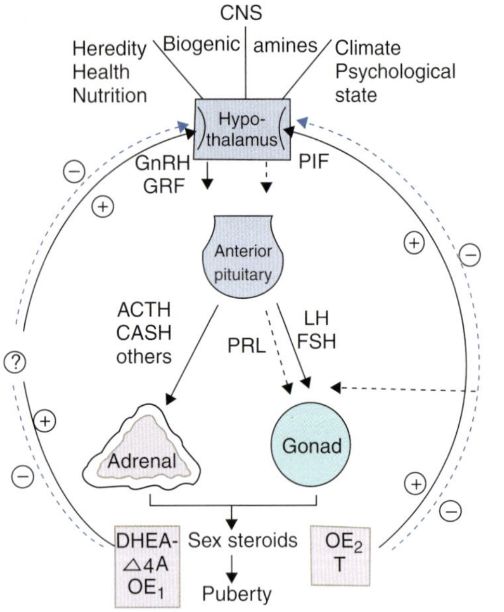

Figure 6.1 Neuroendocrinologic control of puberty. CASH, corticoadrenal-stimulating hormone.

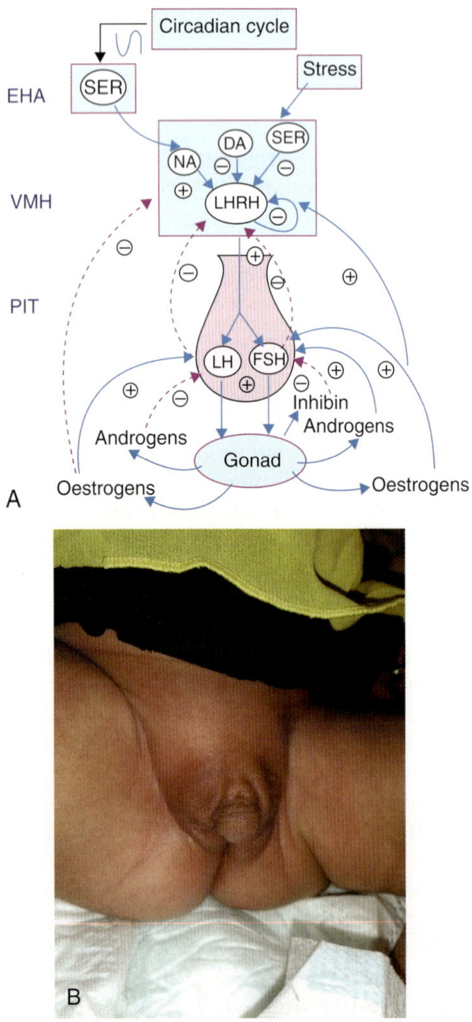

Figure 6.2 **(A)** Hypothalamic–pituitary–ovarian axis regulatory control. EHA, extrahypothalamic areas; VMH, ventral medial hypothalamus; PIT, pituitary; SER, serotonin; DA, dopamine; NA, noradrenalin. **(B)** Abnormal finding of clitoromegaly.

pulsatile frequency enhances, there is a greater rise in LH surges and establishment of the adult pattern of gonadotropin release. The positive feedback to oestrogen develops and the cyclic pattern of gonadotropin release and the normal menstrual cyclicity get established (Figs 6.1 and 6.2A).

THE NEWBORN FEMALE INFANT

History and physical examination – the newborn: The best time to begin documenting clinical observations is at birth. General examination should assess the gestational maturity of the neonate and document any abnormal findings such as webbing of the neck, ectopia vesicae, congenital ureteric fistula, imperforate anus, vaginal anus, congenital adrenal hyperplasia, the presence of inguinal hernia, umbilical hernia or abdominal mass suggestive of a genital tract abnormality, a bulging hymen (mucocolpos), clitoromegaly (Fig. 6.2B), ambiguous external genitalia, heterosexuality or true intersex. General physical examination begins with the examination of the breasts. At birth the breast nodule can be felt easily, and on squeezing, some clear to milky secretion can be often seen from the nipples (witch's milk) because of in utero fetus exposure to the high circulating levels of maternal oestrogens during pregnancy. This effect is transient and spontaneously resolves with the passage of time. The external genitalia should be examined under a good light keeping the newborn supine with the thighs well flexed against the abdomen. Once again oestrogen effects on the genitalia are apparent, the labia majora appears thick and full and tend to cover the labia minora, the clitoris appears prominent – the clitoral index (glans width × length) should not exceed 6.0 cm^2. Values exceeding this call for further investigations as clitoromegaly may be due to serious underlying causes such as congenital adrenal hyperplasia, which demands immediate attention and treatment in contrast to other causes such as true hermaphroditism and maternal exposure to androgens (teratogens – drugs having androgenic side effects or androgen-secreting tumours of the adrenals or ovaries).

On separation of the labia, it is not uncommon to observe a white mucoid discharge/blood which may persist for about 7–10 days. The vaginal orifice may be somewhat difficult to visualize, pressure on the vestibule often results in expression of mucous discharge, which confirms patency of the outflow tract; ultrasound examination of the pelvis clarifies the doubt. Assigning the correct sex/gender at birth is crucial.

THE GROWING GIRL CHILD

A young prepubertal girl child may be brought with complaints related to her private parts such as swelling, itching, offensive vaginal discharge, bleeding or injury. The examination of the prepubertal child calls for patient persuasion, gentleness, reassurance and skill and goes a long way in accomplishing a satisfactory examination. Sometimes the clinician may have to resort to sedation or even anaesthesia.

A vaginoscope/colposcope may be used to inspect the lower genital tract. Distension of the vagina with saline can be accomplished by holding the labia tightly around the vulval introitus; this may allow sufficient distension for a satisfactory inspection of the cervix, vaginal vault, health of the vaginal walls, detection of any neoplasm or the presence of any foreign body inserted inadvertently into the vagina. Endoscopic examination may be a satisfactory alternative to a difficult clinical examination.

The preschool girl child is best examined supine with her hips well abducted and the feet apposed (frog leg position), older child is best examined supine with her legs supported in stirrups. In young prepubertal girls, the labia majora appear flattened, the labia minora are thin and relatively prominent and the clitoris is small. On parting the labia or drawing the lower parts of the labia downwards and outwards, the vaginal orifice can be well visualized. The vaginal walls appear thin and congested, the transverse rugae present in adults are not seen, a midline longitudinal ridge may be present. If vaginal discharge is required for testing, this should be collected with a moist cotton tipped applicator, rubbing should be avoided as this not only causes discomfort but also can be traumatic to the thin and delicate vaginal epithelium. In the young prepubertal girl child, the vagina measures 4–5 cm, the cervix is twice the length of the uterus; the ovaries are located high up at the pelvic brim. Endocrine activity of the pituitary, ovaries and adrenal glands increasingly manifest between the ages of 7 and 10 years when increases in oestrogen effects on the genitalia become clinically evident. In case of suspected child sexual molestation or rape, the child may be better examined in the knee-chest position. In this position, the vagina balloons out and the introitus and hymen are easily visualized, the trauma of forced sexual assault is often apparent as laceration or tear of the introitus posteriorly. In this position, it is easier to collect discharge from the vagina for culture and forensic tests. The pelvic examination should be avoided in an adolescent girl, but when required, it is done under sedation of anaesthesia.

The vagina lengthens to 10–12 cm in a fully grown adolescent, the vagina becomes more capacious, the vaginal epithelium is thick with the presence of rugae and covered with a white acidic discharge and the vagina shows the presence of a mixed flora of nonpathogenic organisms. The cervix feels like a knob at the top of the vaginal vault and the uterus to cervix ratio reverses to 2:1. With approaching puberty, the ovaries descend into the pelvis and the ovaries show evidence of commencing follicular function.

COMMON PAEDIATRIC GYNAECOLOGIC PROBLEMS

The prepubertal girl child: The common problems for which medical opinion is sought broadly include following:

- Vulvovaginal infections and leucorrhoea
- Vaginal bleeding
- Ambiguous genitalia
- Abdominal neoplasms
- Sexual abuse
- Teenage – sexuality

The common gynaecologic problems affecting the prepubertal girl child for which consultation may be sought usually involve vulval pruritus, vaginal bleeding or discharge, developmental anomalies, suspected abdominal lump, precocious or late puberty and suspected sexual assault.

Although the genital structures are in the resting state during early childhood, they are not immune to diseases. The prepubertal female genitals are delicate and are prone to infection and bleeding.

Vulvovaginal infections, pruritus and discharge: Irritation or inflammation of the vulva may result from numerous causes. Infections (*molluscum contagiosum,* condylomata acuminata, herpes genitalis and gonorrhoea) may be transmitted through a sexual or nonsexual close contact with the child. Poor personal hygiene may lead to candidal vulvovaginitis, vulval irritation may follow worm infestation such as pin worms or thread worms secondary to anorectal contamination. Poor sexual hygiene may lead to chronic nonspecific vulvovaginitis and irritation leading to vulvitis causing labial adhesions. Exposure to chemicals (deodorants/antiseptics) may cause atopic dermatitis leading to a chronic discharge, vulvar skin excoriation and over time cause labial adhesions or eczematoid changes.

Vaginal discharge: This is generally the result of infection caused by nonspecific causes, generally resulting from poor hygiene or as a result of specific infections. Sometimes, it is caused by an inadvertent insertion of a foreign body by the child.

Nonspecific vulvovaginitis: This is best treated by initially improving perineal hygiene such as warm sitz baths, cleaning the perineal area with a bland olive oil followed by soap and water, keeping the parts dry and the use of clean cotton undergarments. Often these measures suffice. Vulvar medications should be prescribed sparingly as the skin of the genital region is very sensitive in children. In case of an unsatisfactory response in 2–3 weeks, consider topical application of an oestrogenic cream (Premarin/Dienesterol/Evalon). This brings about a thickening of the vaginal mucosa, lowers the vaginal pH and encourages growth of lactobacilli which in turn helps overcome offending bacterial infection. Oestrogen also helps to improve the vulvovaginal vascularity and produce rapid clinical improvement. Nonspecific vulvovaginitis can sometimes cause a copious foul-smelling blood-stained discharge secondary to anorectal contamination with *Escherichia coli, Streptococcus faecalis* or by *Shigella* organisms or by *intestinal parasites* such as thread worms or pin worms which respond to antihelminthic drugs. Finally, any offensive vaginal discharge that follows retention of a *foreign body* responds promptly to its removal.

Specific vulvovaginitis: Diagnosis should precede treatment. Sexually transmitted disorders require a specific treatment. Early diagnosis and treatment prevent sequelae. These infections have been specified in chapter on Sexually Transmitted Diseases. Labial adhesions caused by infection can be effectively managed by manual separation and local oestrogen cream.

Vaginal bleeding: This can be the result of simple treatable causes or be indicative of a more serious underlying cause requiring thorough investigation and a timely treatment.

Diagnostic approach: A history of the nature of bleeding and a general physical examination are essential to begin with. Smear and culture of the discharge if serosanguinous or purulent blood-stained and offensive are of fundamental importance. Smear of the discharge for cytologic evaluation is necessary whenever a neoplasm is suspected.

In difficult cases where localization of the cause of bleeding is not possible, a thorough examination under anaesthesia under a good light, and if necessary a direct endoscopic visualization using a paediatric cystoscope/hysteroscope helps to clear the diagnosis.

Common causes include endocrine causes, trauma, prolapsed urethra and neoplasms.

Endocrine causes include transient neonatal vaginal bleeding as a result of maternal circulating oestrogens in the newborn. Precocious puberty has been reported as early as the age of 6 years; however, the presence of other endocrine stigmata helps to resolve the diagnosis. Accidental ingestion of the mother's oral contraceptive (OC) pills resulting in bleeding has also been reported.

Trauma may be accidental; straddle-type injuries resulting from falling astride a sharp object may result in minor injuries such as lacerations, or a blunt injury may result in a vulval haematoma; the injuries caused by penetrating objects may be serious and may result in peritoneal trauma involving internal viscera requiring laparotomy. Self-inflicted during play or following sexual abuse may not be reported by the child for fear of remonstration. Examination under a good light coupled with a detailed history help to arrive at the cause. Precautions must be taken to ascertain and exclude the possibility of foreign body inserted in the vagina being overlooked.

Prolapsed urethra may follow undue physical exertion when the child complains of painful micturition, vulvar pain and bleeding. Separation of the labia reveals a mulberry-like protrusion at the site of the urethral orifice. It is possible to pass a soft rubber catheter through the centre of the mass and the bladder decompressed. The catheter may be left in situ for a few days, suitable antibiotic cover and analgesics should be prescribed. The oedematous mass may subside or undergo necrosis when after a few days it can be excised at the line of demarcation with a cutting cautery knife.

Condylomata acuminata are warty or granular lesions may bleed at times in a prepubertal child.

Sarcoma botryoides also known as grape-like sarcoma is a rare and highly malignant tumour of childhood carrying a serious prognosis.

Ambiguous genitalia: The recognition of genital abnormalities at an early age is important to determine the sex of rearing of the infant, and to chalk out plans for their correction, long-term management, prognosis and parental counselling.

The examination of the external genitalia is of primary importance. An enlarged phallus at birth raises the first doubt about ambiguous genitalia and the need for proper assigning of the sex of the child. The commonest cause of ambiguous genitalia (>90% cases) is adrenal hyperplasia which can have a serious prognosis if not promptly recognized and treated. The immediate concerns of the clinician in the salt-wasting type are to prevent rapid dehydration leading to fluid and electrolyte imbalance. The parents should be counselled that the external genitalia are incompletely formed and further investigations are warranted. As a working clinical rule, the presence of a midline frenulum on the phallus is strongly indicative of the infant being a genetic male, whereas paired attachment of the labia to the phallus suggests a genetic female. Clitoral enlargement with ambiguous genitalia at birth may be due to female pseudohermaphroditism, mixed gonadal dysgenesis, male pseudohermaphroditism and rarely true hermaphroditism. Usually the more pronounced the ambiguity, the simpler it is to raise the child as a female regardless of its genetic sex. History and clinical physical examination often throw considerable light on the possible cause – for example, history of administration of large doses of progestogens to the mother in early first trimester, or a family history of sexual ambiguity in other female relatives or a maternal aunt or another female relative who suffered from amenorrhoea or infertility with ambiguous genitalia is indicative of the possibility of a recessive genetic disorder. A history of surgery for inguinal hernia in early infancy with the unexpected finding of an undescended testis helps to identify the underlying aetiology.

The importance of examination of the newborn should include a rectal examination to determine the presence of the uterus at birth. Visualization of the hymen and testing its patency as discussed earlier is important. In case of doubt, sex chromatin studies and karyotype, imaging studies using ultrasound or MRI, hormone assays of gonadotropins (FSH and LH), 17-ketosteroids and 17 α-hydroxyprogesterone (which is elevated in 21-hydoxylase deficiency) are indicated for formulating a diagnosis. Estimations of serum electrolytes and blood glucose are important in the management of the salt-wasting variety of adrenal hyperplasia. Other investigational aids which may be of use include vaginoscopy, colpogram and laparoscopy. Rarely is an exploratory laparotomy required for diagnostic purposes alone. It is advisable to adopt a multidisciplinary approach to tackle the long-term management of the child. In the newborn infant, the diagnosis of the salt loosing adrenal hyperplasia as early as possible is important to institute a prompt treatment to avoid a serious outcome.

An imperforate hymen needs to be tackled at the time of puberty to forestall hydrocolpos/haematocolpos. Vaginal anomalies detected at birth do not call for immediate surgical intervention. Let the child grow up to the age of puberty. If pelvic imaging shows the presence of a well-developed uterus and ovaries, then the consideration for plastic surgery for an artificial vaginal reconstruction (partial or complete) becomes mandatory; however, in case of congenital absence of the vagina, in the absence of the uterus, postponing of the surgical procedure until the time of marriage is important, as coital frequency helps to maintain the patency of the vagina.

It must be remembered that in the case of suspected hermaphroditism, the undescended testis in the inguinal canal or intraabdominal situation should be surgically removed at puberty as it is prone to a malignant change with advancing age.

Tumours of gynaecological origin in children: The role of the gynaecologist is to be aware of the possible occurrence of tumours in childhood, and to be familiar with the investigations to arrive at the proper diagnosis and management plan. A large variety of swellings and tumours of diverse origins have been recognized in infancy and childhood. Many of these are not strictly of gynaecologic origin but enter the domain of differential diagnosis or are seen by the gynaecologist first, hence the need about their awareness. These include sacrococcygeal tumour, duplication cysts of the gastrointestinal tract (GI tract), urachal cyst, umbilical hernia, Wilms tumour, single pelvic kidney, lymphoma, haemangioma, chordoma, neuroblastoma, meningioma and hamartoma. Sarcoma botryoides is a rare and highly malignant tumour of childhood, it generally presents as a polypoidal of grape-like neoplasm protruding through the vulva. However, germ cell tumours of ovary are commonest tumours seen in this age group. Other common ovarian tumours are teratoma, yolk sac tumour, granulosa cell tumour.

A distended urinary bladder can present as a swelling in infancy and childhood. Ovarian tumours, both cystic and solid, are known to occur in children, and account for 1.0% of all neoplasms in premenarcheal children. Girls with ovarian neoplasms generally present with abdominal enlargement and pain. In the prepubertal child, the bulk (greater than 60%) of these tumours are of germ-cell origin (dermoids are the commonest; however, immature teratomas, embryonal cell tumours, endodermal sinus tumours, dysgerminomas, choriocarcinomas and gonadoblastomas have been recognized in childhood, many of these are malignant). Many of these tumours secrete substances such as alpha fetoproteins, carcinoembryonic antigen and human chorionic gonadotropin hormone which serve as tumour markers and help to arrive at a diagnosis. With approaching adolescence, the incidence of epithelial cell tumours of the ovary begin to make their appearance, so that in adult life epithelial tumours of the ovary predominate and account for almost 80% of all ovarian neoplasms. In India, the incidence of ovarian neoplasms in people younger than 20 years accounts for about 4%–14% of all ovarian neoplasms. About a third of the tumours tend to be malignant. Bulk of these is the germ cell tumours (dysgerminomas predominant); endodermal sinus tumours, teratomas and mixed cell types have a dismal outlook. The survival rates are encouraging in girls treated early for the disease.

Ultrasound examination of the abdomen and pelvis and CT/MRI scans are useful in establishing the diagnosis of ovarian neoplasms and assessing areas of solid and cystic components. Areas of calcification in degenerated parts of these tumours are not infrequent. A rare tumour of the lower genital tract namely sarcoma botryoides also affects children; it is a tumour posing a grave prognosis and should be tackled in a paediatric oncologic setting.

In general, all treatments should aim at conserving reproductive potential as far as possible without jeopardizing the patient's life. This is important to enable the growing child to achieve maturity and preserve future childbearing potential. The ovarian tumours have been detailed in chapter on Benign and Malignant Ovarian Tumours.

Child sexual abuse: Two basic forms of sexual abuse are recognized. The first involves victimization by a stranger; it may involve any form of sexual activity brought about by enticement, coercion or force. Such acts are usually reported by the child. This situation must be handled very tactfully. Appropriate medical examination and tests should be performed, counselling should be offered and efforts should be undertaken to bring the offender to book. The second form of sexual abuse rampant in society, and underreported is incest.

Incest occurs frequently in families with social problems of alcoholism, drug abuse, physical abuse, broken homes, violence, delinquency, mental retardation and an atmosphere of violence. Father–daughter relationships are the commonest, but it may involve any close male relative. Among children of incestuous relationship only 10% have normal psychological development. Anger, guilt feelings, mood swings, depression, lying, cheating and stealing are some bad habits these children develop; poor school performance often follows and unexplained physical complaints, sleep disturbances and aggressive behaviour are frequent manifestations. Rape leads to an immediate emotional shock and a feeling of anger all around. Tactful handling and timely psychiatric help give the child the best chance of coming out of the experience unscathed.

Sex education and female sexuality: Fifty years ago, parental supervision and early marriages prevented young individuals from experimenting with sexuality. Changes in societal behaviour, freer interaction between the sexes, influence of the media and greater involvement of women in the workforce have led to changing moral and ethical values and altered adolescent behaviour. The fact that almost 10% of pregnancies occur in teenagers, nearly 5%–8% of reported medical termination of pregnancy (MTPs) are in teenagers and 6% of all deaths from unsafe abortions occur in teenagers emphasizes the need for imparting sex education to senior school and college-going adolescents to prevent unwanted pregnancies, MTPs, sexually transmitted diseases (STDs) and HIV (Mukherjee, 1999).

PUBERTY AND ADOLESCENCE

BIOLOGICAL SEQUENTIAL EVENTS OBSERVED DURING PUBERTY

Adolescence is the age between 10 and 19 years. Puberty is the period of transition from childhood to adult sexual maturation. It is the process of biological, psychological and physical development through which sexual reproduction becomes possible. Progression occurs through sequential changes described as thelarche → adrenarche → peak growth spurt → menarche → ovulation. The interval between the breast development and menarche is 2–3 years. Hormonal events earlier described play a key role in orchestrating this transition. Profound bodily changes, sexual development and altered emotional and behavioural changes are observed during this maturational period. Besides endocrinal influences, genetic, nutritional and other environmental factors play an important role during this transitional period of life.

Insulin-like growth factors peak level coincides with E_2 level. Initially FSH is released at night at first followed later by an LH pulse. The level of growth hormones doubles during this growth period.

Endocrine mechanisms underlying puberty: These have been highlighted in the following:

- Early in puberty, the sensitivity of the gonadostat to the negative effects of low estradiol (E_2) gradually decreases.
- Late in puberty, maturation of positive E_2 feedback initiates the LH surge.
- Basal levels of pituitary gonadotropins increase throughout puberty due to an enhanced hypothalamic GnRH pulse amplitude rather than frequency.

Age of onset of puberty: The age of onset is influenced by nutritional status, genetic and environmental influences including racial and cultural background, climate and residence. Hence a great deal of variations is observed in the evolution of puberty changes. Normal age of puberty varies between 9 and 13 years, and the duration lasts 2–3 years. Although the beginning of puberty is subtle and cannot be dated precisely, the end point is menstruation (menarche).

Over the last century, the age of menarche has progressively lowered; this has been very evident in the developed world including the West and Japan. Also menarche occurs later in women residing at higher altitudes as seen in Eskimos. A critical body mass has to be achieved prior to menarche, obesity predisposes to earlier age of menarche (minimum of 45 kg).

When environmental factors are optimal, puberty is controlled by genetic factors as witnessed by the fact that the age interval between the times of menarche in identical twins is 2.2 months that between dizygotic twins is 8.2 months.

FACTORS AFFECTING TIME OF ONSET OF PUBERTY

- Genetics
- Race. The African-American girls enter puberty about 1–1.5 years earlier than the White American girls
- Nutritional status. Puberty sets in earlier in moderately obese girls and is delayed in malnourished girl. Leptin (peptide) secreted by the fat cells stimulate GnRh secretion and induce early puberty. Minimum of a 45 kg body weight is required to induce pubertal changes. Macrosomic babies tend to grow obese and have early menarche thereby.
- General health status
- Altitude. Delayed in Eskimo girls compared to girls living in the tropics
- Psychological state. Exposure to education, media
- Exposure to light (blind individuals enter puberty earlier than sighted individuals)

Growth spurt and menstruation: The starting of the physical growth curve is soon followed by a typical sequence of development of female secondary sexual characteristics, which include thelarche, adrenarche, continuing growth spurt genital organ growth and menarche. These will hereafter be discussed at length.

Tunner and Marshall described five stages of pubertal changes – these are in the following sequences (Fig. 6.3A):

- Physical growth and weight gain
- Development of breasts
- Pubic and axillary hair
- Development of ovaries and genital organs
- Growth spurt and menstruation

Gordon et al. (2002) depicted the physical changes occurring during puberty as follows:

A comparison of the growth rates in male and female growing children reveals a similar curve until the age of 10.5 years (the male growth being somewhat ahead throughout, thereafter the growth spurt in the female child overtakes that of the male child for 1–2 years before it plateaus out). However, the growth curve in the male child demonstrates the final spurt a couple of years later before plateauing. Thus, the average mean height of a fully grown man is greater than that in woman as shown in Fig. 6.4.

PHYSICAL GROWTH AND BODY WEIGHT

The growth in the height and weight in the female child begins on average around the age of 10.5 years (average of 9–11 years) and is completed by the age of 14 years. During this period, the height growth that stabilizes at 4–10 cm/year before puberty doubles during puberty (5–10 cm/year). Growth is attributed to growth-promoting hormone of the anterior pituitary, and also by insulin-like growth factor (IGF-1). The body shape also takes on the feminine configuration. The bone mass during adolescence increases by 50%, emphasizing the importance of providing adequate calcium, iron and nutritional needs during the growing years of adolescence. Iron requirement increases by 15%.

SECONDARY SEX CHARACTERS (SSC) – TANNER CLASSIFICATION OF THE SEQUENCE OF DEVELOPMENT

THELARCHE

The first sign of puberty is the development of the breasts. Breast budding usually appears between the ages of 9 and 11 years; it is indicative of the competency of the hypothalamic–pituitary–ovarian axis. The adolescent breast development is divided into five stages:

B1 – denotes the prepubertal breast. At this infantile stage only the papilla is elevated.

B2 – denotes thelarche. The breast buds are palpable, areola enlarges and the breast is elevated like a small mound.

B3 – there is further enlargement of the breast and its areola without separation of its contours.

B4 – preferential growth of the areola and nipple leads to formation of a secondary mound over the mound of the breast.

B5 – formation of the mature adult breast. There is recession of the areola into the general contour of the breast because of greater growth of the breast tissue (Fig. 6.3B).

ADRENARCHE

The adrenals are the main source of androgens, which are responsible for the growth of pubic and axillary hair. Pubic hair generally make its appearance about 6 months after thelarche at the B4 stage. Axillary hair generally make their appearance 1–2 years after pubarche. Rarely axillary hair development precedes pubic hair development.

PUBIC HAIR DEVELOPMENT

The stages of pubic hair growth are as follows:

P1 – prepubertal stage when there are no coarse pubic hair present, the vellus hair present over the pubic area are similar to the ones seen over the abdominal wall.

P2 – pubarche denotes the appearance of long or slightly curved and pigmented hair sparsely over the labia.

P3 – darker, coarser and curly hair are seen spread over the mons pubis.

P4 – the preadult stage when thick dark growths of curly hair are seen covering the area short of the inverted triangle.

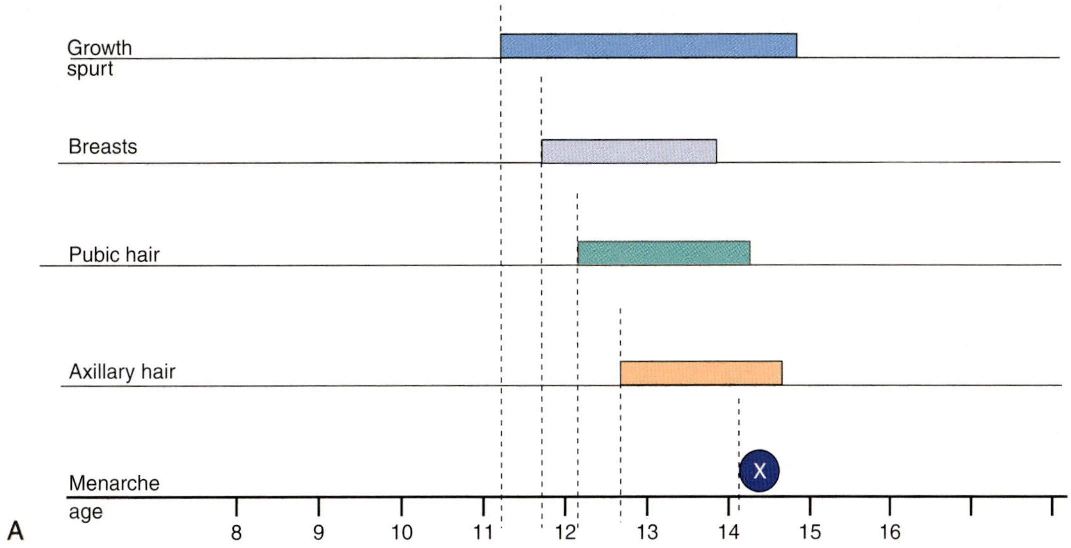

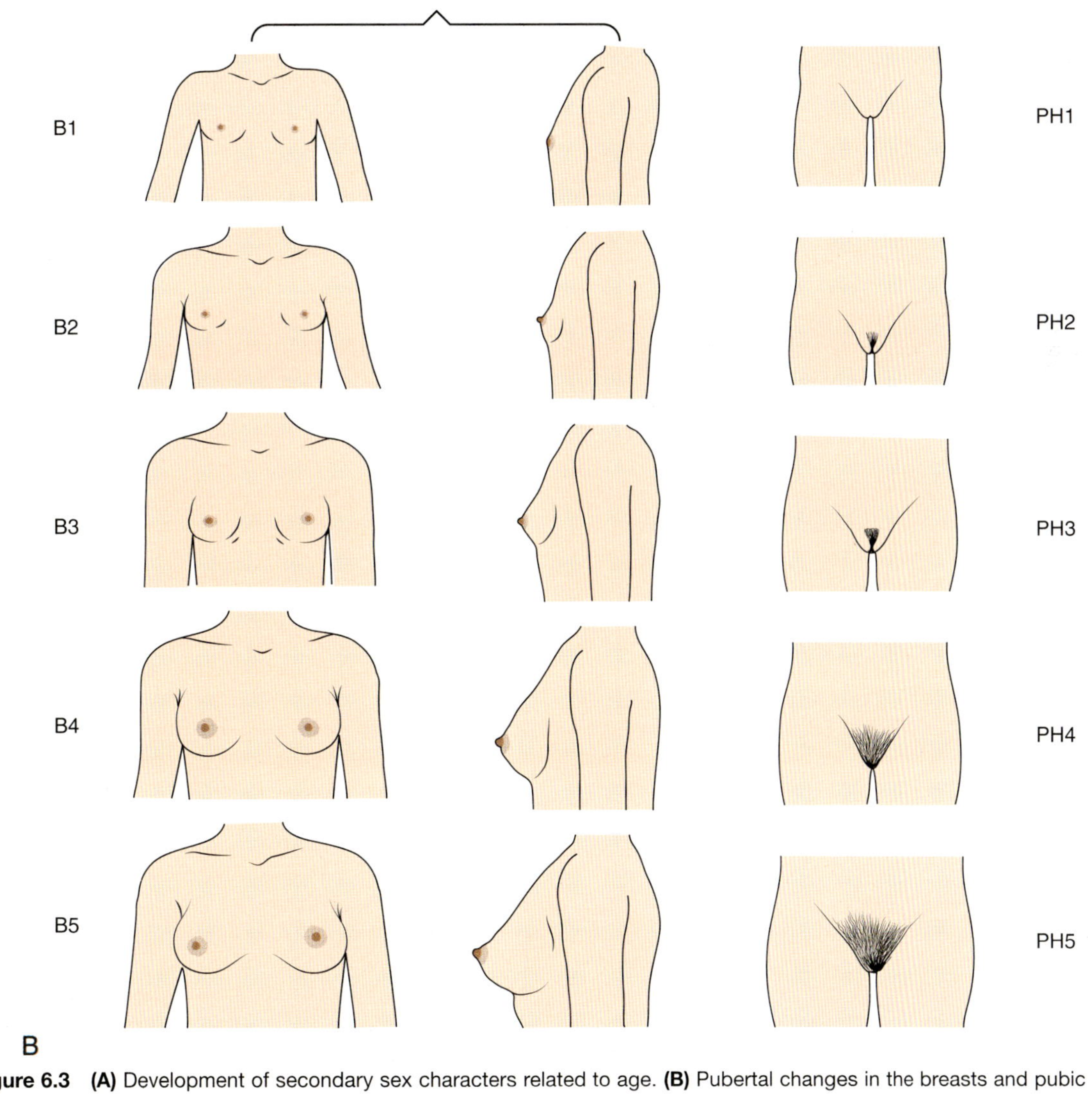

Figure 6.3 **(A)** Development of secondary sex characters related to age. **(B)** Pubertal changes in the breasts and pubic hair.

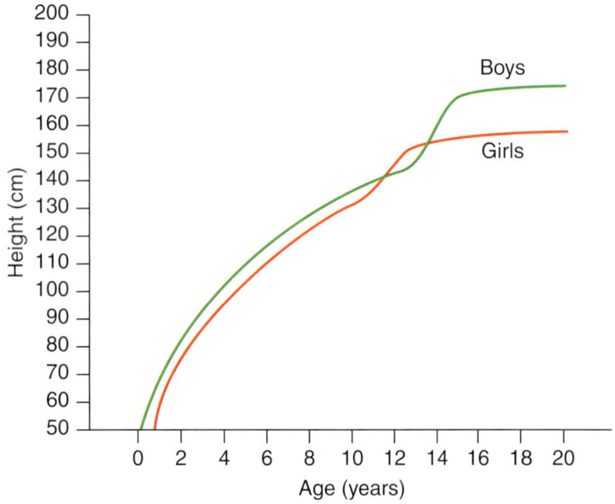

Figure 6.4 Height attained growth curves for boys and girls showing growth spurt.

P5 – adult inverted triangular distribution of thick, coarse, dark curly hair spreading out towards the medial aspects of the thighs is evident.

Increased secretion of dehydroepiandrosteronesulphate (DHAS) is responsible for growth of pubic hair.

AXILLARY HAIR DEVELOPMENT

The sequence of axillary hair development is as follows:

A1 – prepubertal stage. No axillary hair present.
A2 – appearance of sparse axillary hair.
A3 – adult distribution of thick, coarse and dark pigmented hair.

GENITAL ORGANS

- Vulva – vulval skin under the influence of oestrogen becomes keratinized and resistant to infection. Fat is deposited in the labia majora.
- Vaginal mucosa becomes multilayered with the formation of superficial layer containing glycogen and PH is maintained at 4.5 by Döderlein's bacillus acting on glycogen.
- The uterus grows rapidly, and prepubertal ratio of uterus/cervix of 1:1 changes to 2:1 or 3:1.
- The ovaries start developing primordial follicles into Graafian follicles. However, a dominant follicle with ovulation occurs in 50% cases. Rest take 1–2 years for ovulatory cycles to occur.

MENARCHE

The first menstrual period generally follows thelarche by about 2 years, when growth development is almost complete and breast development reaches the adult mature stage. The initial menstrual cycles are generally anovulatory for about 12–18 months after menarche, presenting with irregular cycles without dysmenorrhoea.

SKELETAL AGE

Sexual maturation correlates more with bone age than chronological age.

Determination of bone age provides a better marker for prediction of the remaining growth potential and the final adult height.

MANAGEMENT

Although puberty is a transitional physiological period, lack of knowledge regarding various physical changes and fear of future impose stress and anxiety in these adolescent girls, though lately they have acquired a better knowledge than before. Psychological and emotional changes need to be taken note of and adequately managed.

- Sex education is very useful in schools. The knowledge regarding STD, HIV and risk of pregnancy will dissuade them from indulging in premarital sex. Where promiscuity prevails, contraceptives should be encouraged. Barrier method protects against STD, and oral pills protect against pregnancy.
- Nutrition from protein, calcium and iron are required for the growth and maintaining haemoglobin; calcium need increases by 50% and iron by 15%.
- Lately, HPV vaccination is strongly recommended for adolescents, especially if they indulge in sexual activity.
- Quadrivalent vaccine is given at 0, 2, 6 months.
- Bivalent vaccine is given at 0, 1, 6 months.

PUBERTY – ANOMALIES OF GONADAL FUNCTION

Delayed puberty is defined when the secondary sexual characters do not appear by the age of 14 and menarche is not established by 16 years of age (10%).

Primary amenorrhoea and delayed puberty: Causes for these conditions can be broadly divided into hypogonadal and eugonadal varieties. Patients with hypogonadism may have hypergonadotropism secondary to ovarian failure (Turner) or hypogonadism as a result of failure of maturation of the hypothalamic–pituitary–ovarian relationship. The eugonadal variety consists of patients with evidence of steroidogenesis but delayed menarche. In this group the possibility of primary amenorrhoea due to other causes such as Müllerian developmental anomalies leading to outflow obstruction, less commonly testicular feminization syndrome (androgen insensitivity), failure of development of the positive feedback mechanism in spite of adequate endogenous oestrogen production and hyperprolactinaemia often resulting from a pituitary neoplasm (prolactinoma) should be suspected. Malnutrition and anorexia nervosa are other causes. Details are described in chapter on Amenorrhoea.

Aetiology of delayed puberty:

- Commonly, it is familial or idiopathic (60%).
- Kallmann syndrome – Hypothalamic and pituitary inadequacy. CT, MRI of sella turcica, FSH, LH level confirm the diagnosis.
- Ovarian causes – Turner syndrome, Swyer syndrome, resistant ovary, autoimmune disease, testicular feminizing syndrome, high FSH.
- Polycystic ovarian disease.

- Development of secondary sexual characters, but no menstruation – absent uterus or cryptomenorrhoea, obstruction in the lower genital tract.
- Malnutrition, anorexia nervosa, childhood illness and vigorous exercise.
- Hypothyroidism.

Investigations and management – see chapter on Primary and Secondary Amenorrhoea.

Anorexia nervosa is being increasingly recognized and treated with the help of a psychiatrist. Identification of the group of patients who exhibit pubertal maturation but fail to develop a positive feedback system for establishing appropriate LH surges required for triggering ovulation. In the long term, these individuals with chronic anovulation are at risk of developing endometrial hyperplasia and malignancy.

Approach to diagnosis: All patients after the age of 14 years manifesting the absence of breast development and oestrogen effects need to be investigated. Besides a detailed history and physical examination including record of height in centimetres and weight in kilograms, the following investigations are recommended:

1. Serum FSH, LH, PRL and TSH, steroid hormone assays including androgens
2. CT scan of the skull
3. Buccal smear for sex chromatin determination
4. Karyotype, G-banding, polymerase chain reaction and fluorescent Y testing
5. Ultrasound to detect uterine anomalies and the presence of the ovary
6. Laparoscopy in selected patients

TREATMENT OF DELAYED PUBERTY

1. Treat the cause following investigations and diagnosis.
2. When no cause found, oestrogen and progestogen initiate menstruation and regular cycles, allow proper growth and height, secondary sexual characteristics and also prevent osteoporosis. Most respond well and have no adverse effect on future reproduction.

Precocious puberty: This is defined as the appearance of any of the secondary sexual characteristics before the age of 8 years or the occurrence of menarche before the age of 10 years (Fig. 6.5). It is not a common clinical entity. Broadly speaking, precocious puberty can be divided into two types. The first variety (known as true, complete or isosexual precocious puberty) results from the premature activation of the endocrine pathway comprising the hypothalamic–pituitary–ovarian axis. In such girls, the total growth spurt and potential increase in height is not achieved, hence it is necessary to identify the possibility early and advocate a prompt treatment to delay the maturation process to enable the child to achieve increase in height. In contrast, the second variety known as the pseudo or incomplete precocious puberty is the result of sex steroid stimulation independent of the above axis.

True precocious puberty: When there is premature maturation of hypothalamic–pituitary axis with increased production of GnRH, it is called true precocious puberty. There is cyclical ovulation in these girls. Such girls are at a risk of pregnancy and sexual abuse. At least 85% cases of precocious puberty belong to this variety. This is mostly as a result of constitutional factor or CNS disorders.

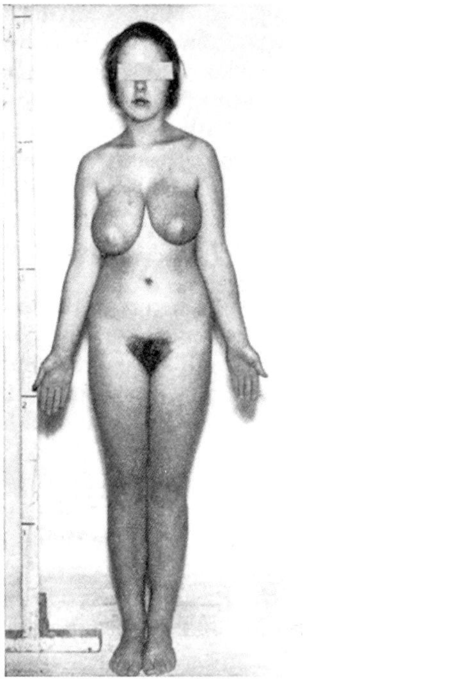

Figure 6.5 Precocious puberty – a girl aged 11 years. Note well-marked breast development and adult pubic hair growth.

Pseudoprecocious puberty: Elevated level of oestrogen, and other hormones because of ovarian or adrenal tumours or intake of hormone containing tablets results in pseudoprecocious puberty. This variety is associated with vaginal bleeding and other changes but there is no cyclical ovulation or risk of pregnancy.

Aetiological classification of precocious puberty: The various causes are as follows:

1. *Complete precocious puberty:*	a) Idiopathic, familial or sporadic, genetic (75%) b) Congenital lesions of the *hypothalamus–pituitary* Acquired lesions – trauma, infection, neoplasm – tuberculosis (TB) meningitis in childhood c) Part of a specific syndrome – McCune–Albright (5%), von Recklinghausen's neurofibromatosis d) Other causes – endocrine/ metabolic disorders
2. *Incomplete precocious puberty:*	a) Premature thelarche b) Premature adrenarche c) Premature menarche
3. *Pseudoprecocious puberty: (GnRH independent)*	a) Feminizing ovarian tumours (10%) (hormone secreting) b) Adrenal hyperplasia/ neoplasm – 20% c) Hypothyroidism d) Hepatoblastoma producing gonadotropins e) Iatrogenic–oestrogen administration

In more than 90% of cases, no organic lesion is detected. The hypothalamus–pituitary–ovarian axis and the adrenal functions mature early resulting in precocious puberty.

Pregnancy in a young girl aged 6 years has been recorded. Investigations reveal that gonadotropins and ovarian steroid hormones are secreted in adult quantities.

A number of skull problems such as rickets can cause precocious puberty. Tumours at the base of the brain such as craniopharyngioma, pituitary tumours, optic glioma, teratomas and astrocytomas may be contributory causes. Infections such as encephalitis, meningitis and hydrocephalus have also been implicated.

Clinical features of precocious puberty: The commonest variety termed constitutional precocity tends to run in families. It must be borne in mind that this diagnosis is one of exclusion. Long-term follow-up is recommended as some of the cerebral conditions come to light only in adulthood. Sexual precocity is consistent with a normal reproductive function, and is not related to early onset of menopause. In these children, the sequence of events of sexual maturation follows the normal standard pattern. The growth spurt occurs at an earlier age, so there is a transient but short-lived increase in height. As the epiphysis of the long bones fuse early under premature oestrogen effects, there is an eventual stunting of the height. Intellectual, psychosexual and emotional development correspond to the chronological age; hence, these youngsters and their families have to face potentially difficult social and emotional situations.

McCune–Albright syndrome affects about 5% of children with precocious puberty. Multiple cystic bone lesions are seen. Café-au-lait spots on the skin may be evident at birth. Menstruation sets in early independent of the customary sequence events of thelarche and adrenarche preceding menarche. This is attributed to the autonomous production of oestrogens by the ovaries. Eventual fertility remains unimpaired and the adult height attained.

In every case of sexual precocity, the possibility of an underlying functional hormone-secreting tumour of the ovary must be entertained and its possibility excluded.

Investigations: The following investigations are recommended:

1. Radiograph of the wrist to establish bone age.
2. Thyroid function tests – T_3, T_4, and TSH. TSH stimulates FSH receptors.
3. EEG and CAT/MRI scan of the skull.
4. Adrenal function tests to exclude heterosexual precocity.
5. Pelvic sonography to exclude pelvic neoplasms.
6. GnRH test to exclude autonomous ovarian cysts from those secondary to gonadotropin stimulation. GnRH test – i.v. 20 mcg/kg GnRH – estimate LH level 30 minutes later; level $>$ 9.2 IU/L indicates true precocious puberty (GnRH related).
7. FSH, LH, oestrogen levels.

Management: Precocious puberty is a disturbing development for the parents and child. All efforts must be undertaken to detect the underlying cause. However, the cause may not be apparent and may be detected only later in life. Parents should be counselled accordingly. Parents should be warned that the child is vulnerable to sexual assault and needs careful supervision.

A proper treatment should be instituted for hypothyroidism, adrenal hyperplasia and surgical intervention for tumours of the ovary, adrenals or of neurological origin.

Drug treatment of constitutional precocity includes:

1. Inj. depot medroxyprogesterone acetate (DMPA) 100–200 mg, i.m. every 2–4 weeks to induce regression of these changes and cessation of menstruation. It is however not very efficient in inhibiting bone growth. Treatment depresses adrenocortical and hypothalamic–pituitary activities. Instead of injection, daily or cyclical progestogen avoids injections, but are not convenient.
2. Cyproterone acetate exerts antiandrogenic and antigonadotropin effects. Oral administration of 70–150 mg/m^2/day has been found to be superior to DMPA. It also helps in increase of height and stature. Adrenal suppression is a known side effect.
3. GnRH agonists (Buserelin) form the mainstay of the treatment in present-day practice.

The monthly administration of depot preparations allows pubertal development to be arrested temporarily until the full height potential has been achieved and the child reaches the appropriate age for the onset of puberty.

- Buserelin 100 mcg nasal spray daily.
- Leuprolide 7.5 mg monthly. A single implant of histrelin – effect lasts for 1 year.
- Triptorelin 11.25 mg 3 monthly for 1 year with calcium and vitamin D to prevent osteoporosis 20 mcg.

In precocious puberty, future reproductive capacity is not compromised and premature menopause is not documented.

Calcium and vitamin D supplementation is required to prevent drug-related osteoporosis.

ADOLESCENT CONTRACEPTION

This is a complex subject. Cultural, religious, socioeconomic and educational factors impact it. Understanding adolescent sexuality and the emotional need of youth help in the proper and effective implementation of this increasingly important social and health goal. Teenage sex can be viewed as a normal behaviour development and milestone, or a risk behaviour pattern which may lead to serious consequences beyond the adolescent's comprehension.

Children from poor socioeconomic strata of society, living in crowded localities, disrupted families and states of depression and unhappiness as well as teenagers from the affluent classes are prone to experiment with sex.

Premarital sex can end in acquiring STDs and unwanted pregnancy.

Recommended contraceptive methods: Adolescents should be informed about sexuality, the importance of self-control and abstinence until a more responsible age. However, growing adolescents resent sermonizing and are more responsive when their individuality is respected. Information about contraception is necessary to equip them to face real-life situations.

OC are in general preferred as these safeguard the adolescent girl against any unwanted pregnancies. These OC pills also confer the advantage of regular periods with modest flow, and freedom from discomfort. In case of girls in an unstable relationship with a male partner, insistence on the additional use of barrier contraception by the male partner is desirable to protect her against STDs.

Emergency contraception should be made available in case of contraception failure such as condom slippage/condom bursting/forgotten use. The contraceptives for adolescents have been detailed in chapter on Temporary and Permanent Methods of Contraception.

MTP services. Access to these back-up services should be available to unmarried adolescents

MISCELLANEOUS PROBLEMS

Apart from the more pertinent problems discussed earlier, adolescents are subject to other health problems which will be discussed briefly hereafter.

1. ***Puberty menorrhagia:*** Soon after the menarche, the early menstrual cycles tend to be irregular and often prolonged leading to severe anaemia.
2. ***Dysmenorrhoea:*** In adolescents, the menstrual cycles tend to be irregular and anovulatory to begin with, however, in the following 12–18 months, with maturing of the endocrine axis, the cycles become more regular, ovulation sets in and the periods become painful. Spasmodic dysmenorrhoea can be severe enough to require medication. Drugs such as mefenamic acid 500 mg, twice daily, help to control the pain. This drug acts by virtue of inhibiting the enzyme prostaglandin synthetase.
3. ***Hirsutism:*** The causes of the masculine distribution of coarse hair can be psychologically disturbing to the individual. The causes can be broadly classified as follows:
   (a) Idiopathic
   (b) Ovarian
      (i) Polycystic ovarian disease
      (ii) Pure gonadal dysgenesis
      (iii) Virilizing ovarian tumours such as arrhenoblastoma, hilar cell tumour, gynandroblastoma, lipoid cell tumour
   (c) Adrenal
      (i) Congenital adrenal hyperplasia of the delayed variety
      (ii) Virilizing adrenal tumours
      (iii) Cushing syndrome
   (d) Iatrogenic
      (i) Anabolic agents
      (ii) Androgenic drugs such as danazol
4. ***Endometriosis:*** Thought to be of ***rare occurrence*** in India, recent investigational advances such as pelvic sonography and laparoscopy have revealed that this disease can also occur in adolescence and be the cause of severe dyspareunia, dysmenorrhoea and chronic pelvic pain.

Acne is common among adolescent girls. For treatment, refer to chapter on Diseases of the Ovary.

KEY POINTS

- Puberty is a transition from childhood to adulthood and involves physical, biological, endocrinological and psychological changes.
- Normal age of puberty in females is 9–14 years. Puberty is precocious when the secondary sexual characters appear before the age of 8 years and menstruation begins before the age of 10 years. The most common type of precocious puberty is constitutional, but other causes should be excluded. It is desirable to suppress menstruation until the appropriate age is reached to allow the girl to reach the height.
- Delayed puberty is the absence of features of puberty by the age of 16 years may be familial or idiopathic, but requires investigations.
- Puberty menorrhagia can cause anaemia needing blood transfusion and supportive treatment.
- Acne may be due to PCOD and should be treated.

SELF-ASSESSMENT

1. Describe the endocrinology of puberty.
2. Describe Tanner classification of development of female secondary sex characteristics.
3. Describe the causes of delayed puberty.
4. Write short notes on adolescent contraception.
5. Discuss the problems of teenage pregnancies.
6. Discuss the causes and management of abnormal uterine bleeding in adolescence.
7. What are the common causes of hirsutism in female adolescents?

SUGGESTED READING

The American College of Obstetricians and Gynecologists. Health Care for Adolescents. Washington, D.C., ACOG, 2003 Education Pamphlets.

Berek JS, Adashi EY, Hillard PA (eds). On Puberty. Novak's Gynaecology. 12th Ed. Philadelphia, Williams & Wilkins, 1996.

Delamarre-von de-Waal HA. Regulation of puberty. Best Pract Res Clin Endocrinol Metab 2002; 16: 1.

Droegemueller W, Herbst AL, Mishell DR, Stenchever MA (eds). Pediatric gynecology. Comprehensive Gynecology. 1st Ed. USA, CV Mosby & Co. 1987; 231.

Gordon JD, Speroff L. Abnormal puberty and growth problems. Handbook for Clinical Gynecologic Endocrinology & Infertility. Philadelphia, Lippincott-Raven, 2002; 199.

Kaplowitz P. Clinical Characteristics of 104 children referred for evaluation of precocious puberty. J Clin Endocrinol Metab 2004;89(8): 3644.

Palmer MR, Boepple PA. Variations in timing of puberty. Clinical spectrum and genetic investigation. J Clin Endocrinol Metabol 2001;86: 2364.

Speroff L, Glass RH, Kase NG (eds). Normal and abnormal sexual development. Clinical Gynecologic Endocrinology and Infertility. 4th Ed. Philadelphia, Williams & Wilkins, 1999; 379.

7 Menopause and Related Problems

CHAPTER OUTLINE

INTRODUCTION

Menopause is a physiological and natural event in the life of a woman. It is characterized by the permanent cessation of menstruation. Most women anticipate such an event as age advances. However, few women develop a sense of fear with approaching menopause thinking that it might lead to a loss of femininity, lack of interest by husband and fear of ageing.

The process leading to the final onset of menopause is determined by the number of oogonia present in the ovaries at birth, the rate of atresia during reproductive years and the hormonal interplay regulated by the hypothalamic–pituitary–ovarian axis.

PERIMENOPAUSE (CLIMACTERIC)

Perimenopause is a period of 3–4 years before actual menopause is characterized by a number of changes in body due to declining levels of hormones produced by the ovary. These changes may be in the form of mood changes, hot flushes, generalized weakness and alterations in menstrual pattern. Most women accept these changes and anticipate the onset of actual menopause in near future. However, for some women such changes produce anxiety, fear of cancer, etc. A careful and sympathetic counselling by health care provider may allay her fears and prepare her mentally for approaching menopause. A general physical examination, pelvic examination and common investigations are reassuring for patient.

Perimenopause is followed by 1 year of amenorrhoea. This period is associated with a mild ovarian hormonal deficiency leading to anovulation and menstrual disorders, especially menorrhagia, and sometimes obesity.

Apart from general health check-up to rule out cardiovascular disorder, diabetes and hypertension, a pelvic examination mammography, ultrasound, bone density and Pap smear may be advisable to assure the woman of her good health.

Management comprises the following:

- Diet, advice on smoking and alcohol, calcium supplementation and exercise will help. Smoking is toxic to the follicles and causes rapid metabolism of oestrogen in the liver and is, hence antiestrogenic.
- Counselling on contraception will help. Intrauterine contraceptive devices and oral combined pills are not recommended on account of irregular bleeding and risk of thrombosis, respectively. Surgical method is not required for a short period of fertility. Progestogen-only pills may cause irregular bleeding. Barrier contraceptive is the safest method.
- If a woman has fibroids, a short course of GnRH or Mirena IUCD can shrink the fibroid and avoid hysterectomy. Dysfunctional uterine bleeding requires investigations.
- The woman needs guidance on menopausal symptoms. The need for hormone replacement therapy (HRT) will be discussed later.

DIAGNOSIS OF APPROACHING MENOPAUSE

1. A fall in the level of inhibin B (not inhibin A) causes a rise in follicle-stimulating hormone (FSH) level. FSH> 40IU/L is reported.
2. Rise of FSH level and leutinizing hormone (LH) level elevated more than normal values.
3. A fall in the level of anti-Müllerian hormone suggests a low ovarian reserve and low antral follicular count.

Study of FSH level on day 2–5 after the last menstrual period detects premenopausal stage.

MENOPAUSE

Menopause is defined as the cessation of ovarian function resulting in permanent amenorrhoea. It takes 12 months of amenorrhoea to confirm that menopause has set in, and therefore it is a retrospective diagnosis.

Climacteric is the phase of waning ovarian activity, and may begin 2–3 years before menopause and continue for 2–5 years after it. The climacteric is thus a phase of adjustment between the active and inactive ovarian function and occupies several years of a woman's life, and it involves physical, sexual and psychological adjustments.

DEMOGRAPHY

Sixty million women in India are older than 55 years. With women living longer than before, a majority would spend one-third of their life in the postmenopausal stage. The health problems cropping up during this period and their relationship to oestrogen deficiency of menopause are now obvious and better understood. It is important therefore to address all these menopause-related diseases and apply prophylactic measures so that these women can lead an enjoyable and healthy life. An average Indian woman now lives up to 65 years, whereas in the developed countries a lifespan up to 80 years is possible.

AGE

Menopause sets in when the follicular number falls below 1000. Menopause normally occurs between the ages of 48 and 52 years, the average age being 49 years. It is not uncommon, however, to see a woman menstruate well beyond the age of 50 years. This delayed menopause may be related to good nutrition and better health. Late menopause is also common in women suffering from uterine fibroids and those at high risk of endometrial cancer. Menopause setting before the age of 40 years is known as **premature menopause.**

Menopausal age is not related to menarche, race, socioeconomic status, number of pregnancies and lactation or taking of oral contraceptives. It is however directly associated with smoking and genetic disposition. Smoking induces premature menopause. Most reliable predictor of age of menopause may be the age of menopause in her sister and mother.

PATHOPHYSIOLOGY

During climacteric, ovarian activity declines. Initially, ovulation fails, no corpus luteum forms and no progesterone is secreted by the ovary. Therefore, the premenopausal menstrual cycles are often anovulatory and irregular. Later, Graafian follicles also fail to develop, oestrogenic activity is reduced and endometrial atrophy leads to amenorrhoea. The cessation of ovarian activity and a fall in the oestrogen and inhibin levels cause a rebound increase in the secretion of FSH and LH by the anterior pituitary gland. The FSH level may rise as much as 50-fold and LH three- to fourfold. Menopausal urine has become an important commercial source of human menopausal gonadotropin (hMG). With further advancing years, gonadotropin activity of the pituitary gland also ceases, and a fall in FSH level eventually occurs.

HORMONE LEVELS

There is 50% reduction in androgen production and 66% reduction in oestrogen production at menopause. The oestrogen level may remain low at 10–20 pg/mL. Some oestrogen comes directly from the ovary, but most of it is oestrone (E_1) derived from peripheral conversion of androstenedione secreted by the ovary, and its level varies between 30 and 70 pg/mL. The ovary also secretes a small amount of testosterone which causes mild hirsutism at menopause. The FSH appears in high concentration in the urine (more than 40 IU/L). E_2/E_1 ratio maintained greater than 1 in the premenopausal period is reduced to less than 1 after menopause, causing an oestrogen deficiency state. Oestrogen level greater than 40 pg/mL exerts protective bone and cardiotropic effect, but the level less than 20 pg/mL may predispose to osteoporosis and ischaemic heart disease (Table 7.1). Low level of growth hormone also causes ovarian failure.

Risk factors for menopause-related diseases are as follows:

- Early menopause.
- Surgical menopause or radiation.
- Chemotherapy especially alkylating agents.
- Smoking, caffeine, alcohol.
- Family history of menopausal diseases (genetic).
- Drugs such as GnRH, heparin, corticosteroids and clomiphene (antioestrogen) when given over a prolonged period (more than 6 months) can lead to oestrogen deficiency.
- Diabetes.

ANATOMICAL CHANGES

The genital organs undergo atrophy and regression. The ovaries shrink and their surfaces become grooved and furrowed. The tunica albuginea thickens. The menopausal ovary measures less than 2 × 1.5 × 1 cm in size (8 mL in volume) as seen on ultrasound. Fifteen years later, it should not measure more than 2 mL. The plain muscle in the fallopian tube undergoes atrophy, cilia disappear from the tubal epithelium and the tubal plicae are no longer prominent.

The uterus becomes smaller because of atrophy of its plain muscle, so that the connective tissues are more conspicuous. The endometrium is represented by only the basal layer with its compact deeply stained stroma, and a few simple tubular glands. The lymphoid tissue and the functional layer disappear. The cervix becomes smaller and its vaginal portion is represented by a small prominence at the vaginal vault. The cervical stenosis and pyometra are not uncommon.

Table 7.1 Hormone Levels in a Menopausal Woman

E_2	5–25 pg/mL
Oestrone	20–70 pg/mL – more in obese women
FSH	> 40 mIU/mL
Androgen	0.3–1.0 ng/mL
Testosterone	0.1–0.5 ng/mL
LH	50–100 mIU/mL
Androstenedione	800 pg/mL
Growth hormone Inhibin B Anti-Müllerian hormone	Low

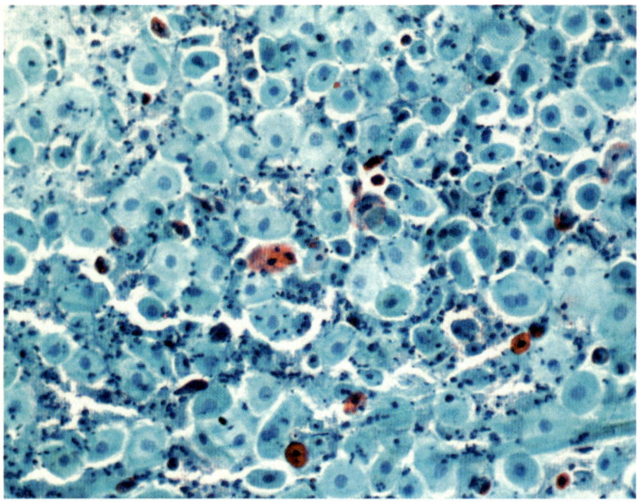

Figure 7.1 Cytology of senile vaginitis. (*Courtesy*: Dr Sandeep Mathur, AIIMS.)

The vaginal fornices gradually disappear as the cervix shrinks after the menopause. The vagina becomes narrow and its epithelium becomes pale, thin and dry and gets easily infected causing senile vaginitis (Fig. 7.1). The vulva atrophies and the vaginal orifice narrows and this can cause dyspareunia. The skin of the labia minora and vestibule becomes thin, pale and dry, and there is considerable reduction in the amount of fat contained in the labia majora. The pubic hair is reduced and becomes grey. The red patches seen around the urethra and introitus are caused by senile vulvitis, and a urethral caruncle may form. The pelvic cellular tissue becomes lax and the ligaments that support the uterus and vagina lose their tone, and these changes predispose to prolapse of the genital organs, stress incontinence of urine and faecal incontinence.

Apart from the atrophy of the genital organs, general disturbances that develop are almost certainly caused by alterations in the endocrine balance maintained during the childbearing period. Fat is deposited around the breasts, hips and abdomen. Although the mammary glandular tissue atrophies, deposition of fat often makes the breasts more pendulous. Glandular tissue constitutes 30% of the breast volume, it is reduced to only 5% after the menopause. The skin wrinkles and hair grow around the chin and lips. Hypertension, cardiac irregularities and tachycardia are at times noticed after menopause. Arthritis and osteoporosis of the vertebral bones, upper end of the hip joint and wrist are related to oestrogen deficiency after menopause.

Tooth decay, keratoconjunctivitis and cataract are related to menopausal oestrogen deficiency.

MENOPAUSAL SYMPTOMS (Table 7.2)

MENSTRUAL

The three classical ways in which the menstrual period ceases are as follows:

- Sudden cessation
- Gradual diminution in the amount of blood loss with each regular period until menstruation stops
- Gradual increase in the intervals between periods until they cease for at least a period of 1 year

Table 7.2 Early Features of Menopause

- Hot flushes
- Sweating
- Insomnia
- Headache
- Psychological
- Cancer phobia
- Dyspareunia, decreased libido
- Pseudocyesis
- Irritability
- Depression, insomnia, tiredness
- Lack of concentration, loss of memory
- Urinary stress incontinence, dyspareunia

Although by definition, menopause is said to have set in if amenorrhoea lasts for a year, a woman who bleeds after a gap of 6 months is considered to have postmenopausal bleeding and should be thoroughly investigated. Continuous bleeding, menorrhagia or irregular heavy bleeding in the perimenopausal period are considered abnormal and should be investigated for malignancy of the genital tract.

HOT FLUSHES

It is the most common symptom experienced by women after menopause. Almost 60%–70% women go through their menopausal period without problems. The rest need guidance and treatment. The most common and the most noticeable symptoms of hot flushes and sweating are the hallmark of the climacteric in 85% women. Hot flushes are the waves of vasodilation affecting the face and the neck, and these last for 2–5 minutes each. These are followed by profuse sweating. These flushes occur several times in a day, but are more severe during the night, and can disturb sleep. The hot flushes are sometimes preceded by headache. Palpitation and anginal pains may be felt. Mental depression due to disturbed sleep or otherwise, irritability and lack of concentration are noticed. With the passage of time, the frequency and severity of flushes diminish over a period of 1–2 years. Hot flushes are caused by noradrenaline, which disturbs the thermoregulatory system. Oestrogen deficiency reduces hypothalamic endorphins, which release more norepinephrine and serotonin. This leads to an inappropriate heat loss mechanism.

Other causes that can be associated with the symptom of hot flushes include thyroid disease, epilepsy, pheochromocytoma, carcinoid syndromes, autoimmune disorders, mast cell disorders, insulinoma, pancreatic tumours and even leukaemias.

The vasomotor symptoms are more severe in surgical menopause than natural menopause.

OTHER SYMPTOMS

Some women develop a condition of pseudocyesis, when they fear pregnancy and attribute amenorrhoea and increased abdominal girth to pregnancy.

Cancer phobia may also develop; the woman starts worrying over her looks.

NEUROLOGICAL

Vasomotor symptoms and paraesthesia may take the form of sensations of pins and needles in the extremities.

LIBIDO

Sexual feeling and libido may increase in some, if they feel happy to get rid of menstruation and fear of pregnancy. Many however notice decreased libido after menopause (15%; lack of orgasm and arousal).

The symptoms which develop little later are as follows:

- Urinary symptoms such as dysuria, stress and urge incontinence, recurrent infection (urethral syndrome)
- Genital symptoms such as dry vagina, dyspareunia, loss of libido
- Faecal incontinence
- Thyroid dysfunction

URINARY TRACT

Oestrogen deficiency can cause urethral caruncle, dysuria, with or without infection, urge and stress incontinence. The stress incontinence is caused by poor vascularity and tone of the internal urinary sphincter. These urinary symptoms are clubbed together under the term 'urethral syndrome'.

GENITAL

Atrophic vagina reduces vaginal secretion, and dry vagina can cause dyspareunia. Loss of libido adds to sexual dysfunction. Rarely, senile vaginitis can cause vaginal bleeding (Fig. 7.1). Prolapse of genital tract and stress incontinence of urine and faeces are mostly menopausal related.

NEUROLOGICAL

Depression, loss of memory, irritability, poor concentration and tiredness, poor sleep and predementia.

LATE EFFECTS OF MENOPAUSE

Menopausal women with chronic oestrogen deficiency are liable to develop the following:

- Arthritis, osteoporosis and fracture, backache
- Cardiovascular accidents such as ischaemic heart disease, myocardial infarction, atherosclerosis and hypertension.
- Hypothyroidism and diabetes.
- Stroke
- Skin changes
- Alzheimer disease
- Ano-colonic cancer
- Tooth decay
- Prolapse of genital tract, stress incontinence of urine and faecal incontinence
- Cataract, glaucoma and macular degeneration

Locomotor system disorders: Menopausal arthropathy, osteoarthritis, fibrositis and backache may be age related.

Osteoporosis (Fig. 7.2)

It is an incipient slowly progressing skeletal disorder characterized by microarchitectural deterioration of bone mass resulting in increased fragility and predilection to fracture in the absence of significant trauma. About 15% of elderly women suffer from osteoporosis and almost three times as many suffer from osteopenia (deficient bone mass). Both osteopenia and osteoporosis predispose to fractures. These constitute a significant cause of morbidity such as pain, deformity and impaired respiratory and other bodily functions. Hip fractures are often associated with a high rate of mortality. Wrist and hip joints are particularly affected.

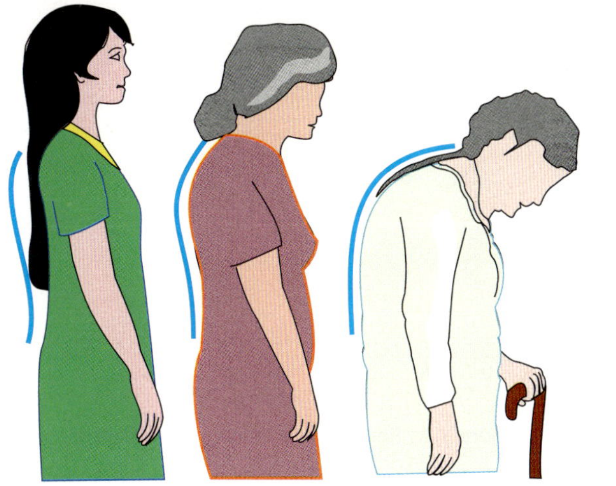

Figure 7.2 Osteoporosis of the vertebral column.

With increasing longevity of women in India, the medical practitioners will be called upon more often to care for osteoporosis-related problems.

Osteoporosis is defined as a condition in which there is a fall in bone mass exceeding 2.5 standard deviations (SD) below the mean for young adults. World Health Organization (WHO) has defined low bone mass as *osteopenia* and *osteoporosis* on the basis of axial skeleton BMD (bone mineral density) to facilitate screening and identification of individuals at risk. These definitions apply specifically to T-scores derived from the use of dual-energy X-ray absorptiometry (DEXA) of the lumbar spine. WHO defines osteopenia as a BMD between 1 and 2.5 SD below the young adult mean peak bone mass and osteoporosis as BMD which is 2.5 SD or more below the standard adult mean values. These changes begin 2 years before menopause.

Pathophysiology. Bone is not an inert supporting tissue. *Bone remodelling* takes place constantly. At the cellular level, bone remodelling is a balance between bone resorption (osteoclastic activity) and bone formation (osteoblastic activity), whereas the main functions of the osteocytes and lining cells are metabolic, subserving the nutrition of bone and the maintenance of calcium homeostasis. After the cessation of adult growth, the skeleton consolidates to reach peak bone mass (PBM) at the age of 35–40 years. Thereafter, a slow subsequent age-related loss of bone mass occurs in everyone at the rate of 0.4% annually, but women are additionally exposed to an accelerated rate of bone loss during the perimenopausal age and the initial 5–8 years of the early menopause (2% cortical bone and 5% trabecular bone). Oestrogen deficiency is the dominant factor contributing to osteoporosis in women. Additional contributing factors such as calcium and vitamin D deficiency also need consideration. At the age of 40 years, bone calcium amounts to 1200 g. When the level drops below 750 g, fracture of the bone is likely to occur.

Fig. 7.3 shows that women live a third of their lifespan after menopause. Elderly women suffer from vertebral fractures leading to gibbus formation, a bent spine and shortening of height.

The other high-risk factors for osteoporosis are as follows:

- Family history of osteoporosis.
- Low calcium intake in diet.

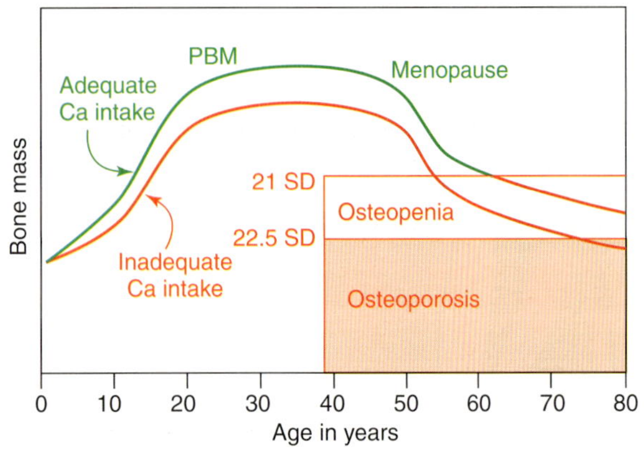

Figure 7.3 Bone mineral density – age related.

- Smoking and excess of caffeine and alcohol intake.
- Early menopause.
- Low weight.
- Surgical menopause following hysterectomy with or without oophorectomy. It is now believed that even if the ovaries are conserved, the disturbance in their vascularity may lead to ovarian atrophy.
- Radiation menopause.
- Woman on GnRH, heparin, corticosteroids, danazol, clomiphene.
- Thyrotoxicosis.
- Sedentary lifestyle, diabetes.

Diminished BMD can be assessed by DEXA and single- or dual-photon absorptiometry for spine, neck of the femur and radius. This technique detects bone loss of as little as 1%–5% compared to plain radiography, which shows a loss of bone mass only at 30% loss.

Cardiovascular Diseases

Oestrogen is cardioprotective by maintaining a high level of high-density lipoprotein (HDL) and lowering the low-density lipoprotein (LDL) and triglycerides. Oestrogen deficiency therefore predispose to atherosclerosis, ischaemic heart disease and myocardial infarction. Obese women with hypertension and previous thromboembolic episodes are likely to experience to cardiovascular accidents. Oestrogen prevents atherosclerosis through its antioxidant property.

Stroke

The incidence of stroke also increases in menopausal women.

Skin

Collagen content is reduced, causing skin to wrinkle. The 'feminine forever' thought applies to oestrogen cream to delay the age-related skin changes. However, it is observed that after a few months the skin actually thins out, and oestrogen cream may be beneficial temporarily and only in the initial phase of treatment.

Alzheimer Disease

It is believed that Alzheimer disease is precipitated by oestrogen deficiency at menopause, and hormonal therapy is beneficial in preventing or delaying its onset. It is beneficial only if given in the perimenopausal age or soon after menopause. Giving hormone later is not effective.

Endocrine System

Mild virilization as seen in the form of hirsutism is probably because of adrogens produced from the adrenals and obesity, particularly deposition of fat around the hips. Hypothyroidism with a low basal metabolic rate (BMR), high cholesterol level, dryness of skin, brittleness of hair and lack of concentration are noticed in some menopausal women.

Pyometra

Years after menopause, a woman may develop senile pyometra caused by cervical stenosis, and needs drainage by cervical dilatation under general anaesthesia.

APPROACH TO A MENOPAUSAL WOMAN

- History of various symptoms.
- General examination includes blood pressure recording, palpation of the breasts, weight and hirsutism.
- Pelvic examination, Pap smear.
- Blood sugar, lipid profile, ECG.
- Mammography, pelvic ultrasound.
- Bone density study. DEXA is a quick test with less radiation.
- Oestrogen (E_2) and FSH levels to decide on the need of HRT.
- Endometrial biopsy in women on HRT and tamoxifen.

MANAGEMENT

The clinician should adopt a holistic approach towards management of health problems of menopausal women and selectively prescribe hormone therapy according to the requirement. Minimal required dose avoids risks while conferring the beneficial effects.

COUNSELLING

The woman often develops phobia about pregnancy and cancer. It is the duty of the gynaecologist to convince her, after thorough examination and investigations, that all is well with her. It is a good practice to document baseline recordings of pelvic ultrasound, which includes the ovarian size and the endometrial thickness, mammography as well as E_2 and FSH levels, when HRT is considered. Regular counselling may be required until the woman is well settled in menopause.

The advice on contraceptives is necessary. Until menopause is well established and amenorrhoea has lasted for 12 months, the couple is advised to use barrier method. Hormonal pills may not be safe from the point of view of thromboembolism. Progestogen pills or depot injections may be the alternative, but they cause irregular bleeding and depression.

Diet should include at least 1.2 g of calcium, vitamin A, C, E and 400 I.U. of vitamin D. Soya beans are good source of phytoestrogen (discussed later). Weight-bearing exercises (walking and aerobic) delay the onset of osteoporosis.

MILD TRANQUILLIZERS

These relieve woman's anxiety, sleeplessness and depression. Antidepressants such as sulpiride may be needed.

Antidepressant drugs – Venlafaxine 30–150 mg daily, Paroxetine 10–20 mg daily, Gabapentin 300 mg three times a day.

HORMONE REPLACEMENT THERAPY

Not all women require HRT. Besides, HRT does not suit all, and it may cause complications and can be harmful. However, it is logical to prescribe HRT and not withhold it when one needs it in the minimal effective dose for the shortest needed duration under supervision.

Earlier, every menopausal woman was advised to have HRT as soon as menopause set in, to be taken for several years. Newer researches and their observations reveal that only a few women need prophylactic and therapeutic HRT. 70%–85% of women remain healthy and need only good nutrition and healthy lifestyle.

Who Needs HRT?

- Symptomatic women who suffer from oestrogen deficiency (therapeutic).
- High-risk cases for menopause-related complications such as a cardiovascular disease, osteoporosis, stroke, Alzheimer disease and colonic cancer (prophylactic).
- Premature menopause, spontaneous or following surgery (hysterectomy, tubectomy). The surgical procedures disturb and compromise the blood supply to the ovaries. Menopause caused by radiotherapy and chemotherapy for cancer, especially alkylating agents (prophylactic).
- Gonadal dysgenesis in adolescents (therapeutic).

The type of hormone, route of administration and duration of treatment depend upon the purpose for which it is used, i.e. prophylactic or therapeutic.

Symptomatic women who suffer vasomotor symptoms, urinary symptoms and sexual disharmony because of dyspareunia, as well as psychosomatic problems need to be treated with HRT on a short-term basis for a period varying between 3 and 6 months. Most improve by the end of 6 months after which the woman usually gets adjusted and settles down well in the menopausal phase of life.

The high-risk cases for osteoporosis have already been mentioned. The women with atherosclerosis, hypertriglyceridaemia and ischaemic heart disease may benefit from cardioprotective effect of prophylactic oestrogen. However, HRT is not recommended for women who are already suffering from ischaemic heart disease.

Recently, it was proved that prophylactic HRT may delay or prevent the occurrence of Alzheimer disease and allow the woman at risk to lead a comfortable life for years.

There are women who are healthy and at no risk of the above diseases. They do however feel inclined to take HRT with the belief that they will have the feeling of well-being and can lead an enjoyable life. These women need a proper screening before prescribing the hormones. They should be counselled regarding the benefit, side effects and the cost, and the need for periodic check-up while on hormones. Certain contraindications to be noted for oestrogen therapy are as follows:

- Breast cancer, uterine cancer or family history of cancer
- Previous history of thromboembolic episode
- Liver and gall bladder diseases
- Uterine fibroids – the fibroids may enlarge in size

Hypertension, diabetes and smoking are not contraindications, provided they are regularly monitored. Rather cardiac disease, stroke and smoking may be the indications for oestrogen therapy to derive benefit and improve their health from oestrogen deficiency.

Uses of HRT

- **Short term** – hot flushes, vasomotor symptoms
  - Dyspareunia, libido
  - Urethral syndrome
- **Long term** – osteoporosis
  - Cardiovascular
  - Alzheimer disease

OSTEOPOROSIS

HRT is the cornerstone in the prophylaxis and treatment of osteoporosis. After menopause, the woman loses on an average 3% BMD every year causing osteopenia and eventually osteoporosis and fracture of the vertebra, femur and the wrist. The trabeculated bone is most affected. The morbidity arising from pelvic fractures is considerable. The benefit of HRT is proved beyond doubt in preventing or delaying bone resorption. When to start HRT remains a controversial point, although earlier it was recommended in the perimenopausal age or soon after menopause, the poor compliance over a long period, the cost and the limited benefits restrict their use for a short period of time. For optimal benefits of HRT, natural oestrogen, progestogen, tibolone and raloxifene are beneficial in osteoporosis, if prescribed early in menopause. Osteoporosis occurring late in menopause benefits from bisphosphonates, as primary treatment.

It is observed that benefit of HRT lasts while the woman continues to take HRT, and the bone loss resumes once she stops taking drugs. The prolonged therapy beyond 8–10 years is not beneficial but at times harmful, so most gynaecologists now follow-up the woman for osteopenia and prescribe HRT when osteopenia occurs.

Oestrogens delays or protects against osteoporosis in 50% of all skeletal bones, and is not restricted to trabecular bones of spine, wrist and upper hipbones.

PROPHYLAXIS OF OSTEOPOROSIS

- Oestrogen hormone therapy – ERT (hysterectomized)
- Oestrogen + progesterone (HRT)
- Tibolone
- Raloxifene
- Soya extracts
- Bisphosphonates for late osteoporosis
- Calcitonin
- Hormone
- Diet

CARDIOPROTECTIVE EFFECT OF HRT

Oestrogen deficiency increases the risk of atherosclerosis, ischaemic heart disease and angina in a postmenopausal woman. Oestrogen is therefore cardioprotective in prevention of cardiovascular disease. It also increases HDL and decreases LDL, cholesterol and triglycerides. Oestrogen is most effective when taken orally as far as its effect on a lipid profile is concerned. Oestrogen and tibolone are strongly cardioprotective in menopausal women. However, a woman with previous ischaemic heart disease does not benefit from HRT and its use is not recommended.

DRUGS, DOSAGE AND ROUTE OF ADMINISTRATION

Oestrogen Therapy

Short-term therapy is required to relieve the woman of hot flushes, night sweats, palpitations and disturbed sleep. Oestrogen should however be given in the smallest effective dose for a short possible period of 3–6 months. Natural oestrogens are preferred. Oral Premarin (E_1 – natural equine-conjugated oestrogen) in the dose of 0.375 mg or 0.625 mg daily, increasing to 1.25 mg if necessary, ethinyl oestradiol 0.01 mg, micronized oestrogen (1–2 mg) or Evalon 1–2 mg are effective. Progestogen such as Duphaston/medroxyprogesterone 10 mg or Primolut N 2.5 mg daily for 10–12 days each month should be added to prevent endometrial hyperplasia and carcinoma. This therapy can still cause endometrial hyperplasia in 5% and atypical hyperplasia in 0.7% cases. Because of this, some prefer to give a combined hormone therapy (Femet) containing 2 mg 17β-oestradiol and 1 mg of norethisterone acetate, which is known to cause endometrial atrophy. Progesterone is not required in a hysterectomized woman. Cyclical combined HRT causes cyclical bleeding. Period-free HRT can be attained if the combined hormones are taken continuously.

Dyspareunia, urethral syndrome and senile vaginitis respond well to local oestrogen cream, which is preferred over oral therapy. Oestriol base cream 1/2 g is applied every day for 10–12 days each month for a period of 3–6 months until the symptoms disappear. ESTRING (vaginal ring) releases 5–10 mcg oestrogen and is 90% effective over a period of 3 months.

Long-Term Therapy. Long-term oestrogen therapy is beneficial in delaying osteoporosis and reducing the risk of a cardiovascular disease in a postmenopausal woman. However, it is observed that extending the medication beyond 8–10 years does not confer any further benefit.

Oral Route. Orally administered oestradiol gets extensively metabolized into oestrone in the intestine and liver so that only 10% reaches the systemic circulation as oestradiol. Larger doses therefore need to be given orally compared to the nonoral route (Table 7.3). This metabolism in the gut and the liver is known as 'first-pass' effect, and this also increases certain liver proteins, alters the clotting factors and increases the secretion of renin. However, given orally, it improves the lipid profile except serum triglyceride and improves the cardioprotective effect. Very recently, however, the controversy has been raised regarding its protective role in a woman already suffering from a cardiovascular disease, and HRT is not recommended for them.

Transdermal Patch (Estraderm). It avoids the first-pass effect of liver metabolism, and the hormone reaches the systemic circulation as oestradiol. The risk of thromboembolic episode and probable hypertension is eliminated. It reduces serum triglyceride levels as well.

Estraderm patch contains 3–4 mg of oestradiol releases 50 mcg per day. The disadvantage of skin reaction with alcohol-based patch is now avoided by newer transdermal system, but it cannot be reapplied after being taken off the skin during bath. The patch needs to be changed twice a week. The cost prohibits many women from using them. It should be applied away from the breasts, on the arms, legs and thighs.

Table 7.3 Advantages and Disadvantages of Oral and Transdermal Route of Oestrogen

Oral	Transdermal
Advantages	**Advantages**
• Cheap	• Low-dose oestradiol
• Easy to take	• Avoids first-pass effect and liver metabolism
• Can be withdrawn quickly in presence of side effects	• Reduces triglycerides
• Good for a lipid profile and cardiovascular protection	• No thromboembolic risk or hypertension
Disadvantages	**Disadvantages**
• Higher dose required	• Costly
• First-pass effect in liver	• Not tolerated in warm climates
• Daily intake	• Variable absorption
• Tablet contains lactose, and not suited to women who are allergic to lactose	
• High incidence of side effects	
• ↑ Hypertension	
• ↑ Thromboembolism	

Gel (100 mg contains 60 mg β-oestradiol) is applied to the skin for improving the collagen content and avoid wrinkles (two measures of 0.75 mg oestradiol). The plasma level is maintained at 60–80 pg/mL.

Vaginal Cream. Oestriol cream is used in urethral syndrome and dry vagina. About 1/2 g is applied daily for a few days each month on a short-term basis. Premarin is also available as cream.

Vaginal Ring. Oestrogen supplementation can also be effectively achieved by inserting a vaginal ring that releases 0.0075 mg of 17β-oestradiol daily for 90 days. This form of medication should be considered in the management of menopausal vaginal symptoms.

Implant. Implant containing 25–50 mg oestradiol is effective for 6 month each, and maintains the E_2 level at 50–60 pg/mL. A minor operation is required for insertion and removal. It is suitable in hysterectomized women.

Intranasal 300 mcg of oestrogen raises the level of hormone in 30 minutes, and becomes effective. However, breakthrough bleeding, sneezing and itching occur in 1%–3% cases and 55% have stopped the therapy by the end of 1 year.

The oestrogen therapy reduces the incidence of fracture by 50% at the end of 5 years (90% vertebra and 50% hip). Similarly, cardiovascular complications have been reduced by 40%–50% with oestrogen therapy.

Unfortunately, compliance of long-term use of hormone therapy is marred by vaginal bleeding. To overcome this problem, 'period-free' HRT is now produced by the combination of oestrogen and progesterone taken continuously instead of cyclically. Not only continuous progestogen suppresses oestrogen-stimulated endometrium, it also allows a smaller dose of oestrogen and progestogen and lesser side effects. Even then, vaginal bleeding may occur up to

6 months of this regime, followed by amenorrhoea. Any bleeding after that requires investigations.

Risks of HRT Usage:

- Endometrial cancer
- Breast cancer
- Ovarian cancer
- Thromboembolism
- Lipid profile dysfunction
- Gall stones, liver dysfunction
- Vaginal bleeding with continuous HRT (period-free HRT) is more common if the therapy is started within 1 year of menopause, and may last up to 6 months. After the first year of menopause, there is less risk of vaginal bleeding. Persistent vaginal bleeding requires endometrial biopsy. The bleeding can however be avoided by decreasing oestrogen dose or increasing the dose of progestogen. With 'period-free' HRT, 75%–100% women become amenorrhoeic by the end of 1 year.

Gabapentin is a nonhormonal anticonvulsant that reduces hot flushes by 50% if given in a dose of 900–2400 mg daily. Dizziness (14%) drowsiness (12%), tiredness, headache, blurred vision, dry mouth and memory problem gradually disappear after a week or so.

- Thromboembolism.
- Endometrial cancer if E_2 is taken alone and the risk lasts for 10 years after stoppage of therapy.
- Breast cancer is due to progestogen if HRT is taken for more than 5 years.
- The possibility of a coronary heart disease in a woman with a cardiovascular disease has caused a great concern regarding the use of HRT in these women. HRT is contraindicated in these cases.
- Increased risk of ovarian cancer.

Progestogens

Progestogens are used for 10–12 days in each cycle to avoid the risk of endometrial hyperplasia and cancer in nonhysterectomized women. The risk of endometrial hyperplasia is reduced to 4%, if given for 12 days in each cycle. It does so through enzyme 17β-hydroxy dehydrogenase, which inactivates E_2 and controls the mitotic activity within the endometrial cells. They do reduce the bone resorption, but not to the extent seen with oestrogen therapy. Some of them have an adverse effect on a lipid profile (Fig. 7.4).

The drugs used are Norethisterone 2.5 mg, medroxyprogesterone and Duphaston, 10 mg. Progestogen implants are also available for those intolerant to oestrogen. Progestogens cause bloated feel, weight gain and depression and may adversely alter the lipid profile. Medroxyprogesterone has no adverse effect on lipids but reduces the bone density. To avoid the systemic side effects and poor compliance with oral progestogen, Mirena IUCD containing levonorgestrel is inserted for 5 years in HRT programme. Micronized progesterone is not useful in HRT.

Drospirenone, a new progestogen, has no androgenic and adverse lipid effect. A dose of 3 mg combined with 30 mcg oestradiol (Yasmin, Janya, Tarana) has been tried in menopausal women, but more research is needed.

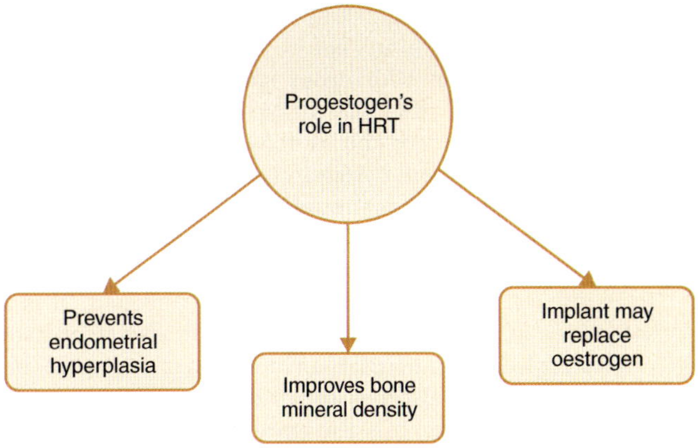

Figure 7.4 Role of progestogen in HRT.

Testosterone implant and combined tablet with oestrogen are used to improve libido. The role of Viagra to improve libido is controversial at present.

Yohimbine resembles reserpine, an indole alkyl amine alkaloid derived from the bark of tree *Rauwolfia.* It improves libido. A dose of 6–10 mg daily at night is prescribed. Tolerance develops with this drug. Risk of hirsutism should be borne in mind. Recently Flibanserin, and serotonin-2A antagonist in a dose of 100 mg at bed time has been approved for a loss of libido.

Other Drugs

1. **Tibolone** (Livial) is a synthetic derivative of 19-nortestosterone and has a weak oestrogenic, progestogenic and androgenic action. The tablet containing 2.5 mg does not cause endometrial hyperplasia but causes irregular bleeding in 15% cases. It also elevates the mood, relieves the vasomotor symptoms, improves the sex drive and reduces bone resorption. Its main action is cardioprotection by reducing the level of triglycerides. Side effects include weight gain, oedema, tenderness in the breast, gastrointestinal symptoms and vaginal bleed (15%). The greasy skin and increased hair growth are due to androgenic action. It should be initiated only after 1 year of menopause to avoid vaginal bleeding.
2. **Raloxifene,** a nonsteroidal compound (Evista), is a selective oestrogen receptor modulator (SERM), which reduces the risk of fracture by 50%, especially in vertebra by increasing BMD by 2%–3%. It causes 10% reduction in total cholesterol and LDL and raises HDL level. It does not raise the levels of triglycerides. It is therefore cardioprotective in long term. It has a very low risk of endometrial and breast cancer. It is beneficial in reducing osteoporosis and is given 60 mg daily with calcium and vitamin D. It is absorbed from the gastrointestinal tract (60%), following which glucuronidation occurs in the liver and is excreted in the faeces. Toremifene 20 mg daily is effective dose in 60% cases. *Side effects* are hot flushes, cramps, increased incidence of venous thrombosis and retinopathy. It does not control vasomotor symptoms. Newer SERMs: Ospemifene, Lasofoxifene and Arzoxifene are being tried. Contraindications are as follows:
   - Venous thrombosis.
   - It should not be given with oestrogen.

- Hepatic dysfunction.
- Stop the drug 72 hours before surgery.
- Not to be given with drugs such as indomethacin, naproxen, ibuprofen and diazepam.

3. **Soya.** Soya beans contain isoflavone (phytoestrogens, genistein and daidzein). About 11 g soya contains 2–4 mg phytoestrogens, which is strongly oestrogenic, though it is a nonsteroidal plant product. About 45–60 mg soya daily is protective without the potential risk of breast cancer, liver disease and other side effects of oestrogen. It is a safe alternative to hormonal therapy. It also decreases cholesterol, LDL and triglycerides with a marginal increase in HDL. It also has antiviral, antifungal and anticarcinogenic effects. It is also present in lentil and chick peas.
4. **Bisphosphonates** such as etidronate and tiludronate reduce bone resorption through the inhibition of osteoclastic activity. Etidronate 10 mg/kg body weight (approximately 400 mg orally daily) is given for 2 weeks followed by a gap of 2–3 months (3-month course), and this course is repeated for 10 such cycles. The drug should not be given with calcium, because its absorption is reduced. Calcium should be taken in the morning and etidronate swallowed (not chewed) in the afternoon, on an empty stomach with a glass of water in the upright position; stay upright for half an hour. This reduces the oesophageal irritation. The tablet should not be swallowed with coffee, tea or juice. Overdose causes hypocalcaemia. Milk and antacid can reduce gastric irritation. It is recommended that HRT should be prescribed in early menopausal age. After 60 years, osteoporosis should be managed with bisphosphonates. **Alendronate** is given as either 5 mg daily or 35 mg weekly. Overdose causes hypocalcaemia. **Risedronate** has reduced gastric side effects and is effective in a dose of 5 mg daily or 35 mg once a month. **Zoledronic acid** is used therapeutically once a year as intravenous infusion of 5 mg over 15 minutes, but osteonecrosis of the jaw and visual disturbances are the major side effects, though very rare. Ibandronate sodium is given 2.5 mg daily or 150 mg monthly orally or 3 mg intravenously 3 monthly. **Calcitonin** is a peptide produced by thyroid C cells. It inhibits osteoclast activity and inhibits bone resorption. It is given as a nasal spray at a single dose of 200 IU daily for 3 months. Nasal spray can cause flushes, rhinitis, allergic reaction and nasal bleeding. It reduces the incidence of fracture by 30%. **Subcutaneous injection** of calcitonin is also available, but gastrointestinal symptoms, anaemia and inflammation of joints cause poor compliance, as does the high cost. **Teriparatide** is the recombinant formation of parathyroid hormone. About 20 mcg once-daily subcutaneous injection decreases vertebral fracture by 65% and others by 50% if used less than 2 years. Nausea and headache are the complications. **Strontium ranelate** given 1–2 g daily orally increases BMD by 50%. However, it is very expensive and not easily available. **Clonidine** is an imidazoline derivative used to treat hot flushes. It is also effective in hypertensive women not responding to oestrogen. Clonidine lowers blood pressure in addition to relieving hot flushes. Dose of 0.2–0.4 mg daily suffices. It acts centrally. Side effects are dry mouth, dizziness and nausea. Androgens improve libido, but carries the risk of hirsutism.

SUGGESTIONS FOR HRT

- Not every menopausal woman needs HRT.
- A symptomatic woman due to oestrogen deficiency requires HRT for 3–6 months. The duration and route of HRT depend upon the purpose for which the therapy is prescribed.
- Total duration of a prophylactic therapy beyond 8–10 years has not proved beneficial, but side effects may harm the woman.
- The benefit of a therapy should be balanced against the risks of breast and endometrial cancers and venous thromboembolism.
- Phytoestrogen is available as 'Femarelle', one tablet to be taken twice a day.
- Therapy should be individualized according to the need.

Lately, once a month oral ibandronate is made available which improves bone density (ibandronate is marketed as IDROFOS – 150 mg).

The drug increases the BMD by 5%–10% and also prevents recurrence of fracture. Nonresponse is seen in 10% cases.

Alendronate is the third generation of bisphosphonates (nonhormonal) and is 1000 times more potent than etidronate with no side effects. It is marketed as Osteofos (5, 10, 35 and 70 mg).

HORMONE REPLACEMENT THERAPY AND RISK OF BREAST CANCER

- The risk of breast cancer is not increased up to 3 years of HRT and 5 years of oestrogen alone replacement therapy.
- Lower risk is seen with use of dydrogesterone in HRT.
- HRT can cause recurrence of breast cancer and is therefore contraindicated in a woman who has been treated for breast cancer. Tibolone is safe.
- HRT increases the density of breast tissue and impedes screening programme of mammography subsequently.
- Breast cancer developing following HRT is of low grade with good prognosis.

HORMONE REPLACEMENT THERAPY AND ENDOMETRIAL CARCINOMA

- ERT can cause well-differentiated carcinoma of endometrium.
- Minimum of 12 days of progesterone added to ERT reduces the risk of endometrial cancer to 2%.
- Combined oestrogen and progesterone provides a better protection against endometrial cancer.
- Tibolone is a safe drug and does not cause endometrial hyperplasia.
- Raloxifene, unlike tamoxifen exercises antioestrogen action on endometrium.
- The risk of cancer with ERT is dose and duration dependent.

PREMATURE MENOPAUSE (PREMATURE OVARIAN FAILURE)

Premature menopause is defined as ovarian failure occurring before the age of 40 years. It is clinically defined as secondary amenorrhoea for at least 3 months with raised FSH level, raised FSH/LH ratio and low E_2 level in a woman younger than 40 years.

The incidence is 1%. Before the age of 30 years the incidence is 1:1000, at 35 it is 1:250 and just before 40 years it is 1%.

AETIOLOGY

Some known causes of premature menopause are as follows:

- Fewer germ cell migration from the yolk sac
- More apoptosis of germ cells
  1. Genetic disorders such as chromosomal abnormalities are reported in 10%–20% of cases involving X chromosomes. Autosomal dominant sex-linked inheritance is also known. Ovarian dysgenesis is seen in 30% cases.
  2. Autoimmune diseases are reported in 30%–60% cases. Mumps, thyroid dysfunction, hypoparathyroidism and Addison disease may account for a few cases. The ovarian biopsy shows infiltration of the follicles with plasma cells and lymphocytes. Raised CD_8 count and low CD_4 count suggest an autoimmune disease. Antiovarian antibodies are present.
  3. Tuberculosis of the genital tract involving the ovaries can cause secondary amenorrhoea and ovarian failure.
  4. Smoking is known to induce premature menopause, and the age when it occurs depends upon the degree of smoking. It is toxic for the follicles.
  5. Radiation and chemotherapy can cause premature menopause, but the effect is reversible and the ovary may resume ovulation and menstruation after about a year of amenorrhoea. Alkylating agents are strong inducers of premature menopause.
  6. Ovarian failure following hysterectomy is known to occur in 15%–50% cases even when ovaries are retained and is caused by kinking and blockage of ovarian vessels. Tubectomy can also produce a similar effect.
  7. Prolonged GnRH therapy may lead to ovarian suppression and failure.
  8. Enzyme defects such as 17α-hydroxylase deficiency and galactosemia have adverse effect on oocytes, but more often cause primary amenorrhoea.
  9. Resistant ovary: This terminology is used less frequently these days and it is presumed that the follicles fail to respond to gonadotropin stimulation.
  10. Induction of multiple ovulations in infertility can cause premature menopause when the follicles get exhausted.

PATHOPHYSIOLOGY

Either exhaustion of primordial follicles in ovary or lack of receptors and presence of antibodies has been described as a cause of premature ovarian failure.

CLINICAL FEATURES

Hot flushes and sweating occur in 75% cases and may be more severe than seen in natural menopause. Libido is diminished in 10%–20% cases. Vaginal dryness and urinary symptoms are less complained.

INVESTIGATIONS

- FSH level: 40 mIU/mL or more
- E_2 level: 20 pg/mL or less
- Thyroid function, calcium level, chromosomal study and thyroid antibodies
- Blood sugar
- MRI pituitary fossa for presence of tumour.
- BMD study is not always necessary
- Ovarian biopsy
- Ultrasound
- Prolactin level

COMPLICATIONS

The risks of osteoporosis and cardiovascular diseases increase in premature menopause.

MANAGEMENT

1. The cause of premature menopause should be ascertained and should be treated. Follicular maturation, ovulation and menstruation have been restored following the treatment of the cause.
2. Oophoropexy and ovarian shield during radiotherapy can protect ovaries.
3. Corticosteroid therapy is effective in an autoimmune disease if antibodies to sex hormones are present in the blood. Plasmapheresis has also been attempted.
4. A woman with hypo-oestrogenism may require HRT or other drugs to prevent osteoporosis. Oestrogen implant with oral progesterone or Mirena IUCD offers long-term HRT.

Specific management according to the need is as follows:

1. An older woman or a parous woman not interested in pregnancy or menstrual functions may require HRT if she develops menopausal symptoms. She may require prophylactic HRT if she is a high-risk case of cardiac complication, or osteoporosis.
2. Libido improves with testosterone and E_2 therapy.
3. A woman not interested in pregnancy, but requests for restoration of menstrual cycles, should recieve combined oestrogen-progesterone cyclical therapy.
4. A young woman interested in pregnancy should be offered either ovulation induction therapy (if an ovarian reserve present) or be offered donor eggs for in vitro fertilization.
5. In a young woman with a diminished ovarian reserve, Dehydroepiandrosterone (DHEA) 25 mg + folic acid (OVOSTORE) three times a day for 4–6 months and stimulation of ovary improves the pregnancy rate (30%–50%) by increasing the oocyte and embryo quality. It also reduces aneuploidy in embryos.

LATE MENOPAUSE

It is defined as a condition in which menstruation continues beyond 52 years. Late menopause occurs in women with fibroids and is seen in women who develop endometrial cancer. Often it is constitutional. Beyond 52 years, endometrial biopsy is required to rule out endometrial pathology.

Benefits of late menopause are:

- Late ageing – better quality of life
- Cardioprotective, delay in osteoporosis

Disadvantages – increased risk of breast, uterine and ovarian malignancies.

POSTMENOPAUSAL BLEEDING

Postmenopausal bleeding is defined as any bleeding from genital tract after 1 year of menopause. Normally a 1-year period of amenorrhoea after the age of 40 is considered as menopause. However, vaginal bleeding occurring anytime after 6 months of amenorrhoea in a menopausal age should be considered as postmenopausal bleeding and investigated. Even without amenorrhoea or irregular bleeding, if a woman older than 52 years continues to menstruate, she needs investigations to rule out endometrial hyperplasia and malignancy of the genital tract. Malignancies of genital tract remains a cause of concern in woman with postmenopausal bleeding and need to be ruled out.

CAUSE OF POSTMENOPAUSAL BLEEDING

Several causes account for genital tract bleeding in a postmenopausal woman (Table 7.4):

1. **Vulva** – trauma, vulvitis, benign and malignant lesions.
2. **Vagina** – foreign body such as ring pessary for prolapse, senile vaginitis, vaginal tumour (benign as well as malignant) and postradiation vaginitis.
3. **Cervix** – cervical erosion, cervicitis, polyp, decubitus ulcer in prolapse and **cervical malignancy.**
4. **Uterus** – senile endometritis, tubercular endometritis, endometrial hyperplasia (10%), polyp, **endometrial carcinoma** and sarcoma and mixed mesodermal tumour.
5. Uterine polypi and **endometrial hyperplasia.**
6. **Fallopian tube** malignancy.
7. **Ovary** – benign ovarian tumour such as Brenner tumour**, granulosa** and **theca cell** tumour and **malignant ovarian tumour.**
8. Blood dyscrasia.
9. **Urinary tract** – urethral caruncle, papilloma and carcinoma of the bladder may be mistaken for genital tract bleeding.
10. **Bowel** – bleeding from haemorrhoid, anal fissures and rectal cancer may be misleading.

Table 7.4 Cause of Postmenopausal Bleeding

1. Malignancies: Carcinoma of the endometrium Carcinoma of the cervix Carcinoma of the ovary Carcinoma of the vulva and vagina Sarcoma of the uterus
2. Benign causes: Endometrial hyperplasia Endometrial polyps Fibroids Decubitus ulcer
3. Infections: Pyometra Tuberculosis Senile vaginitis Senile endometriosis
4. Bleeding from urinary tract or anal canal
5. Irregular intake of HRT

An important reason for postmenopausal bleeding is indiscriminate or prolonged use of oestrogen unopposed by progestogens, and HRT when applied cyclically. Tamoxifen causes endometrial hyperplasia and cancer.

Twenty to thirty per cent of postmenopausal bleeding is attributed to malignancy of the genital tract, the most common being endometrial cancer, cervical cancer and ovarian tumours. Common benign conditions are endometrial hyperplasia and polypi and dysfunctional uterine bleeding. Postmenopausal bleeding due to oestrogen and tamoxifen are not uncommon, others are rare.

CLINICAL FEATURES

HISTORY

The age of menopause, history of taking oestrogen and tamoxifen should be elicited. Abdominal pain and foul-smelling discharge are noted in malignant tumours. Urinary and rectal symptoms are also important features to be noted.

EXAMINATION

1. Blood pressure.
2. General examination includes BMI and obese women are prone to endometrial cancer.
3. Abdominal palpation will reveal a tumour or ascites.
4. Speculum and bimanual examination may reveal an obvious cause in the lower genital tract such as cancer cervix.

INVESTIGATIONS

Excluding malignancy is the main aim of investigations:

1. Blood count and smear will reveal blood dyscrasia.
2. Blood sugar levels.
3. Cervical cytology or cervical biopsy from obvious lesions. Endometrial tissue sampling.
4. Sonosalpingography for endometrial polyp.
5. Ultrasound – endometrial thickness of more than 4 mm indicates the need of endometrial biopsy.
6. CA 125 serum levels.

Several methods are now available to obtain endometrial tissue for histological examination. Although many endometrial benign lesions cause bleeding, the main objective is to exclude malignancy:

- Dilation and curettage (D&C) – fractional curettage comprising of separate scrapings of endometrium and endocervix not only allows the exact site of malignancy if present but also detects the extent of spread of the

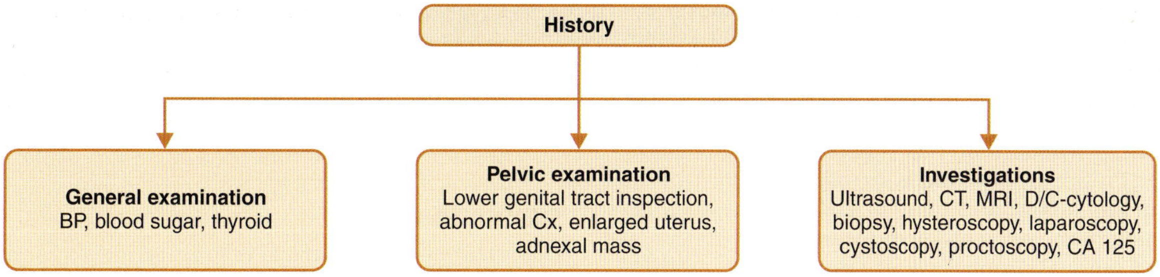

Figure 7.5 Flowchart of postmenopausal bleeding.

tumour and staging. The curettage requires general anaesthesia and hospitalization.

- Uterine cavity aspiration for endometrial sampling may be done as an outpatient procedure and has the additional advantage of avoiding anaesthesia.
- Hysteroscopy + EA

Vibra aspirator, Gravlee's jet washer, Isaac's aspirator and Pipelle aspirator are used to obtain endometrial sampling.

Aspiration is mainly employed in screening women on HRT and tamoxifen. D&C is best to rule out cancer when postmenopausal bleeding is reported.

None of these methods are 100% foolproof, and in some cases, we may fail to detect the cause of bleeding.

1. Hysteroscopic visualization: To improve the predictive value of endometrial study, **hysteroscopic inspection** and selective biopsy are now considered the gold standard in the diagnosis of endometrial lesion, though 1%–3% false-negative findings are reported.
2. Ultrasound, CT and MRI. Transvaginal ultrasound is an adjunct to other investigations, in detecting the endometrial thickness and irregularity and pelvic tumour. In case endometrial cancer is detected, CT and MRI are useful preoperative investigations and these detect the extent of spread of the tumour to the myometrium and the lymph nodes. Doppler ultrasound with increased diastolic blood flow and low resistant index suggest malignant growth.
3. When the genital tract as a cause of bleeding has been excluded, cystoscopy and proctoscopy may discover the cause of bleeding in bladder or rectum.

Detection of a benign lesion should not deter further investigations to rule out malignancy of the genital tract, as both may coexist. Postmenopausal bleeding is explained in Figs 7.5 and 7.6.

MANAGEMENT

1. Treat the cause.
2. When no cause is found, and if there has been only one bout of bleeding, the patient should be kept under observation. About 80% of these cases do not bleed again. If the woman continues to bleed, or bleeding recurs, it is advisable to perform a laparotomy and hysterectomy. An undiagnosed small tumour may be discovered and dealt with appropriately. Otherwise abdominal hysterectomy with bilateral salpingo-oophorectomy should be performed and the specimen should be sent for histopathological study.

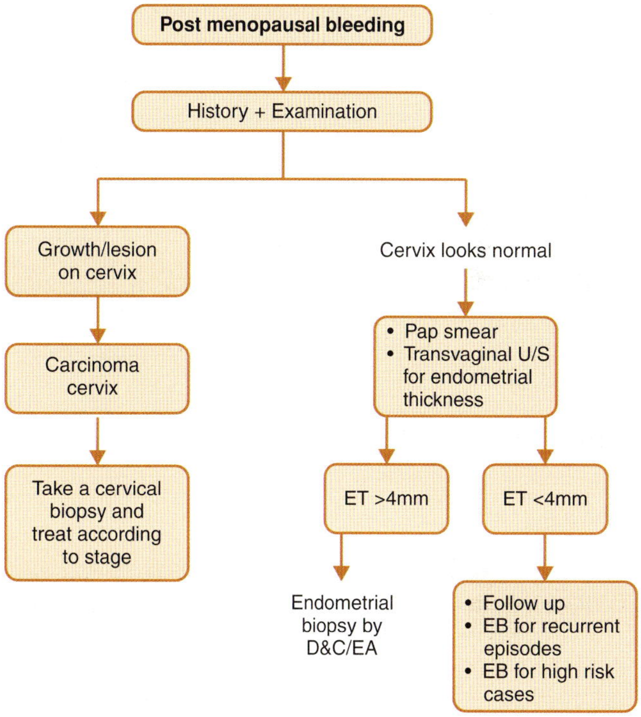

Figure 7.6 Flowchart for investigating post menopausal bleeding. ET: endometrial thickness, EB: endometrial biopsy.

KEY POINTS

- Normal menopause sets in around 48–52 years.
- Premature menopause before 40 years can cause menopausal symptoms, osteoporosis and cardiovascular diseases. Late menopause is a high-risk factor for uterine malignancy and breast cancer.
- In 20%–30% of postmenopausal bleeding is caused by genital cancers, and needs detailed investigations.
- Urethral syndrome, dry vagina with dyspareunia and menopausal symptoms require short-term oestrogen therapy.
- Long-term HRT is protective against osteoporosis, cardiovascular accidents, stroke, Alzheimer disease and colon cancer.
- A proper diet, exercise and HRT help in delaying menopausal diseases. Oestrogen cream, oral tablets with progestogen and skin patches are available. The implants and Mirena have recently been introduced in HRT. Other optional drugs are tibolone (Livial), raloxifene (SERM), phytoestrogens and bisphosphonates.

- Not all require HRT. Rational thinking and recommendation is 'selective use of HRT' with minimal dose for minimum required period. The side effects and contraindications to hormone therapy should be known. A regular follow-up is necessary in women on HRT. Proper counselling is mandatory. The type of hormone, dosage and route of HRT is prescribed according to the need of the individual.
- Nonhormonal prophylactic therapy may be used instead of HRT.
- A woman may spend one-third of her life in oestrogen deficiency state and this may pose health problems. High-risk cases need monitoring and prophylactic therapy so that she leads a healthy life.

SELF-ASSESSMENT

1. Define menopause. Describe the anatomical changes and alterations in the hormonal profile that characterize menopause.
2. Enumerate the symptoms associated with the onset of menopause.
3. Describe the pathophysiology of postmenopausal osteoporosis and its management.
4. Describe the commonly prescribed regimes of HRT. Enumerate its advantages and limitations.
5. Briefly describe the use of medications prescribed in the management of osteoporosis.

SUGGESTED READING

Cauley JA, Seeley DG, Ensrud K, et al. Estrogen replacement therapy and fractures in older women. Study of Osteoporotic Fractures Research Group. *Ann Intrn Med.* 1995;122:9-16.

Colditz GA, Hankinson SE, Hunter DI, et al. The use of estrogens and progestins and the risk of breast cancer in postmenopausal women. *N Eng J Med.* 1995;332:1589-1593.

Jazmann LJB. Epidemiology of the climacteric syndrome. In: Campbell S, (ed). *Management of the Menopause and Post-menopausal Years.* Lancaster, England: MTP Press Ltd; 1976:12.

Lind T, Cameron EC, Hunter WM, et al. A prospective controlled trial of six forms of hormone replacement therapy given to postmenopausal women. *Br J Obstet Gynaecol.* 1979;86:1.

Lobo RA, Picker JH. Wild RA, et al. Metabolic impact of adding medroxyprogesterone acetate to conjugated estrogen therapy in postmenopausal women. The Menopause Study Group. *Obstet Gynecol.* 1994;84:987-995.

Newcombe PA, Longnecker MP, Storer BE, et al. Long-term hormone replacement therapy and risk of breast cancer in postmenopausal women. *Am J Epidemiol.* 1995;142:788-795.

Utian WH, Schiff I. NAMS-Gallup survey on women's knowledge, information, sources and attitudes to menopause and hormone replacement therapy. *Menopause.* 1994;1:39-48.

Breast and Gynaecologist

8

CHAPTER OUTLINE

The breast is an essential part of gynaecological examination and should be included in the general examination of every woman coming with a gynaecological problem.

A routine breast examination may discover a breast lump, hitherto not recognized by the woman. Breast examination becomes mandatory in an ovarian tumour suspected to be a metastatic growth. During infertility work-up, galactorrhoea may point to hyperprolactinaemia as a cause of infertility. In primary amenorrhoea, ill-developed breasts suggest hypothalamic–pituitary cause whereas well-developed secondary sex characters indicate a local genital cause for amenorrhoea. Regular breast examination is essential in a woman on hormonal replacement therapy (Figs 8.1–8.3).

HORMONAL EFFECTS ON THE BREASTS

Breast tissues, glandular, ductal as well as the stroma respond to and remain sensitive to ovarian hormones throughout the reproductive period and also after menopause. Therefore, excess of ovarian hormones and antihormones play a major role in breast diseases.

CONGENITAL DEFORMITIES

Congenital deformities include an absent or an extra nipple, supernumerary breasts, aplasia or hypoplasia, sometimes unilateral.

In Turner syndrome, and in some cases of primary amenorrhoea, oestrogen therapy may develop breasts and reduce the risk of osteoporosis.

Trauma and infection are mainly confined to breastfeeding puerperal women. Cracked nipples will be healed with Masse cream. Mastitis requires analgesic, hot fomentation and antibiotics. An abscess will require incision and drainage.

MASTALGIA

Painful breast seen in young women is often cyclical, but in older women it is usually acyclical. Cyclical mastalgia is the breast pain occurring for a few days before menstruation. Severe mastalgia lasts more than 7 days, requires drugs and interferes with the woman's activities. Chronic mastalgia is described when pain lasts for more than 6 months, and requires investigations.

TREATMENT

Treatment (Fig. 8.4) comprises the following:

- Analgesics – nonsteroidal anti-inflammatory drugs (NSAIDs).
- Evening primrose oil capsule (Wellwomen capsule) containing gamma linoleic acid or gamolenic acid 3 g daily relieves pain in 70%. Occasional nausea and headache are the side effects.
- Danazol 100 mg b.i.d. produces severe androgenic side effects in some, and is expensive. Although it is 70% effective, cost and side effects may preclude some woman taking them. Vitamin B_6 benefits few women.
- Bromocriptine 2.5 mg b.i.d.: Nausea, vomiting and giddiness may occur, and because of these side effects, compliance is poor with danazol and bromocriptine. About 45% success is reported. *Cabergoline is long-acting with less side effects.* (Dostinex 0.25 mg twice a week.)
- Tamoxifen 10 mg has less side effects, but endometrial hyperplasia and in rare cases, cancer has been reported.

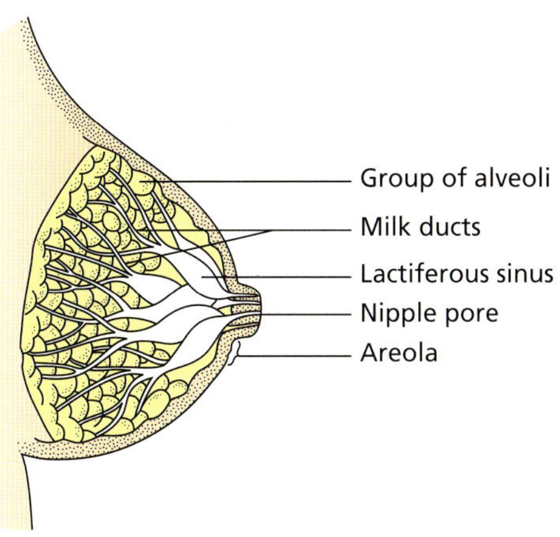

Figure 8.1 Milk-producing structures and ducts in the human breast (simplified cross-section).

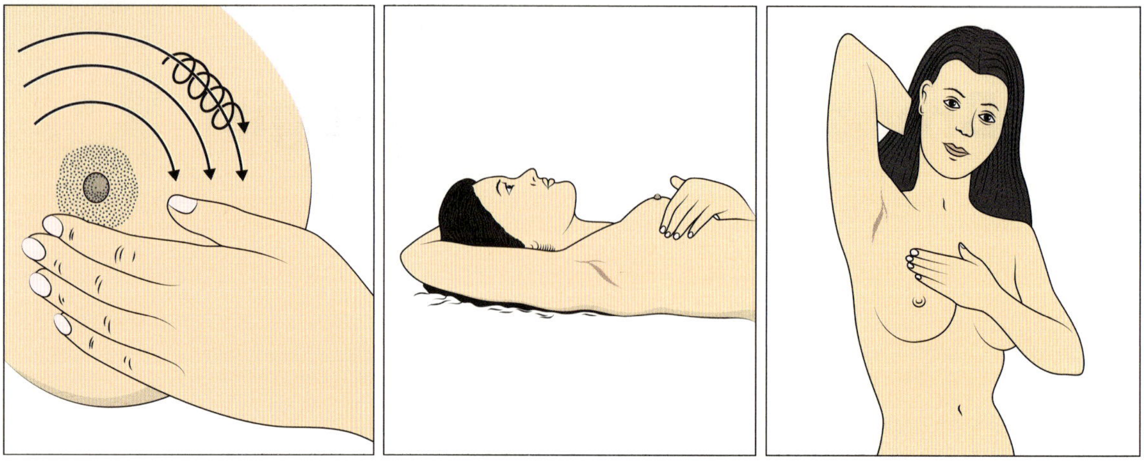

Figure 8.2 Self-palpation of breasts.

- Gonadotropin-releasing hormone (GnRH) analogue (goserelin) 3.6 mg as monthly depot injection is effective but influences the menstrual cycle (amenorrhoea) and causes osteoporosis on prolonged use. Short-term therapy is useful, but very expensive.
- Testosterone undecanoate (Restandol) 40 mg b.i.d. is effective. Androgenic side effects after 3 months of treatment are often the limiting factor in its use.

Noncyclical mastalgia is seen in older women and may be a symptom of breast cancer. This requires investigations to find out the underlying cause. Some women suffer from chest wall pain (Tietze syndrome). If this is the cause, NSAIDs usually relieve pain. If not, injection with an anaesthetic–steroid combination locally has shown 75% response.

BREAST LUMP

Less than 10% women presenting with a breast lump have breast cancer. Nevertheless, systematic examination and investigations are required to rule out malignancy. *Symptomatic lump (pain or growing) requires surgery.*

Cystic swelling. A single cyst is often benign. Multiple cysts can become malignant. Fine-needle aspiration cytology (FNAC), mammography and ultrasound will identify the cyst. *Blood-stained fluid, recurrence after aspiration and multiple cysts should be treated surgically. In young women, simple aspiration and cytology will be adequate. Breast abscess* is an acute disorder affecting women of childbearing age. It can be either lactational or nonlactational. Lactational breast abscess is more common and may be secondary to cracked nipple or trauma while feeding the baby. *Staphylococcus aureus* is the predominant organism found in these cases. Nonlactational abscess occurs in women of older age group as compared to lactational abscess. They are associated with diabetes and history of smoking in females.

Periductal mastitis occurs in older women. Nipple discharge and retracted nipples are clinical features often associated with smoking, although the cause is not clear. Perhaps it alters the bacterial flora in the ducts, with a preponderance of *E. coli* and anaerobic organisms, and this leads to infection. Another possibility is direct toxic action of smoking on the vascular structure of ductal epithelium. Antibiotics and excision of the lesion are required.

Nipple discharge can be hormonal, but blood-stained discharge is due to ductal papilloma and periductal mastitis, rarely due to malignancy. Cytology and mammography are not always useful. Resection of the lobe is the recommended treatment.

GALACTORRHOEA

Galactorrhoea is caused by hyperprolactinaemia and pituitary adenoma. Prolactin level more than 25 ng/mL can cause galactorrhoea, but not all hyperprolactinaemias produce galactorrhoea. The condition is associated with amenorrhoea, oligomenorrhoea and infertility. The macroadenoma can cause pressure on optic nerve. The management of galactorrhoea is described in chapter on Primary and Secondary Amenorrhoea.

Other causes are hypothyroidism, chest wall injury, herpes zoster, stress, and oestrogen and dopamine receptor-blocking agents.

BENIGN TUMOURS

FIBROADENOMA

This is a benign tumour and occurs at any age. It is usually a single tumour, rarely grows more than 5 cm and accounts for 15% of all breast tumours. Before the age of 30 years, the tumour runs a benign course, and if the investigations prove the benign nature of the tumour, it is safe to leave it behind. However, after this age the possibility of malignant change cannot be ruled out, and excision biopsy is recommended. If the benign tumour in a young woman becomes tender or increases in size, surgery is a wise decision.

Fibroadenosis in young women responds to danazol.

Progestogen-only pill (mini pill) reduces the incidence of benign breast disease by 35%–40% but increases the risk of cancer.

Duct papilloma causes blood-stained discharge. The cytology of the discharge, mammography and ultrasound locate the lesion. Ductoscopy confirms the nature of the lesion. It can turn malignant and requires excision.

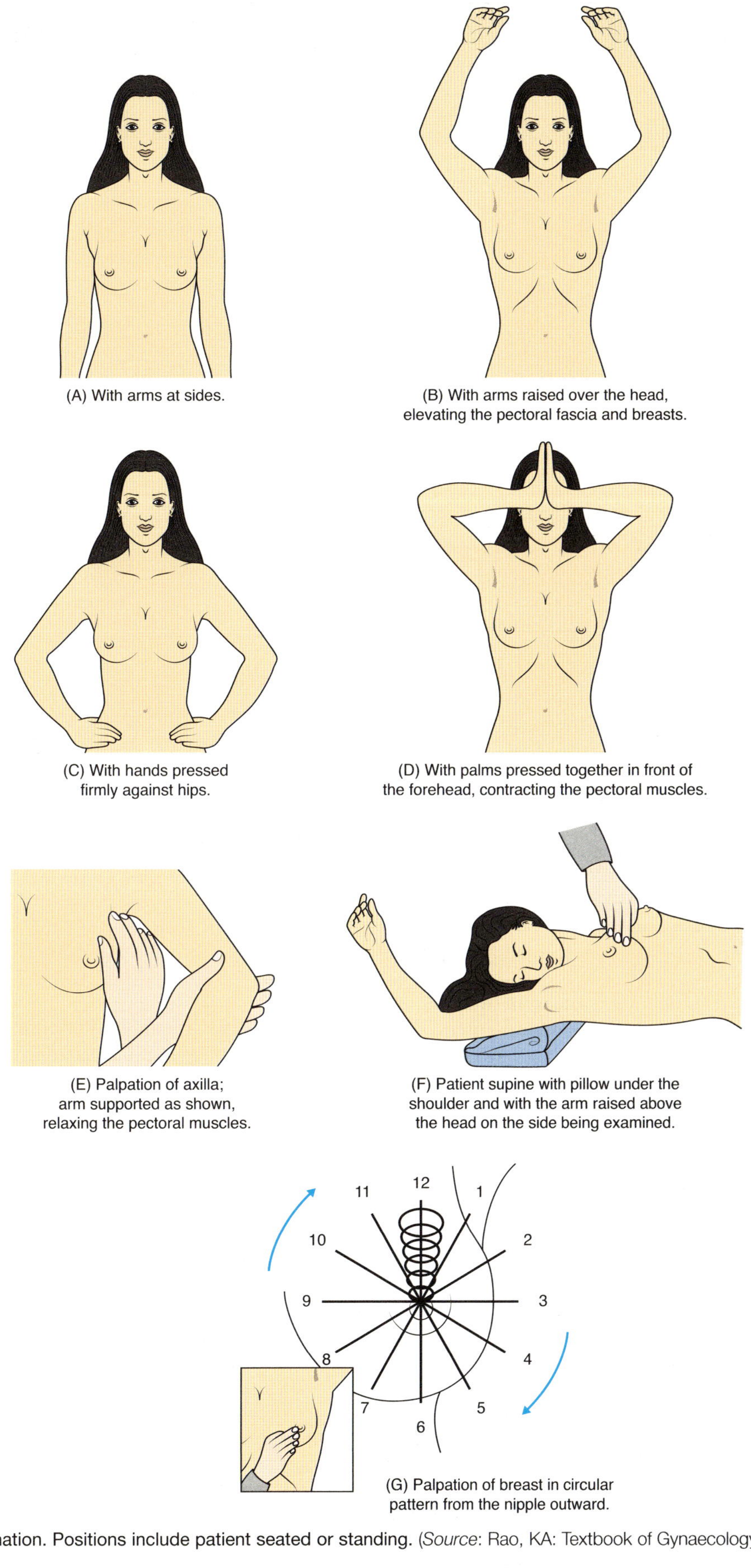

(A) With arms at sides.

(B) With arms raised over the head, elevating the pectoral fascia and breasts.

(C) With hands pressed firmly against hips.

(D) With palms pressed together in front of the forehead, contracting the pectoral muscles.

(E) Palpation of axilla; arm supported as shown, relaxing the pectoral muscles.

(F) Patient supine with pillow under the shoulder and with the arm raised above the head on the side being examined.

(G) Palpation of breast in circular pattern from the nipple outward.

Figure 8.3 Breast examination. Positions include patient seated or standing. (*Source*: Rao, KA: Textbook of Gynaecology, India: Elsevier, 2008.)

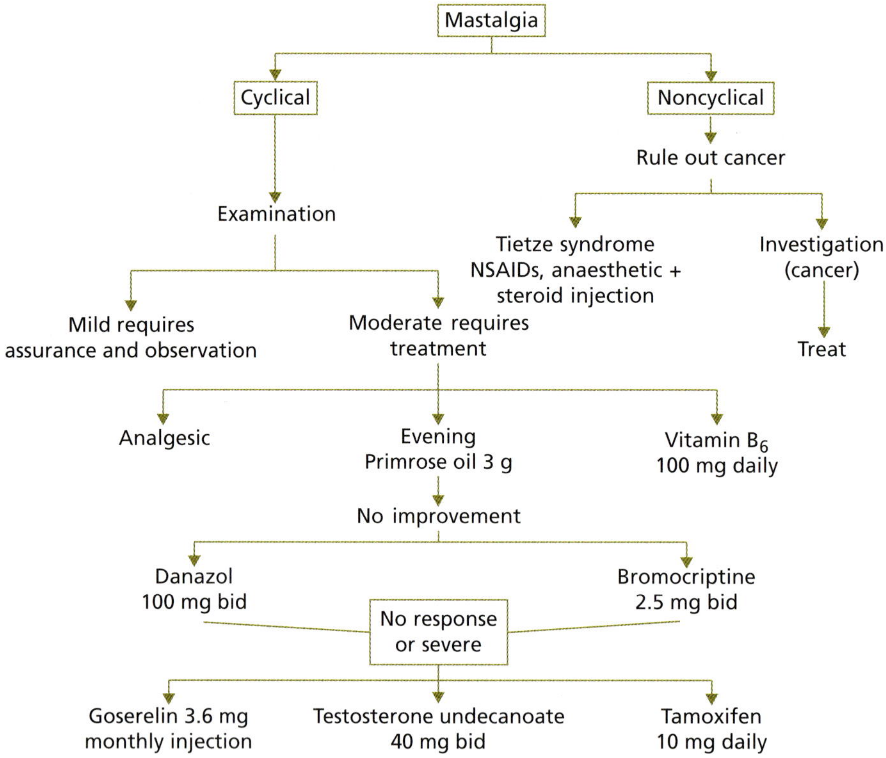

Figure 8.4 Treatment of mastalgia.

PREMENSTRUAL MASTALGIA

It is treated with toremifene, which is an selective estrogen receptor modulator and belongs to the tamoxifen group of drugs; 60 mg daily is given only in the luteal phase. It improves mastalgia in 60% cases. It has lesser side effects as compared to tamoxifen (Fig. 8.4).

BREAST CANCER

Breast cancer is the commonest cancer in woman and accounts for 10% of all breast problems presented at the clinic. Breast carcinoma is more prevalent in elderly women, and needs prompt investigations and treatment comprising surgery followed by radiotherapy and chemotherapy, as the need be. Certain high-risk cases have been recognized and will need regular screening. These are as follows:

- *Familial history.* A family history of breast cancer in first, second degree relatives suggest that genetic factor is responsible for development of breast carcinoma. BRCA1 and BRCA2 genes mutations may be found in 3-8% cases. Presence of these mutations indicates a higher risk of development of breast cancer in other family members.
- A woman with ovarian cancer is at a high risk of breast cancer and vice versa. Both malignancies share common aetiological factors and have common oncogens.
- A woman with ovarian cancer should be screened for breast tumour, as the ovarian tumour could be a metastasis from the breast.
- *Age.* After the age of 60 years, 50% breast lumps prove to be malignant. In childbearing age, 15% of lumps are malignant.
- *Parity.* Nulliparity, late first pregnancy (after age of 30 yrs) and nonlactation are the high-risk factors.
- Obese women too have a propensity for breast cancer.
- Early menarche and late menopause with greater number of menstrual cycles and shorter cycles expose the breast tissues to oestrogen hormones and make them susceptible to the development of breast cancer. Endogenous as well as exogenous oestrogens are carcinogenic. Lately, progestogens also have proved carcinogenic.
- The risk of breast cancer is high in young women on oral contraceptive pills. The risk decreases 10 years after the stoppage of hormones. However, cancer is well differentiated in these women.
- *Smoking.* It encourages periductal mastitis and atypical growth. It is also immunosuppressive. Alcohol too may be a factor.
- *Hormones.* It is strongly suspected that combined oral contraceptives (COC) containing high-potency progestogen given for more than 4 years to a woman younger than 25 years and before her first pregnancy may predispose her to breast cancer at a later age and the risk is two- to fivefold. One should be careful in prescribing COC to young women. Progestogen-only pill (POP), while protecting against benign tumours, increases the risk in elderly women. The risk decreases after 10 years of stoppage of oral contraceptive pills. Low-dose COC may have a lower risk. The risk is related to the duration of COC intake. Lately, COC is considered a higher risk factor than oestrogen alone because of progestogen content.

Breast cancer is the main concern while prescribing hormone replacement therapy (HRT) to a menopausal woman. A woman on HRT should be screened regularly for breast lump, and mammography should be done every 1–2 years. HRT should not be administered for more than 10 years.

Fortunately, breast cancer following HRT is of low malignant "potential" with good prognosis.

It may be prudent not to recommend HRT to a woman treated for breast cancer. It is equally important to carefully monitor a woman on tamoxifen for breast and uterine cancers. It is suggested that vitamin A may be protective. Obesity increases the risk of cancer because of peripheral conversion of oestrogen. Raloxifene is safe against endometrial cancer but causes thrombosis.

CLINICAL FEATURES

Very often, the first thing a woman feels is a lump in her breast. Nipple discharge and pain come later.

The lump feels firm, irregular and fixed in the later stage. Axillary lymph nodes become palpable in the advanced stage. The other breast should also be palpated.

INVESTIGATIONS (Figs 8.5–8.7)

Clinical palpation is not 100% accurate for detecting cancer. In patients younger than 40 years, 50% cases can be missed. Between the age of 40 and 49 years, accuracy is 80%; between 50 and 59 years, 90%; and over 60 years, accuracy is 95%. Self-examination increases the awareness in a woman and brings her to the doctor at an early stage for the treatment. Examination by physician supplements self-examination (Figs 8.2 and 8.3).

Mammography is indicated in the following cases:

- Older and high-risk women.
- To assure normality when a woman has cancer phobia.
- If a lump is present.
- Prior to HRT; Yearly/2-yearly screening between the age of 45 and 60 years is cost-effective.

Contraindications. Mammography is contraindicated in pregnancy because of the risk of radiation.

Using only mammography as an investigation tool is unreliable in 50% women below the age of 40 years because of dense breast tissue. Mammography identifies cancer in 75% cases between 40 and 49 years of age, and reliability increases with age. It must be mentioned that interpretation of mammography findings may be difficult if a woman had previous breast surgery. Similarly, HRT also interferes with mammographic screening. Mammography should include two views of both breasts: *mediolateral oblique view* and *craniocaudal view.* Regular mammography can reduce the mortality of cancer by 30%. The findings include:

- Alteration in density of breast tissue
- Microcalcification
- Thickening of skin
- Presence of fibrous streaks
- Nipple alteration
- Detection of fibroadenoma, lymph nodes, galactocele
- Cysts and solid tumour.

Ultrasound imaging, using 10-MHz probe, is useful in all age groups, especially before the age of 35 years when mammography may not be reliable. Ultrasound differentiates cystic from solid malignant tumour. It is required in young women, pregnant and lactating woman, and in duct papilloma. Ultrasound, however, fails to identify microcalcification, which is the hallmark of

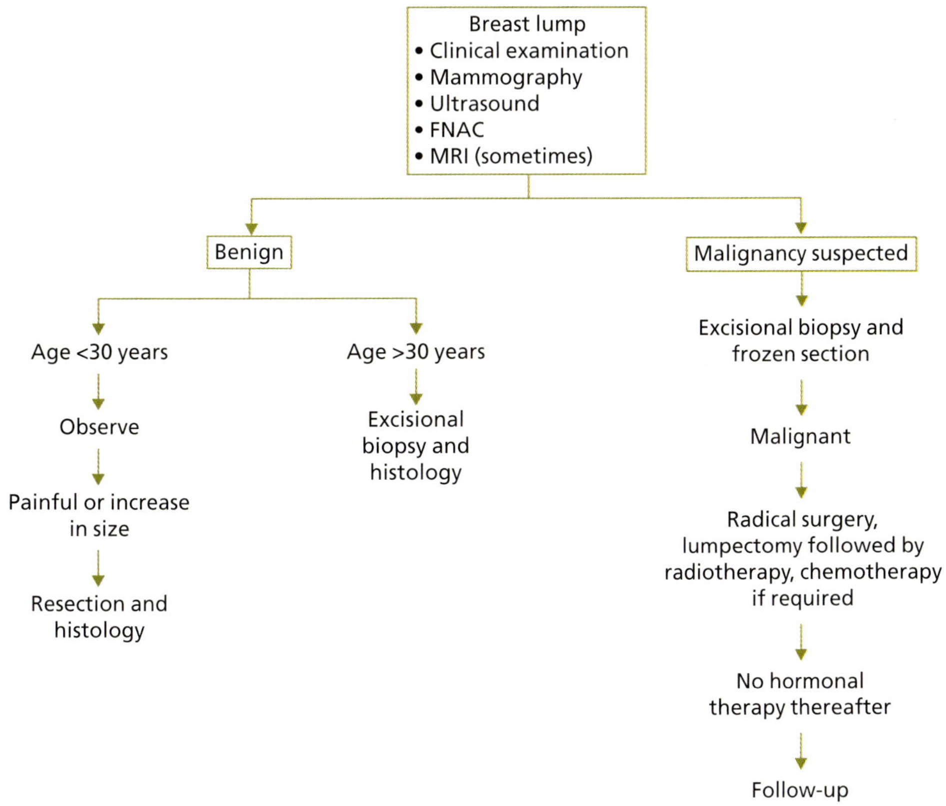

Figure 8.5 Investigation and treatment of breast lump.

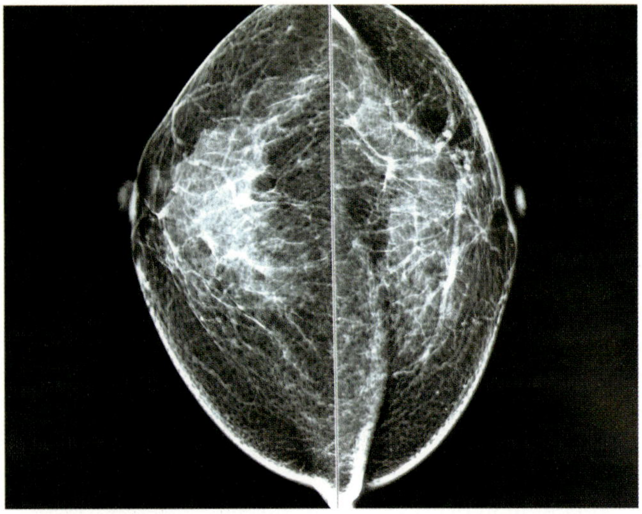

Figure 8.6 CC view – mammography craniocaudal view.

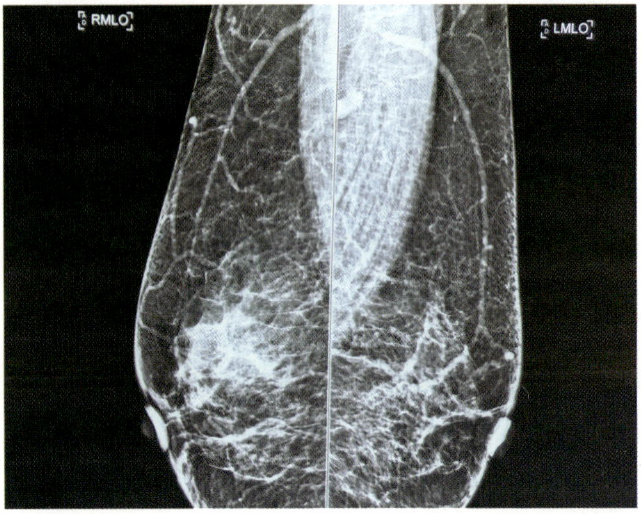

Figure 8.7 MLO – mammography mediolateral oblique view.

early cancer. In the cancer of breast, ovarian screening by ultrasound is important, as one cancer spreads to the other.

- *Doppler ultrasound* displays vascular pattern of a tumour and indicates the probability of malignancy.
- *Computer-aided detecting diagnosis* (CADD) and electrical impedance imaging are new technologies.
- *Ductoscopy and cytology* when duct papilla is suspected.
- *X-ray chest*, CT brain and abdominal ultrasound for metastasis.
- *MRI* gives the most accurate measurement of tumour size of invasive cancer, and helps in staging. It also predicts the response to primary chemotherapy. It is useful in young women and in women who had previous breast surgery.
- *FNAC* under ultrasound or clinical guidance yields the cellular study of lump. Ultrasound/mammography should be performed prior to FNAC because haematoma sometimes caused by aspiration can obscure the image (90%–95% specific).
- Clinical examination, combined with mammography, FNAC and ultrasound can identify cancer in 99.5% cases.
- *Tru-cut biopsy* removes a core of tissue for frozen section, histology and receptor study. A big tumour requires excisional biopsy.

SCREENING

Screening is an important tool to identify women at higher risk of developing breast cancer. It allows for early detection and timely channelization of modalities of treatment best suited for the patient. A patient must be evaluated on the basis of certain risk factors to determine whether referrals are needed for genetic testing and for consideration of chemoprevention and/or prophylactic surgery.

Major factors used to determine a risk category, based on a patient's history, are as follows:

- Personal history of ovarian, peritoneal (including tubal) or breast cancer
- Family history of breast, ovarian or peritoneal cancer
- Genetic predisposition (if the patient's BRCA status is known)
- Radiotherapy of the chest between the age of 10 and 30 years

AVERAGE RISK

- **Age under 40 years** – No screening for average-risk women who are younger than 40 years. Among women younger than 40 years, the incidence of breast cancer is low.
- **Age between 40 and 49 years** – For women who decide to initiate screening in their 40s, a screening mammography every 2 years is performed.
- **Age between 50 and 74 years** – Breast cancer screening with mammography for average-risk women aged between 50 and 74 years. We typically screen every 2 years.
- **Age 75 years and older** – Women older than 74 years should be offered screening only if their life expectancy is at least 10 years.

HIGH RISK

As per American College of Obstetrics and Gynaecology (ACOG) guidelines 2011, for women who test positive for BRCA1 or BRCA2 mutations or have a lifetime risk of 20% or greater, screening should include twice yearly clinical breast examination, annual mammography, annual breast MRI and breast self-examination.

For women who received thoracic irradiation between the age of 10 and 30 years, screening should include annual mammography, annual MRI and screening and clinical breast examination every 6–12 months beginning at 8–10 years after radiation treatment or at the age of 25 years.

As per the American Society of Cancer guidelines 2015, women who are at high risk of breast cancer based on certain factors (such as having a parent, sibling or child with a BRCA1 or BRCA2 gene mutation) should get an MRI and a mammogram every year.

TREATMENT

Treatment comprises the following:

- Excisional biopsy and frozen section followed by definitive surgery as required

- Lumpectomy
- Simple mastectomy
- Radical mastectomy
- Postoperative radiotherapy and chemotherapy

Lumpectomy yields similar results as radical mastectomy. Axillary lymph nodes are removed in the advanced stage.

Radiotherapy may be required as an adjunct in advanced cases. Reconstructive prosthesis is done in the same sitting or at a later date.

Adjuvant chemotherapy reduces the risk of recurrence by 30%. Tamoxifen 20 mg daily or raloxifene 60 mg daily reduces the risk of recurrence in contralateral breast by 50% for about 5 years, but is teratogenic in pregnancy and causes atropic vaginitis. Anastrozole (aromatase inhibitor) is better tolerated than tamoxifen (1–2 mg).

CHEMOTHERAPY

- Four cycles of adriamycin and cyclophosphamide
- Six cycles of 5-FU, adriamycin and cyclophosphamide
- Six cycles of 5-FU, epirubicin and anthracycline

Taxane improves survival. A woman should not conceive for 2 years after stoppage of chemotherapy.

PROGNOSIS

Prognosis is based on staging, E_2 receptors in the tissues and axillary lymph node involvement. Metastasis is treated with chemotherapy.

Ovarian ablation may be required to prevent recurrence.

HRT and COC are contraindicated in a woman who is treated for breast cancer. However, severe menopausal symptoms may require a low-dose therapy. Under supervision, raloxifene is safe, does not cause endometrial hyperplasia and osteoporosis, although risk of thrombosis needs to be watched for. Lactation is also contraindicated in a woman treated for breast cancer because of the risk of developing cancer in the opposite breast.

Breast cancer occurring during pregnancy is known. Surgery and radiotherapy are not contraindicated during pregnancy, provided adequate shielding is provided. If, however, chemotherapy is considered postoperatively, termination of early pregnancy is necessary because of teratogenicity of the drugs. Late in pregnancy, chemotherapy can be delayed until after delivery.

PROPHYLAXIS

Tamoxifen and raloxifene for 5 years:

- Reduce the incidence of contralateral breast cancer by 50%.
- Prolongs disease-free interval.
- Reduces the risk of recurrence.

KEY POINTS

- Examination of the breasts should form part of the routine examination of all patients undergoing gynaecological examination.
- Examination may reveal congenital developmental anomalies such as absent or extra nipple, hypoplasia, mastalgia, mastitis in nursing mothers, cracked nipples, galactorrhoea of significance in infertile women, presence of benign neoplasms such as freely mobile fibroadenomas, presence of cysts such as galactocele, irregular nodularity in chronic cystic mastitis, hard indurated nodule suggestive of breast cancer or the presence of blood-stained nipple discharge indicative of a possible underlying cancer.
- Breast lumps may be benign or malignant. Mammography and ultrasound examination, Doppler studies and MRI reveal presence of solid or cystic neoplasms. FNAC and cytological examination of the aspirate may help to establish early diagnosis of cancer.
- Breast cancer carries a worse prognosis if it occurs during pregnancy and lactation because of immunosuppressive condition.
- HRT is contraindicated in a woman treated for the cancer of breast. However, tibolone and bisphosphonates can be offered to prevent osteoporosis.
- Tamoxifen is teratogenic.
- Increasing awareness among clinicians of the importance of breast examination and teaching patients about the art of self-examination promote early diagnosis of cancer.
- A baseline mammography in all menopausal patients starting HRT is a desirable precaution. Use of oestrogens and progestogens should be withheld in women with a strong family history of breast cancer.

SELF-ASSESSMENT

1. Describe the benign lesions of the breast.
2. A 50-year-old woman presents with a lump in the left breast. How will you manage this case?
3. A 22-year-old nullipara presents with galactorrhoea. How will you manage this case?

SUGGESTED READING

Gradishar WJ, Anderson BO, Balassanian R, Blair SL, Burstein HJ, Cyr A, et al. NCCN Guidelines Insights Breast Cancer, Version 1.2016. J Natl Compr Canc Netw. 2015;13(12):1475–85.

Mango V, Bryce Y, Morris EA, Gianotti E, Pinker K. ACOG practice bulletin July 017: breastcancer risk assessment and screening in average-risk women. Br J Radiol. 2018;24:20170907.

Speroff L, Fritz MA. Clinical Gynecologic Endocrinology and Infertility. 8th ed. Philadelphia: Lippincott Williams & Wilkins, 2011:621-672.

Sule EA, Ewemade F. Management of pregnancy associated breast cancer with chemotherapy in a developing country. Int J Surg Case Rep. 2015;17:117–20.

9 Sexual Development and Disorders of Sexual Development

CHAPTER OUTLINE

Sex differentiation is a complex process comprising a cascade of events that begin with the undifferentiated (potentially bisexual) gonad up to the 6th week of intrauterine life and end up with the development of the specific gonads and their corresponding internal and external genital organs. *Genetic and hormonal influences are the main determinants in the development of sex, although other factors may modify its development.* The environmental and teratogenic factors, such as ionizing radiation, viral infection, chemical agents, immunological disturbances, hormones and nutritional deficiencies, play a role in sexual differentiation.

New insights into the biology of sexual development and advances in chromosome analysis have encouraged clinicians to determine sex of the individual at an early age and institute prompt treatment of the intersexual state to enable the individual to lead a more normal life.

The expanding knowledge and recognition of intersexual states have helped to develop a classification of abnormal sexual development based on gonadal and genital anatomy, chromosomal findings and specific identifiable genetic/metabolic defects.

The knowledge of embryology is necessary to understand how congenital malformations occur in 1% of female population.

PRINCIPLES OF SEXUAL DEVELOPMENT (Fig. 9.1)

The development of normal male and female genital organs and tracts is determined by several factors, all of which are time specific during embryogenesis. In the 5th week of intrauterine life, the undifferentiated gonad contains cortex and medulla. The critical period for gonadal development is at 6–7 weeks of embryogenesis when Y chromosome promotes male gonadal development. The external genital organs (phenotype) start developing at 10th week and reach completion by 16th week.

The genetic sex is determined at fertilization, but the gonads remain undifferentiated until 6 weeks of intrauterine life. First, the sex chromosomes determine whether the indifferent gonad (urogenital ridge) will differentiate into a testis or an ovary. Y chromosome develops a male gonad and absence of Y and presence of XX chromosome develop ovaries. If the gonad is male, genes associated with the Y chromosome interact with other components of the somatic cells in the primitive gonad and initiate development along the male lines. The elaboration of the H–Y antigen complex in the short arm of Y chromosome, known as sex-determining region Y (SRY), induces testicular development. Sertoli cells in the developing testis produce Müllerian-inhibiting substance (MIS) that causes regression of the Müllerian (paramesonephric) ducts. In the absence of MIS, the Müllerian ducts develop passively to form the fallopian tubes, uterus and upper vagina. Female internal organs and external genitalia develop partially without the need of ovarian hormones and differentiate even in the absence of gonads unless interrupted by the regressive influence of MIS. Differentiation of the Müllerian ducts proceeds cephalocaudally to form the female internal genital organs. In the absence of the masculinizing effects of dihydrotestosterone (DHT) of testicular origin, the undifferentiated external genital anlage develops along feminine lines (vulva). The genital tubercle develops into the clitoris and the genital folds into the labia majora. Only if the female fetus is exposed to elevated levels of androgen before the 10th to 12th week of gestation, does any degree of masculine developments occur. In such situations, the external genitalia may appear ambiguous. If the androgens are not elevated until after the 20th week, the only masculine effect is an enlarged clitoris as the external genitalia have fully formed by that time.

In Turner's syndrome, the germ cells fail to migrate to the ovary by 6th week, causing streak ovaries. Two XX chromosomes are required for the ovarian development. The cortex of undifferentiated gonad develops into ovary.

SUMMARY OF SEX ORGANS DEVELOPMENT

GONADS

1. Formation of testis occurs in the presence of Y chromosome (46XY).

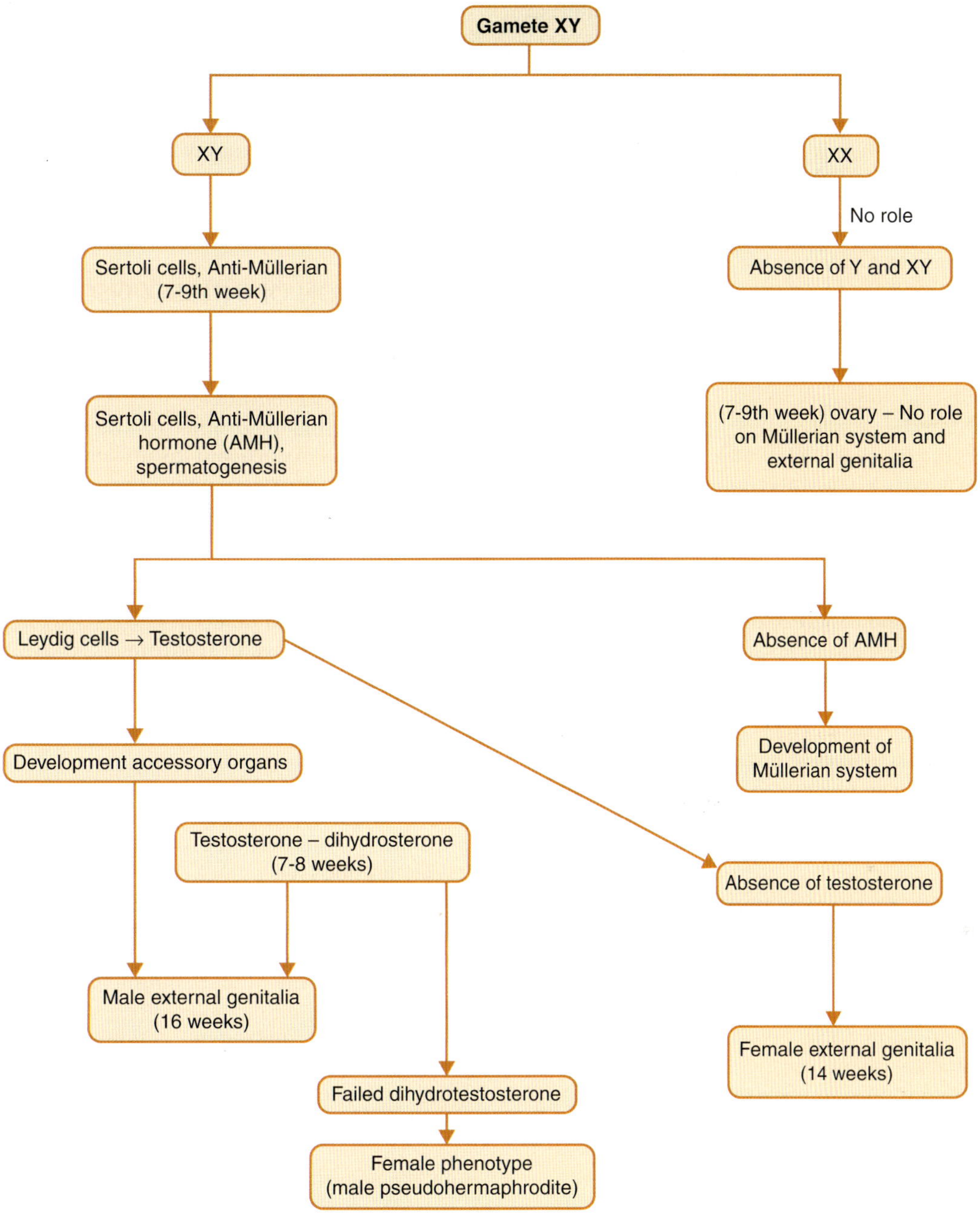

Figure 9.1 Development of male and female reproductive organs.

2. Formation of ovary occurs in the absence of Y chromosome and in the presence of second X chromosome. XX chromosomes are required for ovarian development. One X chromosome causes ovarian dysgenesis or Turner syndrome.
3. Development of the gonads begins between 6 and 7 weeks of gestation.

Testicular determinants: SRY gene of the short arm (p) of the Y chromosome is the gene involved in testis determination. At first, the germ cells appear followed by Sertoli cells that secrete Müllerian-inhibiting factor (MIF) and prevent development of female genital tract.

Sertoli cells also secrete testosterone-binding protein that binds to testosterone; as a result, testosterone concentration in the testis is higher than in serum, and this is necessary for spermatogenesis from primitive germ cells.

A week later (8th week), Leydig cells start secreting testosterone under the influence of human chorionic gonadotropin (hCG) which has LH like activity and develop accessory organs (Wolffian duct).

Peripheral conversion of testosterone to DHT is responsible for male external genitalia (male phenotype); genital tubercle enlarges to form penis by 20th week.

Ovarian determinants: Unless SRY is expressed, ovarian development ensues in the presence of XX karyotype.

The ovary has no role in the development of Müllerian system and external genital organs.

INTERNAL GENITALIA

Wolffian ducts under the influence of testosterone (testes) form epididymis, vas deferens and seminal vesicles (male internal genitalia). MIS from the Sertoli cells suppresses the development of female internal genitalia from the Müllerian ducts. Müllerian ducts in the absence of MIS form fallopian tubes, uterus and upper vagina (female internal genitalia).

Müllerian and Wolffian development begins at the same period of embryogenesis; these are local phenomena occurring ipsilaterally depending on the presence or absence of testosterone and MIS.

EXTERNAL GENITALIA

DHT determines the development of male external genitalia. It is produced in adequate amounts from 7–8 weeks of gestation until term. hCG stimulates Leydig cells of the fetal testis to produce increasing amounts of testosterone, which develops male organs such as vas deferens, epididymis and seminal vesicles. Feminization of the external genitalia is completed by 14 weeks of gestation, whereas masculinization is completed by 16 weeks of gestation. Descent of the testis is mediated by testosterone, insulin-like 3 ligand and its receptor. Masculinization of cloaca occurs only if testosterone is converted via 5-alpha-reductase to DHT. In the absence of this enzyme, the Wolffian system develops normally but external genitalia will be of female phenotype. Similarly, exposure to androgen in utero causes masculinization of external genitalia in a female, but the Müllerian system develops normally.

FACETS OF SEXUAL DIFFERENTIATION

These can be broadly classified as follows:

1. Gonadal development
2. Genital differentiation
3. External genitalia – phenotype.
4. Behavioural differentiation: Sexual/gender identity as male or female is consciously appreciated by an individual by the age of 2–3 years, derived through internalization of cues based on external genitalia. Patients with 5-alpha-reductase deficiency or 17-beta-hydroxysteroid dehydrogenase deficiency may change their identity from male to female at puberty, suggesting a hormonal role in sexualization. Sexuality is influenced by libido driven by testosterone and intimacy driven by oestradiol (Table 9.1).

CLASSIFICATION OF INTERSEX DISORDER

GENDER IDENTITY DISORDERS ASSOCIATED WITH NORMAL SEX CHROMOSOME CONSTITUTIONS

Female pseudohermaphroditism:
- Adrenogenital syndrome (testosterone overproduction due to adrenocorticoid insufficiency)
- 21-alpha-hydroxylase deficiency
- 11-beta-hydroxylase deficiency
- Treatment of mother with progestins or androgens
- Ovarian virilizing tumour

Male pseudohermaphroditism:
- Primary gonadal defect
- Testicular regression syndrome
- Leydig cell agenesis
  - Defective hCG–luteinizing hormone (LH) receptor
- Defect in testosterone synthesis
  - 20,22-desmolase deficiency
  - 3-beta-hydroxylase dehydrogenase deficiency
  - 17-alpha-hydroxylase deficiency
- Male pseudohermaphroditism (testosterone insufficiency only)
  - 17,20-desmolase deficiency
  - 17-beta-hydroxysteroid (17-ketosteroid reductase) dehydrogenase deficiency
  - Defect in the Müllerian-inhibiting system

End-organ defect:
- Disordered androgen action (cytosol androgen receptor-binding defect)
  - Androgen insensitivity syndrome (testicular feminization)

Table 9.1 Chronological Order of Sexual Development

Time in Weeks	Organ	Male	Female
At fertilization	Genetic determinant (XX or XY)	XY and SRY antigen in the short arm of Y chromosome induce testicular development	XX or absence of Y chromosome induces ovarian development
7–8 weeks	Gonads are formed	Testes - seminiferous tubules	Ovarian cortex medulla-rete ovarii
10–12 weeks	Internal and external genitalia	Wolffian duct develops into vas, epididymis, seminal vesicles and external genitalia	Müllerian duct develops into fallopian tube, uterus, cervix and upper three-fourths of vagina; external genitalia
At birth		Appropriate external genitalia	Appropriate external genitalia
Puberty		Continuous GnRH releases testosterone secretion and development of male secondary sex characters	Pulsatile secretion of GnRH releases FSH, LH and ovarian hormones Development of secondary sex characters

    - Incomplete androgen insensitivity syndrome (Reifenstein syndrome)
- Disorders of testosterone metabolism
    - 5-alpha-reductase deficiency

GENDER IDENTITY DISORDERS ASSOCIATED WITH ABNORMAL SEX CHROMOSOME CONSTITUTIONS

Sexual ambiguity infrequent:

- Klinefelter syndrome (XXY)
- Turner syndrome (XO)
- XX male
- Pure gonadal dysgenesis (some forms)

Sexual ambiguity:

- Mixed gonadal dysgenesis (MGD), including
    - Some forms of pure gonadal dysgenesis
    - Dysgenetic male pseudohermaphroditism
- True hermaphroditism

FACTORS INFLUENCING DESIGNATION OF SEX

GENETIC SEX

In each individual, the nuclei of humans contain a diploid number of chromosomes, 22 pairs of autosomes and 1 pair of sex chromosomes, making a total of 46 chromosomes. During maturation, a reduction division results in each ovum or spermatozoon containing only the haploid set of 22 unpaired autosomes and 1 sex chromosome. In the ovum, the sex chromosome is always X, but in the sperm, it is either X or Y.

The relative number of X- and Y-carrying spermatozoa is equal. As the spermatozoon carries either an X or a Y chromosome, fertilization results in a 46-chromosome pattern carrying either an XX or XY – a genetic female or a genetic male, respectively. Thus, the original diploid number of chromosomes is restored (22 pairs of autosomes plus the paired sex chromosomes – 46 in all).

The genetic sex of an individual is determined at fertilization. In the fertilized egg, the Y chromosome directs the development of the undifferentiated gonads into testes and absence of Y into ovaries 2 weeks later. The ovaries do not participate in sexual development. Y chromosome contains on its short arm H–Y antigen (surface SRY cell antigen), which is responsible for the development of testes. The autosomes also take part. This Y chromosome has no further influence beyond the development of the gonads.

The germ cells arise in the endodermal wall of the primitive gut near the yolk sac, from where they migrate along the dorsal mesentery into the gonadal site. Leydig cells (interstitial cells) produce testosterone that develops the Wolffian duct and urogenital sinus into male genital organs and external genitalia respectively. The Sertoli cells of the testes also secrete a nonsteroidal substance known as the MIF, which is responsible for inhibiting the growth of the Müllerian system in males.

The embryo bearing XX chromosome develops along the female line and turns the undifferentiated gonad into ovaries. The absence of testosterone will cause atrophy of the Wolffian duct, and the absence of MIF will permit the growth of the Müllerian system along the female line.

It must be emphasized that it is the absence of Y chromosome with its H–Y antigen that directs the gonads and the Müllerian system into the female pattern. Recently, it has been reported that it is the sex-determining region located on the short arm of Y chromosome (SRY), which controls the development of testes. Its absence leads to the development of female gonads. In a rare case when the Sertoli cells fail to secrete MIF, the individual will develop Müllerian structures in addition to the Wolffian derivatives and grow as a hermaphrodite.

Similarly, castration of male gonads in early embryos will cause atrophy of the Wolffian duct but will permit growth of the Müllerian system along the female lines. Unilateral castration has enabled one-sided growth of the Wolffian system and growth of the Müllerian duct on the castrated side.

The testicular differentiation starts at the 6th week of intrauterine life. First, the Sertoli cells appear followed by the seminiferous tubules. Under hCG influence, Leydig cells secrete testosterone (peak level at 15–18 weeks). In absence of Y chromosome, the ovary develops 2 weeks later.

Chromosomal sex can be determined by the study of the leucocytes or by simply taking a smear from the buccal mucosa (Fig. 9.2). The nuclei of female cells contain a small stainable body called the sex chromatin; hence, female cells are termed as *chromatin positive.* In epithelial cell nuclei, this small, peripherally situated, darkly staining nodule is called the 'Barr body'. Male cell nuclei lack this body and are therefore termed as chromatin negative. This chromatin nodule has been shown to consist of deoxyribonucleic acid (DNA). It measures 1 micron in diameter and is present in approximately 75% of the female cells. A distinctive and similar type of nuclear appendage shaped like a drumstick is seen attached to the nuclear substance of female neutrophils. It is also possible to determine sex from eosinophils. The culture of the fetal cells allows the chromosomal pattern study (Fig. 9.3). The sex of the fetus can be determined in utero by examining fetal

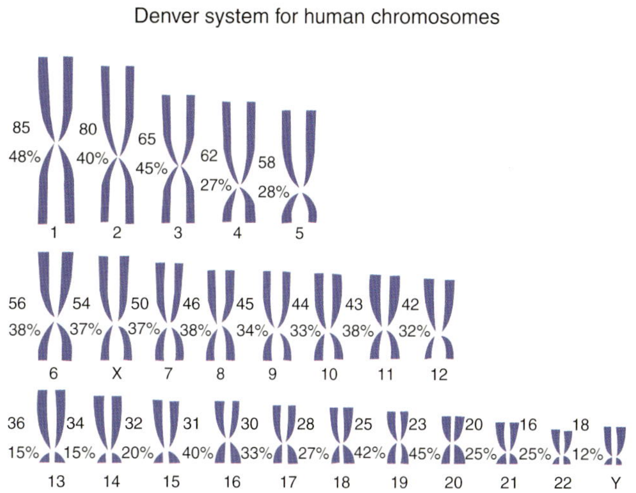

Figure 9.2 An idealized chromosome set, numbered according to the internationally agreed Denver system. Note that only one of each pair is represented. The small figures besides each chromosome indicate approximately the relative length of the whole chromosome and the proportion of the total length occupied by the short-term arm (*Source*: By permission of Dr Bernard Lennox and the Lancet.)

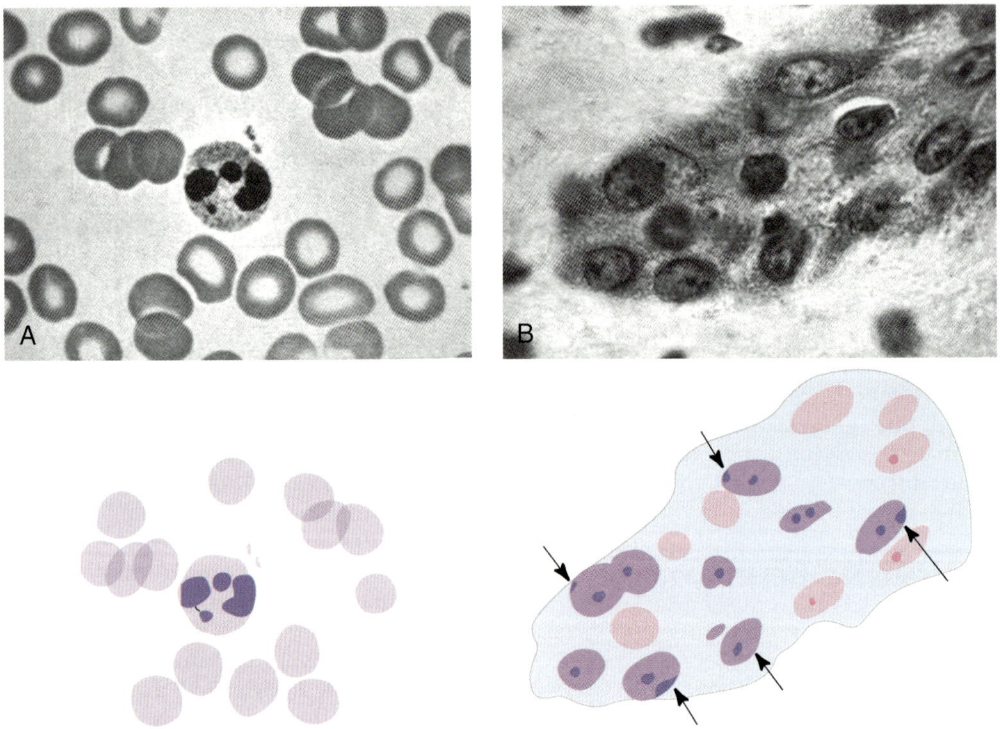

Figure 9.3 **(A)** A typical chromatin nodule in a neutrophil leucocyte in female. The nodule measures 1.4 microns and red cells measure 7.3 microns. **(B)** Typical nodules in the nuclei of the epithelial cells of the skin. The nucleus is 1.6 × 0.9 microns.

desquamated epithelium in the liquor amnii. Chorionic villus biopsy (CVB) either through cervical route in early pregnancy or transabdominally in the second trimester has recently become the well-established technique of determining the fetal sex.

The latest noninvasive technique of studying fetal sex is polymerase chain reaction (PCR) staining of fetal cell-free nuclei in the maternal blood of a pregnant woman.

EXTERNAL ANATOMICAL SEX

The shape of the body contours, the development of the musculature, the characteristics of the bones (notably the pelvis), the distribution of hair on the face and body, breast development and the external genitalia are strong presumptive evidence of either sex.

INTERNAL ANATOMICAL SEX

The presence of a recognizable uterus, fallopian tubes and ovaries is the evidence that the individual is a female. The rare exception is the true hermaphrodite.

GONADAL SEX

Gonadal sex depends on the histological appearance of the gonad from the study of a biopsy or the removal of the organs. It is not entirely diagnostic as in the case of an ovotestis in which both female and male elements are histologically demonstrated. Also, it is possible to have a rudimentary testis on the one side and a rudimentary ovary on the other. Such findings are, however, so rare that the sex of the gonad is a reasonably reliable guide to the true sex of an individual.

HORMONAL INFLUENCES

In a female pseudohermaphrodite, an excess production of androgenic hormone by adrenal cortical hyperplasia can modify the external genitalia of a genetic female. Hypertrophy of the phallus and fusion of the labia majora may cause the parents to consider their child to be a male. The virilizing tumours of the ovary, such as arrhenoblastoma, can cause hirsutism, hypertrophy of the clitoris, deepening of the voice, masculine body contours and amenorrhoea. The presence of oestrogen in the male can cause gynaecomastia (Fig. 9.4). These are all examples of how hormones, natural or exogenous, can modify the sexual organs and secondary sexual characteristics.

PSYCHOLOGICAL SEX

Many men and women are psychologically dominated towards sexual inversion, a persistence of the childhood tendency. Behaviour, speech, dress and sexual inclination proclaim this fact. Transvestism and effeminate behaviour are the most obvious and complete examples where men dress in women's clothes and assume that gender role and vice versa.

ENVIRONMENT AND UPBRINGING

Environment and upbringing decide the sex of rearing. There are many examples of genetic males and females being reared by their parents in the mistaken sexual category, and who have acquired over the years the habits and mental inclination of the opposite sex to a sufficient degree to pass off as members of the opposite sex. Fig. 9.5 shows the development of gonads and genital organs.

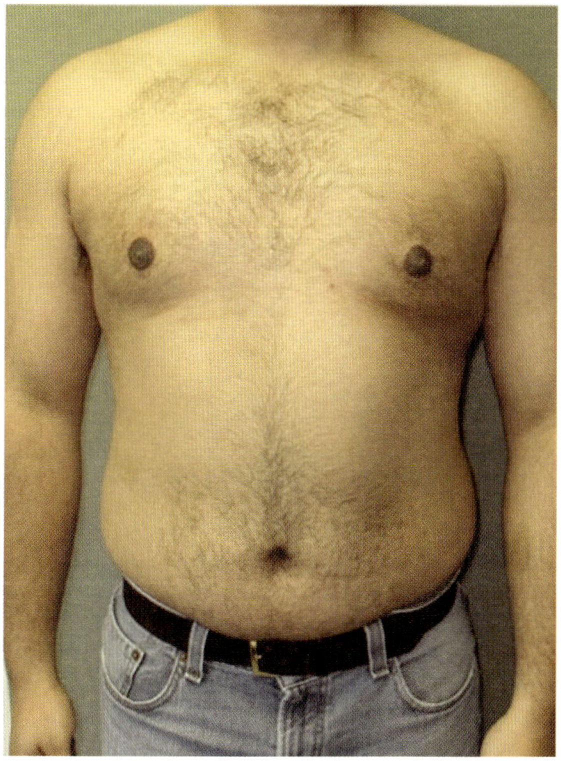

Figure 9.4 Gynaecomastia in an otherwise obvious male. (*Source*: https://www.harleystreetskinclinic.com/en/treatment/gynaecomastia/)

CLINICAL DIAGNOSIS OF SEX

Some of the abnormalities are seen at birth, but most are discovered at puberty.

EXTERNAL APPEARANCE

Most men look like men, and women like women because of their so-called secondary sexual characteristics. A man is broad shouldered, he is more hirsute, especially about the face and chin, his scalp hair is coarser, his nature is more aggressive and robust, his voice deep and his sexual instincts inclined to the heterosexual. A woman has narrow shoulders, broad hips, is rarely hirsute, has fine abundant scalp hair, more delicately modelled features, and a typical pattern of pubic hair, triangular, with the apex downwards and a flat base at the upper level of the mons, her voice is softer, her nature is supposed to be less self-assertive and aggressive than the male and her sexual instincts are heterosexual; a well-developed breast is probably the strongest external evidence of femininity.

EXTERNAL GENITALIA

In the male, the phallus is well developed from genital tubercle, the urethra opens in the glans by 12th week, the scrotum is rugose because of presence of the dartos muscle – an almost exclusively male possession – and the testicles are in the scrotum. In the female, the phallus (clitoris) is rudimentary, the urethra opens into the vestibule, the labia majora are smooth and bifid and do not possess a dartos muscle and a vagina is present.

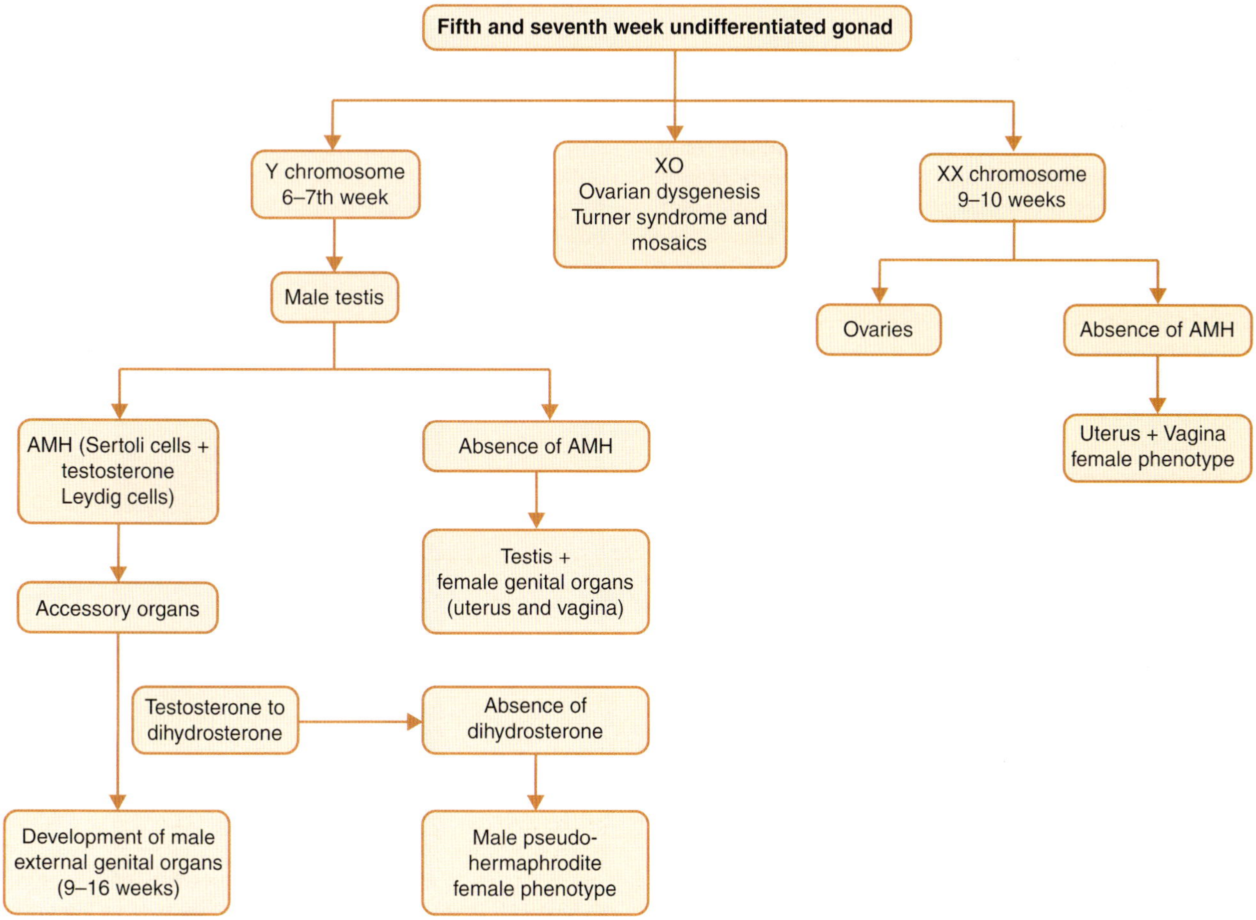

Figure 9.5 Development of gonads and genital organs.

INTERNAL GENITALIA

Bimanual examination discloses the presence of a uterus and appendages in the female.

SIGNS OF FEMINISM IN THE MALE

EXTERNAL APPEARANCE

Feminine figure, poor musculature, a tendency to obesity, high-pitched voice, absence of hirsutism, feminine personality and sexual inclinations and gynaecomastia (Fig. 9.4).

EXTERNAL GENITALIA

Hypospadias (urethra opening below the phallus), underdevelopment of the phallus, a split scrotum and undescended testicles.

Grey areas exist in the biological spectrum ranging from pure masculine to pure feminism.

CLINICAL EXAMPLES

Intersex is classified as follows:

- Chromosomal abnormalities
- Gonadal abnormalities
- Masculinization of female
- Partial or incomplete masculinization in a male

DISORDERS OF FEMALE SEXUAL DIFFERENTIATION

SWYER SYNDROME

This syndrome is a male pseudohermaphrodite, a pure 46XY gonadal dysgenesis with the presence of uterus and the cervix but with hypo-oestrogenism and poorly developed breasts. Undeveloped testes do not secrete testosterone and MIF, resulting in the development of female genital organs and female phenotype. The woman presents with primary amenorrhoea, absence of secondary sex characters and female external genitalia. Cyclical oestrogen and progestogen can induce menstruation. Conception with in vitro fertilization (IVF) using donor eggs is a possibility. The gonads (testes) have 30% risk to develop malignancy and should be removed.

TURNER SYNDROME

Incidence of Turner syndrome is 1:2000 to 1:5000 live born girls. About 70%–90% of pregnancies with XO chromosome abort in early weeks of gestation. In this syndrome, either the short arm of X chromosome is deleted or the nucleus possesses only 45 chromosomes, i.e. 22 pairs of autosomes plus a sex chromosome XO. The absence of Y chromosome resembles the female, but these patients are, like males, chromatin negative, i.e. their nuclei contain no nuclear satellite body and no drumsticks in the neutrophils. It should be explained here that the presence of a Barr body is dependent on the presence of the second X chromosome, and if the chromosome pattern is XXX or XXXY, the extra X complement renders the eccentric chromatin nodule either larger in size or in number.

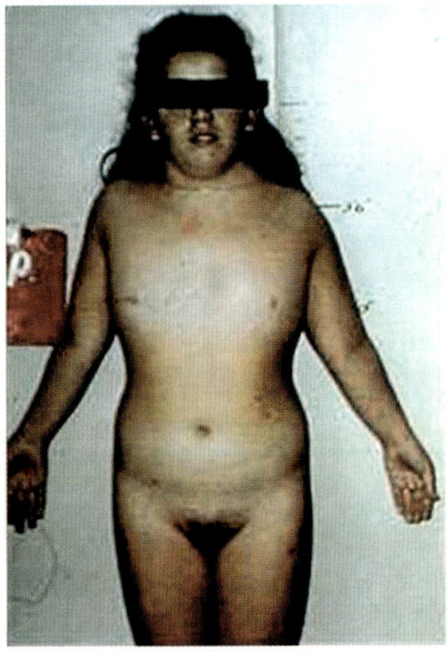

Figure 9.6 Turner syndrome. Note the marked cubitus valgus. (*Source*: Neena Khanna, Illustrated Synopsis of Dermatology and Sexually Transmitted Diseases, Sexual Growth and Development, 4th ed. Elsevier, 2012.)

Turner syndrome has also been called ovarian agenesis or gonadal dysgenesis because at laparotomy the gonad is found to consist of undifferentiated stroma with absence of sex cells, a mere pale strip of fibrous tissue attached to the back of the broad ligament, the so- called streak gonad. The follicles grow up to 20th week of fetal life but become atretic due to absence of one X sex chromosome. In some, germ cells fail to migrate to the genital ridge from the yolk sac. These ovaries do not contain Graafian follicles, so oestrogen is not produced. The patients are clinically of short stature, though not actual dwarfs, the trunk is muscular, the neck is short and webbed, and cubitus valgus is notable. The breasts are not developed; pubic and axillary hair are scanty or absent (Figs 9.6 and 9.7). Exaggerated epicanthic folds may be present, one of the obvious defects first noticeable on examining the patient. The vagina and uterus are present but underdeveloped. Other gross congenital abnormalities are present such as coarctation of the aorta and deformities of the digits are also seen. Other stigma of Turner syndromes includes shield chest, high palate,

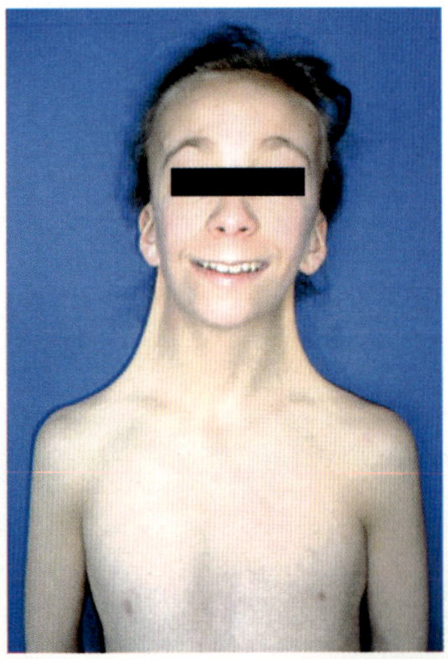

Figure 9.7 Turner syndrome. Note the webbing of the neck and aplasia of breasts.

low-set ears, lymphoedema of the extremities at birth and deafness. The stigma is due to chromosomal deficiency in the short arm of X chromosome and is not always present (seen in 20%–30%), and the percentage of stigma depends on the percentage of abnormal X chromosome.

The classical case of Turner syndrome as described should have a chromosomal pattern of XO. However, there are variants in which mosaicism of XO/XX or even XO/XY produce less clear-cut syndromes, e.g. a normal-appearing female apart from gonadal dysgenesis. When a young girl with Turner's syndrome presents with primary amenorrhoea and serum follicule-stimulating hormone (FSH) is above 40mIU/mL and E2 is below 25 pg/mL, ostrogen therapt with intermittent progesterone is advised to prevent osteoporosis. Artificial vagina may be needed at a later date for sexual function. Administration of growth hormone 0.05 mg daily for 5 years near puberty will improve the height. A pregnancy can occur with donor egg in IVF programme if the uterus is present. If few follicles persist after puberty, menstruation and pregnancy is possible (15%).

SUPERFEMALE (TRIPLE X CHROMOSOME)

The presence of an extra X is not uncommon because it is quite compatible with complete feminine normality. There is, however, a well-recognized triple X syndrome in which the patient, who is often mentally subnormal, suffers from scanty or irregular menstruation and infertility. Clinical examination may reveal hypoplasia of the genital tract. The importance of chromosomal studies in such a patient is obvious, and its determination plays an important role in the investigations and management.

MALE PSEUDOHERMAPHRODITE

Testicular feminizing syndrome, initially described by Norris in 1953, is now designated as either complete androgen insensitivity syndrome (CAIS) or partial androgen insensitivity syndrome (PAIS), and this reflects the aetiology. Incidence is 1:2000 to 1:60,000.

AETIOLOGY

The peripheral receptors for testosterone are absent or are scanty or they fail to respond to testosterone. The external genitalia are of female phenotype. Chromosome is XY, and the testes are located along its line of descent in the abdominal cavity or in inguinal canal, and are maldeveloped. The Wolffian duct fails to develop because of absence of testosterone receptors. Testes produce MIF, so the Müllerian system fails to develop. However, the lower portion of the vagina derived from sinovaginal bulb appears as a dimple of 1–2 cm in length. There is often a strong familial tendency to this disorder, and several cases may appear in the same family and in different generations, and the condition is attributed to X-linked recessive gene.

Unless there is a family history, or childhood inguinal hernia containing the testis, the condition is not diagnosed until puberty. The girl is typically feminine and tall. The pubic and axillary hair are scanty, but the breasts are developed because of oestrogen derived from peripheral conversion of androstenedione. The girl presents with primary amenorrhoea. Ovaries and uterus are absent.

Ultrasound reveals absence of ovaries and uterus. Testosterone is present (>200 ng/mL). LH is raised, but FSH is normal. Chromosome study reveals XY chromosomes (Fig. 9.8A and B).

MANAGEMENT

- Once diagnosed, it is important to trace the location of the testes and perform gonadectomy, because testes are liable to undergo malignancy in 10%–30% cases. The controversial point is as to when to perform gonadectomy. It is preferred to remove the testes in puberty when the correct diagnosis is made (16–18 years).

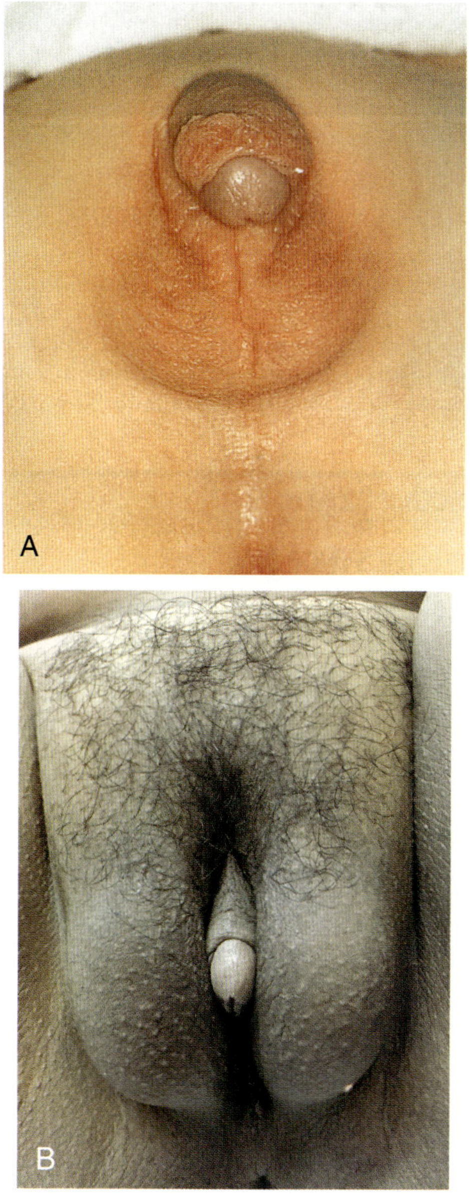

Figure 9.8 **(A)** Ambiguous genitalia in a child with XY karyotype and partial androgen insensitivity. **(B)** Male pseudohermaphrodite showing micropenis with labioscrotal gonads. (*Source* **(A):** Hacker NF, Gambone JC, Hobel CJ, Hacker and Moore's Essentials of Obstetrics and Gynecology, 5th ed. Philadelphia: Elsevier, 2010. *Courtesy*: **(B)** Dr Sunesh kumar, AIIMS)

- These patients will require oestrogen therapy for the development of the breasts and to prevent osteoporosis.
- If she plans to marry, vaginoplasty should be done. If sufficient length of vagina prevails, vaginal dilators may be effective in stretching its length.

The reproductive function is not possible with absent ovaries and uterus.

PARTIAL ANDROGEN INSENSITIVITY SYNDROME

In PAIS, few receptors respond to testosterone, and the clinical features are variable. Some present at birth with ambiguous genitalia, and chromosome study reveals XY chromosomes. Others present at puberty with lack of virilization in a boy, or signs of virilization in a girl with primary amenorrhoea.

The treatment is based on the sex in which the child is reared, psychological behaviour and the amount of virilization. If the child is reared as female, it is best to perform gonadectomy in childhood to avoid virilization. In a boy, testosterone will help. The reproductive function remains poor.

ENZYME ERRORS IN ANDROGEN PRODUCTION

The production of testosterone from the testes requires enzymes, the most important of which is 5-alpha-reductase. This enzyme converts testosterone into DHT, which is capable of acting on peripheral target tissues to produce male phenotype. Absence of this enzyme results in female phenotype and male pseudohermaphroditism.

MASCULINIZATION

KLINEFELTER SYNDROME

Klinefelter syndrome is seen in 1:500 males. The patient with this rare disorder externally resembles a male in general body conformity, the penis is small or normal in size; the testes are small, but as a rule are normally placed. Sterility is common, gynaecomastia is frequently present (Fig. 9.4), the voice may be high pitched, and the appearance may be eunuchoid. The patient is often mentally defective or delinquent. Most of these individuals are sex chromatin positive like females because of the extra X chromosome. Genetic analysis reveals their karyotype to be 47XXY. Testicular biopsy usually reveals hyaline degeneration of the seminiferous tubules and overgrowth of Leydig cells, as a result of which sterility is so often the presenting symptom (Fig. 9.9). Sole-to-pubic length is more than normal. The person should be bred as male and should not be told about chromosomal abnormality. Testosterone may help. The breasts may need surgical excision.

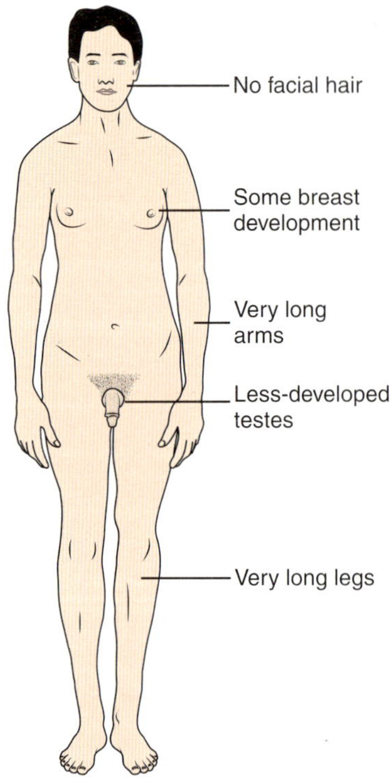

Figure 9.9 Klinefelter syndrome. Note the superficially normal male genitalia, gynaecomastia and feminine distribution of the pubic hair.

VIRILISM

Virilism is characterized by hirsutism and some of the male appearances, and atrophy of the breasts.

In patients exhibiting virilism, the chromosomal and gonadal sex is female and the accessory sex organs of Müllerian origin are also feminine. The external genitalia, however, resemble the male.

CLINICAL FEATURES

The body conformity is largely male with good muscular development and broad shoulders. The voice is deep and the thyroid cartilage is prominent. Hirsutism is present to a remarkable degree, with a male distribution of hair. The psychological sex is often but not invariably male.

The external genitalia show hypertrophy of the clitoris and fusion of the labia majora due to failure of the cloacal membrane to divide in congenital variety. The vagina is often absent if the cause is congenital (Figs 9.10 and 9.11). The breasts are underdeveloped. Other signs are frontal, temporal and vertex baldness, hoarseness of voice, diminished size of breasts, hirsutism, clitoral enlargement, acne and amenorrhoea. Adrenal tumour and male hormone secreting ovarian tumor are responsible for virilism.

CLINICAL VARIETIES

ADRENOGENITAL SYNDROME

Adrenogenital syndrome occurs due to hyperplasia of the adrenal cortex and is of two types. This condition is also known as congenital adrenal hyperplasia (CAH).

Congenital or Intrauterine Adrenogenital Syndrome

Congenital or intrauterine adrenogenital syndrome (CAS) is the condition in which the primary defect is a block in the conversion of progesterone to deoxycorticosterone due to enzyme failure of 21-hydroxylase. The normal adrenal cortex produces three C21 compounds: hydrocortisone,

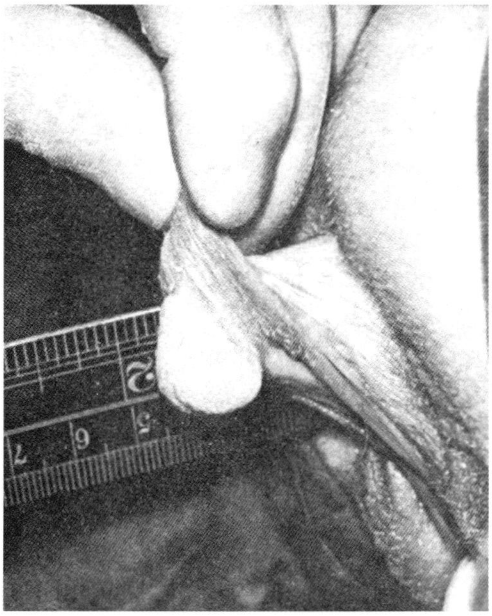

Figure 9.10 Female hermaphrodite showing hypertrophy of the phallus, masculine appearance of the glans and rudimentary scrotal sac.

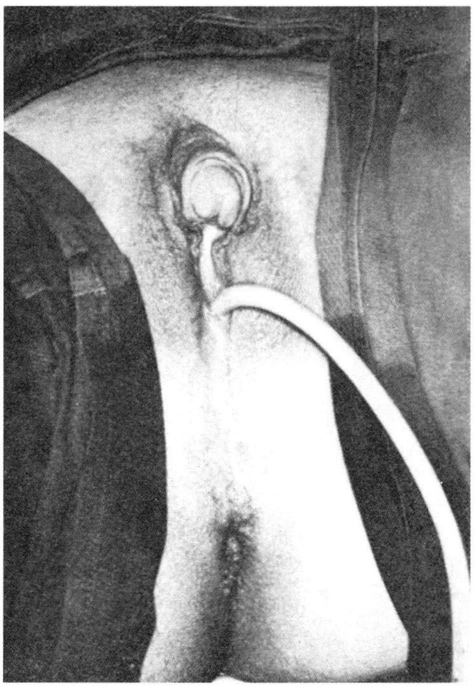

Figure 9.11 Patient with a catheter in the immature vagina.

corticosterone and aldosterone and in addition certain androgen C19 compounds. The production of 17-hydroxyprogesterone, which is mildly androgenic in action, is controlled by adrenocorticotropic hormone (ACTH), and this, in turn, is controlled by the reciprocal action of hydrocortisone. If, therefore, the hydrocortisone–ACTH interaction is upset by a deficiency of hydrocortisone, the pituitary gland produces an excess of ACTH, which in turn leads to adrenal cortical hyperplasia and excess output of androgens, notably 17-hydroxyprogesterone. The main androgenic activity of 17-hydroxyprogesterone is due to its conversion into D4-androstenedione and hence to other orthodox androgens. These androgens are responsible for phallus of the female pseudohermaphrodite showing hypertrophy, the masculine appearance of the glans, and the persistence fusion of the labia majora to resemble a scrotum (Fig. 9.10). The miniature vagina opens into the urogenital sinus and the external appearance is that of a male with hypospadias (Fig. 9.11). The diagnostic feature is the very high value of 17-ketosteroids and 17-hydroxyprogesterone (>8 mg/mL) excreted. As expected, the chromosomal pattern in these girls is XX. Ultrasound should be done to look for ovarian and adrenal tumours. Electrolytes should be monitored, as there is a possibility of hyperkalaemia and hyponatraemia.

The treatment of this condition consists in the administration of cortisone or hydrocortisone or the newer synthetic corticosteroids such as prednisone or prednisolone (2.5 mg twice daily is an adequate maintenance dose for adult and will restore the output of 17-ketosteroids to normal). The continued use of these drugs carries certain dangers of adrenal deficiency due to suppression of ACTH, and this especially operates at times of stress such as when a patient needs an anesthetic. At these times, cortisone coverage should be given to tide over the period of stress (i.e. 1 day before, on the day of operation and for 3 days afterwards). Dose of cortisone is 0.15 mg/kg in four divided doses for child. In a child with salt-losing condition, fludrocortisone 50–100 mcg daily with intravenous (i.v.) saline is recommended.

The vulval abnormality is corrected by a small plastic operation, and as a rule, it is wise to amputate the hypertrophied clitoris between 5 and 10 years of age. Clitoroplasty with conservation of glans is preferred to amputation. Fusion of labial folds should be corrected at puberty. Menarche is often delayed and fertility is reduced in these girls.

Cases of virilization of the fetus in utero have been reported following the use of progesterone in the pregnant mother. In fact, all synthetic progestogens except 17-hydroxyprogesterone have some degree of androgenic effect. If progestogen is to be used in pregnant woman it should be devoid of any androgenic effect.

The effect on the fetus depends largely on the duration of the pregnancy at the time of administration and the dosage employed. If progestogens are given before the 12th to 14th weeks of gestation, the neonatal picture may be similar to that of the intrauterine adrenogenital syndrome, i.e. enlarged phallus and imperforate perineal membrane. The virilism is, however, nonprogressive.

Postnatal Adrenogenital Syndrome

This can be due to excessive output of ACTH from a basophil adenoma of the anterior pituitary gland (Cushing syndrome) which gives rise to adrenal cortical hyperplasia. An adrenal tumour that can be benign or malignant has the same effect. An adrenal tumour is not dependent on influence of pituitary gland. In an undiagnosed case, initial accelerated skeletal maturation is followed by early epiphyseal fusion and stunted height. Precocious puberty and increased libido with aggressive behaviour is reported in a few cases. Sterility is common. Cortisol therapy can avoid these undesirable effects. Males with this syndrome also present with these features.

VIRILIZING TUMOURS AND OTHER CONDITIONS OF THE OVARY

The virilizing tumours and other conditions of the ovary, such as arrhenoblastoma, hilus cell tumour, polycystic ovary and hyperthecosis, are causes of virilism and produce a clinical picture somewhat similar to the postnatal adrenogenital syndrome and are due to excess of testosterone secreted by the ovary. In the postnatal variety of virilism, the genital tract is normal, but the clitoris enlarges, the uterus atrophies with the resulting amenorrhoea, the voice deepens, hirsutism is marked and the breasts atrophy. Excretion of 17-ketosteroids is raised only if the adrenal is hyperplastic or neoplastic, whereas with a virilizing ovarian tumour, it is unaltered.

TREATMENT

FEMALE PSEUDOHERMAPHRODITISM

- If the fault is an enzyme block at the level of 17-hydroxyprogesterone, the administration of cortisone or synthetic corticosteroids will effectively control the excess production of ACTH. The external genitalia can be restored to a feminine pattern by plastic surgery, e.g. the formation of an artificial vagina by McIndoe's operation. Cortisone therapy, if successful, may restore menstruation in a patient with amenorrhoea. It is important in such patients to correct any anatomical defects of the lower genital tract in order to obviate the complications of retained menstrual products such as haematocolpos or haematometra.
- If the virilism is due to a tumour, surgical removal is needed. This also applies to ovarian androgenic tumours.
- A regular maintenance dose of oestrogen is usually effective in restoring some of the secondary sex characteristics, e.g. breast development. Additional intermittent progesterone therapy prevents breast and uterine malignancy.
- The most effective treatment of facial hirsutism is shaving and cosmetics.

INVESTIGATIONS AND MANAGEMENT OF AN INTERSEXUAL PATIENT

In the determination of a patient's sex, the following investigations are required:

- Genetic, chromosomal or nuclear sexing. It is simple and reliable from a study of buccal smear, skin biopsy or neutrophil examination.
- The external genitalia should be examined, preferably under anaesthesia, when, for example, a vagina may be discovered concealed by the fusion of labia majora. Contrast radiography is sometimes helpful. Magnetic resonance imaging (MRI) is most helpful in these cases.
- Gonadal biopsy of testes in an apparent male.
- Laparotomy or laparoscopic-directed gonadal biopsy in an apparent female provides an opportunity for examination of internal genitalia. The presence of rudimentary or underdeveloped Müllerian structures strongly suggests a female sex. It is important to note that during a laparoscopic biopsy of a streak ovary, the ureter that is in close proximity is vulnerable to injury.
- Ultrasound is an alternative to laparoscopy. It may also throw light on some accompanying Wolffian anomalies.
- Estimation of oestrogen, 17-ketosteroids, testosterone and 17-hydroxyprogesterone in the serum or urine may be done. Dehydroepiandrostenedione (DHEA) level >700 mcg/dL and total testosterone >200 mcg/dL is abnormal.
- Estimation of serum electrolytes.
- I.v. pyelogram to detect any coexisting renal anomalies, MRI for suspected adrenal neoplasm, radiography of the pituitary fossa and the skeleton.
- Psychological assessment of the patient's sexuality.

The gynaecologist often needs help of endocrinologist and psychiatrist before finally declaring the sex of the person, the diagnosis and the treatment is best deferred till puberty when an individual declares, i.e. the sex towards which the individual shows greater inclination and attitude. During this consultation, the parents should be available as their cooperation and intelligent supervision are vital for the ultimate interest of an intersex individual (Fig. 9.12).

HIRSUTISM

Hirsutism is defined as the presence of coarse hair in a female at sites normally present in males, i.e. upper lip, chin, chest, lower abdomen and thighs. Hirsutism may or may not be associated with menstrual disturbances such as oligomenorrhoea and amenorrhoea. Virilization refers to a condition of hirsutism associated with other male characteristics such as temporal baldness, hoarse voice, clitoromegaly and muscle enlargement as well as defeminization such as amenorrhoea and breast atrophy.

ENDOCRINOLOGY

In a woman, androgens are secreted by the ovaries and the adrenal glands in varying proportions. To some extent, they are produced by the peripheral conversion of androstenedione in the fat. The androgens produced are as follows: 25% comes from the adrenal glands, 25% from ovaries and rest from the peripheral conversion of androstenedione.

1. *Testosterone*, 0.2–0.3 mg daily – 50% comes from ovaries (0.2–0.8 ng/mL blood level) and remaining from adrenal glands.
2. *DHEA*, 20 mcg daily (serum level 130–980 ng/mL) and rest from adrenal glands.
3. *Androstenedione*, 3 mg daily (1.5 mg from ovaries).
4. *Dehydroepiandrosterone sulphate* (DHEAS), 0.5–2.8 mcg/mL (adrenal gland). Higher levels suggest possibility of CAH, 17-hydroxyprogesterone >800ng/dL is present in congenital adrenal hyperplasia (CAH).

Testosterone is bound to serum hormone-binding globulin (SHBG). SHBG production in the liver is inhibited by androgens and increased by oestrogen and thyroid hormone. Low oestrogen and thyroid hormone cause fall in SHBG level, and this results in some testosterone being

	Normal female	Simple constitutional masculinism	Adreno-genital masculinism	Female homosexual	Female transvestism	Female intersex 1 without adrenal disorder	True hermaph-roditism	Turner's syndrome	Swyer's syndrome	Male intersex II testicular feminization syndrome	Klinefelter's syndrome	Male transvestism	Male homosexual	Adreno-genital feminism	Simple constitutional feminism	Male with hypospadias	Normal male
NUCLEAR SEX CHROMATIN	+	+ but lesser% in polymorphs	+	+ occasionally – in polymorphs	+	+	+ or –	– rarely +	–	–	+ rarely –	+ rarely –	–	–	–	–	–
GONADS	○ ○	○ ○	○ ○	○ ○	○ ○	○ ○	○ ●		?	● ●	● ●	● ●	● ●	● ●	● ●	● ●	● ●
HORMONES: OESTROGENS	normal F.			normal F.	normal F.	normal F.			high	normal M.	not increased	n. to n. for male	normal M.	probably > n. for male		normal M.	normal M.
HORMONES: ANDROGENS	normal F.	increased for female	increased for female ++	normal F.	normal F.	normal F.	normal or low	low	normal	normal M.	< normal	deficient for male	normal M.	increased ++	diminished for male	normal M.	normal M.
EXTERNAL ANATOMY	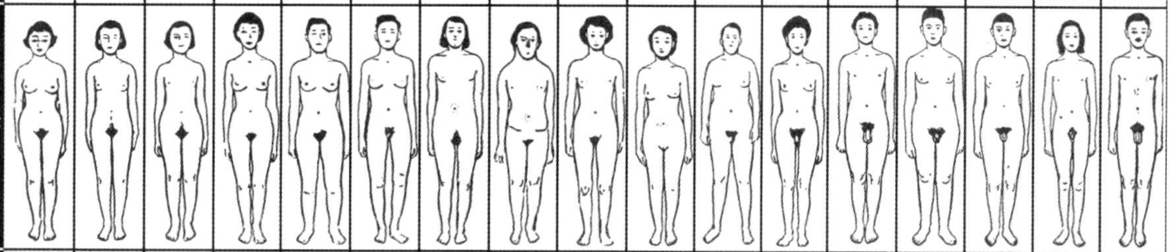																
PHALLUS: PENIS / CLITORIS	normal size	normal size	enlarged	normal to enlarged	normal to enlarged	enlarged ++	normal penis or enlarged clitoris	normal size	normal to enlarged	normal size	small to moderate size	small	normal size	normal size	small	small (often mistaken for enlarged clitoris)	normal size
MICTURITION	♀	♀	♀	♀	♀	♀	♀	♀	♀	♀	♂	♂	♂	♂	♂	♀	♂
MENSTRUATION	normal	irregular or amenorrhoea	absent	normal or irregular	normal or irregular	normal	usually absent	absent	amenorrhoea	absent							
FERTILITY	+	+ or –	–	+	+	–	–	–	–	–	–	– or +	+	–	+	–	+
PSYCHOLOGICAL SEX	F.	F.	F.	M. or F.	Neutral or M.	F. or M.	F. or M.	F.	F.	F.	Neutral or M.	Neutral or F.	M., F. or both	M.	M. or rarely F.	M.	M.
AETIOLOGY	genetic	genetic or hormone	genetic or hormone	genetic or psychological	genetic	genetic	genetic	genetic	genetic	genetic	genetic	genetic	genetic psychological	hormone	genetic or hormone	genetic	genetic

Figure 9.12 The spectrum of sex: possible sexual aberrations in diagrammatic and tabular forms.

released into the blood circulation as free testosterone, which can cause hirsutism. Similarly, obesity causes fall in SHBG as well as more peripheral conversion of androstenedione to testosterone.

Ferriman and Gallwey described a scoring system for hirsutism in nine body areas on a scale of 0–4 and quantified hair growth. A score >8 is labelled as hirsutism.

CAUSES OF HIRSUTISM

- Genetic and ethnic.
- Excess androgen or increased sensitivity of the pilosebaceous unit to testosterone
- Liver disease when the SHBG level drops.
- *Ovarian.* Polycystic ovarian disease (PCOD), hyperthecosis, masculinizing ovarian tumours, e.g. arrhenoblastoma, hilus cell tumour.
- *Adrenal.* Congenital adrenal hyperplasia, Cushing syndrome, adrenal tumour (1%–2% cases).
- *Drugs.* Androgens, progestogens with androgenic effect, e.g. 19-norsteroids, and levonorgestrel anabolic steroids, phenytoin, danazol and minoxidil.
- *Others.* Obesity, hypothyroidism, anovulatory hypo-oestrogenism, idiopathic – 15%, hyperprolactinaemia.
- *Hirsutism occurs early in congenital adrenal hyperplasia, around puberty in PCOD and in elderly women at menopause.*
- Idiopathic increased sensitivity of end organ to 5 alpha reductase.

CLINICAL FEATURES

- **PCOD** accounts for 80% cases of hirsutism and is characterized by oligomenorrhoea, obesity, hirsutism and often infertility. Both ovaries are enlarged and covered with a thick, smooth, fibrotic, pearly white capsule. Multiple small cysts, 2–9 mm in size, are present at the periphery of the ovary, and the ovarian stroma is increased due to theca cell hyperplasia. Ultrasound reveals the ovarian morphology clearly, and diagnosis can be accurately established. LH level is raised even in the preovulatory phase of the menstrual cycle, causing a high LH/FSH ratio (more than 1). This results in anovulation and high oestrogen level, but absence of progesterone. About 50% of women with PCOD will show raised levels of androgens (testosterone, androstenedione and DHEA). Testosterone level although raised, remains below 200 ng/dL, unlike that in ovarian tumour (see also Chapter 24).
- **Masculinizing ovarian tumours** cause defeminization such as breast atrophy and amenorrhoea besides hirsutism, hoarseness of voice and muscular development. Clinical examination may not always detect small tumour.

Laparoscopy, ultrasound and MRI may be required to locate the tumour. Testosterone level is raised above 200 ng/dL. Removal of the tumour restores the menstrual cycle, but hoarseness of voice and existing hirsutism may require appropriate management.

- **Congenital adrenal hyperplasia** is diagnosed and treated before puberty. It is due to deficiency of enzyme 21-hydroxylase. 17-Hydroxyprogesterone plasma level is raised more than 8 ng/mL. Cortisol deficiency occurs at times of stress. To diagnose, dexamethasone suppression test is done by giving 1 mg of dexamethasone at night and studying a single plasma cortisol level in the morning. The level should be less than 130 nmol/L (100 mcg) – this test has low false-positive finding. Computed tomography (CT) scan of abdomen and pituitary fossa may be required.
- **Cushing syndrome** occurs due to overproduction of ACTH by pituitary gland or adrenal tumour. The diagnosis is established by dexamethasone suppresion test, ACTH level estimation and CT scan of the pituitary and adrenal glands. DHEA and androstenedione levels are raised in this syndrome.
- **Hyperprolactinaemia** may be due to enlargement of the pituitary gland or due to a pituitary tumour. Prolactin levels exceed 100 ng/mL. An MRI will help in the diagnosis; mild hyperprolactinaemia occurs in PCOD.

INVESTIGATIONS

HISTORY

The onset and speed of progression help to determine the cause of hirsutism and virilism. Change in the voice, breast atrophy and amenorrhoea indicate defeminization and possibility of an ovarian tumour. History of drug intake should be ellicited. Infertility may be due to anovulation, and points towards PCOD.

EXAMINATION

Degree of hirsutism should be noted, including any change in voice. Breast palpation, search for any abdominal tumour, clitoral enlargement and pelvic mass by bimanual examination should be carried out.

HORMONAL STUDY

This includes study of testosterone, DHEA and androstenedione levels and that of thyroid hormones. Preovulatory LH and FSH levels need to be estimated. In PCOD, LH level exceeds 10 IU/L; testosterone > 2.5 nmol/L and SHBG < 30 nmol/L. Testosterone level > 6 nmol/L is seen in ovarian tumour and hyperthecosis. Normal prolactin level is up to 25 ng/mL. Cortisol level should be <100 mcg/mL.

In adrenal tumour, DHEAS levels are raised >700–800 mcg/dL. It is a better estimate than 24-hour urine estimation of 17-ketosteroid.

17-Alpha hydroxyprogesterone > 800 ng/dL is seen in CAH, and plasma testosterone > 200 ng/dL is seen in ovarian and adrenal tumours.

ULTRASOUND SCAN

It may help to detect an ovarian tumour, PCOD and adrenal tumour.

CT scan and MRI are needed in case pituitary or adrenal tumour is suspected.

Laparoscopic visualization of pelvic organs, dexamethasone and ACTH tests are often necessary.

MANAGEMENT

1. **Treat the cause.** Removal of ovarian and adrenal tumour will stop further hirsutism. Existing facial hair needs treatment. Virilization will cease following removal of a masculinizing ovarian tumour, but hoarseness of voice may persist. Menstrual cycles are restored and breasts start growing. This is preferably done under video pelviscopic vision. Infertility will need ovulation induction drugs, and an older woman should receive cyclical progestogen therapy to prevent endometrial hyperplasia and cancer developing from unopposed oestrogen stimulation. Metformin 500 mg t.i.d. for 8 weeks reduces hyperinsulinaemia seen in PCOD.
2. **Drugs.** Dexamethasone 0.25–0.5 mg daily at night will control adrenal hyperplasia if DHEA is raised. Sometimes combined oral contraceptive pills (OCPs) may be needed in addition to dexamethasone to suppress androgens. *Suppression of androgens* with combined OCPs not containing androgenic progestogen such as norethisterone and levonorgestrel will suppress ovarian androgens. Oestrogen is not only antiandrogenic but by stimulating production of SHBG will bind circulating free testosterone to SHBG, thus suppressing its peripheral action on the hair follicles. Antiandrogens used are (1) spironolactone and (2) cyproterone acetate.
   - Spironolactone in a dose of 100–200 mg daily blocks the androgen receptors, reduces its production and increases its metabolism, and thus prevents hirsutism in a further 60% of cases. It is best given with combined oral pills to avoid irregular menstruation, and prevents conception, thus preventing possible feminization of a male fetus, lest the woman concieves. The side effects include transient diuresis, menstrual irregularity (polymenorrhagia 10%) and breast enlargement. Occasionally, hyperkalaemia and hyponatraemia may occur. Maintenance dose after 6–12 months is 50-mg spironolactone with OCPs (see also chapter on Hormonal Therapy in Gynaecology). Drospirenone 3 mg with 30-mcg oestradiol (Yasmin, Janya, and Tarana) used cyclically for 3 weeks is found very effective in hirsutism in PCOD.
   - Cyproterone acetate is a potent progestogen with antiandrogenic activity, a synthetic derivative of 17-alpha-hydroxyprogesterone; it inhibits DHT binding to its receptors at the periphery and has a weak corticosteroid effect. It is given combined with oestrogen as 50–100-mg cyproterone daily for the first 10 days of the menstrual cycle with 30–50 mcg of ethinyl oestradiol (EE) for 21 days. After 6–12 months, a maintenance dose of 5–10-mg cyproterone acetate with EE will be effective in preventing recurrence of hirsutism. The effect becomes apparent after 4 months of treatment. Oral contraceptives regularize the cycle and prevent pregnancy. Oestrogen present in the pills avoids menopausal symptoms and also raises the serum hormone-binding capacity, which binds the free

androgens and reduces insulin-like growth factor. Side effects are weight gain, nausea and headache, rarely liver damage.

3. **Weight reduction** will increase SHBG levels and bind free testosterone, thus reducing its peripheral action on hair follicles.
4. **Cosmetics.** Bleaching, waxing, shaving and laser are useful in removal of facial hair. Electrolysis is highly satisfactory in treating hirsutism.
5. **New drugs** available are
   - *Flutamide* (nonsteroidal) 250 mg b.d. for 3 weeks cyclically with oral contraceptives for 6 months blocks the androgen effect at the receptor level. Side effects are dry skin, oligomenorrhoea and liver damage. It is faster acting than spironolactone.
   - *Finasteride* 5 mg daily for 6 months blocks the conversion of testosterone to potent androgen and is safer than flutamide. It reduces conversion of testosterone to DHT.
   - Dutasteride (AVODART), 5-reductase inhibitor, is under trial.

Polycystic ovarian disease is detailed in chapter on Diseases of the Ovary. Summary of causes and management of hirsutism is explained in Table 9.2.

Table 9.2 Summary of Causes and Management of Hirsutism

Cause	Mechanism	Diagnostic Information	Treatment
Ovarian androgens	Androgen-producing tumours (Sertoli, Leydig cell, hilar cell tumours)	• Rapid progress • High testosterone level • Pelvic mass present • Clitoromegaly	• Surgical excision of functioning tumour
	Polycystic ovary syndrome	• Long-term duration • Mild elevation of testosterone • Elevated LH/FSH ratio • Anovulation • Infertility • Irregular menstruation/amenorrhoea • Obesity	• Oral contraceptive pills, antiandrogens • Weight control • Metformin • Changes in life style • Laparoscopic ovarian drilling • Assisted reproductive technology (ART) procedures
	Luteoma of pregnancy/ theca lutein cysts	• Onset during pregnancy	Conservative management
Adrenal androgens	Androgen-producing tumour	• Rapid onset • High DHEAS • Abdominal mass present • Clitoromegally	• Remove tumour
	• Congenital adrenal hyperplasia (late onset) 21-hydoxylase deficiency	• Elevated serum 17-dihydroxy progesterone	• Glucocorticoid replacement and suppression
	• Cushing syndrome	• Elevated plasma cortisol	• Varies as to cause
Exogenous androgens	• Hormonal drugs	• Methyltestosterone • Anabolic steroids • Danazol	• Withdraw offending drug
Hair follicle sensitivity	• Excessive conversion of DHT in hair follicle	• Long duration • Family history • Racial trait	• Spironolactone • Cyproterone acetate • Flutamide • Depilatories • Electrolysis • Cosmetic treatments – waxing/shaving
Exogenous causes of hypertrichosis	• Nonhormonal medications	• Phenytoin • Diazoxide • Minoxidil • Streptomycin • Penicillamine	• Withdraw offending medications
	• Pathological states	• Hypothyroidism • Anorexia • Dermatomyositis • Porphyria	• Treat the cause
	• Normal states	• Old age • Ethnic trait • Pregnancy	• Observation • Cosmetic therapy

ACNE

Acne is a mild form of hirsutism seen in young girls. This should be treated with Dianette pill containing 35-mcg E_2, 2-mg cyproterone acetate starting on the first day of cycle for 21 days in each cycle. Cimetidine 1.5 mg daily also helps, but it can cause galactorrhoea and the drug is very expensive. Vaniqa (eflornithine) 11.5% cream is also effective; antibiotic creams such as clindamycin 1%, erythromycin 2% and retinoids also help. Vaniqa cream is applied twice daily for 24 weeks – some develop allergic dermatitis and mild burning sensation.

- Isotretinoin suppresses sebaceous gland secretion.
- Dutasteride (Avodart) is 5-alpha-reductase inhibitor is under trial. It inhibits DHT production in 99% cases. It is contraindicated in pregnancy.

TRUE HERMAPHRODITE

True hermaphrodite is an individual with ovotestes or ovary on one side and testes on the other. The uterus and vagina develop and the person menstruates. In addition, the external genitalia is of male phenotype. The individual is brought up as a male until puberty, so it may be prudent to retain the male gender and do mastectomy and hysterectomy. Testosterone therapy helps to develop secondary sexual characters of the male phenotype. Plastic surgery on the phallus may be required, and sexual function is possible. Fertility, however, may remain low.

PSYCHOLOGICAL SEX

Homosexuality, transvestism and transsexuality are abnormal sexual behaviour. Transsexuality is defined as a disturbance of gender identity in which a person anatomically of one gender has an intense and persistent desire for medical, surgical and legal change of sex and lives as a member of the opposite gender. These are psychosexual patients and need careful handling and a lot of counselling before taking and accepting the individual's decision. Initially, hormone therapy followed by surgery will be needed to reconstruct the body phenotype of the desired gender. Oestrogen for a male and progestogen for a female will reduce the secondary sexual characters over a period of 1–2 years. This makes reconstructive surgery easier, apart from the fact that it gives the individual to assert her/his decision over the change of sex.

KEY POINTS

- Intersexuality is a difficult gynaecological problem to tackle because the condition is extremely rare and the experience of a gynaecologist is limited.
- Detailed knowledge on genetic sex, hormonal influences coupled with investigations are required to make the accurate diagnosis and conduct the appropriate management.
- Hirsutism is now increasingly encountered in young women as the incidence of PCOD has increased. Other causes are idiopathic, adrenal, drug administration, hypothyroidism and hyperprolactinaemia.
- Ultrasound and hormonal profile study are necessary.
- Various drugs used in hirsutism are cyproterone acetate, spironolactone, finasteride and combined hormonal pills.
- Acne is a cosmetic problem and demands treatment.
- Varieties of intersex now can be diagnosed based on chromosomal study. Surgical management allows an individual to live near-normal life as possible.
- Virilism requires immediate management; otherwise, certain masculinizing features will persist despite treating the cause. These persistent features are deepening of voice and baldness.

SELF-ASSESSMENT

1. Describe the phenotypic appearances of individuals with sex chromosomal abnormalities.
2. Enumerate the components contributing to determination of sex.
3. What are the common causes of hirsutism? Describe their management.
4. Describe the features of Swyer syndrome, Turner syndrome and Klinefelter syndrome.
5. Define Virilism. Describe its clinical features, types and management of this disorder.

SUGGESTED READING

Ehrmann DA. Polycystic ovary syndrome. N Eng J Med 2005;352: 1223–36.

Hiort O, Birnbaum W, Marshall L, Wünsch L, Werner R, Schröder T, et al. Management of disorders of sex development. Nat Rev Endocrinol. 2014;10(9):520–9.

Linden MG, Bender BG, Robinson A. Intrauterine diagnosis of sex chromosome aneuploidy. Obstet Gynecol 1996;87:468–75.

Norman RJ. Metformin – comparison with other therapies in ovulation induction in polycystic ovary syndrome. J Clin Endocrinol Metab 2004;89:4797.

Ostrer H. Disorders of sex development (DSDs): an update. J Clin Endocrinol Metab. 2014;99(5):1503–9.

Speroff L, Fritz MA. Clinical Gynecologic Endocrinology and Infertility. 8th ed. Philadelphia: Lippincott Williams & Wilkins, 2011;331-389.

Speroff L, Fritz MA. Hirsutism in Clinical Gynecologic Endocrinology and Infertility. 7th ed. Philadelphia: Lippincott Williams & Wilkins, 2004;465–98.

Studd J. Progress in Obstetrics and Gynaecology. 3:197.

SECTION 2

DISORDERS OF MENSTRUATION

SECTION OUTLINE

10 Common Disorders of Menstruation

CHAPTER OUTLINE

MENSTRUAL CYCLE IRREGULARITIES

Menstruation is the end point in a series of events which begins in the cerebral cortex and hypothalamus and ends at the uterus in the hypothalamic–pituitary–ovarian–uterine axis. Any break in this axis creates menstrual problems.

Excessive or inappropriately timed menstruation and amenorrhoea are the most common complaints for which women seek advice from medical health care providers.

As described in Chapter 4, normal menstruation requires integration of the hypothalamic–pituitary–ovarian (H–P–O) axis with a functional uterus, a patent lower genital outflow tract and a normal genetic karyotype of 46XX.

Abnormal menstruation can be a harbinger of a sinister pelvic pathology or denote a relatively minor problem; therefore, a thorough investigation into the problem is called for in every patient presenting with this complaint.

In normal healthy women, menarche occurs between the age of 10 and 16 years, mean age of menarche being around 12.5 years. Cyclic menstruation persists throughout the reproductive era of life with an average rhythm of 28 ± 7 days, inclusive of 4–6 days of bleeding (except pregnancy and lactation). It is not uncommon for minor variations to occur from time to time.

VARIOUS TYPES OF MENSTRUAL CYCLE IRREGULARITIES

Except amenorrhea rest are the discarded terminology not used now a days.

- **Amenorrhoea** indicates the absence of menstruation. It is a symptom and not a disease entity.
- **Oligomenorrhoea** denotes infrequent and irregularly timed episodes of bleeding usually occurring at intervals of more than 35 days.
- **Polymenorrhoea** denotes frequent episodes of menstruation, usually occurring at intervals of 21 days or less.
- **Menorrhagia** denotes regularly timed episodes of bleeding that are excessive in amount (>80 mL) and/or duration of flow (>5 days).
- **Metrorrhagia** refers to irregularly timed episodes of bleeding superimposed on normal cyclical bleeding.
- **Menometrorrhagia** means excessive and prolonged bleeding that occurs at irregularly timed and frequent intervals.
- **Hypomenorrhoea** refers to regularly timed but scanty episodes of bleeding.
- **Intermenstrual** bleeding refers to bleeding (usually not excessive) that occurs between otherwise normal menstrual cycles.
- **Precocious** menstruation denotes the occurrence of menstruation before the age of 10 years.
- **Postcoital bleeding** denotes vaginal bleeding after sexual intercourse.

HEAVY MENSTRUAL BLEEDING (HMB)

The term 'heavy menstrual bleeding' defined as excessive blood loss interfering with physical, social, emotional and or material quality of life. It is generally caused by conditions affecting the uterus or its vascularity, rather than any disturbance of function of the H–P–O axis. Whenever the uterine endometrial surface is enlarged, the bleeding surface is increased, contributing to excessive bleeding. Such conditions prevail in uterine fibroids, adenomyosis, uterine polyps, myohyperplasia and endometrial hyperplasia.

HMB is also seen in women with increased uterine vascularity such as in chronic pelvic inflammatory disease (PID) and pelvic endometriosis. The uterus is often retroverted in position with restricted mobility. Such a uterus tends to be bulky and congested. The presence of an intrauterine contraceptive device (IUCD) often leads to heavy and prolonged bleeding. Lastly, menorrhagia may be the result of bleeding disorders like Von Willebrand disease or an arteriovenous aneurysm.

A normal menstrual blood loss is 50–80 mL and does not exceed 100 mL. In menorrhagia, the menstrual cycle is unaltered, but the duration and quantity of the menstrual loss are increased. Menorrhagia is essentially a symptom and not in itself a disease. It affects 20%–30% of women at sometime or other with significant adverse effects on the quality of life in terms of anaemia, cost of sanitary pads and interference with day-to-day activities. Several causes may prevail in a few cases and attribute to excess bleeding. In a few cases, the underlying cause may be difficult to detect.

OLIGOMENORRHOEA AND HYPOMENORRHOEA

OLIGOMENORRHOEA

In some women, the pattern of menstruation extends to cycle lengths exceeding 35 days without any impairment of their fertility. This is compatible with normal reproductive capacity within the limits of its own infrequent ovulation, so it requires no treatment. However, if the cycles are very erratic and infrequent, medical attention is called for. The causes and findings of clinical investigations are similar to those of amenorrhoea. Many of these women are obese, hirsute with poorly developed secondary sexual characteristics, genital hypoplasia and ovarian subfunction. Amenorrhoea is often the continuum of oligomenorrhoea. This condition is often encountered in women at the extremes of reproductive life and in some lactating women. Other causes are genital tuberculosis and polycystic ovarian disease.

HYPOMENORRHOEA

In some women, menstruation lasts for only 1–2 days, and the blood loss is so scanty that she may need a change of just one to two sanitary pads. Scanty menses, which is otherwise regular, may not be pathological because its regularity presupposes a normal H–P–O relationship. In these women, the uterine end organ may be at fault. A small hypoplastic uterus, genital tuberculosis and partial Asherman syndrome also cause hypomenorrhoea and need investigation and treatment. *Oral combined pills also cause* hypomenorrhoea. Scanty periods may precede menopause.

POLYMENORRHOEA OR EPIMENORRHOEA

Women with polymenorrhoea (epimenorrhoea) suffer from shortened cycles. Menorrhagia often goes hand in hand with this complaint. It is more frequent in adolescent girls and in perimenopausal women. The exact aetiology of this problem is not known. In most of these women, the follicular phase of the cycle is accelerated, resulting in shorter cycles. The ovaries often appear hyperaemic and may contain haemorrhagic follicles. Myohyperplasia of the uterus is a common accompaniment. The lining endometrium is generally of normal thickness; however, in women suffering from polymenorrhagia, the lining endometrium may appear thickened. The cause of ovarian overactivity seems to be the result of a disturbed endocrine axis.

Polymenorrhagia is frequently observed when women resume menstrual activity after a delivery. It is attributed to the persistence of the activity of the anterior lobe of the pituitary gland initiated during pregnancy into the postnatal phase. The excessive stimulation by the gonadotropins causes frequent ovulation and menstruation. In a substantial number of women, associated pelvic pathology, such as PID, endometriosis and fibroids, is also encountered. Treatment should then be directed to the cause. When no definite cause is identified, treatment with cyclic hormone therapy restores the normal menstrual pattern.

METRORRHAGIA

The preferred term 'intermenstrual bleeding' is used to define any acyclic bleeding from the genital tract. In strict terms, the term should be restricted to bleeding arising from the uterus only. The bleeding may be intermittent or continuous. It is superimposed on a normal menstrual cycle.

Intermenstrual bleeding may be physiological, occurring at the time of ovulation when hormonal changes triggering ovulation take place. These women complain of midmenstrual bleeding (Mittelschmerz) lasting from a few hours to 1 day, a profuse sticky discharge and intermittent cramping pain of short duration. These episodes coincide with ovulation, and this fact can be confirmed by basal body temperature (BBT) charts/sonography. All that is required is to provide an explanation to the patient of the underlying cause and alleviate her anxiety. *A few months of combined oral pills will cure ovulation bleed.*

Particularly in elderly women, postcoital bleeding should not be brushed aside lightly. It may be the earliest symptom of a neoplasm; a meticulous search should be instituted to exclude such a possibility. Besides a thorough clinical examination of the lower genital tract, speculum examination of the cervix in good light for a polyp, vascular erosion, endocervicitis, cancer of the cervix and the presence of an IUCD should be looked for, along with lower genital tract ulcers and growths. *A Pap smear examination should be obtained.* A diagnostic hysteroscopy and an endometrial curettage for histological study of the endometrial tissue are important. A pelvic sonography to evaluate the pelvic organs is recommended. Refer to Table 10.1 for a brief summary of the types of uterine bleeding.

Table 10.1 Types of Abnormal Uterine Bleeding

Terms in Clinical Usage	Menstrual Pattern
Oligomenorrhoea	Cycle length > 38 days
Polymenorrhoea	Cycle length < 24 days
Menorrhagia	Increased menstrual flow/increased duration at regular cycles
Hypomenorrhoea	Scanty bleeding and shorter days of bleeding
Metrorrhagia	Irregular bleeding in between the cycles
Menometrorrhagia	Increased menstrual flow as well as irregular bleeding between the cycles

DYSMENORRHOEA

DEFINITION

Dysmenorrhoea means cramping pain accompanying menstruation.

AETIOLOGY

Patients can be classified into groups for understanding the pathogenesis of this distressing condition.

TYPES

1. *Primary dysmenorrhoea* refers to the one that is not associated with any identifiable pelvic pathology. It is now clear that the pathogenesis of pain is attributed to a biochemical derangement. It affects more than 50% postpubescent women in the age group of 18–25 years with ovulatory cycles.
2. *Secondary dysmenorrhoea* refers to the one associated with the presence of organic pelvic pathology, i.e. fibroids, adenomyosis, PID and endometriosis. Unilateral dysmenorrhoea occurs in a rudimentary horn of a bicornuate uterus. It is also seen in some women wearing IUCD and in cases of cervical stenosis.

VARIETIES

Dysmenorrhoea is described under three clinical varieties:

1. *Spasmodic dysmenorrhoea* is the most prevalent one and manifests as cramping pains, generally most pronounced on the first and second day of menstruation.
2. *Congestive dysmenorrhoea* manifests as increasing pelvic discomfort and pelvic pain a few days before the start of menses. Thereafter, the patient rapidly experiences relief in symptoms. This variety is commonly seen in PID, IUCD wearers, pelvic endometriosis and fibroids. It is also experienced by women having varicosity of pelvic veins.
3. *Membranous dysmenorrhoea* is a special group in which the endometrium is shed as a cast at the time of menstruation. The passage of the cast is accompanied by painful uterine cramps. This is a rare variety.

AETIOLOGY OF PAIN (Fig. 10.1)

Spasmodic pain is attributed to myometrial contractions due to increased $PGF_2\alpha$ secreted under progesterone effect. Increased peristaltic action is seen in the subendometrial zone on ultrasound scan and this causes myometrial activity. The pelvic venous congestion as recognized on Doppler ultrasound explains congestive dysmenorrhoea. Relief from dysmenorrhoea following cervical dilatation and vaginal delivery is attributed to damage to sympathetic nerves around the cervix.

Vasopressin by increasing $PGF_2\alpha$ secretion in primary dysmenorrhoea is also held responsible. Similarly, endothelin by increasing $PGF_2\alpha$ contributes to dysmenorrhoea.

CLINICAL FEATURES (Table 10.2)

Primary dysmenorrhoea is widely prevalent; more than 50% of teenagers and 30%–50% of menstruating women suffer from varying degrees of discomfort. The severe incapacitating type, which interferes with a woman's daily activities, affects only about 5%–15% of the population. Its prevalence is higher amongst the more intelligent and sensitive working-class

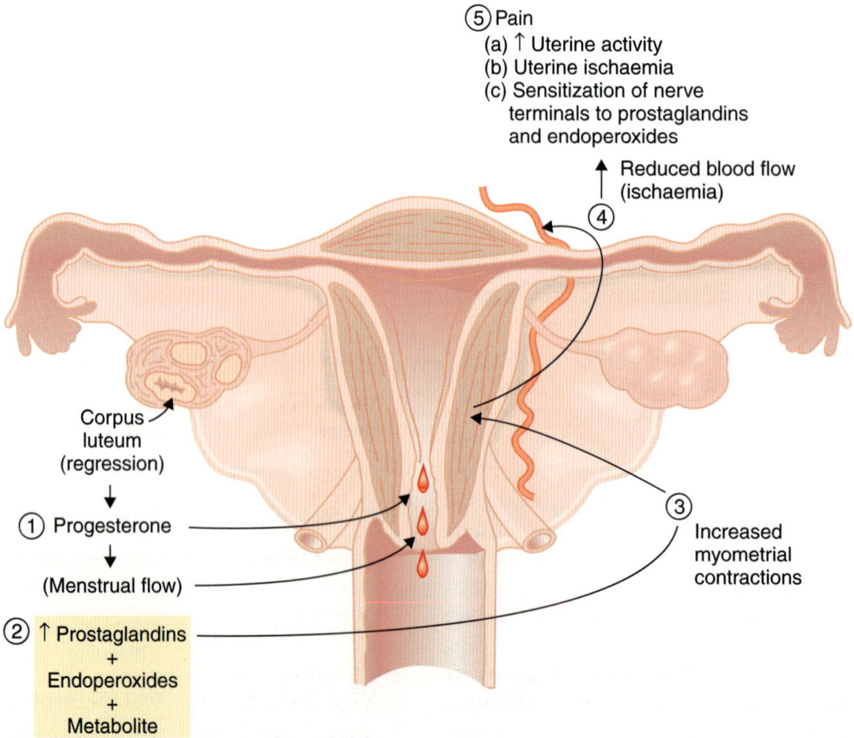

Figure 10.1 Postulated mechanism in the generation of pain in dysmenorrhoea. (*Source*: Hacker NF, Gambone JC, Hobel CJ. Hacker and Moore's Essentials of Obstetrics and Gynecology, 5th ed. Philadelphia: Elsevier, 2010.)

Table 10.2 Differentiating Features of Primary and Secondary Dysmenorrhoea

Differentiating Features	Primary	Secondary
Onset	Within 2 years of menarche	20–30 years, maybe pre- and postmenstrual
Description	Cramping – hypogastrium, back, inner thighs	Variable dull ache
Symptomatology	Nausea, vomiting, diarrhoea, headache, fatigue	Dyspareunia, infertility, menstrual disorders
Pelvic findings	Normal	Variable, depending on cause
Aetiology	Excessive myometrial contraction, ischaemia, excessive prostaglandin production	Endometriosis, PID, adenomyosis, fibroids, pelvic vein congestion
Management	Reassurance, analgesics, NSAIDs, antispasmodics, OC pills, in rare cases, surgery – Cotte's operation or laparoscopic uterosacral nerve ablation (LUNA)	Treatment directed to the cause

women. Both local and systemic symptoms are apparently the result of increased levels of prostaglandins ($F_2\alpha$) in the menstrual fluid. This results in uterine cramping, nausea, vomiting, backache, diarrhoea, giddiness, syncope and fainting. It is responsible for the highest incidence of absenteeism, resulting in loss of work hours and economic loss.

Primary dysmenorrhoea occurs in ovulatory cycles; hence, it makes its appearance a few years after menarche with at least 6–12 months of painless periods. It is most intense on the first day of menses and progressively lessens with menstrual flow. It often lessens with passage of time and after childbirth. Pelvis findings are normal. Pain may be accompanied by nausea, vomiting, headache and fainting.

INVESTIGATIONS

In women suffering from secondary dysmenorrhoea, tests to confirm the clinical diagnosis and unravel the extent and type of underlying pathology should be carried out. These commonly include the following:

- Pelvic sonography followed by CT scan or MRI scan, if indicated
- Diagnostic hysterosalpingogram/sonosalpingography
- Endoscopy – diagnostic hysteroscopy/laparoscopy

TREATMENT

Treatment includes counselling, psychotherapy to modify patient's perception of her problem and alter behavioural attitude, medical measures and surgical interventions.

MEDICAL MEASURES

Therapy for primary dysmenorrhoea consists of measures to relieve pain and suppress ovulation if the woman desires contraception additionally.

- Analgesics such as paracetamol 500 mg t.i.d./piroxicam 20 mg b.i.d.
- Antispasmodics such as hyoscine (Buscopan) compounds t.i.d./camylofin (Anafortan) t.i.d./drotaverine (Drotin) t.i.d., diclofenac t.i.d.
- Prostaglandin synthetase inhibitors are cyclooxygenase inhibitors. Nonsteroidal anti-inflammatory drugs (NSAIDs), such as mefenamic acid 250–500 mg/q.i.d., provide relief in 80–90% cases. Indomethacin 25 mg three to six times daily provides relief in 70% cases. Naproxen 275 mg t.i.d. relieves about 80% cases/ketoprofen 50 mg t.i.d. is successful in 90% cases. Ibuprofen 400 mg 6–8 hourly is also effective. The advantage of the above regimes is that medication is restricted to the symptom days alone, and it does not interfere with ovulation. Meloxicam has no gastric side effects. The side effects of these drugs are nausea, vomiting, blurred vision, nephrotoxicity and gastric ulcer on prolonged use.
- Glyceryl trinitrate (nitroglycerine), a nitric oxide donor, relieves pain by relaxing smooth muscles of the uterus.
- Progestogen-containing IUCD (Mirena, Progestasert) relieves pain in addition to providing contraceptive measures and reducing bleeding.
- Oral contraceptives (OCs) administered cyclically suppress ovulation and are useful in relieving dysmenorrhoea. The advantages of regularity of periods, modest bleeding and desired contraception make this the treatment of choice in many young women. The drugs also cure Mittelschmerz pain.
- Pelvic endometriosis may be treated with increasing doses of danazol/OCs/gonadotropin-releasing hormone GnRH agonists (leuprolide, buserelin and nafarelin).
- Vitamin E, 200 mg b.i.d., starting 2 days before and 3 days during periods claims to reduce dysmenorrhoea.

SURGERY

Surgery is rarely undertaken if medical measures fail to provide relief and in women with secondary dysmenorrhoea to treat the underlying pelvic pathology. Surgical interventions may be diagnostic to begin with, followed by definitive treatment based on severity of symptoms, patient's age, desire for childbearing, menstrual functions and the patient's perception of her problem. Surgical interventions include the following:

- Diagnostic hysteroscopy followed by dilation and curettage (D&C), excision of polyp or uterine septum. Dilatation of cervix – it damages the nerves.
- Diagnostic laparoscopy followed by lysis of pelvic adhesions, myomectomy, draining of chocolate cyst, cautery or

laser vaporization of islands of endometriosis, excision of adnexal masses, laser-assisted uterosacral nerve ablation (LUNA) for spasmodic dysmenorrhoea.
- Laparotomy followed by excision of chocolate cysts, eradication of endometriosis, myomectomy, excision of localized adenomyoma, presacral neurectomy (Cotte's operation).
- Hysterectomy in elderly woman is the last resort.
- Transcutaneous electrical nerve stimulation (TENS) is effective in 45% cases.

PREMENSTRUAL SYNDROME

Premenstrual syndrome (PMS), also described as premenstrual tension (PMT), is a symptom complex recognized primarily by cyclic changes associated with ovulatory cycles. It occurs 7–14 days prior to menstruation and resolves spontaneously after menses. It is frequently encountered in middle-aged women. It is important for two reasons, firstly because the symptoms of PMT are responsible for socioeconomic loss, and secondly because of associated legal and women's rights issues that have arisen in conjunction with personal accountability during the premenstrual period. It comprises physical, psychological and behavioural changes not associated with organic lesion (Table 10.3). It is prevalent in 5% women.

AETIOLOGY

The exact cause of PMS is not known. It has been postulated that it represents a syndrome which is the result of multiple biochemical abnormalities. Amongst these, the following have been implicated: (i) oestrogen excess or progesterone deficiency in the luteal phase; (ii) increased carbohydrate intolerance in the luteal phase; (iii) pyridoxine deficiency – this vitamin plays a role in oestrogen synthesis and also in dopamine and serotonin production; (iv) increased production of vasopressin, aldosterone, prolactin and systemic prostaglandins which adversely affect renal function and contribute to fluid retention and bloating; and (v) fluctuations in opiate peptide concentrations affecting endorphin levels. However, biochemical estimations do not bear these out. Hence, at present it is not yet clear whether PMS is an abnormal response to normal hormonal fluctuation or a result of hormonal abnormalities. *A woman with hysterectomy but conservation of ovaries may also suffer from PMT, suggesting that the ovarian hormones have a role in PMT.*

Low level of β-endorphins (neurotransmitters) in the brain and low level of serotonin are probably responsible for psychiatric disorders. Genetic predisposition is also recognized in a few cases.

CLINICAL FEATURES

The syndrome may be mild, moderate or severe.

Symptoms of PMS are myriad and not associated with organic lesion in the pelvis. The classic description includes increasing breast tenderness, abdominal bloating, headache, sleeplessness, fatigue, emotional lability, mood swings and depression, irritability, fluid retention and weight gain beginning 7–14 days prior to menses. As menstruation approaches, psychological abnormalities such as irritability and hostility increase. The dominant symptom in different groups varies from anxiety, to depression, to fluid retention, bloating, headache and breast pain, to increased appetite and craving for sweet foods. About 5% suffer from severe symptoms which influence daily activity. The body weight increases by 1 kg and breast volume by 20% due to oedema and increased vascularity. PMT does not occur before puberty, during pregnancy or after menopause. It may, however, occur if the postmenopausal woman goes on hormone replacement therapy (HRT).

DIAGNOSIS

Diagnosis depends on history and careful questioning. Temporal correlation of symptoms with the premenstrual phase of the cycle as documented in a menstrual diary helps to arrive at a rational diagnosis. No organic pelvic lesion is detected, and no definite test is available to confirm the diagnosis.

TREATMENT (Table 10.4)

- For psychological symptoms (psychotherapy), counselling and reassurance alone suffice for the milder cases. Vitamin B_{12} 5–50 mcg, vitamin B_6 100 mg and vitamin E 200 mg daily help PMS cases.
- For breast symptoms alone, beneficial therapies include (i) Danazol 100–200 mg in divided doses during the luteal phase. However, adverse masculinizing effect following long-term usage is a drawback. (ii) GnRH analogues

Table 10.3 Various Symptoms of Premenstrual Tension

1. Pain	Headache, breast pain, abdominal cramps, muscle stiffness, backache, generalized body ache
2. Water retention	Breast pain, bloating, weight gain
3. Behavioural changes	Low performance, difficulty in concentration, irritability, depression, forgetfulness, low judgement, anxiety, loneliness, feeling like crying
4. Autonomic changes	Dizziness, faintness, nausea, vomiting, hot flushes

Table 10.4 Management of Premenstrual Syndrome

Psychosomatic	Vitamins B_1, B_6, E Selective serotonin reuptake Inhibitor, sertraline, citalopram anxiolytics
Breast pain	Danazol, bromocriptine GnRH
Pelvic pain and bloatedness	Yasmin, primrose Prostaglandin inhibitors OC, progestogen Mirena IUCD

provide relief, but long use causes menopausal (antioestrogenic effects) symptoms and osteoporosis. Besides, the drugs are expensive. The following drugs are used:
- Goserelin (Zoladex) 3.6 mg subcutaneously, 4 weekly
- Leuprorelin acetate (Prostap) 3.75 mg i.m., 4 weekly
- Triptorelin (Decapeptyl) 3.75 mg i.m., 4 weekly
- Buserelin (Suprefact) 200–500 mcg daily subcutaneously three times a day for 6 months. Oestrogen and progestogen as add-back therapy to GnRH prevents side effects of oestrogen deficiency.
- Bromocriptine 0.25–2.5 mg relieves breast tenderness but has side effects such as nausea, dizziness, weight gain and swelling.

- For bloatedness, weight gain, fluid retention and headaches (i) salt and fluid restriction and (ii) spironolactones 100 mg and diuretics may help. Buspirinone 7.5-15 mg daily or drospirenone may be used. Yasmin containing 3 mg of spironolactone and 30 mcg of EE2, is used cyclically as combined oral pills. Evening primrose oil (Primosa) 500 mg t.i.d.; it is nonhormonal and contains polyunsaturated essential fatty acids. It diverts harmful PGE2 to PGE1 and replenishes CNS PGE1. By this, it suppresses irritability and depression as well as reduces fluid retention and mastalgia. Gold prim contains Primosa with vitamin and minerals (six capsules a day).
- *Prostaglandin inhibitors*: Mefenamic acid and naproxen improve mood and physical symptoms. These drugs cause gastrointestinal (GI) upsets and rashes. Cyclooxygenase inhibitor (cox-2) has fewer side effects than NSAID. Ibuprofen 400 mg 6–8 hourly is also useful.
- Anxiolytics (alprazolam) 0.25 mg and antidepressants (tricyclics) do provide some relief from PMS, but the benefits of therapy must be weighed against the side effects.
- γ-Aminobutyric acid (GABA) suppresses anxiety level in the brain. Therefore, GABA agonists are effective. Selective serotonin re-uptake inhibitors (SSRI) such as fluoxetine 20 mg daily and sertraline 50 mg have been beneficial in treating physical as well as behavioural symptoms (60% curative). The side effects include headache, drowsiness, insomnia, sexual dysfunction and GI disturbances.
- Sertraline 50–150 mg and citalopram 20–40 mg daily are also used in the premenstrual phase. Vitamin B_6 (60–100 mg) and magnesium (200 mg) are cofactors in the synthesis of neurotransmitters serotonin and dopamine. One gram calcium daily also helps to relieve neurological symptoms. Venlafaxine is a combination of sertraline and noradrenaline reuptake inhibitor.
- Micronized progesterone pessary 200–400 mg daily in the premenstrual phase. Mirena IUCD is now used instead of oral progestogens.
- OCs render the cycles anovulatory and provide relief.
- Oestrogen skin patch releasing 100 mcg daily or 50 mg oestrogen implant with 100-mg testosterone is also employed.
- General measures such as exercise, relaxation and hobbies, meditation and yoga are likely to be beneficial.
- Hysterectomy with removal of ovaries is a last resort. In a younger woman, oophorectomy will need in vitro fertilization (IVF) programme with donor eggs.
- Reassurance, counselling, psychotherapy and selective use of drugs help to control the symptoms.

KEY POINTS

- Normal menstruation occurs as a result of fine coordination between hypothalamus, interior pituitary gland and ovarian functions, resulting in cyclical maturation of endometrium and finally its shedding.
- A number of variations in normal menstruation are seen due to underlying diseases of uterus, ovaries, pituitary gland and systemic diseases. These symptoms may be in the form of menorrhagia, polymenorrhoea, polymenorrhagia, metrorrhagia and dysmenorrhoea.
- Although these terms such as menorrhagia, metrorrhagia, polymenorrhoea/polymenorrhagia are in common use in clinical practice, recently a newer classification system for abnormal uterine bleeding given by the International Federation of Gynecology and Obstetrics (FIGO) (PALM-COEIN) recommends the use of term abnormal uterine bleeding (AUB) in place of these terms.
- Spasmodic dysmenorrhoea is common in adolescents and young women. Congestive dysmenorrhoea is often associated with PID, fibroids and pelvic endometriosis.
- Secondary dysmenorrhoea is a manifestation of organic uterine pathology such as fibroids and adenomyosis.
- Premenstrual syndrome is a functional disorder found in educated and economically well-to-do middle-aged women, and requires treatment.

SELF-ASSESSMENT

1. Describe commonly used terms for menstrual irregularities.
2. Describe the management and clinical features of premenstrual syndrome.

SUGGESTED READING

Bonnar J. Recent Advances in Obstetrics and Gynaecology. 2003;15:169.

Speroff L, Fritz MA. Clinical Gynecologic Endocrinology and Infertility. 8th ed. Philadelphia: Lippincott Williams & Wilkins, 2011: 567-589.

Studd J. Progress in Obstetrics and Gynaecology Volume 3, 11:189.

Ussher JM, Perz J. PMS as a process of negotiation: women's experience and management of premenstrual distress. Psychol Health. 2013; 28(8):909–27.

Vigod SN, Ross LE, Steiner M. Understanding and treating premenstrual dysphoric disorder: an update for the women's health practitioner. Obstet Gynecol Clin North Am. 2009;36(4):907–924, xii.

11 Abnormal Uterine Bleeding (AUB)

CHAPTER OUTLINE

INTRODUCTION

Menstrual irregularities and abnormal heavy menstruation account for up to 25%–33% of women attending gynaecological outpatient department. Although woman of any age group can be affected with abnormal uterine bleeding (AUB), it is more commonly experienced by women of 35–45 years of age. It is also commonly seen among young girls soon after attaining menarche. There have been a number of classification systems to classify causes of AUB but recently International federation of gynaecologists and obstetricians has suggested newer classification popularly known as 'PALM–COEIN' classification to define cause of AUB. Further, AUB is divided into acute and chronic AUB, depending on the duration of the problem persisting in the woman. Chronic AUB is defined as bleeding that is abnormal in volume, regularity and/or timing for the past 6 months. It does not usually require immediate intervention. Acute AUB is an episode of heavy menstrual bleeding of sufficient quantity to require immediate intervention to prevent further loss. It can be seen with existing chronic AUB.

About 10%–25% of women experience episodes of AUB at some time during the reproductive years of their lives. It is common during the extremes of reproductive life, following pregnancy and during lactation. It has been shown that 55.7% of adolescents experience abnormal menstrual bleeding in the first year or so after the onset of menarche because of the immaturity of the hypothalamic–pituitary–ovarian (H–P–O) axis leading to anovulatory cycles. It generally takes 18 months to 2 years for regular cycles to be established.

It is not uncommon for a premenopausal woman to develop menorrhagia, and this is often due to anovulatory cycles in 80% of cases. However, endometrial malignancy should be ruled out before deciding the type of treatment.

The term 'dysfunctional uterine haemorrhage' was specifically used when menorrhagia was not associated with any genital tract abnormalities, general or endocrinological diseases. In this case, a hormonal imbalance is considered the root cause of hyperplasia of the endometrium that causes menorrhagia; this often happens in anovulatory cycles with excessive or unopposed influence of oestrogen on the endometrium. This term is now replaced by Abnormal uterine bleeding.

In some cases, abnormal endometrial haemostasis is the cause of abnormal excessive bleeding.

NORMAL CONTROL OF MENSTRUAL BLEEDING

Once the menstrual bleeding starts, the platelet aggregation forms clots in the opened vessels. Prostaglandin $F_2\alpha$ ($PGF_2\alpha$) causes myometrial contractions and constricts the endometrial vessels. The repair and epithelial regeneration begin on the third and fourth day of period, by the growth of epithelial cells from the open endometrial glands aided by the vascular endothelial, epidermal and fibroblast growth factors.

In excessive bleeding with regular menstrual cycles, the H–P–O axis is intact, but endometrial changes get altered. It is observed that, in these cases, PGE_2 (prostacyclin), which is a local vasodilator, is increased compared to $PGF_2\alpha$ in the endometrial tissue.

CAUSES OF ABNORMAL UTERINE BLEEDING (TABLE 11.1)

The causes can be divided into following: (i) those due to general diseases, (ii) those which are local in the pelvis, (iii) those caused by endocrine disorders, (iv) contraceptives and (v) iatrogenic. The new classification of causes of AUB is shown in Figs 11.1–11.4.

To view the lecture notes scan the symbol or log in to your account on www.MedEnact.com

Table 11.1 Aetiology of Menorrhagia

General Causes	Pelvic Causes	Contraceptive Use	Hormonal/AUB
• Blood dyscrasia	• PID, pelvic adhesions	• IUCD	• Ovulatory: irregular ripening or irregular shedding
• Coagulopathy	• Uterine fibroids, endometrial hyperplasia • Adenomyosis	• Posttubal sterilization	• Anovulatory: resting endometrium – 80% • Metropathia haemorrhagica
• Thyroid dysfunction	• Feminizing tumour or the ovary	• Progestogen-only pills	
• Genital TB	• Endometriosis • Pelvic congestion, varicose veins in the pelvis		

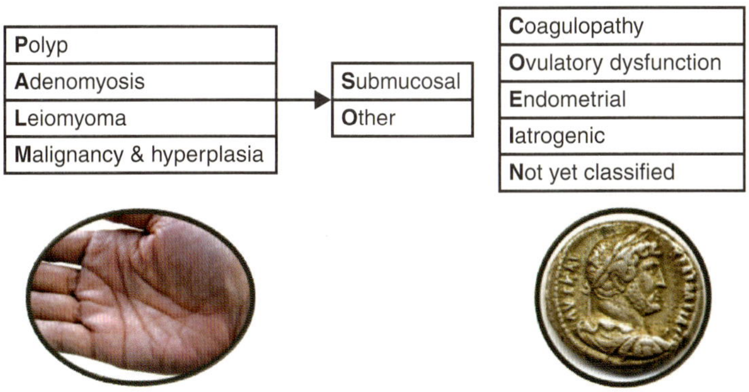

Figure 11.1 Basic FIGO classification system for causes of AUB in the reproductive years. The system includes four categories that are defined by visually objective structural criteria (PALM: polyp, adenomyosis, leiomyoma, malignancy or hyperplasia); four unrelated to structural anomalies (COEI: coagulopathy, ovulatory dysfunction, endometrial, iatrogenic); and one (N) that includes entities not yet classified. (*Source:* From Figure 1. Malcolm G Munro: Obstetrics and Gynecology Clinics. Vol 38(4): 703–731, 2011.)

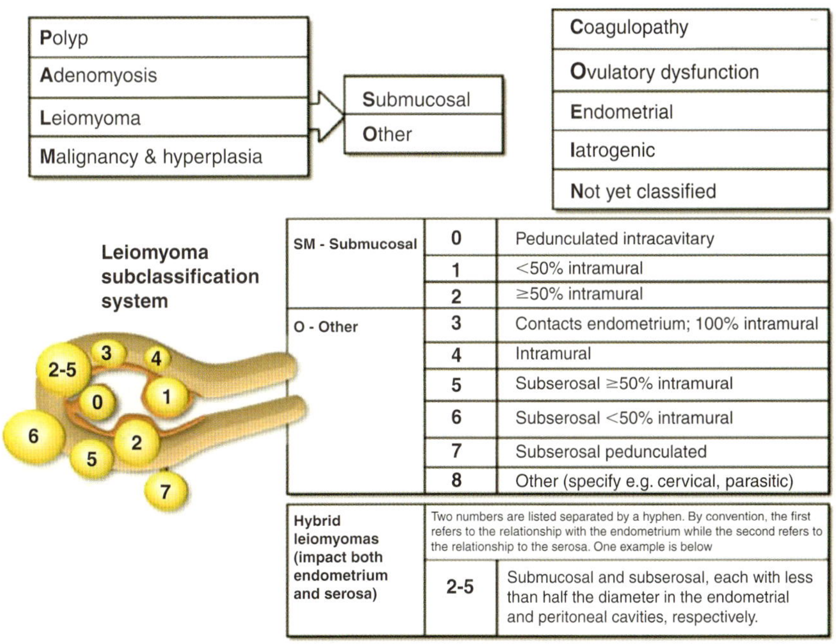

Figure 11.2 FIGO classification system including the leiomyoma subclassification. The classification of leiomyomas categorizes the submucosal (SM) group according to the Wamsteker system 12 and adds categorizations for intramural, subserosal and transmural lesions. Intracavitary lesions are attached to the endometrium by a narrow stalk and are classified as type 0, whereas types 1 and 2 require that a portion of the lesion is intramural, with type 1 being 50% or less and type 2 more than 50%. Type 3 lesions are totally extracavitary but abut the endometrium. Type 4 lesions are intramural leiomyomas that are entirely within the myometrium with no extension to the endometrial surface or to the serosa. Subserosal (types 5–7) myomas include type 5, which are more than 50% intramural; type 6, which are 50% or less intramural, and type 7 being attached to the serosa by a stalk. Lesions that are transmural are categorized by their relationships to both endometrial and serosal surfaces. The endometrial relationship is noted first, whereas the serosal relationship is second (e.g. type 2–5). An additional category, type 8, is reserved for myomas that do not relate to the myometrium at all and include cervical lesions, those that exist in the round or broad ligaments without a direct attachment to the uterus, and other so-called parasitic lesions. (*Source:* From Figure 2. Malcolm G Munro: Obstetrics and Gynecology Clinics. Vol 38(4): 703–731, 2011.)

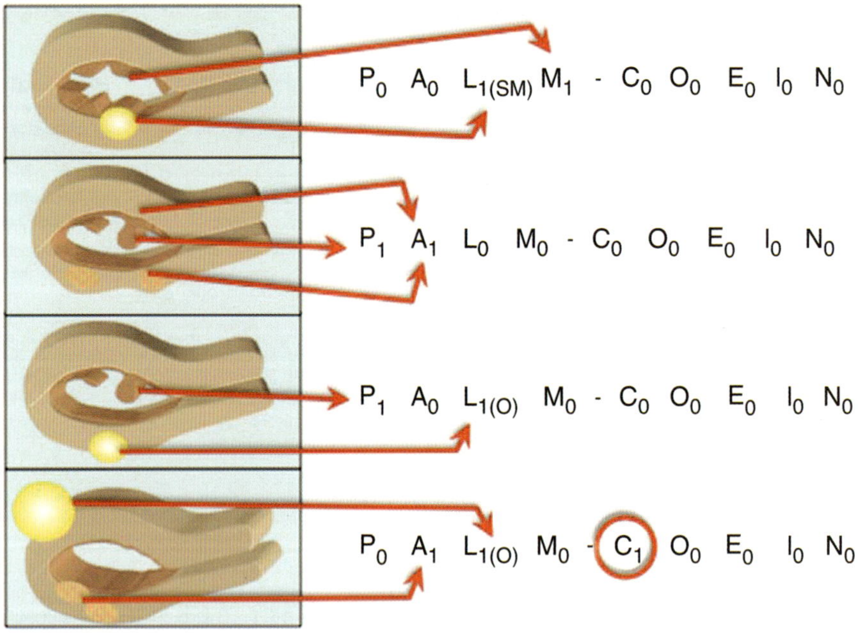

Figure 11.3 FIGO classification system for causes of abnormal uterine bleeding in the reproductive years. FIGO, International Federation of Gynecology and Obstetrics. (*Source:* From Figure 1. Malcolm G Munro, Hilary OD Critchley and Ian S Fraser: American Journal of Obstetrics and Gynecology, Vol 207(4): 259–265, 2012.)

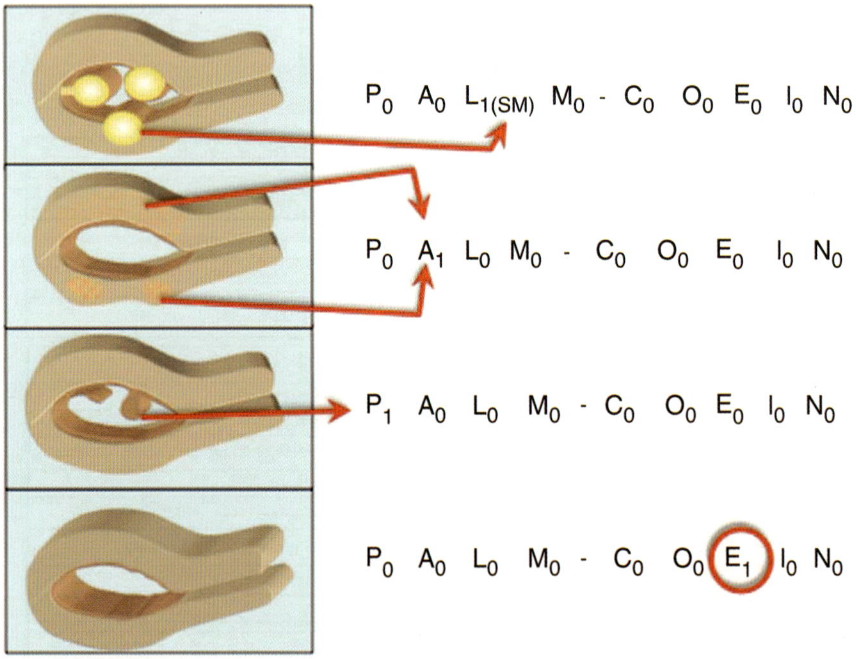

Figure 11.4 Notation for FIGO classification system. FIGO, International Federation of Gynecology and Obstetrics. (*Source:* From Figure 2. Malcolm G Munro, Hilary OD Critchley and Ian S Fraser: American Journal of Obstetrics and Gynecology Vol 207(4): 259–265, 2012.)

GENERAL DISEASES CAUSING HEAVY MENSES

General diseases causing heavy menstrual blood loss are as follows:

- Blood dyscrasia, i.e. leukaemia, coagulopathy, thrombocytopenic purpura, severe anaemia; coagulation disorders are seen in 20% of adolescents; Von Willebrand disease.
- Thyroid dysfunction – Hypothyroidism and hyperthyroidism in the initial stages.
- General tuberculosis may cause menorrhagia initially, but in the advanced state, amenorrhoea ensues.

LOCAL PELVIC CAUSES

These include following:

- **Uterine causes**: Uterine fibroids, fibroid polyp, adenomyosis, endometrial hyperplasia.

- **Ovarian causes:** Chocolate cyst, ovarian feminizing tumours, polycystic ovarian disease (PCOD), endometriosis.

Tubo-ovarian causes: Salpingo-oophoritis, pelvic inflammatory disease (PID), genital TB, varicose veins in the pelvis (Fig. 11.5).

- **Arteriovenous malformations:** Uterine arteriovenous fistula and varicosity of vessels (rare) – This may be congenital, but quite often it is traumatic following dilatation and curettage (D&C).
- Immediate puerperal and postabortal periods.
- Iatrogenic causes: Irregular use of oral contraceptive pills and other hormonal contraceptives.

INTRAUTERINE CONTRACEPTIVE DEVICE

Intrauterine contraceptive device (IUCD) has provided yet another aetiological factor. About 5%–10% of women wearing the device suffer menorrhagia in the first few months. Poststerilization menorrhagia is reported in 15% of cases, but the aetiology is not clear.

No obvious cause is seen in 40%–50% of the cases. In the past these cases were labelled as dysfunctional uterine bleeding (DUB).

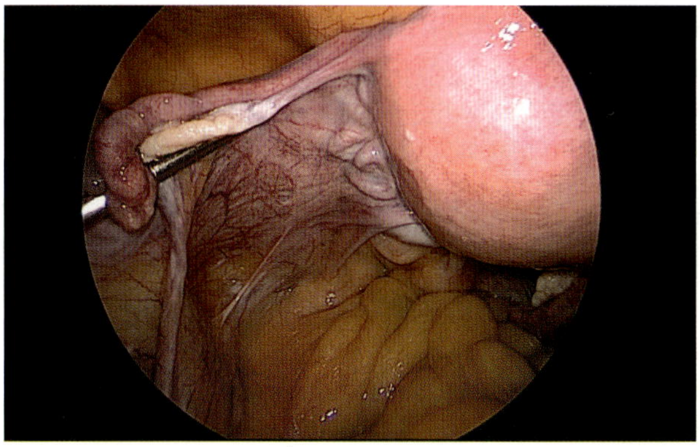

Figure 11.5 Laparoscopic view of varicose uterine vessels. (*Courtesy:* Dr Vivek Marwah, New Delhi.)

INVESTIGATIONS

AUB patients should be completely investigated. Besides physical examination, the following tests are advised:

- Complete haemogram.
- Bleeding time and clotting time.
- Thyroid profile as indicated.
- Pelvic sonography.
- Diagnostic hysteroscopy.
- Endometrial tissue sampling by D&C or endometrial aspiration.
- Diagnostic laparoscopy.
- Sonosalpingography can delineate a submucous fibroid clearly.
- Pelvic angiography is required when the cause of menorrhagia is not detected by other means. This shows varicosity and arteriovenous fistula.

MANAGEMENT

Management consists of the following (Fig. 11.6):

- General measures to improve the health status of the patient. Advice regarding proper diet, adequate rest during menses, oral administration of haematinics, vitamins and protein supplements and to maintain a menstrual calendar noting duration and extent of blood loss.
- Treat the cause.

In women suffering from menorrhagia, consider the following:

- In ovulatory cycles, oral nonsteroidal anti-inflammatory drugs (NSAIDs) such as mefenamic acid 500 mg t.i.d. along with antacids. Other drugs in this category include naproxen, and ibuprofen. Blood loss is reduced by 30%–40%. These drugs are effective in ovulatory bleeding and

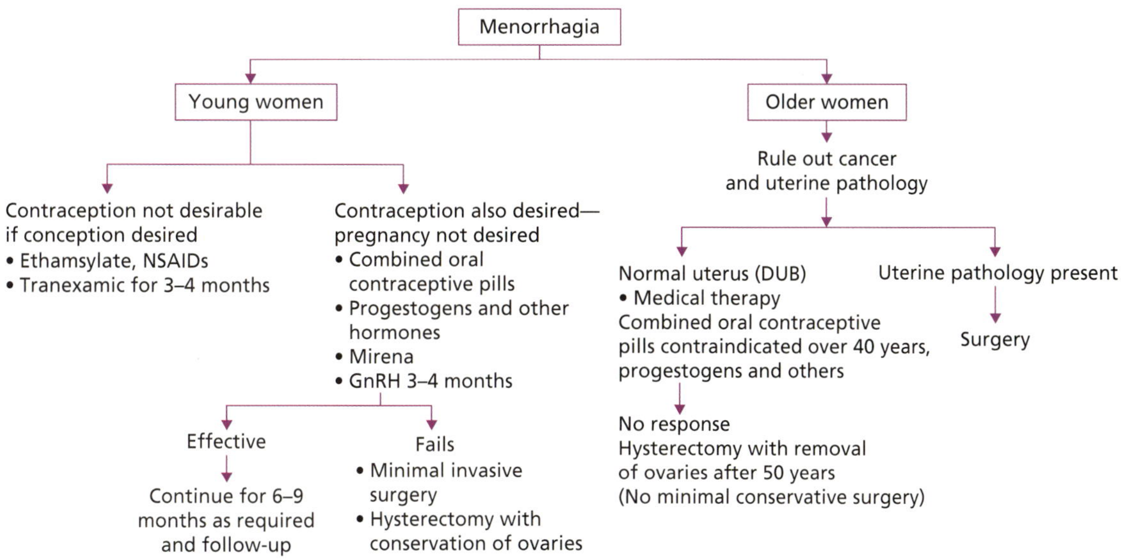

Figure 11.6 Management of menorrhagia.

in IUCD users. They are antiprostaglandins and inhibit cyclooxygenase activity. They decrease the menstrual bleeding, but have no effect on the duration of menstrual bleeding. These drugs should be taken only during menstruation, which is an advantage, over cyclical hormone therapy.

- Tranexamic acid is currently the most commonly prescribed drug for the control of excessive menstrual bleeding. Given in a dose of 500–1000 mg two or three times a day during the phase of heavy menses, this drug reduces blood loss by 35%.
- Cyclic oral contraceptive pills.
- Progestogens in endometrial hyperplasia.
- Mirena IUCD.
- Minimal invasive surgery includes endometrial thermal ablation, endometrial resection and others (see later).
- Hysterectomy in selected cases.
- GnRH analogues: They are not effective in immediate control of bleeding; however, their use can induce amenorrhoea. In women manifesting obvious pathology, corrective measures for the same are called for, depending on her age and the desire for retaining menstrual and childbearing functions. Therapeutic measures include following:
- Removal of an IUCD, if medical therapy fails.
- Myomectomy/hysterectomy for uterine fibroids.
- Adenomyomectomy/hysterectomy for adenomyosis of the uterus.
- Laparoscopic lysis of adhesions for chronic PID.
- Electrocautery or laser vaporization of endometriosis and drainage of chocolate cysts in pelvic endometriosis.
- Hysterectomy with or without removal of the adnexa according to the age and the individual needs of the patient.
- In patients suffering from bleeding disorders, a haematologist's opinion should be sought.
- Uterine artery embolization in varicose vessels.
- Von Willebrand disease; intravenous desmopressin.

AUB is of two following types:

1. Anovulatory cycles (80%)
2. Ovulatory cycles (20%)

PALM-COEIN CLASSIFICATION

DUB was coined to describe abnormal heavy menstrual bleeding when no structural genital tract abnormality or a general cause was detected, in a woman of reproductive age in the absence of pregnancy. This condition is due to several causes that make the standard methods of investigations and management inconsistent and difficult. Several causes may be attributed to AUB in an individual, whereas none may be detected in some. In some, the lesion detected may not be the real cause of AUB, i.e. an uterine fibroid may be a coincidental finding, asymptomatic and not the true cause of AUB.

For this reason, FIGO in 2011 came forward with the new nomenclature of AUB instead of DUB, and a new classification system to define its cause. This classification is named 'PALM–COEIN' system. It stands for polyp, adenomyosis, leiomyoma, malignancy, coagulopathy, ovulatory dysfunction, endometrium, iatrogenic and nonclassified. The first four are related to visually objective structural uterine abnormalities that can be measured visually with imaging modalities and by a histopathological study. The others are nonstructural and attributed to coagulation disorders and hormonal dysfunction. N stands for not yet specified.

PALM–COEIN classification is further subdivided into secondary and tertiary subclassification according to the findings detected.

Contrary to the PALM group, the COEIN group cannot be detected by imaging and histopathology. This category refers to coagulopathy, ovarian steroid dysfunction, either endogenous or by administration of hormones, for various conditions (oral contraceptives, IUCD, drugs).

AUB may be acute or chronic. Acute bleeding may occur sporadically de novo or may be superimposed on chronic AUB, and requires an immediate treatment. Chronic AUB is described as abnormal menstrual bleeding related to volume, timing, regularity and duration of bleeding that lasts for 6 months (minimum 3 months), and requires thorough investigations.

AUB does not include the bleeding caused by lesions in the lower genital tract.

PALM–COEIN CLASSIFICATION

The classification is stratified into nine basic categories that are arranged according to the acronym PALM–COEIN (polyp, adenomyosis, leiomyoma, malignancy and hyperplasia endometrium, coagulopathy, ovulatory disorders, endometrium, iatrogenic and nonclassified).

POLYP – (AUB-P)

It is categorized and defined by ultrasound, saline sonography, hysteroscopy with or without histopathology.

P category is subdivided according to number, size, location and histology.

ADENOMYOSIS (AUB-A)

It is diagnosed by ultrasound and MRI. MRI is expensive and not available in many centres. In such cases, ultrasound alone is used for the diagnostic purpose. The category is subdivided depending on the depth of endometrial myometrial invasion. It is important to remember that many cases of adenomyosis are asymptomatic and only diagnosed on hysterectomy specimens.

LEIOMYOMA (AUB-L)

Many leiomyomas are coincidental findings and are not the cause of AUB. Because of the number, different locations and size, this group is divided into primary, secondary and tertiary group.

The primary classification reflects only the presence or absence of leiomyomas as determined by ultrasound. In the secondary classification, it is necessary to distinguish myomas that involve the uterine cavity, as these are the ones that are likely to cause AUB – the ones away from the endometrium are unlikely to do so.

The tertiary classification involves submucosal growths. It also includes number, size and location of myomas.

MALIGNANCY AND PREMALIGNANT LESIONS (AUB-M)

This group is rare in the reproductive age, but may occur in a woman with a PCOD and chronic anovulation. The diagnosis is by histopathological examination of the endometrium (D&C, biopsy) or by hysteroscopic biopsy.

COAGULOPATHY (AUB-C)

It consists of a spectrum of systemic disorders of haemostasis that can cause AUB in around 13%–20% women of reproductive age. The most common is von Willebrand disease. However, many of these may be asymptomatic and not related to AUB.

OVULATORY DISORDERS (AUB-O)

About 80% are anovulatory cycles with unpredictable, irregular menstrual cycles, some with heavy bleeding. About 20% are ovulatory but may be a consequence of 'luteal-out-of phase' (LOOP) events with deficient progesterone. Some of these are caused by hypothyroidism or hyperprolactinaemia.

ENDOMETRIAL CAUSES (AUB-E)

The mechanism regulating local endometrial 'haemostasis' secondary to abnormal secretion of prostaglandins is as explained earlier. In rare cases, it is due to tubercular endometritis or infection, particularly chlamydial infection. There are no tests available, except for infections, to estimate the local causes, and the case is placed in this category by exclusion of other causes.

IATROGENIC (AUB-I)

This is caused by steroidal hormones administered as contraceptives, especially in low dose, IUCD, copper-T may cause unscheduled 'breakthrough bleeding' or menorrhagia. The drugs that are responsible are anticoagulants, phenothiazine and tricyclic antidepressants which affect dopamine metabolism.

NOT CLASSIFIED (AUB-N)

Rare causes not well defined or diagnosed are arteriovenous malformations, varicose veins of the uterine vessels or myohyperplasia. In others, no cause is discernible by the existing investigations. They are all clubbed in this group of unclassified AUB. As and when better investigations become available, they may be allocated to a new category in future.

ABNORMAL UTERINE BLEEDING IN REPRODUCTIVE AGE AND PREMENOPAUSAL WOMEN

The menstrual cycles, which are painless in most cases, are anovulatory cycles. One point to be emphasized here is that D&C and endometrial study are important in premenopausal women to rule out endometrial carcinoma. In younger women, D&C is done when medical therapy fails. Instead of D&C, uterine aspiration or hysteroscopic biopsy is chosen by some to study the endometrial lining and to detect small polypi that can be missed on ultrasound and to diagnose tubercular endometritis.

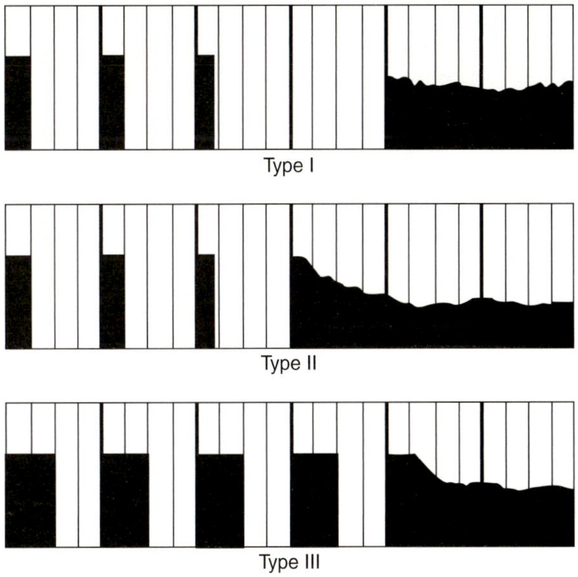

Figure 11.7 Menstrual history in cases of metropathia haemorrhagica. Continuous uterine bleeding is the most constant symptom, and most frequently this is preceded by amenorrhoea of about 8–10 weeks' duration. Sometimes, the bleeding follows upon a normal period, while at other times, the continuous bleeding may be preceded by menorrhagia.

METROPATHIA HAEMORRHAGICA

It is a specialized form of anovulatory AUB, seen in women between 40 and 45 years. It is not related to parity.

The symptoms are typical. The woman develops continuous painless vaginal bleeding, sometimes starting at the onset of menses, or preceded by 6–8 weeks of amenorrhoea (Fig. 11.7). Occasionally, the woman reveals a history of menorrhagia before this. The uterus is slightly bulky. This condition may simulate abortion and ectopic pregnancy, if amenorrhoea precedes bleeding, but pain is conspicuously absent.

PATHOLOGY

A mild degree of myohyperplasia with the uterine wall measuring up to 25 mm, and a uniformly enlarged uterus is seen in metropathia haemorrhagica. The endometrium is thick, polypoidal, and thin slender polypi project into the uterine cavity (Fig. 11.8). The endometrium shows characteristics of cystic glandular hyperplasia (Figs 11.9 and 11.10). The Swiss cheese pattern is another name given to describe this endometrium. The second feature is the absence of secretary endometrium with the absence of cock-screw glands. Areas of necrosis as seen during menstruation can be seen in the superficial surface. One or both ovaries may contain a cyst not larger than 5 cm, but corpus luteum is absent.

INVESTIGATIONS

- A history of the onset, duration and amount of bleeding should be noted. Antecedent causes such as IUCD, pills, pregnancy, abortion, drug therapy are also pertinent in these cases.
- General examination, with special reference to anaemia and thyroid function, blood count, coagulation profile, is carried out. Pelvic examination is done.

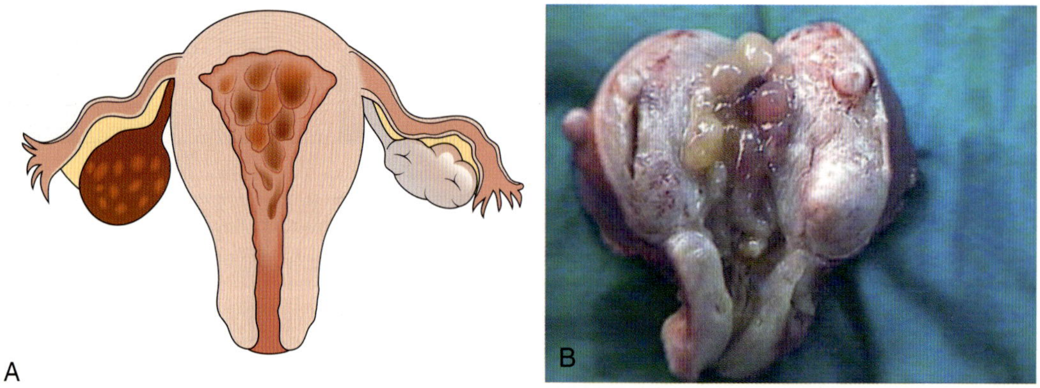

Figure 11.8 **(A)** Metropathia haemorrhagica. Note that the right ovary is cystic and that the endometrium shows diffuse polyp due to hyperplasia. **(B)** Cut section of the uterus showing thickened myometrium (myohyperplasia) and thickened polypoidal endometrium.

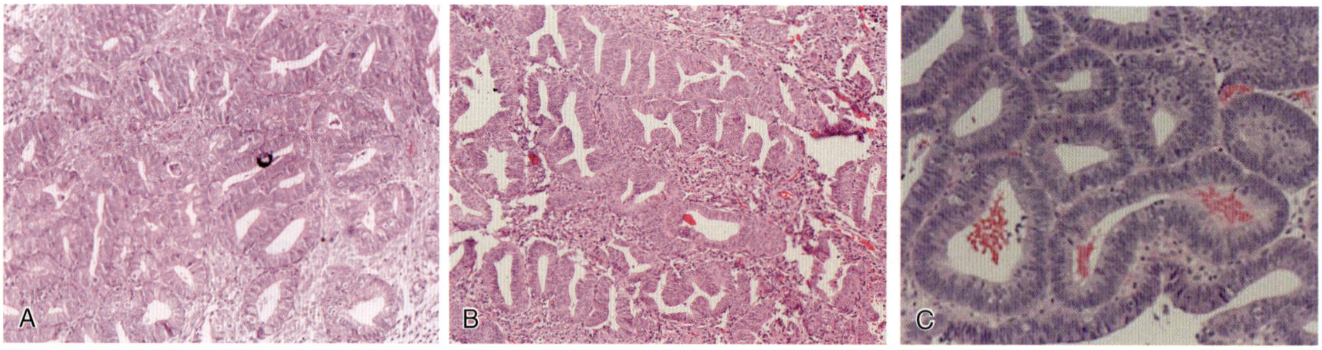

Figure 11.9 Endometrial biopsies of normal proliferative endometrium. **(A)** Simple endometrial hyperplasia without atypia. **(B)** Complex endometrial hyperplasia with **(C)** cellular atypia. (*Courtesy* **(B):** Dr Sandeep Mathur, AIIMS. **(C):** Hacker NF, Gambone JC, Hobel CJ, *Hacker and Moore's Essentials of Obstetrics and Gynecology, 5th ed.* Philadelphia: Elsevier, 2010.)

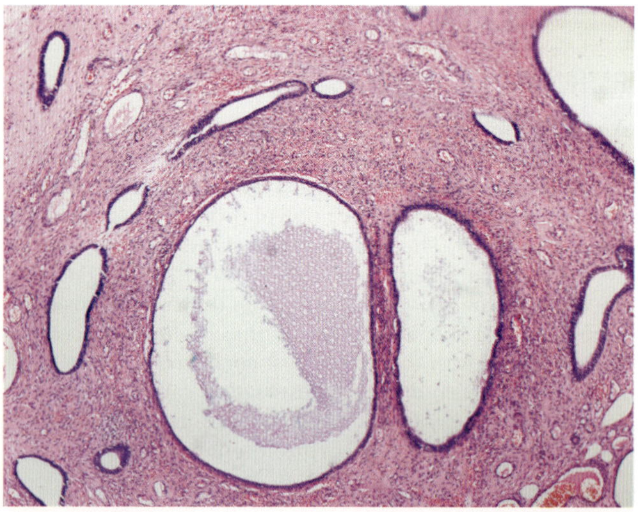

Figure 11.10 Metropathia haemorrhagica. Endometrium showing superficial necrosis. This necrosis resembles that seen on the first day of menstruation. The glands, however, do not show any secretory change (×110).

- Ultrasound to study pelvic organs and to rule out pelvic organic disease.
- Endometrial study by curettage, uterine aspiration or hysteroscopic biopsy is mandatory in premenopausal women, and necessary in a few younger women suspected to have endometrial tuberculosis.
- Doppler ultrasound to study endometrial vascularity may help in the diagnosis.
- Hysterosalpingography and saline salpingography may be employed, if hysteroscopic facilities are not available.

History, Examination (H/o Hormones/Drugs, Rule Out Pregnancy)

↓

Investigations

↓

Blood Test	Structural abnormalities	Histology
• Complete blood cell count • Coagulation profile	• Ultrasound • MRI as needed • Hysteroscopy	• Dilatation and curettage • Hysteroscopic endometrial biopsy • Endometrial aspiration biopsy

TREATMENT OF ABNORMAL UTERINE BLEEDING

- Treat the cause. Menorrhagia without any organic or general disease should be treated as follows:
  A wide variety of treatment modalities are now available. The treatment should be based on the age of the woman, her desire to retain fertility, previous treatment and severity of menorrhagia.
- Anaemia should be treated simultaneously. *The first line of treatment is medical therapy.* If that fails, D&C may be helpful mainly for diagnostic purpose, but a few women may benefit from it therapeutically. If hormonal treatment causes side effects, many now prefer to insert a Mirena IUCD. Failing this, decision has to be taken regarding a conservative surgery or hysterectomy. Lately, conservative surgeries have reduced the number of hysterectomies for AUB, and are cost-effective with quick recovery.

CONSERVATIVE TREATMENT

If the menorrhagia is not heavy and the woman is not anaemic, menstrual chart for a few months should be observed. Spontaneous cure is possible and can be awaited. Anaemia can be treated appropriately, if it exists.

HORMONE THERAPY (Table 11.2)

1. Oestrogen therapy alone is not recommended because of the risk of endometrial and breast cancer. Oral combined pills are effective in only select women and not safe after the age of 35 years, in smokers and obese women.
2. Progestogens are the main hormones used in AUB. Progestogen induces oestradiol 17β-dehydrogenase which converts oestradiol to weak oestrone which in turn suppresses E_2 receptors, DNA synthesis and has antimitotic activity. Thus, progestogens cause endometrial atrophy. A high initial dose of 10–30 mg a day should arrest bleeding in 24–48 hours, after which 5 mg daily is given for 20 days. Withdrawal bleeding occurs 2–5 days after stopping the drug, and normal blood loss is expected. A further course of 5 mg daily for 20 days is started on the second or third day of the periods cyclically for 3–6 months (given at night to reduce side effects). Dydrogesterone (10 mg) does not suppress ovulation in women who desire pregnancy, and it does not influence lipoproteins. Progestogens used commonly are norethisterone, Dydrogesterone, DMPA or newer progestins. *Gestrinone*, a derivative of 19-nortestosterone, is effective in an oral dose of 2.5 mg twice weekly or 5 mg vaginal tablets thrice weekly for 6 months. Instead of a 3-week cyclical therapy, giving progestogen only in the luteal phase is not effective.
   Three-monthly Depo-Provera is also now recommended to reduce the number of menstruations in a year. Instead of cyclical administration of progestogens, continuous oral progestogens daily for 3 months with a break of 1 week reduces the number of menstrual cycles to four in a year which many women welcome.
   Fibroplant implant releasing 14 mcg daily of levonorgestrel is under trial.
3. Danazol has a limited role when oral contraceptives and progestogens are not suited to a woman. It has androgenic side effects. Danazol 200 mg daily for 3–4 cycles is recommended.
4. Clomiphene is advocated, if pregnancy is desired.
5. Ethamsylate reduces capillary fragility, 500 mg four times a day from 5 days before anticipated period, up to 10 days reduces menorrhagia by 50% (Table 11.2) in ovulatory cycles.
6. NSAIDs taken during menstruation for 4–5 days control menorrhagia by 70% in ovulatory cycles, post-IUCD and poststerilization menorrhagia. These drugs inhibit cyclooxygenase and prostaglandin productions.

Table 11.2 Medical Therapy

Drugs	Dosage	Side Effects
Combined oral contraceptives	20–30 mcg EE_2 + progestogen monthly seasonale – 3 monthly (4 cycles in a year)	Nausea, headache, hypertension, hyperglycaemia, thrombosis, liver and gall bladder disease, breast cancer
Progestogens	5–10 mg tablet (10–30 mg daily) for 3 weeks cyclically • Continuous 3 monthly • 3 monthly injections • Implant	Weight gain, depression, headache, acne, abnormal lipid profile, breast tumours
Gestrinone Danazol	2.5 mg twice weekly 100–200 mg daily	Acne, hirsutism, weight gain, reduced high density lipoprotein, cholesterol
GnRH analogues	4 weekly injections	Menopausal symptoms, osteoporosis, loss of libido
Tranexamic acid	1 g, 6 hourly	Nausea, vomiting diarrhoea, headache, visual disturbances, intracranial thrombosis
NSAIDs	Mefenamic acid 500 mg t.i.d.	Nausea, vomiting, dyspepsia, gastric ulcer, diarrhoea, thrombocytopenia
Ethamsylate	500 mg four times daily	Nausea, headache, rash
Mirena IUCD	52 mg levonorgestrel	Less than those of oral progestogen – because its action is local resulting in endometrial suppression; however, it takes 2–3 months to reduce menorrhagia and the effect lasts for 5 years
Ormeloxifene	60 mg twice weekly	

7. Antifibrinolytic agents – Tranexamic acid, 1–2 g four times a day for 6–7 days during menstruation is effective in 50% of the cases. Ethamsylate combined with 250 mg tranexamic acid is also advocated. Combined tranexamic acid with mefenamic acid is now available (Trapic-MF).
8. GnRH is employed, if the above fails. Depot injection 3.6 mg given monthly for 4–6 months or 6.6 mg implant is nearly 100% successful. A longer duration of treatment with its antioestrogenic action causes menopausal symptoms and osteoporosis. This can be counteracted by 'add-back therapy' by giving 5–10 mg norethisterone (not Medroxyprogesterone acetate since it is not bone protective) or tibolone, and this allows longer administration of GnRH (more than 6 months). GnRH takes 4 weeks to act and is therefore not effective in acute episodes of bleeding.
9. **SERM** (selective oestrogen receptor modulator) – A new drug ormeloxifene, nonhormonal centchroman 60 mg twice weekly for 12 weeks to 6 months and thereafter weekly, is 50% effective. It does not cause breast or uterine cancer because of its antioestrogenic effect. It is also agonist to the cardiovascular system and bone protective. It sometimes lengthens the follicular phase and delays menstruation. It can cause a functional cyst, dyspepsia and headache at times.
10. When oestrogen is not contraindicated and a woman also needs contraception, a new drug Seasonale (combined oestrogen and progestogen) is used daily for 84 days with a gap of 6 days in a 3-monthly treatment. Menstruation occurs during the tablet-free period. It is welcomed by women because of infrequent periods.

MIRENA

To avoid side effects of hormonal therapy, Mirena IUCD is now employed to control menorrhagia. It directly suppresses endometrium with minimal side effects. It has no action on the ovaries; therefore, E_2 and progesterone levels remain normal (Fig. 11.11). It reduces blood loss by 70%–90% in 3 months, and acts as a contraceptive for those who do not desire pregnancy.

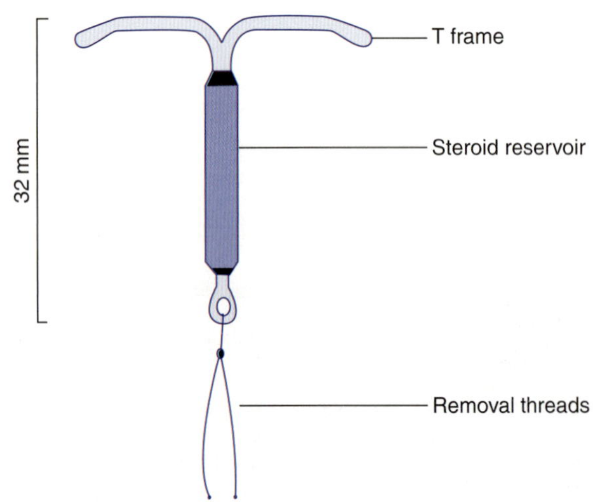

Figure 11.11 Mirena IUCD.

Mirena can be retained for 5 years. However it may cause irregular bleeding during the first 3 months, and the woman is advised to persevere retaining Mirena and not get it removed on this account. About 25% of women become amenorrhoeic at the end of 1 year. A quick return of fertility is noted following its removal. About 80% conceive by 12 months. Mirena is also useful in women with menorrhagia and dysmenorrhoea associated with uterine fibroid, adenomyosis.

Disadvantages of Mirena

The following are the disadvantages of Mirena:

- Slightly difficult to insert.
- Takes 3 months before it becomes effective.
- Amenorrhoea occurs in 20%–25%, which is not desirable in younger women.
- Ectopic pregnancy is reported in 0.2 per 100 women.
- Hysterectomy is required in 25% by the end of 3 years because of recurrence of menorrhagia.

MINIMAL INVASIVE SURGERY (MIS) (Table 11.3)

- D&C and endometrial study are required, if genital tuberculosis or endometrial cancer is suspected or the medical therapy fails. Though mainly performed for a diagnostic purpose, 30%–40% are relieved of menorrhagia at least for a short period of time.

Ablative Techniques

The idea of endometrial ablation arose from oligomenorrhoea occurring in Asherman syndrome due to synechiae. These procedures are safe, effective with lesser morbidity than hysterectomy, as well as cost-effective with quicker recovery. Hysterectomy is avoided in many cases. The endometrium is destroyed upto the basal layer.

Fertility is not possible following ablative therapy. Therefore, these procedures are mainly suitable for women who wish to preserve the uterus, avoid hysterectomy, but are not interested in pregnancy.

The method should destroy 2–3 mm of myometrium, if recurrence of menorrhagia has to be avoided.

Various procedures have been developed. These are as follows:

- First generation – Hysteroscopic endometrial ablation by resectoscope, loop, rollerball coagulation and laser (transcervical endometrial resection [TCRE])
- Second generation – Radiofrequency-induced thermal ablation, Cavaterm balloon therapy, microwave endometrial ablation (MEA), laser therapy

Table 11.3 Minimal Surgical Methods of Treating Menorrhagia

Ablative technique
First generation
• Hysteroscopic ablation endometrium resectoscope, roller ball laser (TCRE)
Second generation
• RITEA, balloon therapy, microwave ablation
• Uterine tamponade in acute bleeding
• Bilateral uterine artery embolization

- Uterine tamponade
- Bilateral uterine artery embolization

Hysteroscopic Endometrial Ablation. These procedures should be performed soon after the menstrual period or the endometrium is thinned out by giving progestogens, danazol or GnRH for 4–6 weeks before the procedure. The patient needs to be selected and contraindications are as noted below:

- Uterine size > 12 weeks (12 cm) (volume > 30 mL)
- Uterine fibroid
- Scarred uterus (previous surgery)
- Young woman desirous of pregnancy
- Adenomyosis – TCRE can cause dysmenorrhoea
- Genital infection
- Uterine cancer or preinvasive cancer, atypical hyperplasia

TCRE under general anaesthesia using hysteroscope destroys 4–5 mm endometrium and forms uterine synechiae. The earlier monopolar electrode is replaced by a bipolar electrode (VERSAPOINT™).

Complications are as follows:

- Anaesthetic complications.
- Fluid imbalance with fluid overload (glycine 1.5%), pulmonary oedema, hypertension, hyponatremia, anaphylactic reaction with dextran, haemolysis and at times death.
- Uterine, bowel and bladder injury with burns and vaginal fistula.
- Embolism, infection and haemorrhage.
- Menorrhagia recurs in 25% cases by the end of 3 years and needs repeat TCRE or hysterectomy.
- Dysmenorrhoea in a few women, and haematometra due to cervical stenosis.

Radiofrequency-Induced Thermal Endometrial Ablation. It is a blind procedure using radiofrequency electromagnetic thermal energy which destroys the endometrium at 66°C. A 0.6-mm metallic probe is inserted transcervically under general anaesthesia and rotated over 360° for 20 minutes. About 85% get cured and 30% develop amenorrhoea by the end of 1 year. It is cheaper compared to TCRE, does not require hysteroscope and complications of distending media are avoided. Contraindications and complications are similar to those of TCRE.

Advantages of RITEA

- Less skill required to perform the procedure. Hysteroscopy not required.
- Less risk with this procedure.

An occasional uterine perforation, vaginal heat leading to vesicovaginal fistula has been reported.

Cavaterm Balloon Therapy (Fig. 11.12). First invented by Neuwirth in 1994, this instrument comprises a central computer system, battery and a disposable silicon rubber balloon catheter 5 mm in diameter. Under local anaesthesia, the catheter is inserted transcervically into the uterine cavity, and the balloon is distended with 15–30 mL sterile solution such as 5% glucose or 1.5% glycine. The heating element in the balloon raises the temperature to 87°C (187°F) and this temperature is maintained for 8 minutes over a pressure of 160–180 mm Hg to exert a tamponade effect. The catheter has an inherent safety design related to time, pressure and temperature, and it gets automatically deactivated to avoid complications. About 6 mm of endometrium gets destroyed, so preoperative endometrium thinning is not required. Approximately, 70%–90% resume normal cycles and 15% become amenorrhoeic by the end of 1 year. Hysteroscopy is not required. Failure in retroverted uterus is due to unequal distribution of heat over the endometrium. Cramping felt in the first few hours is treated with NSAIDs and antibiotics are given. Contraindications are endometrium thicker than 11 mm and others similar to TCRE. This technique is easy to learn.

Microwave Endometrial Ablation. It utilizes magnetic energy and works at the frequency of 9.2 GHz. It is an OPD procedure, done under local anaesthesia. It uses an 8 mm

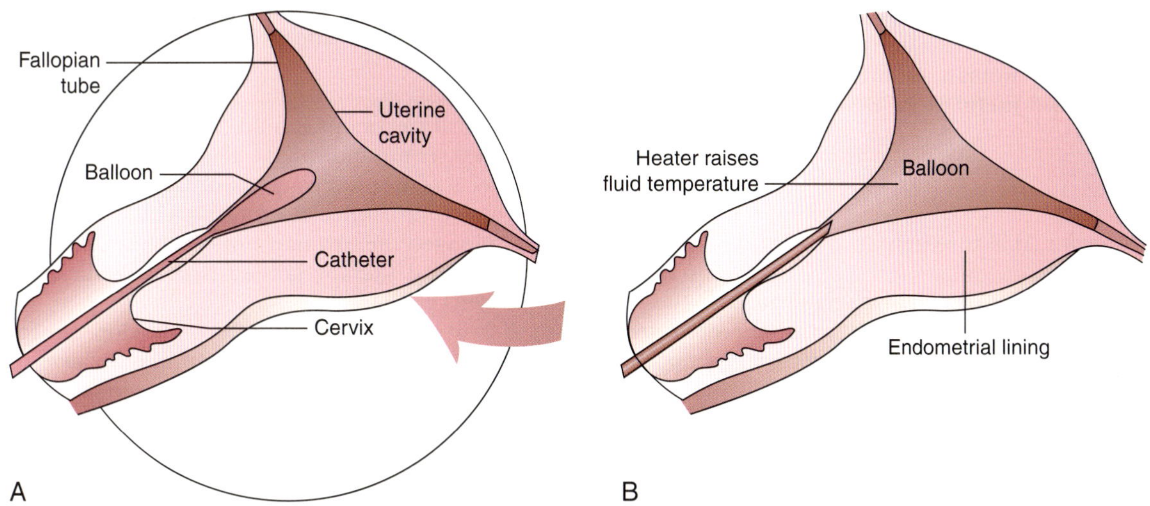

Figure 11.12 Cavaterm balloon. **(A)** Balloon inside the uterus. **(B)** Using the syringe, fluid is injected through the catheter-inflating balloon.

applicator with no need of preoperative endometrial thinning. Temperature of 80°C is maintained for 3 minutes. About 50% become oligomenorrhoeic and 40% amenorrhoeic. Up to 6 mm endometrium gets ablated. No earthing is required unlike TCRE. Total operating time is 12 minutes. Hysteroscopy is also not required. The contraindications and complications are similar to other ablative procedures.

Vesta System. This system uses a single-use multielectrode intrauterine balloon to ablate the endometrium. The silicon inflatable electrode carrier has a triangular shape, which unfolds when its insertion sheath is withdrawn. The controller unit is connected to a standard electro surgical generator. It regulates energy to each balloon electrode plate. The temperature is set at 75°C. The balloon is inflated with air following cervical dilatation up to No 9. The procedure takes 5 minutes under local anaesthesia. About 90%–94% are cured of menorrhagia. The instrument is very expensive and sufficient data are not available to assess its outcome.

Uterine Tamponade. Goldrath advocated uterine tamponade in acute episodes of bleeding by inserting a Foley catheter, distending with 30 mL fluid and leaving the catheter for 24 hours.

NovaSure (impedance-controlled endometrial ablation) is the latest and most safe procedure, taking just 90 seconds. It uses bipolar radiofrequency and vaporizes endometrium up to myometrium.

Endometrial laser intrauterine thermotherapy (ELITT) is a new laser therapy that destroys the entire endometrium as well as 1–3.5 mm of myometrium. It is done as an OPD procedure, and takes 7 minutes. The machine is known by the name 'GyneLase'. Both touch and non-touch technique can be employed.

The second-generation ablative techniques are simpler than TCRE; they are more effective, safe OPD procedures; they are cost-effective and save hysterectomy in several women. They do not require pre-operative preparations, easy to learn and perform quickly without the risk of fluid imbalance.

Bilateral Uterine Artery Embolization. Primarily used in uterine fibroids, this technique is extended in intractable AUB in a young woman to preserve her reproductive function. It is also useful in AUB complicated by varicose uterine vessels.

HYSTERECTOMY

Hysterectomy for AUB is required:

- If medical/MIS fails or menorrhagia recurs.
- In older women more than 40 years not desirous of childbearing, and who opt for hysterectomy as a primary treatment or ablation fails.

Initially performed by abdominal route, it was replaced by laparoscopic hysterectomy or laparoscopic-assisted vaginal hysterectomy (LAVH) for its quick recovery, less pain, less abdominal adhesions and avoidance of abdominal scar. Lately, many gynaecologists have shifted to vaginal hysterectomy for undescended uterus which may even be enlarged. This trend is adopted because of lesser morbidity, and lesser postoperative complications of adhesions, scar hernia and pulmonary complications.

Vaginal hysterectomy is contraindicated if:

1. Uterus is grossly enlarged.
2. Previous surgery with possible adhesions, fixity and limitation of uterine mobility.
3. Presence of endometriosis or adnexal mass.

Nulliparous women or women with a very narrow vagina. In a woman less than 50 years of age, ovaries should be conserved unless they are diseased.

Sequelae or Delayed Complications of Hysterectomy

Although hysterectomy is a one-time procedure, safe and cures AUB, delayed complications are known to occur. These are as follows:

- Ovarian atrophy due to devascularization; the woman develops menopausal symptoms and its complications.
- Adhesions of the ovaries to the vaginal vault causing an ovarian residual syndrome, dyspareunia and chronic pelvic pain.
- Vault prolapse.
- Sexual dysfunction – dyspareunia due to a short vagina.
- Chronic abdominal pain due to postoperative pelvic adhesions.
- Urinary and bowel symptoms due to denervation.
- Psychological disturbances.

NEW SYSTEMS

VERSAPOINT™ bipolar electrosurgical system works in normal saline, is cheap, has excellent haemostasis and causes instantaneous tissue vaporization.

Advantages of Mirena IUCD over ablative techniques are as follows:

- Low cost
- OPD procedure – no hospitalization
- Preservation of fertility after its removal

Pregnancy occurs within a year. The only disadvantage is occasional systemic side effects of progestogen.

SUMMARY

1. Medical treatment should be the first line of treatment, unless contraindicated. The drawbacks are the side effects of hormones and the fact that symptoms sometimes return once the hormone therapy is stopped. A prolonged therapy may not be desirable.
2. If medical therapy fails or is contraindicated, consider Mirena IUCD.
3. If Mirena fails or side effects develop, go for ablative techniques. The second-generation ablative techniques are safer, quick to perform and are equally effective.
4. When the above methods fail, consider hysterectomy.

IRREGULAR RIPENING

It is an ovulatory bleeding due to deficient corpus luteal function. The breakthrough bleeding occurs before the actual menstruation in the form of a spotting or brownish discharge. Progestogen given during the late luteal phase cures the spotting.

IRREGULAR SHEDDING (HALBAN DISEASE)

It is rare and self-limited. Irregular shedding is due to persistent corpus luteum. The menstruation comes on time, is prolonged but not heavy. Progestogen can suppress the bleeding, but needs to be taken on a tapering dose for 20 days to complete the cycle.

ADENOMATOUS ENDOMETRIAL POLYP

This form of polyp is really a localized area of endometrial hyperplasia when area or areas of thickened endometrium project into the cavity of the endometrium to look like polyp. The polyp may be single or multiple, small or large enough to protrude through the cervical canal. Mostly, they are sessile and small.

This type of polyp occurs in following:

- Endometrial hyperplasia (anovulatory cycles)
- Metropathia haemorrhagica (diffuse polyposis)
- A woman on tamoxifen
- Some cases of fibroid

PATHOLOGY

A polyp is covered by cubical epithelium and contains endometrial glands that do not respond to hormones.

CLINICAL FEATURES

These polypi cause menorrhagia, metrorrhagia or postmenopausal bleeding. The uterus is normal in size or slightly enlarged uniformly. Ultrasound, sonosalpingography and hysterosalpingography detect these polypi, but may miss them, if they are very small. Hysteroscopic visualization and resection is the best treatment, and hysterectomy can be avoided. Histopathology is mandatory to rule out a malignant change.

Adenomyomatous polyp resembles adenomatous polyp, but it contains muscle tissue in the stroma. The symptoms and management are similar in both conditions.

ENDOMETRIAL HYPERPLASIA

This occurs in following cases:

- Anovulatory cycles with unopposed oestrogen acting on the endometrium
- Metropathia haemorrhagica
- Obese women
- PCOD
- A woman on tamoxifen
- A menopausal woman on hormone replacement therapy without progestogen
- Feminizing ovarian tumours

Hyperplasia may be simple hyperplasia, glandular or atypical.

Two per cent women with simple hyperplasia are at a risk of endometrial cancer, and 4%–10% women with glandular hyperplasia develop the cancer. Atypical hyperplasia, however, has the tendency to develop into carcinoma in as much as 60%–70% cases.

While 80% cases of simple hyperplasia without atypia respond to progestogens, response of atypical hyperplasia is only 50%, but with the risk of malignancy. For this reason, atypical endometrial hyperplasia should be treated by hysterectomy and not merely by an ablative technique. A small portion of endometrium left behind and undergoing malignancy may not be easily detected following ablative treatment.

Surprisingly, Mirena is not effective against endometrial hyperplasia caused by tamoxifen.

ABNORMAL UTERINE BLEEDING IN ADOLESCENTS

The commonest cause lies in the H–P–O dysfunction (50%). Immature development of these organs results in anovulation in the 1-5 years following menarche, unopposed estrogen causing endometrial hyperplasia. As the girl matures, the normal menstrual cycles are established.

- Blood dyscrasia – Coagulation disorders, thrombocytopenia purpura, Von Willebrand disease, leukaemia account for 20% of cases.
- Hypothyroidism – 4% of cases.
- PCOD – 10%–12% of cases.
- Genital tuberculosis – 4% of cases.
- Liver disorders.
- Feminizing ovarian tumours – granulosa cell and theca cell tumours.
- Adrenal hyperplasia.

CLINICAL FEATURES

Menorrhagia may be noticed from the start of menarche, but often the initial cycles may be normal. It takes the form of heavy regular cycles, or normal bleeding lasting for several days, but dysmenorrhoea is invariably absent in anovulatory cycles. Anaemia may supervene. The pelvic findings by ultrasound scanning are normal except in ovarian tumour.

It is important to rule out other causes of menorrhagia before instituting hormonal therapy.

INVESTIGATIONS

- Blood profile – Hb%, bleeding and clotting time, coagulation factors; blood film.
- X-ray chest for tuberculosis.
- Thyroid function tests.
- Pelvic ultrasound to rule out PCOD, early fibroid.
- If medical treatment fails, D&C should be done to rule out endometrial tuberculosis by PCR test.

MANAGEMENT

Aim is to:

- Control menorrhagia.
- Prevent or treat anaemia.
- Prevent recurrence.
- Treat the cause.

- Anovulatory cycles
  - In an acute episode of bleeding, i.v. Premarin 25 mg 6–8 hourly will control bleeding in 24–48 hours. Thereafter, oestrogen for 21 days with progestogen added for 10 days for 3–6 cycles will regularize the cycles.
  - In chronic menorrhagia, oral combined pills or cyclical progestogen is the first line of treatment. About 70%–80% responds well. Medical treatment is detailed below.
- NSAIDs: Mefenamic acid 250–500 mg t.i.d. during periods. Naproxen, ibuprofen.
- Androgens (danazol) are not recommended, though effective, because of androgenic effects in young girls.
- GnRH therapy takes 4 weeks to act, so not useful in acute episode. The drug is expensive and a prolonged treatment more than 4–6 months can cause osteoporosis.
- If progestogens cause side effects, Mirena IUCD for a few months can control menorrhagia.
- Arterial embolization is required in case of varicosity of uterine vessels.
- When the above treatments fail, uterine tamponade using Foley catheter for 24 hours can control bleeding in the acute episode.
- Anti-TB treatment in endometrial tuberculosis.

Blood transfusion may be required to correct anaemia.

Lately, the trend is to give intravenous tranexamic acid 1 g with 25 mg of oestrogen, and then continue with oestrogen and progesterone as mentioned above. Desmopressin analogue of arginine vasopressin is given intravenously or by a nasal spray (1.5 mg/mL – total 150-300mcg diluted in 30mL saline) in van Willebrand syndrome.

Tranexamic acid inhibits tissue plasminogen activator which is a fibrinolytic enzyme, whose level increases in AUB.

KEY POINTS

- AUB may be due to general systemic causes, local pelvic pathology such as fibroid, adenomyosis, endometrial polyp, PID, feminizing ovarian tumours and pelvic endometriosis.
- The management of AUB is based on the age of the woman and her parity, and the cause.
- Medical therapy comprising various hormones and drugs should be employed in young women as the first line of treatment. When this fails, Mirena, conservative minimal surgery or hysterectomy should be considered.
- Medical therapy is effective and is the first-line treatment. Some, however, develop side effects with a prolonged therapy; Mirena IUD is the next choice.
- Mirena is a nonsurgical effective method to control menorrhagia, and may help avoid hysterectomy in many women. Ablative therapy was popular in the past. Hysterectomy is the last choice in AUB.
- In perimenopausal women, D&C is mandatory to rule out malignancy. If histology is benign, either hormonal therapy, Mirena or hysterectomy will be required.
- Hysterectomy can be done by abdominal, vaginal route or laparoscopic hysterectomy. Endometrial hyperplasia may be simple or glandular without atypia whose malignant potential is low. It can be treated conservatively with hormones or minimal invasive procedures.
- Atypical endometrial hyperplasia has 28%–30% risk of malignancy and should be managed by hysterectomy.

SELF-ASSESSMENT

1. Enumerate the causes of AUB.
2. How would you investigate and manage a case of AUB. Define AUB. How would you manage an adolescent with AUB?
3. Describe the alternatives of minimally invasive surgery in the management of AUB.
4. Discuss the medical management of AUB in a 35-year-old woman.
5. Describe puberty menorrhagia and its management.
6. A 38-year-old woman presents with polymenorrhagia. The uterus is 12 weeks size. Discuss the management.
7. Write short notes on the following:
   - Metropathia haemorrhagia
   - Endometrial hyperplasia

SUGGESTED READING

Aberdeen Endometrial Ablation Trials Group. A randomized trial of endometrial ablation versus hysterectomy for the treatment of dysfunctional uterine bleeding; outcome of four years. Br J Obstet Gynaecol 1999;106:360–66.

Breitkopf DM, Fredrickson RA, Snyder RR, et al. Detection of benign endometrial masses by endometrial stripe measurement in premenopausal women. Obstet Gynecol 2004;104(1):120.

Farquhar CM, Lethaby A, et al. An evaluation for risk factors for endometrial hyperplasia in premenopausal women with abnormal utrine bleeding. Am J Obstet Gynecol 1999;181(3):585.

Khrouf M, Terras K. Diagnosis and Management of Formerly Called "Dysfunctional Uterine Bleeding" According to PALM-COEIN FIGO Classification and the New Guidelines. J Obstet Gynaecol India. 2014;64(6):388–93.

Kouides PA, Phatak PD, Burkart P, et al. Gynecological and obstetrical morbidity in women with type-I von Willebrand disease: Results of patient survey. Hemophilia 2000;6(6):643.

Laberge P, Leyland N, Murji A, Fortin C, Martyn P, Vilos G, et al. Endometrial ablation in the management of abnormal uterine bleeding. J Obstet Gynaecol Can. 2015;37(4):362–79.

Munro MG, Critchley HOD, Fraser IS, FIGO Menstrual Disorders Working Group. The FIGO classification of causes of abnormal uterine bleeding in the reproductive years. Fertil Steril. 2011; 95(7):2204–8, 2208.e1-3.

Pinion SB, Parkin DE, Abamrovich DJ, et al. Randomised trial of hysterectomy, endometrial laser ablation and transcervical endometrial resection for dysfunctional uterine bleeding. Br Med J 1994;309: 979–83.

Speroff L, Fritz MA. Clinical Gynecologic Endocrinology and Infertility. 8th ed. Philadelphia: Lippincott Williams & Wilkins, 2011: 591-62.

Studd J, Seang Lin Tan, Frank A Chervenak. Progress in Obstetrics and Gynaecology. 1996;12:309.

Studd J, Seang Lin Tan, Frank A Chervenak. Progress in Obstetrics and Gynaecology. In: Ablative Procedures in Abnormal Uterine Bleeding and Medical Management. 2000;14.

Studd J, Seang Lin Tan, Frank A Chervenak. Progress in Obstetrics and Gynaecology. MIRENA 2005;16:389.

Studd J, Seang Lin Tan, Frank A Chervenak. Progress in Obstetrics and Gynaecology. Minimal Invasive Surgery 2006;17:259.

Vilos GA, Tureanu V, Garcia M, Abu-Rafea B. The levonorgestrel intrauterine system is an effective treatment in women with abnormal uterine bleeding and anticoagulant therapy. J Minim Invasive Gynecol. 2009;16(4):480–4.

Primary and Secondary Amenorrhoea

12

CHAPTER OUTLINE

AMENORRHOEA

The initiation of menstruation is an important milestone in the reproductive lives of women.

Amenorrhoea denotes the absence of menstruation. It may be *physiological* or *pathological*.

Its onset may be *primary* or *secondary*.

Physiological amenorrhoea naturally prevails before the onset of puberty, during pregnancy and lactation and after menopause.

Pathological amenorrhoea is the result of genetic factors, systemic diseases, endocrinopathies, disturbance of the hypothalamic–pituitary–ovarian–uterine axis, gynatresia, nutritional factors, drug usage, psychological factors and other rarer causes.

Primary amenorrhoea refers to the failure of the onset of menstruation beyond the age of 16 years, regardless of development of secondary sexual characters.

Secondary amenorrhoea refers to the failure of occurrence of menstruation for 6 months or longer in women who have previously menstruated.

Normally, menarche occurs between 10-16 years of age, with a mean age of 12.5 years.

PRIMARY AMENORRHOEA

Primary amenorrhoea at the age of 14 years behoves the clinician to undertake investigations for the cause of failure of occurrence, and institute a timely therapy. However, in the presence of well-developed secondary sexual characteristics, investigations may be delayed until the age of 16 years with the hope that spontaneous menstruation will eventually ensue in due course of time. *This occurs in delayed puberty.*

In the vast majority of cases, a detailed evaluation of growth charts, height and weight records, chronology of development of secondary sexual characteristics, body habitus, history of cyclic abdominal pain, administration of drugs, history of illnesses such as tuberculosis, thyroid disease, juvenile diabetes, mumps and any previous surgery may be important in revealing the possible aetiological cause. Physical examination should include documentation of the height–weight ratio, stature, Tanner evaluation for maturation status of the secondary sexual characteristics and observation of any genetic or endocrine stigmata. The presence of the uterus and vagina must be established by ultrasound scanning of the pelvis. In all patients presenting with primary amenorrhoea, estimation of the levels of serum follicle-stimulating hormone (FSH), oestradiol and prolactin is important. Serum FSH levels help to differentiate between the central nervous system (CNS) aetiologies and gonadal failure. A baseline radiological evaluation of bone age and a simple skull film or CT to exclude pituitary macroadenoma should precede further investigations. Genetic karyotyping is strongly indicated in all subjects revealing serum FSH levels elevated more than 40 mIU/mL. A few selective investigations such as thyroid function profile, renal function tests and androgen estimation must be done when indicated.

CLASSIFICATION

The spectrum of diagnosis presenting clinically as primary amenorrhoea can be conveniently classified according to the status of her serum FSH levels into hypergonadotropic (FSH > 40 mIU/mL), eugonadotropic or hypogonadotropic (Table 12.1).

HYPERGONADOTROPIC PRIMARY AMENORRHOEA

- Gonadal dysgenesis: 45OX (Turner syndrome) mosaics, abnormal X.
- 46XX pure gonadal dysgenesis.
- 46XY gonadal dysgenesis – Swyer syndrome, testicular feminizing syndrome.
- Gonadotropin-resistant ovary syndrome – Savage syndrome.

EUGONADOTROPIC PRIMARY AMENORRHOEA

A. Absence of Müllerian development:
- Androgen insensitivity syndrome (testicular feminization).

Table 12.1 Classification of Primary Amenorrhoea

Secondary sexual characteristics normal
- Imperforate hymen
- Transverse vaginal septum
- Absent vagina and functioning uterus
- Absent vagina and nonfunctioning uterus (Mayer–Rokitansky–Küster–Hauser syndrome [MRKH])
- XY female – androgen insensitivity
- Resistant ovary syndrome
- Constitutional delay

Secondary sexual characteristics absent
- Normal stature
  - Hypogonadotrophic hypogonadism
    - Congenital
      - Isolated gonadotrophin-releasing hormone deficiency
      - Olfacto–genital syndrome
    - Acquired
      - Weight loss/anorexia
      - Excessive exercise
      - Hyperprolactinaemia
  - Hypergonadotrophic hypogonadism
    - Gonadal agenesis
    - Chromosomal aberrations resulting from XX-agenesis
  - Gonadal dysgenesis
    - Turner mosaic
    - Other X deletions or mosaics
    - XY enzymatic failure
    - Ovarian failure
    - Galactosaemia
- Short stature
  - Hypogonadotrophic hypogonadism
    - Congenital
      - Hydrocephalus
    - Acquired
      - Trauma
      - Empty sella syndrome
- Tumours
  - Hypergonadotrophic hypogonadism
    - Turner syndrome
    - Other X deletions or mosaics

Heterosexual development
- Congenital adrenal hyperplasia
- Androgen-secreting tumour
- 5α-reductase deficiency
- Partial androgen receptor deficiency
- True hermaphrodite
- Absent Müllerian inhibitor

- Müllerian agenesis – the absence of uterus/vagina. Rokitansky–Küster–Hauser syndrome.

B. Normal Müllerian development:
- Female or true intersex.
- Polycystic ovary syndrome.
- Adrenal or thyroid diseases.

C. Cryptomenorrhoea – imperforate hymen, vaginal septum, cervical atresia.

D. Tubercular endometritis.

E. Constitutional delay – nutrition.

HYPOGONADOTROPIC PRIMARY AMENORRHOEA

A. Hypothalamic causes:
- Delayed menarche and puberty.
- Hypothalamic hypogonadism (Kallmann syndrome); gonadotropin-releasing hormone (GnRH) deficiency syndrome.
- Psychogenic causes, weight loss, stress, anorexia nervosa and malnutrition.

B. Pituitary causes:
- Pituitarism causes short stature, obesity, genital dystrophy, mental retardation, polydactyly and retinitis pigmentosa.
- Neoplasms – prolactinomas, craniopharyngiomas, adenomas and empty sella turcica.
- Hypopituitary states – Simmond disease, Chiari–Frommel syndrome, Forbes–Albright syndrome and pineal gland tumour.

C. Severe systemic diseases such as tuberculosis, syphilis.

D. Other endocrinal disorders – thyroid or adrenal gland.

AETIOLOGY

According to the location of cause of amenorrhoea aetiology is as follows:

- Delayed puberty.
- Pregnancy before menarche is extremely rare, but not impossible.
- Cerebral cortex – stress, emotional disturbances, infection, trauma, tumour.
- Hypothalamus – Kallmann syndrome, vigorous exercise, weight loss.
- Pituitary gland – empty sella turcica, Fröhlich syndrome, Laurence–Moon–Biedl syndrome, Cushing disease, pineal tumour, prolactinaemia, galactosaemia.
- Ovary – Turner syndrome, primary ovarian failure (Savage syndrome), polycystic ovarian disease (PCOD), 17-hydroxylase deficiency.
- Genital tract – absent uterus, (Mayer–Rokitansky–Kuster–Hauser [MRKH] syndrome. Testicular feminizing syndrome), refractory endometrium, obstruction in the lower genital tract, genital tuberculosis, Asherman syndrome (uterine adhesion).
- Chromosomal – intersex, Turner syndrome, testicular feminizing syndrome, Swyer syndrome.
- Other endocrine glands – juvenile diabetes, thyroid, adrenal glands.
- Drugs – tranquillizers, antihypertensives, antidepressants, metoclopramide, oestrogen.
- Nutrition – overweight, weight loss, tuberculosis, malnutrition.

ANOREXIA NERVOSA

Anorexia nervosa is a psychological somatic self-imposed eating disorder mainly affecting adolescents and young women more than men. It is the failure to maintain body weight for age and height. For menstruation to occur, minimal fat should constitute 22% of body weight. Loss of weight > 15% causes amenorrhoea. Leptin in the fat initiates GnRH secretion. When weight reduction falls below required body fat, GnRH and gonadotropin secretions fail. Clinically, fasting, excessive exercise with or without purging and self-induced vomiting cause atrophy or nondevelopment of breasts and amenorrhoea (Fig. 12.1).

Hypoestrinism thus induced following causes:

- Mortality through cardiac failure, arrhythmia (15%).
- Amenorrhoea, infertility, decreased libido.
- Osteoporosis.

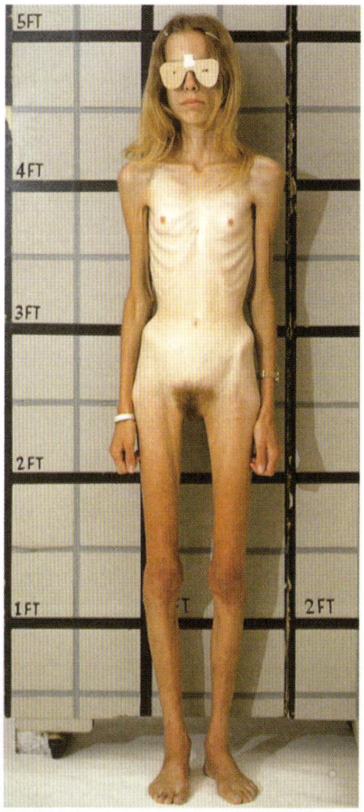

Figure 12.1 Anorexia nervosa. (*Source*: Lawrence A. Schachner, Ronald C Hansen. Pediatric Dermatology. Cutaneous manifestations of endocrine, metabolic, and nutritional disorders. Mosby, 2011.)

- Hypercortisolism, decreased muscle mass, low IGF-1, hypothyroidism, anaemia, granulocytopenia, neutropenia.
- Psychiatric problems.

Management

- Psychological
- Psychotherapy
- Nutritional
- GnRH to initiate hypothalamic–pituitary–ovarian (H–P–O) axis
- Hormonal therapy: To initiate or complete H–P–O axis

About 70% improve with treatment.

KALLMANN DISEASE

This disease occurs in 1:50,000 girls. Low or absent GnRH is due to either autosomal dominant or an X-linked autosomal recessive gene. The condition is characterized by anosmia and maldevelopment of neurons in the arcuate nucleus.

Management

- GnRH and pituitary hormones to induce menstruation, ovulation.
- Oestrogen and progestogen cyclically to induce menstruation.

CLINICAL APPROACH

The clinician is required to make an assessment of the cause of primary amenorrhoea on the basis of history, clinical examination and tests that are most likely to provide the answers to the underlying cause. Such information will provide the basis to offer a reasonable prognosis and initiate rational treatment. Table 12.2 offers clinical guidelines for management of primary amenorrhoea.

Some believe in clinical classification based on the presence/absence of secondary sex characters, stature and heterosexual development.

Important features to be noted are as follows:

1. History of diabetes, TB, mumps.
2. Family history of PCOD, delayed puberty, testicular feminizing syndrome.
3. Height, weight, breast development – certain stigmas.
4. Thyroid enlargement.

Table 12.2 Clinical Approach to Primary Amenorrhoea

Clinical Features	Presumptions	Distinguishing Tests
Breasts absent; uterus present	Lack of breasts indicates lack of oestrogen production from gonads (causes – H-P-O failure, lack of ovarian follicles, lack of two active X chromosomes, Turner syndrome [Fig. 12.2]); presence of uterus indicates that the Y chromosome is absent	**FSH level** identifies cause of oestrogen lack; high FSH (ovarian failure), low FSH indicates hypothalamic–pituitary failure; GnRH distinguishes hypothalamus (LH ↑) from pituitary cause (no LH response)
Breasts present; uterus absent	Presence of breasts indicates presence of gonadal oestrogen; absent uterus indicates Müllerian agenesis, or presence of Y chromosome or testicular feminizing syndrome	Serum testosterone levels high in androgen insensitivity (Y chromosome), but normal in 46XX with Müllerian agenesis; karyotyping confirms genetic sex. Gonadectomy advised for androgen sensitivity syndrome, Müllerian syndrome.
Breasts absent; uterus present	Absent breast suggests lack of oestrogen; because of gonadal agenesis, the absence of gonads, gonadal enzyme defects; absent uterus indicates the presence of Y chromosome with testes that suppresses Müllerian development; the presence of normal female external genitals indicates the absence of testes, hence no testosterone present when external genitals were developing	Karyotyping – 46XY, high FSH and testosterone – normal female range suggests gonadal agenesis/absence; gonadal biopsy to detect enzyme deficiency
Breasts present; uterus present	The presence of breasts indicate oestrogen present; uterus present indicates Y chromosome is absent	Investigations include following: progesterone challenge test, S. prolactin and thyroid profile, tests to exclude genital TB; urine test for the presence of β-hCG and UPT and USG to be done to rule out pregnancy

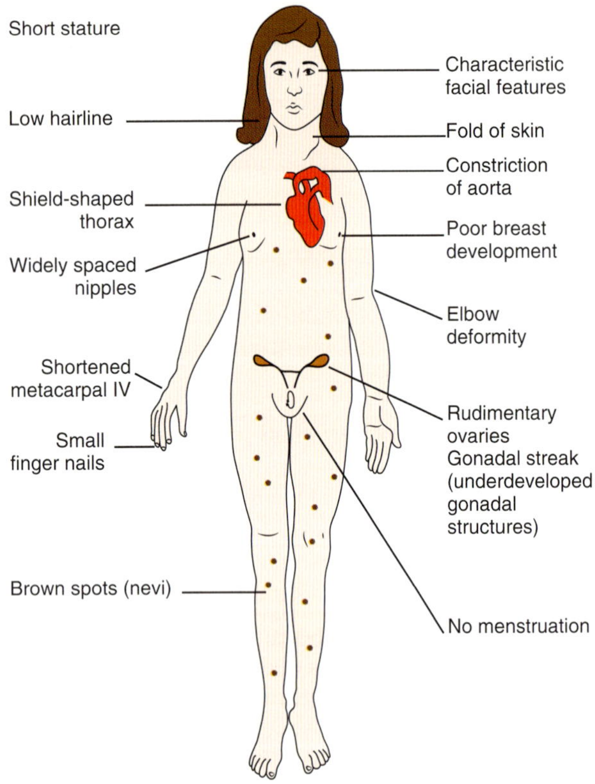

Figure 12.2 Clinical features of Turner syndrome.

5. Abdominal mass.
6. Ultrasound for presence of uterus, haematometra, presence of ovaries.
7. Chromosomal study

MANAGEMENT

HYPERGONADOTROPIC PRIMARY AMENORRHOEA

Hypergonadotropic primary amenorrhoea patients have gonadal failure. Various forms of gonadal dysgenesis account for these cases. These women have streak ovaries with the absence of ovarian follicles, there is no oestrogen production and they have elevated levels of FSH (>40 mIU/mL) and low oestradiol levels (<25 pg/mL). The sexual development is prepubertal with no endometrial proliferation; *hence, the progesterone challenge test is negative.* Chromosome studies reveal 45XO chromosomes (Turner syndrome).

Some patients with mosaicism or minor structural abnormalities of the X chromosome may have a few functional follicles capable of inducing menstruation, stray ovulation and pregnancy. *Chromosome study is relevant.*

Gonadectomy is indicated in patients with testicular feminizing syndrome, as these male gonads are prone to malignancy. Intersex is discussed in Chapter 9.

Women with streak ovaries are infertile, but they can bear children with oocyte donation. All women in this group must be treated with cyclic oestrogen and progestogen to promote feminization and secondary sexual characteristics and prevent osteoporosis. Women with resistant ovarian syndrome have normal ovaries on histology, they show the presence of primordial follicles, but there is probably a deficiency of receptors for FSH. They are not amenable to treatment.

Savage syndrome is due to a receptor defect of gonadotropic hormones in ovaries, and resembles autoimmune disease and resistant ovary syndrome. The height is normal, ovaries contain follicles but serum FSH is raised.

EUGONADOTROPIC PRIMARY AMENORRHOEA

If the FSH levels are within a normal range, the women have normal breast development; but due to abnormal Müllerian development, the uterus may be rudimentary or absent because of insensitivity to androgens.

In women with testicular feminization syndrome, the phenotype is a female with a karyotype of 46XY chromosomes. The gonads are testes often present in the inguinal canal and produce testosterone and Müllerian-inhibiting factor, but because of androgen insensitivity at target organs (due to deficient androgen receptors or lack of enzymes to convert testosterone to the more active dihydrotestosterone) these patients present with lack of axillary hair and pubic hair, absent uterus and upper vagina. They have a blind pouch of the lower vagina. Breast development appears normal because of peripheral conversion of androgen to oestrogen. These gonads are prone to malignancy; therefore, as soon as full sexual development is achieved by the age of 18–20 years, a prophylactic gonadectomy should be advised, followed by oestrogen therapy to maintain feminization. A vaginoplasty may be contemplated at an appropriate time in the future.

On the contrary, women with simple Müllerian agenesis and a karyotype of 46XX present with normal secondary sexual characters and functional ovaries (Rokitansky syndrome). They reveal a normal hormone profile. This syndrome is associated with renal and skeletal abnormality in 30% of the cases. These women do ovulate, and appropriate management requires creation of a functional vagina for coital purposes. If they plan to have children, it may be through surrogacy.

In women with cryptomenorrhoea presenting as primary amenorrhoea, the common cause is an intact hymen or vaginal septum. A history of cyclic abdominal colicky pain, retention of urine, the presence of a palpable abdominal lump and the visualization of a tense bluish bulging membrane on separation of the labia enables the diagnosis. Ultrasound scan of the pelvis confirms it. A simple cruciate incision of the hymen permits free drainage of the collected menstrual blood and leads to a normal reproductive function.

Septate vagina or atresia vagina requires excision and vaginoplasty.

The vaginal septum is recognized from the imperforate hymen by a pinkish concave covering in contrast to the bluish convex bulge in the latter. The vaginal septum, i.e. atresia, requires more extensive dissection and vaginoplasty. The atresia in the upper vagina and cervix often restenosis after surgery and eventually requires hysterectomy.

- Polycystic disease is described in the chapter on Ovarian Tumours.
- 17-hydroxylase deficiency causes deficient cortisol secretion and raised levels of adrenocorticotropic hormone. This causes hypertension, hypernatraemia, hypokalaemia and amenorrhoea.
- Endometrial nonresponsiveness and amenorrhoea are due to absent hormonal receptors. Hormonal profile remains normal.
- Tubercular endometritis requires anti-TB treatment.

HYPOGONADOTROPIC PRIMARY AMENORRHOEA

These women have FSH level less than 40 mIU/mL. Hypogonadotropinaemia leading to hypogonadism is usually the result of hypothalamic dysfunction, pituitary failure or systemic illnesses. Administration of GnRH helps to differentiate hypothalamic dysfunction from pituitary failure. In the latter, GnRH stimulation will not raise Luteinizing Hormone (LH) level.

Empty sella turcica is characterized by herniation of subarachnoid membrane into the pituitary sella turcica and may exist with pineal gland tumour as prolactin adenoma. The absence of pituitary gland causes absence or low level of FSH and LH. Gonadotropin hormone therapy is required.

OTHER HORMONAL DYSFUNCTIONS

Both hypothyroidism (cretinism) and hyperthyroidism can cause amenorrhoea. Congenital adrenal hyperplasia and tumour are also responsible for primary amenorrhoea, so also juvenile diabetes.

Premature ovarian failure seen in 1% of the cases is due to poor germ cell migration from the yolk sac during fetal development or due to an accelerated rate of depletion (apoptosis) of unknown reason. In this condition, FSH level is more than 40 mIU/mL, and E_2 level is below 20 pg/mL. Karyotyping is required. The woman presents menopausal symptoms. She needs hormone replacement therapy (HRT).

NUTRITION

Excessive weight, anorexia nervosa and malnutrition with loss of weight are also responsible for amenorrhoea in young girls.

The most common cause of hypothalamic dysfunction is related to psychogenic effects, anorexia nervosa, weight loss and inappropriate secretion of neurotransmitters leading to lack of GnRH synthesis (Kallmann syndrome). Women with Kallmann syndrome manifest isolated deficiency of GnRH associated with olfactory dysfunction and anosmia.

Pituitary failure generally follows hypopituitarism, neoplasms or empty sella turcica. Skull radiography or preferably MRI, estimation of prolactin levels and ophthalmic evaluation of the fields of vision help to arrive at a diagnosis. Fröhlich syndrome consists of short stature, lethargy, obesity, genital dystrophy and amenorrhoea. In Laurence–Moon–Biedl syndrome, polydactyly, retinitis pigmentosa and mental deficiency are the additional features.

In all such women, cyclic administration of oestrogen and progestogen to maintain femininity and prevent osteoporosis is essential. In case the woman desires to conceive, induction of ovulation with gonadotropins is warranted. In women with neoplasms, appropriate neurological consultation followed by treatment with bromocriptine for prolactinomas or surgery should be planned.

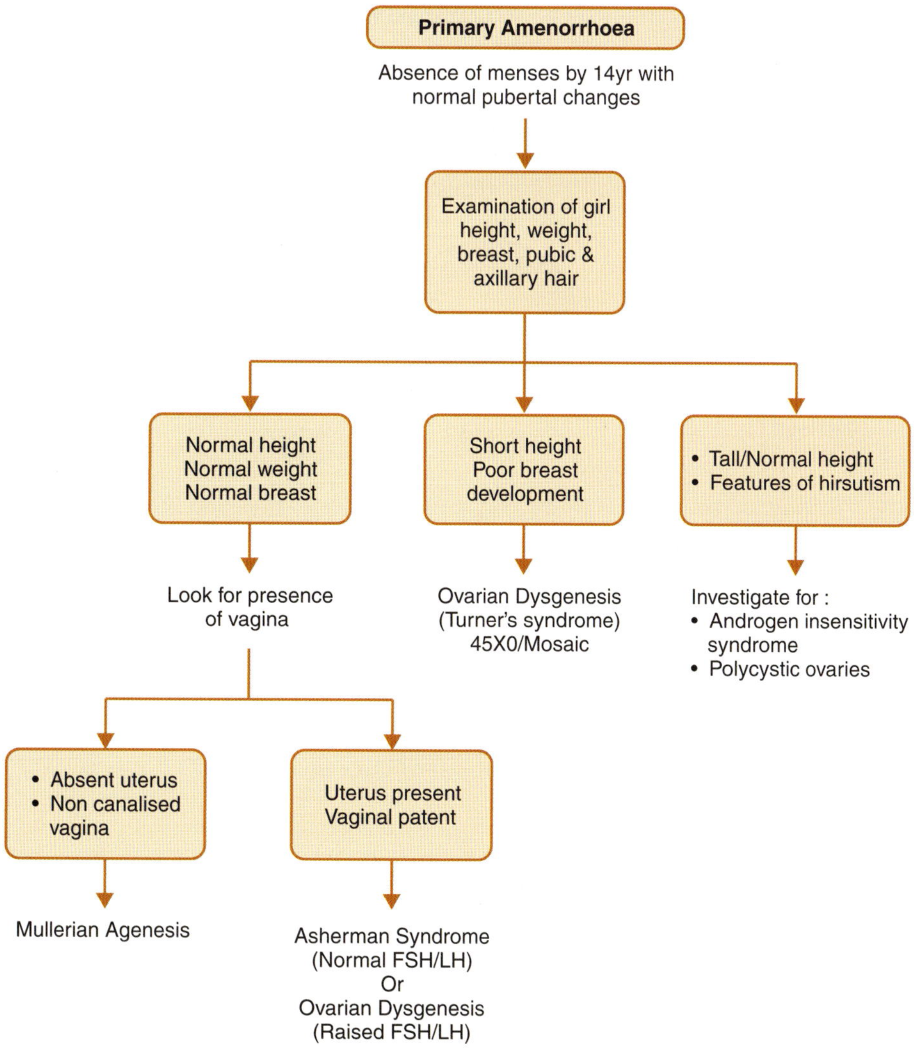

SUMMARY

Müllerian agenesis: Absent/blind vagina, normal breasts, normal FSH/LH.
Asherman syndrome: Normal uterus, normal vagina, normal FSH/LH but fail to have withdrawal bleeding with oestrogen + progesterone.
Ovarian dysgenesis: Normal/short height, poor breast development, raised FSH/LH, karyotype abnormality.
Androgen insensitivity syndrome: Tall, normal breasts, blind vagina, absent uterus, 26XY pattern.
PCOD: Obese, hirsutism, normal FSH/LH, increased LH.

SECONDARY AMENORRHOEA

Secondary amenorrhoea is defined as amenorrhoea of 6 months or more in a woman with previous normal menstrual patterns in the absence of pregnancy and lactation (2%–3% women).

However, in clinical practice, patients seek advice earlier and it is prudent to begin with simpler investigations and reassurance and await the outcome.

AETIOLOGY (Fig. 12.3)

Many causes are similar to those of primary amenorrhoea. However, the emphasis is somewhat different. Dysfunction of the hypothalamic–pituitary–ovarian–uterine axis accounts for the majority of cases of pathological secondary amenorrhoea.

The causes can be classified as follows:

- **Physiological**
  1. Pregnancy
  2. Lactation
- **Pathological**
  1. Genital tract
     - Acquired obstruction (gynatresia) of cervical canal causing severe stenosis or atresia follows electrocauterization, chemical burns, cervical amputation in a Fothergill repair operation, conization for cervical dysplasia or cervical intraepithelial neoplasia (CIN) and genital tuberculosis.
     - Vaginal atresia due to scarring following a traumatic delivery.

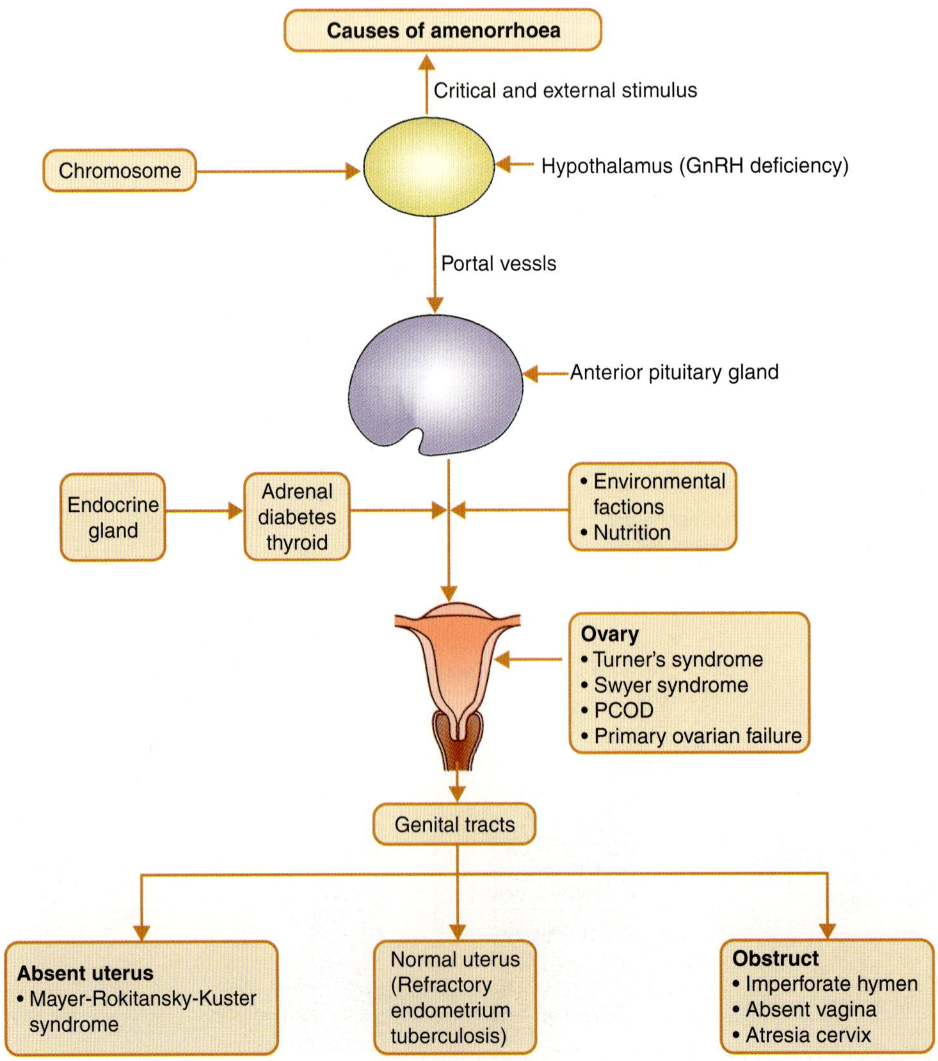

Figure 12.3 Causes of amenorrhoea.

- Asherman syndrome following excessive curettage, uterine infection or endometrial tuberculosis, transcervical resection of endometrium for abnormal uterine bleeding (see Chapter 21) and uterine packing in postpartum haemorrhage.
- Vesicovaginal fistula – cause unknown.

2. Ovarian causes
   - Surgical extirpation.
   - Radiotherapy.
   - Autoimmune disease (thyroid, diabetes).
   - Induction of multiple ovulation in infertility – leading to premature menopause.
   - PCOD.
   - Resistant ovarian syndrome – due to absent FSH receptors.
   - Infections – mumps, tuberculosis, and in rare cases, pyogenic infections.
   - Masculinizing ovarian tumours.
   - Premature menopause – premature ovarian failure.
3. Nutritional causes
   - Anorexia nervosa, bulimia (Fig. 12.1).
   - Extreme obesity.
   - Excessive weight loss in athletes and ballet dancers.
4. Pituitary causes (Figs 12.4–12.9)
   - Insufficiency as in Simmond disease, Sheehan syndrome.

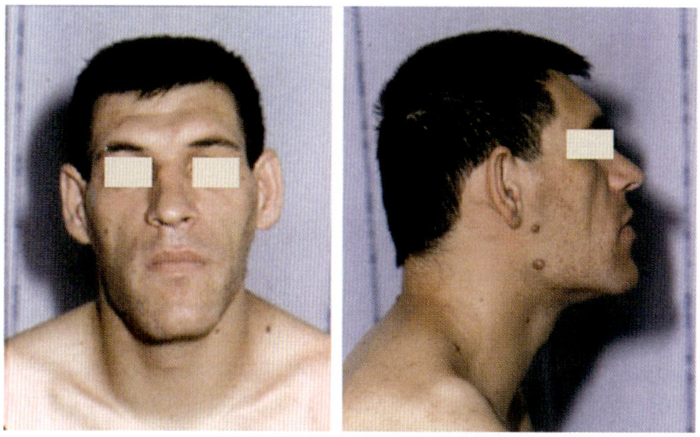

Figure 12.4 Acromegaly. Note the broad enlargement of the nose and coarse facies. (*Source*: Wikimedia commons.)

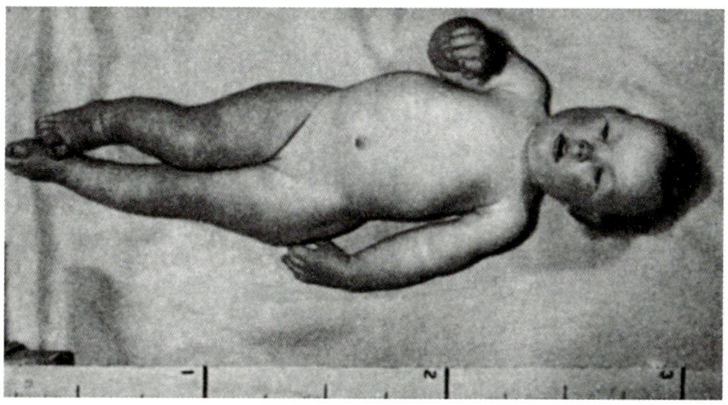

Figure 12.5 Gigantism. Child aged 1 year, measuring more than 3 feet in height.

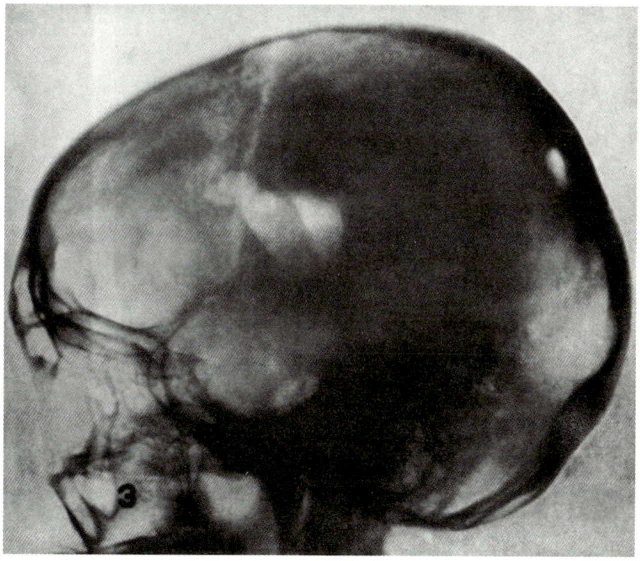

Figure 12.6 X-ray of pituitary fossa showing extreme bone expansion due to pituitary tumour.

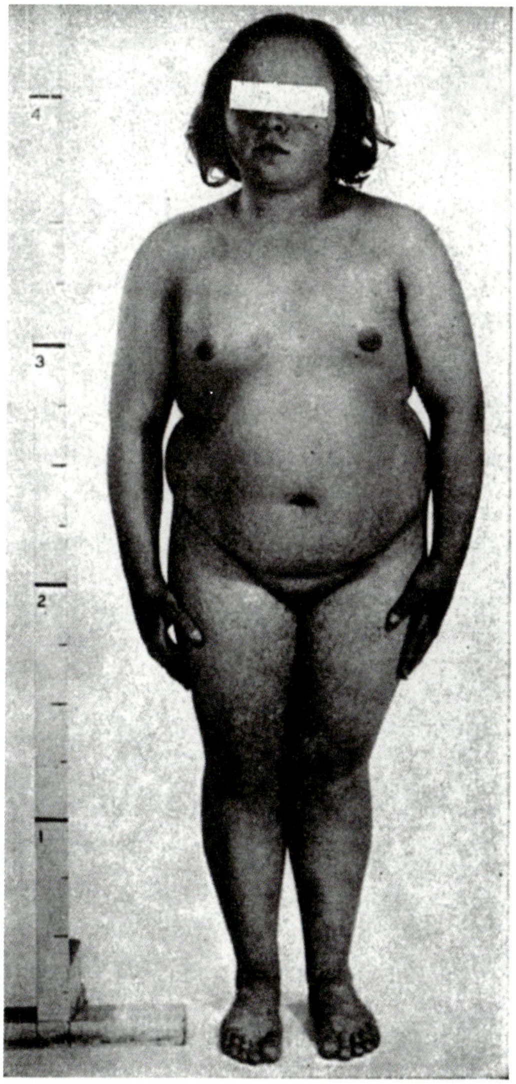

Figure 12.7 Fröhlich syndrome.

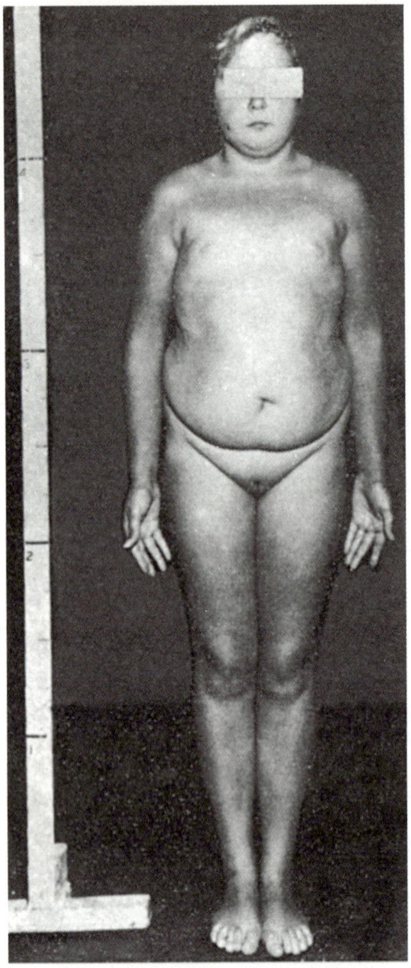

Figure 12.8 Pituitary infantilism, patient aged 17 years. Note obesity, aplasia of breasts, absence of pubic hair and short stature.

- Hyperprolactinaemia.
- Tumours such as prolactinomas and chromophobe adenomas and Cushing disease.
- Empty sella syndrome.
- Drugs – tranquillizers, oral contraceptive (OC) pills, metoclopramide, dopamine blockers, antihypertensives, antidepressants, cimetidine and phenothiazine.

5. Hypothalamus.
   - GnRH deficiency.
   - Vigorous exercise – stress, obesity.
   - Pseudocyesis.
   - Brain tumours.
   - Anorexia nervosa.
6. Suprarenal causes
   - Addison disease.
   - Adrenogenital syndrome.
   - Suprarenal tumour.
7. Thyroid
   - Hypothyroidism, chest wall lesions.
   - Graves disease.
8. Other causes
   - Diabetes.
   - Tuberculosis – liver disease.

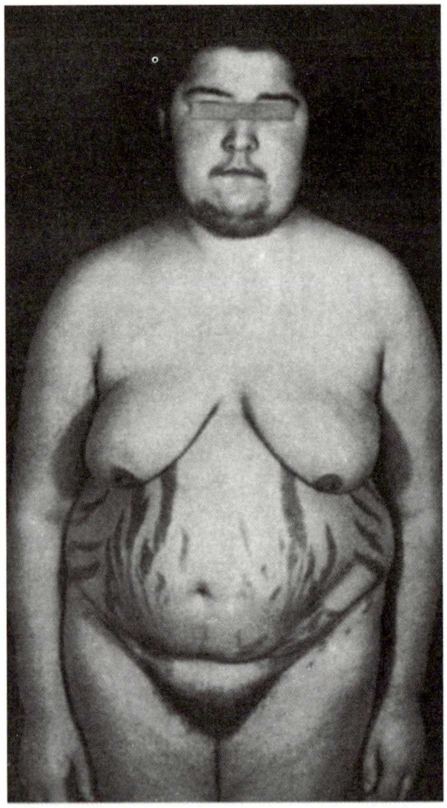

Figure 12.9 Cushing syndrome. Note hirsutism of face, obesity and striae.

- Renal disease – due to reduced excretion of LH and prolactin.
- Severe anaemia, malnutrition.
- Idiopathic, genetic.

RESISTANT OVARIAN SYNDROME

In resistant ovarian syndrome and autoimmune disease, ovaries fail to respond to gonadotropin hormones and cause amenorrhoea. The ovaries show plasma cells and lymphocyte infiltration. Biopsy, however, is not necessary for the diagnosis. FSH level is high. It may be prudent to study antithyroid, rheumatoid factors and antinuclear antibodies to establish autoimmune disease. Pregnancy with a donor egg in in vitro fertilization (IVF) is possible.

SIMMOND DISEASE

Simmond disease related to pregnancy and Sheehan syndrome following severe postpartum haemorrhage cause pituitary necrosis by thrombosis of its vessels, and panhypopituitarism. The woman fails to lactate following delivery, remains lethargic and shows signs of hypothyroidism and cortisol deficiency. She requires appropriate hormonal support. A young woman may require ovulation induction drugs to achieve conception.

In the management of secondary amenorrhoea, the clinician must attempt to answer the following six questions sequentially to arrive at a diagnosis quickly and economically.

- Is the patient pregnant?
- Is her serum prolactin level elevated?

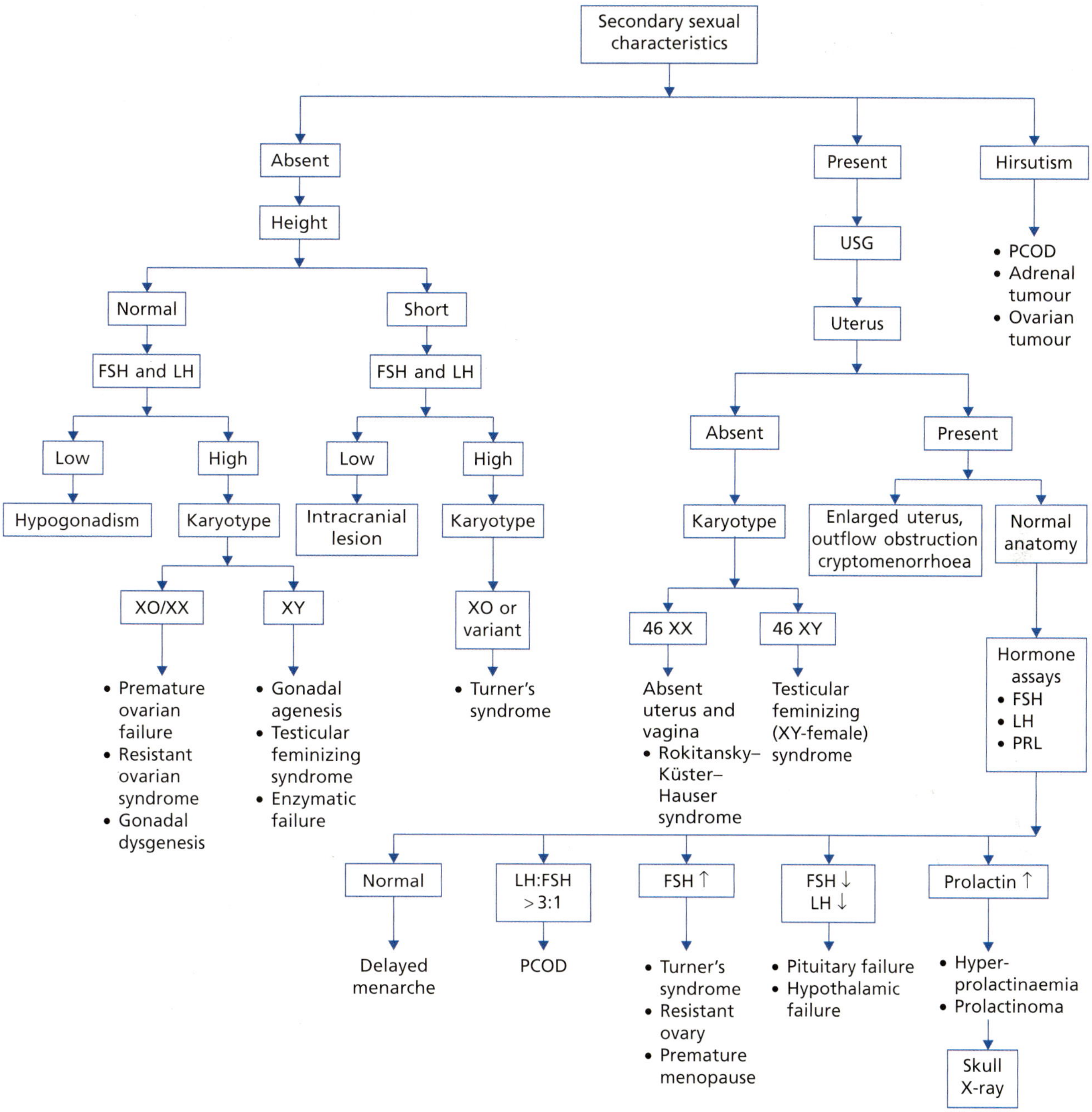

Figure 12.10 Investigations in amenorrhoea.

- Is there clinical evidence of oestrogen deficiency?
- Does she have a positive response to the progesterone challenge test?
- Is it premature menopause?
- What are the levels of her serum FSH and LH?

The importance of each of the above questions is analysed in detail below. Detailed history is important.

INVESTIGATIONS (Fig. 12.10)

PREGNANCY

This is the most common cause of secondary amenorrhoea. Hence, its exclusion must precede all further investigations. Clinical examination, urine pregnancy test and sonographic scan of the pelvis should help to establish the diagnosis beyond doubt.

ELEVATED LEVELS OF SERUM PROLACTIN

Prolactin secreted by the anterior pituitary gland is normally under the inhibitory effect of hypothalamus by the prolactin-inhibitory factor dopamine. It is stimulated by oestrogen and suckling. It is also present in the decidua and amniotic fluid. Prolactin levels fluctuate periodically; therefore, several measurements may be necessary to confirm hyperprolactinaemia which is defined as persistent high level of prolactin in a nonpregnant and nonlactating woman.

Causes

Apart from the physiological condition of pregnancy and lactation, it occurs in the following cases:

- During sleep, stress, nipple stimulation and chest wall injury such as herpes zoster.
- Empty sella turcica.
- Hypothalamic tumour, pituitary tumour and head injury (acromegaly, Cushing disease, Addison disease).
- Twenty per cent cases of PCOD and in some cases of endometriosis.
- Hypothyroidism because of the stimulating effect of raised thyroid-stimulating hormone (TSH).
- Liver and chronic renal disease because of altered metabolism and delay in excretion.
- Drugs such as neuroleptics, narcotics, antidepressants, phenothiazine, antihypertensives, calcium channel blockers, prolonged use of OCs, oestrogen (in high doses), cocaine, amphetamine, cimetidine, haloperidol, metoclopramide. Serotonin and opiates reduce the level of dopamine and cause hyperprolactinaemia.

The woman presents with oligomenorrhoea culminating in amenorrhoea due to suppression of FSH and LH. About 50% of the cases develop galactorrhoea. Infertility and abortion through corpus luteal phase defect are other features. Headache and visual disturbances occur when the tumour presses upon the optic nerve. In males, it causes loss of libido, impotency and infertility. The normal level of prolactin is 25 ng/mL. Levels up to 100 ng/mL suggest hyperprolactinaemia and more than 100 ng/mL occurs in the presence of a tumour. CT, MRI and visual check-up are necessary in the diagnosis and follow-up. Thyroid functions need to be checked.

Treatment

- Treat the cause.
- Drug-induced hyperprolactinaemia requires stoppage of drug or alternative therapy.
- Bromocriptine and long-acting derivatives are effective in most cases. Menstrual cycles are restored in 3-month time. About 90% ovulate and 70%–80% conceive.
- Quinagolide 25–150 mg daily in divided doses with a maintenance dose of 75 mg daily.
- The drugs are discussed in detail in the chapter on Hormonal Therapy.
- Macroadenoma (more than 10 mm) and microadenoma not responding to drugs require transsphenoidal adenectomy or radiotherapy 4500 cGY for 25 days. However, 30% recurrence rate is reported within 6 years, and prolonged follow-up is necessary.

EVIDENCE OF OESTROGEN DEFICIENCY

Hot flushes, loss of breast mass, dyspareunia and dryness of vagina are suggestive of lack of oestrogen and premature menopause. It requires oestrogen replacement therapy.

POSITIVE PROGESTERONE CHALLENGE TEST

This test depends on the presence of oestrogen-primed endometrium in the uterine cavity. The test is considered positive, if the patient responds to the administration of oral tablet medroxyprogesterone (Provera/Modus/Deviry) 10 mg daily for 5 days or injection progesterone in oil 100 mg intramuscularly or Primolut-N 5 mg three times a day for 3 days. Withdrawal bleeding occurs within 2–7 days. A positive test indicates amenorrhoea secondary to anovulation. The common underlying causes are hypothalamic dysfunction and polycystic ovary syndrome.

A negative test requires giving oestradiol 0.02 mg or conjugated oestrogen 1.25 mg for 25 days and progestogen from 16th to 25th day. A negative test suggests endometrial unresponsiveness in the presence of normal FSH.

Pituitary. In Simmond disease due to panhypopituitarism, the woman is lethargic, blood sugar and thyroid functions are low. When postpartum haemorrhage causes vascular thrombosis of the pituitary vessels, panhypopituitarism is known as Sheehan syndrome. CT and MRI detect a tumour. FSH and LH are required.

Hypothalamic dysfunction is the most frequent cause of secondary amenorrhoea. Although in the majority of cases no specific cause can be found, a careful history may reveal a precipitating factor. *Stress and drugs* may contribute to amenorrhoea. Stress situations are often poorly recognized by the patient (examinations, change of jobs, economic problems, breaking up of relationships, etc.). A prolonged use of phenothiazines and tricyclic antidepressant drugs affect dopaminergic systems in the CNS and are associated with raised levels of prolactin hormone. *Postpill amenorrhoea* (1%) following the use of OC pills is also the result of hypothalamic dysfunction. The diagnosis is made only if spontaneous menses do not resume after 6 months of stopping the pill. In such women, changeover to an OC pill with a higher oestrogen content (ethinyloestradiol 0.05 mg daily for 21 days cyclically, for a few cycles) helps to restore normal cycles. *Weight change and amenorrhoea* are not uncommonly seen in clinical practice. Young adolescent girls and working women are often the subjects of this disorder. A weight loss exceeding 15% of the ideal weight may predispose the woman to menstrual disturbances. Investigations at this stage may reveal normal FSH and LH values and the patient will respond positive to a progesterone challenge test. However, as the weight loss further increases (anorexia nervosa) to 25% or more, low levels of hormones namely gonadotropins and oestrogens are observed, and these are often accompanied by thyroid dysfunction. Proper counselling and advice to regain weight often suffices. However, there is a subgroup of patients who resist advice and may need psychiatric treatment. An excessive weight gain may also be accompanied by menstrual irregularities. Obesity is often a manifestation of a stress situation leading to a compulsive eating disorder. Successful weight reduction often restores regular menstruation. *Polycystic ovary syndrome* is associated with an abnormal gonadotropin secretion revealing an increased ratio of LH:FSH exceeding 3:1, which differentiates patients of PCOD from patients with hypothalamic dysfunction. In patients with PCOD, ovarian steroidogenesis is abnormal, leading to an increased production of androstenedione and testosterone, which in turn predisposes the patient to hirsutism, acne and menstrual irregularity. The diagnosis is established on the basis of clinical suspicion, an increased LH:FSH ratio and sonography revealing enlarged ovaries with multiple peripheral cystic follicles. Laparoscopy reveals bilateral enlarged ovaries with thickened tunica albuginea and multiple cystic follicles.

Ultrasound scanning helps in the diagnosis of PCOD, ovarian tumour and uterine lesions such as haematometra and Asherman syndrome.

Specific treatment will depend on the cause and the patient's desire for fertility at the time of consultation. If she desires fertility, the treatment of choice is induction of ovulation with clomiphene citrate or gonadotropins. On the contrary, if the patient does not desire fertility, she may be advised a progestational agent (medroxyprogesterone or dydrogesterone) for 7–10 days every 2 months or so to induce periods. This treatment protects the patient against the ill-effects of endometrial hyperplasia, adenomatous hyperplasia and endometrial carcinoma due to prolonged unopposed oestrogen action on the endometrium. These patients should be advised to use some form of contraception (condoms/diaphragm) to safeguard them against any unwanted pregnancy resulting from a stray ovulation or spontaneous recovery of menstrual function. Premature menopause requires HRT to protect against osteoporosis and avoid menopausal symptoms.

A hysterosalpingogram or preferably a diagnostic hysteroscopy helps to establish the diagnosis of Asherman syndrome, first described in 1948. Operative hysteroscopy to lyse the synechiae, followed by cyclic hormonal therapy with high doses of conjugated oestrogens of 2.5–5.0 mg/day for 3–6 months, results in the restoration of menstruation in about 50% of cases. Some surgeons prefer to insert an intrauterine device in the uterine cavity after lysis of adhesions to ensure keeping the cavity patent and prevent recurrence of adhesions. Hypo-oestrogenic subjects of secondary amenorrhoea have serum oestradiol levels of less than 30 pg/mL and benefit with oestrogen and progesterone therapy. Asherman syndrome is caused by dilatation and curettage (D&C), medical termination of pregnancy (MTP), uterine packing in postpartum haemorrhage, uterine infection and tubercular endometritis. It causes amenorrhoea, oligomenorrhoea, dysmenorrhoea, habitual abortion and infertility depending upon the extent of uterine cavity obliteration.

SUMMARY

Ovarian failure: Raised FSH/LH, no withdrawal bleeding with progestin but get withdrawal bleeding with Oestrogen + Progestin

Asherman syndrome: Normal FSH/LH, no withdrawal bleeding with Progestin. No withdrawal bleeding with Oestrogen + Progestin combination

Hyperprolactinaemia: Galactorrhoea, raised serum prolactin levels get withdrawal bleeding with Oestrogen + Progestin

Anorexia nervosa: Low FSH/LH, no withdrawal to Progestin

PCOD: Normal FSH, raised LH, feature of hirsutism, withdrawal bleeding to Progestin.

FSH AND LH CONCENTRATIONS

Women with hypo-oestrogenic amenorrhoea have either ovarian failure or hypothalamic–pituitary dysfunction. Serum concentrations of FSH and LH of more than 40–50 mIU/mL are diagnostic of ovarian failure. Serial assessments may be necessary because of the pulsatile nature of pituitary gonadotropin secretion. Most women younger than 40 years belonging to this category have premature ovarian failure, about 10%–15% have gonadotropin-resistant ovaries (Savage syndrome) and another 10%–15% have autoimmune ovarian failure. The last two entities have their normal complement of primordial follicles, but their granulosa cells do not respond to FSH. There are no other clues to suggest the gonadotropin-resistant ovarian syndrome. However, evidence of any other autoimmune disorder (myasthenia gravis, rheumatoid arthritis, systemic lupus erythematosus – SLE) are suggestive of autoimmune ovarian failure with hypergonadotropic amenorrhoea. Hypothalamic–pituitary dysfunction or failure may occur with a weight disorder (<85% or >125% of ideal body weight), a tumour of the hypothalamus or pituitary gland, after head injury, following infiltrating lesions, after surgery or irradiation. Most often the cause is not known. A CT scan or MRI should be asked for if there is evidence suggestive of a central mass lesion. In women with FSH and LH values less than 5 mIU/mL, measurements of thyroid function tests (T_3, T_4 and TSH) and serum cortisol concentrations are important to exclude panhypopituitarism involving other tropic hormones additionally. Such women will require concurrent thyroid and corticosteroid replacement therapy as well. HRT for premature menopause is warranted along with supplementary oral calcium and advice on change of lifestyle. In women with hypothalamic failure, therapy should begin with preliminary priming with GnRH administered in pulsatile fashion with a pump or subcutaneously for several weeks until the circulating levels of serum oestradiol of greater than 600 pg/mL are achieved, before initiating gonadotropin therapy for induction of ovulation in women desiring pregnancy.

See Table 12.3 for aetiology of amenorrhoea according to anatomic sites and recommended diagnostic work-up. The management of secondary amenorrhoea is shown in Fig. 12.11.

Sequela of secondary amenorrhoea

1. Menopausal symptoms, osteoporosis.
2. Infertility in a young woman.
3. Psychological effects, loss of libido.

Management

- HRT for menopausal symptoms and prophylaxis.
- Induction of ovulation, IVF for infertility.
- Induction of menstrual cycles.
- Treat the cause.

Table 12.3 Aetiology of Amenorrhoea According to Anatomic Sites and Investigations

Anatomic Level	Anatomic Site	Pathology	Gonadotropin Level	Diagnostic Methods
1.	Hypothalamus	Tumours, Kallmann syndrome, weight loss, exercise	Low	Clinical evaluation MRI/CT scan
2.	Anterior pituitary	Panhypopituitarism, Sheehan syndrome	Low	History, examination, GnRH stimulation test
3.	Ovary	Gonadal dysgenesis, Turner syndrome, ovarian failure (premature, radiation, mumps, surgical excision, chemotherapy), steroidogenic defect (adrenal hyperplasia)	High	History, karyotyping, gonadal biopsy
4.	Anovulation	PCOD, hyperprolactinaemia, weight loss, stress, exercise, drugs, chest wall stimulation	Normal	History, progesterone challenge test, USG/MRI/CT scan
5.	Uterus or endometrium	Müllerian agenesis, RKH syndrome, Asherman syndrome, tuberculosis, radiotherapy, androgen insensitivity	Decreased FSH, Increased LH, increased prolactin	History, examination, karyotyping, USG, laparoscopy, hysteroscopy
6.	Outflow tract	Imperforate hymen, vaginal agenesis, cervical atresia	Normal	History and pelvic examination/USG

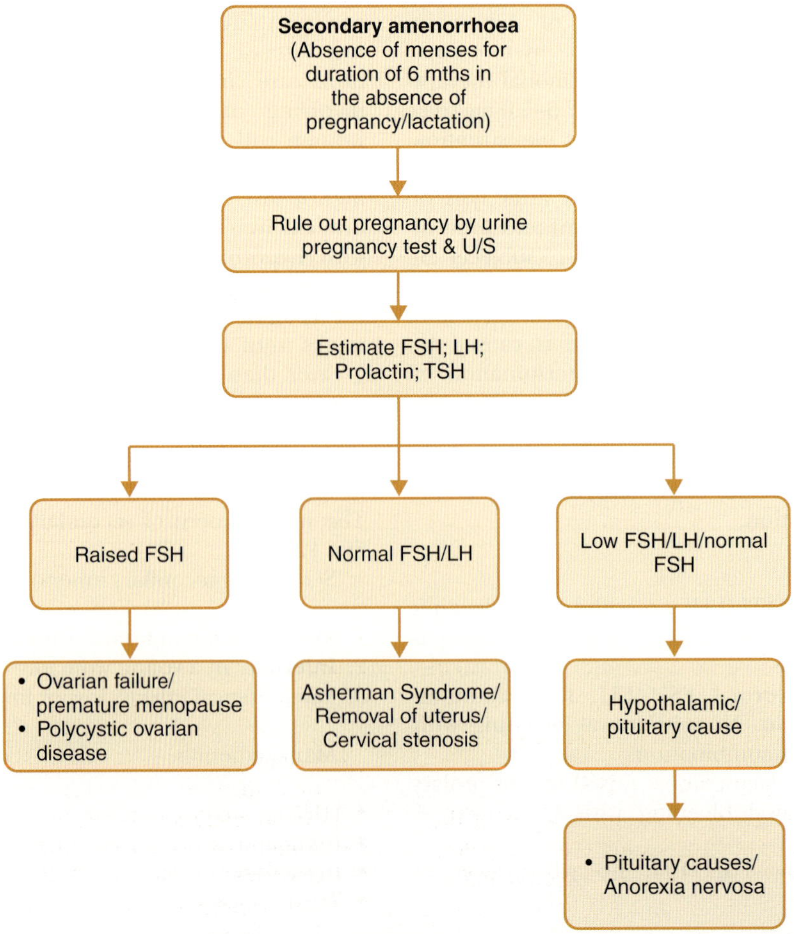

Figure 12.11 Management of secondary amenorrhoea.

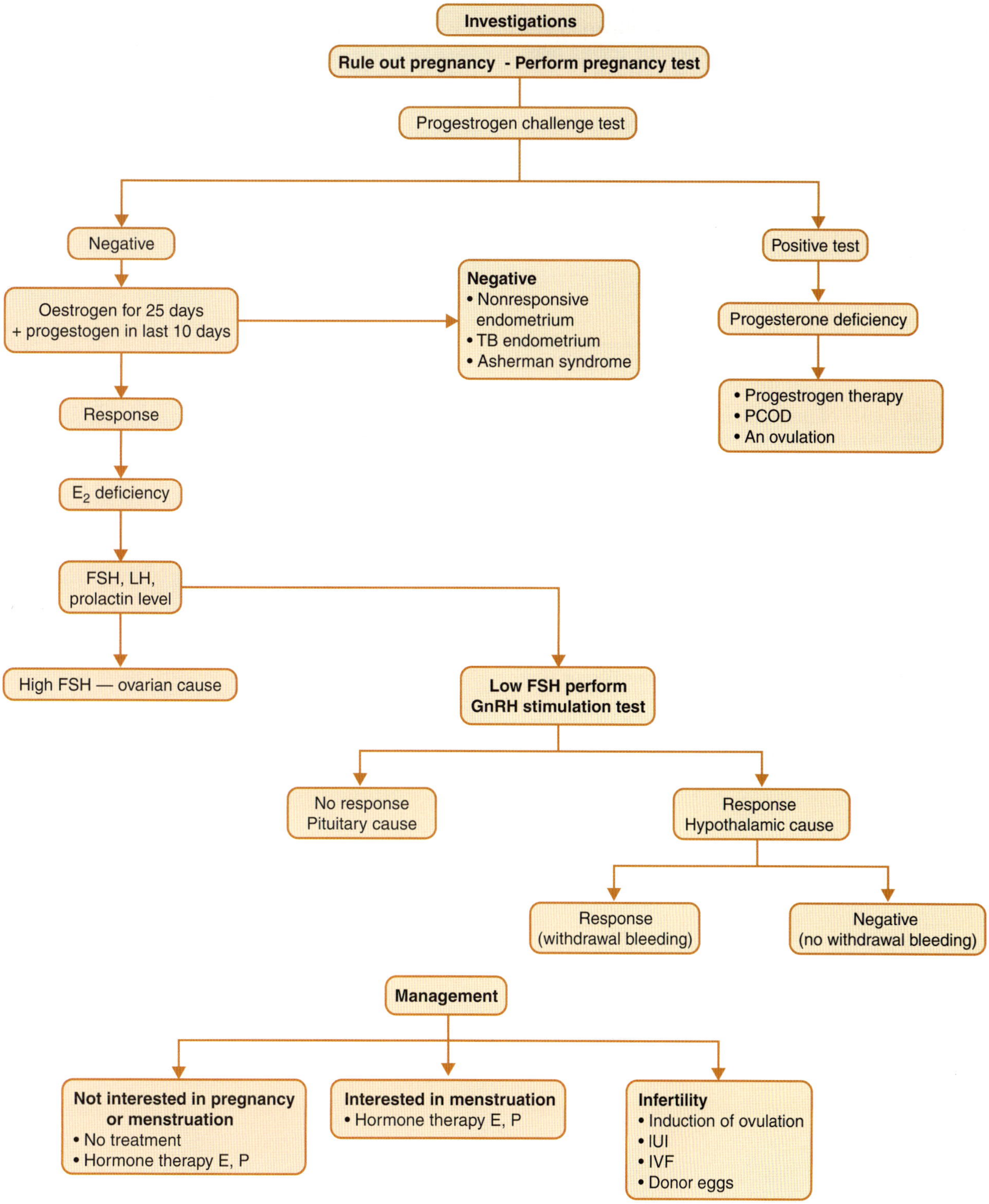

Figure 12.11, cont'd

KEY POINTS

- Normal menstruation requires the integration of the H–P–O axis with a normal functioning uterus, a patent outflow tract and a normal genetic karyotype of XX.
- Menarche occurs between the ages of 10 and 16 years, with a mean age of 12.5 years.
- Failure to achieve puberty by the age of 13–14 years or failure to achieve menarche by the age of 15–16 requires investigations.
- Amenorrhoea may be due to a hormonal functional disorder or be an early symptom of genital tract abnormalities, hence, the need for thorough investigation.

- Clinical examination, hormone assays, ultrasonography, endoscopic procedures and genetic testing may be required for the diagnosis of amenorrhoea.
- In India, tuberculous endometritis and Asherman syndrome may cause hypomenorrhoea or secondary amenorrhoea.
- Treatment of amenorrhoea depends upon the cause. Hormonal therapy on a long-term basis may be required for proper growth and to maintain menstrual functions.

SELF-ASSESSMENT

1. Classify the causes of primary amenorrhoea.
2. Describe the management of primary amenorrhoea.
3. What are the causes of secondary amenorrhoea. How would you manage such cases?
4. How would you diagnose and manage a case of premature ovarian failure?

SUGGESTED READING

Aiman J, Smentek C. Premature ovarian failure. Obstetrics and Gynecology 1985;66(1):9–14.

Carlson KJ, Schiff I. Alternatives to hysterectomy for menorrhagia. N Engl J Med 1996;335:198–99.

Chuong CJ, Brenner PF. Management of abnormal uterine bleeding. Am J Obstet Gynecol 1996; 175:787–92.

De Arce MA, Costigan C, Gosden JR, et al. Further evidence consistent with Yqh as an indicator of risk of gonadal blastoma in Y-bearing mosaic Turner syndrome. Clin Genet 1992; 41:28.

Gise LH, Kase NG, Berkowitz RL (eds). Contemporary Issues in Obstetrics and Gynecology. The Premenstrual Syndromes. Vol. 2. New York: Churchill Livingstone; 1988.

Hasin M, Dennerstein L, Gotts G. Menstrual cycle related complaints: A cross-cultural study. J Psychosom Obstet Gynecol 1988;9:15–42.

Knobil E. The neuroendocrine control of the menstrual cycle. Recent Progr Horm Res 1980;36:53–88.

Krasna IH, Lee ML, Smilow P, et al. Risk of malignancy in bilateral streak gonads: the role of the Y chromosome. J Pediatr Surg 1992; 27:1376.

Laitinen EM, Vaaralahti K, Tommiska J, et al. Incidence, phenotypic features and molecular genetics of Kallmann syndrome in Finland. Orphanet J Rare Dis 2011; 6:41.

Lukusa T, Fryns JP, Kleczkowska A, Van den Berghe H. Role of gonadal dysgenesis in gonadoblastoma induction in 46, XY individuals. The Leuven experience in 46, XY pure gonadal dysgenesis and testicular feminization syndromes. Genet Couns 1991; 2:9.

Martin KA, Hall JE, Adams JM, Crowley WF Jr. Comparison of exogenous gonadotropins and pulsatile gonadotropin-releasing hormone for induction of ovulation in hypogonadotropic amenorrhea. J Clin Endocrinol Metab 1993; 77:125.

Practice Committee of the American Society for Reproductive Medicine. Current evaluation of amenorrhea. Fertil Steril 2006; 86:S148.

Reindollar RH, Byrd JR, McDonough PG. Delayed sexual development: a study of 252 patients. Am J Obstet Gynecol 1981; 140:371.

Santoro N, Filicori M, Crowley WF Jr. Hypogonadotropic disorders in men and women: diagnosis and therapy with pulsatile gonadotropin-releasing hormone. Endocr Rev 1986; 7:11.

Treloar AE, Boynton RE, Benn BG, et al. Variation of the human menstrual cycle through reproductive life. Int J Fertil 1967;12(1):77–126.

Trunell EP, Turner CW, Kaye WR. A comparison of the psychological and hormonal factors in women with and without premenstrual syndrome. J Abnorm Psychol 1988;97:429–36.

Warren MP. The effect of exercise on pubertal progression and reproductive function in girls. J Clin Endocrinol Metab 1980;51:1150–57.

Weiss MH, Teal I, Gon P, et al. Natural history of microprolactinomas: Six year follow-up. Neurosurgery 1983; 12:180–83.

Fibroid Uterus

13

CHAPTER OUTLINE

FIBROMYOMAS

Fibromyomas (leiomyoma, fibroma, fibroids) are the commonest benign neoplasm arising from uterus. They are commonly seen in women of reproductive age, incidence varies from 5%–20% of women depending upon age group. They tend to be multiple in numbers. Size may vary from peanut size to often as big as size of a head of a newborn. Small fibroids may be palpable only on vaginal examination, but once uterus is enlarged, they may become palpable per abdomen. All fibroids begin in myometrium but some may grow more towards endometrial cavity (submucous type), or others may grow towards the serosal surface of uterus (subserous type). However, most tend to remain in myometrium (interstitial type).

Fibromyomas (leiomyomas, fibroids or simply myomas) are the commonest benign uterine neoplasms, commonly encountered in gynaecological practice (5%–20% of women in the reproductive age group). They are slow-growing tumours and take 3–5 years to be clinically palpable unlike ovarian tumours. They tend to be multiple in numbers, but some may grow large in size.

AETIOLOGY

A myoma is derived from smooth muscle cell rests, either from vessel walls or uterine musculature.

Although oestrogen, progesterone growth hormone and human placental lactogen have been implicated in the growth of myomas, the evidence in support of oestrogen and progesterone dependence for their growth is impressive:

- Myomas are rarely found before puberty, and they generally cease to grow after menopause.
- New myomas rarely appear after menopause.
- The association of fibroids in women with hyperoestrogenism is evidenced by endometrial hyperplasia, abnormal uterine bleeding and endometrial carcinoma.
- Myomas are known to increase in size during pregnancy and with oral contraceptives usage and shrink after delivery.
- Treatment with mifepristone to shrink the fibroid proves that progesterone, like oestrogen, is responsible for the growth of the fibroid. GnRH also shrinks the fibroma.
- Risk factors are early menarche, nullipara or low parity.

Unusual forms of leiomyomas include intravenous leiomyomatosis, which is characterized by polypoid projections of smooth muscle tumours into the veins of the parametrium and broad ligaments. During surgery these appear as worm-like cords of benign fibrous tissue when pulled out of the veins. Fragments of tumour emboli can cause obstruction of blood flow from the atrium and sudden death. Similarly, a rare form of disseminated intraperitoneal leiomyomatosis involving large areas of subperitoneal surfaces is seen during pregnancy and while on oral contraceptives. The fibroids are often associated with adenomyosis, pelvic endometriosis and pelvic inflammatory disease.

PATHOLOGY

Grossly myoma is a well-circumscribed tumour with a whorled appearance and a pseudocapsule. It is firm in consistency. The cut surface is pinkish white and has a whorled appearance. The capsule consists of connective tissue which surrounds the tumour in the myometrium. The vessels that supply blood to the fibroid lie in the capsule and send radial branches into the tumour. Because of this arrangement of blood supply, the central portion of the fibroid receives the least blood supply, and degeneration is noticeable early and most often in this part of the fibroid. On the other hand, calcification begins at the periphery and spreads inwards along the vessels. The vessels are best seen over the subserous myoma whereas in the case of large intramural growth, they can be seen beneath the peritoneal covering of the uterus – this serves to distinguish the enlargement of the uterus due to a myoma from a normal intrauterine pregnancy.

Microscopically, the tumour consists of bundles of plain smooth muscle cells, separated by varying amount of fibrous strands. Areas of embryonic muscle tissue may be present in a myoma.

To view the lecture notes scan the symbol or log in to your account on www.MedEnact.com

The tumour may grow symmetrically, remaining within the myometrial wall, when it is called 'intramural' or 'interstitial'. If the tumour grows outwards towards the peritoneal surface, it shows itself as a bossy growth and is termed as 'subserous'. Further extrusion outwards with the development of a pedicle makes it a pedunculated fibroid. In rare cases, such a tumour gets attached to a vascular organ and is cut off from its uterine origin (parasitic fibroid). Uterine contractions may force the myoma towards the cavity where it is covered only by a thin endometrium, it is then called 'submucous' myoma. This myoma may force itself downwards towards the vagina by a pedicle, and become a 'submucous myomatous polyp'. The distribution of myoma in the body of the uterus is broadly classified as follows (Fig. 13.1A):

- Intramural (interstitial) 75%
- Submucous 15%
- Subserous 10%

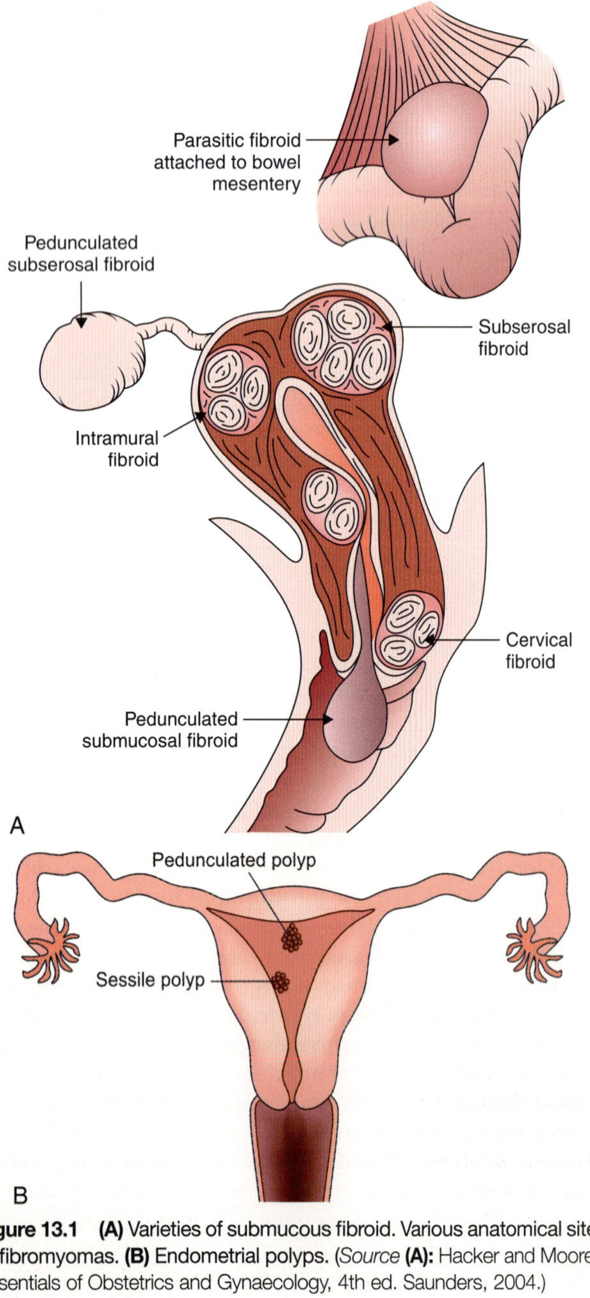

Figure 13.1 (A) Varieties of submucous fibroid. Various anatomical sites of fibromyomas. **(B)** Endometrial polyps. (*Source* **(A):** Hacker and Moore's Essentials of Obstetrics and Gynaecology, 4th ed. Saunders, 2004.)

The majority of myomas arise in the uterus but they may also arise from the round ligament, the utero-ovarian and uterosacral ligaments, the vagina and the vulva. Tumours can therefore be classified as uterine and extrauterine – the uterine myomas are further divided into those that arise from the body and those that arise from the cervix (Figs 13.2–13.7). Subserous and cervical myomas contain

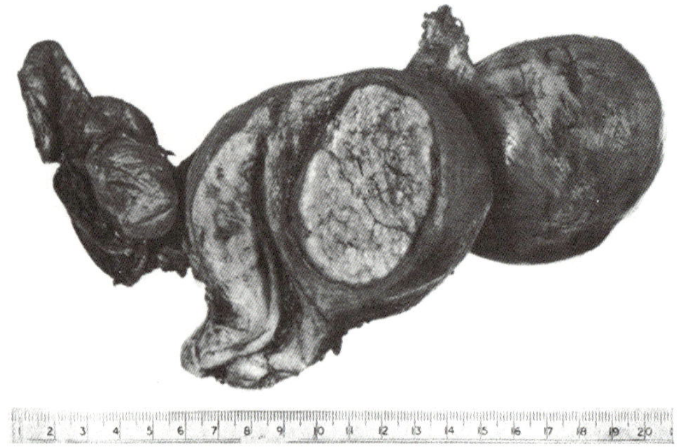

Figure 13.2 Calcified intramural fibroid and subserous fibroid on the right of the picture.

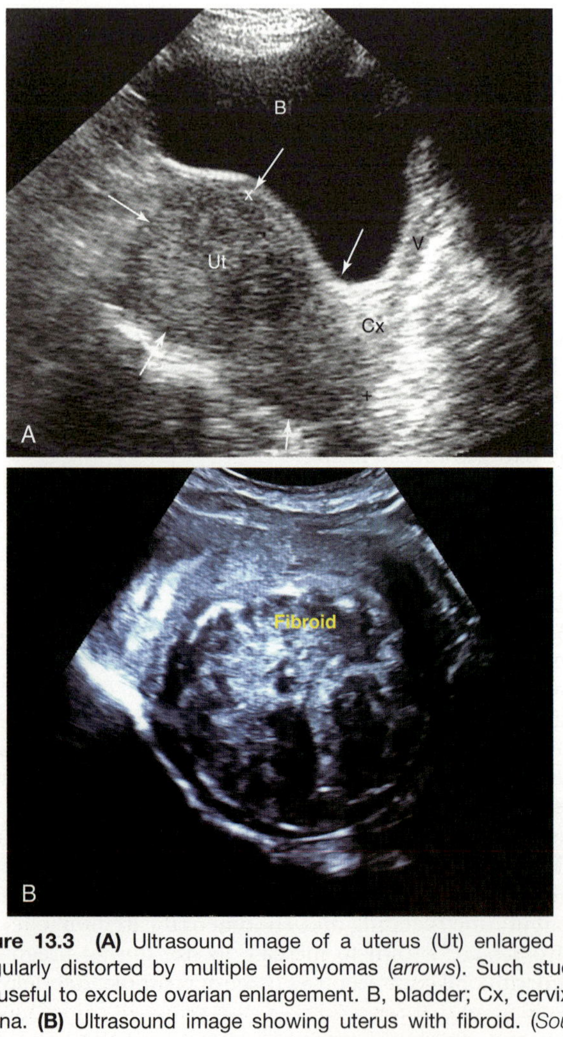

Figure 13.3 (A) Ultrasound image of a uterus (Ut) enlarged and irregularly distorted by multiple leiomyomas (*arrows*). Such studies are useful to exclude ovarian enlargement. B, bladder; Cx, cervix; V, vagina. **(B)** Ultrasound image showing uterus with fibroid. (*Source* **(A)**: Hacker NF, Gambone JC, Hobel CJ. Hacker and Moore's Essentials of Obstetrics and Gynecology, 5th ed. Philadelphia: Elsevier, 2010.)

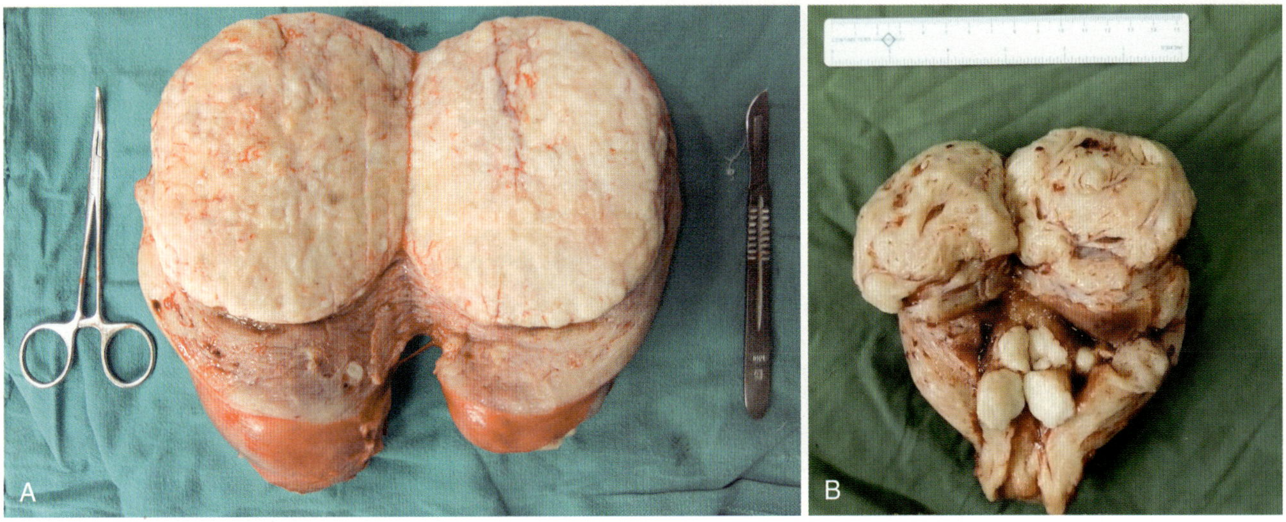

Figure 13.4 **(A)** Interstitial fibroid uterus. **(B)** Uterus showing multiple fibroids: submucous, intramural and subserosal fibroids.

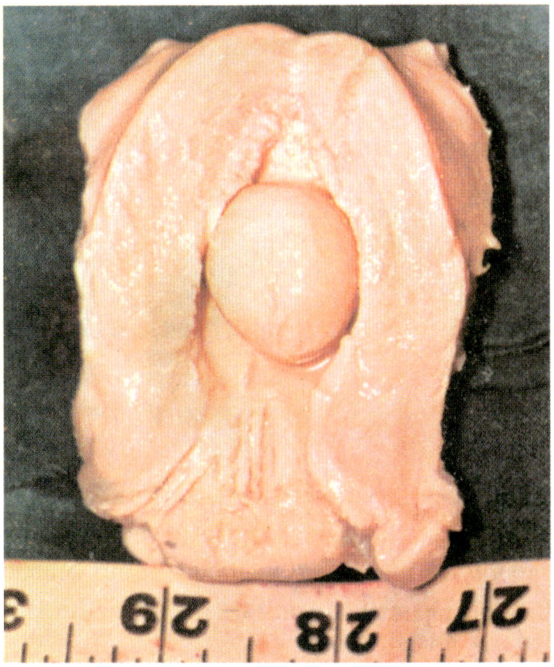

Figure 13.5 Submucous myoma.

more fibrous tissue and less of muscle as compared to other varieties of uterine myomas.

The presence of myoma causes hyperplasia of the myometrial wall. The cavity of the uterus is often distorted and enlarged. The endometrium tends to be thicker due to endometrial hyperplasia. The ovaries at times are enlarged, cystic and hyperaemic with an evidence of salpingo-oophoritis in about 15% cases.

Cervical, submucous and broad ligament fibroids are usually single. Interstitial and subserous fibroids may be single or multiple, varying in size from a seedling fibroid to a huge neoplasm.

CERVICAL FIBROID

Cervical fibroids account for 1%–4% of all fibroids. These may develop as a central, anterior, posterior fibroid or grow laterally in the broad ligament (Fig. 13.8).

PSEUDO-MEIGS SYNDROME

Penduculated fibroid can cause right-sided hydrothorax and ascites mimicking malignant ovarian tumour. This is known as pseudo-Meigs syndrome and this disappears spontaneously following removal of the tumour.

SYMPTOMS

A cervical fibroid exerts pressure on the bladder, ureter and in rare cases on the rectum. A woman may feel a lump in the lower abdomen. During pregnancy, it can cause retention of urine. Obstructed labour occurs if the cervical fibroid lies below the presenting part. The other clinical features are those of uterine fibroids.

Other Sites of Fibroids

Occasionally, fibroids may be found at the following uncommon sites.

Broad ligament fibroids: These fibroids are mostly uterine fibroids which extend laterally in the broad ligament (pseudo broad ligament fibroid). Rarely fibroids may arise de nova within broad ligament either from wall of a vessel or some other structure, and then these are called true broad ligament fibroids. Although fibroid from uterus extending into broad ligament displaces ureters and vessels laterally and downwards, true broad ligament fibroids displace ureter and vessels medially and upwards.

Round ligament fibroids: Occasionally, a fibroid may arise from round ligament.

Ovarian ligament fibroids: Fibroids attached to ovarian ligament may arise from this structure, but is uncommon.

Parasitic fibroids: When a fibroid is found in a structure such as omentum or surface of intestine, they may arise from uterus, and subsequently because of blood supply

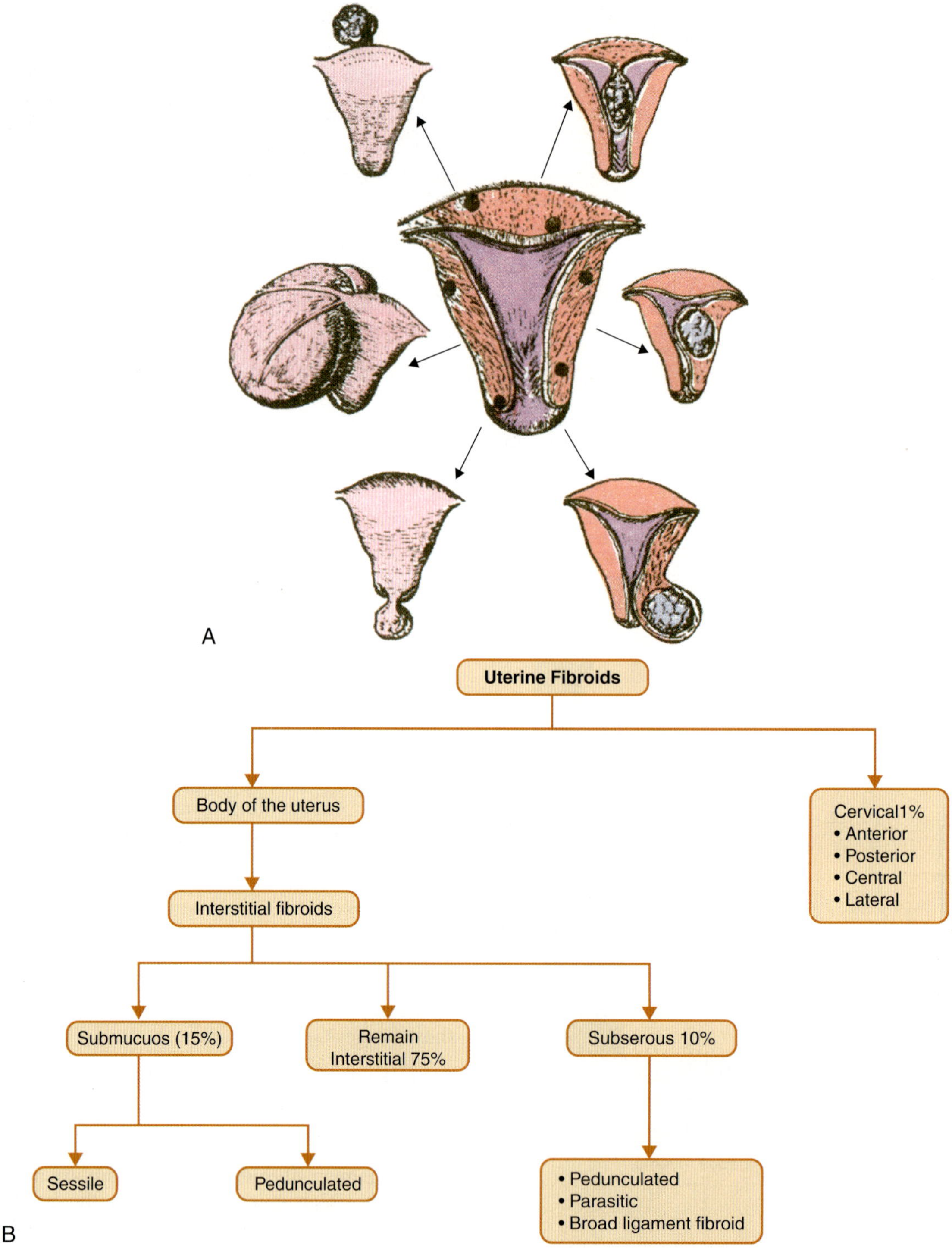

Figure 13.6 **(A)** Development of different types of uterine myomas. **(B)** Types of fibroids.

from these structures, loose their attachment to uterus and appear to arise from omentum or intestine.

SECONDARY CHANGES IN FIBROIDS (Table 13.1)

Atrophy

As a result of diminished vascularity after menopause, there is shrinkage in the size of the tumour, which becomes firmer and more fibrotic. A similar change occurs in myomas after delivery, when a tumour easily palpable during pregnancy may be difficult to define. Temporary shrinkage by 50% occurs following GnRHa therapy, but regrows after stoppage of therapy.

Hyaline, cystic and fatty degenerations that occur in the central areas of fibroids are of no clinical significance and are caused by diminished vascularity in large fibromyomas (Figs 13.9 and 13.10).

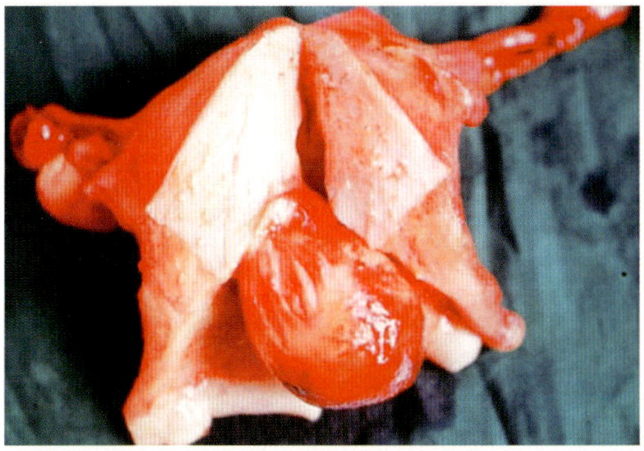

Figure 13.7 Submucous fibroid polyp protruding through the cervix. (*Courtesy*: Dr Narayan M Patel, Ahmedabad.)

Table 13.1 Secondary Changes and Complications in Fibromyomas

- Hyaline change, cystic degeneration and atrophy
- Calcareous degeneration, osseous degeneration
- Red degeneration
- Sarcomatous change
- Torsion, haemorrhage
- Infection/ulceration, particularly in the dependent part of a submucous polyp
- Inversion of the uterus
- Endometrial carcinoma associated with fibromyoma
- Endometrial and myohyperplasia
- Accompanying adenomyosis
- Parasitic fibroid

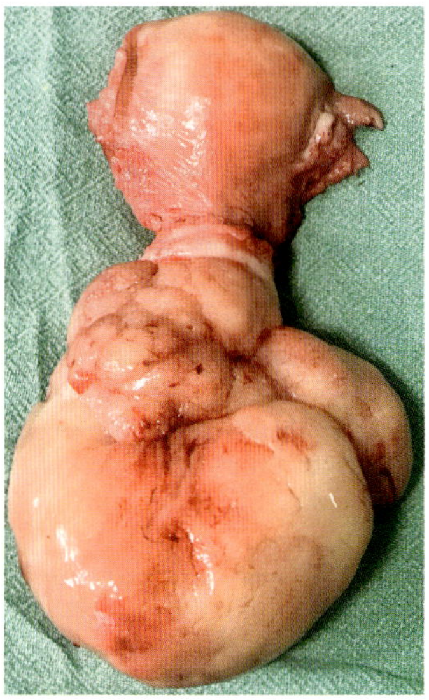

Figure 13.8 Cervical Fibroid.

Calcareous Degeneration

In calcareous degeneration, phosphates and carbonates of lime are deposited in the periphery along the course of the vessels. The best examples of calcareous myomas are those in old patients with long-standing myomas. They are like 'wombstones' in graveyards. Calcareous tumours are easily identified on a plain X-ray of abdomen (Figs 13.11 and 13.12).

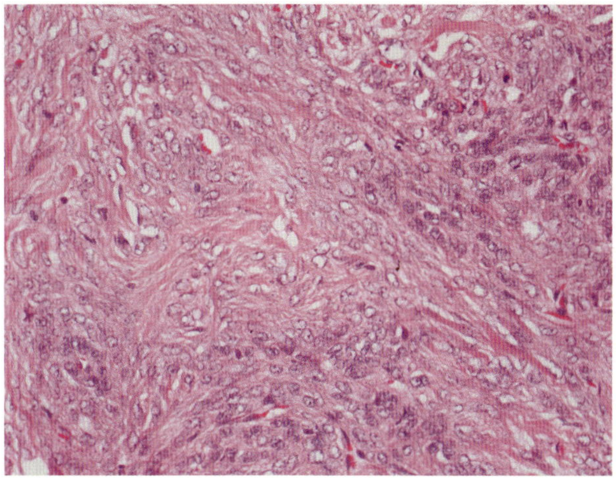

Figure 13.9 Fibroid with hyaline degeneration: smooth muscle cells arranged in fascicles with marked hyalinization. (*Courtesy*: Dr Sandeep Mathur, AIIMS.)

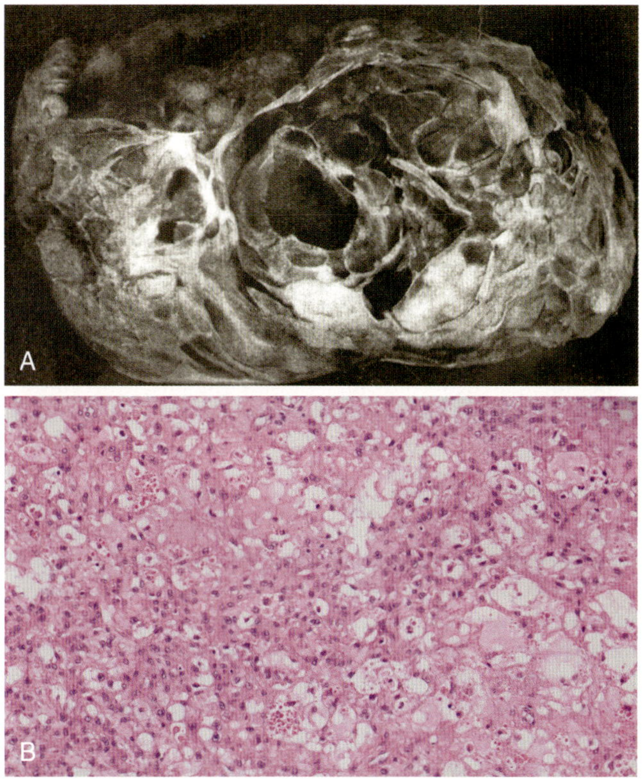

Figure 13.10 **(A)** Cystic degeneration in a fibroid. **(B)** Leiomyoma with cystic change: Leiomyoma with presence of prominent cystic areas, oedema and vascular congestion. (*Courtesy*: Dr Sandeep Mathur, AIIMS.)

Red Degeneration

This complication of uterine myomas develops most frequently during pregnancy, although it is not rare in cases of painful myomas in women older than 40 years. The myoma becomes tense and tender and causes severe abdominal pain with constitutional upset and fever. The tumour itself assumes a peculiar purple red colour and develops a fishy odour. If the tumour is carefully examined, some of the large veins in the capsule and the small vessels in the substance of the tumour will be found thrombosed.

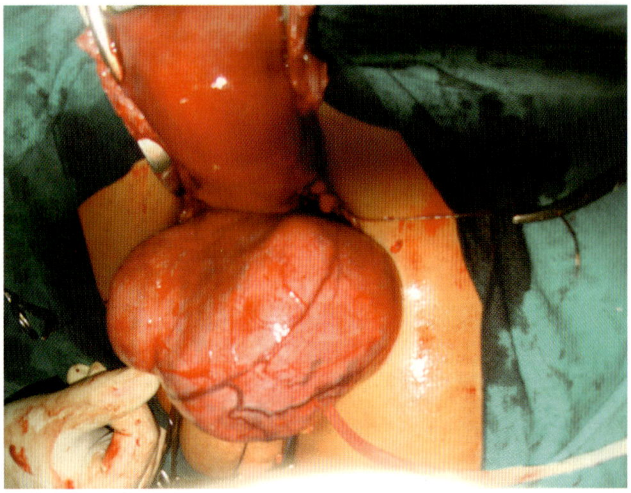

Figure 13.11 Laparotomy finding of uterus with an anterior cervical fibroid.

The discolouration is possibly caused by diffusion of blood pigments from the thrombosed vessels. Histologically, apart from thrombosis, no specific appearances have been identified. Little is known of the exact aetiology, and particularly, as of why only the myoma is involved and not the myometrium. Although the patient is febrile with moderate leucocytosis and raised ESR, the condition is an aseptic one (Fig. 13.13). It needs to be differentiated from appendicitis, twisted ovarian cyst, pyelitis and accidental haemorrhage. Ultrasound is useful in the diagnosis.

Pseudomeig Syndrome

A pedunculated fibroids may cause light side hydrothorax and ascitic mimicking malignant tumour. Removal causes automatic regression of these fluids.

Sarcomatous Change

Sarcomatous change in a myoma is extremely rare, and the incidence is not more than 0.5% of all myomas. Intramural and submucous tumours have a higher potential for sarcomatous change than subserous tumours. It is rare for malignant change to develop in a woman younger than 40 years. It is more commonly seen in a postmenopausal woman when it is observed that the tumour grows suddenly, causing pain and postmenopausal bleeding. To the naked eye, a sarcomatous myoma is yellowish grey in colour and haemorrhagic. The consistency is soft and friable and not firm like a simple myoma (Fig. 13.14). Another important sign is the nonencapsulation of the tumour. Sarcomas are highly malignant and spread via the bloodstream.

OTHER COMPLICATIONS OF MYOMAS

Torsion

A subserous pedunculated myoma may undergo rotation at the site of its attachment to the uterus. As a result, the veins are occluded and the tumour becomes engorged with blood. Very severe abdominal pain is experienced. In very rare cases, the rotated tumour may adhere to an adjacent viscera, obtain a fresh blood supply from these adhesions and finally gets detached completely from the uterus – the so-called 'wandering fibroid' or parasitic fibroid. Axial torsion of a subserous myoma is a rare phenomenon.

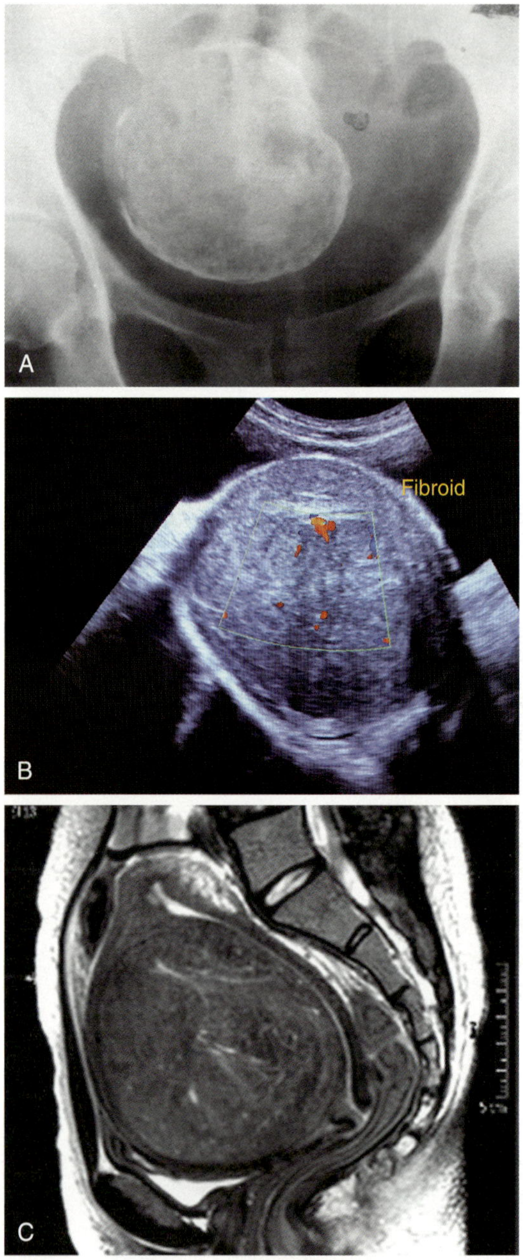

Figure 13.12 (A) Radiograph showing large calcified myoma. **(B)** Ultrasound showing fibroid uterus. **(C)** MRI showing degenerative fibroid. (*Courtesy*: Dr Parveen Gulati, New Delhi.)

Axial rotation of the whole uterus with myoma itself is a very rare occurrence. In such cases, a large subserous myoma is usually attached near the fundus; the uterus itself being only slightly enlarged, and the site of rotation is in the neighbourhood of the internal os, at about the level of Mackenrodt's ligaments; the symptoms are comparable with those developing with torsion of a subserous myoma.

Inversion

Inversion of the uterus caused by a submucous fundal myoma has been described in the chapter on Displacements of the Uterus.

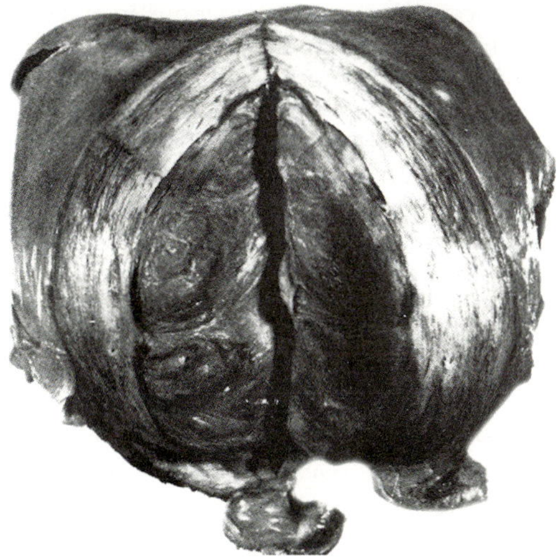

Figure 13.13 Red degeneration of a myoma. Note that the encapsulated tumour shows uniform dark discolouration.

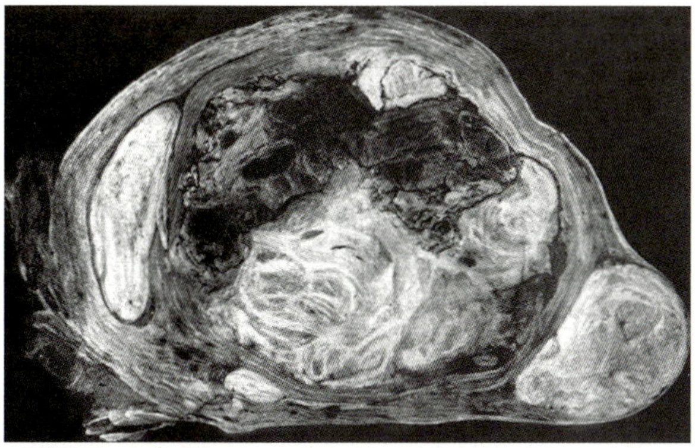

Figure 13.14 Sarcomatous change in a uterine myoma. The dark irregular areas in the substance of the myoma, which lie in the middle of the specimen, represent areas of sarcomatous change.

Capsular Haemorrhage

If one of the large veins on the surface of a subserous myoma ruptures, profuse intraperitoneal haemorrhage can cause acute haemorrhagic shock.

Infection

Infection is common in submucous and myomatous polyps if they project into the cervical canal or the vagina.

An infected polyp can cause blood-stained purulent discharge. Infection is more likely in the postpartum and postabortal state. If the tumour causes delayed postpartum haemorrhage (PPH) or sepsis, it may have to be removed.

Associated Endometrial Carcinoma

Endometrial carcinoma is associated with fibromyoma in women older than 40 years in 3% cases. Hyperoestrogenism explains the coexistence of these two conditions (Fig. 13.15 and Table 13.1).

SYMPTOMS (Table 13.2)

- Menorrhagia, polymenorrhoea, metrorrhagia, continuous or postmenopausal bleeding
- Infertility, recurrent abortions

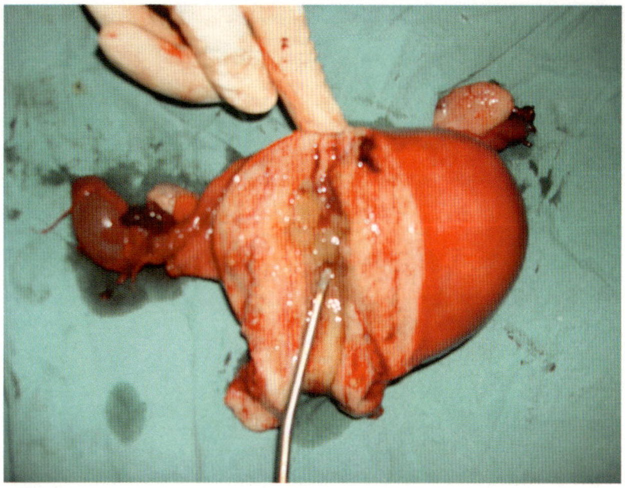

Figure 13.15 Myomas with concomitant carcinoma of endometrium. (*Source*: Nirmala Duhan, Daya Sirohiwal. European Journal of Obstetrics and Gynecology. Uterine myomas revisited. Elsevier, 2010.)

Table 13.2 Clinical Symptomatology and Complications Associated with Uterine Fibromyomas

- Menstrual disturbances – menorrhagia, polymenorrhagia, intermenstrual bleeding, continuous bleeding, postmenopausal bleeding
- Infertility
- Pain – spasmodic dysmenorrhoea, backache, abdominal pain
- Lump in the abdomen or mass protruding at the introitus
- Pressure symptoms on adjacent viscera – bladder, ureters and rectum
- Pregnancy losses, postpartum haemorrhage, uterine inversion
- Vaginal discharge

- Pain
- Pressure symptoms
- Abdominal lump
- Vaginal discharge

Not all fibroids cause symptoms.

As many as 50% women are asymptomatic. These fibroids are detected during gynaecological check-up or ultrasound done for unrelated symptoms. The woman may have a variety of symptoms depending upon the number, size and location of the fibroids. Fibroids are seen in women of childbearing age, and rarely may be seen in younger women. Woman may be nulliparous or of low parity (only 20%–30% women are multiparous). Delayed menopause is observed in a woman with fibroids. Occasionally, woman complains of postmenopausal bleeding.

MENSTRUAL DISTURBANCES

Progressive menorrhagia seen in intramural and submucous myoma is due to increased vascularity, endometrial hyperplasia and enlarged uterine cavity. Further away from the cavity, lesser is the possibility of menorrhagia. For this reason, subserous and pedunculated fibroids do not cause menorrhagia.

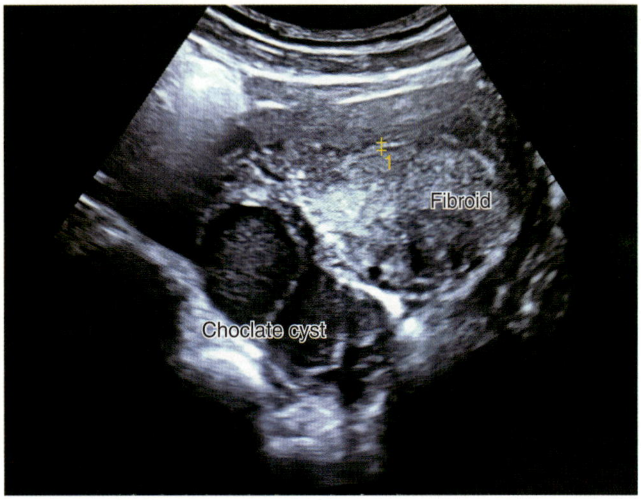

Figure 13.16 Fibroid with endometriosis.

Polymenorrhoea occurs when cystic ovaries and pelvic inflammatory disease (PID) coexist with fibromyomas.

Metrorrhagia is common with submucous fibroids. An infected polyp will also cause purulent discharge. Metrorrhagia in a woman older than 40 years requires dilation and curettage (D&C) to rule out endometrial cancer, which may be associated with fibroids in 3% cases.

INFERTILITY

Fibroids can be responsible for infertility (Fig. 13.16). Infertility is either due to associated PID, endometriosis or anovulatory cycles or due to distortion of the uterine cavity causing obstruction to sperm ascent, poor nidation or cornual tubal block. A fibroid bigger than 4 cm in size can cause infertility.

Submucous myomas are more likely to be responsible for infertility and recurrent pregnancy loss in up to 20% cases.

PAIN AND DYSMENORRHOEA

Most women complain of heaviness in the lower abdomen. Congestive and spasmodic dysmenorrhoea is often symptoms of fibroids or associated pelvic diseases. A submucous fibroid often causes spasmodic dysmenorrhoea.

Acute pain is seen when a fibroid is complicated by torsion, haemorrhage and red degeneration. Pain in a rapidly growing fibroid in an elderly woman may be due to sarcomatous change.

PRESSURE SYMPTOMS

Anterior and posterior fibroids in the lower segment or cervix can cause increase in the frequency and retention of urine, more often premenstrually because premenstrual congestion results in enlargement of the fibroids. Broad ligament fibroids can cause hydroureter and hydronephrosis, changes which are reversible following surgery.

Constipation and intestinal obstruction are rare, but if it occurs, it may be due to a loop of intestine adherent to fibroid.

ABDOMINAL LUMP

A large fibroid may be present as an abdominal tumour which has been growing slowly over a long period. A rapid growth only occurs during pregnancy due to oral contraceptive hormones and malignancy. A pedunculated fibroid feels separate from the uterus and gives the impression of an ovarian tumour.

Other symptoms are due to anaemia such as dyspnoea and palpitation. A rare condition of pseudo-Meigs syndrome has been described with a pedunculated fibroid causing ascites and right hydrothorax. Haemorrhagic shock due to intraperitoneal haemorrhage is rare.

VAGINAL DISCHARGE

Excessive vaginal discharge is a symptom associated with pedunculated submucous fibroid.

Acute emergency condition: Acute clinical conditions associated with uterine fibroids are as follows:

- Acute retention of urine and acute abdominal pain with red degenerative fibroids during pregnancy.
- Retention of urine, torsion of a pedunculated fibroid, haemorrhage infection and sarcomatous change cause severe abdominal pain.
- Rare case of thromboembolism.

PHYSICAL SIGNS

Anaemia may be noted. An abdominal lump may be felt arising from the pelvis with well-defined margins, firm in consistency and smooth or bossy surface. The tumour is mobile from side to side unless fixed by its own large size or adhesions, or by broad ligament fibroid. Ascites is rare.

Bimanual examination will reveal an enlarged uterus, regular or bossy, depending upon the number and size of fibroids. The cervix moves with the movement of mass which is not felt separate from the uterus unless it is pedunculated. In a cervical fibroid, the normal uterus is perched on top of the fibroid. A broad ligament fibroid displaces the uterus to the opposite side.

In a myomatous polyp, the cervical os is open and its lower pole is felt. The uterine fundus cannot be palpated if inversion is associated with fundal submucous fibroid polyp. The uterus is uniformly enlarged in submucous fibroids. Intravascular and disseminated peripheral fibroids rarely exist but are often diagnosed only at laparotomy.

DIFFERENTIAL DIAGNOSIS (Table 13.3)

PREGNANCY

A cystic degenerated fibroid causing a soft enlarged uterus can be mistaken for pregnancy. The breast sign, soft cervix, urine pregnancy test and ultrasound resolve the doubt.

HAEMATOMETRA

Haematometra, caused by cervical stenosis, causes enlarged uterus and secondary amenorrhoea. Ultrasound and urine pregnancy test are useful.

ADENOMYOSIS

Adenomyosis shares the same clinical features as uterine fibroma. The uterus of more than 12 weeks size or an

Table 13.3 Differential Diagnosis in a Patient with Suspected Uterine Fibromyomas

• Haematometra/pyometra	• Full bladder
• Pregnancy	• Bilateral tubo-ovarian masses
• Adenomyosis	• Pelvic endometriosis
• Bicornuate uterus	• Endometrial carcinoma
• Endometriosis	• Uterine sarcoma
• Ectopic pregnancy	• Ovarian neoplasms
• Chronic PID	• Paraovarian cysts
• Ovarian tumour	• Pelvic kidney
• Chronic inversion	

irregularly enlarged uterus favours the diagnosis of fibroma. Besides, adenomyomatous uterus is often tender. Ultrasound confirms the diagnosis. Doppler ultrasound shows peripheral vessels in a fibromyoma, but for adenomyosis, the vessels are diffused inside.

BICORNUATE UTERUS

Bicornuate uterus can be diagnosed by hysterogram, hysteroscopy and ultrasound.

ENDOMETRIOSIS, CHOCOLATE CYST

The clinical features are similar, but the uterus is normal in size and adherent to the pelvic mass.

ECTOPIC PREGNANCY

Chronic ectopic pregnancy with pelvic haematocoele can give the clinical impression of a fibroid. However, the history is different – ultrasound will clear the doubt.

CHRONIC PID

The history and clinical findings may be identical, but inflammatory masses are slightly tender and the uterus is of normal size and fixed.

BENIGN OVARIAN TUMOUR

A subserous or pedunculated fibroid may resemble an ovarian tumour. Menorrhagia may not be present in all cases of fibroids. Ultrasound will show the nature of tumour, but at times the true nature of the tumour is revealed only by laparotomy.

MALIGNANT OVARIAN TUMOUR

One of the serious errors is to mistake a malignant ovarian tumour for a uterine fibroid. Laparotomy should be performed in case of doubt.

ENDOMETRIAL CANCER

Endometrial cancer and myoma coexist in elderly women. Abnormal bleeding requires curettage of endometrium to rule out malignancy.

MYOMATOUS POLYP

Myomatous polyp protruding through the os may be mistaken for products of conception and cervical cancer. The history and tissue biopsy establish the diagnosis.

CHRONIC INVERSION OF UTERUS

Chronic inversion of uterus is often associated with fibroid polyp. The sounding of uterine cavity and laparoscopy are mandatory before surgical excision if uterine perforation is to be avoided.

Pelvic Kidney

Rarely, a pelvic kidney may be mistaken as a fibroid. The history is unlike uterine fibroids. The tumour is fixed, behind a normal-size uterus. Ultrasound will reveal absence of the abdominal kidney, and IVP will locate the pelvic kidney.

INVESTIGATIONS

In a majority of cases, the clinical features are clear-cut, and detailed investigations are not required. The following investigations may be carried out:

- Haemoglobin and blood group are required for management
- Ultrasound (see Fig. 13.3). A fibroma shows specific features of a well-defined rounded tumour, hypoechoic with cystic spaces if degeneration has occurred. Ultrasound can also identify adenomyosis as a diffuse growth with intramural cystic spaces, ovarian tumour, ectopic and adnexal mass. Preoperative ultrasound checks the number, location and size of the fibroids, and helps to reduce overlooking small fibroids during surgery, which might lead to persistence or recurrence of symptoms. Ultrasound is useful in the follow up of fibroids after menopause and while following GnRH therapy. However, it does not recognize sarcomatous change in a fibroid – MRI does. Three-dimensional ultrasound is very useful in deciding the management. Doppler ultrasound shows vascularity of the uterus and fibroids. Besides, it can differentiate between fibroids and localized adenomyosis. *The blood flow surrounds a fibroid but diffuses through adenomyosis.* The 3D ultrasound is precise in locating the site and type of fibroids.
- Hysterosalpingography and sonosalpingography identify a submucous myoma and check the patency of fallopian tubes in the presence of infertility (Fig. 13.17).
- Hysteroscopy not only identifies a submucous polyp but also allows its excision under direct vision.
- D&C is required to rule out endometrial cancer. It is necessary in a woman complaining of menstrual disorder and postmenopausal bleeding. Histopathology of the endometrium gives clue to its aetiology and rules out endometrial cancer.
- Laparoscopy is required in rare situations such as inversion of uterus while excising a myomatous polyp and to detect associated PID and endometriosis.
- Radiography has been superseded by ultrasound. Calcification seen as a peripheral calcified area is also seen in certain ovarian tumours, TB mass, calcified mucocoele of appendix and bony tumour. MRI is very useful in virgins and old women when pelvic examination clinically is not desirable in the former and hysteroscopy may be difficult due to narrow cervix.
- CT scan is not very useful, but MRI is accurate in identifying adenomyosis and sarcoma (Fig. 13.18A and B).

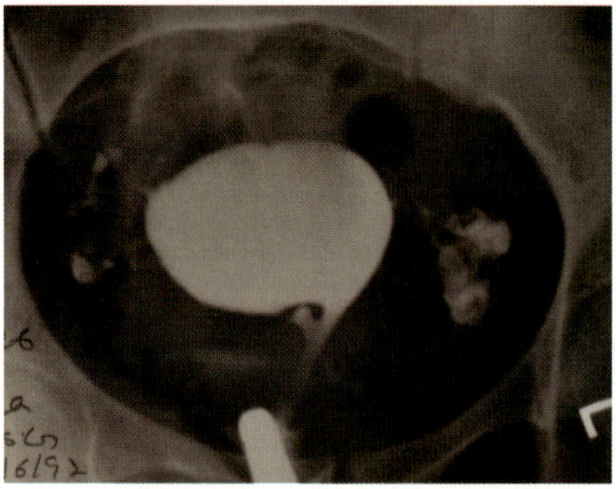

Figure 13.17 Hysterosalpingogram showing uterine cavity is enlarged in size with a diverticulum in the uterocervical junction in the right wall. Cavity was enlarged due to large interstitial fibroid. (*Courtesy*: Dr K.K. Saxena, New Delhi.)

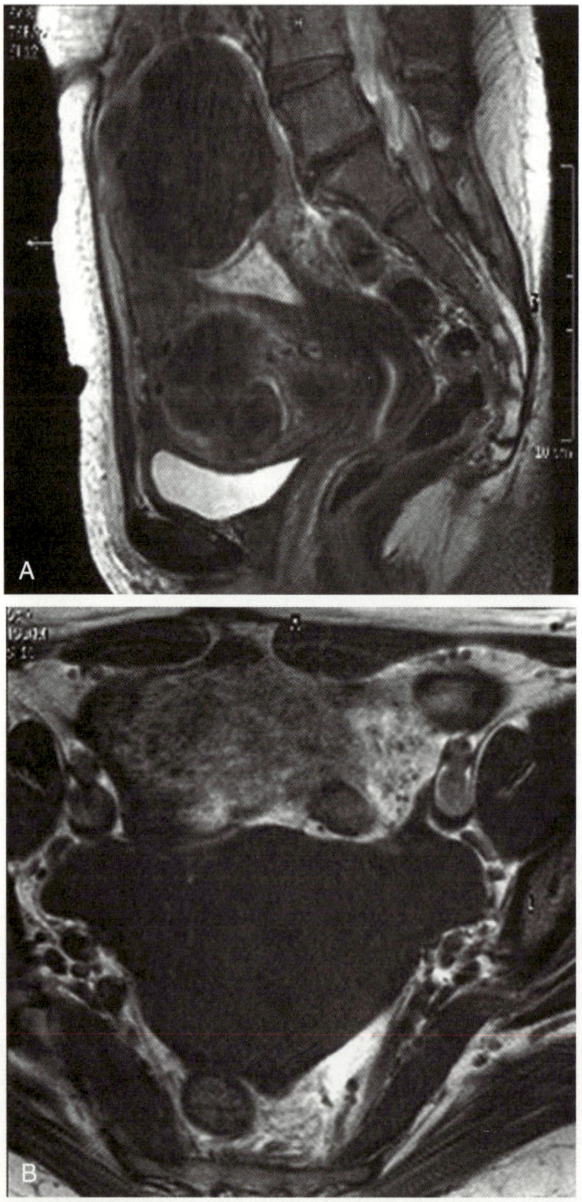

Figure 13.18 **(A)** MRI shows multiple uterine fibroids. **(B)** MRI showing submucous fibroid. (*Courtesy*: Dr Parveen Gulati, New Delhi.)

- Intravenous pyelography may be required for broad ligament fibroids to check the anatomy and course of ureter and to identify a pelvic kidney.
- With the development of minimal invasive surgery, it is very important to know the exact location of a fibroid. The 3D sonography is important in this connection, although MR provides more valuable information than 3D to interventional radiologist.

TREATMENT

Small and asymptomatic uterine fibroids do not require removal or medical treatment. They can be observed every 6 months. It is needless to emphasize that malignant lesion should be ruled out, and diagnosis of fibromyoma should be certain. A young woman should be informed about the presence of this tumour so that she understands the possibility of growth and red degeneration during pregnancy. Similarly, a perimenopausal woman should realize the importance of regular follow-up. *Also, it should be noted that tumour can grow if a menopausal woman is on* HRT.

During pregnancy, surgery is contraindicated, except in the case of a pedunculated fibroid if it undergoes torsion. Acute retention of urine is treated by continuous catheterization for 48–72 hours, when the growing uterus rises above the pelvic brim. Red degeneration merits conservative treatment.

Similarly, myomectomy is not advisable during caesarean section because of the uncontrolled bleeding that may ensue, except for a pedunculated fibroid.

Indications for treatment in an asymptomatic fibroid are as follows:

- Infertility caused by a cornual fibroid blocking the tube, and habitual abortions due to a submucous fibroid. Other causes of infertility and abortions should be ruled out before myomectomy is undertaken.
- A fibroid of more than 12 weeks size and a pedunculated fibroid which can cause torsion.
- An asymptomatic fibroid causing pressure on the ureter, that is, broad ligament fibroid and pressure on the bladder, leaving residual urine and causing urinary infection.
- Rapidly growing fibromyoma in a menopausal woman, implying impossible malignancy.
- When the nature of tumour cannot be ascertained clinically (laparotomy is needed in this situation).
- All symptomatic fibroids.

Faced with a woman having symptoms, it is important to determine whether the fibroids are really responsible for these symptoms, or are they mere 'innocent bystanders'. If so, they can be followed up and the cause of symptoms managed appropriately. Performing surgery for fibroids in such a woman may not relieve her symptoms.

Treatment may be as follows (see Table 13.4):

- Expectant – wait and observe (6 months for growth)
- Medical
- Nonsurgical – uterine artery embolization (UAE) and MRI
- Minimal invasive surgery
- Surgery

Table 13.4 Advantages and Disadvantages of Medical and Surgical Treatment

Advantages	Disadvantages
Medical • Avoids anaesthesia and surgical risks • Cures menorrhagia and controls anaemia, cures pressure symptoms • Reduces the size of tumour and blood supply; therefore, less operative bleeding and allows Pfannenstiel incision • Allows laparoscopic myomectomy by reducing vascularity and size	• Side effects of the drugs do not allow treatment over indefinite period (see GnRH therapy) • Failure of treatment • Recurrence of symptoms and regrowth after stoppage of treatment • Surgery may still be required
Surgery • Removes fibroids and cures symptoms in one sitting • Improves fertility in 40% cases • Risk of malignancy eliminated	• Risks of anaesthesia and surgery (bleeding and trauma) • Risk of postoperative adhesions • Recurrence of fibroids due to growth of seedling fibroids (5%–10%) • Persistence of menorrhagia in 5%–10% due to congestion, enlarged uterine cavity

Table 13.5 Management of Uterine Fibromyoma

Asymptomatic	Symptomatic	Cervical 1%

• Observation with regular follow-up
  • Size < 12 weeks
  • Uncomplicated pregnancy with fibroid
• Surgery
  • Size > 12 weeks
  • Cornual fibroid causing infertility
  • Pedunculated cornual fibroid
  • Pregnancy with torsion of pedunculated fibroid
	• Medical
	  • Hormones to shrink the fibroid – surgery
	  • Uterine artery embolization
	  • Myomectomy
	  • Lap myomectomy
	  • Lap myolysis
	• MRI-guided ablation
	  • Total/subtotal abdominal hysterectomy
	  • Vaginal hysterectomy
	  • Total laparoscopic hysterectomy
	  • Lap hysterectomy
	  • Laparoscopic-assisted vaginal hysterectomy
		• Vaginal polypectomy or myomectomy
		• Myomectomy
		• Laprascopic myomectomy
		• MRI-guided myolysis
		• Vaginal hysterectomy
		• Total abdominal hysterectomy

MEDICAL TREATMENT (Table 13.5)

- Iron therapy for anaemia. Blood is rarely used preoperatively.
- The drugs used to control menorrhagia have been described in Chapter 11. Mirena controls menorrhagia, provided the uterus is not enlarged beyond 12 weeks.
- The purpose of medical therapy is to control menorrhagia and improve haemoglobin before surgery, or to shrink the fibroid before surgery.
- In older women, successful medical therapy will allow women to reach menopause when the fibroid will shrink and cease to be a problem.

RU486 (mifepristone) 10–25 mg daily for 3 months causes amenorrhoea and shrinkage of tumour by 50% (recently, 5 mg daily is found effective). Danazol 400–800 mg daily for 3–6 months reduces the size of tumour by 60%. However, development of hirsutism and other side effects, as well as the cost, preclude its routine use. Regrowth of fibroid is reported following stoppage of the drug.

Low-dose oral contraceptives, such as gestrinone 2.5 mg thrice a week, are also effective. Asoprisnil, selective progesterone receptor modulator, is better than mifepristone. Recently, ulipristal, a selective progesterone receptor modulator, has been used.

GnRH THERAPY

GnRH analogues used for 6 months reduce the size of tumour by 50%–80%. This treatment in premenopausal women and young women with infertility may eliminate the need for surgery. It is also useful in reducing vascularity besides size preoperatively, and by causing amenorrhoea or reducing menorrhagia restores the haemoglobin level. Shrinkage of fibroid allows Pfannenstiel incision in abdominal operation, minimal invasive surgery or a vaginal hysterectomy instead of an abdominal hysterectomy, and also reduces bleeding. Monthly depot injection of 3.6 mg should not be extended beyond 6 months to avoid menopausal symptoms and osteoporosis. *One should remember that the tumour can regrow after stoppage of the drug.*

Instead of monthly injection, 3-monthly leuprolide acetate, 11.23 mg, may be convenient to administer. Pure antioestrogen (Faslodex) may be effective for the same purpose. These hormones, however, do not relieve dysmenorrhoea. Other anti-E_2s, such as raloxifene and aromatase inhibitor fadrozole, are under trial.

The disadvantages of GnRH therapy preoperatively are that the fibroid capsule may thin out, making enucleation rather difficult. Small fibroids become invisible at surgery, but recur later. *Mirena IUCD can be used to control menorrhagia and dysmenorrhoea due to fibroids.* GnRH analogues are expensive and need to be injected subcutaneously.

Add-back therapy with oral combined pills, tibolone or progesterone with GnRH, can reduce the side effects and allow longer use of GnRH. GnRH antagonists are better than agonists, as they avoid initial 'flare-up' effect and act faster.

Isoprisinol (selective progesterone receptor modulator) is under trial. *HRT should not be offered to a menopausal woman with fibroids.*

Aromatase inhibitors, such as letrozole, have been employed. They inhibit conversion of androgens to oestrogen in the ovaries and in peripheral fat, and shrink the fibroid by 50%.

SURGERY

The techniques used are conventional myomectomy and hysterectomy by laparotomy or laparoscopically.

Myomectomy

Myomectomy refers to the removal of fibroids, leaving the uterus behind. It is indicated in an infertile woman or a woman desirous of childbearing and wishing to retain the uterus. It is done by open surgery, laparoscopically, vaginal or through hysteroscopic route.

Preoperative Requisites

- Haemoglobin should be restored.
- Autotransfusion arranged a few days before surgery is preferred to donor transfusion at surgery to avoid transmission risk of HIV, malaria and hepatitis B.
- In infertility, other causes of infertility should be excluded.
- Signature for hysterectomy is required in difficult unforeseen circumstances.
- Myomectomy should be performed in preovulatory menstrual cycle to reduce blood loss during surgery.
- Endometrial cancer to be ruled out by D&C.
- Bowel preparation avoids bowel injury.

Technique of myomectomy (Fig. 13.19)

- Opening the abdominal cavity by Pfannenstiel incision is possible if the uterus is less than 16–20 weeks size, and is mobile. If difficulty is anticipated as with a large uterus, fixed uterus with adhesions, associated PID and endometriosis, a vertical paramedian incision is safer.
- Care should be taken not to injure the bladder while incising the parietal peritoneum, as the bladder may be elevated in cervical and low-lying anterior wall fibroids.
- The pelvic organs should be carefully inspected and the feasibility of myomectomy confirmed.
- An incision over the anterior uterine wall is preferred whenever possible and as many fibroids removed through minimal tunnelling incisions.
- Haemorrhage should be controlled with the myomectomy clamp. The clamp should be applied from the pubic end of the abdominal wound and the round ligaments which will include the uterine vessels should be gripped. The ovarian vessels may be temporarily occluded with a sponge forceps. If the myomectomy clamp cannot be applied as in cervical fibroids, a rubber tourniquet will serve the purpose. Local injection of dilute vasopressin also helps to reduce blood loss.

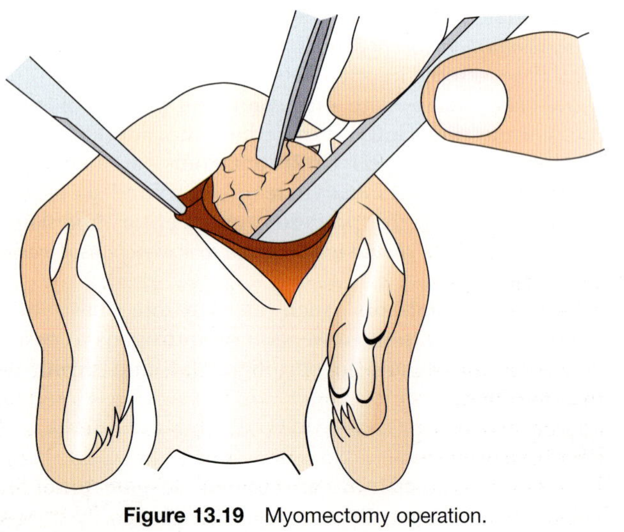

Figure 13.19 Myomectomy operation.

- The capsule should be incised and the fibroid enucleated. This will minimize bleeding and avoid trauma to the bladder and ureter. Myomectomy screws help during enucleation (Figs 13.20–13.22).
- Following enucleation, the haemostasis is secured and the cavity obliterated with several catgut sutures. This will avoid scar rupture during subsequent pregnancy and labour.
- The clamp should be released and haemostasis confirmed.
- The raw visceral area should be well peritonized to prevent postoperative adhesions. Hydroflotation also

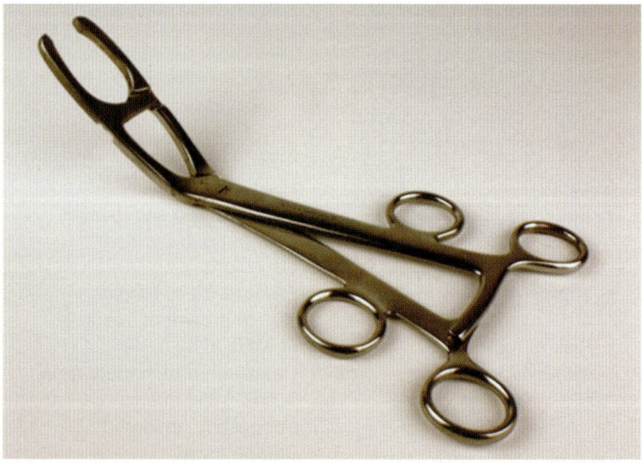

Figure 13.20 Bonney's myomectomy clamp.

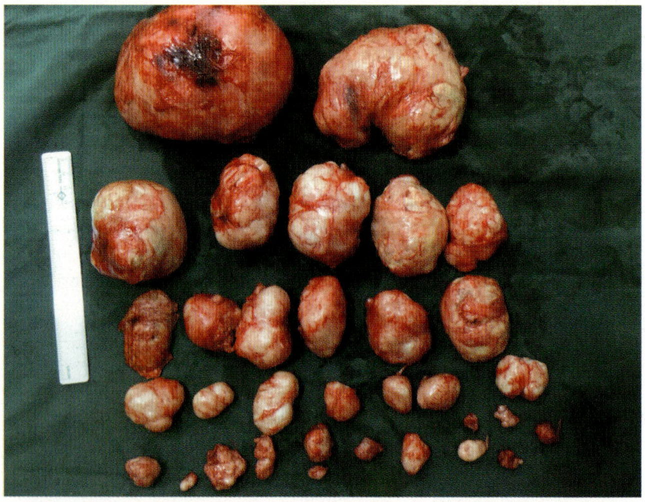

Figure 13.21 Multiple fibroid removed by open myomectomy.

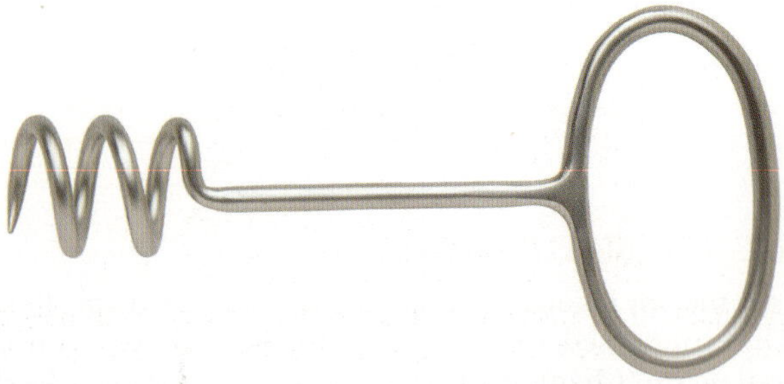

Figure 13.22 Myoma screw.

reduces adhesions. The uterus remains bulky following myomectomy and requires to be anteverted by plicating the round ligaments with nonabsorbable sutures.

Results. Pregnancy rate of 40%–50% has been reported following myomectomy, and pregnancy loss reduced. However, 10%–15% continue to suffer from menorrhagia. Recurrence of fibroids in 5%–10% cases is due to overlooking seedling fibroids at the time of surgery.

Complications. The complications that may result from myomectomy are as follows:

- Primary, reactionary and secondary haemorrhage
- Trauma to the bladder, ureter and bowel during surgery
- Infection
- Adhesions and intestinal obstruction
- Recurrence of fibroids and persistence of menorrhagia

Vaginal myomectomy (Fig. 13.23): It is indicated in submucous fibroid polyps. Vaginal myomectomy is possible in cervical fibroids and pedunculated fibroid polypus and if more than 50% submucous fibroids project into the cavity.

Hysteroscopic myomectomy: Hysteroscopic myomectomy has become possible for submucous fibroids not removable easily by the vaginal route. The fibroid is excised either by cautery, laser or resectoscope. It is best done under laparoscopic guidance to avoid uterine perforation. Complications of hysteroscopic myomectomy are as follows:

- Cervical trauma, uterine perforation
- Thermal injury
- Bleeding – Foley catheter can be used as tamponade to stop bleeding
- Infection
- Failure
- Uterine adhesions
- Complications of distending media : Water overload or pulmonary oedema

Laparoscopic myomectomy: Laparoscopic view of various fibroids is shown in Figs 13.24 and 13.25.

Laparoscopic myomectomy (Fig. 13.26A–I) is feasible in:

- A pedunculated fibroid

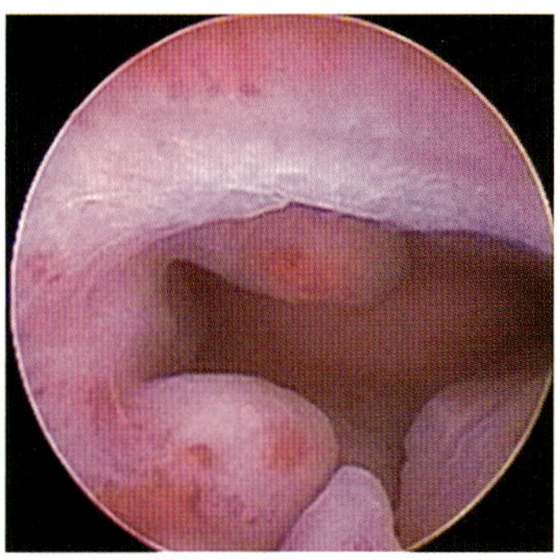

Figure 13.23 Hysteroscopy reveals multiple endometrial polyps. (*Source:* From Figure 2A. Chunxia Cheng, Ting Zhao, Min Xue, et al. In: Use of suction curettage in operative hysteroscopy. Journal of Minimally Invasive Gynecology, Volume 16(6): 739–742, 2009.)

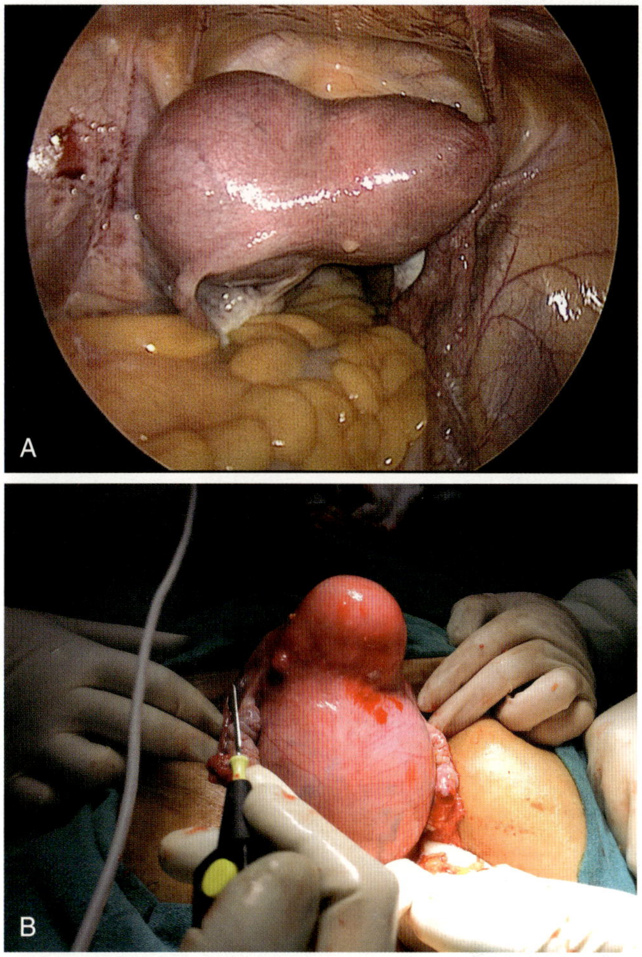

Figure 13.24 **(A)** Subserous fibroid seen on laparoscopy. **(B)** Central cervical fibroid (lantern on the dome of St. Paul's Cathedral) seen on laparotomy. (*Courtesy* **(A):** Dr Vivek Marwah, New Delhi.)

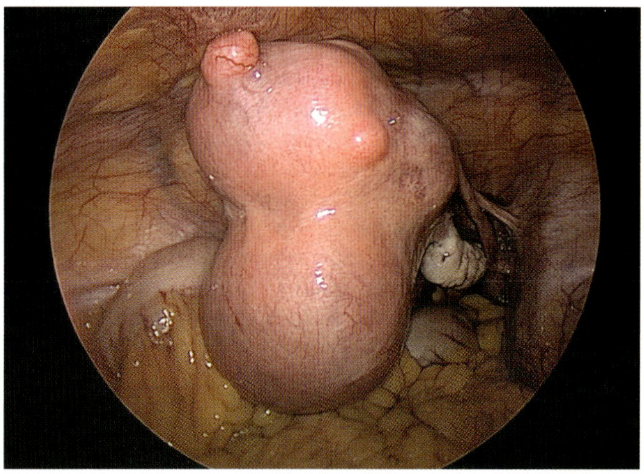

Figure 13.25 Multiple uterine fibroids. (*Courtesy*: Dr Vivek Marwah, New Delhi.)

- Subserous fibroid not exceeding 10 cm in size and not more than four in number. Multiple fibroids of any size should be approached by laparotomy. Unipolar, bipolar cautery and laser have been employed to remove the fibroma and obtain haemostasis. The fibroma is retrieved through posterior colpotomy, minilaparotomy or by morcellation. Myolysis, a

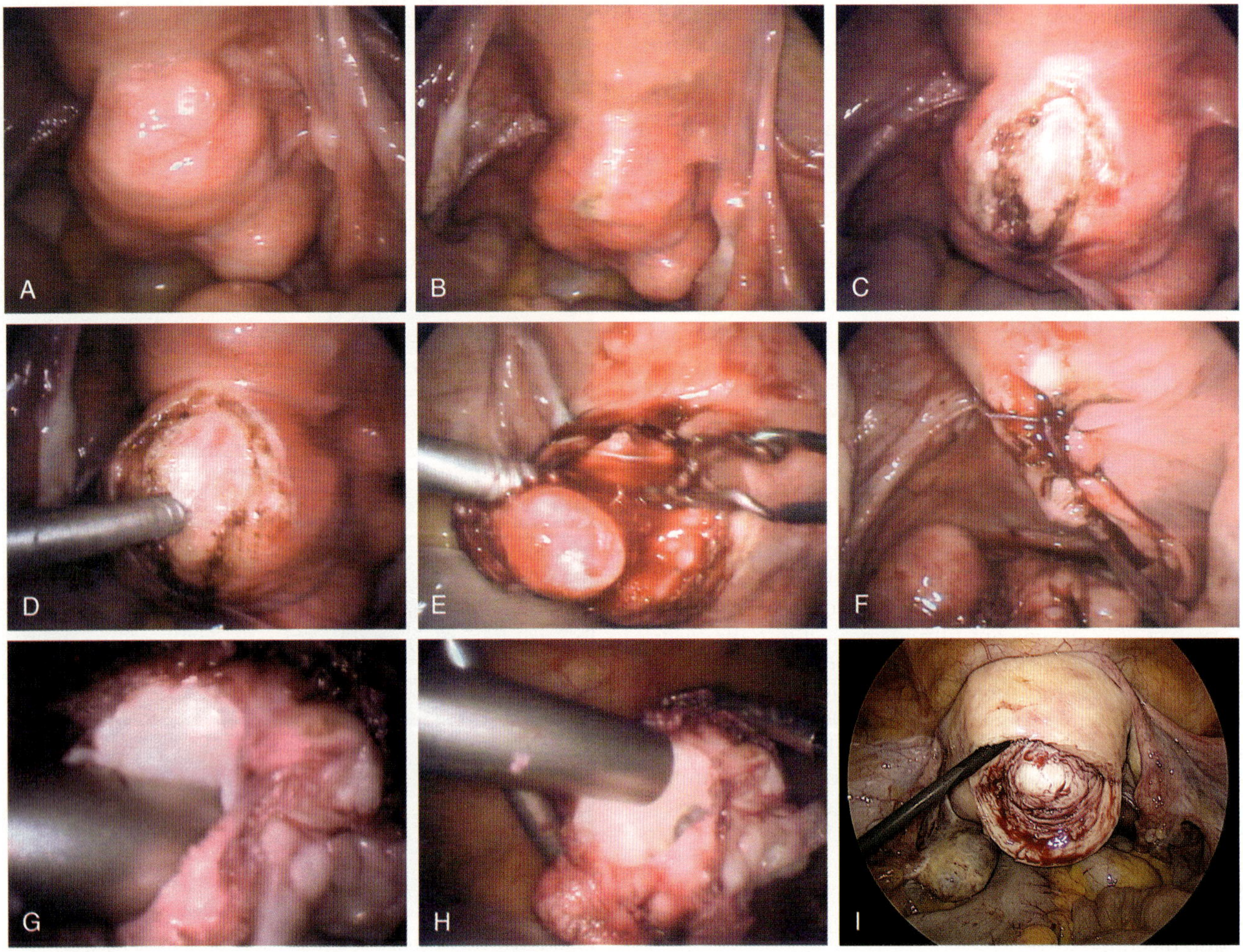

Figure 13.26 Laparoscopic myomectomy – steps of operation. **(A)** Fibromyoma uterus. **(B)** Incision taken on the fibromyoma. **(C)** Fibromyoma exposed. **(D)** Myoma screw inserted to steady the myoma. **(E)** Myoma dissected from its bed. **(F)** Edges of myoma bed approximated with interrupted Vicryl sutures. Removed myoma seen in POD. **(G)** Myoma being morcellated. **(H)** Tunnel in myoma after removal of cylindrical mass. **(I)** Laparoscopic myomectomy. (*Courtesy*: Dr Vivek Marwah, New Delhi.)

technique of destruction of myoma tissue by laser or cautery, is a sophisticated technology practised by endoscopists.
- Laparoscopic-assisted vaginal hysterectomy (LAVH) enables vaginal hysterectomy to be completed from below in the presence of pelvic pathology.

Laparoscopic myomectomy is made easier and faster by newer instruments, morcellator, newer energy sources and newer suture materials. The bleeding is controlled by infiltration of myoma with vasoconstrictors and bilateral uterine artery ligation before myomectomy.

Disadvantages of Laparoscopic Myomectomy

Although a minimal invasive surgery, and without an abdominal scar, laparoscopic myomectomy can cause more bleeding because of nonapplicability of a haemostatic clamp, and being an adhesiogenic procedure, it takes longer to perform. Postoperative adhesions can increase the infertility rate. Scar rupture is also reported in late pregnancy and during labour. Some use intercede (oxidized regenerated cellulose) to prevent or reduce adhesions. The major complication is rupture of the myomectomy scar during pregnancy or labour due to imperfect or inadequate suturing of the myomectomy wound. *Laparoscopic myomectomy may therefore not be safe in an infertile woman*, except for small fibroids. The recurrence rate is reported higher than that in laparotomy.

Newer minimal invasive procedures successfully introduced in recent years are:

- UAE
- MRI-guided laser ablation
- Laparoscopic myolysis

Uterine Artery Embolization

In 1991, Jacques Ravina, a French gynaecologist, first performed UAE preoperatively to reduce vascularity and the size of fibroid. Improvement in symptoms cancelled definitive surgery is some cases. Menorrhagia was relieved in 80%–90%, pressure symptoms in 40%–70%; the volume decreased by 50% at the end of 3 months, by 60% at 6 months and by 75% at the end of 1 year. Thus, this technique is now employed successfully in selective cases.

Contraindications

- *Subserous and pedunculated fibroids.* Necrosis and fall of the tumour into the peritoneal cavity can occur. Big fibroids are not suited for UAE.

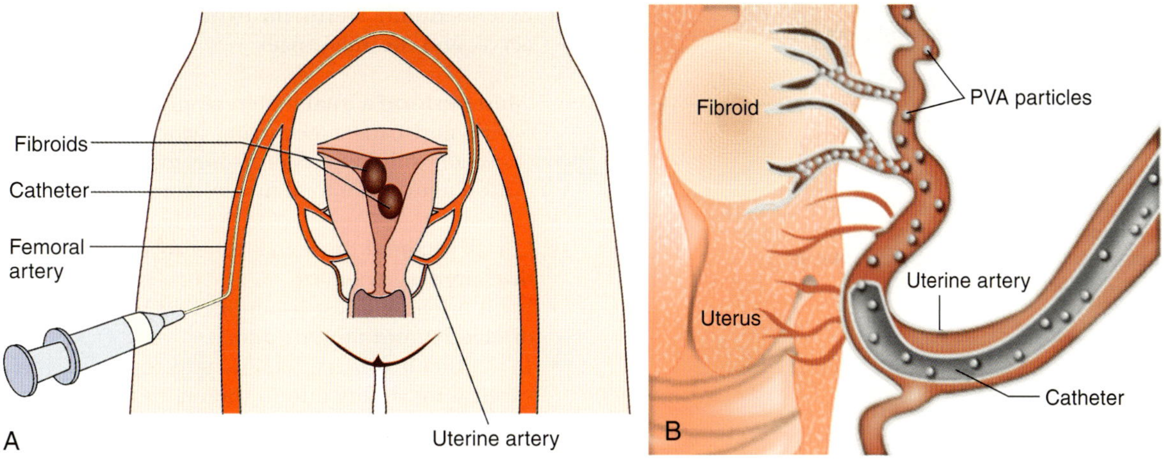

Figure 13.27 (A) Transfemoral catheterization of uterine arteries. **(B)** Injection of polyvinyl alcohol particles. (*Source*: Rao, K. A. Textbook of Gynaecology, India: Elsevier, 2008.)

- Submucous fibroid is not cured.
- Infertility rate may increase following this technique because of postembolization pelvic adhesions.
- Calcified fibroid cannot shrink with this technique.
- Associated inflammatory disease may also preclude the employment of this technique.

Technique. Under local sedation, bilateral UAE is approached through percutaneous femoral catheterization. It is done using polyvinyl alcohol (PVA), gel foam particles or metal coils. Embolization reduces vascularity and the size of fibroid in 3–4 months (Fig. 13.27) (40% at 6 weeks and 75% at 1 year). Pregnancy should be postponed for at least 6 months.

The symptoms are relieved in 70%–80% women. The following are the postoperative complications:

- Fever and infection
- Vaginal discharge and bleeding (5%)
- Ischaemic pain suggests successful therapy but can be unbearable and requires analgesia
- Pulmonary embolism
- Ovarian failure following accidental ovarian vessel blockage and premature menopause (up to 30%)
- Fertility rate is reduced due to adhesions
- Failure due to inadequate embolization caused by arterial spasm or tortuosity of the vessels
- Expulsion of a fibroid into the peritoneal cavity (10%)
- Allergic reaction and contrast induced renal failure
- Radiation exposure
- Haematoma at the femoral site
- Extrusion of a subserous fibroid into the peritoneal cavity which requires retrieval.
- Intraperitoneal adhesions

Proper selection of patients is key to clinical success and avoiding complications. A follow-up with ultrasound 6 months later is also necessary to observe the shrinkage of the fibroid, and to register success or failure of this treatment.

Other indications for UAE besides fibroids are as follows:

- Arteriovenous aneurysm or increased uterine vascularity causing menorrhagia
- Postpartum haemorrhage
- Placenta accreta to reduce bleeding before placental removal, or caesarean delivery

Laparoscopic localized uterine artery occlusion using clips or electrodessication is being tried. This avoids ovarian devascularization.

UAE is the most suited procedure for menorrhagia in a multiparous woman.

The following are the advantages of UAE:

- No major surgery
- No intraoperative bleeding
- Short hospital stay
- Less abdominal adhesions
- 75%–80% women are satisfied

MRI-guided percutaneous laser ablation using high-intensity focused ultrasound (HIFU) has been recently attempted with success. This generates heat, 55°C, at the focused point on the fibroid for few seconds. It ablates the vessels as well as the tumour. The woman is able to return to work in 2 days time. This technique may also find a place in the treatment of adenomyosis.

MRI-Guided Focused Ultrasound

This is a noninvasive technique and uses high-intensity focused ultrasound beam that heats and destroys fibrous tissues. MRI guides in targeting the beam path towards the fibroid.

A large fibromyoma can be treated in two sessions, or the fibroid is reduced in size with monthly GnRH injections for 3–4 months before treatment.

Side effects are as follows:

- Skin burn
- Pain
- Nerve damage (rare)

Advantages

1. Noninvasive technique
2. Local anaesthesia – takes 1–2 hours to do
3. No hospitalization
4. No scar
5. Quick recovery
6. Fertility preservation technique

Table 13.6 Indications for Hysterectomy

Abdominal	Vaginal
Benign	Prolapse
Menorrhagia	Carcinoma in situ
Uterine fibromyoma	Cancer cervix + lymphadenectomy
Adenomyosis	Menorrhagia
Tubo-ovarian mass	Uterine fibroid
carcinoma in situ	Genital prolapse
atypical endometrial hyperplasia	
Endometriosis	
Malignant	
Carcinoma of the cervix	
Carcinoma of the endometrium	
Carcinoma of the ovary	
Uterine sarcoma-mixed mesodermal tumour	
Choriocarcinoma (rare)	
Obstetric	
Rupture uterus	
PPH, molar pregnancy	
Carcinoma of the cervix	

Contraindications

1. Calcified fibroid
2. Degenerated fibroid
   - Interstitial laser ablation is done laparoscopically by inserting laser fibres into the myoma.

Laparoscopic Myolysis

This is an optional surgery using Nd:YAG laser, CryoProbe or diathermy to coagulate a subserous fibroid. It is used in a multiparous woman. The contraindications and complications are similar to those of UAE.

Hysterectomy (Table 13.6)

Hysterectomy, the removal of the uterus, is indicated in a woman older than 40 years, a multiparous woman or when associated with malignancy. Uncontrolled haemorrhage and unforeseen surgical difficulties during myomectomy may also necessitate hysterectomy. Hysterectomy guarantees removal of all fibroids and relief from symptoms. Normally, the aim is total hysterectomy. However, subtotal hysterectomy may be performed in the presence of PID, endometriosis and any technical problem when the cervix is left behind. Prior cervical cytology is desirable.

Types of Hysterectomy

- Abdominal hysterectomy
- Vaginal hysterectomy
- Laparoscopic hysterectomy

Abdominal Hysterectomy

Abdominal hysterectomy includes:

- Total hysterectomy
- Subtotal hysterectomy when the cervix is retained
- Panhysterectomy (TAH with B/L Salpingo Oopherectomy) when ovaries are also removed
- Extended and Wertheim hysterectomy in cancer of the cervix and uterine cancer

Most perform a total hysterectomy, as it prevents chronic cervicitis and cancer occurring at a later stage. However, occasionally, subtotal hysterectomy may have to be resorted.

Advantages of subtotal hysterectomy are as follows:

- Cervix retained for sexual function. The normal cervical discharge is beneficial.
- Vault prolapse is less common. Less bleeding and less risk of bladder and ureter trauma.
- In a difficult surgery, total hysterectomy may increase the surgical morbidity due to trauma to the bladder and denervation, causing difficult micturition and incontinence.

Pap smear before surgery ensures that the cervix is normal.

What about the ovaries?

In benign conditions, the ovaries should be retained to avoid menopausal symptoms in a premenopausal woman, provided they look normal.

Disadvantage of conserving the ovaries:

- Benign or malignant ovarian tumour may develop in 1% cases.
- Residual ovarian syndrome is known to occur in some cases and cause dyspareunia.
- Atrophy of the ovaries has been reported due to kinking of the ovarian vessels within 3–4 years of hysterectomy; they become nonfunctional and cause early menopause.

Total Abdominal Hysterectomy

Hysterectomy is straightforward in most cases of fibroids. However, in case of a cervical, low anterior wall and a posterior fibroid, and one encroaching into the broad ligament where bladder, ureter and rectum are displaced from their normal anatomical position, they are at risk of injury. In a cervical and large anterior wall fibroid which is close to the bladder, it is prudent to perform myomectomy first. This allows a clear view of vaginal vault and safeguards against bladder injury. Thereafter, hysterectomy can be performed. Similarly, in a low posterior fibroid, the upper portion of the broad ligament may not be accessible until the fibroid is first enucleated.

In a central cervical fibroid, and a huge posterior fibroid, hemisection of the uterus and enucleation of the fibroid will allow safe hysterectomy.

Vaginal Hysterectomy

Vaginal hysterectomy is possible if the uterus is mobile, uterine size is less than 14 weeks with no previous surgery or there is no other pelvic pathology; in all other cases, abdominal hysterectomy is performed. The ovaries may be conserved in a woman younger than 50 years, provided they are healthy. Vaginal hysterectomy is not a good approach in nulliparous women with narrow vagina.

Lately, vaginal hysterectomy is being done for uterine size more than 12 weeks, provided the uterus is not fixed by adhesions, adnexal inflammatory mass or endometriosis by performing:

- Previous laparoscopy to confirm the absence of pelvic adhesions, size of the uterus and rule out pelvic pathology

- Bisection of uterus, and removing each half separately
- Myomectomy and enucleation of fibroid first
- Morcellation

Laparoscopic-Assisted Vaginal Hysterectomy (LAVH). This avoids an abdominal scar, minimizes pain and shortens the recovery period and hospital stay.

Contraindications to LAVH are as follows:

- Uterus more than 14–16 weeks in size.
- The fibroid is located in the broad ligament, cervical fibroids and extensive pelvic adhesions, endometriosis.

Complications of Hysterectomy

- Primary, reactionary and secondary haemorrhage
- Trauma to the bladder, ureter and bowel may occur in cervical and broad ligament fibroma; associated PID and endometriosis expose the ureter to injury
- Sepsis
- Anaesthetic complications
- Paralytic ileus, intestinal obstruction due to postoperative adhesions
- Thrombosis, pulmonary embolism, chest infection
- Burst abdomen, hernia
- Postoperative infection such as wound infection, peritonitis, pelvic infection and embolism – chronic pelvic pain
- Abdominal adhesions cause chronic abdominal pain
- Dyspareunia
- Vault prolapse
- Residual ovarian syndrome and atrophy of the ovaries due to decreased vascularity, causing premature menopause in 2–3 years
- Ovarian cancer in 1% if ovaries are left behind during hysterectomy
- Urinary dysfunction due to denervation of bladder
- Granulation tissue at the vault prolapse of the fallopian tubes

Management of uterine fibromyoma is summarized in Table 13.5.

Contraception. A young woman with uterine fibroids may seek contraceptive advice. Oral hormonal contraceptives should not be prescribed because the fibroid may grow in size under hormonal influence. Intrauterine contraceptive device (IUCD) can cause menorrhagia and dysmenorrhoea and is therefore not suitable in this woman. She can choose between a barrier method and centchroman.

CERVICAL FIBROID

Surgery for cervical fibroids, either myomectomy or hysterectomy, is associated with a greater risk of injury to bladder and ureters besides increased blood loss during surgery. To decrease risk of injury to bladder or ureters, it may be desirable to first enucleate fibroid and then proceed with rest of the surgery.

FIBROIDS COMPLICATING PREGNANCY

Pregnancy associated with fibroids is associated with the increased chances of complications. Pregnancy generally causes an increase in the size of fibroids (Fig. 13.28); there is an increase in their vascularity and a higher tendency to undergo degenerative changes such as hyaline change and cystic degeneration. Red degeneration is a result of softening of the surrounding supportive connective tissue. The capillaries tend to rupture and blood effuses out into the myoma, causing a diffuse reddish discolouration of the same. Such a patient complains of severe pain in the abdomen and may present as an emergency for acute abdominal pain; examination reveals the pain to be restricted to the uterus around the site of the fibroid, and all other parameters remain stable. Such a patient is treated conservatively with bed rest and analgesics, until the pain subsides. On rare occasions, when laparotomy is carried out, the myoma is seen to be dusky in appearance; its cut section has an appearance of cooked meat and is known to emit a fishy odour. Fibroids by their sheer size may cause respiratory embarrassment, retention of urine or obstructed labour. They are sometimes known to adversely affect the outcome of pregnancy and there is an increased risk of abortion, preterm labour, abnormal presentation, accidental haemorrhage, dystocia in labour, PPH, puerperal sepsis and uterine inversion.

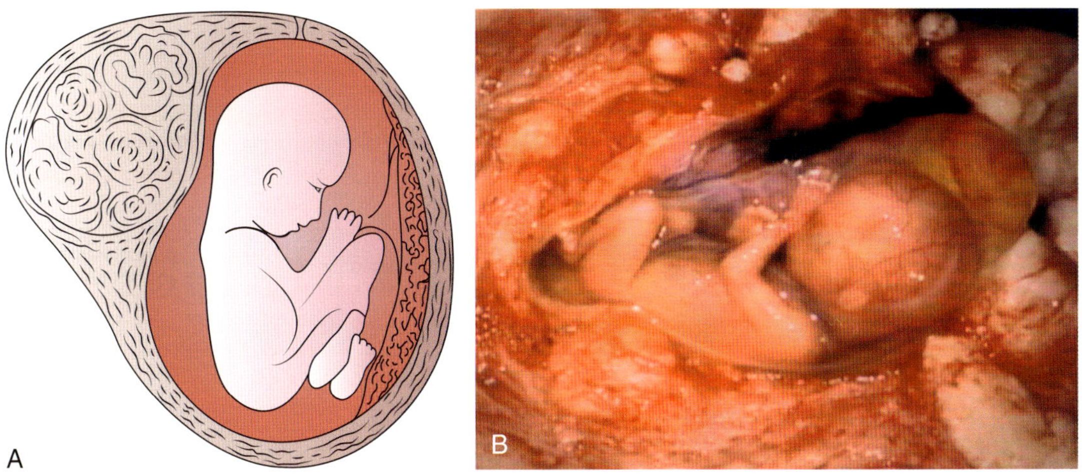

Figure 13.28 **(A)** Subserous fibroid associated with uterine pregnancy. **(B)** Uterus studded with multiple fibroids and pregnancy.

ENDOMETRIAL POLYPS

UTERINE POLYPS

Uterine polyps are usually benign comprising endometrial, fibroid, adenomyomatous and placental polyps. Cervical polyps are mucous and fibroadenomatous polyps arise from the endocervix.

ENDOMETRIAL POLYPS

Endometrial polyps mostly arise from hyperplasia of the endometrium, some part of the endometrial lining protruding into the uterine cavity as polyps. They may be single or multiple; they appear as pink swellings, 1–2 cm in diameter, with a pedicle. The polyp is composed of endometrial glands and stroma covered with a single layer of columnar epithelium. Secondary malignant change may occur in a benign polyp; thus, it is mandatory to study its histology.

In a malignant polyp arising ab initio, the entire polyp shows malignancy, including its base whereas secondary malignancy is seen at the apex of the polyp – the base or the pedicle shows no such change. Adenomyomatous polyp has smooth muscle as well as endometrial elements. Tamoxifen can cause endometrial hyperplasia and polyps.

A *fibroid polyp* is a submucous fibroid developing a pedicle and protruding into the uterine cavity or projecting through the os with a long pedicle. It is pale looking, firm with infection and necrosis at the base if it protrudes through the cervix. It can be sessile or a pedunculated cervical fibroid.

PLACENTAL POLYPS

Placental polyps are formed from retained placental tissue, thus causing secondary PPH or intermittent vaginal bleeding following an abortion or a normal delivery.

CLINICAL FEATURES

Uterine polyps can cause menorrhagia, metrorrhagia or postmenopausal bleeding. If these protrude through the os, may cause postcoital bleeding or continuous bleeding in a young woman after they are asymptomatic.

Clinically, the uterine polyp may not be evident as the uterus may or may not be enlarged; it is easy to diagnose when the polyp protrudes through the cervical canal. Ultrasound can detect uterine polyp, so also saline sonosalpingogram or hysterosalpingogram *(HSG)*.

Hysteroscopy is both diagnostic and therapeutic.

MANAGEMENT

D&C can scrape the polyp. Hysteroscopic removal of multiple polyps may be desirable to ensure their complete removal.

Endocervical polyps have been dealt with in the chapter on inflammation of the uterus and the cervix.

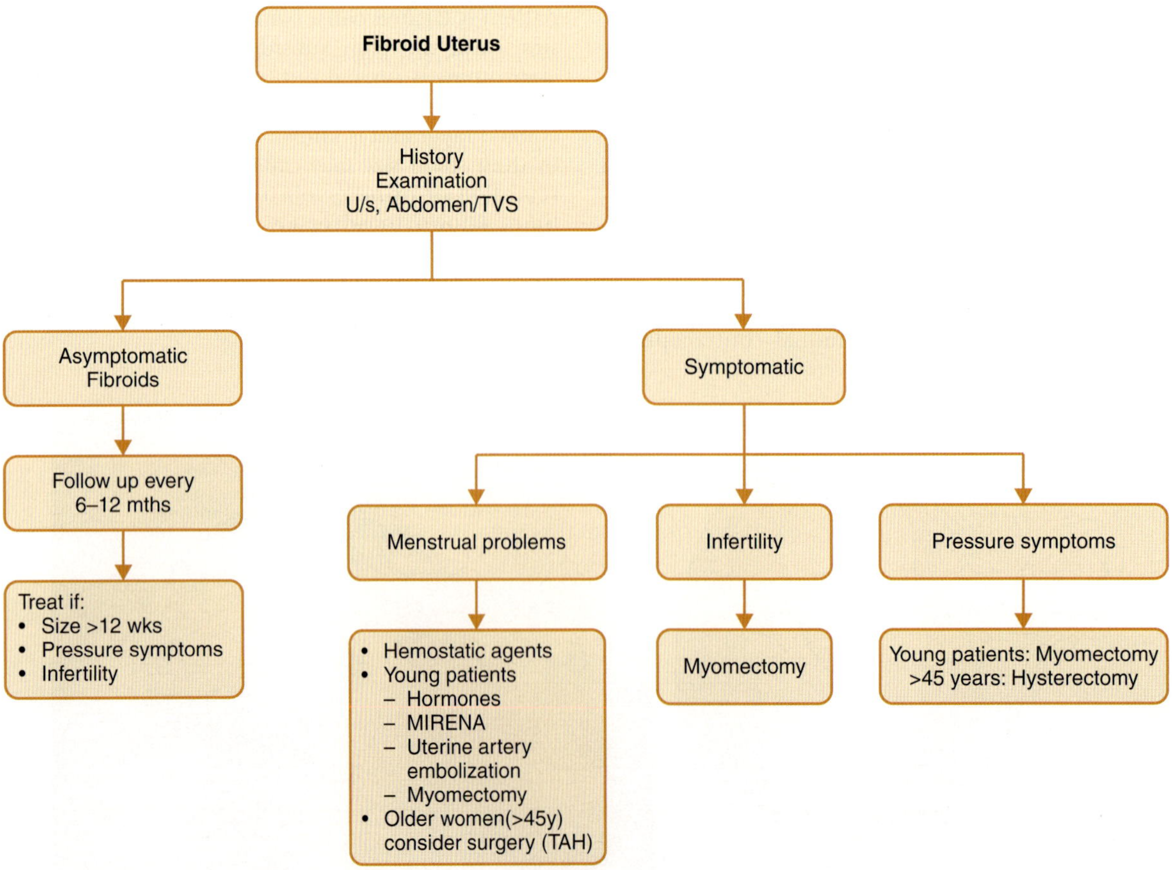

Management of Fibroid uterus

KEY POINTS

- Fibromyomas are benign neoplasms of the uterus affecting 5%–20% of women in the reproductive age group.
- Fibromyomas may be present without symptoms. However, depending on their size and location, they may contribute to menstrual irregularities, dysmenorrhoea, infertility, pain in the abdomen, abdominal fullness, pressure symptoms and complications during pregnancy.
- Ultrasonography, CT/MRI, laparoscopy and hysteroscopy help in establishing the diagnosis of uterine fibromyomas. They are also useful to determine the number, location and size of tumours. This helps in planning the treatment.
- Asymptomatic tumours often do not require treatment but follow-up is recommended.
- Symptomatic fibroids require treatment. Myomectomy is indicated in younger women desirous of retaining the childbearing function whereas in elderly women, hysterectomy is the procedure of choice.
- Medical treatment helps to relieve menorrhagia. GnRHa and SERM are adjuvants to surgery when a huge fibroid or multiple fibroids are encountered. They shrink the fibroids and reduce the blood loss during surgery.
- Endoscopic procedures enable the removal of moderate-size myomas.
- Hysterectomy is advised in elderly and multiparous women.
- Laparoscopy, hysteroscopy and arterial embolization provide minimal invasive surgery and have reduced the number of abdominal hysterectomy in women with uterine fibroids. MRI-guided high-frequency ultrasound is now possible.
- UAE is not recommended in women with infertility because of pelvic adhesions and risk of scar rupture during pregnancy or in labour.
- Location, size and number of fibroids decide the route of operation.

SELF-ASSESSMENT

1. Discuss the clinical features of uterine fibroids.
2. How will you manage a case of uterine fibroids in a 32-year-old, para 1 woman?
3. Discuss the management of uterine myoma in a nulliparous woman.
4. A woman, 38-year-old, presents with menorrhagia. She shows three fibroids on ultrasound. How will you manage the case?

SUGGESTED READING

Arulkumaran S. Acute complications of fibromyoma. Clin Obstet Gynaecol 2009;5:23.

Baird DD, Garrett TA, Laughlin SK, et al. Short-term change in growth of uterine leiomyoma: tumor growth spurts. Fertil Steril 2011; 95:242.

Baird DD, Harmon QE, Upson K, et al. A Prospective, Ultrasound-Based Study to Evaluate Risk Factors for Uterine Fibroid Incidence and Growth: Methods and Results of Recruitment. J Womens Health (Larchmt) 2015;24:907.

Borah BJ, Laughlin-Tommaso SK, Myers ER, et al. Association Between Patient Characteristics and Treatment Procedure Among Patients With Uterine Leiomyomas. Obstet Gynecol 2016;127:67.

Brucker SY, Huebner M, Wallwiener M, et al. Clinical characteristics indicating adenomyosis coexisting with leiomyomas: a retrospective, questionnaire-based study. Fertil Steril 2014;101:237.

Cardozo ER, Clark AD, Banks NK, et al. The estimated annual cost of uterine leiomyomata in the United States. Am J Obstet Gynecol 2012; 206:211.e1.

Committee on Practice Bulletins—Gynecology. Practice bulletin no. 128: diagnosis of abnormal uterine bleeding in reproductive-aged women. Obstet Gynecol 2012;120:197. Reaffirmed 2016.

Donnez J, Donnez O, Matule D, et al. Long-term medical management of uterine fibroids with ulipristal acetate. Fertil Steril 2016;105:165.

Duncan J, Shulman LP (Eds). Yearbook of Obstetrics and Gynaecology 2010;379.

Reyes C, Murali R, Park KJ. Secondary Involvement of the Adnexa and Uterine Corpus by Carcinomas of the Uterine Cervix: A Detailed Morphologic Description. Int J Gynecol Pathol 2015;34:551.

Sengupta, Chattopadhyay, Varma. Textbook of Gynaecology for Postgraduates and Practitioners. Elsevier, 2007.

Shiota M, Kotani Y, Umemoto M, et al. Deep-vein thrombosis is associated with large uterine fibroids. Tohoku J Exp Med 2011;224:87.

Stewart EA. Clinical practice. Uterine fibroids. N Engl J Med 2015; 372:1646.

Studd J (Ed). Embolization of fibroid. Progr Obstet Gynaecol 2006;17:333.

Studd J (Ed). Progress in Obstetrics and Gynaecology 2005;16:277.

Sturdee, et al. (Eds). Yearbook of Obstetrics and Gynaecology 2009;9.

Velez Edwards DR, Hartmann KE, Wellons M, et al. Evaluating the role of race and medication in protection of uterine fibroids by type 2 diabetes exposure. BMC Womens Health 2017;17:28.

Wise LA, Laughlin-Tommaso SK. Epidemiology of Uterine Fibroids: From Menarche to Menopause. Clin Obstet Gynecol 2016;59:2.

14 Endometriosis and Adenomyosis

CHAPTER OUTLINE

ENDOMETRIOSIS

Endometriosis is the presence of endometrium at a site outside endometrial lining. This condition was first described by Carl Von Rokinstasy in 1860. Since its original description, this condition is being increasingly recognized in women with infertility, chronic pelvic pain (CPP) and menstrual irregularity. These islands of endometriosis are composed of endometrial glands surrounded by endometrial stroma, and are capable of responding to a varying degree to cyclical hormonal stimulation. The disease although a benign proliferative growth process yet having some of the features of cancer like the propensity to invade the normal surrounding tissues, causing extreme pain and tendency for recurrences. Whereas cancer can kill the women, endometriosis cripples her life.

The reported incidence is about 10%, but incidence is increasing on account of greater use of diagnostic laparoscopy. Amongst infertile women, incidence is 20%, and it is 15% in women with CPP. The incidence is very high amongst Japanese women.

Characteristics of endometriosis

- The ectopic endometrial tissue responds to ovarian hormones.
- Although proliferative endometrium is always seen, secretory endometrium depends upon the presence of progesterone receptors in the tissues.
- Blood oozing during menstruation in ectopic endometrium causes local adhesions in the pelvis.
- Malignancy is extremely rare, though endometrial tissue is highly proliferative.

AETIOLOGY

Endometriosis is a proliferative hormone-dependent disease of the childbearing period. It is extremely rare before menarche and disappears after menopause. Its incidence appears to be on the increase partly due to improvement in diagnostic techniques and partly due to changing social patterns such as late marriage and limitation of family size. It tends to occur more amongst the affluent class, and is frequently associated with infertility. Genetic susceptibility and familial tendency are seen in 15% cases.

Several theories have been propounded to explain endometriosis; chief among these are the following.

IMPLANTATION THEORY

Sampson's pioneering work in 1922 attributed endometriosis to reflux of menstrual endometrium through the fallopian tubes and its subsequent implantation and growth on the pelvic peritoneum and the surrounding structures. Sampson observed that in cases of uncomplicated endometriosis, the fallopian tubes were usually patent. Several workers then questioned the viability of desquamated endometrium and its capacity to implant and grow. Convincing support to Sampson's theory of retrograde menstruation, implantation and spread has been provided by the experimental work of Scott, Te Linde and Wharton. The occurrence of scar endometriosis following classical caesarean section, hysterotomy, myomectomy and episiotomy further supports this view.

Lately, it has been suggested that hypotonia of the uterotubal junction influences the quantity of retrograde spill and occurrence of pelvic endometriosis. The occurrence of endometriosis in young girls with cryptomenorrhoea, and retrograde collection of menstrual fluid, is also a proof of Sampson's implantation theory.

COELOMIC METAPLASIA THEORY

Meyer and Ivanoff (1919) propounded that endometriosis arises as a result of metaplastic changes in embryonic cell rests of embryonic mesothelium, which are capable of responding to hormonal stimulation. Embryologically, Müllerian ducts arise from these same tissues; hence, such a transformation in later life seems plausible.

METASTATIC THEORY

Although the above theories can explain the occurrence of endometriosis at the usual sites, they found it difficult to explain its occurrence at less accessible sites such as the umbilicus, pelvic lymph nodes, ureter, rectovaginal septum, bowel wall, and remote sites such as the lung, pleura, endocardium and the extremities. Hence, it was suggested by Halban et al. (1924) that embolization of menstrual fragments occurs through vascular or lymphatic channels, and this leads to the launching of endometriosis at distal sites. Endometrial tissue has been retrieved in pelvic lymphatics in 20% women with endometriosis.

HORMONAL INFLUENCE

Whatever be the initial genesis of endometriosis, its further development depends on the presence of hormones, mainly oestrogen. Pregnancy causes atrophy of endometriosis chiefly through high progesterone levels. Regression also follows oophorectomy and irradiation. Endometriosis is rarely seen before puberty and it regresses after menopause. Hormones with antioestrogenic activity also suppress endometriosis and are used therapeutically.

Cyclical hormones stimulate its growth, but continuous hormone secretion or therapy suppresses it. Smoking reduces oestrogen level, thereby the incidence of endometriosis proliferation.

IMMUNOLOGICAL FACTOR

The peritoneal fluid in endometriosis contains macrophages cytokines and natural killer (NK) cells which clear blood spilled into the peritoneal cavity. Impaired T cell and NK cell activity and altered immunology in a woman may increase the susceptibility to proliferation and growth.

OTHER FACTORS

Other factors implicated in the occurrence of endometriosis are genetic, multifactorial, vaginal or cervical atresia encouraging retrograde spill. The more frequent the cycles, and the more the bleeding, greater is the risk of endometriosis. Prostaglandins secreted by endometriotic tissue may exacerbate chronic pain and dysmenorrhoea.

Risk factors are polymenorrhagia, retroverted uterus, which increases the risk of retrograde spill. A woman who has undergone tubectomy rarely develops endometriosis. History of familial tendency is reported in 15% cases.

Genetic basis accounts for 10% of endometriosis; and incidence in first-degree relative is sevenfold. It may be that several factors are involved in the aetiology of endometriosis at different sites and none of the above theories fits into the development of endometriosis in a particular category.

The incidence is lower in multi paras and those on oral contraceptives.

SITES OF ENDOMETRIOSIS (Table 14.1)

Endometriosis is found widely dispersed throughout the lower pelvis, and below the level of umbilicus. The common sites are the ovaries, the pouch of Douglas, including the uterosacral ligaments, peritoneum overlying the bladder, sigmoid colon, back of the uterus, ovarian fossa, intestinal coils and appendix. Endometriosis is seen in the umbilicus following an operation, in laparotomy scars, in tubal stumps following sterilization operation, in the amputated stump of the cervix and in the scars of the vulva and perineum (Fig. 14.1). Scar endometriosis following lower segment caesarean section is seen in only 0.2%, but is high following classical caesarean section.

Rectovaginal septal endometriosis has a different origin and is described later in this chapter.

Table 14.1 Sites of Endometriosis

- Pelvic endometriosis
- Pelvic peritoneum, pouch of Douglas, uterosacral ligament
- Rectovaginal endometriosis
- Ovarian endometriosis
- Chocolate cyst of ovary
- Other sites – appendix, pelvic lymph nodes; metastatic – lungs, umbilicus and scar endometriosis

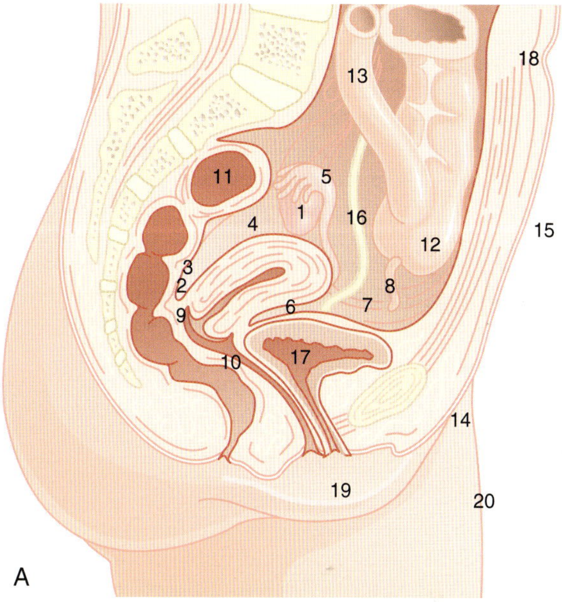

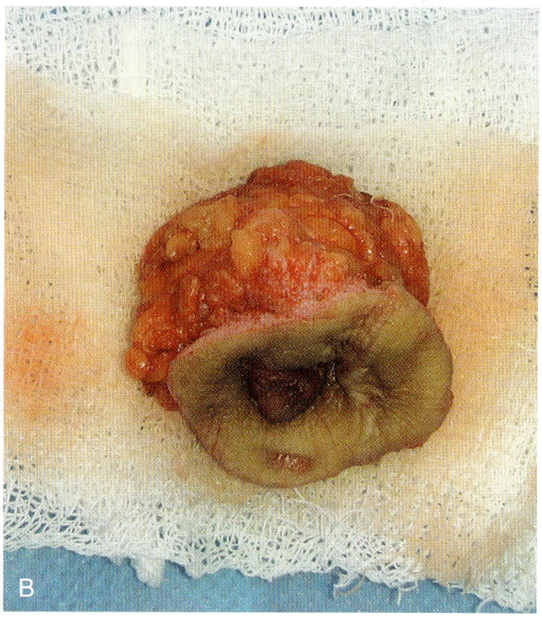

Figure 14.1 **(A)** Common sites of endometriosis in decreasing order of frequency: (1) ovary, (2) cul-de-sac, (3) uterosacral ligaments, (4) broad ligaments, (5) fallopian tubes, (6) uterovesical fold, (7) round ligaments, (8) vermiform appendix, (9) vagina, (10) rectovaginal septum, (11) rectosigmoid colon, (12) cecum, (13) ileum, (14) inguinal canals, (15) abdominal scars, (16) ureters, (17) urinary bladder, (18) umbilicus, (19) vulva and (20) peripheral sites. **(B)** Scar endometriosis. (*Source* **(A):** Hacker NF, Gambone JC, Hobel CJ. Hacker and Moore's Essentials of Obstetrics and Gynecology, 5th ed. Philadelphia: Elsevier, 2010.)

PATHOLOGY

There are three common types of endometriosis.

- Pelvic endometriosis may be localized or diffused and scattered over the pelvic peritoneum, pouch of Douglas and uterosacral ligaments.
- Ovarian endometriosis or chocolate cyst.
- Rectovaginal endometriosis.

Each category has a different mode of development.

PELVIC ENDOMETRIOSIS

Early lesions appear papular and red vesicles are filled with haemorrhagic fluid with surrounding flame-like lesions. With age, these vesicles change colour and *endometriotic areas* appear as dark red, bluish or black cystic areas adherent to the site where they are lodged. Scarring around the endometriosis gives it a puckered look. Lately, atypical lesions such as nonpigmented areas or yellowish-white thick plaques have been noticed, which are healed lesions. Peritoneal cavity contains yellowish-brown fluid in the cul-de-sac, and this contains prostaglandin responsible for pain. Powder-burnt areas are inactive and old lesions are seen scattered over the pelvic peritoneum.

Sometimes, healed areas of endometriosis appear as small peritoneal defects (windows) or white patches.

CHOCOLATE CYSTS OF OVARY

Chocolate cysts of the ovaries represent the most important manifestation of endometriosis. To the naked eye, the chocolate cyst shows obvious thickening of the tunica albuginea, and vascular red adhesions are well marked on the undersurface of the ovary. The inner surface of the cyst wall is vascular and contains areas of dark brown tissue. The chocolate cyst lies between the ovary and the lateral pelvic wall (Figs 14.2–14.4).

Histology fails to reveal endometrial tissue in most chocolate cysts. The lining epithelium is usually columnar with a tendency to form papillae. Beneath the epithelium, a zone of tissue containing large cells with brown cytoplasm, polyhedral

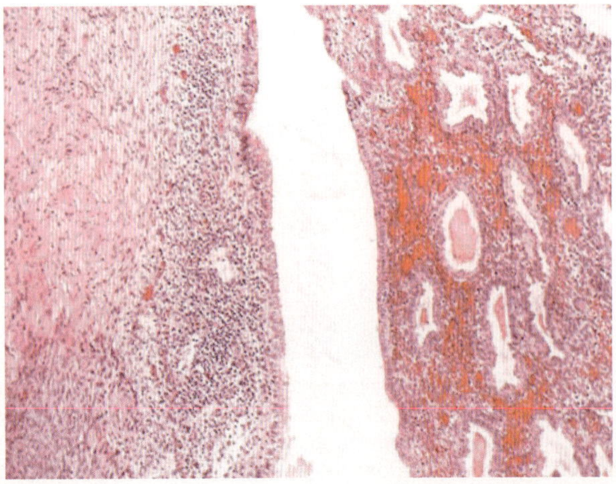

Figure 14.2 Typical endometriotic cyst lining containing endometrial glands (right) or a more attenuated lining with sparse stroma (left). (*Source:* From Figure 22-48. Christopher P Crum, Marisa R Nucci and Kenneth R Lee: Diagnostic Gynecologic and Obstetric Pathology. Elsevier: Saunders, 2011.)

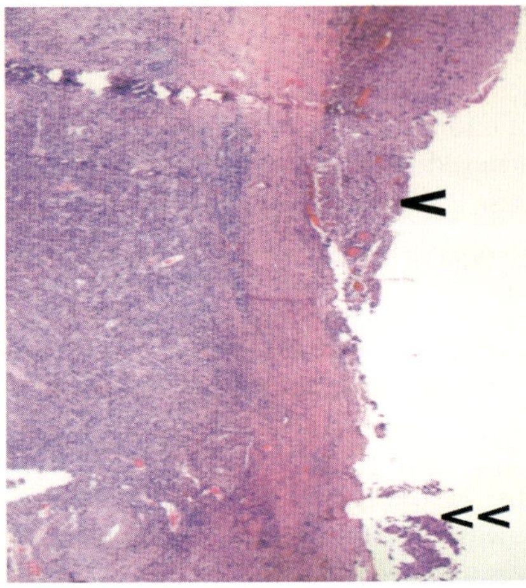

Figure 14.3 Lining of the primary squamous cell carcinoma of the ovary showing endometriosis at the top (<) and carcinoma at the bottom (<<) (magnification ×4). (*Source:* From Figure 1. *International Journal of Gynecology and Obstetrics.*In: Primary squamous cell carcinoma of the ovary associated with endometriosis. Pages 16–20, 2009.)

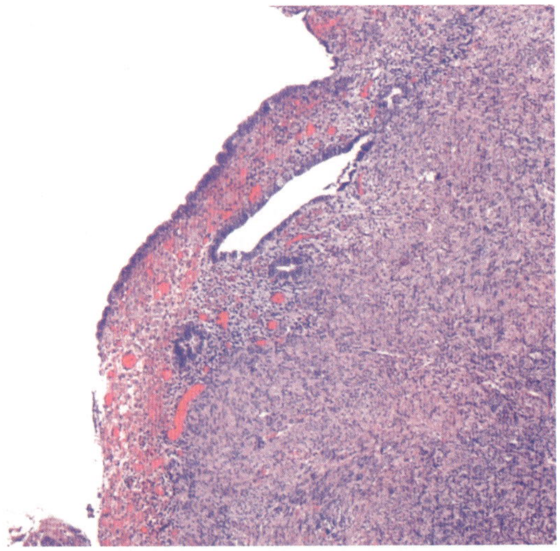

Figure 14.4 Focus of ovarian endometriosis adjacent to carcinoma (magnification ×10). (*Source:* From Figure 1. International Journal of Gynecology and Obstetrics. In: Primary squamous cell carcinoma of the ovary associated with endometriosis. Pages 16–20, 2009.)

in shape and resembling lutein cells is nearly always seen. These pseudoxanthoma cells are probably large macrophages or scavenger cells, and their brown colouration is due to ingested blood pigments such as haemosiderin. The chocolate cyst develops as an invagination into the ovarian cortex. Circular peritoneal defects over the broad ligament and uterosacral ligaments reveal endometriotic tissue by biopsy in 50% cases, and they are healed areas of endometriosis. The levels of tumour necrosis factor and matrix metallo-proteinase inhibitors are raised in pelvic endometriosis.

STAGING OF ENDOMETRIOSIS

The current classification (Table 14.2) is based on the appearance, size and depth of peritoneal and ovarian implants, presence and extent of adnexal adhesions and

Table 14.2 American Society for Reproductive Medicine Revised Classification of Endometriosis (1996)

Patient's Name	**Age/Date**		
Stage I	(Minimal)	Score 1–5	Laparoscopy/laparotomy/photography
Stage II	(Mild)	Score 6–15	Recommended treatment
Stage III	(Moderate)	Score 16–40	
Stage IV	(Severe)	Score > 40	
Total	*Prognosis*		
Peritoneal endometriosis	<1 cm	1–3 cm	>3 cm
Superficial	1	2	4
Deep	2	4	6
Ovarian endometriosis	<1 cm	1–3 cm	>3 cm
Right side – superficial	1	2	4
Deep	4	16	20
Left side – superficial	1	2	4
Deep	4	16	20
Posterior cul-de-sac obliteration	Partial		Complete
	4		40
Ovarian adhesions	<1/3 Enclosure	1/3–2/3 Enclosure	>2/3 Enclosure
Right side – flimsy	1	2	4
Dense	4	8	16
Left side – flimsy	1	2	4
Dense	4	8	16
Tubal adhesions[a]	<1/3 Enclosure	1/3–2/3 Enclosure	>2/3 Enclosure
Right side – flimsy	1	2	4
Dense	4	8	16
Left side – flimsy	1	2	4
Dense	4	8	16

[a]If the fimbriated end of the fallopian tube is completely closed, change the assignment to 16.
Note additional endometriosis. Note presence of any associated pathology. (*Source:* Reproduced from *Fertility and Sterility* 1985; 43: 351–52.)

the degree of obliteration of the pouch of Douglas. It does not take into account complaints such as infertility or pain; however, it forms the acceptable basis for comparison of therapeutic outcomes in relieving symptoms and improving fertility.

Availability of laparoscopic procedures has made it possible to diagnose with confidence small and early lesions, which are often asymptomatic, assess the extent and severity of the disease and allow an accurate classification prior to initiating of therapy. The classification described by the American Fertility Society (1985) is based on the size and location of the endometriotic lesion and is classified as minimal, mild, moderate and severe (Fig. 14.5). This classification is correlated with fertility outcome rather than pain symptoms.

Minimal. Small spots of endometriosis seen at laparoscopy, but no clinical symptoms.

Mild. Scattered fresh superficial lesions. No scarring or retraction. No adnexal adhesions.

Moderate. Ovaries are involved, with some scarring and retraction. They contain endometriomas not more than 2 cm in size. There are minimal peritubal and periovarian adhesions. Endometriotic lesions in the anterior and posterior peritoneal pouch with some scarring and retraction may be seen.

Severe. Ovaries are involved, with the size of the endometriomas exceeding 2 cm. Dense peritubal and periovarian adhesions severely restrict mobility. The uterosacral ligaments are thickened and involved, and lastly, there may be evidence of involvement of the bowel and urinary tract.

Laparoscopic findings vary with the duration of the lesion, size and location. 'Powder-burn' – puckered black spots, red vascular, bluish, blackish cysts, chocolate cysts and dense adhesions in the pelvis as well as yellow-brown peritoneal fluid are the findings. Biopsy of the lesion may be necessary to confirm the diagnosis in doubtful cases. Early

Stage I (Minimal)

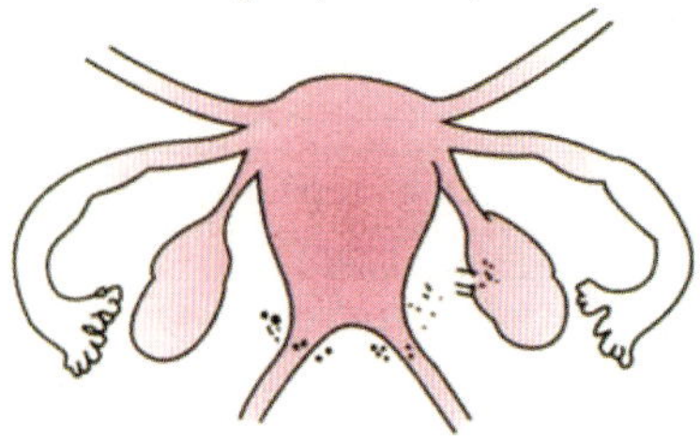

Peritoneum		
Superficial endo	– 1–3 cm	2
R. ovary		
Superficial endo	– <1 cm	1
Filmy adhesions	– <1/3	1
Total points		4

Stage II (Mild)

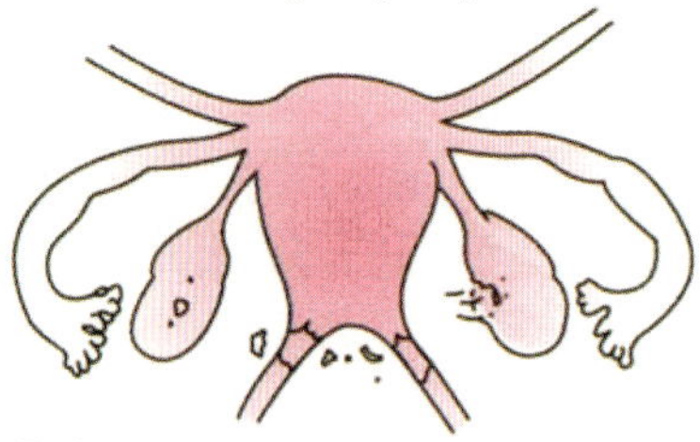

Peritoneum		
Deep endo	– >3 cm	6
R. ovary		
Superficial endo	– <1 cm	1
Filmy adhesions	– <1/3	1
L. ovary		
Superficial endo	– <1 cm	1
Total points		9

Stage III (Moderate)

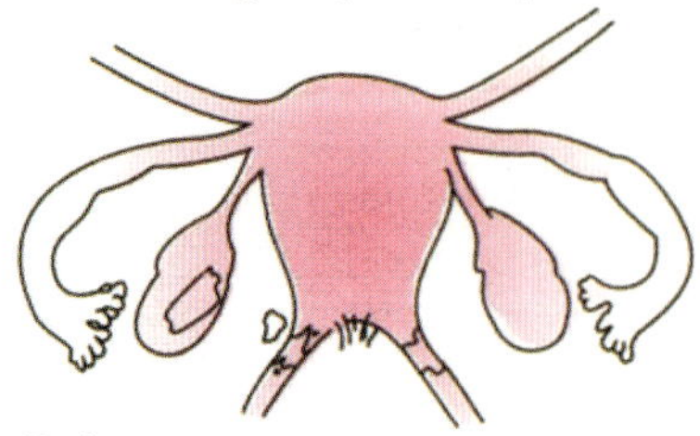

Peritoneum		
Deep endo	– >3 cm	6
Cul-de-sac		
Partial obliteration	– <1 cm	4
L. ovary		
Deep endo	– <1–3 cm	16
Total points		26

Stage III (Moderate)

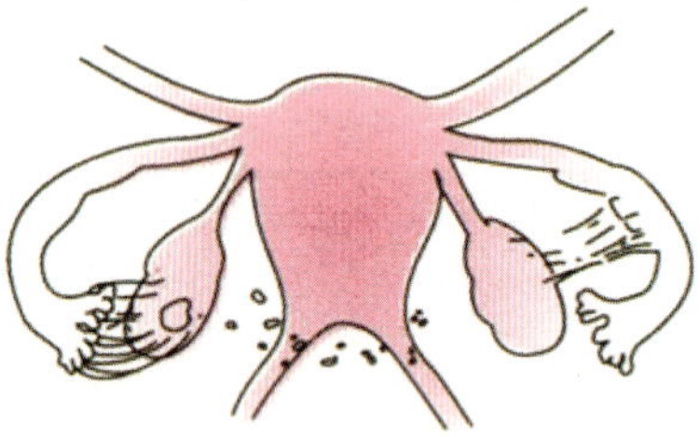

Peritoneum		
Superficial endo	– >3 cm	3
R. tube		
Filmy adhesions	– <1/3	1
R. ovary		
Filmy adhesions	– <1/3	1
L. tube		
Dense adhesions	– <1/3	16•
L. ovary		
Deep endo	– <1 cm	4
Dense adhesions	– <1/3	4
Total points		29

Stage IV (Severe)

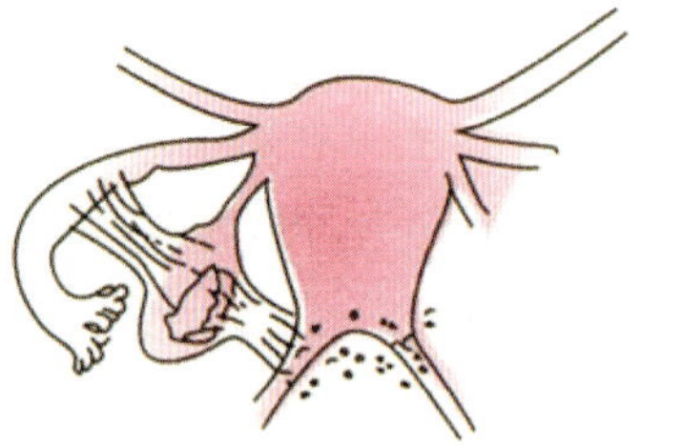

Peritoneum		
Superficial endo	– >3 cm	3
L. ovary		
Deep endo	v <1–3 cm	32••
Dense adhesions	– <1/3	8••
L. tube		
Dense adhesions	– <1/3	8••
Total points		51

•Point assignment changed to 16
••Point assignment doubled

Stage IV (Severe)

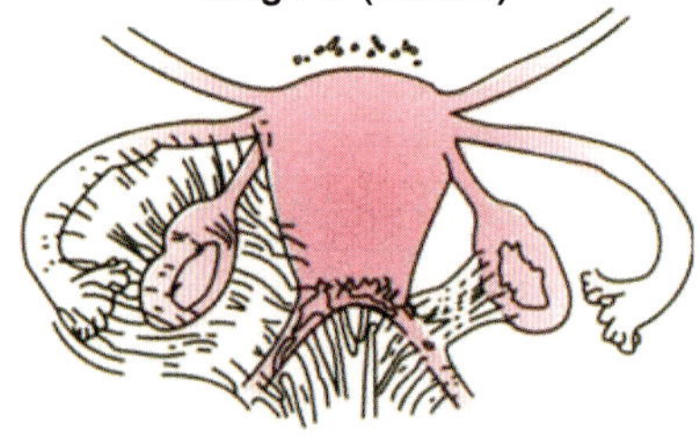

Peritoneum		
Deep endo	– >3 cm	6
Cul-de-sac		
Complete obliteration		40
R. ovary		
Deep endo	– <1–3 cm	16
Dense adhesions	– <1/3	4
L. tube		
Dense adhesions	– >2/3	16
L. ovary		
Deep endo	– 1–3 cm	16
Dense adhesions	– >2/3	16
Total points		114

Figure 14.5 American Society for Reproductive Medicine Revised Classification of Endometriosis (endo, endometriosis).

and fresh lesions appear red flame-like raised areas, whereas older and healed lesions present yellow brown patches and white plaques over the peritoneum and peritoneal windows. The lesions are more marked on the left side because the sigmoid colon forms a conduit for the tissue to grow. It is not surprising for laparoscopy to reveal pelvic endometriosis in an asymptomatic woman.

Poor correlation between the naked eye appearance and histology is well documented. Therefore, biopsy of the suspicious areas becomes necessary to prove the presence of endometriosis.

CLINICAL FEATURES

Endometriosis affects women in the reproductive age, i.e. around 30 years of age. It may occur in an adolescent if obstruction in the lower genital tract causes cryptomenorrhoea and retrograde spill of menstrual fluid. A rare case of endometriosis has been reported in a postmenopausal woman on hormone replacement therapy (HRT).

SYMPTOMS

The symptoms vary according to the site, depth of lesion and do not always correlate well with the extent of disease. The classic symptom complex includes dysmenorrhoea, dyspareunia, menorrhagia and infertility. About 30% of the patients are asymptomatic. Overlapping of symptoms is common. The following are the common symptoms.

DYSMENORRHOEA

This is the most common symptom. About 70% pain begins before the onset of menstruation, builds up continuously until the flow begins, and thereafter it declines gradually. The character of pain can be very variable, from a dull ache to grinding or crushing pain, colicky pain or a bearing-down pain. Backache is a common accompaniment. Sometimes, there may be radiating pain along the sciatic nerve. With passage of time, the intensity and duration of pain increases and dysmenorrhoea may persist for a few days after menstruation. Pain of endometriosis is chiefly related to the location and not the extent of the lesion. Deeper lesions cause more pain than superficial ones. The peritoneal fluid contains prostaglandin, which is supposed to cause dysmenorrhoea and abdominal pain.

ABDOMINAL PAIN

Lower abdominal pain of varying intensity may appear at any time but is usually common around menstruation. It is a dull ache culminating in dysmenorrhoea. Occasionally, the pain suddenly becomes very severe, presenting as an acute abdomen necessitating immediate surgery. At laparotomy, a ruptured chocolate cyst is observed.

DYSPAREUNIA

Endometriotic involvement of the cul-de-sac and the uterosacral ligaments may produce adhesions and fixation of the uterus and nodular thickening of the uterosacral ligaments. Movements of the cervix elicit tenderness. Dyspareunia and backache may be the result of this pathology. These patients are often reluctant to attempt intercourse, and this adds to the magnitude of infertility (25%–50%).

INFERTILITY

Endometriosis affects fertility at all stages of the disease but in asymptomatic women with mild disease, infertility is difficult to explain. Although about one-fifth of all women who are infertile tend to suffer from endometriosis, the incidence of infertility amongst women suffering from endometriosis ranges between 30% and 40%. Endometriosis possibly interferes with tubal motility and function. It may inhibit ovulation, ovum pick-up by the fimbria, and because of dyspareunia there is reduced frequency of sexual intercourse. Other causes of infertility are luteinized unruptured follicular (LUF) syndrome, increased prolactin and corpus luteal phase defect, nonovulation and tubal blockage as well as poor oocyte quality. Prostaglandin affects the tubal motility and also causes corpus luteolysis. The activated macrophages in the peritoneal fluid engulf the sperms or immobilize them.

MENSTRUAL SYMPTOMS

Menorrhagia (20%) is common with adenomyosis, and irregular bleeding may occur with cervical and vaginal lesions. Polymenorrhoea is noted with ovarian involvement (10%–30%).

CHRONIC PELVIC PAIN

Endometriosis is one of the important causes of CPP. Brownish-yellow peritoneal fluid containing prostaglandin E_2 is responsible for this pain. Nerve entrapment in endometriosis tissue may also be responsible for pain.

OTHER SYMPTOMS

Urological symptoms such as increase in frequency, dysuria and, in rare cases, haematuria during menstruation may result from bladder or ureteral involvement. Obstruction of the ureter directly or as a result of kinking by adhesions leads to hydronephrosis and renal infection. Bowel symptoms are often the result of direct involvement of the sigmoid colon and rectum causing painful defecation, diarrhoea and melaena around menstruation. Occasionally, pelvic endometriotic adnexal masses can cause obstructive symptoms of constipation and present with a painful abdominal mass or as an acute abdomen simulating peritonitis, appendicitis or an ectopic pregnancy. Scar endometriosis causes cyclical pain and enlargement, and pulmonary lesion causes cyclical haemoptysis.

PHYSICAL FINDINGS

Abdominal examination may reveal a cystic swelling which simulates an ovarian tumour in a chocolate cyst of the ovary. The swelling is often fixed and may be slightly tender. Speculum examination may reveal bluish or blackish puckered spots in the posterior fornix, and these spots may be tender to touch. The presence of these puckered spots is pathognomonic of endometriosis. Vaginal examination reveals a tender fixed retroverted uterus. A fixed tender cystic mass or bilateral masses may be felt in the pelvis. If the uterosacral ligaments and the pouch of Douglas feel thickened and shotty with multiple small nodules palpable through the posterior fornix, the diagnosis becomes reasonably certain. These are described as cobblestone feel of uterosacral ligaments. During vaginal examination, tenderness in the lateral fornices indicates the possible existence of endometriosis even in the absence of any adnexal mass.

ENDOCRINOLOGICAL ABNORMALITIES

Endometriosis is often associated with anovulation, abnormal follicular development, luteal insufficiency and premenstrual spotting. Luteinization of the unruptured follicle is known to occur, and hyperprolactinaemia with associated galactorrhoea are noted findings. However, no definite correlation between these endocrine events and the degree of endometriosis has been established. Cortisol and prolactin may be slightly raised.

DIFFERENTIAL DIAGNOSIS

Because of varied clinical features, endometriosis poses a diagnostic challenge at times.

- Chronic pelvic inflammatory disease (PID) closely mimics endometriosis in its symptoms and signs. Both the conditions produce pelvic pain, congestive dysmenorrhoea, menorrhagia and sterility. Endometriosis may, if there is leakage of blood contents, produce leucocytosis, raised erythrocyte sedimentation rate (ESR) and moderate fever. Both also have similar physical signs. Laparoscopic visualization of the pelvis will reveal the true pathology.
- Uterine myomas, unless degenerate, are painless and the uterus is not fixed. Ultrasound and laparoscopic visualization will differentiate one condition from the other.
- Ovarian malignant tumour with metastatic deposits in the pouch of Douglas can be mistaken for endometriosis. History, pain, age of the patient and other symptoms suggestive of endometriosis are against the diagnosis of cancer, but the physical signs, apart from tenderness, are very similar to those of an ovarian neoplasm.
- Rectosigmoid involvement will cause rectal symptoms which resemble the symptoms of rectal carcinoma. It may be impossible to make an accurate diagnosis until sigmoidoscopy and biopsy are performed.
- If the chocolate cyst ruptures, all possibilities of an acute abdominal catastrophe must be considered, including a ruptured tubal gestation, though the most frequent error is to operate for acute appendicitis.
- Chronic pelvic congestion syndrome due to other causes must be excluded by ultrasound, CT, magnetic resonance imaging (MRI) and laparoscopy.

Table 14.3 Investigations

Laparoscopy – diagnostic and therapeutic. Gold standard.
CA 125 > 35 U/mL
Ultrasound – mass, echogenic areas
MRI:
Colour Doppler – increased blood flow
Cystoscopy – Urinary cause
Sigmoidoscopy – rectal cause
Antiendometrial antibodies

INVESTIGATIONS (Table 14.3)

LAPAROSCOPIC FINDINGS

These have already been described earlier. Laparoscopy should be employed not merely for diagnostic purposes; the endoscopist should be able to proceed with minimal invasive surgery (see below) in the presence of this pathology. Laparoscopy is the gold standard in the diagnosis of endometriosis. The diagnosis should be validated by peritoneal and tissue biopsy (Fig. 14.6) because corpus luteal haematoma can resemble a chocolate cyst.

Role of laparoscopy

- To detect and diagnose pelvic endometriosis.
- Locate the site of endometriosis and staging.
- To take biopsy.
- To surgically treat endometriosis by ablation and removal.

CA-125, glycoprotein and cell surface antigen, is raised to more than 35 U/mL in 80% cases of endometriosis and the level is directly proportional to the extent of the disease. The level is not specific, because it is also raised in abdominal tuberculosis, PID, malignant epithelial ovarian tumour, chronic liver disease and in 2% normal women, especially during menstruation. Although CA-125 estimation may not be helpful in the initial diagnosis, once the diagnosis is established, raised level of CA-125 indicates either persistence or recurrence of the disease in the follow-up.

ULTRASOUND AND MRI

Transvaginal ultrasound reveals an echo-free cyst, low-level echoes or clumps of high-density level echoes representing clots. The cyst wall is thick and irregular, and multiple cysts in different phases of evolution may be observed. Ultrasound is 83% sensitive and 98% specific, as small nodules may not be picked up by ultrasound.

CT and MRI give identical picture as in ultrasound, and are not more useful in the diagnosis of endometriosis (Figs 14.7 and 14.8).

- Colour Doppler flow shows increased vascularity but does not confirm the diagnosis – vascularity is diffuse; in a fibroid, blood vessels are seen in the periphery.
- Cystoscopy will identify involvement of the bladder.
- Sigmoidoscopy is required if the woman develops bowel symptoms. A biopsy is required if malignancy is suspected.
- Antiendometrial antibodies are identified in the serum, peritoneal fluid and endometriotic fluid as well as in normal endometrial tissue. However, as yet, these are not measured to be of screening value and used as a tissue marker. These may also not be sensitive and specific.
- Tumour necrosis factor is raised proportionately to the severity of the disease.
- MRI reveals thickening of ligaments and nodules.

PROPHYLAXIS

- Low-dose oral contraceptive pills reduce the menstrual flow and protect against endometriosis. Three monthly oral pills are convenient to take and are effective.
- Tubal patency tests should be avoided in the immediate premenstrual phase to avoid spill.
- Operations on the genital tract should be scheduled in the postmenstrual period.
- Classical caesarean section and hysterotomy operation which cause scar endometriosis are now rarely performed.

MANAGEMENT

Minimal asymptomatic cases should be observed over 6–8 months. Infertility should be investigated and treated as necessary (Fig. 14.5).

All symptomatic women need treatment. The treatment (Fig. 14.9) depends upon the age of the patient, need for preserving reproductive functions, severity of the symptoms, extent of the disease, response to medical treatment, relief obtained with any previous conservative surgery and the attitude of the patient towards her problem. The objective of the treatment should be to eradicate the lesion and avoid recurrence of the disease process, alleviate symptoms, facilitate childbearing and enable the patient to lead a comfortable life. Therefore, the treatment should be individualized. The treatment comprises medical and surgical and a combination of both.

DRUG TREATMENT

Drug treatment should aim at causing atrophy of the ectopic endometrium with minimal side effects, improving symptoms, fertility rate and avoiding or delaying recurrence.

Endometriosis is oestrogen dependent. Hormones act on receptors in the endometriotic tissue and cause their atrophy and shrinkage. The purpose of administration of various hormones is to act as antioestrogens; the drugs produce a hypo-oestrogenic effect. Superficial lesions respond better than the deeper ones. However, one must note that hormonal therapy suppresses endometriosis for the duration of therapy; it does not prevent recurrence once the therapy is stopped. Moreover, the hormones delay pregnancy by their contraceptive effect and cause side effects on prolonged therapy, besides the drugs being expensive. The drugs are best suited for multiparous women.

1. **Combined oral contraceptives (OCP).** It is used as a primary treatment or preoperatively to shrink endometriosis. Administered intermittently or continuously, oral contraceptives may alleviate the disease. However, high incidence of side effects and risk of thromboembolism

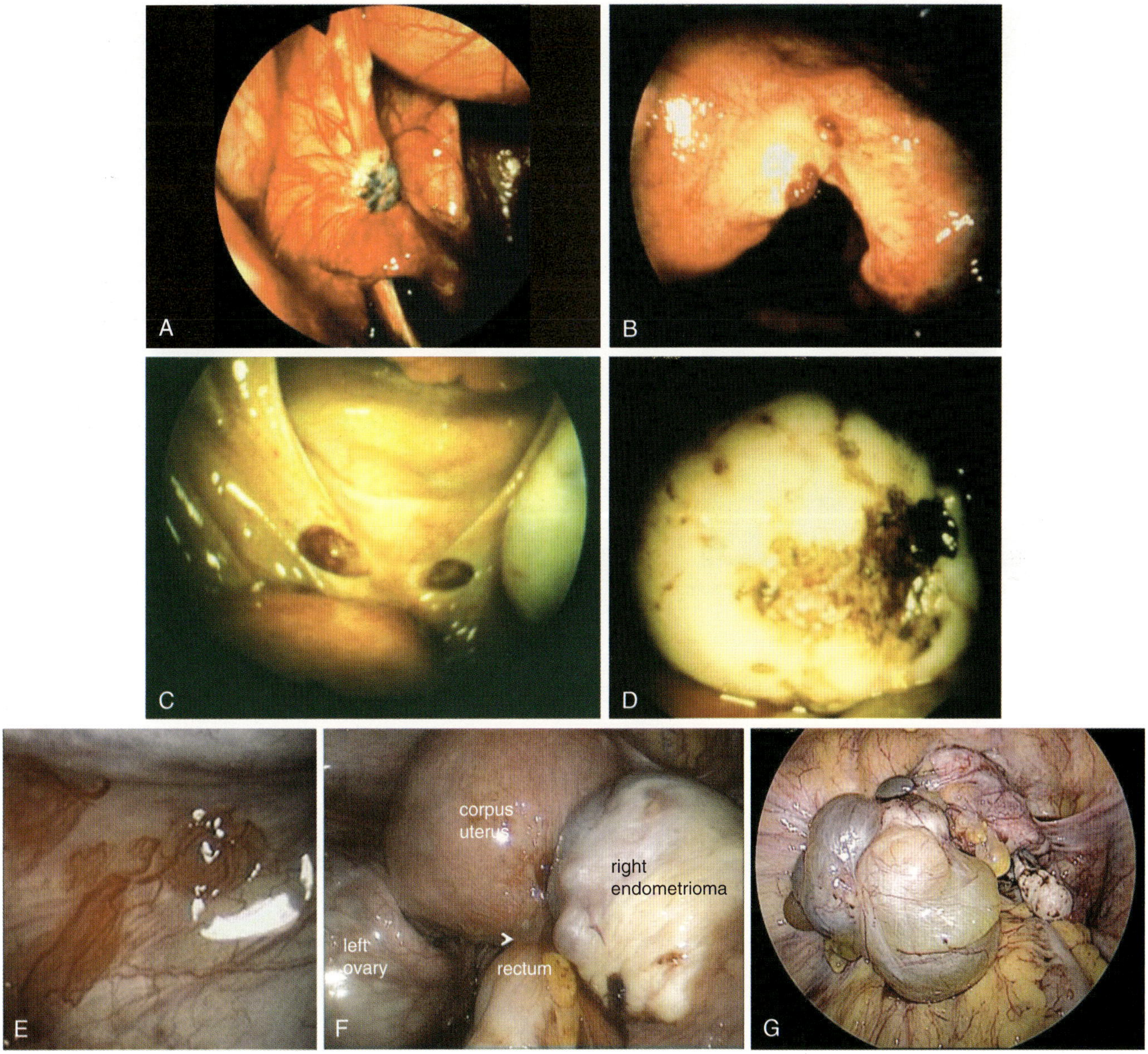

Figure 14.6 **(A–D)** Appearance of old endometriosis with 'tattooing' (blue-grey lesions), and red, brown and black raised lesions of active endometriosis at the time of laparoscopy. **(E)** Pelvic endometriosis showing red lesions on laparoscopy. **(F)** Complete obliteration of the pouch of Douglas (white arrowhead) was noted during diagnostic laparoscopy. **(G)** Laparoscopic view of bilateral endometriosis. (*Source* **(A–D):** Hacker NF, Gambone JC, Hobel CJ. Hacker and Moore's Essentials of Obstetrics and Gynecology, 5th ed. Philadelphia: Elsevier, 2010.) (*Courtesy* **(G):** Dr Vivek Marwah, New Delhi.)

limit their prolonged use. About 30% pregnancy rate is reported following this treatment. OCP delay pregnancy. Seasonale OCP for 84 days, with 6 days tablet-free, reduces the menstrual periods to just four cycles in a year and may be suited in endometriosis.

2. **Oral progestogens.** These drugs exert an antioestrogenic effect and their continuous administration causes decidualization and endometrial atrophy. The treatment over a period of 6–9 months produces a state of pseudopregnancy, which ultimately causes regression of the disease. The drugs in common use are norethisterone, 5.0–20.0 mg daily, or dydrogesterone 10–30 mg daily. Dydrogesterone 40–60 mg daily in the luteal phase relieves symptoms. *This hormone does not prevent ovulation and is suitable for a woman trying to conceive.* It also has less toxic side effects. Instead of restricted luteal phase administration, it can be given 10 mg b.d. from day 5–25 for three cycles. Tibolone is also useful in endometriosis. Medroxyprogesterone acetate may be administered as a long-acting depot preparation, 50 mg i.m. weekly, 100 mg i.m. every 2 weeks for 3 months, followed by 200 mg monthly for 3–6 months or oral 30 mg daily. About 50%–70% symptomatic relief and pregnancy rate of 40%–50% have been reported. Weight gain and irregular bleeding are the side effects of progestogens. Other side effects include reduced libido, mental depression, breast tenderness and decreased high-density lipoprotein (HDL). Moreover, fertility is impaired for 2 years after prolonged

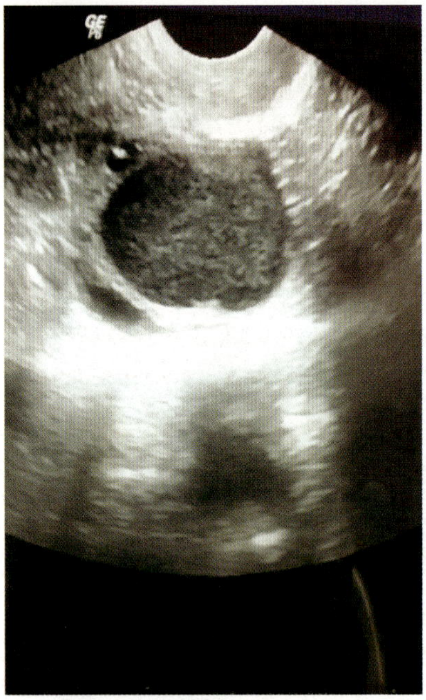

Figure 14.7 Ultrasound showing endometrioma.

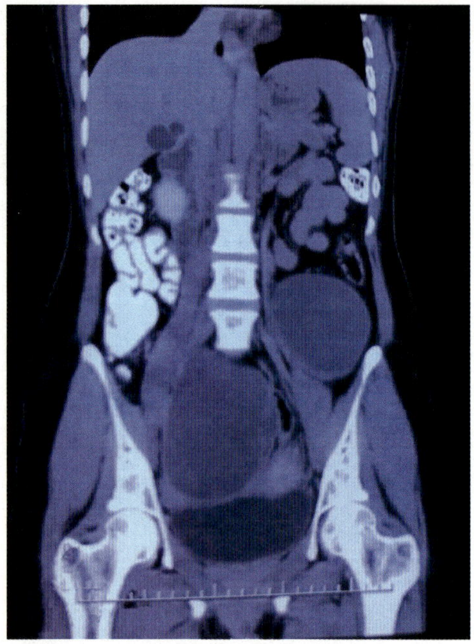

Figure 14.8 MRI showing endometrioma.

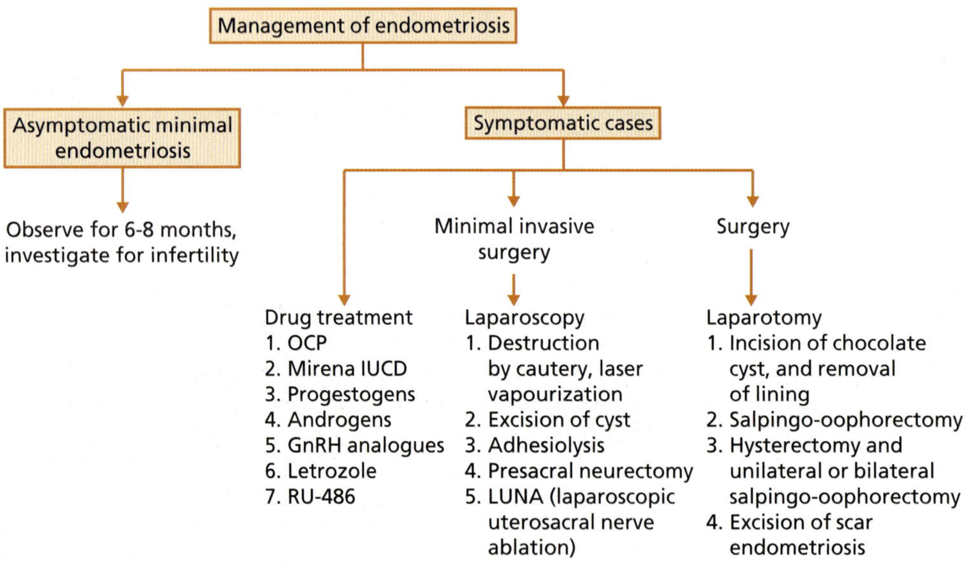

Figure 14.9 Management of endometriosis.

hormone therapy. The side effects are dose and duration related. *Mirena IUCD reduces dysmenorrhoea and menorrhagia in endometriosis.* It is a one-time treatment lasting for 5 years with minimal systemic side effects. Danacrine, an anabolic drug, does not cause menopausal symptoms, as E_2 level does not drop below 50 pg/mL. The progesterone level rises in 15 minutes, peaks in a few hours and stabilizes thereafter. It causes endometrial gland atrophy, and decidualization of stromal cells. It is ideal to relieve pain and menorrhagia in premenopausal women who have completed their families.

3. **Dydrogesterone** 40–60 mg daily in the luteal phase or 10 mg daily from 5th–25th day improves symptoms and the fertility rate.
4. **Danazol**, a synthetic derivative of ethinyl testosterone, inhibits pituitary gonadotropins. It is mildly anabolic, antioestrogenic and antiprogestational. It reduces sex hormone–binding globulin SHBG and releases free testosterone. It is a very effective, though an expensive drug, and is administered in doses of 200–800 mg daily for 3–6 months starting on the first day of menses. It causes symptoms simulating menopause if used in higher doses over 6–8 months. The lesions regress remarkably, but many patients suffer from side effects such as weight gain, hirsutism, excessive sweating, muscle cramps, depression, atrophy of breasts and vaginal epithelium, lowering of HDL, and liver and renal damage. The resulting amenorrhoea promptly corrects itself on withdrawal of the drug.

The chances of successful pregnancy following this therapy range from 30% to 50%. It is reported that 80% of endometrial implants resolve with danazol. Recurrence, however, is likely after stoppage of the drug (30%). It is contraindicated in liver dysfunction, and pregnancy should be avoided as it is teratogenic. Recently, danazol is implicated in the development of ovarian cancer, and many gynaecologists are now reluctant to use this drug.

Gestrinone is a 19-nortestosterone derivative similar to danazol in action, but it has fewer side effects and is long-acting. It reduces the LH surge and SHBG. Dose is 2.5–5 mg twice weekly. About 85%–90% patients experience amenorrhoea. Anti-inflammatory drugs, such as mefenamic acid 500 mg three times a day during menstruation, relieve dysmenorrhoea in 70%–80% patients. Other antiprostaglandin and anti-inflammatory (nonsteroidal) drugs such as naproxen are also useful.

5. **Gonadotropin-releasing hormone (GnRH).** This hormone is administered continuously to downregulate and suppress pituitary gonadotropins; it causes atrophy of the endometriotic tissue in 90% cases. The synthetic analogue of GnRH is given in doses of 10–20 mg i.v., twice daily, or 200–400 mg intranasally daily for 6 months. Monthly depot injection (Zoladex) of 3.6 mg is also available. Discontinuation of GnRH and danazol causes recurrence of endometriosis within a year in 50% cases. GnRH is better tolerated than danazol. However, prolonged GnRH therapy over 6 months causes hypo-oestrogenism and menopausal symptoms such as hot flushes, dry vagina, urethral syndrome and osteoporosis. To avoid this, add-back therapy with progestogens and tibolone or etidronate is recommended. This also allows prolonged therapy with GnRH for 2 years.

   Other drugs available are as follows:
   - Buserelin and leuprolide (nonapeptides).
   - Nafarelin and goserelin (decapeptide). The superficial lesions respond better than the deep-seated lesions.
   - Cetrorelix (GnRH antagonist) – 3 mg weekly × 8 weeks.
   - Goserelin 3.6 mg monthly subcutaneously.
   - Leuprolide 3.75 mg i.m. monthly or 11.25 mg 3 monthly.
6. **Aromatase inhibitors.** Aromatase inhibitors available are letrozole (2.5 mg), anastrozole (1–2 mg) and rofecoxib (12.5 mg) daily for 6 months. These are antioestrogen and should be given with vitamin D (400 g IU) and calcium (1 g) to prevent osteoporosis. Nausea, vomiting and diarrhoea are the other side effects. Anastrozole is less osteoporotic than others. They block aromatase activity by preventing the conversion of androgen to oestrogen. They may be combined with 2.5 mg norethisterone.
7. **RU486** (antiprogestogen) is also tried in a dose of 10–25 mg daily for 3 months. It reduces pain and delays recurrence.

   The failure and recurrence following medical therapy is due to the following:
   - The drug cannot penetrate the fibrotic capsule.
   - Ectopic endometrium responds less to hormones as compared to normal endometrium.
   - *Side effects* – Hormones prevent conception besides other consequences.

MINIMAL INVASIVE SURGERY

Hormones delay pregnancy, so primary surgery is preferred in infertile women. Recent advances in gynaecology have introduced laparoscopy in the management of pelvic endometriosis in young women. This offers the advantages of conserving the ovaries and the fallopian tubes, and improving fertility.

The methods employed are as follows:

- Aspiration of peritoneal fluid in cul-de-sac: It removes PGE_2 and relieves dysmenorrhoea, pelvic pain and improves pregnancy rate.
- Destruction of endometriotic implants less than 3 cm by diathermy cauterization, or vaporization by CO_2 or Nd:YAG laser. Superficial lesions are easier to destroy and yield better fertility results than the deep implants. Laser has the advantage of controlling the depth of destruction by adjusting the power density. It does not cause adhesions and fibrosis. It can be applied to the bowel and bladder.
- Larger lesions and chocolate cyst can be excised. The residual lesion can be dealt with by hormonal therapy. Cauterization of the cyst wall is preferred in young women. It avoids ovarian destruction with peeling off of the cyst wall but recurrence is slightly high.
- Role of surgery
  - Failed medical therapy
  - Infertility
  - Recurrence
  - Chocolate cyst of ovary
- The consensus of opinion is that cystectomy is more beneficial in extent of pain relief, longer recurrence time and longer pain-free intervals. However, the excision of the cyst wall deprives the patient of potential ova and thereby reduces her fertility potential. In older women, excision of the cyst wall is recommended.
- Laparoscopic lysis of adhesions in the pelvis relieves dysmenorrhoea and pelvic pain. It also restores patency of the fallopian tubes and ovulation. Presacral neurectomy can be performed simultaneously. Bleeding and haematoma are its complications. Pregnancy rate following minimal invasive surgery is around 30%–50%.
- Laser uterine nerve ablation (LUNA) for midline pain in endometriosis is effective in some cases.
- Pregnancy rate following conservative surgery is 40%, 50% and 70% in severe, moderate and mild endometriosis, respectively.
- Prolapse of genital tract and bladder dysfunction are noted with LUNA. It is advisable to postpone laparoscopic technique for 3 months if hormone therapy has already been given to avoid under diagnosis.

OTHER MODALITIES OF TREATMENT IN AN INFERTILE WOMAN ASSOCIATED WITH PELVIC ENDOMETRIOSIS (Fig. 14.10)

Ultrasonic-guided chocolate cyst aspiration followed by mifepristone for 6 months is also tried.

- *Mild endometriosis.* Surgery followed by superovulation and IUI/IVF (aspiration of endometriosis cyst).
- Advanced endometriosis involving the fallopian tube. The choice is between tuboplasty and IVF. Alternatively, 3 months of medical therapy followed by IVF.
- Postoperative medical therapy to deal with the residual tissue and prevent recurrence.

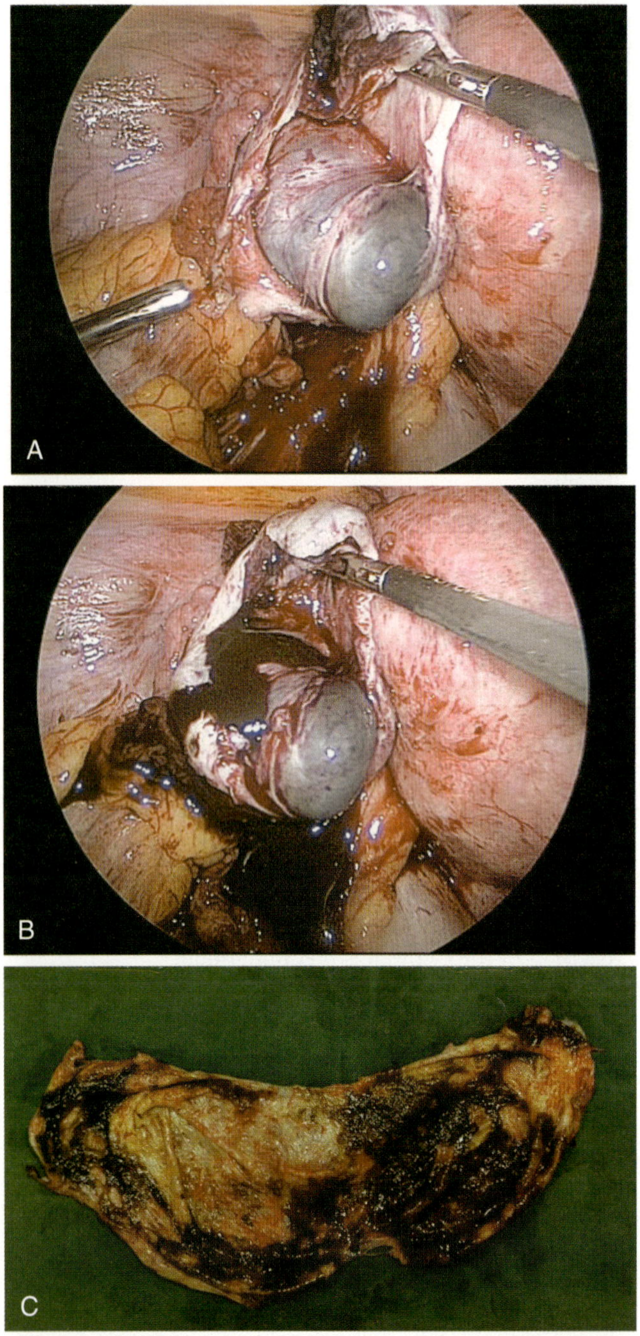

Figure 14.10 **(A)** Endometriotic cyst (chocolate cyst). **(B)** Same as (A), except that the cyst has burst. **(C)** Cut section of endometriotic cyst. (*Courtesy* **(A)** and **(B):** Dr Vivek Marwah, New Delhi.)

- Dydrogesterone 40 mg in the luteal phase relieves pain without compromising infertility, as it does not prevent ovulation.
- Pre- and postoperative hormonal therapy may alleviate symptoms but delay pregnancy.

SURGERY

Recurrence following conservative surgery may be seen in 10% at the end of 1 year and 25% at the end of 3 years. Adhesions form in 10%, more with cauterization than laser. These women may require second surgery, which may be technically difficult. Therefore, some prefer laparotomy over laparoscopy when repeat surgery is required. Indications for open surgery are as follows:

- Advanced stage of disease detected
- Large lesion – can be dealt with
- Medical therapy fails or is intolerable
- Recurrence occurs
- In elderly parous women

LAPAROTOMY

Laparotomy is also required in advanced stages and for larger lesions if medical therapy fails or hormones cannot be tolerated and for recurrence.

- Dissection and excision of a chocolate cyst.
- Salpingo-oophorectomy.
- Abdominal hysterectomy and bilateral salpingo-oophorectomy. Surgery can be difficult due to adhesions in pelvis.

Mirena IUCD is an alternative to a repeat surgery.

A premenopausal woman may need HRT after the radical surgery; tibolone is safer than E_2 P therapy. Scar endometriosis requires excision or danazol.

HRT following bilateral ovarian removal in young women may be prescribed under strict monitoring, as the risk of recurrence remains. Calcium and vitamin D are added to HRT. It may be better to delay HRT by 1–3 months to reduce risk of recurrence.

As mentioned before, tibolone 2.5 mg daily is better than E_2 and progestogen.

COMBINED THERAPY

Combined therapy is indicated in the following conditions.

- Preoperative GnRH monthly for 3 months reduces the size and extent of the lesions, softens the adhesions and makes the subsequent surgery easier and more complete.
- Postoperative hormonal therapy may be required if the surgery has been incomplete, and some residual lesion is left behind due to technical difficulty. It also reduces the recurrence rate.

ENDOMETRIOSIS OF THE RECTOVAGINAL SEPTUM

Rectovaginal endometriosis with obliteration of the pouch of Douglas involves the uterosacral ligaments, posterior fornix and anterior wall of the rectum and sigmoid colon. The aetiology of this condition differs from that of pelvic endometriosis. It is not caused by deep infiltration of pelvic endometriosis and retrograde menstruation but according to Nicolle et al., it is derived from embryologically derived Müllerian tissue and the theory of Müllerian metaplasia applies here. Rectovaginal endometriosis contains more fibrous tissue than glandular tissue with flame-like appearance. Laparoscopically, it is seen as a yellowish-white appearance with small haemorrhagic areas and dense fibrotic adhesions.

CLINICAL FEATURES

The woman is often of reproductive age. She complains of dysmenorrhoea, dyspareunia abdominal pain, backache and menorrhagia. If the rectum is involved, rectal pain, constipation and occasional diarrhoea may occur. Cyclical rectal bleeding is also reported. Ureteric compression with uterosacral ligament involvement causes renal damage.

Speculum examination is painful. Red spots are seen in the posterior fornix. Bimanual examination reveals thickening of the posterior fornix and uterosacral ligaments. Rectal examination should be performed to assess the rectal involvement.

DIFFERENTIAL DIAGNOSIS

The clinical features mimic PID, diverticulitis, colonic cancer and inflammatory bowel syndrome.

INVESTIGATIONS

Investigations include ultrasound using rectal probe, CA-125 (may be raised), MRI, but are nonspecific and unrewarding. Proctoscopy and sigmoidoscopy rule out malignancy. IVP needs to be done if ureter appears involved. Laparoscopy is both diagnostic and therapeutic, and biopsy should confirm the diagnosis.

MANAGEMENT

Poor hormonal response makes laparoscopic surgery the treatment of choice. Bowel preparation preoperatively is necessary in case bowel is involved and needs resection. Ablative and excisional techniques are employed depending upon the degree of involvement. Normally, bowel mucosa is spared, but in case stricture has formed, resection of bowel mandates the involvement of anorectal surgeon. Mirena IUCD is very effective in relieving symptoms.

PROGNOSIS

Morbidity and quality of life are influenced by CPV, dysmenorrhoea, dyspareunia and renal damage.

Malignant change is rare (1:150) and manifests as endometrioid cancer.

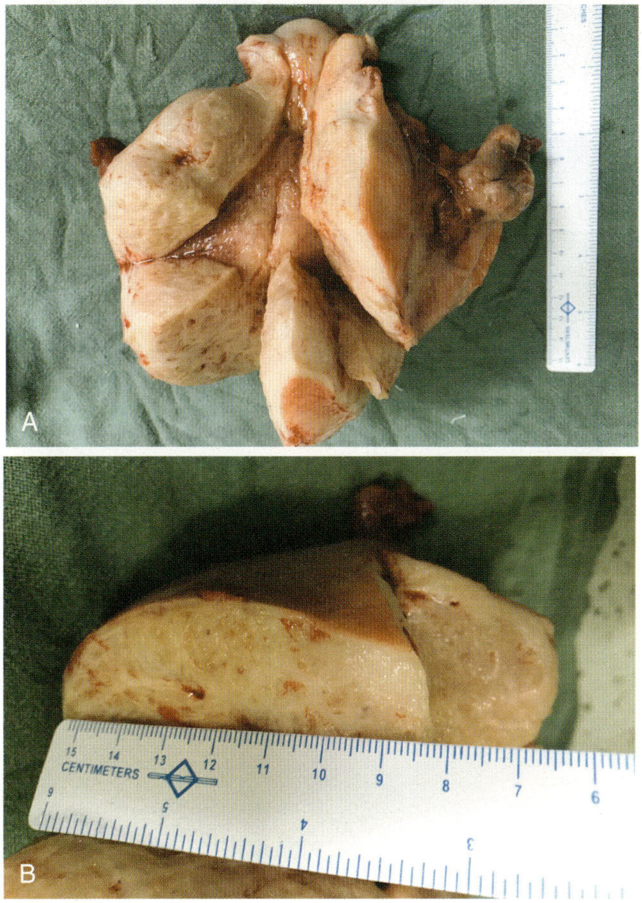

Figure 14.11 **(A)** Adenomyosis of the uterus. **(B)** Adenomyosis of the uterus showing cystic spaces and myohyperplasia.

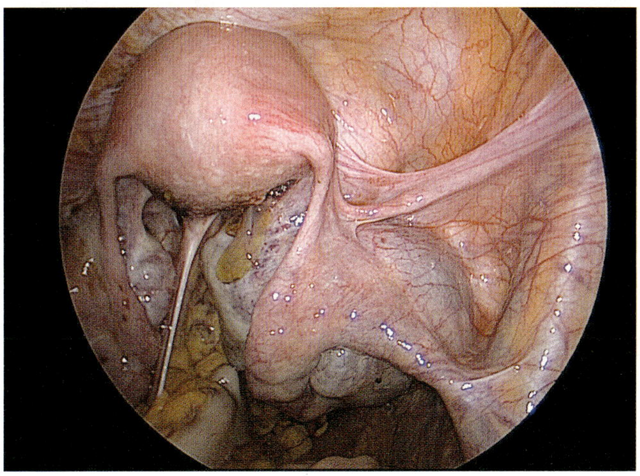

Figure 14.12 Laparoscopic view of adenomyosis of the uterus. (*Courtesy*: Dr Vivek Marwah, New Delhi.)

ADENOMYOSIS

Adenomyosis, also labelled as uterine endometriosis, is a relatively common condition in which islands of endometrium are found in the wall of the uterus. It is observed frequently in elderly women. More than one-third of the hysterectomy specimens from women aged 40 years and above reveal the presence of adenomyosis, irrespective of the indications for hysterectomy. The disease often coexists with uterine fibromyomas, pelvic endometriosis (15%) and endometrial carcinoma.

Grossly, the uterus appears symmetrically enlarged to not more than 14 weeks size. The cut section may show only a localized nodular enlargement. Most of the time, the affected area reveals a peculiar, diffuse, striated and noncapsulated involvement of the myometrium, mostly the posterior wall, with tiny dark haemorrhagic areas interspersed in between (Fig. 14.11).

Laparoscopy reveals a uniformly enlarged uterus (Figs 14.12 and 14.13). Histological examination reveals islands of endometrial glands surrounded by stroma in the midst of myometrial tissue at least two low-power fields beyond the endomyometrial junction (Fig. 14.14), more than 2.5 mm beneath the basal endometrium.

These women are usually parous, aged around 40 years. Some are asymptomatic, others present with menorrhagia and progressively increasing dysmenorrhoea. Pelvic discomfort, backache and dyspareunia are the other symptoms of adenomyosis. Clinical examination reveals a symmetrical

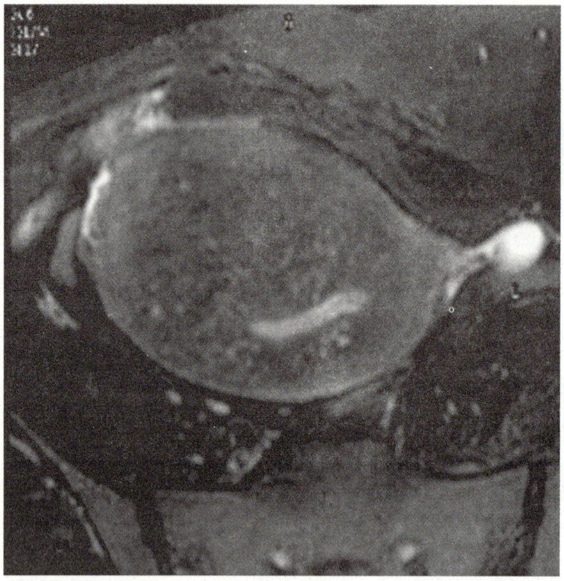

Figure 14.13 MRI showing adenomyosis of the uterus. (*Courtesy*: Dr Parveen Gulati, New Delhi.)

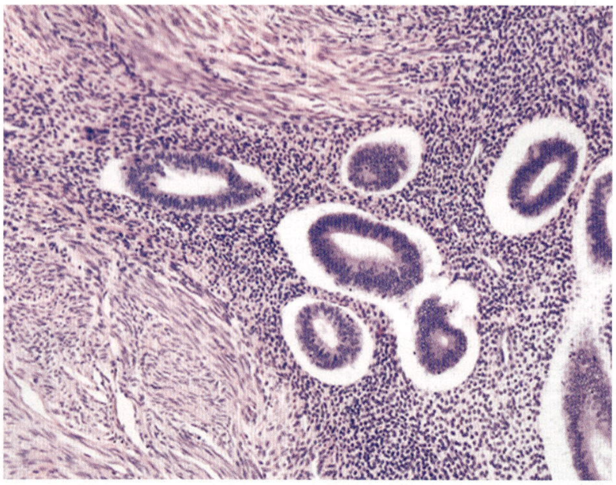

Figure 14.14 Adenomyosis uteri. Note the island of endometrial glands with associated stroma deep in the myometrium (×33). (*Source*: Wikimedia commons.)

enlargement of the uterus if the adenomyosis is diffuse and the uterus is tender. The uterine enlargement rarely exceeds that of a 3-month pregnancy and is often mistaken for a myoma. If a patient gives a history of menorrhagia with accompanying dysmenorrhoea, one should always consider the possibility of adenomyosis. If the adenomyosis is localized, the enlargement is asymmetrical and the resemblance to a myoma is closer. A myoma of this size is rarely painful. Therefore, a painful, symmetrical enlargement of the uterus should suggest the correct diagnosis. MRI is superior to ultrasound showing hypo- or anechoic area in the uterine wall. Ultrasound shows ill-defined hypoechoic areas, heterogeneous echoes in the myometrium, asymmetrical uterine enlargement and subendometrial halo thickening (Fig. 14.15). It also shows endometrial infiltration into the myometrium.

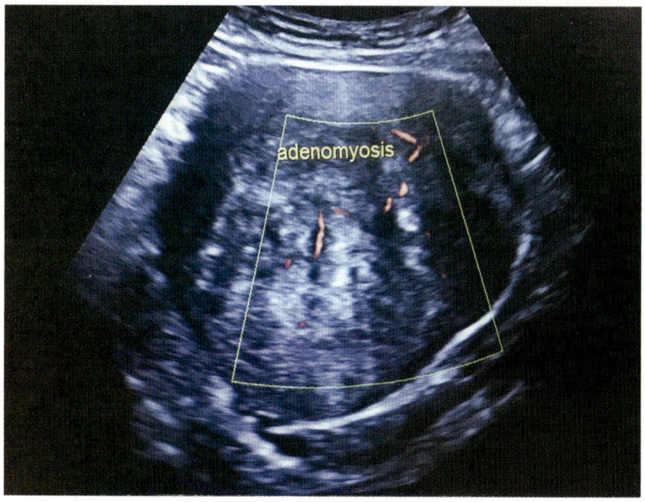

Figure 14.15 Adenomyosis with chocolate cyst.

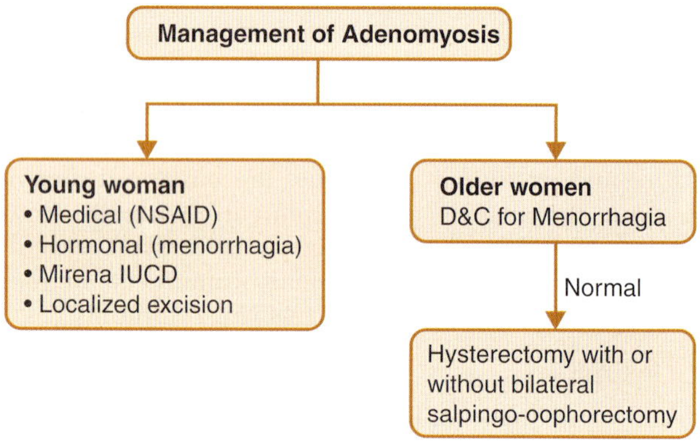

Figure 14.16 Management of adenomyosis.

TREATMENT (Fig. 14.16)

A diagnostic hysteroscopy combined with a curettage is the initial step in the management of adenomyosis because of menorrhagia. Most women are elderly and past the child-bearing age, total hysterectomy is the treatment. In younger women, in whom a localized adenomyosis is found confined to one part of the uterus, a localized excision is sometimes feasible, and this conservative resection is reasonable if the patient is particularly anxious to have a child. The possibility of scar rupture should be borne in mind.

Nonsteroidal anti-inflammatory drugs (NSAIDs) and hormonal therapy are employed with some success in women reluctant to undergo hysterectomy, but the overall results are not satisfactory. Drugs used are danazol, GnRH and Mirena IUCD for menorrhagia and pain. Transcervical resection of endometrium (TCRE) is effective for about 2 years. Unlike fibroid, uterine artery embolization has no effective role in adenomyosis. Mirena has been increasingly used in adenomyosis.

Unlike endometriosis, adenomyosis does not respond well to hormone therapy. MRI-guided ultrasonic-focused surgery and resection is under trial, and is desirable in young women.

STROMAL ENDOMETRIOSIS

It is a rare type of endometriosis, when only stromal tissues without glandular elements are present in ectopic sites. The stromal cells penetrate the uterine wall and spread via lymphatics and veins into the broad ligaments. The symptoms are similar to endometriosis and the uterus appears enlarged. Hysterectomy is recommended. The ovaries may be retained. Local recurrence is common and the tumour behaves like a malignancy. In case it recurs, radiotherapy is the treatment of choice.

New drugs under trial:

- Aromatase inhibitors and selective oestrogen receptor modulator (SERM)
- Dopamine agonist cabergoline, Pentoxifylline

KEY POINTS

- Endometriosis refers to the presence of ectopic endometrial tissue outside the cavity of the uterus.
- Theories of origin include retrograde menstruation and implantation of menstrual blood into the peritoneal surfaces and organs, coelomic metaplasia, vascular embolization and lymphatic permeation.
- Endometriosis manifests as islands of flame-shaped chocolate deposits or appears like powder-burn marks. It can cause extensive adhesions between the ovaries, back of the uterus and the pouch of Douglas, obliterating the same and causing dense rectal adhesions. Many appear as a cystic ovarian enlargement or ovarian endometriomas (chocolate cyst).
- The patient presents with pelvic pain, dysmenorrhoea, dyspareunia, menstrual disturbances and infertility. Symptoms related to other organs depend on the extent of spread of the disease.
- Laparoscopy is the most useful tools in establishing the diagnosis.
- Medical treatment consists of analgesics to control pain. Hormonal therapy and GnRH analogues provide relief from pain and help regression of disease, but delays fertility. For women desirous of childbearing, operative laparoscopy with electrocauterization/laser ablation of endometriosis, evacuation of large endometriomas with cautery, peeling out of its lining and surgery to restore tubo-ovarian relationship help to improve fertility status.
- Medical treatment is the first line of treatment in mild and moderate endometriosis. All hormones are equally effective. One should choose the drug that is cost-effective and has less side effects.
- Recently, a long-acting progesterone, Endoreg, has been found to be effective and a useful alternative in the treatment of endometriosis.
- Dydrogesterone does not prevent ovulation and is preferred in infertile women.
- Pre- and postoperative hormonal therapy relieves pain and symptoms, but do not improve fertility rate.
- Laparoscopy causes less postoperative pelvic adhesions and is preferred over laparotomy in young women.
- For adenomyosis and extensive disease, a hysterectomy with or without bilateral salpingo-oophorectomy brings relief to middle-aged patients.
- The relationship between mild endometriosis and infertility cannot be explained on the basis of anatomical alterations alone.
- Both laparoscopy and laparotomy yield similar pregnancy rate, but laparoscopy has less morbidity and causes less postoperative adhesions.
- Infertility is best treated surgically. IVF has a therapeutic role when other measures fail.
- Rectovaginal endometriosis is a separate entity and requires surgery, but Mirena is also found useful.
- Malignant change in a long-standing endometriosis has been reported in the form of clear cell carcinoma or endometroid carcinoma of ovary.
- Malignancy kills a woman; endometriosis cripples her.

SELF-ASSESSMENT

1. Discuss the clinical features and management of pelvic endometriosis in a young nulliparous woman.
2. A woman, para 1, presents with dysmenorrhoea, menorrhagia and chronic abdominal pain. A tender mass is felt in the right fornix. How will you investigate and manage the case?
3. A 35-year-old woman presents with menorrhagia, dysmenorrhoea. The uterus is 14 weeks enlarged. Discuss the differential diagnosis and management.
4. Short notes on:
    - Chocolate cyst of ovary
    - Endometriosis of rectovaginal septum

SUGGESTED READING

Anaf V, et al. Hum Reprod 1999;57:514.
Bonnar J. Recent Adv Obstet Gynecol 2003;21:101.
Chakravarti BN. Bull Inst Reprod Med 2002;41:9.
Desai S. Elsevier Clinical Advisory Board (ECAB) Clinical Update – Sadhana Desai. 2010.
De Cicco C, Corona R, Schonman R, et al. Bowel resection for deep endometriosis: a systematic review. BJOG 2011; 118:285.
Donnez J, et al. Fertil Steril 1999;62:63.
Duncan J, Shulman (Eds). Yearbook of Obstetrics and Gynecology. 2010;347.
Dunselman GA, Vermeulen N, Becker C, et al. ESHRE guideline: management of women with endometriosis. Hum Reprod 2014; 29:400.
Eltabbakh GH, et al. Minerva Ginecol 2008;60:323.
Greenblatt RB. Ferti Steril 1971;22:102.
Jaime TJ, Jaime TJ, Ormiga P, et al. Umbilical endometriosis: report of a case and its dermoscopic features. An Bras Dermatol 2013; 88:121.
Kennedy SH, et al. Greentop Guidelines 2006; 24.
Mechsner S, Kaiser A, Kopf A, et al. A pilot study to evaluate the clinical relevance of endometriosis-associated nerve fibers in peritoneal endometriotic lesions. Fertil Steril 2009; 92:1856.
Medeiros LR, Rosa MI, Silva BR, et al. Accuracy of magnetic resonance in deeply infiltrating endometriosis: a systematic review and meta-analysis. Arch Gynecol Obstet 2015; 291:611.
Morales Martínez C, Tejuca Somoano S. Abdominal wall endometriosis. Am J Obstet Gynecol 2017; 217:701.
Nezhat F, Datta MS, Hanson V, et al. The relationship of endometriosis and ovarian malignancy: a review. Fertil Steril 2008; 90:1559.
Oliveira FR, Dela Cruz C, Del Puerto HL, et al. Stem cells: are they the answer to the puzzling etiology of endometriosis? Histol Histopathol 2012; 27:23.
Studd J (Ed). Progress in Obstetrics and Gynecology 1991;9:273.
Sturdee J (ed). Yearbook of Obstetrics and Gynecology 2009;9:226.
Vercellini P, Fedele L, Aimi G, et al. Association between endometriosis stage, lesion type, patient characteristics and severity of pelvic pain symptoms: a multivariate analysis of over 1000 patients. Hum Reprod 2007; 22:266.
Vercellini P, Viganò P, Somigliana E, Fedele L. Endometriosis: pathogenesis and treatment. Nat Rev Endocrinol 2014; 10:261.
Vercellini P, et al. Curr Opin Obstet Gynecol 2005;17:359.
Yap C, et al. Cochrane Database Syst Rev 2004;(3): CD003678.

15 Hormonal Therapy in Gynaecology

CHAPTER OUTLINE

Hormonal therapy is extensively used in gynaecological practice today. A few of these hormones are available in their natural form in adequate quantity, but most of them are now synthesized, and effectively and safely used in infertility, contraception, menopause and menstrual disorders. Lately, hormonal therapy has reduced the number of hysterectomies in abnormal uterine bleeding. Various hormonal assays and availability of a large range of synthetic hormones have enabled the application of correct dosage, optimal route and the suitable hormone for each individual condition. Different routes have been employed to cater to individual needs, convenience as well as their effectiveness. They are used for both diagnostic and therapeutic purposes.

Broad groups of common hormonal preparations are discussed in this chapter.

OESTROGENS

Oestrogens are naturally occurring C-18 steroidal sex hormones produced by the ovaries, adrenal glands and the placenta during pregnancy. In the ovaries, the luteinizing hormone (LH) induces theca cells to produce androstenedione, which is aromatized to oestrogen by the granulosa cells. Adipose tissue in the peripheral areas and liver also contain aromatase, which converts androstenedione to oestrone. The biologically active oestrogen is oestradiol. It is synthesized during pregnancy in the placenta. It is also synthesized from cholesterol and metabolized in the liver to conjugates of oestradiol, oestriol and oestrone, which are excreted in the urine. Oestriol and oestrone are biologically weak oestrogens. After menopause, the source of oestrogen is adrenal glands, and oestrone is synthesized in the body fat mass peripherally by conversion of epi-androstenedione secreted by the ovary to oestrone. Oral oestrogen is extensively metabolized in the walls of the small intestine and liver and only 10% reaches the circulation as oestradiol (Table 15.1). The rest is converted to oestrone and oestradiol glucuronide. *These are weaker oestrogens; therefore, a large dose is required if the oral route is chosen. This effect is known as the 'first pass effect' in the liver.* Oestrogen increases the sensitive proteins in the liver, such as sex hormone–binding globulin (SHBG), corticosteroid, thyroxine-binding globulin, renin substrate and various coagulation and fibrinolytic factors. *The risk of hypertension and thrombosis therefore increases with oral hormones.* However, high-density lipoprotein (HDL) also increases and oral route is cardioprotective. Although the nonoral route avoids the 'first pass effect' and the above complications, they do not protect the patient from cardiovascular risks. Synthetic oestrogens are derived from the extracts of soya and Mexican yam, are inexpensive, effective and have found a wide application in clinical therapeutics.

PHYSIOLOGY

During the reproductive years of life, natural oestrogens are produced principally by the Graafian follicles in response to

Table 15.1 Advantages and Disadvantages of Oral Oestrogens

Advantages	Disadvantages
1. Easy to take	1. Daily dose
2. Cheaper	2. First pass effect in the liver
3. Can be withdrawn quickly if side effects develop	3. Causes hypertension and thrombosis
4. Cardioprotective	4. Large dose is required because of the first pass effect

pituitary gonadotropins. Oestrogen is responsible for the development of secondary sex characters, including the breasts, provides the negative feedback signal to the pituitary gland and hypothalamus and maintains adequate mineralization of the bones.

The liver and adipose tissue also contain aromatase, which converts androstenedione to oestrone. Sixty per cent of circulating oestrogen gets bound to SHBG and 38% to albumin. The rest is left as free hormones circulating in the blood. About 60% is excreted in the urine, of which 20% is oestradiol and the rest are its metabolites. About 10% is excreted in the faeces, and the fate of the rest is not known. Oestrogen binds to the cytoplasmic receptors and then translocated to the nucleus and influences the target tissues.

Oestrogenic preparations (Table 15.2) are used singly or in combination with progestogen in various gynaecological disorders.

COMMONLY USED OESTROGENS

1. *Ethinyl oestradiol* (EE2) *and mestranol* are given orally in the form of a skin patch and gel. It has a half-life of 12–14 hours, reaching the peak level in 4 hours. It is a common component in oral combined contraceptive pills (OCP) and is used in abnormal uterine bleeding (AUB) to regulate and control the amount of bleeding. Realizing that the side effects of breast cancer and thromboembolism in contraceptive pills were due to a high dose of oestrogen, the dose of EE2 in OCP is now reduced to 20–30 mcg of oestrogen in each pill. Synthetic oestrogens are most potent.
   Ethinyl oestradiol (EE2) dose is 0.01–0.05 mg. Oestradiol valerate and succinate tablet 1–2 mg.
   Mestranol 0.01–0.05 mg.
   Mestranol is no more used in combined pills because of increased risk of thrombosis.
2. *Conjugated oestrogen* is a natural oestrogen derived from mare's urine. *It is used in menopausal women to promote bone mineralization and cardioprotective effect.* It is also effective in controlling profuse bleeding of puberty menorrhagia when given as 25 mg i.v. or as an oral tablet Premarin containing 0.625 and 1.25 mg oestrogen.
3. *Dienoestrol cream* is nonsteroidal oestrogen (oestriol) *for topical use in senile vaginitis (vaginal), kraurosis vulva and urethral syndrome in menopausal women.* Gel is also available. The cream is applied once or twice daily for 2–10 days each month for 3–4 months. It has no protection against bones.
4. *Implants* are used as part of a long-term hormonal replacement therapy (HRT) in spontaneous or surgically induced menopausal women. Although providing a good compliance, its surgical insertion and removal, if side effects develop, are the disadvantages.
5. *Oestrogen patch* is a transdermal patch applied over the outer aspects of the buttocks or lower abdomen, but not over the breasts, in HRT. By avoiding the first pass effect in the liver, the side effects are minimized; it lowers triglycerides. The skin patch can cause skin irritation. The gel gets absorbed in 2 minutes and does not cause skin irritation.
6. *Micronized oestrogens* are used orally.
7. Stilboestrol – synthetic nonsteroid is used in prostatic cancer.

CONTRAINDICATIONS

Oestrogen is contraindicated in:

- Suspected malignancy of the genital tract
- Breast cancer
- History of thromboembolism
- Liver and gall bladder disease
- Cardiac, hypertensive and diabetic women
- Lactation – reduced milk production
- Sickle cell anaemia because of thrombosis
- With rifampicin, barbiturates, phenytoin and anticoagulants, as these drugs interfere with its metabolism and reduce its efficacy

INDICATIONS

- Short-term use for menopausal symptoms. Premarin 0.625 mg or Evalon 1–2 mg orally daily for 3–4 months is effective (see Chapter 7). Oestrogen cream is prescribed

Table 15.2 Oestrogen Preparations in Therapeutics

Generic Name	Doses in Common Use	Indications
1. Oral		
• Ethinyl oestradiol	0.01, 0.02, 0.03, 0.05, 1.0 mg	Irregular menses, OC pills
• Conjugated equine oestrogen (Premarin)	0.325, 0.625, 1.25 mg	HRT puberty
• Micronized oestrogen (E_2)	1–2 mg	Menorrhagia, irregular menses
• Combined pills		Contraceptives
2. Injectable		
• Conjugated equine oestrogen	25.0 mg slow i.v.	Puberty Menorrhagia
3. Topical vaginal		
• Dienoestrol cream, Evalon cream	0.01% in cream base	Senile vaginitis, urethral syndrome
4. Transdermal patches		
• 17 β -oestradiol (3–7 days)	0.03–0.1 mg	HRT
• Combined E + MPA	0.625 mg + 5.0 mg	HRT
• Oestradiol implant	25, 50, 100 mg	Long-acting HRT - 6-monthly

for local symptoms such as dry vagina and urethral syndrome.

- Long-term HRT prevents or delays osteoporosis and is also cardioprotective (see Chapter 7).
- Oestrogen cream is prescribed in vulvovaginitis in children, senile vaginitis and urethral syndrome in menopausal women.
- Oral contraceptives – see chapter on Contraception.
- Abnormal uterine bleeding – see Chapter 11.
- *Intersex.* Patients suffering from Turner syndrome and testicular feminizing tumour should receive oestrogen combined with progestogens cyclically throughout life to develop secondary sex characters, avoid cardiovascular accidents and osteoporosis.
- Oestrogen is used in prostatic cancer.
- Supresses lactation.
- Improves mood in postpartum and menopausal depression.
- Premenstrual tension syndrome.

SIDE EFFECTS

- Nausea and vomiting when given orally.
- Mastalgia, water retention and increase in weight.
- Thromboembolism and cerebral thrombosis.
- Endometrial and breast cancer if given for a long period without progestogen.
- Hepatic adenoma and gall bladder disease.

Tibolone and selective oestrogen receptor modulators (SERMs) have both oestrogenic and antioestrogenic action. They have antioestrogenic action on the breast tissue but agnostic action on the endometrium and bones. They can cause endometrial hyperplasia and cancer.

PROGESTERONE

Progesterone is the natural hormone produced by the theca cells of the corpus luteum and the placenta. It is metabolized in the liver and excreted in the urine as sodium pregnanediol glucuronide. Natural progesterone is not active orally and is given only by intramuscular injection in an oil base. Progesterone acts on target tissues only when the latter are primed with oestrogen, as oestrogen produces progesterone receptors.

A large number of synthetic compounds which can be taken orally have been marketed in recent years.

PREPARATIONS

Progestogens are synthetic compounds belonging to two main groups – the oestrone or 19-norprogestins, which are structurally similar to testosterone, and pregnane or 17-acetoxy compound structurally similar to progesterone. The oestrone compounds are mainly incorporated in oral contraceptive pills, and pregnane compounds are used in pregnancy and AUB.

CLASSIFICATION

- Pure progesterone – Oral and vaginal micronized progesterone have no adverse effects on lipid profile.
- Pregnane (derived from progesterone molecule), lynestrenol (allyloestrenol), medroxyprogesterone, megestrol acetate.
- Estrane (derivative of testosterone) – Norethisterone, norethandriol (first generation).
- Gonane – Levonorgestrel, norgestrel (second generation). They reduce the level of SHBG, have androgenic and anti-E effects.
- Third-generation progesterone (desogestrel, gestodene and norgestimate). These are less androgenic and cause less metabolic disorders but increase the risk of thrombosis.
- Hybrid drospirenone (3 mg equivalent to 25-mg spirinone) now used in oral pills for acne and PCOS. Yasmin contains 30 mcg of EE_2 (21 days), Janya contains 20 mcg EE_2 for 24 days in a cycle.
- Hybrids (drospirenone) have antiandrogens, and antimineral corticosteroid effect; are used in premenstrual tension; causes hyperkalaemia by decreasing potassium excretion in the urine, less water retention and weight gain.

These have no influence on lipid profile and have a very good control of menstrual cycles. Micronized progesterone – oral tablet (100 mg) causes vomiting, giddiness and liver damage. Micronized vaginal tablet (100 mg) is without these oral side effects but causes vaginal irritation.

Progestogens are administered:

- Orally – singly or with oestrogen
- Intramuscular injection monthly, three-monthly as contraceptives
- Implants – Norplant (contraceptives)Intrauterine contraceptive device (IUCD) impregnated with levonorgestrel (Progestasert, Mirena)
- Vaginal tablet and rings
- Skin patches

Crinone 8% (90 mg) vaginal gel is a micronized progesterone in dilute emulsion system.

THERAPEUTIC APPLICATIONS

- Pure progesterone as injection in oil or micronized vaginal or oral capsules is used in threatened and recurrent abortions, and in corpus luteal-phase deficiency (CLPD).
- High doses of injections are used in advanced endometrial cancer.
- Contraception – Oral in combination with oestrogen, mini-pills and injectables are used as contraceptives. Implants (Norplant) are effective over 5 years (see chapter on Contraception). IUCDs impregnated with progesterones are available (Mirena). Mirena is effective for 5 years.
- Abnormal uterine bleeding (see Chapter 11).
- Dysmenorrhoea, premenstrual tension syndrome.
- *Endometriosis.* Although Danazol is the drug of choice, but owing to cost and hirsutism, progestogens continue to be employed in endometriosis.
- Endometrial ablation in AUB. Before the transcervical resection of endometrium (TCRE), endometrial shrinkage is achieved by progestogens given over 4–6 weeks.

- *Amenorrhoea.* Progesterone challenge test – A single injection of 100 mg progesterone will induce withdrawal bleeding if endometrium is primed by oestrogen (see Chapter 12). Oral tablets also work. (Primolut-N 5 mg t.i.d. × 3 days.)
- Postcoital pill – Levonorgestrel 0.75 mg tablet given within 72 hours of unprotected coitus and repeated 12 hours later will prevent pregnancy in 98% cases.
- With oestrogen in HRT (see Chapter 7).
- Postponement of menstruation – 5-mg norethisterone t.i.d. for 4–5 days or longer will delay the onset of menstruation (starting 3 days before anticipated period).
- Allyl progesterone is used in abortions.
- Progestogens are used as 'add-back' therapy with gonadotropin-releasing hormone (GnRH) to prevent osteoporosis and allow prolonged GnRH therapy.

CONTRAINDICATIONS

- Undiagnosed vaginal bleeding
- Breast cancer, breast tumour
- Thromboembolism

SIDE EFFECTS

- Nausea, vomiting
- Headache, mastalgia, water retention, cramps in the legs, weight gain
- Hirsutism in androgen-related compounds
- Depression
- Increased low-density lipoproteins and cardiovascular accidents
- Deep venous thrombosis, pulmonary embolism with desogestrel and gestodene
- Breast tumours, cancer
- Medroxyprogesterone acetate causes bone loss
- Increase in low-density lipoprotein (LDL) and decrease in HDL

ANDROGENS (Fig. 15.1)

Androgens are 19 carbon steroids derived from cholesterol and formed in the adrenal gland, ovaries and also peripherally.

TYPES

- Testosterone – Potent (T)
- Dihydrotestosterone by conversion of (DHT) testosterone by 5α-reductase – Most potent hormone acting at the target organs, i.e. hair follicles
- Androstenedione – Weak androgen
- Dehydroepiandrosterone (DHEA) – Weak androgen
- Dehydroepiandrosterone sulphate (DHEAS) – Weak androgen

Testosterone is a natural androgen hormone secreted by the ovarian stroma and the adrenal glands. The normal level is 0.2–0.8 ng/mL. Its use in modern gynaecology is limited on account of hirsutism and availability of synthetic progestogens, which have similar biological effects. About 50% androgen in women is derived from the ovaries and 50% comes from the adrenal cortex. About 90% is bound to SHBG and some to albumin and remains inactive, and the rest (1%) circulates in the blood. At the target tissues, it is converted to dihydrotestosterone, which is biologically active and causes acne and hirsutism in excess as seen in polycystic ovarian syndrome.

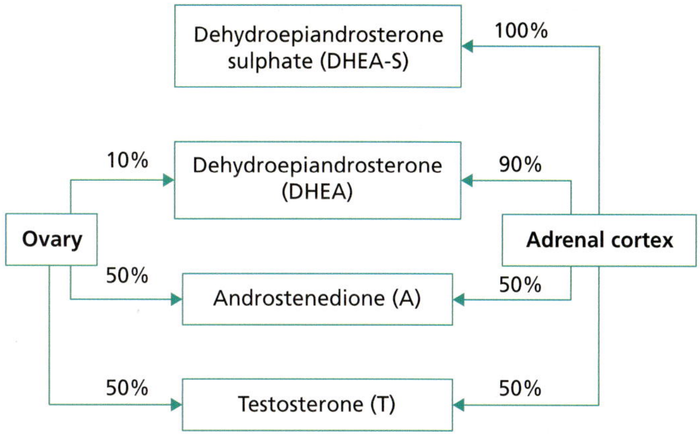

Figure 15.1 Sources of androgens.

DHEA – 90% from adrenal gland; 10% from the ovary

DHEA > 8000 ng/mL is seen in the adrenal cortex tumour. The compound is quickly metabolized and cannot be estimated clinically. Its normal level is 40–340 mcg/dL. Plasma level of more than 700 mcg/dL occurs in adrenal tumours. Serum 17-hydroxyprogesterone level of more than 5 ng/mL is seen in adrenal hyperplasia. Ovarian production of testosterone is 0.2–0.3 mg daily and is responsible for 50% of total testosterone, the other 50% is derived from the adrenal gland. Androstenedione contribution is 50% each from ovaries and adrenal gland.

DHEAS comes exclusively from the adrenal gland.

LH stimulates production of ovarian testosterone hormone in the ovarian stromal tissue as in PCOS. Insulin resistance is often the cause of LH stimulation to produce ovarian androgens.

It is used orally, i.m. or as a 6-month implant.

Androgens cause masculinizing effect such as

- Moustache, beard, hair on the chest
- Frontal baldness
- Acanthosis nigricans is often associated with insulin resistance

USES

- Endometriosis – Danazol is effectively used.
- Male infertility – Oligospermia.
- Decreased libido – 100 mg implant for 6 months is available for menopausal women to improve libido.
- In mastalgia and fibrocystic disease of the breast.

SIDE EFFECTS

Virilization and hirsutism

DANAZOL

Danazol is an isoxazole derivative of 17-alpha-ethinyl testosterone. It acts directly on the endometrium causing atrophy by displacing oestrogen receptors in the endometrium. Its indirect suppressive action on the pituitary gland also reduces oestrogen and progesterone secretion. By reducing the SHBG, it frees bound testosterone into circulation. It has androgenic and anabolic properties.

Uses

- It is largely used in endometriosis either as a primary treatment or following surgery to eradicate residual tumour and prevent recurrence. The oral dose varies from 400 to 800 mg daily in divided doses. About 75%–90% improvement is seen within 6 months.
- *Abnormal uterine bleeding.* Danazol should not be offered to young women in view of risk of hirsutism, but in older women, it is used when oestrogen is contraindicated and progestogens fail to cure menorrhagia. With the availability of several drugs such as nonsteroidal anti-inflammatory drugs (NSAIDs) and antifibrinolytics, the role of Danazol is limited in this disorder.
- Danazol is given in a dose of 200 mg daily for 4–6 weeks before transcervical resection of endometrium in AUB to produce endometrial thinning and atrophy.
- Danazol is effective in cyclical mastalgia: 100 mg twice daily will improve 60% cases.
- Fibrocystic disease of breasts is also treated with Danazol.
- Gynaecomastia.
- It improves libido in menopausal women.
- It shrinks fibroid and is used before surgery.
- Improves spermatogenesis in male infertility.

Side effects

Danazol should not be given for more than 6–9 months at a time because of antioestrogenic action and virilizing effect.

Other side effects:

- Weight gain, headache, water retention and oedema.
- Acne, hirsutism and muscle cramp.
- Breast atrophy, amenorrhoea; deepening of voice, which is irreversible.
- Liver damage, increased LDL, lowers HDL with its associated cardiovascular complications.
- It is teratogenic in early pregnancy, causing masculinization of a female fetus.
- Glucose intolerance.
- Contraindicated in liver disease and prostate cancer.

GESTRINONE

Gestrinone is a trienic 19-norsteroid derivative of testosterone, which has androgenic, antioestrogenic, antiprogestogenic and antipituitary action. Its mode of action is similar to Danazol, and its clinical applications are also similar, but it is more expensive.

Oral dose of 2.5–5 mg twice weekly to be taken at the same time and the same day in the week will induce amenorrhoea in 85% cases of AUB. Its side effects are milder and are therefore preferred to Danazol. Vaginal tablet 2.5 mg is applied weekly.

ANTIOESTROGENS

Apart from androgens, which are antioestrogenic (inhibit the ovarian function through the pituitary gland and oppose the action of oestrogens on the target organs), the drugs which antagonize oestrogens at the receptor level are clomiphene and tamoxifen.

CLOMIPHENE CITRATE

In 1956, Greenblatt first introduced clomiphene in gynaecology for inducing ovulation.

Clomiphene citrate is a nonsteroidal compound related to diethylstilbestrol (DES). It is a mixture of two isomers, cis (now known as zuclomiphene) and trans (now known as enclomiphene citrate). Cis fraction is responsible for inducing ovulation. Clomiphene citrate contains 38% cis and 63% trans isomers. It has a half-life of 5 days. It is metabolized in the liver and excreted in bile and faeces.

MODE OF ACTION

Clomiphene is the first drug of choice for inducing ovulation. By competing with cytoplasmic oestrogen receptors in the hypothalamus, it blocks the negative feedback of circulating endogenous oestrogen. This allows release of GnRH into the pituitary portal system and stimulates LH and follicle-stimulating hormone (FSH) secretion. Starting on the 2nd day of the cycle and given for 5 days, E_2 level starts increasing 5–6 days after stopping the drug and induces maturity of the Graafian follicle and ovulation with LH surge. The best action is seen if a certain amount of oestrogen is present in the body. However, it exerts anti-E action on the endometrium and cervical mucus, causing slight decrease in the fertility rate.

INDICATIONS

Clomiphene is indicated in:

- Anovulatory infertility
- Polycystic ovarian syndrome (PCOD) associated with infertility
- In in vitro fertilization: Gamete intrafallopian transfer (GIFT) technique and assisted reproduction therapy (ART)
- 25 mg orally for 25 days each month for 3–6 months to stimulate spermatogenesis

CONTRAINDICATIONS

Clomiphene is contraindicated in:

- Ovarian cyst – The cyst can increase in size.
- Chronic liver disease, because it is metabolized in the liver.
- Scotoma.

If the woman suffers from amenorrhoea, clomiphene can be started any day. In normal cycles, the drug is started on the 2nd day of the period in a dose of 50 mg daily for

5 days. Monitoring is done by serial ultrasound from the 10th day onwards until the signs of ovulation are observed. Normally, the follicle increases in size daily by 1–2 mm. When the dominant follicular size reaches 20 mm, human chorionic gonadotropin (hCG) 5000 IU is injected intramuscularly. Ovulation occurs about 36–40 hours after injecting hCG – the couple is advised intercourse around this time. Not only does the hCG injection indicate the precise time of ovulation, it also compensates for CLPD caused by clomiphene.

On clomiphene administration, 80% ovulate and about 50% conceive. This low pregnancy rate may be attributed to the antioestrogenic effect of clomiphene on cervical mucus, CLPD on endometrium. The cyclical therapy is recommended for 6 months, after which a break is given for 2–3 months. Further attempt to induce ovulation is repeated after that. If ovulation fails to occur and follicular size does not attain 20 mm, the dose of clomiphene is increased by 50 mg in each cycle to the maximum of 150 mg daily. Alternately, the tablets may have to be taken for 7 days in each cycle. If this too fails, the patient is offered FSH/LH therapy.

To reduce the peripheral antioestrogenic action and improve the fertility rate, clomiphene is lately replaced by letrozole 2.5 mg daily for 5 days. However, the drug can cause drowsiness.

In endometriosis, 30% conceive, and in PCOS, although 80% ovulate, 40% become pregnant.

In PCOS, the high level of DHEAs reduces the pregnancy rate. Adding 0.5 mg dexamethasone lowers DHEA levels and improves conception rate.

SIDE EFFECTS

The side effects are (i) ovarian enlargement in 10%, (ii) hot flushes, sweating due to oestrogen deficiency, osteoporosis, (iii) nausea, vomiting, (iv) visual disturbances, blurring, scotoma, (v) headache, dizziness, urticaria, (vi) hair loss 3%, (vii) weight gain, (viii) antioestrogenic effect on cervical mucus and endometrium (ix) CLPD, (x) hyperstimulation syndrome, (xi) two- to threefold increased risk of neural tube defect has been reported by many, although not proved, (xii) multiple ovulation and multiple pregnancy in 10%, (xiii) abortion rate 25%–40% due to CLPD, (xiv) ovarian malignancy if the treatment is extended beyond 1 year and (xv) premature ovarian failure, caused by exhaustion of follicles through multiple ovulation.

Incidence of unruptured luteinized follicle is increased.

OVARIAN HYPERSTIMULATION SYNDROME

Ovarian hyperstimulation syndrome (OHSS) (Fig. 15.2 and Table 15.3) is a complication of assisted reproductive technologies and an iatrogenic complication occurring in the luteal phase or early pregnancy. It is a potentially life-threatening condition, occurring in 1%–10%. It results from induction of ovulation in infertility cases. It is more common in FSH/LH therapy than clomiphene and pulsatile GnRH drugs. Its incidence is higher in PCOS and anovulatory infertility as compared to infertility caused by amenorrhoea. Raised LH in PCOS is responsible for hyperstimulation, and hCG should not be included in the therapy in these cases. Administration of hCG increases the risk, so also the dose of drugs, size and number of ovarian follicles. It is also common in a conceptional cycle if multiple ovulation occurs. It is characterized by ovarian enlargement, pleural and peritoneal effusion, oliguria, liver damage and thromboembolism. Severe form of OHSS occurs if the woman conceives during that cycle.

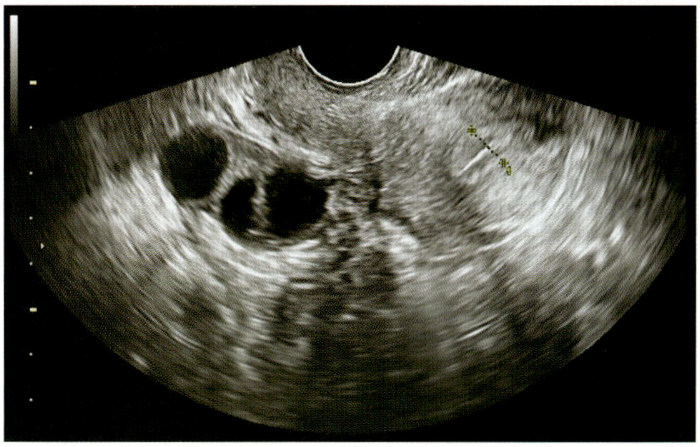

Figure 15.2 Ultrasound showing multiple maturing follicles.

Table 15.3 Varieties of SERMs and Comparison of their Therapeutic Effects

Therapy	Hot Flashes Insomnia	Genital Atrophy	Endometrial Proliferation	Ovulation	Osteoporosis	Breast Cancer	CVD
Oestrogen[a] ERT/HRT	↑	↑	NA	NA	↑	↑	↑
Clomifen	NA	↑	↑	↑	NA	NA	NSC
Tamoxifen	↑	↑	↑	NA	↑	↑	↑
Raloxifene	↑	NSC	↑	NA	↑	↑	↑
Genistein	↑	↑	NSC	NA	↑	NSC	↑
Centchroman	NA	NSC	NSC	NSC	↑	↑	NSC

[a]Estrogen alone are used following hysterectomy.
CVD, cardiovascular disease including deep venous thrombosis; NA, not applicable in the clinical situation; NSC, no significant change.

Pathogenesis

The main reason for OHSS is the increased vascular permeability leading to fluid shift from intravascular to extravascular space. This causes decreased blood volume and albumin as well as electrolyte levels. It leads to accumulation of fluid such as ascites and hydrothorax. The increased vascular permeability is due to prostaglandin, cytokines and growth factors secreted by multiple growing follicles.

The risk factors for OHSS are as follows:

- Young age of the woman.
- PCOS.
- Previous OHSS.
- Increased oestradiol level, >3000 pg/mL.
- 20 or more small follicles.
- Increased renin and angiotensin factors.
- Vascular endothelial growth factor (VEGF) causes neovascularization of granulosa cells and increased E_2 level.
- PCOS, high LH/FSH ratio, hCG and pregnancy in stimulated cycle.
- FSH/LH causes higher incidence of OHSS (30%) than clomiphene (10%) and GnRH (1%).

OHSS can be predicted by high level of E_2 (>3000 pg/mL), more than 20 follicles on ultrasound and increased Doppler blood flow. There is increased release of renin and angiotensin.

Complications

Complications of OHSS are as follows:

- Vascular – cerebrovascular accidents, thromboembolic phenomenon, deep venous thrombosis
- Coagulopathy
- Liver dysfunction
- Adult respiratory distress caused by ascites/hydrothorax
- Renal failure due to hypovolaemia
- Gastrointestinal – Related to E_2 level
- Torsion and haemorrhage in the ovarian cyst

Prevention

hCG should be withheld in a cycle if more than 20 follicles are seen on ultrasound and E_2 level rises to 3000 pg/mL. In PCOS, it is prudent to withhold hCG. Albumin 5% infusion in 500 mL lactated Ringer's solution during and after oocyte retrieval prevents OHSS. Dopamine agonist cabergoline 0.5 mg daily for 8 days starting on day 1 of hCG avoids OHSS.

Ovarian hyperstimulation syndrome occurs with smaller than larger follicular size 5–8 days after hCG administration. It is an iatrogenic condition of increased vascular permeability resulting in exudation of fluids from the intravascular to the extracellular compartment. Progesterone support helps.

Treatment

Ovarian hyperstimulation syndrome requires hospitalization. Medical therapy includes:

- *IV fluids for hypovolaemia.* Colloids, plasma expanders or human albumin infusion 5% in 500 mL Ringer's lactate. Half-life of albumin is 3–10 days. Fifty grams of albumin (25% albumin in 50 mL) raises blood volume to 500 mL. Human albumin 20% with 2 L of dextrose may be needed. Gelofusine for hypovolaemia may be required – continuous autotransfusion of ascitic fluid (CATAF) is performed for 5 hours each day.
- Diuretics and NSAIDs should be avoided because of hypovolaemia and poor renal perfusion except in pulmonary oedema and to correct electrolytes.
- High thigh venous support stocking prevents deep venous thrombosis.
- Immunoglobulins i.v. may prove to be effective.
- Glucocorticoids.
- Anticoagulants – heparin.
- Dopamine improves renal blood flow, oliguria and prevents renal failure.
- Correction of electrolytes.

Investigation and Monitoring

- Investigation and monitoring are done by
- Hb%, WCC, platelet count – TLC 15,000 and haematocrit.
- Urea, electrolyte estimation, serum protein level.
- Repeat ultrasound to monitor size of ovarian cyst and ascites.
- Weight recording.
- Renal function tests.
- Liver function tests.
- Coagulation profile.
- Central venous pressure recording.
- X-ray chest for pleural effusion.

Surgery is required if the ovarian cyst ruptures, undergoes torsion or haemorrhages. Aspiration of ovarian cyst, ascites, pleural and pericardial effusion may be required.

AROMATASE INHIBITORS

LETROZOLE

Letrozole (nonsteroidal aromatase inhibitor) is used in the induction of ovulation. It has a half-life of 45 hours and is eliminated through kidneys. It prevents conversion of androstenedione to oestrone. A dose of 2.5 mg daily for 5 days in a cycle has the following advantages over clomiphene:

1. It has no antioestrogenic action on the endometrium and the cervix – yields better pregnancy rate.
2. It induces monofollicular stimulation, adequate LH surge and avoids multiple pregnancy.
3. Better implantation.
4. No hyperstimulation syndrome. It is suited in cases of PCOS. Lately, a single dose of 20 mg on day 3 is being tried. It is contraindicated in hepatic dysfunction.

It can, however, cause drowsiness and liver dysfunction. Anastrozole is useful in endometriosis (1 mg a day).

SELECTIVE OESTROGEN RECEPTOR MODULATORS ACTING AS ANTIOESTROGEN (Table 15.3)

TAMOXIFEN

(Tamoxifen, cytofen, eldtam, mamofen and oncomox)

Tamoxifen is a nonsteroidal antioestrogenic drug. It acts by binding to and reducing the availability of oestrogen receptors. It is mainly used in the palliative treatment of advanced breast cancer in postmenopausal women. It has also been used successfully in cases of PCOD. Tamoxifen is effective in primary and secondary prevention of breast cancer; it prevents spread to the other breast, and recurrence by 50% and mortality by 25%. It is also bone and cardioprotective. Primary chemoprevention is indicated in $BRCA_1$ and $BRCA_2$ gene positive women, usually first relatives of breast cancer patients.

Side effects (two-fold increase) are hot flushes, vaginal dryness (anti-E_2 action), endometrial hyperplasia, polyp, endometrial carcinoma and sarcoma.

Hyperglyceridaemia, deep venous thrombosis, ischaemic heart disease and retinopathy are other complications to watch for during tamoxifen therapy.

Progestogens do not protect against tamoxifen-induced endometrial hyperplasia.

DOSAGE

The dose is 10–20 mg twice daily for not more than 5 years in breast cancer because it becomes ineffective after that.

PRECAUTIONS

Tamoxifen enhances the effects of warfarin. It is known to cause endometrial hyperplasia and cancer. It is mandatory to monitor endometrial growth by serial sonography and uterine aspiration.

An important second-generation SERM is raloxifene, which has less beneficial action on the breast than tamoxifen. It is cardioprotective, maintains bone density and has no adverse effect on the endometrium unlike tamoxifen. However, it is antioestrogen and does not cure menopausal symptoms such as hot flushes.

The dose is 60 mg daily. It is mandatory to discontinue therapy before, during and after surgery, to avoid the risk of superficial and deep venous thrombosis.

Raloxifene, 60 mg daily used in endometriosis do not cause endometrial hyperplasia.

ORMELOXIFENE (CENTCHROMAN)

It is a nonsteroidal antioestrogen developed for its contraceptive potential. Due to its long half-life, it is available in Indian market as a 'weekly nonsteroidal pill'. It is free from adverse effects on the breast, endometrium, ovary, liver and coagulation factors. It does not inhibit ovulation and exerts contraceptive effect on implantation. It has antioestrogen activity on endometrium (also see chapter on birth control).

ANTIPROGESTERONE

An antiprogesterone in common use is mifepristone (RU486).

MIFEPRISTONE

Mifepristone – RU486 (Mifegest and Mifeprine)

Mifepristone is a 19-norsteroid derivative of the synthetic progestogen norethindrone. The drug binds to the receptors in the cell nucleus and blocks progesterone action at the target organs. It also binds to glucocorticoid and androgen receptors. About 85% of the drug is absorbed after oral therapy. Peak level is reached in 1–2 hours. The half-life of the drug is 24 hours. It is excreted in bile and faeces. Bioavailability is 60%.

Administration of the drug (150 mg) during the first 3 days of the follicular phase has no effect on the menstrual cycle. Drug administration in the late follicular phase suppresses LH surge, and ovulation fails to occur. A single dose of the drug given within 2 days of the LH surge does not alter menstruation. Late administration in the luteal phase causes luteolysis and prevents pregnancy. Epostane is another progesterone synthesis inhibitor.

THERAPEUTIC APPLICATIONS

This drug has been approved for medical termination of pregnancy (MTP) up to 49 days. Successful abortion occurs in about 85% of cases. Usually, the abortion takes place within 5 days of drug administration; however, one has to wait for 28 days to judge success. In 15% cases, when abortion fails to occur or is incomplete, or the patient continues to bleed, surgical evacuation becomes necessary. The drug is administered in the form of three tablets (200 mg each), followed by two tablets of misoprostol 200 mcg, each orally or preferably vaginally 48 hours later. Just 200 mg mifepristone has also been proved effective. Lately, MTP extended up to 9 weeks of gestation with mifepristone and misoprostol has proved successful. By reducing the level of β-hCG, it causes necrosis of the decidua and death of the embryo.

- It is useful in ripening of the cervix before prostaglandin induction of mid-trimester abortion. A dose of 200–600 mg RU486 followed by prostaglandin 24–48 hours later (400 mcg) shortens induction–abortion interval, and reduces the dose and the side effects of prostaglandin.
- It is effective in missed abortion (same dose as in MTP).
- Ectopic pregnancy – mifepristone injected into the unruptured ectopic pregnancy causes its resolution (see Chapter 17 on Ectopic Gestation).
- Cushing syndrome – because of its antiglucocorticoid therapy.
- Postcoital contraception – 10 mg given within 72 hours of unprotected coitus is used as a postcoital contraception.
- It has some beneficial influence on the shrinkage of fibroids and endometriosis (10–25 mg daily for 3 months).

SIDE EFFECTS

- Headache (5%).
- Gastrointestinal symptoms of nausea, vomiting (3.5%). Occasional diarrhoea.
- Faintness, skin rash.
- Adrenal failure if massive dose is employed.
- Teratogenic. If medical method fails with RU486, pregnancy should be terminated.
- Endometrial hyperplasia by reducing progesterone effect.
- Low potassium level, increase in creatinine level.

ANTIANDROGENS

CYPROTERONE ACETATE (DIANETTE AND ANDROCUR)

Cyproterone, chemically related to progesterone, is derived from 17-alpha-hydroxy progesterone and exerts a mild progestation activity. It is a potent antiandrogen, and competes with dihydrotestosterone for intracellular androgen receptor sites – it inhibits its binding. It has a weak corticosteroid effect. Small doses have no effect on the pituitary function, but large doses cause amenorrhoea, loss of libido, suppression of spermatogenesis and gynaecomastia in males. By lowering LH level, it also reduces production of androstenedione in the ovary.

It is used in the treatment of hirsutism. A dose of 50–100 mg cyproterone acetate is given during the first 10 days of the cycle along with 30 mcg of ethinyl oestradiol (EE_2) given cyclically for 3 weeks every month. *The effects begin to be seen only after 3 months of therapy.* Cyclic administration should continue for 6–12 months, followed by a maintenance dose of 5–10 mg of cyproterone acetate with EE for a prolonged period to prevent recurrence of hirsutism. Combination with EE is necessary to prevent pregnancy and thereby avoid teratogenic effects; it also regulates the cycles. In cases of PCOS, treatment regularizes menstruation, increases the levels of serum sex-binding globulins which bind the free testosterone, thereby reducing hair growth, acne and dry skin. On stopping therapy, results of induction of ovulation protocols improve. The drug is also useful to treat acne. The dose for acne is 2 mg with EE_2 to be taken daily for 21 days of each cycle (also see Chapter 9).

SPIRONOLACTONE

Spironolactone is an aldosterone antagonist and was used as a diuretic. Its antiandrogenic properties have been put to use in the treatment of hirsutism. Its beneficial effects are observed after 3–4 months of therapy. The drug blocks the androgen effect at the receptor level in the hair follicles. It also reduces the 17-alpha-hydroxylase activity, lowering the plasma levels of testosterone and androstenedione (see Chapter 9).

DOSAGE

A daily dose of 150 mg along with the cyclic administration of EE provides relief in about 60% of the cases. It is useful in cases of PCOS. The maintenance dose of 50 mg is continued after 6–12 months of therapy.

SIDE EFFECTS

Transient diuresis; polymenorrhoea is encountered in 10% of users; breast engorgement; and electrolyte disturbances (hyperkalaemia) when high doses are used.

FLUTAMIDE

(Cytomid-250, Drogenil, Flutacare, Prostamid and Flutide)

Flutamide is a substituted anilide. It is a nonsteroidal, antiandrogenic drug blocking the action of androgen at the receptor levels.

DOSAGE

A dose of 125–250 mg twice daily for 6 months along with OC pills are useful in the treatment of hirsutism. In males, it has been used in the treatment of prostatic hyperplasia and cancer.

SIDE EFFECTS

Hepatotoxicity, dry skin, oligomenorrhoea and decreased libido.

FINASTERIDE

(Finast, fincar, Fistide and finpecia)

Finasteride is a competitive inhibitor of the enzyme 5-alpha reductase, which converts testosterone to dihydrotestosterone. It has no affinity to androgen receptors. It has no effects on other hormones and it does not influence the hypothalamus–pituitary–gonadal axis.

It is also used in benign prostate hyperplasia.

DOSAGE

A dose of 5.0 mg/daily for 6 months is recommended.

SIDE EFFECTS

Hypersensitivity to the drug; decreased libido; teratogenic effect on the fetus during pregnancy.

GLUCOCORTICOIDS

Dexamethasone 0.25–0.5 mg or prednisone given at night daily for 6 months reduces ACTH secretion and hirsutism. It is contraindicated in obese women. The drug is also used in PCOS, with clomiphene in infertility, and adrenal hyperplasia.

PITUITARY HORMONES

GONADOTROPINS

The anterior pituitary gland secretes FSH, LH and prolactin (PRL). The physiology of their secretion is described in Chapter 4.

FSH is extracted from the urine of menopausal women and is available in injection form. One ampoule contains 75 IU FSH as a frozen dried powder along with a solvent.

Human β-chorionic gonadotropin hormone, which simulates LH in action, is extracted in a similar manner. It is available in 1000, 2000 and 5000 IU as frozen dry powder with an ampoule of solvent.

Both recombinant FSH and recombinant gonadotropin are now available. They are self-administered subcutaneously, very effective and have lesser risk of hyperstimulation.

THERAPEUTIC USES

Gemzell first reported its use in 1958.

Therapeutic uses of gonadotropins are as follows:

- Induction of ovulation in anovulatory infertility. Those who fail to respond to clomiphene are treated with FSH and LH. Infertility caused by pituitary hypofunction also needs this therapy. The dose is adjusted according to

ultrasonic findings of follicular growth and E_2 level. The treatment is started on the second day of the cycle and continued until ovulation occurs.
- Induction of multiple ovulation using hyperstimulation protocols for infertile women going through ART as in in vitro fertilization, GIFT, zygote intrafallopian transfer (ZIFT) and ICSI.
- Hypogonadotrophic hypogonadism in males.
- Cryptorchism.
- In primary and secondary amenorrhoea caused by pituitary failure in hypogonadotropic hypogonadism.
- hCG is used in CLPD, infertility and early abortions.

No teratogenicity is reported.

250 mcg recombinant hCG is equal to 5000 IU of hCG with less local side effects.

SIDE EFFECTS

The side effects are as follows:

- Hyperstimulation syndrome.
- Multiple pregnancy in 10%.
- Local reaction at the site of injection, fever, arthritis.

Anti-FSH and anti-LH are in the process of being developed as contraceptives.

GROWTH HORMONE

Growth hormone (GH) is a polypeptide secreted by the anterior pituitary gland. Its action is to induce and promote linear growth at puberty. The growth of the long bones are indirect and is mediated via insulin-like growth factor I (IGF I), secreted mainly by the liver in response to GH. Subcutaneous administration of GH causes rise in the serum IGF I within 4–6 hours, and IGF I in turn has a direct negative feedback on the pituitary hormones. GH is secreted in a pulsatile fashion during sleep. At puberty, its level rises.

Recombinant GH is available as a subcutaneous injection and is used in Turner syndrome and those with short stature. In adults, it reduces the body fat mass, decreases protein catabolism but increases protein synthesis. It causes carbohydrate intolerance. Side effects include ankle oedema, carpal tunnel syndrome, arthralgia, arthritis and diabetes. It, however, improves osteoporosis.

GONADOTROPIN-RELEASING HORMONE AND ITS ANALOGUES

GnRH is a decapeptide first isolated by Matsuo et al. and Scally et al. in 1971. Pulsatile administration of this hormone or its analogues causes a rapid rise in FSH and LH. The rate and intensity of pulsatile release determines the secretion of pituitary hormones. Continuous administration, however, suppresses the pituitary gonadotropins. It has a half-life of 15 minutes. Because of its inactivation in the gut, parenteral routes (subcutaneous and nasal spray) are employed. Agonists and antagonists are available.

AGONISTS AND ANTAGONIST GNRH: MODE OF ACTION

In in vitro fertilization, GnRH agonists cause an initial rise in FSH and oestrogen called 'flare up' followed by gonadotropin suppression (downregulation). Therefore, it takes longer for induction of ovulation.

Synthetic antagonists (cetrorelix and ganirelix) compete with receptors in the anterior pituitary gland and directly suppress gonadotropin secretion. They, therefore, have the following advantages:

- Smaller amount of gonadotropin required for ovulation.
- Shorter stimulation period with FSH.
- Reduced incidence of OHSS and multiple pregnancy.
- Comparable success as agonists in IVF.

Cetrorelix 0.25 mg is started 6 days after FSH therapy until the time of hCG administration, or a single 3 mg dose given at the end of FSH stimulation.

CLINICAL USES

DIAGNOSTIC

GnRH stimulation test, 50–100 mcg, i.v. causes rise in FSH and LH in hypothalamic failure. In pituitary failure , there is no secretion of FSH and LH. This differentiates between hypothalamic and pituitary gland failure in amenorrhoea.

Synthetic GnRH analogues (buserelin, Factrel and goserelin) have been used in clinical practice as follows:

- Pulsatile GnRH analogues 5–10 mcg i.v. every 90–120 minutes (infusion pump) and pulsatile 15–20 mcg subcutaneously or 200 mcg intranasally every 2 hours have been useful in hypothalamic amenorrhoea to stimulate the hypothalamic–pituitary–ovarian axis and induce cyclical menstruation in delayed puberty.
- Pulsatile GnRH, in the above doses, has been used with success in hypothalamic hypogonadal infertility or in those who fail to respond to FSH/LH. Monitoring of ovulation is done ultrasonically and by estimation of E_2 level and the dose is either reduced or replaced by hCG in the luteal phase following ovulation; 50–100 mcg i.v. induces FSH secretion in 30–60 minutes and LH secretion in 15–30 minutes.
- GnRH analogues are used in downregulation protocol to bring down pituitary hormones before starting on FSH/hCG regime in inducing ovulation.
- GnRH in infertility caused by PCOS and endometriosis yields a lower success rate.
- Cryptorchism in males.

Continuous administration or monthly depot injections (Zoladex 3.6 mg) are useful in the following:

- Precocious puberty to suppress pituitary–ovarian hormones until such time that normal puberty is desired.
- Contraception, but administration is difficult and expensive. Buserelin 6.6 mg implants suppress E_2 for 6 months.
- Abnormal uterine bleeding if other measures fail.
- Endometriosis.
- To shrink the size of uterine fibroid preoperatively. Depot injection of 3.6 mg injected i.m. every 28 days for

3 months shrinks the volume and vascularity by 50%–80%. The size of the fibroid starts growing again after stoppage of the drug; therefore, surgery should be undertaken soon after the therapy.
- To shrink the endometrium before transcervical resection of endometrium in menorrhagia.
- Breast cancer to suppress oestrogen.
- Prostatic cancer, cryptorchidism.

When given intravenously or subcutaneously in a pulsatile manner, a special infusion pump is used and the site of infusion changed every 2–3 days.

SIDE EFFECTS

The following are the side effects:

- Hyperstimulation syndrome is reported between 0.6% and 14% (normally 1%).
- Multiple pregnancy is the same as in the general population, i.e. 1%.
- Abortion rate may be slightly increased.
- In gynaecological use, prolonged administration for more than 6 months causes hypo-oestrogenic state and menopausal symptoms, osteoporosis. For this reason and considering the high cost, GnRH therapy should not be given beyond 6 months at a time; 'add-back therapy' can be used.

ADD-BACK THERAPY

The concept of add-back therapy is to counteract the hypo-oestrogenic side effect without affecting the condition for which GnRH therapy is employed. This allows prolonged use of GnRH therapy. The drugs used in add-back therapy are oestrogen, progestogens, tibolone and bisphosphonates especially to prevent osteoporosis. Norethisterone 5–10 mg daily is better than MDPA, as the latter causes osteoporosis. Tibolone is also effective.

Agonists as well as antagonists are now available in GnRH therapy. Antagonists, such as cetrorelix and ganirelix, act faster (3–4 days) against agonists, which may take 3 weeks, and carry some advantage in certain situations.

Other side effects are as follows:

- Insomnia, nausea, decrease in breast size, myalgia, dizziness, decreased libido, LDL, HDL and increased cholesterol.
- Allergic reaction and infection at the site of injection or spray, bronchospasm.
- Drugs used are:
- Nafarelin 400 mcg intranasally for 6 months. Half-life is 4.4 hours.
- Buserelin 300 mcg t.i.d. subcutaneously or intranasally for 3–6 months or 6.6 mg 3-monthly injection (nanopeptide).
- Goserelin (Zoladex) 3.6 mg implant or i.m. monthly (nanopeptide).
- Leuprolide 3.75 mg 4 weekly for 3–6 months or 10.8 mg 3-monthly.
- Superfact 200–500 mg subcutaneously daily.
- Buserelin implant 6.6 mg suppresses ovarian hormones for 3 months.
- Triptorelin 3–7 mg i.m. 4-weekly.

Antagonists of GnRh:

- Antarelix
- Cetrorelix
- These prevent premature LH surge. Advantages of antagonists over agonists are as follows:
- They are cost-effective.
- Short durations of drugs are required compared to prolonged therapy with agonists.
- Smaller doses are required.

Disadvantage: Weekly subcutaneous injection against monthly and 3-monthly injections of agonists.

PROLACTIN

PRL is a polypeptide hormone resembling GH and human placental lactogen. It contains 198 amino acids and is secreted by pituitary lactotrophs in a pulsatile manner. Extra pituitary sites for prolactin production are endometrium, decidua, hypothalamic neurons, intestine, lungs and certain tumors like renal cancer. Prolactin is normally under the inhibitory influence of prolactin-inhibiting factor, dopamine, which acts directly on lactotrophs. Prolactin exists in three forms, little PRL, big PRL and big big PRL. Native or little PRL (50%) which is biologically most active, a big PRL which is elevated in pregnancy and a big big PRL which is inactive.

Stimulating factors for prolactin:

- Prolonged lactation.
- Thyroid-releasing hormone.
- Oestrogen promotes PRL release by inhibiting dopamine of hypothalamic level as well as by directly stimulating lactotrophs.
- Endorphins, tricyclic antidepressants methyldopa phenothiazine stress.
- Sleep increases its secretion.
- Empty sella turcica and pituitary tumours, craniopharyngioma.
- Some cases of endometriosis.
- Some cases of PCOS.
- Liver and renal diseases reduce its excretion.

Clinical features of hyperprolactinaemia are oligomenorrhoea, amenorrhoea, galactorrhoea, infertility and recurrent abortions through CLPD (see Chapters 10 and 12 also).

Normal prolactin level determined by radio-immunoassay (RIA) is up to 25 ng/mL. It is up to 100 ng/mL in hyperprolactinaemia, but level crosses 100 ng/mL in the presence of a tumour. Apart from CT and MRI to detect a brain tumour, visual examination is necessary to detect pressure on the optic nerve.

Treatment is by antiprolactin drugs or surgery for macroadenoma. Antiprolactin drugs are bromocriptine and other derivatives.

Drugs are used in:

- Hyperprolactinaemia
- Microadenoma < 10 cm
- Macroadenoma (>10 cm) to shrink tumour before surgery

BROMOCRIPTINE

Bromocriptine, a synthetic ergot derivative (lysergic acid derivative of ergoline) and a powerful dopamine agonist, was discovered in 1971. It suppresses prolactin while promoting the secretion of gonadotropins. It thus induces menstruation, ovulation and promotes pregnancy. It also suppresses lactation.

Bromocriptine is available as parlodel, proctinal, cabergoline and serocrip tablets.

Pergolide is now also available as a vaginal tablet and intramuscular injection by the name of parlodel-LAR (glycolipid microspheres).

CONTRAINDICATIONS

Hypertension and cardiovascular disease

THERAPEUTIC APPLICATIONS

Bromocriptine's therapeutic uses:

- Suppression of lactation – 2.5–5 mg daily orally.
- Cyclical mastalgia.
- Anovulatory infertility caused by hyperprolactinaemia.
- Treatment of microadenoma and preoperatively in macroadenoma to shrink the tumour before surgery.

In infertility due to hyperprolactinaemia, 70%–90% ovulate and menstruation is established, 70% pregnancy rate is also encouraging. If pregnancy follows, the treatment should be discontinued, though no teratogenic effect is reported in the fetus.

In pregnancy, the level of prolactin rises and the follow-up is mainly by fundus examination, which suggests optic nerve pressure by the tumour. Bromocriptine can be continued during pregnancy if the tumour appears to increase in size as suggested by fundus examination. Cabergoline is safe during pregnancy.

DOSE

The dose starts with 1.25 mg at bedtime and gradually increases to 2.5 mg b.i.d. or more as required. The effect lasts for 12 hours.

In patients who cannot tolerate the oral drug, or in resistant cases, the vaginal tablet or cream is to be used daily. Alternately, the long-acting tablet in the name of cabergoline (Dostinex) is available. Starting with an initial dose of 0.25 mg twice weekly, the dose is gradually built up to 1 mg twice weekly. It acts at a D_2 receptor site.

Parlodel-LAR monthly intramuscular injection, used in the initial dose of 50 mg increasing to 100 mg if necessary, causes acute reduction in prolactin level by 30%–80%, reduction in tumour volume by 25% with minimal side effects.

Quinagolide 25–150 mcg daily in divided doses followed by a maintenance dose of 75 mcg daily.

SIDE EFFECTS

The following side effects are seen in 10%:

- Nausea, vomiting; the patient is advised to take the tablet at night.
- Hypotension and dizziness due to postural hypotension.
- Nasal congestion, headache, constipation.

RESULTS

The drugs normalize prolactin level in 86% of idiopathic hyperprolactinaemia and 77% in microadenoma. The macroadenoma shrinks in 70%. Some require surgery.

HUMAN CHORIONIC GONADOTROPIN

hCG is a glycoprotein containing two linked subunits alpha and beta. Alpha unit contains 92 amino acids similar to LH, FSH and thyroid-stimulating hormone. Beta unit contains 145 amino acids, and has a specific biological activity in pregnancy and ectopic pregnancy.

hCG starts rising soon after fertilization and is detected in the serum 1 week before the due menstrual period. The level doubles every 2–3 days, peaks on the 100th day and then declines gradually. The hormone secreted by the syncytiotrophoblast is luteotropic, and corpus luteum secretes progesterone until the 10th week when the placenta takes over the hormonal functions. With progesterone, it provides endometrial support to the embryo.

Role of hCG

- It supports early pregnancy.
- In ectopic pregnancy and missed abortion, the level is low and does not double every 2–3 days. In hyperemesis and in hydatidiform mole, the level is high, so also in multiple and diabetic pregnancy.
- Although the level is high in trisomy 21 (Down syndrome), it is low in a fetus with trisomy 18.
- Its role in ovarian stimulation in anovulatory infertility has already been described.
- hCG is detected by
- Urine pregnancy test.
- Quantitative test in serum is useful in monitoring ectopic pregnancy and follow-up of molar pregnancy.
- In management decision-making in ectopic pregnancy.

THERAPEUTIC APPLICATIONS

- In habitual abortion, it provides support to the embryo.
- IVF programme: hCG given when the follicular size reaches 20 mm causes follicular rupture 36–38 hours following injection, and provides support in implantation and endometrial vascularization.
- In CLPD.

KEY POINTS

- Oestrogen preparations in clinical use include ethinyl oestradiol used in contraceptive pills, and conjugated oestrogens in HRT in menopausal and urethral syndrome. Implants are mainly employed for long-term use. Vaginal cream is effective in atrophic vaginitis and urethral syndrome.
- Progesterone as injectable in oil or micronized preparation is used in CLPD and early pregnancy support.
- Progestogens are used in abnormal uterine bleeding and as combined contraceptive pills and as mini-pills. They are required in HRT.
- Androgens (Danazol) are effective in the treatment of endometriosis and fibrocystic disease of the breasts.

- Clomiphene and tamoxifen are employed in infertility. Tamoxifen is mainly useful in breast cancer.
- Mifepristone (anti-P) is recently introduced in the termination of early pregnancy.
- Antiandrogens are used to treat hirsutism in PCOS.
- Hypothalamic gonadotropin-releasing hormones (GnRH) are employed in various gynaecological conditions for not more than 6 months. However, add-back therapy allows prolonged use of GnRH therapy.
- Bromocriptine and cabergoline are useful in hyperprolactinaemia and suppression of lactation.
- The side effects of all hormonal preparations should be known and avoided in clinical practice.
- hCG hormone is used in the induction of ovulation and pregnancy support in early gestation.
- Antiprolactin drugs are employed in hyperprolactinaemia and microadenoma. They induce menstruation and ovulation, and improve pregnancy rate. Macroadenoma may require surgery.
- FSH and HCG are used in the induction of ovulation if clomiphene fails, and in IVF to induce multiple ovulation.

SELF-ASSESSMENT

1. Describe the physiological role of oestrogens in the body. Enumerate the indications and the commonly used oestrogenic medications in clinical practice.
2. Classify progestogens and their clinical applications.
3. Name the androgenic medications and their clinical applications.
4. Name the pituitary gonadotropins and their role in therapeutics.
5. What are GnRH analogues? What is their role in clinical practice?
6. A woman, 28-year old, complains of galactorrhoea. How will you investigate and manage this case?
7. Discuss the drugs used in anovulatory infertility.

SUGGESTED READING

ACOG Committee on Gynecologic Practice. ACOG Committee Opinion #322: Compounded bioidentical hormones. Obstet Gynecol 2005; 106:1139.

ACOG Practice Bulletin No. 141: management of menopausal symptoms. Obstet Gynecol 2014; 123:202.

Amar AP, Couldwell WT, et al. Predictive value of serum prolactin levels after transphenoidal surgery. J Neurosurg 2002;97(2): 307.

Arulkumaran S. Clinics in Obstetric and Gynecology 2009;23:5.

Bergendal A, Kieler H, Sundström A, et al. Risk of venous thromboembolism associated with local and systemic use of hormone therapy in peri- and postmenopausal women and in relation to type and route of administration. Menopause 2016; 23:593.

Canonico M. Hormone therapy and thromboembolism amongst postmenopausal women: Impact of the route of administration of estrogen and progestogens: The ESTHER study. Circulation 2007;115(7): 840–845.

Carr B, Breslau N, Givens C, et al. Oral contraceptive pill, GNRH agonists, or use in combination in the treatment of hirsutism. J Endocrinol Metab 1995;60(4):1169–1173.

Cicarelli E, Cammani F. Diagnosis and drug therapy of prolactinomas. Drugs 1996;51(6):954.

Crandall CJ, Hovey KM, Andrews CA, et al. Breast cancer, endometrial cancer, and cardiovascular events in participants who used vaginal estrogen in the Women's Health Initiative Observational Study. Menopause 2018; 25:11.

Duncan J & Shulman P. Yearbook of Obstetrics, Gynaecology and Women's Health, 2010;207.

ECAB (GnRH). Clinical Update in Obstetrics Gynaecology, 2010.

Felson DT, Zhang Y, Hannen MT, et al. The effect of postmenopausal estrogen therapy on bone density in elderly women. N Engl J Med 1993;329:1141–1146.

Fruzzetti F, Bersi C, Parrini D, et al. Treatment of hirsutism: Comparisons between different antiandrogens with central and peripheral effects. Fertil Steril 1999;71:445.

Grodstein F, Manson JE, Stampfer MJ, Rexrode K. Postmenopausal hormone therapy and stroke: role of time since menopause and age at initiation of hormone therapy. Arch Intern Med 2008; 168:861.

Kaunitz AM. Clinical practice. Hormonal contraception in women of older reproductive age. N Engl J Med 2008; 358:1262.

Legro RS, Barnhart HX, Schlaff WD, et al. Clomiphene, metformin or both for infertility in polycystic ovarian syndrome. N Engl J Med 2007;356(6):551–566.

Lunenfeld B, Insler V. Human gonadotropins. In Wallach EE, Zacur HA (eds) Reproductive Medicine and Surgery. St. Louis: Mosby – Year Book 1995;611–638.

Marjoribanks J, Farquhar C, Roberts H, et al. Long-term hormone therapy for perimenopausal and postmenopausal women. Cochrane Database Syst Rev 2017; 1:CD004143.

Obstet Gynecol Clin N Am

Petiti DB. Combination estrogen progestin oral contraceptives. N Engl J Med 2003;349(14):1443–1440.

Rosen CJ. Postmenopausal osteoporosis. N Engl J Med 2005; 353 (6):595–603.

The NAMS 2017 Hormone Therapy Position Statement Advisory Panel. The 2017 hormone therapy position statement of The North American Menopause Society. Menopause 2017; 24:728.

Worsley R, Davis SR, Gavrilidis E, et al. Hormonal therapies for new onset and relapsed depression during perimenopause. Maturitas 2012; 73:127.

SECTION 3

COMMON CONDITIONS IN GYNAECOLOGY

SECTION OUTLINE

16 Infertility - Male and Female

CHAPTER OUTLINE

Procreation or desire to have one's own offspring is the greatest desire among human beings. Since inception of civilization, failure to have one's own baby or infertility has affected countless couples both rich and poor alike. Infertility besides being a health issue is more of a social problem which affects personal, social and mental health of affected person. It is estimated that 10%–15% of married couples suffer from infertility. Due to changing social system, professional life and academic achievement more and more couples face this problem. In India commonly held notion about infertility is that it is due to female partner; however, in actual life both partners contribute equally to infertility. Following section discusses physiology of reproduction, common causes of infertility, modes of investigation and therapeutic approaches for infertility.

PHYSIOLOGY OF FERTILIZATION

Conception results from the fertilization of the ovum by a spermatozoon. Much information is now available about the biological process whereby the spermatozoon enters the ovum as fertilization can be studied in, in vitro fertilization (IVF) programme.

The mechanism whereby spermatozoa pass along the uterus is not properly explained. As ciliary movement of the cervical and endometrial epithelia is downwards, the spermatozoa must migrate against the ciliary current. It can only be assumed that spermatozoa, which live in an attractive alkaline medium of the seminal fluid (pH 8), find the acid environment of the vaginal secretion (pH 4.5) lethal in a matter of 2–4 hours. The cervix has the same pH as the seminal fluid and is undoubtedly and demonstrably attractive to the spermatozoa. Spermatozoa are powerful, fast swimmers, and from the time of ejaculation to the time of arrival in the ampulla of the tube, it takes about 60 minutes for the spermatozoa to cover the intervening 20 cm. This distance compared to the size of a spermatozoon represents a rapid and purposeful travel. The subendothelial layer of the endometrium exhibits increased upward peristalsis during the follicular phase near ovulation time, and this may hasten the migration of sperms into the fallopian tube.

It is now generally accepted that though a spermatozoon after ejaculation may remain motile for a long period, its useful life span is limited to 24 hours, and after this short interval, it is less capable of performing its biological duty. The period of survival of a mature ovum is probably even shorter than that of a spermatozoon, and the time which elapses after its escape from a ripe Graafian follicle and its entry into the fallopian tube during which it is potentially fertilizable is estimated at 12 hours and rarely up to 24 hours. The significance of this statement is that coitus, to be capable of fertilization, must take place in the 24-hour period around ovulation. Ovulation most commonly occurs 14 days before the onset of the next period, though variations are known.

The fimbriae of the fallopian tube by muscular contraction spread out over the ovary at the time of ovulation, a movement which simplifies the transport of the discharged ovum into the lumen of the fallopian tube. Furthermore, the musculature of the fallopian tube undergoes rhythmical contractions, especially at the time of ovulation. It is most likely the peristaltic contraction of the fallopian tube that determines the transport of the ovum towards the cavity of the uterus. The sperm that reaches the ovum first penetrates the zona pellucida and normally inhibits entry by other sperms. By the time the fertilized egg enters the uterine cavity, the endometrium has grown under the effect of progesterone into secretory endometrium and is ready to receive the egg for implantation and provide its nutrition.

On general biological principles, the blame of infertility should be shared between the two partners. It is not uncommon for patients to complain of difficulty during coitus when they have little knowledge of the correct method to be employed. During sexual intercourse, the erectile tissues around the vaginal orifice become engorged and the vaginal orifice becomes more patulous. There is a discharge of mucous from the ducts of Bartholin's glands, which acts as a lubricant. The female orgasm is induced by stimulation of the clitoris partly during the penetration of the penis and partly as the result of the clitoris being rhythmically pressed against the penis after penetration. The importance of the extragenital areas of sexual stimulation must not be forgotten. These erogenic areas vary with the individual and their susceptibility to stimulation is equally variable, but their aggregate response is cumulative and plays a vital part in the ultimate achievement of an orgasm. There is some evidence that the mucous secretion contained in the cervical canal is extruded into the vagina during the orgasm. The seminal fluid is mainly deposited in the posterior fornix of the vagina, but it is possible that some of it is ejaculated directly into the cervical canal. It is also believed that the contractions of the uterus and the fallopian tubes during the female orgasm cause seminal fluid to be aspirated into the cavity of the uterus, and it is possible that this aspiration effect is responsible, in part at least, for the migration of spermatozoa upwards into the fallopian tubes. A more likely suggestion is that rhythmic contractions of the pelvic muscles direct the seminal ejaculate towards the cervix, where the propulsive power of the spermatozoa provides the forward momentum. The female orgasm is not essential for conception, and it is not uncommon to see women who have conceived without full consummation of the marriage and in whom the hymen is intact. In such cases the spermatozoa, having been deposited around the hymen, migrate through their own motility along the whole length of the vagina and uterus.

INFERTILITY

According to World Health Organization (WHO), positive reproductive health of a woman is a state of complete physical, mental and social well-being and not merely the absence of disease related to reproductive system and functions.

Infertility implies apparent failure of a couple to conceive, while sterility indicates absolute inability to conceive, for one or more reasons. If a couple fails to achieve pregnancy after 1 year of 'unprotected' and regular intercourse, it is an indication to investigate the couple. This is based on the observation that 80% of normal couples achieve conception within a year. It is observed that 50% conceive within 3 months following regular, unprotected intercourse, 75% in 6 months and 80%–85% conceive within a year. Infertility is termed as **primary,** if conception has never occurred, and **secondary**, if the woman fails to conceive after having achieved a previous conception. The incidence of infertility in any community varies between 5% and 15%.

Optimal age for conception is 20–35 years in a woman. After the age of 40 years, the fertility rate is reduced, and there is an increased risk of chromosomal abnormalities and other malformations in the fetus. For a man age is less important, but after 50 years, decreased libido and sexual dysfunction reduce fertility and predispose to malformed fetus Therefore, it may be prudent to proceed with investigations of apparent infertility in a woman near or after the age of 35 years, instead of waiting for a year, if she seeks gynaecological help.

Conception is the result of successful fertilization of the female egg by the sperm. Hence, the couple should be counselled individually and then together because both partners contribute varyingly to the occurrence of the infertile state. It is mandatory to investigate both the partners simultaneously, carry out the necessary tests and adopt appropriate measures to enhance the fertility potential of each individual partner.

ISSUES INVOLVED

The major goals involved in the comprehensive investigations of the infertile couple are as follows:

- Identification and correction of causes contributing to the infertile state over a short span of time.
- Providing accurate information, education and counselling to both the partners, and explaining the nature of therapy and the cost.
- Counselling about alternative management of infertility if pregnancy fails or is not possible (sterility) should be provided. This may include discussions on the roles of assisted reproductive techniques, artificial insemination and the option of adoption. Prognosis and success rate of each should be discussed. It is also important to realize the futility of repeating the same investigations by different doctors which may be frustrating to the couple apart from the expense incurred. It may be prudent on the part of the doctor to study the previous records before asking for a repeat test.

Prognosis

The advance age of the woman, long duration of infertility and previous failed medical and surgical treatment are associated with poor prognosis.

INITIAL COUNSELLING

During the initial counselling, it is important to explain to both the partners, in simple words, the process of reproduction with the help of charts and models. Explain that it is possible to find a faulty function in both partners, and often overlapping causes exist, hence the need to evaluate and treat both the partners concurrently.

MALE INFERTILITY

DEVELOPMENT AND GROWTH IN A MALE

SPERMATOGENESIS

Spermatogenesis occurs in the seminiferous tubules of the testis. The primordial germ cells appear in the yolk sac in the 3rd week of embryo and migrate along the dorsal mesentery to the genital ridge. These germ cells divide by mitosis into 1300 primordial cells or spermatogonia by the 6th week. These remain quiescent in the seminiferous tubules throughout childhood.

Near puberty, spermatogonia divide by mitosis into primary spermatocytes. Meiosis occurs only at puberty and smaller secondary spermatocytes containing haploid number of chromosomes are formed. These develop into spermatids. The spermatozoa develop by acquiring an acrosome cap, elongation and condensation of sperm nucleus and a tail. The development of sperms take 72 days (Fig. 16.1) and entire spermatogenesis including transit time in the duct takes 3 months.

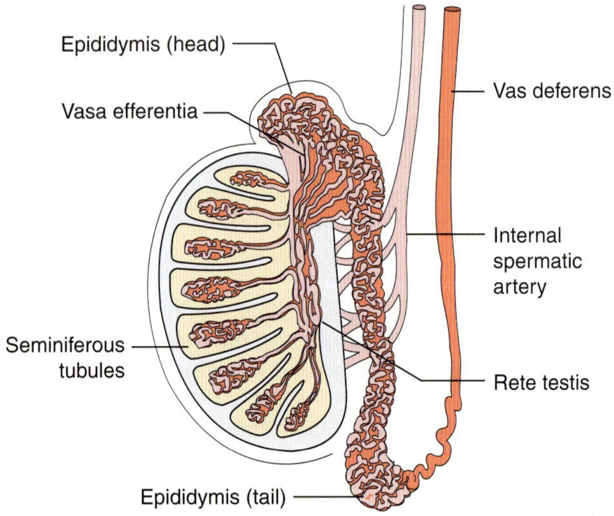

Figure 16.1 Normal anatomy of the testes.

STRUCTURE OF THE SPERM (Fig. 16.2)

The mature sperm has a head with an acrosome covering, midpiece and a tail which allows motility. Acrosome membrane contains enzyme hyaluronidase, acrosin and other proteases, which allow acrosin reaction, break down of acrosome membrane and penetration of sperm into zona pellucid. Hyaluronidase dissolves corona radiata cells. The sperms are stored in the epididymis. One spermatocyte produces four spermatids, and one spermatid produces four spermatozoa.

Spermatogenesis beginning at puberty is a continuous process unlike ovulation, which occurs once a month, and continues with senescence though with less efficiency. The testes show germ cells in different stages of maturation at any given time, and the sperms mature in the testes as well as the accessory organs, and undergo capacitation in the cervix before they are capable of fertilization.

The seminiferous tubules are lined by germ cells and Sertoli cells lying adjacent to germ cells. The Sertoli cells produce androgen-binding protein by follicle-stimulating hormone (FSH) and bind testosterone to this protein causing a high level of testosterone within the testes compared to that in the blood. The interstitial cells (Leydig cells) produce testosterone by luteinizing hormone (LH).

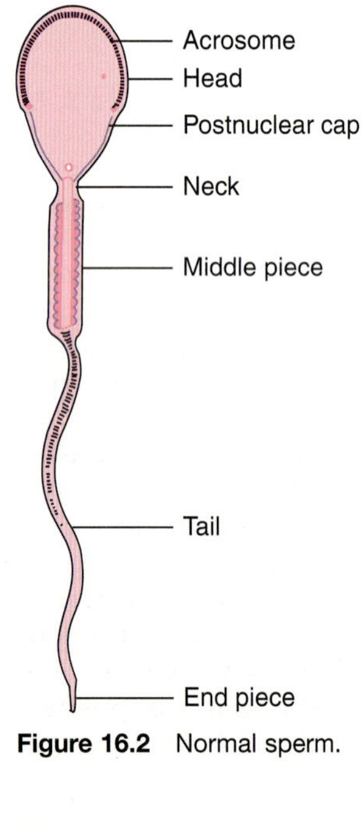

Figure 16.2 Normal sperm.

ENDOCRINE CONTROL

Hypothalamus is critical in the development of male organs and spermatogenesis. Gonadotropin-releasing hormone (GnRH) in males is produced continuously, unlike in a pulsatile fashion in females. FSH is not essential for spermatogenesis; it acts on the Sertoli cells and produces androgen-binding protein mentioned above. The Sertoli cells also produce Müllerian inhibiting hormone (MIH) and inhibin which inhibit FSH. MIH inhibit development of Müllerian system. LH stimulates testosterone secretion by the Leydig cells.

Hypothalamic failure leads to loss of spermatogenesis and testosterone production.

The sperms are formed in the lining epithelium of the seminiferous tubules from the germinal cells – spermatogonia (Fig. 16.3).

Spermatogonia are diploid germinal cells which divide by mitosis into spermatocysts. These undergo reduction division (meiosis I) into haploid secondary spermatocysts, which by meiosis II develop into spermatids. These spermatids develop into compact, virtually cytoplasm-free sperms with condensed DNA in the head, capped by apical acrosome and a tail (Fig. 16.2). These sperms are incapable of fertilization after they undergo capacitation in the female cervical canal. The entire process of spermatogenesis takes 74 days, and if we include transport in the ductal system it takes 3 months. They are present in the testes in different stages of development at any given time. The testes produce 200–300 million sperms daily.

Capacitation can also be induced following incubation in a culture media in IVF. Cervix plays the following role in reproduction:

1. Nutrition to the sperms.
2. Alkaline medium for survival of sperms.

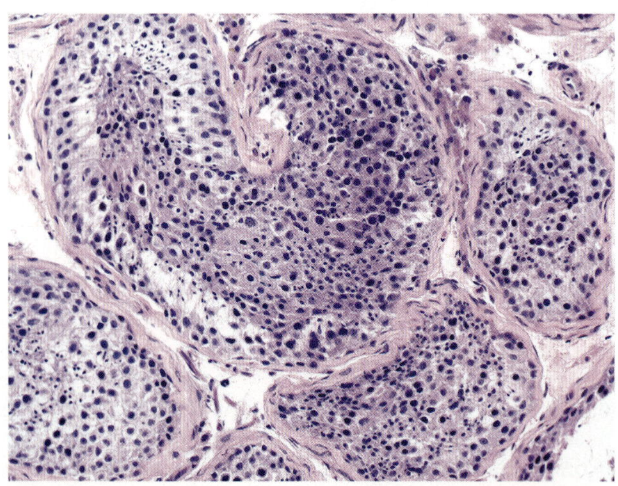

Figure 16.3 Testicular biopsy. Normal seminiferous tubules. Note spermatozoa in lumen (×250). (*Source*: Dharam Ramnani, MD, Richmond, VA, http://www.webpathology.com/image.asp?case=27n=1)

3. Sieves out abnormal sperms.
4. Causes capacitation of sperms. Storage until upward propulsion of sperms.

Acrosome reaction is an important component of capacitation for zona penetration into the oocyte. Acrosome is a modified lysosome over the sperm head, under its action the overlying membrane becomes unstable, breaks down and releases hyaluronidase enzyme, which allows the penetration of corona radiata and zona pellucida.

The Sertoli cells line the seminiferous tubules and extend from the base of the membrane to the lumen. They support the spermatids and possess receptors for FSH and testosterone. The tropic effect of FSH and testosterone on spermatogenesis is mediated via the Sertoli cells. There are four sperms per Sertoli cell. The Sertoli cells produce Müllerian inhibitory factor which prevents the development of Müllerian system. The Sertoli cells also produce testosterone-binding protein which maintains high level of testosterone within the testis. This is necessary for continuous spermatogenesis.

ENDOCRINE CONTROL OF SPERMATOGENESIS

The spermatogenesis depends on the hypothalamic–anterior pituitary–testicular functions. GnRH stimulates the anterior pituitary gland to secrete FSH and LH. FSH acts on the Sertoli cells, and LH triggers testosterone secretion by the Leydig cells (interstitial cells). The concentration of testosterone is higher in the testes than in the plasma. The testosterone in turn exerts a negative feedback on the pituitary gland, as well as the hypothalamus.

A total of 60% of serum testosterone is bound to sex hormones binding globulin (SHBG) and 20% to albumin. A small portion is converted to oestrogen. Two per cent free testosterone is converted to dihydrotestosterone by 5-alpha reductase enzyme which acts on hair follicles and is responsible for male phenotype.

The Sertoli cells also secrete inhibin B which in turn inhibits FSH but stimulates LH secretion.

Fertilization

Following capacitation, a mature sperm meets the ovum in the ampullary portion of the fallopian tube. By acrosomal reaction and hyaluronidase release, it penetrates the zona pellucida, which in turn prevents entry of other sperms (polyspermia). It is possible to aspirate the polar body or a blastocyst cell for genetic study of the embryo, without disturbing further development of the embryo.

MALE FACTOR INFERTILITY

In one-third of all cases, the male is directly responsible, in one-third both partners are at fault and in the remaining third the cause of failure is attributed entirely to the female. These figures are perhaps extremes and it might be more appropriate to distribute the fault evenly between the two partners.

Faults in the Male

Following factors in males contribute to infertility:

- Disorders of spermatogenesis – 50%
- Obstruction of the efferent ducts – 30%
- Disorders of sperm motility – 15%
- Sexual dysfunction
- Unexplained – 15%

For adequate spermatogenesis, the testicle must lie in its correct position in the scrotum, where the temperature is slightly cooler than elsewhere in the body. The factors which raise the scrotal temperature can adversely influence spermatogenesis, e.g. the occupation of men who work as stokers or in blast furnaces and are subjected to excessive heat, the wearing of a tight scrotal support and the presence of a varicocele. The ectopic or undescended testicle provides the best example of the adverse effect of temperature on spermatogenesis. The collecting apparatus of the epididymis may be damaged by trauma or inflammatory disease, notably gonorrhoea or tuberculosis. The vas deferens itself may be occluded, and this is specially to be suspected if there is a herniorrhaphy scar and doubly so if the scar is bilateral. Chronic inflammatory diseases of the prostate and seminal vesicle may be associated with male infertility. Congenital lesions of the penile urethra such as hypospadias provide an obvious mechanical explanation for imperfect insemination. A history of mumps, venereal disease, diabetes, thyroid or tuberculosis may suggest testicular atrophy or obstruction. The occupation of the male, history of excessive smoking, indulging in excessive alcohol consumption and chewing tobacco and *gutka* may also suggest poor spermatogenesis. Accidental or operative trauma, e.g. blow on the testicle with haematoma formation and subsequent atrophy, or operation for hernia, varicocele or hydrocele may suggest a degenerative lesion of the testes or obstruction to the vas. About 1%–2% males suffer from genetic defects such as Klinefelter syndrome with 47XXY chromosomes.

Aetiological Classification

1. Genetic – abnormal Y chromosome and XXY in Klinefelter syndrome. Mutation of short or long arm Y chromosome.
2. Disorders of spermatogenesis.
   A. Hormonal (pretesticular):
      - Hypothalamic disorder, Kallmann syndrome.
      - Pituitary secretion of FSH, LH.
      - Hyperprolactinaemia causing impotence or diminished libido.
      - Hypothyroidism, adrenal gland disorder and diabetes.
   B. Primary testicular disorders (testicular):
      - Idiopathic, varicocele, absent germ cells.
      - Chromosomal defect, i.e. Klinefelter syndrome.
      - Cryptorchidism.
      - Drugs, radiation, calcium channel blocker, anticonvulsants, antihypertensives, spironolactone and cimetidine.
      - Orchitis (traumatic, mumps, TB, gonorrhoea).
      - Chronic illness.
      - Immunological disorders (5%).
      - Immotility due to the absence of dynein arms. Absent cilia in Kartagener syndrome (15%).
3. Duct obstruction (post-testicular). Congenital absence, inflammatory block (gonococcal, tubercular), surgical trauma, Young syndrome (inspissated mucous) associated with sinusitis and bronchiectasis. *Escherichia coli*,

staphylococci, chlamydial infection. Mycoplasma genitalis causes DNA fragmentation of sperms, decreased motility and apoptosis. Accessory gland disorders: Prostatitis, vesiculitis and congenital absence of vas in cystic fibrosis.

4. Disorders of sperms and vesicular fluid:
   - Sperm antibodies and low fructose in seminal plasma. Immotile cilia syndrome (Kartagener syndrome).
   - Sperm acrosome defect.
   - Zona pellucida binding defect.
   - Zona pellucida penetration defect.
   - Oocyte fusion defect.
5. Sexual dysfunctions:
   - Low-coital frequencies – wrong time, low libido.
   - Impotence, hypospadias.
   - Premature ejaculation.
   - Retrograde ejaculation.
6. Psychological and environmental factors such as smoking, alcohol consumption, tobacco chewing, diabetes and drugs – antihypertensive, antipsychotics, cimetidine, sex steroids (excess testosterone and anabolic used by athletes) chemotherapy, nitrofurantoin, beta-blockers, spironolactone, oestrogen.
7. Obesity increases peripheral conversion of androgen to oestrogen and affects fertility.
8. Chronic illness.

INVESTIGATIONS

1. **History.** History includes age of the male partner, previous marriage, duration of infertility and any contraception practiced and for how long. This gives a true picture of the duration of infertility.
   - The coital frequency and timing related to ovulation.
   - The occupation – a frequent traveller or working in a hot place.
   - Habit of smoking, alcohol, tobacco and other drugs usage.
   - History of tuberculosis, sexually transmitted infection, diabetes and chronic illness. Diabetic neuropathy can cause impotence and retrograde ejaculation. Fever of any cause can suppress spermatogenesis for as long as 6 months. Chronic respiratory disease.
   - Operation on the scrotum, undescended testis or hernia repair.
   - Any coital problem such as premature and retrograde ejaculation, failure to ejaculate.
2. **General examination** in a standing posture to look for size of the testis, the presence of varicocele, thickening of the vas and a per rectal examination for obvious prostate enlargement or tenderness in seminal vesicle. A normal report rules out any major general or local cause for male infertility. One can move on to further investigations. Abnormal semen analysis calls for general and local examination of a male partner.
   - General: height increased in Kallmann and Klinefelter syndrome is due to late closure of epiphyses of the bones.
   - Weight and obesity may point to be hormonal defects.
   - The secondary sex characters are abnormal in Klinefelter syndrome, i.e. gynaecomastia associated with Turner-like stigmata.
   - Thyroid enlargement, enlarged breasts and hirsutism may be noted. Blood pressure should be checked.
3. **Local examination** includes examination of penis and scrotum, and surgical scar. The normal testicular volume is 15–35 mL (average 18 mL). Testicular volume of less than 6 mL is seen in atrophic testes and in Klinefelter syndrome. The testes should be well placed in the scrotum. The epididymis should be palpated for enlargement and thickness. The vas feels thickened in inflamed conditions. Rectal examination includes the prostate examination. The presence of varicocele (more often on left side) can be demonstrated when male is examined in a standing posture, and on Doppler ultrasound.

   Special investigations comprise the following:

- Semen analysis.
- Hormonal assays.
- FNAC from testis
- Testicular biopsy – for histology, genetic study and cryopreservation in assisted reproduction (intracytoplasmic sperm insemination).
- Immunological tests.
- Patency of vas.
- Chromosomal study.

Not all of the above investigations are required in a male. Stepwise investigations will not only save time but also avoid unnecessary and elaborate tests which may turned out to be not only expensive but stressful and frustrating for the male partner.

Semen Analysis

The most important part of the male investigation is the semen analysis, and certain points regarding the method and timing of collection of the specimen are noteworthy. The best specimen is one obtained by masturbation in the vicinity of the laboratory, because this guarantees its freshness, and avoids changes due to temperature variation. If this is not possible, coitus interruptus into a wide necked bottle may be employed. Another method is the postcoital test described later. The production of a condom specimen is to be discouraged as the condom contains spermicidal chemicals and a false low reading may thereby be obtained. The best specimen will be produced if a short period of abstinence of 3–5 days is observed. A more prolonged period of abstinence does not yield better results. A typical normal specimen should show the following features when examined within 2 hours of production (earlier the better). The semen should coagulate soon after ejaculation due to enzyme in the seminal vesicle, but liquefy in 30 minutes because of prostatic enzyme. The semen is greyish white in colour.

In 2010, WHO laid down the latest criteria for normal semen quality and reference (Table 16.1).

- Volume: 2 mL (1.5 mL)
- pH: 7.2–7.8
- Viscosity: <3 (scale 0–4)
- Sperm concentration: 15 million/mL
- Total sperm count: >40 million/per ejaculate or more

Table 16.1 Latest WHO Recommendations for Normal Semen Analysis Reference Values.

Latest WHO standard for semen analysis – 2010:

- Volume: 1.5–5.0 mL
- pH: >7.2
- Viscosity: <3 (scale 0–4)
- Sperm concentration: >15 million/mL
- Total sperm number: >39 million/ejaculate
- Per cent motility: >32%
- Forward progression: >2 (scale 0–4)
- Normal morphology: > 4%
- Round cells: <1 million/mL
- Sperm agglutination: <2 (scale 0–3)

Source: WHO guidelines.

- Motility: >50% or more with at least 25% progressively motile.
- Morphology: >at least 4% normal in morphology
- Viability: >75% or more (50%)
- White blood cells: <1 million/mL
- Round cells: <5 million/mL
- Sperm agglutination: <2

Low volume may be due to following:

- Incomplete collection, poor abstinence
- Abnormalities in the seminal vesicles
- Partial vas obstruction
- Retrograde ejaculation
- Hypogonadism

Pus cells should be absent. The seminal fluid is normally viscous with a pH of 7.2–7.8, and contains fructose.

Aspermia – means no semen.
Azoospermia – implies no sperm in semen.
Oligospermia – low sperm count.
Asthenospermia – no motile sperm or diminished motility.
Necrospermia – dead sperms.
Teratospermia – abnormal morphology of sperms.

A normal sperm is motile, 50 microns in length, half the size of ovum and consists of a head covered by an acrosomal cap, neck, body and tail.

Hypospermia means low volume, less than 1.5 mL. This may be due to improper collection or retrograde ejaculation.

Hyperspermia with more than 5.5 mL means prolonged abstinence or inflammation of seminal vesicle.

The most important factor is the density of the sperm, and counts below 15 million/mL are usually associated with infertility. Oligospermia is mild when the count is 10–20 million, moderate when 5–15 million and severe when less than 5 million/mL sperms are seen.

If one report shows abnormal findings, the patient should be instructed to produce another specimen after a month or so. During this time, the patient should be advised to take a good nutritional diet and restrict smoking and consumption of alcohol. He should take cold or tepid bath and discard tight underwear. Only after two negative or below average counts, he should be proclaimed azoospermic or oligospermic. If so, chromosomal study should be done

A few normal sperms and normal testosterone suggest retrograde ejaculation. Centrifuged specimen can be used for intrauterine insemination (IUI), IVF.

Postcoital Test (*Sims' or Huhner's Test, PCT*)

The couple is advised intercourse close to ovulation time preferably in the early hours of the morning. The woman presents herself at the clinic within 2 hours after the intercourse. The mucous is aspirated from the cervical canal and spread over a glass slide. Another smear made from the posterior fornix serves as a control. Normally 10–50 motile sperms are seen per high-power field in cervical mucous. If there are less than 10 sperms, proper semen analysis should be undertaken. The sperms should show progressive, but not rotatory movements. The presence of antispermal antibodies in the cervical mucous leads shaky or rotatory movements to the sperms or may totally immobilize them. The cervical mucous is simultaneously examined for its quantity, viscosity and fern test. The advantage of this test is that the cervical mucous can be simultaneously studied for oestrogenic effect and ovulation, its capability to allow sperm penetration and the presence of any antisperm antibodies. The test is useless in the presence of cervical infection, which should be treated before performing the postcoital test. Immunological factor is encountered in 5% cases. This test is less employed lately, and many gynaecologists consider this obsolete. This is because they resort to IUI, if semen analysis is abnormal.

A test called the *Miller–Kurzrok* test consists of placing ovulation mucous on a glass slide alongside the specimen of the husband's semen and studying the penetration of sperms under the microscope. Normal cervical mucous permits invasion by motile sperms. Penetration less than 3 cm at 30 minutes is abnormal.

Sperm Penetration Test

The physiological profile of the sperms can be studied in vitro by using the zona-free hamster egg, which resembles the human ovum. A normal sperm is capable of penetrating the zona-free hamster egg, showing its fertilizing capacity. The test is expensive and not reliable.

Sperm agglutination tests, immobilization tests and immunoglobulin specific assays are available to detect immunological defects in the semen.

Semen–cervical Mucous Contact Test

Equal quantity of semen and mucous is mixed, so that there is no interface. In the presence of antibodies more than 25% sperms show jerky or shaky movements by 30 minutes. The cross-check with the donor semen will indicate the source of antibodies, whether it is cervical or seminal antibodies.

Testicular biopsy. Testicular biopsy is indicated in azoospermia to distinguish between testicular failure and obstruction in the vas deferens. It also reveals whether the seminiferous tubules are normal but unstimulated by the anterior pituitary gland, or whether they are incapable of function due to primary gonadal failure. Testicular biopsy will establish which of the factor is at fault (Figs 16.3 and 16.4). The biopsy can also diagnose genital tuberculosis. The tru-cut biopsy under local anaesthesia is simple to

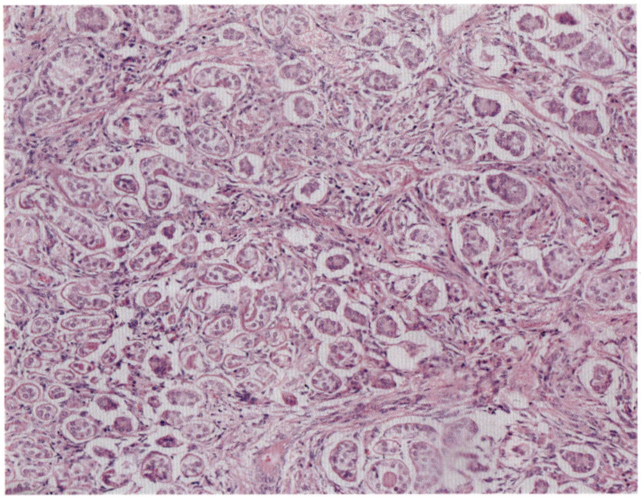

Figure 16.4 Testicular biopsy. Tubular atrophy showing the Sertoli cells only (×250). (*Courtesy*: Dr Sandeep Mathur, AIIMS.)

perform. One to three per cent males have endocrine dysfunction. *In recent times, the testicular biopsy has a very big role to play. Apart from chromosomal and histological study, the testicular tissue provides cryopreservation in assisted reproduction.* The spermatozoa as well as spermatids extracted from the testicular tissue can be used in intracytoplasmic semen insemination (ICSI) in assisted reproduction. Sperm morphology is studied by preparing a slide, air-drying, fixing it with 70% alcohol and staining with Pap stain.

FSH level. A high FSH level denotes primary gonadal failure. A normal level in azoospermia suggests obstructive lesion in the vas or epididymis. A low FSH level indicates pituitary or hypothalamic failure and a need for FSH/LH/GnRH treatment. Prolactin level more than 30 ng/mL indicates hyperprolactinaemia requiring treatment. Low testosterone level indicates low LH or Leydig cell dysfunction. No response to GnRH suggests pituitary failure.

Chromosomal study. Karyotyping should be undertaken in azoospermic men, as 15%–20% of them have chromosomal disorders. The most common disorder is Klinefelter syndrome with 47XXY karyotype.

Immunological disorders. A recent interest in immunological aspects of infertility has led to the detection of various sperm antibodies, both in the seminal plasma and in the cervical mucous. Immunological factors may be important aetiologically in up to 5% of patients with male infertility. An immunological test is required in case of an abnormal postcoital test, abnormal semen profile and unexplained infertility. ELISA and RIA tests determine antibodies to sperm, seminal plasma and cervical secretion.

Ultrasound scanning. The ultrasound scanning of the scrotum detects scrotal volume and varicocele and is useful in ultrasound-guided biopsy. Colour flow Doppler and scrotal thermography detect varicocele.

- Vasogram. It is required when normal FSH level is associated with azoospermia to rule out obstruction in the vas.
- Urine examination. In suspected retrograde ejaculation, postejaculatory urine is made alkaline and centrifuged. The presence of sperms in the urine proves retrograde ejaculation.
- Fragmentation of sperms suggests infection. Chlamydial and other infections should be investigated.
- Sperm fertilization potential.

In IVF, this test is useful in selecting the best sperm for fertilization. This is called hypo-osmotic swelling test (HOS). The sperms are treated with hypo-osmotic saline. If the sperm membrane is intact, the sperms swell up and coiling occurs. These are the best sperms.

MANAGEMENT OF MALE INFERTILITY

Management is based on the assessment of coital function, semen examination report and the result of the postcoital and immunological tests, as well as hormonal reports (Fig. 16.5).

1. Education. This involves: (i) sexual counselling – coital frequency and timing, (ii) coital position and (iii) masturbation leading to sperm dilution.
2. Substance abuse. Advice on avoidance of tobacco (smoking, chewing), moderation in consumption of alcohol and avoidance of drug abuse. Antioxidants, vitamin E improve semen parameters. Pentoxifylline 400 mg t.i.d. improves sperm motility.
3. Reduce heat around the scrotum. Avoid hot baths, wear loose cotton underwear (cotton clothing to encourage ventilation), avoid strenuous activities and occupation in hot environment and control obesity.
4. Correct endocrinopathies. Prompt attention to diabetes and thyroid disorders.
5. Surgical. Surgical correction of varicocele after the diagnosis has been confirmed on ultrasound scanning helps to improve sperm motility. Though recently percutaneous embolization of varicocele is attempted, damage to the testicular artery and recurrence of varicocele make microsurgery the gold standard and the best option for varicocele. Lately, the beneficial effect of varicocele surgery is questioned by many who feel that the surgery for correction of varicocele has no role in improving male infertility. Surgical correction of the undescended testes in childhood improves the semen quality in 60%–70% cases. The obstruction in the vas by micro surgical vasovasal or vaso-epididymal anastomosis will restore patency. Ephedrine 60 mg orally four times a day for 2 weeks or α-adrenergic drug such as phenylephrine (2.5 mg) is tried in retrograde ejaculation. If this fails reconstruction of the bladder neck is recommended. Vasovasostomy in the reversal of vasectomy operation yields a poor result if an interval of more than 5 years has elapsed since vasectomy, because of the formation of sperm antibodies.
6. Antibiotics. Infection indicates the need for appropriate antibiotics to treat epididymo-orchitis, prostatitis and sexually transmitted diseases. Doxycycline 100 mg b.i.d. for 6 weeks is beneficial for chlamydial infection.
7. Role of oxidating stress on sperm function through pro-oxidants liberated by leucocytes, and abnormal sperms is now realized. Some have observed improved sperm count by prescribing lycopene 2 mg daily and vitamin E. Antioxidants contain vitamin E 100 mg, vitamin C 500–1000 mg, N-acetylcysteine 200–500 mg t.i.d., carnitine 3 g daily, selenium 225 mg, pentoxifylline 400 mg t.i.d. Lycopene 2 mg daily for 6 months is reported to

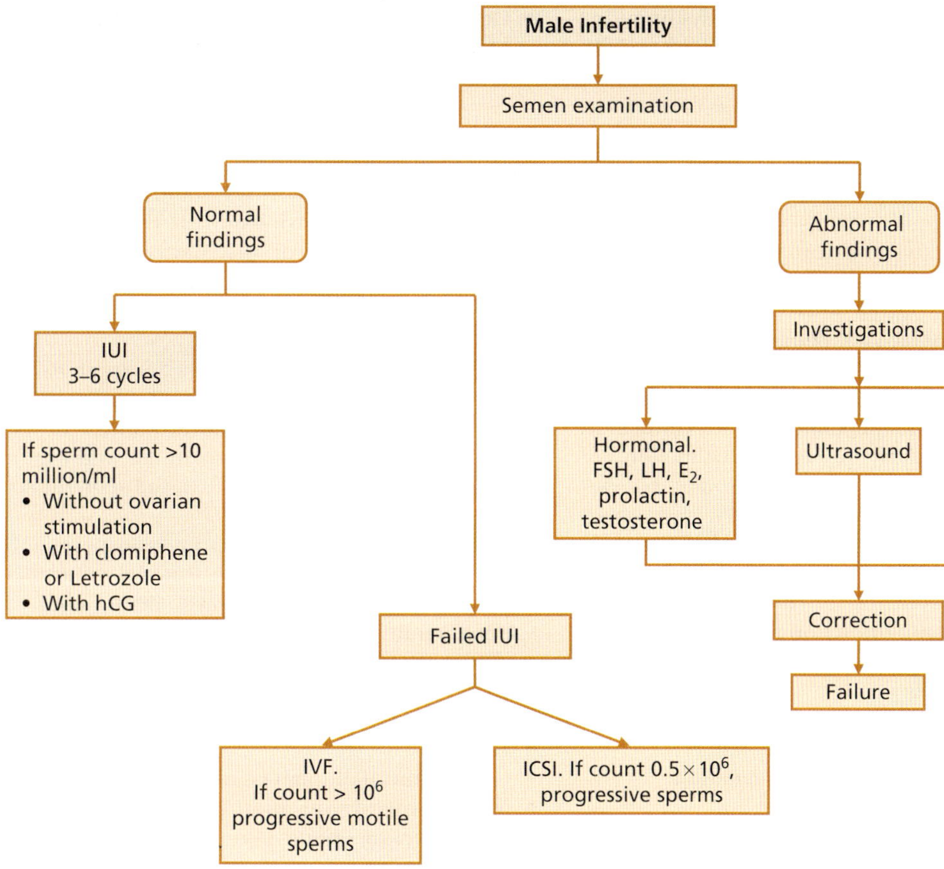

Figure 16.5 Management of male infertility.

improve quality of the sperms and prevent sperm DNA damage, but data-based evidence is lacking at present.

8. Premature ejaculation. Selective serotonin reuptake inhibitors take 2 weeks to reach the therapeutic level, but dapoxetine works within 1 hour; 30–60 mg is taken 1 hour before intercourse.
9. Hormones. Testosterone, pituitary hormones and GnRH have all been tried to improve spermatogenesis with variable results. Bromocriptine is useful in hyperprolactinaemia.

HORMONAL THERAPIES FOR MALE INFERTILITY

1. Human chorionic gonadotropin (hCG) 3000 IU i.m. thrice weekly for 12 weeks. Alternatively, 5000 IU twice weekly may be given. Lately 2500 IU dose has been recommended. Thereafter, 37.5–75 mg FSH subcutaneously is added thrice a week. Follow-up with testosterone level and semen analysis. It takes 6–9 months to produce normal semen counts. Stop FSH, but continue with hCG. About 40% pregnancy rate is reported.
2. Testosterone – An oral daily dose of 25–50 mg improves testicular function. A larger dose of 100–150 mg daily suppresses spermatogenesis. After a 3-month course of treatment, rebound phenomena occur with improved spermatogenesis.
3. Clomiphene – A daily dose of 25 mg for 25 days followed by rest for 5 days is given cyclically for 3–6 cycles. It is recommended in hypogonadal infertility, but is not effective in hypogonadal hypopituitarism. Instead of clomiphene, letrozole 2.5 mg may be employed.
4. Human menopausal gonadotropin (hMG) 150 IU thrice a week for 6 months is recommended in pituitary inadequacy, but it may take as long as 1 year to induce spermatogenesis.
5. GnRH – is indicated in hypothalamic failure.
   GnRH 5–20 mcg subcutaneously 2 hourly for 1–2 years. Nasal spray is also available.
6. Tamoxifen – A daily dose of 10 mg for 6 months has been found effective in some cases.
7. Dexamethasone – A daily dose of 0.5 mg or 50 mg prednisone daily for 10 days in each cycle for 3–6 months is recommended in the presence of spermal antibodies. About 25%–40% pregnancy rate is observed, though avascular necrosis (AVN) of the head of the femur and osteopenia as side effects have to be borne in mind in a prolonged therapy. Cyclosporin A – A daily dose of 5–10 mg/kg for 6 months is better than corticosteroids in T-cell suppression. If corticosteroids are contraindicated, an anti-inflammatory agent such as naproxen 50 mg twice daily may lower the antibody levels.
8. Sildenafil (Viagra) – A dose of 25–100 mg 1 hour before intercourse improves erectile function but recent reports on ischaemic heart disease is alarming, and should be prescribed with care. Colour visual disturbances, headache, rhinitis and dyspepsia have also been reported. It is contraindicated in men on antihypertensive

drugs. Sildenafil dye is used only in erectile dysfunction, and does not improve libido. With 25–100 mg orally 1 hour before intercourse, the effect lasts for 1–2 hours. The drug is effective in 50%–80% cases. It is contraindicated in the following:
- Retinitis pigmentosa.
- Diabetic retinopathy.
- Patient on antihypertensive drugs, nitrates.
- Cardiac disease, previous myocardial infarct, stroke.

Local self-injection of vasoactive drugs for erection is taken 5–10 minutes before intercourse and is 50%–70% effective. Side effects are penile fibrosis, infection and prolonged erection. Prostaglandin E_1 causes penile vasodilatation. Urethral pellets are also available. Penile vascular surgery and penile prosthesis implantation rods are also available for erectile dysfunction.

Penile implant AMS 700 is three-piece inflatable penile prosthesis which is now available.

9. Artificial insemination. An artificial insemination with husband's semen for four cycles has yielded 30% overall success with 10% success per cycle. The results are better if combined with ovulation induction for multiple ovulation, and this is the practice recommended today. It is indicated in the following:
   - Chronic medical disorder.
   - Oligospermia impotency – ejaculatory failure.
   - Premature ejaculation, retrograde ejaculation.
   - Hypospadias.
   - Antispermal antibodies in the cervical mucous.
   - Unexplained infertility.
   - It is also possible to freeze the semen if the husband is a frequent traveller and not available at the time of ovulation for IUI. The semen can also be frozen and used later in case the husband needs to undergo radiotherapy or chemotherapy.
   - HIV-positive male or female.

Techniques used for artificial insemination include (i) intrauterine insemination (IUI) (ii) intracervical, (iii) pericervical and vaginal and (iv) vaginal insemination. The semen is washed, concentrated and its quality improved by the 'swim-up' technique or by use of Percoll gradient. The semen with normal sperms with good motility thus obtained is then inseminated into the female genital tract. Obviously, artificial insemination is done around ovulation. About 1/2 mL of concentrated semen is injected 36 hours after hCG injection when the ovarian follicle reaches 20 mm. Semen washing removes the abnormal sperms, seminal plasma containing antibodies and other debris, as well as prostaglandins.

IUI is normally done once around ovulation, some prefer to do twice in each cycle. IUI is repeated up to 3–6 cycles. The IUI should be done within 90 minutes of collection of semen, for optimal results. Prophylactic progesterone is recommended to the woman in the luteal phase.

The artificial insemination with donor's semen is now legalized in India and should only be undertaken in infertility centres after appropriate counselling and explanation of its implications to both the partners.

Indications are as follows:

- Azoospermia.
- Immunological factors not correctable.
- Genetic disease in the husband. Homozygous Rh-positive husband with previous pregnancy losses.
- Chronic ill health and disease.

The donor for insemination is screened for HIV, sexually transmitted infection and hepatitis B, and good quality of semen confirmed. The frozen semen is stored for 6 months to minimize HIV transmission. If the donor remains HIV negative by the end of this period, the insemination is thawed and used.

Management of Azoospermia

Obstructive azoospermia requires vasogram to study the site and nature of blockage. Vaso-vasal anastomosis has been successful in a few cases. The advantage of surgery over ICSI is that it is a one-time treatment and cost effective, if successful with permanent effect. Subsequent spontaneous pregnancies are possible.

Five per cent males suffer from azoospermia. Depending upon its cause, especially in hormonal deficiencies, GnRH and pituitary hormones have been used to induce spermatogenesis.

Other methods of treatment for male infertility are as follows:

- IVF.
- Gamete intrafallopian transfer (GIFT) technique.
- Microassisted fertilization (MAF) technique.
- Microsurgical epididymal sperm aspiration (MESA) or percutaneous epididymal sperm aspiration (PESA).
- Testicular biopsy, sperm retrieval and MESA supersede other methods in modern treatment of male infertility and with improved success. Even spermatids have been utilized in assisted reproduction.

IVF

In this, induction of ovulation is done with clomiphene, FSH/LH or GnRH depending upon the woman's response to the drug. The aspiration of mature oocytes is done under ultrasonic guidance. The oocytes are kept in the specific culture for a few hours, to complete oocyte maturation. About 50,000 selected sperms are used for insemination.

About 18 hours after insemination, oocytes are observed for the presence of pronuclei (sign of fertilization) and cultured for a further 24 hours. At two- to four-cell stage, two embryos are transferred (embryo transfer [ET]) into the uterine cavity 1 cm below the fundus. The woman is allowed to go home 2–3 hours following ET. The indications for IVF are as follows:

- Idiopathic or unexplained male and female infertility.
- Immunological factor in male and female.
- Blocked fallopian tubes or failed tubal surgery.
- Failed intrauterine or fallopian insemination.
- Mild endometriosis.
- Abnormal semen findings.
- Donor semen or sperm.

The indications for IVF are expected to expand with a rapid improvement in its success and improved technology.

Complications. Apart from hyperstimulation syndrome, multiple pregnancy and its complications, IVF can cause ectopic pregnancy in 5% and heterotropic pregnancy (ectopic + uterine) in 0.4% of cases.

Three to four cycles of IVF yield 15%–30% pregnancy rate. The best results are seen in women with blocked tubes, whereas poor results are seen in oligospermia, teratospermia and asthenospermia. Some clinics claim 40% and above success rate with IVF.

Although IVF avoids laparoscopic surgical procedure and general anaesthesia, and gives considerable information on fertilization process, it requires an expensive and an elaborate laboratory establishment. IVF is a costly therapy not affordable to many couples. Because of multiple pregnancy ensuing from two ETs with associated increased fetal loss through abortion, ectopic pregnancy and preterm delivery, many European centres believe in only one ET at a time, though it takes longer for the woman to conceive. The cost of IVF therapy and the older age of women seeking assisted reproductive therapy in India have compelled the IVF specialists to continue to use two-ET method as of today.

Gamete Intra Fallopian Transfer

GIFT was first described by Asch et al. in 1984. It involves aspiration of oocytes following ovulation induction either laparoscopically or under ultrasound guidance transvaginally. Laparoscopic route is preferred as it is anyway required for sperm and oocyte transfer into the fallopian tube. Two hours before aspiration, the semen is prepared, washed from the seminal plasma and left in culture medium at 37°C. The oocytes (two per tube) are mixed with 50,000 sperms and transferred to each ampullary portion of the fallopian tube 4 cm from the fimbrial end. The volume transferred is 10–20 microns.

GIFT technique allows in vivo fertilization in the natural site (fallopian tube) unlike IVF, but needs laparoscopy technique (invasive). It is not a commonly done procedure now.

Lately, transfer of oocytes and sperms is attempted by transuterine catheterization of the tube (falloscopically) and laparoscopy is avoided.

The *indications* for GIFT are as follows:

- Unexplained infertility.
- Failed IUI.
- Male infertility.
- Immunological factor in male.
- Immunological factors in the cervix.
- Donor semen required (rare).

Both the fallopian tubes must be patent. The results are better with GIFT than IVF, i.e. 45% success versus 15%–20%, but success rate with IVF is improving; besides laparoscopy is not required. Abortion rate of 10%–15%, ectopic pregnancy (7%) and multiple pregnancy (20%–50%) have been reported with GIFT.

Disadvantage – fertilization cannot be confirmed.

MAF *process in vitro.* These sophisticated expensive techniques are needed for the following reasons:

- IVF or GIFT fails due to fertilization failure.
- Immunologically derived infertility.
- Sperm binds to zona pellucida but fails to penetrate due to either spermal antibodies or antibodies to zona pellucida.
- No or weak binding of sperm to zona. This may be caused because of receptor defect on the zona, enzyme digestive defect or defective sperm motility.
- Oligospermia and asthenospermia.

Zona drilling (ZD) to allow spermal penetration has not been successful.

Partial zonal dissection (PZD) or puncture followed by insemination has produced pregnancies, but polygamy and abnormal embryos have occurred.

Subzonal insemination (SUZI) into perivitelline space is useful if the sperms are immotile or have reduced motility.

ICSI is indicated and proved successful in case of immotile sperms and sperm count less than 5 million/mL with a pregnancy rate of 30%–40%. A single sperm is injected into the cytoplasm of the oocyte (under microscope), which is then incubated overnight.

Indications for ICSI are as follows:

- Sperm count less than 5 million/mL.
- Absent or reduced sperm motility.
- Abnormal sperm morphology.
- Previous IVF has failed.
- Unexplained infertility.
- Failure to penetrate zona by sperm as seen in IVF.

Epididymal or testicular aspiration or biopsy. This is the latest technology employed in azoospermia caused by blocked vas. The former can be done under local anaesthesia, but testicular biopsy requires general anaesthesia.

Cryopreservation of semen of the husband and embryos for future fertility is required if the man has to undergo radiation or chemotherapy for malignancy. Alternately, epididymal or testicular aspiration technique is employed. In the latter situation, repeat aspiration can be avoided and sperms cryopreserved. ICSI now supersedes zonal techniques because of following reasons:

- It is more successful in improving fertility.
- Spermatozoa as well as spermatids can be employed.
- Histopathology and karyotype study is possible.
- Cryopreservation saves cost and stress of repeated performance in each cycle.

The low success rate is attributed to older age of the woman undergoing the procedure. Because of the cost and stress of the procedure, women opt for these only if other methods fail.

We have come a long way in male infertility from initial donor insemination, artificial insemination of washed semen to IVF and ICSI with improved success.

Psychological Considerations

The discovery of infertility or sterility can create shock, fear and depression in the couple. Some feel inadequacy and shame of not being able to reproduce (Fig. 16.6). Some lose their self-esteem and feel the social disadvantage. To add to this, the strain of investigations and treatment increase the financial burden not affordable to all. Sympathetic and respectful attitude by the medical personnel will help in dealing with the infertile couple during their consultation.

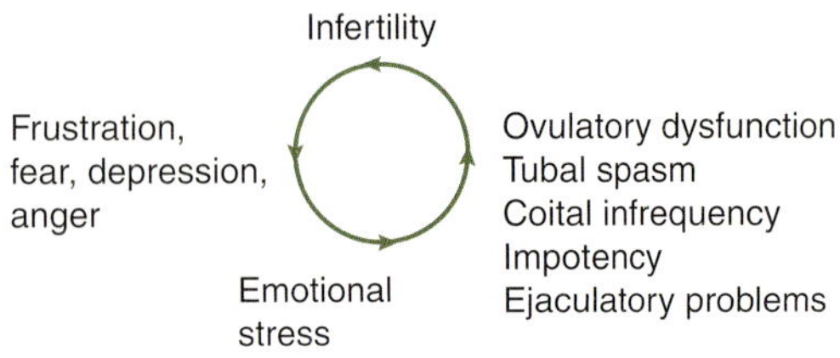

Figure 16.6 Psychological problems in infertility.

Impotence caused by fatigue, drugs, multiple sclerosis and diabetes needs correction. Similarly premature ejaculation needs physiotherapy and psychological counselling.

Erectile failure can be improved by the following methods:

1. Local injection of alprostadil (prostaglandin) into the penile vessel. Erection occurs in 10 minutes and lasts for half an hour. This is painful, can cause infection and fibrosis, besides being clinically impracticable.
2. Vacuum pump is applied to the tip of the penis to draw blood into it.
3. Prostaglandin pellets are inserted in the urethra and the penis is massaged.
4. Silicon cylinder prosthesis is implanted into the penis.

Compared to the above methods, taking Viagra tablet is easy, bearing in mind its side effects and contraindications.

Table 16.2 Female Infertility: Causes, Investigations and Management

Aetiology	Investigations	Management
Tubal cause	• Hysterosalpingography or sonosalpingography • Falloscopy • Salpingography • Laparoscopic chromotubation	• Adhesiolysis (Lap.) • Tuboplasty • Hysteroscopic cannulation and balloonoplasty ↓ If failed or not feasible ↓ IVF/Gif+
Ovulation	• Ovulation monitoring by ultrasound (BBT, BBI) • EB for tuberculosis ↓ Abnormal ↓ Hormonal study • FSH, LH, Prolactin • E_2, P level • Thyroid and diabetes	• Clomiphene, letrozole ↓ Failed ↓ FSH, LH, GnRH ↓ Positive → ↓ Response ↓ No response → ↓ If failed IVF Donor egg → ↓ Adoption
Other causes	Ultrasound, MRI, SSG, hysteroscopy	Treat the cause

FEMALE INFERTILITY

Infertility can be due to some factor in female partner. In case male partner is normal, one begins with investigation of female partner.

AETIOLOGY

The causes of female infertility are shown in Table 16.2 and Fig. 16.7:

1. Dyspareunia and vaginal causes.
2. Congenital defects in the genital tract.
3. Infection in the lower genital tract.
4. Cervical factors.
5. Uterine causes.
6. Tubal factors.
7. Ovulatory dysfunction.
8. Peritoneal causes – adhesions, endometriosis.
9. Chronic ill health – especially thyroid dysfunction.
10. Hormonal – pituitary gland dysfunction, hyperprolactinaemia and hypothalamic disorders.
11. Hypothyroidism.

VAGINISMUS

Vaginismus is regarded as hyperaesthesia which leads to spasm of the sphincter vagina and the levator ani muscles during attempted coitus or when an attempt is made to examine the patient vaginally. In primary vaginismus there is no organic lesion present, whereas in secondary vaginismus some obvious painful lesion in the region of the genital tract can be found on examination. In primary vaginismus, when the patient is being examined and an attempt is made to inspect the vulva by separating the labia, a muscle spasm is induced whereby the thighs are drawn together, the levator muscles become tonically contracted and the patient cries out and endeavours to push the medical attendant away from her. In secondary vaginismus, a minor degree of spasm is induced by painful local lesions such as small infected lacerations of the hymen, urethral caruncle, vulvitis or a sequela of vaginal operations for the repair of prolapse when, as a result of the operation, the calibre of the introitus and the vagina is narrowed. The operation scar is naturally sensitive for some weeks after the repair, and premature attempts at coitus are painful. It is thus easy for organic dyspareunia to lead to a protective spasm in order to avoid the pain of coitus. The spasm is not unlike that seen in primary vaginismus, although it is never of the same degree. Removal of the cause will cure this condition, whereas true vaginismus requires a prolonged therapy and the results are not always satisfactory.

Typical primary vaginismus always has a psychoneurotic basis. Frequently, a history of mental trauma during adolescence can be traced, and in most women with vaginismus, there is a subconscious dread of sexual intercourse. This anxiety neurosis is all too often the result of enthusiastic but a clumsy technique on the part of her husband, dating from the time of the first consummation of her marriage. Sometimes, it dates from a guilt complex engendered by an early, clandestine and extramarital association.

If the patient suffering from vaginismus is examined under an anaesthetic, bimanual pelvic examination will most

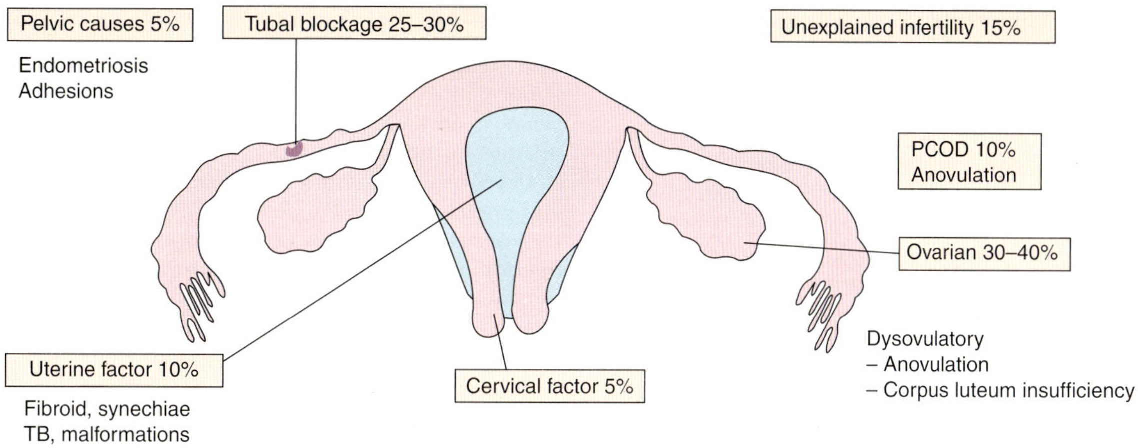

Figure 16.7 Causes of female infertility.

likely reveal no organic abnormality whatsoever. The capacity and calibre of the vagina is normal and it easily admits two fingers. Occasionally, the hymen is incompletely ruptured and the introitus inadequately dilated, but these findings are rare and their correction by plastic enlargement, though logical, does little to relieve the subsequent spasm because it is psychogenic rather than organic. Fortunately, vaginismus is rarely encountered in the recent times.

TREATMENT

The first essential of treatment is to win the confidence and cooperation of both husband and wife, interviewed separately. The interview demands great tact and experience, and is time-consuming, but if conducted correctly is most rewarding. Once the confidence of the couple is won over, the true cause of the trouble will usually be disclosed, and simple instruction in its rectification may often suffice.

If the patient is obsessed with the idea that her genital tract is maldeveloped, she should be examined under an anaesthetic. At this examination, the normality of her lower genital tract is confirmed. The vagina is stretched to three fingers after which a large plastic dilator is inserted.

When the patient recovers from the anaesthetic, this large dilator is removed and its visual presence demonstrates to her beyond argument that her vagina is of a normal capacity. She is then instructed by demonstration to pass a slightly smaller dilator and is supplied with one to be introduced at will every day at home to gain enough confidence and overcome any unfounded fears. The regular passage of the dilator should convince her that there is no obstruction to coitus.

If a rigid hymen appreciated as a sickle-like band resistant to stretching is encountered under anaesthesia, the operation of perineotomy (or Fenton's operation) should be performed. A longitudinal incision is made in the midline through the lower third of the posterior vaginal wall and skin of the perineum. After undercutting the tissues on each side and dividing the superficial muscles of the perineum, the wound is closed by interrupted sutures so that the scar lies transversely. The incision should be made of a length such that the vaginal orifice subsequently admits three fingers. After this operation of plastic enlargement of the introitus, it is useful to pass a medium-sized plastic dilator daily, and the patient is supplied with one for use. Coitus should not be attempted until the perineotomy wound has healed soundly, usually in 3 or 4 weeks.

Botulinum neurotoxin type A injection into levator ani muscle 4 weekly improves vaginismus.

DYSPAREUNIA

The term *dyspareunia* is loosely used for difficult as well as painful coitus. The following classification of the causes of dyspareunia is suggested.

DUE TO THE MALE PARTNER

- Gross congenital abnormality of the penis.
- Impotence, usually partial, e.g. failure to maintain an erection long enough for penetration.
- Premature ejaculation.
- Complete and surprising ignorance in the technique of coitus.

DUE TO THE FEMALE PARTNER

1. Painful lesions in the region of the introitus, such as vulvitis (acute and chronic), urethral caruncle, Bartholin's cyst or abscess, tender scar from obstetric trauma or operation and painful lesions of the anal canal, notably fissures.
2. Obstructive conditions at the vaginal introitus:
   - Rigid or imperforate hymen and painful carunculae myrtiformes giving rise to spasm.
   - Narrow introitus due to congenital hypoplasia, kraurosis or lichen sclerosus – poor lubrication in a menopausal woman.
   - Traumatic stenosis due to obstetric injury followed by scarring, such as painful episiotomy scar, tightly sewn perineal tear or perineorrhaphy operation, mutilation, vulvodynia and vulvar vestibulitis.
   - Cicatrization due to chemical burns.
   - The functional spasm of vaginismus.
   - A large tender Bartholin's cyst is occasionally obstructive to entry.

3. Obstructive conditions above the vaginal introitus:
   - Congenital stenosis and the various maldevelopments – i.e. partial noncanalization of the vagina.
   - Acquired stenosis – chemical burns are rare but the important causes here are the result of surgical operation. Vaginal hysterectomy and prolapse repairs, Wertheim's operation, radium insertion and radiation therapy result in narrowing and shortening of the vagina. Sometimes, the anterior and posterior suture lines of a colporrhaphy become densely adherent and fuse to form a stout septum which allows only partial penetration.
   - Benign and malignant tumours of the vagina are rare causes of obstruction. *Dry vagina in a menopausal woman.*
4. Uterine conditions which are not obstructive but because they are painful give rise to collision dyspareunia:
   - Cervicitis. Chronic inflammatory lesions of the cervix associated with parametritis can cause pain. Deep dyspareunia is due to:
   - Chronic parametritis and parametrial scars.
   - Adenomyosis uterus.
   - A fixed retroversion associated with chronic pelvic inflammatory disease (PID).
5. Lesions of the uterine appendages:
   - Prolapsed ovaries associated with retroversion cause deep dyspareunia.
   - Acute and chronic salpingo-oophoritis. Ovarian residual syndrome.
   - Endometriosis of the pouch of Douglas, rectovaginal septum and uterosacral ligaments.
6. Extragenital lesions in the bowel, such as diverticulitis of the sigmoid colon usually adherent to the left appendages and uterus, and cystitis.

Difficult Coitus

Difficult coitus may be caused by many of the same factors that are responsible for painful coitus. If the cause is insuperable, such as bony ankylosis of the hip in extreme adduction, consummation may be impossible and the correct term is not dyspareunia but apareunia. The latter naturally occurs with severe developmental defects of the vagina such as failure of canalization (vaginal aplasia).

INVESTIGATIONS

Investigations should be conducted along similar lines to that of vaginismus. Clinically, dyspareunia is divided into the following:

1. Superficial: The pain occurs when penetration is attempted and the causative lesion is therefore to be expected at or near the introitus.
2. Deep seated, when the pain is not associated with penetration but is felt only after this has occurred and is usually localized in the depth of the vagina.
3. Postcoital dyspareunia, a less well-known entity, sometimes associated with the deep-seated variety. Here the patient complains of an aching soreness which lasts for several hours after the completion of the act.

Deep-seated dyspareunia is usually organic and is associated with ovarian pathology such as prolapsed and tender ovaries in association with retroversion, endometriosis or chronic PID.

TREATMENT

The treatment consists in dealing with the cause. Local abnormalities at the vulva can usually be cured by an appropriate treatment, but when dyspareunia is caused by abnormalities in the pouch of Douglas, an abdominal operation is necessary. The ovaries may be freed from adhesions, endometriosis and chocolate cysts can be excised and the uterus can be fixed in a position of anteversion by an operation of ventrosuspension. Oestrogen cream is effective in a menopausal woman.

- K-Y Jelly (lubricant) and Rejois vaginal moisturizer two to three times a week relieves dyspareunia due to lower genital tract. A postural change may help.
- Lignocaine ointment is an anaesthetic drug that relieves pain.

When all possible organic causes of the dyspareunia have been eliminated, psychogenic possibilities must be considered; patient enquiry may then elicit the true cause, such as fear of pregnancy, frigidity, marital disharmony or some unhappy sexual experience in the past.

Congenital Defects in the Genital Tract

Absent or septate vagina, hypoplasia and absent uterus are the obvious causes leading to sterility.

Infections in the Vagina and Cervix

Although mild infection may not prevent sperms fast getting into the cervical canal, it is prudent to clear the infection before any therapeutic measures are applied in treatment of infertility.

Chlamydial cervicitis is now recognized to impair sperm functions (fragmentation) besides causing blocked tubes due to PID.

Cervical Mucous

As mentioned earlier, cervical factor can be assessed by the postcoital test. The test also provides an opportunity to assess sperm–mucous interaction and whether satisfactory coitus occurs or not.

- The finding of leucocytes in the mucous is suggestive of infection commonly due to cervicitis. Cultures for gonorrhoea, *Chlamydia trachomatis* and *Ureaplasma urealyticum* may help in selecting the appropriate antibiotic for the treatment of cervicitis. Large erosions are treated with electrocautery/cryocautery. Post-treatment repeat postcoital test often shows marked improvement.
- Nonmotile, nonprogressively motile sperms showing a 'shaking' pattern are highly suspicious of the presence of sperm antibodies and an immunological cause. If an immunological cause is suspected, the patient's serum and cervical mucous can be examined for the presence of antisperm antibodies. If the cervical mucous is found to contain antisperm antibodies, the couple is advised to use a condom or a diaphragm as a barrier method for 3 months. During this period, the antibodies gradually disappear, and once the mucous is found to be normal, conception is attempted. The presence of serum antibodies has a poor prognosis, and IUI, IVF or GIFT technique is offered.

Cervical Factors

The cervix has an active role in the physiology of conception. The position of the cervix and patency of the cervical canal facilitate the entry of sperms into the uterine cavity. The cervical canal acts as a sperm reservoir, and capacitation of sperms occurs here. The cervical mucous is alkaline and is suited for the semen. The ciliated endocervical cells actively select the normal motile sperms and sieve out the abnormal ones by phagocytosis, so that only the healthy fertilizable sperms enter the upper genital tract. The cervical mucous at ovulation exhibits characteristic changes which help in easy sperm penetration. These cervical factors are responsible for about 5% of infertility.

Uterine Causes

Hypoplasia, malformed uterus and incompetent os cause habitual abortion more often than infertility. In pelvic tuberculosis, in addition to blockage of tubes and endometrial tuberculosis causing Asherman syndrome (adhesions) are responsible. Asherman syndrome may also result from other infections, vigorous curettage, postabortal and puerperal infection, as well as packing the uterine cavity to control postpartum haemorrhage.

Asherman syndrome is classified as follows:

- Minimal adhesion involves <25% of the uterine cavity, flimsy adhesions involving the fundus and tubal ostia.
- Moderate adhesion involves 25%–70% of the endometrial surfaces, but no agglutination of the uterine wall.
- Severe > 75% adhesions with agglutination and thick adhesions in endometrial cavity.

The uterine fibroids which may account for infertility are either cornual fibroid blocking the medial end of the fallopian tube, submucous fibroid and cervical fibroid distorting the passage of the sperms and preventing implantation thus resulting in infertility.

Pregnancy rate of 30%–40% following myomectomy proves that other factors may be involved apart from the presence of a fibroid.

Dyssynchrony between the glandular and stromal growth in endometrium or endometrium unreceptive to ovarian hormones can prevent implantation.

Tubal Factors

One of the most important and commonest cause of infertility is tubal factor salpingitis, when as a result of inflammation, adhesions form around the abdominal ostium, while within the lumen of the tube, the plicae become adherent, blocking the passage in the tube. Gonorrhoea and chlamydial infections or salpingitis following septic abortion and puerperal infections are amongst the common causes of blockage of the fallopian tubes. Genital tuberculosis has already been mentioned, and endometrial biopsy shows that 5% asymptomatic infertile women suffer from genital tuberculosis. Apart from tubal blockage, peritubal adhesions and fimbrial end blockage can cause infertility.

Westorm observed that one episode of tubal infection leads to tubal blockage in 12% of cases. The incidence increases to 23% after two episodes of PID and 54% following three episodes.

Ovaries

Anovulation due to endocrine disorders, polycystic ovarian disease (PCOD) and corpus LPDs is one of the important causes of infertility. Periovarian adhesion in pelvic infection and luteinized unruptured follicular (LUF) syndrome in 9% of cases are also responsible. Luteal phase effects either due to deficient progesterone or shorter duration of luteal phase occur in 3%–4% of infertile women. This defect is also seen in IVF programme, pituitary hormone deficiency (defective folliculogenesis), hyperprolactinaemia, excess luteolysis, clomiphene therapy and hypothyroidism.

Corpus luteal phase defect (LPD) is associated with low oestrogen and progesterone levels. Oestrogen is responsible for progesterone receptors in the endometrium, so low Oestrogen and progesterone levels results in poor secretory phase. Thus an inadequate response in endometrium. Corpus LPD means failure of endometrium to exist in the right phase at the right time. In luteal phase defect, histology of endometrium lags behind the day of menstruation by 2 days or more. Retrieval of ova in IVF by puncture can disrupt the granulosa cells. *Duphaston (dydrogesterone) is an effective treatment in corpus LPD without causing any adverse effect on ovulation.*

Subendothelial Layer

A subendothelial layer in the endometrium can be recognized on ultrasound scanning and MRI, and this layer has increased nuclear content and vascularity and is under the influence of ovarian hormones.

Before menarche and after menopause, this zone is indistinct, so also in oral combined pill users and during GnRH therapy. It is prominent in a menopausal woman on hormone replacement therapy (HRT).

In a menstrual cycle with conception, peristalsis of this zone is upwards from cervix to fundus during preovulatory phase and may help in sperm migration. This zone becomes indistinct in the postovulatory period and quiescent and may help in implantation.

In IVF programme, increased activity of this zone may be responsible for failure as well as occurrence of an ectopic pregnancy.

Peritoneal causes. Peritubal and intratubal adhesions by kinking the fallopian tubes can cause blockage of the tubes. More importantly, these adhesions are a result of PID. These adhesions can also impair the peristaltic movements of the fallopian tubes. In pelvic endometriosis, macrophages in the peritoneal fluid may engulf the ovum and sperms, preventing fertilization.

Chronic Ill Health

Hypothalamic and pituitary disease, hypothyroidism and adrenal cortical dysfunction are the important causes of anovulation. Diabetes and tuberculosis may lead to infertility. Smoking is known to impair ovarian function and prevent embryo implantation into the endometrium.

WORK UP OF FEMALE PARTNER

Approach to a female partner of infertile couple comprises the following:

- History.
- Examination.
- Special investigations.

History

Age of the woman, past obstetric history in case of secondary infertility regarding puerperal infection, coital difficulty and menstrual history give clues to the possible cause. History of tuberculosis and previous pelvic infection is important. History of diabetes and thyroid dysfunction may be evident. The duration of infertility and previous use and the type of contraceptive may be linked to infertility.

Examination

This includes height and weight of the woman; blood pressure should be checked. Hirsutism, palpation of thyroid and lymph nodes, palpation of the breasts, the presence of galactorrhoea suggest hormonal dysfunction.

An abdominal swelling may be due to uterine fibroid. Bimanual pelvic examination will reveal an obvious gynaecological cause for infertility.

Tests for Tubal Patency

Hysterosalpingography (HSG) and diagnostic laparoscopy with chromotubation are two commonly used tests for tubal patency. A mere patency of the tubal lumen is not the only criteria to affect fertility. The normal physiological function of the fallopian tube is essential for pregnancy to occur. The endosalpinx is lined by ciliated epithelial cells and the secretory cells. The cilia help in propulsion of the fertilized egg towards the uterine cavity. The secretory cells provide nutrition to the sperms as well as the ovum during their passage across the tube. The peristaltic movements of the fallopian tube are under the influence of oestrogen, progesterone and prostaglandins, and synchronized movements help in propulsion of sperms and the fertilized egg in either direction. The ovarian fimbriae are spread over the ovary at ovulation and bring the ovum into the fimbrial end. The loss of any of these functions could prevent conception.

The testing of tubal patency and detecting tubal pathology are done in the preovulatory phase of the menstrual cycle. If performed in the postovulatory period, insufflation might disturb a fertilized or implanted ovum and may also cause pelvic endometriosis.

Hysterosalpingography

Visualization of the uterine cavity and the fallopian tubes after injecting a radio-opaque dye in uterine cavity should be carried out by screening with the use of an image intensifier in an X-ray room using a Foley catheter, Rubin cannula (Fig. 16.8) or Leech-Wilkinson cannula for insufflation. The investigation is performed between the end of the menstrual period and ovulation (usually the 9th or 10th day of the cycle). After thoroughly cleaning the lower genital tract and with full aseptic precautions, a radiopaque dye is injected with the help of the cannula into the uterine cavity under direct vision under a fluoroscopic screen; 15 mL of the medium is usually adequate to visualize the uterine cavity and the tubes. If the tubes are patent, the medium will be seen to spill out of the abdominal ostia and cover the adjacent bowel. A hydrosalpinx will show as a large confined mass of dye without peritoneal spill. If either of the tube is blocked, the site can be seen. During the examination, radiographic pictures are taken for permanent record of the result. A viscous water-soluble solution, 50% iodine with 6% polyvinyl alcohol in water, is the medium usually employed for HSG. It is rapidly absorbed, and the risk of tissue reaction and adhesion formation in the pelvis is minimal; even when intravasated into the uterine venous system. Although an oil-soluble medium gives a sharper and clearer picture and may have improved therapeutic effect, it is not preferred because of the occurrence of oil granuloma, peritoneal reaction, formation of pelvic adhesions and the need for a delayed film to be taken for detecting peritoneal spill (Figs 16.9–16.12). The pregnancy rate is slightly better with the use of oil-based media. Blockage of tube may be due to fibrosis (stricture), spasms or inspissated amorphous material plugging the lumen.

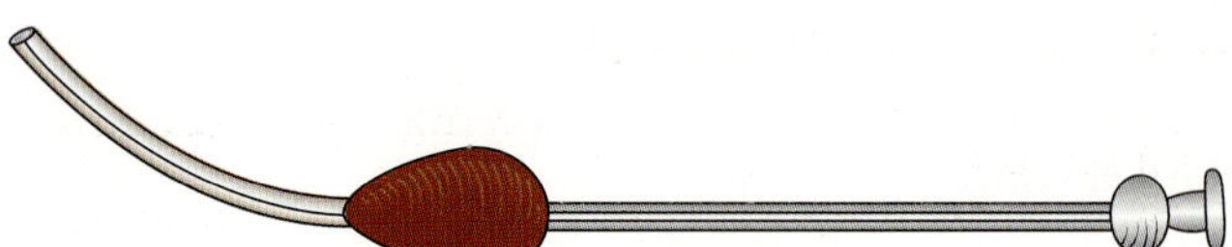

Figure 16.8 Rubin's cannula. It is used in hysterosalpingogram recording: while the dye is instilled into the uterine cavity, the cone prevents retrograde spill into the vagina.

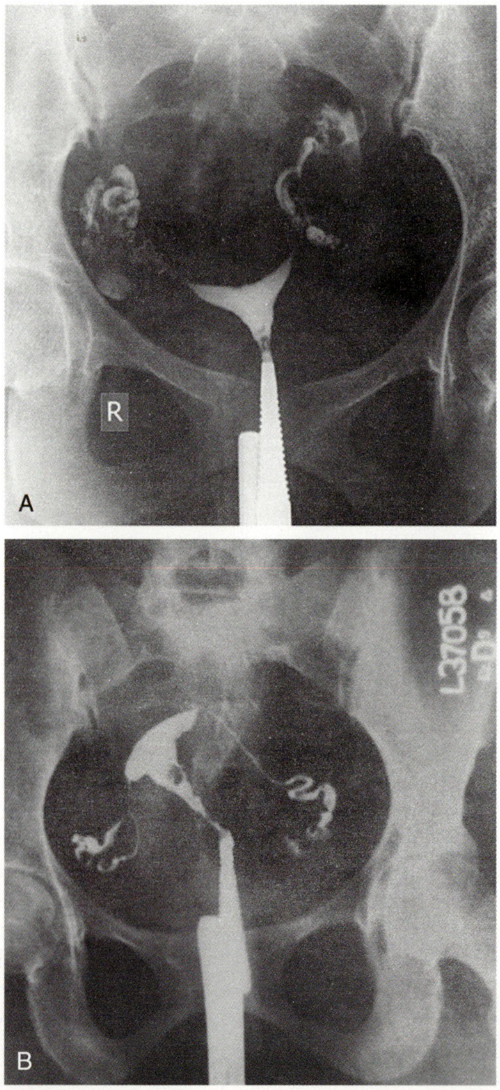

Figure 16.9 **(A)** Normal hysterosalpingogram. Note both the fallopian tubes are patent with spill into the peritoneal cavity. **(B)** HSG showing a filling defect in the uterine cavity which represent a polyp or fibroid. (*Courtesy*: Dr K K Saxena, New Delhi.)

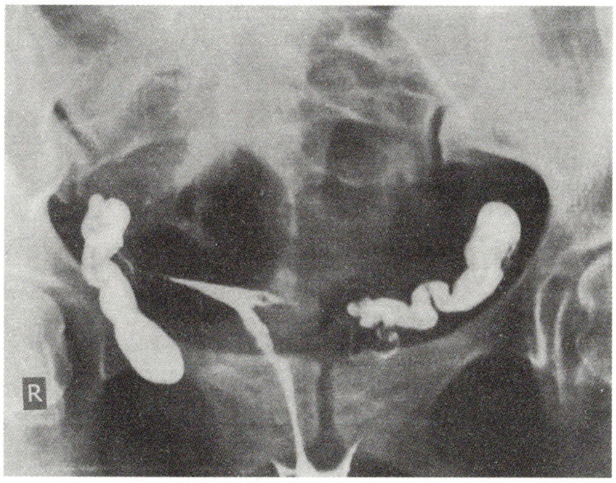

Figure 16.10 HSG showing bilateral dilated fallopian tubes with no free spill suggestive of bilateral hydrosalpinx. (*Courtesy*: Dr K K Saxena, New Delhi.)

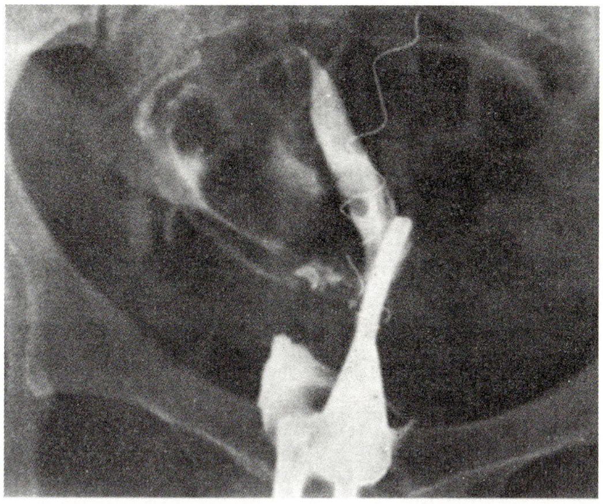

Figure 16.11 Hysterosalpingogram showing unicornuate uterus. The fallopian tube is patent and dye is seen in the peritoneal cavity.

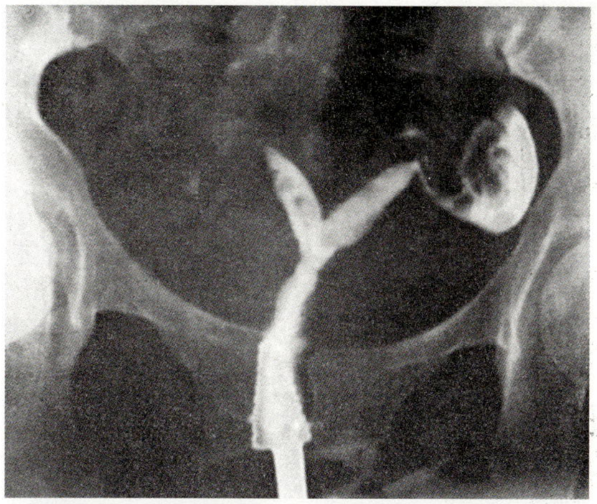

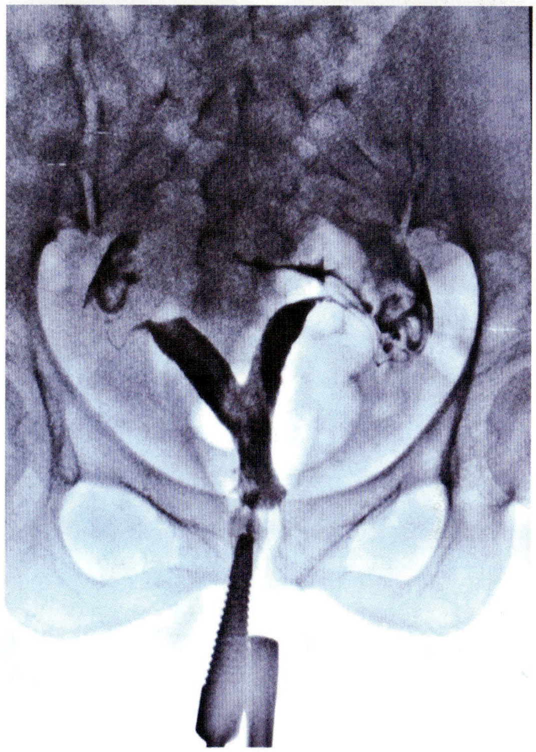

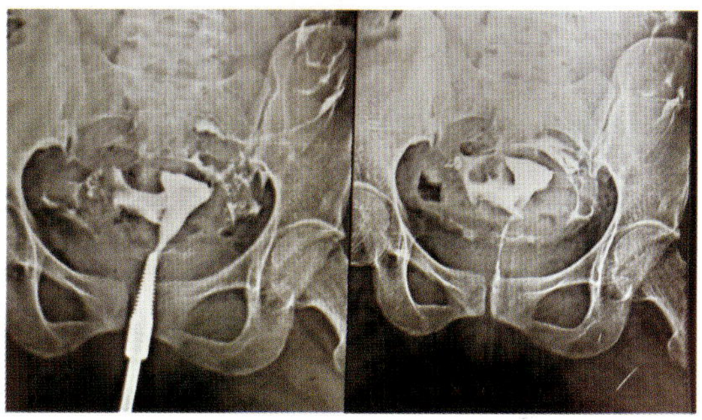

Figure 16.12 Hysterosalpingogram demonstrating a bicornuate uterus. The dye which is present in the peritoneal cavity demonstrates patency of the left fallopian tube.

Bilateral cornual block with extravasation of the dye is highly suggestive of tubercular salpingitis. Other hysterosalpingographic findings in tuberculosis are described in chapter 28.

Apart from tubal anatomy, this examination helps to diagnose congenital abnormalities of the uterus, such as uterus bicornis, arcuate, septate uterus and fibroids. HSG has the advantage that it gives a permanent record and shows the site of tubal blockage. Among its complications are (i) pelvic infection, (ii) pain and collapse which can however be avoided by giving injection atropine half an hour before the procedure and (iii) allergic reaction. HSG should not be performed (i) in the postovulatory period, (ii) in the presence of genital infection and suspected genital tuberculosis and (iii) if the patient is sensitive to iodine. HSG may help to flushing and dislodgement of amorphous material that sometimes blocks its lumen. The amorphous material is an aggregate of histiocytes.

Laparoscopic Chromotubation

It is laparoscopic visualization of the pelvic structures – uterus, fallopian tubes and ovaries and injection of methylene blue through the cervix to visualize the spill of dye. It is indicated in infertility cases to establish patency of the fallopian tubes and to verify the findings when HSG has shown blocked tubes (Fig. 16.13). Apart from visualization of the tubes and ovary, peritubal adhesions and unsuspected endometriosis can be diagnosed. The laparoscopy is indicated in patients with blocked fallopian tubes prior to undertaking tubal microsurgery. In such cases, planning of appropriate surgery can be chalked out and prognosis

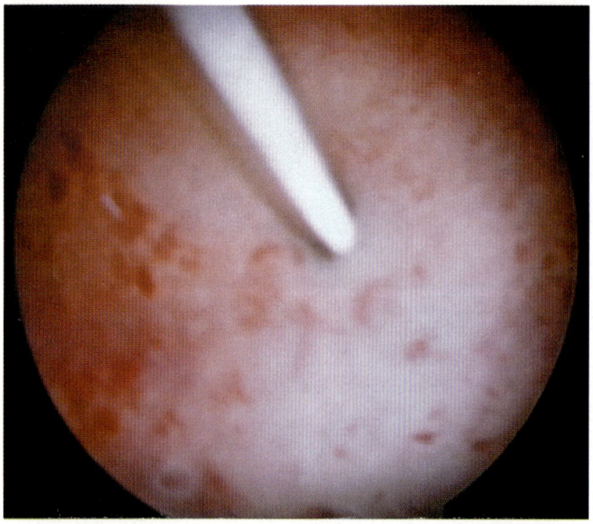

Figure 16.13 Hysteroscopic cannulation of the fallopian tube.

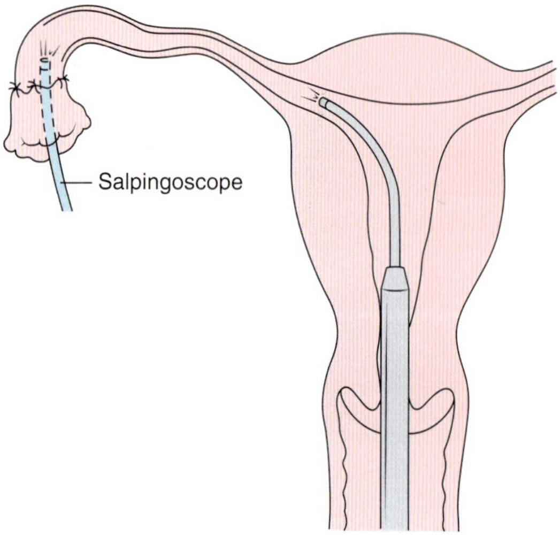

Figure 16.14 Falloposcopy and salpingoscopy. The flexible falloposcope is inserted via a channel in an operating hysteroscope, while salpingoscopy (usually rigid) is performed transabdominally during laparoscopic evaluation of the pelvis.

offered to the couple. Laparoscopy demonstrates the external condition of the fallopian tubes as well as its patency. It is, however, an invasive procedure and requires hospitalization. The greatest advantage of laparoscopy today is that one can proceed with the therapeutic procedure if adhesions or fimbrial block is recognized. Indications for laparoscopy are as follows:

- HSG showing abnormal findings.
- Prior to planning tuboplasty.
- Prior to IUI.
- Prior to induction of ovulation.
- Removal of hydrosalpinx prior to IVF.
- PCOD to puncture the cysts to improve the pregnancy rate of assisted reproduction and avoid hyperstimulation syndrome.
- Suspected cases of endometriosis.

Sonosalpingography (SSG)

It is a safe and practical method of evaluating tubal patency and to study the uterine cavity. Under ultrasound scanning, a slow and deliberate injection of about 200 mL of physiological saline into the uterine cavity is accomplished via a Foley catheter, the inflated bulb of which lies above the internal os and prevents leakage. It is possible to visualize the flow of saline along the tube and observe it issuing out as a shower at the fimbrial end. The ultrasound scan also shows the presence of free fluid in the pouch of Douglas if the tubes are patent. Injecting a small amount of air facilitates the visualization of air-bubble movement in each fallopian tube.

SSG is also a very good technique for detecting submucous fibroid polyp and intrauterine lesions. Many prefer SSG to HSG for following indications:

1. Abnormal uterine bleeding to study the endometrium and detect polypi.
2. Amenorrhoea due to Asherman syndrome.
3. Part of infertility investigation.
4. Repeated pregnancy losses for uterine anomalies.

Newer Modalities of Tubal Tests

Tubal pathology can be assessed by newer diagnostic techniques. These are as follows:

Hysteroscopy and falloscopy. When HSG shows a cornual block, this may be due to tubal spasm (25%, can be avoided by prior atropine injection), mucous or inspissated material (25%), polyp (10%), synechiae or isthmica nodosa. The interstitial end of the fallopian tube is best studied by falloscopy via the hysteroscope.

The mucous plug or inspissated material can be flushed and patency restored. Polypus can be removed. To break synechiae, a soft pliable cannula is passed through hysteroscope and its tip directed at the tubal ostium and gradually advanced while breaking the flimsy adhesions, and the fallopian tube flushed. *Dense adhesions cannot be dealt with in this way* (Fig. 16.14).

Ampullary and fimbrial salpingoscopy. (Fig. 16.15). Salpingoscopy can be utilized to study the mucosa of the

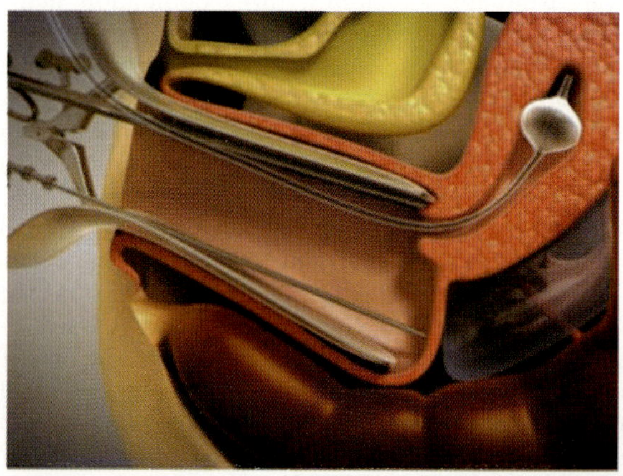

Figure 16.15 Principles of fertiloscopy: Introduction of Veress needle into the pouch of Douglas to study the tubes. (*Source:* From Figure 2. Watrelot A and Chauvin G: Current practice in tubal surgery and adhesion management: a review. Reproductive BioMedicine Online 23, 53–62, 2011.)

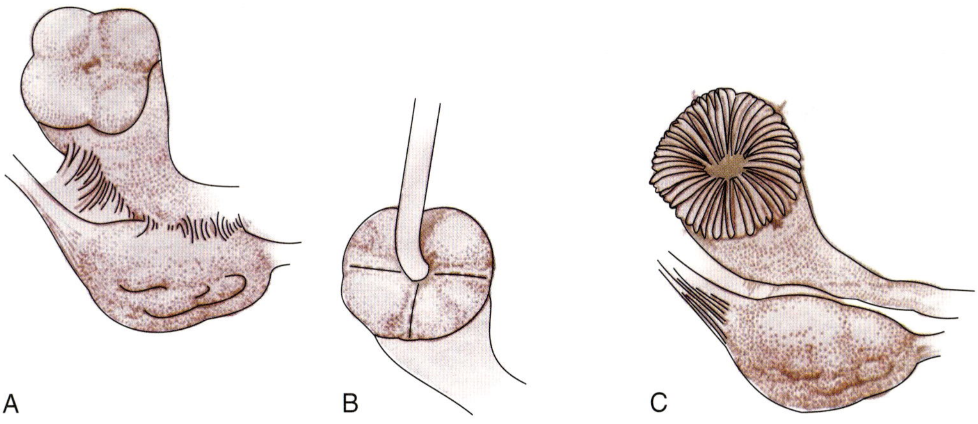

Figure 16.16 Tubal surgery at the fimbrial end (fimbrioplasty).

fallopian tube to choose tubal microsurgery and IVF. Colour Doppler ultrasound for assessing tubal pathology is under study.

A descending test using starch is injected into the pouch of Douglas. The presence of starch in the cervical mucous 24 hours later indicates patency of one or both tubes.

Laparoscopy is now combined with hysteroscopy as a comprehensive one-stop infertility work up, to detect the cause of infertility and treat the cause in one go. This is now considered the gold standard in the investigation of tubal infertility.

Fertiloscopy (Fig. 16.16). Following the initial work by Gordts, fertiloscopy is now introduced as a combined technique parallel to hydropelviscopy, and other methods in infertility work up. It can be done under local or general anaesthesia.

Fertiloscope consists of two introducers, one for uterine cavity and the second to study the genital organs through the pouch of Douglas. The uterine introducer is provided with a balloon for a good seal in the dye test and the vaginal fertiloscopy has three channels.

Technique of fertiloscopy is as follows:

1. Lithotomy position.
2. Local/general anaesthesia.
3. Insertion of Veress needle and creation of hydroperitoneum with saline.
4. Insertion of two fertiloscopes.
5. Chromotubation.
6. Inspection of organs.
7. Therapeutic, if it is needed.

MANAGEMENT OF TUBAL INFERTILITY

Tuboplasty

Tubal microsurgery (Fig. 16.16). It is advocated for tubal blockage. Depending upon the site of block, a number of tuboplasty procedure have been performed with successful pregnancy rates varying from 27% for fimbrial surgery to 50%–60% for isthmic blockage. The success of tuboplasty can be improved with (i) gentle handling of tissues; (ii) use of magnification; (iii) avoiding mopping or rubbing of the tissues but using continuous irrigation and suction to remove the clots, and prevent desiccation of tissues; (iv) haemostasis secured by cautery or laser; (v) use of fine suture material (Vicryl, Proline) and (vi) use of Heparin solution for hydroflotation to prevent postoperative adhesions. Restoration of latency of the fallopian tube should be checked by HSG 3 months later.

The risks of tuboplasty are (i) anaesthetic complications, (ii) postoperative wound infection, chest infection and embolism, (iii) failure and (iv) a subsequent ectopic pregnancy. Other indications for surgery are reversal of tubectomy, conservative ectopic pregnancy and salpingitis isthmica nodosa.

Advantages of tuboplasty:

- One-time therapy.
- Low cost compared to IVF. Successful surgery avoids IVF.
- Saves time of repeated visits to IVF centre.
- Subsequent spontaneous pregnancies possible if surgery is successful.

In-vitro Fertilization

Today, IVF and ET are offered to women in whom tuboplasty has failed or to women with extensive and irreparable tubal damage. The overall success rate of 20%–30% is obtained. This is an expensive therapy, but may be only hope for severe tubal damage. *Contraindications* to IVF are extensive pelvic adhesions and inaccessible ovaries due to adhesions – ova retrieval in such cases may be impossible or dangerous to the bowels. Laparoscopic adhesiolysis followed by IVF may be possible. Normally, three attempts are made and if IVF fails, other MAF processes offered.

Extra embryos can be cryopreserved for subsequent cycles.

Tubal cannulation done through transcervical route under hysteroscopic guidance restores patency in 75% of cases, and pregnancy rate of 40% is reported if tubal blockage is due to flimsy adhesions.

Medial end tubal blockage is seen in 10%–15% cases during HSG. Common causes of medial tubal block are as follows:

- Amorphous material organized as a plug
- Inflammatory exudates

- Tubal spasm
- Polypus
- Fibrosis by PID, endometriosis, isthmica nodosa

Treatment options for proximal and mid tubal block are as follows:

- Tubal cannulation
- Balloon tuboplasty
- Surgery – tuboplasty
- IVF

Pregnancy rate of 20% is reported.
Lateral end block can be treated by following:

- Fimbrioplasty – 50%–60% success rate
- Salpingostomy – 20%–30% success rate
- Adhesiolysis of external adhesions

Uterine causes, such as a septum, Asherman syndrome and a fibroid need surgical correction. Most of these can be treated by operative hysteroscopy carried out under general anaesthesia.

TESTS OF OVULATION

BASAL BODY TEMPERATURE

Basal body temperature (BBT) falls at the time of ovulation by about 1/2°F. Subsequently, during the progestational half of the cycle, the temperature is slightly raised above the preovulatory level, and the rise is of the order of 1/2–1°F. This phenomenon is due to the thermogenic action of progesterone, and is therefore presumptive evidence of the presence of a functioning corpus luteum and hence ovulation. Accurate recordings will therefore indicate whether the ovarian cycle is ovulatory or not and will also denote the timing of ovulation. The patient must be capable of reading the thermometer to 1/10th degree. Oral temperatures are accurate, provided the patient does not take hot or cold drinks before taking the temperature, and this should be done first thing after waking up in the morning. The patient must be instructed to record the temperatures on a graph (Fig. 16.17). BBT is retrospective and does not indicate impending ovulation and is not useful in IVF. It, however, does reveal corpus luteal phase insufficiency and defective folliculogenesis.

BBT has now become obsolete because of following:

1. Tedious daily recording.
2. Not very accurate.
3. Retrospective diagnosis and not useful therapeutically.
4. Better modalities of ovarian monitoring by ultrasound being available.

ENDOMETRIAL BIOPSY

Endometrial biopsy consists of curetting small pieces of the endometrium from the uterus with a small endometrial biopsy curette, preferably 1 or 2 days before the onset of menstruation. The material removed should be fixed immediately in formalin saline and submitted for histological examination. Secretory changes prove that the cycle has been ovulatory. The incidence of anovulation varies

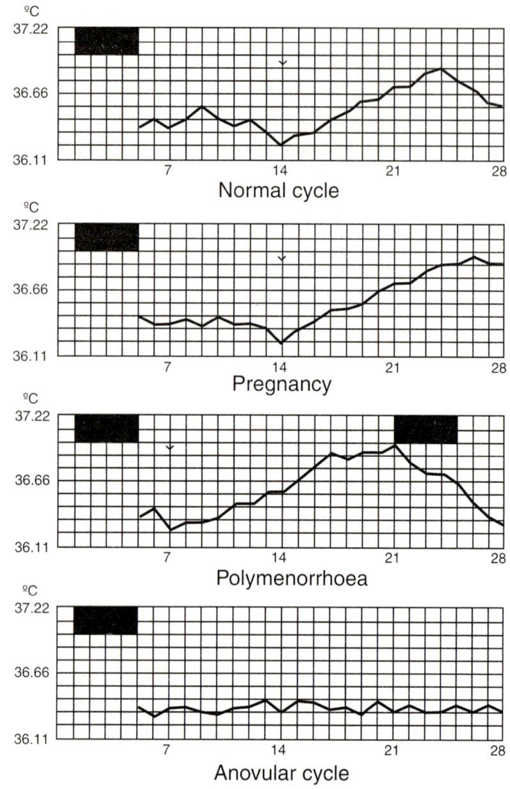

Figure 16.17 Specimen charts of BBT recordings. Arrows indicate ovulation time; the dark zones indicate the days of menstrual bleeding.

between 10% and 25%. Endometrium should be subjected to culture, PCR and staining to rule out genital tuberculosis, which is present in 5%–10% of Indian women complaining of sterility. Corpus LPD can also be diagnosed by endometrial biopsy, which shows a lag of 2–3 days between the calendar and histological dating of the specimen. Endometrial biopsy is now omitted as a routine investigation for infertility and ovulation is monitored by serial ultrasound scanning. *Endometrial biopsy is taken only in suspected tubercular endometritis, and the tissue is subjected to a PCR test as well as culture.*

FERN TEST

A specimen of cervical mucous obtained using a platinum loop or pipette is spread on a clean glass slide and allowed to dry. When viewed under the low-power microscope, it shows, during the oestrogenic phase, a characteristic pattern of fern formation (Figs 16.18 and 16.19). This ferning disappears after ovulation, and if previously present its disappearance is presumptive evidence of corpus luteum activity. The ferning is due to the presence of sodium chloride in the mucous secreted under oestrogen effect. The physical character of cervical mucous also alters with the date of the cycle. At the time of ovulation, the cervical mucous is thin and profuse that the patient may notice a clear discharge, the so-called normal ovulation cascade. This ovulation mucous has the property of great elasticity and will withstand stretching up to 10 cm. This phenomenon is called spinnbarkeit or the thread test for oestrogen activity. During the secretory phase, the cervical mucous becomes tenacious and its viscosity increases so that it loses the

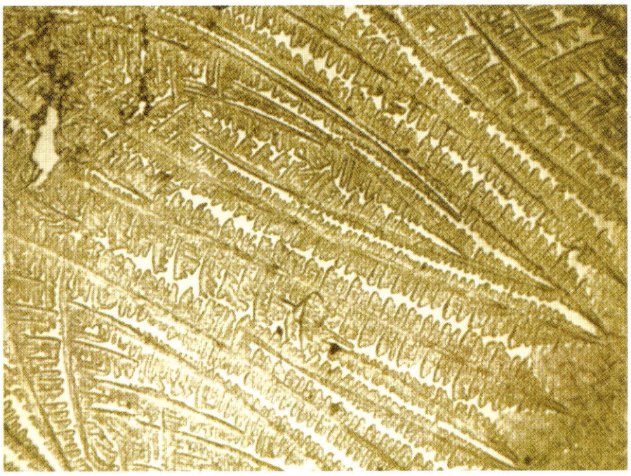

Figure 16.18 Dried cervical mucous showing ferning at the time of impending ovulation.

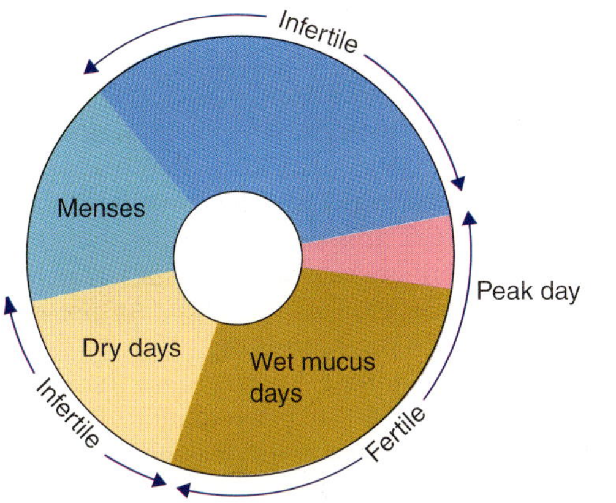

Figure 16.19 Mucous secretion during a menstrual cycle.

property of spinnbarkeit and fractures when put under tension. This property is called tack. The observation of this change in the cervical mucous pattern in a menstrual cycle is another evidence of ovulation (Fig. 16.20). Insler devised a scoring system which takes into account the various cervical mucous properties such as the amount, spinnbarkeit, ferning, viscosity and cellularity. The maximum score is 15 and a score of less than 10 is considered unfavourable. Cervical infection, if any, needs to be treated prior to performing this test. Postcoital test and detection of antibodies in the cervical mucous can be integrated with this test into one composite study. Currently one does not rely much on this test as a test of ovulation.

ULTRASOUND FOLLICULAR MONITORING

Ultrasound has now become the standard and indispensable procedure for monitoring maturation of the Graafian follicle and in detecting imminent ovulation in IVF, IUI and in timing intercourse. This requires daily ultrasonic visualization of ovaries from the 10th to 16th day of the menstrual cycle. It is noninvasive, accurate and safe. Apart from follicular study for ovulation, pelvic pathology if any can be picked up and endometrial thickness measured. The follicle grows at the rate of 1–2 mm daily to reach 20 mm or more when follicular

INFERTILITY

COMPONENTS OF A TYPICAL ART CYCLE

Short (flare) GnRH—a protocol

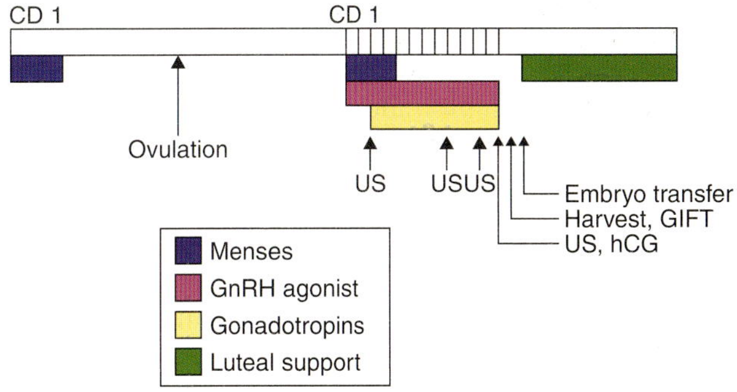

Long (luteal) GnRH—a protocol

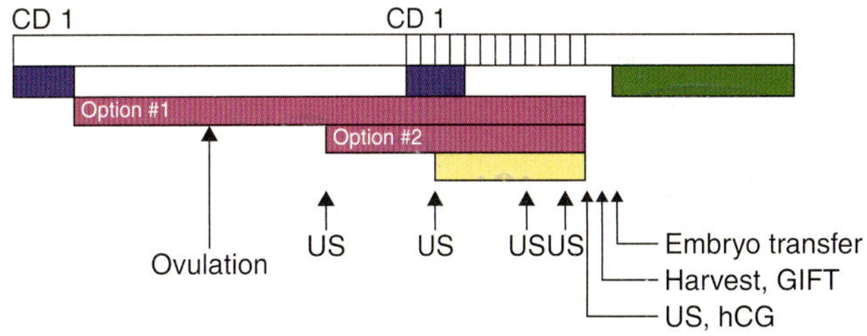

Figure 16.20 GnRH protocols.

rupture and ovulation occur at midcycle. The sudden disappearance of the follicle, presence of free fluid in the pouch of Douglas and growth of corpus luteum are evident. Endometrial thickness of 8–10 mm is the normal response of endometrium to progesterone. A lesser thickness indicates corpus luteal phase deficiency (CLPD).

HORMONAL ASSAYS

Plasma Progesterone

Plasma concentration of progesterone rises after ovulation and reaches the peak of 15 ng/mL at mid-luteal phase (22–23rd day) and then declines as the corpus luteum degenerates. A low level of the plasma progesterone below 5 ng/mL at mid-luteal phase, suggests corpus LPD and prompts hormonal therapy. Use of daily progesterone suppository in the luteal phase or administration of hCG 5000–10,000 IU weekly will help to improve the chances of conception. Oral micronized progesterone 100 mg b.i.d. or 300 mg vaginal pessary twice daily is useful in corpus LPD. Weekly proluton injection (500 mg) and oral dydrogesterone are also used.

Corpus luteal phase deficiency

Aetiology:

- Hypopituitarism with low FSH, LH
- Poor follicular development.
- Hyperprolactinaemia.
- Clomiphene citrate (CC) ovulation induction.
- Retrieval of egg in IVF. CLPD is seen in postmenarchal and premenopause period.

- Poor response of endometrium to endogenous progesterone.

Diagnosis:

- BBT.
- Mid-luteal progesterone estimation (normal 15 ng/mL).
- Endometrial biopsy.

Treatment: Administration of progestogen or hCG administration i.m. weekly.

LH

LH surge from the anterior pituitary gland occurs about 24 hours prior to ovulation. Radioimmunoassay of the morning sample of urine and blood gives the LH results in 3 hours. Not only does the LH surge help in predicting ovulation, but the approximate time of ovulation can be gauged and coitus around this time can improve the chances of conception. Gauging the time of ovulation has therapeutic applications in IVF and in artificial insemination. LH kits are now available.

Hyperprolactinaemia

It is seen in pituitary adenoma, hyperplasia, hypothyroidism and with the usage of drugs, i.e. metoclopramide, cimetidine, methyldopa. Hyperprolactinaemia (more than 25 ng/mL) will require X-ray of pituitary fossa or CT scan, and a fundus examination to exclude a neoplasm. Macroadenomas may require surgery. Microadenomas and hyperprolactinaemia respond to Bromocriptine and allied drugs (see chapter on Hormonal Therapy).

FSH

Raised FSH level is seen in ovarian failure. Low FSH level indicates pituitary dysfunction and anovulation. Normal FSH level in the preovulatory phase is 1–8 mIU/mL, and LH level at ovulation is 1–5 mIU/mL. FSH level > 25 IU/mL clomiphene on day 3 fails ovulation.

Thyroid Tests

These should be done especially in case of hyperprolactinaemia. Hypothyroidism with raised TSH level is related to hyperprolactinaemia.

Ovarian reserve or premature failure includes both qualitative and quantitative estimation of FSH/LH.

MANAGEMENT OF ANOVULATION

Anovulation is a common problem encountered in infertility. Several endocrine disturbances contribute to its occurrence; hence, different drug combinations are required to obtain optimal results.

Following are the commonly used drugs for ovulation induction:

Clomiphene Citrate

Ovulation should be induced with CC, with a dose of 50 mg/day starting from day 2 to day 6 of the cycle for 5 days. Ovulation is monitored by serial ultrasound monitoring of the follicular size, and occurrence of ovulation. If the response to 50 mg CC is not satisfactory, the dose of CC should be increased to 100 mg/day from day 2 to day 6. Further increase in dosage dose of CC, if required, should be undertaken in an infertility set-up, where monitoring facilities by sonography and hormone estimation are easily available. If clomiphene therapy fails following six cycles, other regimen of ovulation induction is recommended. This regime requires constant monitoring, so the treatment should be initiated in special infertility clinics. The risk of multiple ovulations and multiple pregnancies with this regime is around 10%. In hypothalamic disorder, GnRH is given to stimulate the pituitary FSH and LH and the folliculogenesis monitored. The pituitary and hypothalamic stimulation is often employed in in vitro and GIFT techniques to avoid peripheral suppressive oestrogen action on cervical mucous and endometrium by clomiphene, and to improve the fertility rate.

Letrozole

Letrozole 2.5 mg (nonsteroidal aromatase inhibitor) is found superior to clomiphene, which has no such adverse action.

With letrozole, ovulation occurs in 90% of cases and with a pregnancy rate of 40%–50%. Letrozole is given 2.5 mg daily for 5 days starting on the second day of the cycle or 20 mg single dose on day 3.

Letrozole has no adverse peripheral action on endometrium and cervical mucous as with clomiphene (antioestrogen action). It, however, causes drowsiness (no driving). Half-life is 50 hours. It is contraindicated in severe hepatic dysfunction. It enhances the action of FSH, the dose of which is therefore reduced by 50%. At present it is an off-label drug and banned in India.

In case of clomiphene failure, some have tried clomiphene 50 mg with 20 mg Tamoxifen (double dose if necessary) in anovulatory infertility. Tamoxifen, unlike clomiphene, has no anti-oestrogenic action on endometrium and cervical mucous.

In PCOD, if the first line of treatment with clomiphene or other drugs fail, laparoscopic drilling of follicles is done by monopolar cautery or laser.

Octreotide is a peptide (somatostatin analogue) secreted by the hypothalamus; it inhibits the growth hormone and insulin. It enhances the effect of clomiphene and reduces the risk of ovarian hyperstimulation syndrome (OHSS).

In PCOD with insulin resistance, pregnancy rate can be improved by administering metformin 500 mg daily at night for 1 week, and gradually increasing the dose twice a day up to three times a day for 6 months. This avoids vomiting. Progesterone or hCG can be added for pregnancy support.

Combination of CC + hMG

In PCOD, ovulation is ideally induced with a combination of CC and hMG. The patient is advised CC 50–100 mg/day from day 2 to day 6 of the cycle for 5 days. Injecting hMG 75 units intramuscularly is added on day 3, 5 and 7, and more if so required.

Anovulatory women who fail to respond to CC + hMG treatment as well as amenorrhoeic women with low oestrogen levels need to be treated with hMG + hCG as detailed below.

Combination of hMG + hCG

1. Perform baseline oestradiol assay and ultrasound scanning.

2. Administer hMG, two ampoules (75 IU each) per day for 3 days.
3. Repeat oestradiol. If it is doubled, monitor hMG dosage; if not, increase hMG dosage by 50% for 3 days.
4. Repeat step 3 until oestradiol doubles.
5. Perform ultrasound scan every 2–3 days until the dominant follicle is ≥14 mm. Thereafter, daily monitoring till size 20 mm is reached.
6. Administer i.m. injection of hCG 5000 IU. Recommend artificial insemination, otherwise advise natural intercourse.
7. Administer injection of hCG 3000 IU 7 days later.
8. Await onset of menses or perform urine pregnancy test.

GnRH

In hypothalamic dysfunction. This is also used as an alternative to administration of hMG. GnRH is a decapeptide, so it cannot be administered orally. Because continuous administration of GnRH will saturate the receptors and thus inhibit gonadotropin release, GnRH is administered in a pulsatile fashion preferably subcutaneously. Ovulation rates of 75%–85% and pregnancy rates of 25%–30% have been reported. One advantage of GnRH is that the risk of hyperstimulation is greatly reduced (1%) compared to hMG (20%–25%); hence, less monitoring is required. The drug is very expensive (Fig. 16.20).

Prednisolone

In women with anovulation and increased androstenedione, the administration of 5.0 mg prednisolone at night + 2.5 mg every morning is advised until spontaneous ovulation sets in. In case this treatment does not succeed, this can be combined with any other ovulation induction regime.

Hyperprolactinaemia

Hyperprolactinaemia is treated with Bromocriptine 1.25 mg at bedtime daily for 7 days, dose increments of 1.25 mg per week is recommended until the hyperprolactinaemia gets corrected when spontaneous ovulation is likely to occur and pregnancy often follows. Cabergoline 0.5mg twice weekly is more convenient.

Laparoscopic Ovarian Drilling

In women with PCOD in whom induction of ovulation with medical line of treatment fails, laparoscopic ovarian drilling of follicles with monopolar cautery/laser has yielded satisfactory results.

Corpus LPD is treated either with intramuscular progesterone 100 mg or micronized 300–600 mg vaginal tablet daily in the postovulatory phase. Oral micronized progesterone tablets are not recommended. They cause drowsiness, poor absorption and bypass effect in the liver. hCG is also employed.

Poor response to induction of ovulation is indicated by:

- Less than five follicles on day 5.
- Oestradiol level less than 300 pg/mL.

COMPLICATIONS OF OVULATION INDUCTION

- Multiple pregnancy
- OHSS

Table 16.3 Grading of OHSS

Degree	Grade	Clinical Features
Mild stimulation (10%–30%)	Grade I	Abdominal distension, pain
	Grade I + nausea	Vomiting, diarrhoea, ovarian enlargement less than 5 cm
	Grade II	Weight gain < 3 kg
Moderate (3%–4%)	Grade III	Features of mild OHSS + ultrasonic evidence of ascites, hyponatraemia, hypokalaemia, hypoproteinaemia
		Reduced renal output, ovarian size up to 10 cm, weight gain of 10 pound
Severe (0%–5%)	Grade IV	Features of moderate stimulation + clinical ascites and/or hydrothorax, adult respiratory diseases, ovarian size > 12 cm, weight gain > 5 kg
	Grade V	Grade IV + hypovolaemia, hyponatraemia, hyperkalaemia, increased blood viscosity, hypercoagulability, decreased renal perfusion, oliguria, hypotension, hypoproteinaemia, thrombosis, coagulation failure, electrolyte imbalance, leucocytes > 15,000/mm^3, hepatic, renal failure Haematocrit > 55% and serum creatinine > 1.6 mg%

OVARIAN HYPERSTIMULATION SYNDROME

OHSS (Table 16.3) is a complication of assisted reproductive technologies and an iatrogenic complication occurring in the luteal phase or early pregnancy. It is a potentially life-threatening condition, occurring in 1%–10%. **It results from induction of ovulation in infertility cases.** It is more common in FSH/LH therapy than clomiphene and pulsatile GnRH drugs. Its incidence is higher in PCOS and anovulatory infertility compared to infertility caused by amenorrhoea. Raised LH in PCOS is responsible for hyperstimulation, and hCG should not be included in the therapy in these cases. hCG administration increases the risk, so also the dose of drugs, size and number of ovarian follicles. It is also common in a conceptional cycle if multiple ovulation occurs. It is characterized by ovarian enlargement, pleural and peritoneal effusion, oliguria, liver damage and thromboembolism. Severe form of OHSS occurs if the woman conceives during that cycle.

PATHOGENESIS

The main reason for OHSS is the increased vascular permeability leading to fluid shift from intravascular to extravascular space. This causes decreased blood volume and decreased albumin as well as decreased electrolyte levels. It leads to accumulation of fluid such as ascites and hydrothorax. The increased vascular permeability is due to prostaglandin, cytokines and growth factors secreted by multiple growing follicles.

The risk factors for OHSS are as follows:

- Young age of the woman
- PCOS
- Previous OHSS
- Increased oestradiol level > 3000 pg/mL
- 20 or more small follicles
- Increased renin and angiotensin factors
- Vascular endothelial growth factor (VEGF) causes neovascularization of granulosa cells and increased E_2 level
- PCOS high LH/FSH ratio, hCG and pregnancy in stimulated cycle
- FSH/LH causes higher incidence of OHSS (30%) than clomiphene (10%) and GnRH (1%)
- OHSS can be predicted by high level of E_2 (>3000 pg/mL), more than 20 follicles on ultrasound and increased Doppler blood flow. There is increased release of rennin and angiotensin.

COMPLICATIONS

Complications of OHSS are as follows:

- Vascular – cerebrovascular accidents, thromboembolic phenomenon, deep venous thrombosis
- Coagulopathy
- Liver dysfunction
- Adult respiratory distress caused by ascites/hydrothorax
- Renal failure due to hypovolaemia
- Gastrointestinal – Related to E_2 level
- Torsion and haemorrhage in the ovarian cyst

PREVENTION

hCG should be withheld in a cycle if more than 20 follicles are seen on ultrasound and E_2 level rises to 3000 pg/mL. In PCOS, it is prudent to withhold hCG. Albumin 5% infusion in 500 mL lactated Ringer's solution during and after oocyte retrieval prevents OHSS. Dopamine agonist Cabergoline 0.5 mg daily for 8 days starting on day 1 of hCG avoids OHSS.

OHSS occurs with smaller than larger follicular size 5 to 8 days after hCG administration. It is an iatrogenic condition of increased vascular permeability resulting in exudation of fluids from the intravascular to the extracellular compartment. Progesterone support helps.

TREATMENT

OHSS requires hospitalization. Medical therapy includes following:

- *I.v. fluids for hypovolaemia.* Colloids, plasma expanders or human albumin infusion 5% in 500 mL Ringer's lactate. Half-life of albumin is 3–10 days. Fifty grams of albumin (25% albumin in 50 mL) raises blood volume to 500 mL. Human albumin 20% with 2 L of dextrose may be needed. Gelofusine for hypovolaemia may be required – continuous autotransfusion of ascitic fluid (CATAF) is performed for 5 hours each day.
- Diuretics and NSAIDs should be avoided because of hypovolaemia and poor renal perfusion except in pulmonary oedema and to correct electrolytes.
- High thigh venous support stocking prevents deep venous thrombosis.
- Immunoglobulins i.v. may prove to be effective.
- Glucocorticoids.
- Anticoagulants – heparin.
- Dopamine improves renal blood flow, oliguria and prevents renal failure.
- Correction of electrolytes.

INVESTIGATION AND MONITORING

Investigation and monitoring are done by the following:

- Hb%, TLC, platelet count – TLC 15,000 and haematocrit.
- Urea, electrolyte estimation, serum protein level.
- Repeat ultrasound to monitor size of ovarian cyst and ascites.
- Weight recording.
- Renal function tests.
- Liver function tests.
- Coagulation profile.
- Central venous pressure recording.
- X-ray chest for pleural effusion.

Surgery is required if the ovarian cyst ruptures, undergoes torsion or haemorrhages. Aspiration of ovarian cyst, ascites, pleural and pericardial effusion may be required.

PERITONEAL FACTORS

Peritoneal disorders include peritubal adhesions and endometriosis, and are diagnosed on laparoscopy.

Therapy consists of operative laparoscopy for adhesiolysis, ablation of endometriosis, incising the chocolate cyst and removing its lining at laparoscopy. Dilatation of fimbrial phimosis, opening of the terminal end of a hydrosalpinx and microsurgery for restoring tubal patency are also possible with laparoscopic methods.

ENDOMETRIOSIS

Endometriosis, associated with infertility, is treated medically, surgically or as a combination of the two.

LUTEINIZED UNRUPTURED FOLLICULAR SYNDROME

LUF syndrome is seen in 9% cases of infertility and is diagnosed only on ultrasound scanning. Micronized progesterone or hCG is needed in these cases (Table 16.2).

UNEXPLAINED INFERTILITY

Infertility is labelled as unexplained when no obvious factor is found in male and female partner. Approximately 10% of infertility accounts for this subcategory of infertility. However, the more we investigate in depth lesser becomes the proportion of unexplained infertility. Common conditions which may account for unexplained infertility are immunological factors, clinical or subclinical hypothyroidism, hyperprolactinaemia, functional disorders in the partner.

Many a time, infertility is unexplained, but this could be attributed to inadequate or inefficient investigations and inability to detect biological capability of the sperms to fertilize an ovum.

Sperm dysfunction and its biological function are now detected on computer-assisted semen analysis (CASA). Abnormal acrosome reaction and sperm–oocyte fusion defects have been identified by CASA and male infertility problems better understood.

It has been observed that 20% of such unexplained infertile couples succeed in having a baby in due course of waiting. Perhaps newer and advanced technology in this field may yield a better pregnancy rate of 40%–50% in future, albeit at a high cost.

When all fail, and the couple is desperate to have a baby, adoption is recommended.

ASSISTED REPRODUCTIVE TECHNOLOGY: AN OVERVIEW

Assisted reproductive technology (ART) comprises a group of procedures that have in common the handling of oocytes and sperms outside of the body. The gametes or embryos are replaced into the uterine cavity to establish pregnancy.

These procedures, although benefited many infertile couples (20%–40% pregnancies), are stressful and very expensive with complications such as OHSS, multiple pregnancy, abortion and ectopic pregnancies. Although no gross fetal malformations have yet been reported, a long-term study is required to detect subtle and late complications.

DEFINITION

ART refers to any fertility treatment in which the gametes (sperms and ova) are manipulated. Accordingly, ART procedures involve surgical removal of eggs known as *egg retrieval.* IVF is the most common ART procedure. It was first successfully used by Steptoe and Edwards in the UK, leading to the birth of first IVF baby Louise Brown in 1978. Since then, millions of births have been achieved with the successful use of these techniques.

INDICATIONS

The common indications for ART procedures include the following:

- Abnormal fallopian tubes: Blocked tubes or absent tubes (surgical removal).
- Endometriosis-related infertility. Idiopathic or unexplained infertility.
- Male factor infertility.
- Immunologic infertility.
- Failure of ovulation – donor ovum. Bilateral oophorectomy for diseased ovaries, i.e. endometriosis and ovarian cancer.

INVESTIGATIONS PRIOR TO ART

- Semen analysis, semen culture and sensitivity.
- Complete work up including thyroid function tests, blood sugar, serum prolactin level.
- Serum FSH on day 2/3 of cycle. Serum oestradiol on day 2/3 of cycle.
- Test for ovarian reserve: Measurement of anti-Müllerian hormone (AMH) is considered the best test. This is indicated in women older than 35 years, smokers, presence of only one ovary and unexplained infertility. It involves standard day 3 laboratory tests as mentioned above, along with administration of 100 mg clomiphene citrate (CC) from day 5 to day 9, repeat FSH on day 10. FSH values must be the same as on day 3 of the cycle.
- Serologic evidence of chlamydial infection. Zona-free hamster oocyte penetration test to asses fertilizing capacity of sperm (optional).
- Enhanced sperm penetration test using TEST-yolk buffer.
- Testing both partners for antisperm antibodies.
- Assess uterine cavity by hysteroscopy/transvaginal sonography.
- Hydrosalpinx reduces IVF success rates by 50%. Success rate increases to expected rates after surgical tying off or excision of hydrosalpinx. Tying the medial end of the tube also reduces the risk of ectopic pregnancy.
- Diagnostic laparoscopy to assess tubal patency and treat any subtle causes of infertility such as lysis of adhesions, treatment of endometriosis etc. Excision of hydrosalpinx or ligation of medial end of the tube.

TYPES OF ART PROCEDURES IN CURRENT PRACTICE

1. **IVF.** This is the most commonly done ART procedure. It involves ovulation induction, oocyte retrieval and fertilization of the oocytes in the laboratory; embryos are then cultured for 3–5 days followed by their transfer to the endometrial cavity (ET).
2. **GIFT.** This involves ovarian stimulation and egg retrieval, followed by laparoscopically guided transfer of a mixture of two ova and 50,000 sperms into each of the fallopian tubes. This procedure came with a big bang and popularity, however, is no longer in use.
3. **Zygote intrafallopian transfer (ZIFT).** This involves the laparoscopic transfer of day 1 fertilized eggs (zygotes) into the fallopian tube.
4. **ICSI.** This technique was developed in the early 1990s. It aims at helping couples with severe male factor infertility. Under microscopy, one sperm is directly injected into each mature egg prior to intrauterine transfer of the fertilized eggs. The method yields 50%–70% successful fertilization rates.

   Indications of ICSI in male infertility are as follows:

- Sperm count less than 5 million/mL.
- Decreased or absent motility of sperms.
- Many abnormal sperms.
- Previous failed IVF.
- Unexplained infertility.

The sperms are obtained by one of the following sources:

- Semen washing in a normal male.
- Sperms retrieved by testicular sperm aspiration (TESA).
- Percutaneous epididymal aspiration. However, a decreased number of sperms are available (PESA) with this technique. This technique can also cause trauma to the epididymis.
- MESA – the tissue can be cryopreserved for future cycles or future pregnancy.

Cryopreservation

Cryopreservation of embryo, oocytes and sperms avoids need for repeat aspirations, reduces the cost of the procedure and can be used in subsequent cycles as well as for further pregnancies. Cryopreservation is also useful in young men who have to undergo surgery, radiotherapy or chemotherapy for cancer, or are frequent travellers.

1. **Ovum donation.** Donor eggs are offered to women with poor egg numbers or quality and elderly women. An egg donor is screened for HIV and other diseases. She is then subjected to stimulation protocol for inducing superovulation, followed by standard egg retrieval. These eggs are fertilized by the sperms of the patient's male partner and the embryos transferred to the patient's uterus which has been simultaneously prepared as per the standard IVF protocol. Ovum donation is also required if both ovaries are removed or radiated.
2. **Ovarian transplant** is a possibility in future.
3. **Surrogacy and posthumous reproduction** are extensions of ART procedures. However, ethical, legal, religious and social issues of these procedures need clarification and understanding. There are grey areas to be cautious about until legal procedures have been drawn. Hysterectomized woman needs surrogacy.
4. **Adoption.** Considering the cost of ART and the stress involved, adoption can be a suitable alternative for infertile couples. Many, however, prefer to have their own genetic babies and resort to adoption when all other measures fail.

IVF Complications

Short-term complications are as follows:

- Failure.
- Oocyte retrieval can cause bleeding trauma, infection, pain, pelvic abscess.
- Ectopic and heterotopic pregnancy 0.4%.
- Multiple pregnancies and its complications.
- Abortion, Intrauterine Growth Restriction (IUGR).
- OHSS.
- Cost.

Long-term complications are as follows:

- Premature ovarian failure.
- Ovarian cancer – due to repeated ovarian hyperstimulation.
- Breast cancer.

Surrogacy may be indicated for:

- Absent uterus, diseased uterus.
- General condition of the woman precludes pregnancy.
- Repeated pregnancy loss.
- Hereditary disease.
- Failed IVF.

KEY POINTS

- Infertility affects 10%–15% of married couples. Changing lifestyle is associated with increasing incidence of infertility.
- Male and female partners are equally responsible for infertility.
- Investigations of an infertile couple begin with semen analysis, a simple outdoor test. In case of semen abnormalities further detailed work up of male partner is needed in consultation with urologist. Considerable advances have taken place in managing male factor–related infertility.
- In female partner, tubal factor is the most common cause of infertility. HSG followed by diagnostic-laparoscopy are the best techniques to evaluate tubal patency.
- Disorders of ovulation can be responsible for infertility in 15%–20% subjects. Currently ultrasound monitoring of ovary for follicle size is most commonly used test for ovulation. In India, premenstrual endometrial biopsy provides additional information about endometrial tuberculosis.
- Peritoneal factors such as peritubal, periovarian adhesions and pelvic endometriosis can also be responsible for female infertility. Laparoscopy plays a diagnostic and therapeutic role in such conditions.
- ART has offered newer hopes for managing tubal factor infertility, male factor infertility, endometriosis-related infertility and unexplained infertility.

SELF-ASSESSMENT

1. Discuss the causes and management of male infertility.
2. A 28-year-old woman presents with irregular menstrual cycles and primary infertility. How will you investigate this case?
3. A 23-year-old woman presents with primary sterility, hirsutism and oligomenorrhoea. How will you investigate and manage this case?
4. A 32-year-old woman presents with secondary infertility, regular cycles, last delivery was 6 years ago. How will you manage this case?
5. How will you investigate and manage a case of tubal infertility?

SUGGESTED READING

Bonnar J. Recent Advances in Obstetrics and Gynaecology. Ovarian hyperstimulation syndrome. Recent Advances in Obstetrics and Gynaecology 21 Ovarian hyperstimulation syndrome. In: Bonnar J. Recent Advances in Obstetrics and Gynaecology. 6:123, 2000, Churchill Livingstone: Elsevier.

David K. Gardner et al. Textbook of Assisted Reproductive Techniques. 5th edn, Vol 2:2017

Duncan Jeffrey S, Shulman Lee P Duncan, Schuman. Year Book of Obstetrics, Gynaecology, and Women's Health. John Wiley & Sons, 2010.

FOGSI Focus. Intra-uterine insemination. 2010.

Hart R, Norman R. Polycystic ovarian syndrome – prognosis and outcomes. In: Best Practice and Research: Clinical Obstetrics and Gynaecology, Vol 20(5): 751–778, Elsevier, 2006.

K Thomas et al. Surgical treatment of male infertility. In: Studd J. Progress in Obstetrics and Gynaecology, 15:363, 2002, Churchill Livingstone: Elsevier.

PD Sutter. In: Rational diagnosis and treatment in infertility. Best Practice and Research: Clinical Obstetrics and Gynaecology. Vol 20(5): 647–664, 2006.

Shai E Elizur, Ri-Cheng Chian, Hananel EG Holzer, et al. In vitro maturation of oocytes for treatment of infertility and preservation of fertility. In: Studd J, Tan, Chervenak. Progress in Obstetrics and Gynecology, 1st Edition, 18:375, Churchill Livingstone: Elsevier, 2008.

Studd J. In: Gamete intrafallopian transfer (GIFT). Wong PC, Asch RH. In: Progress in Obstetrics and Gynaecology, 15: 233. Churchill Livingstone: Elsevier.

17 Ectopic Gestation

CHAPTER OUTLINE

Implantation of pregnancy at a site other than endometrial lining in body of uterus is called ectopic pregnancy. Normally, the implantation of fertilized ovum takes place in uterine cavity, any factor that interrupts the successful migration of conceptus to the endometrium results in ectopic pregnancy. In pathological conditions, implantation may occur anywhere outside the normal uterine cavity, the subsequent gestation being called ectopic. In about 95% of such cases, ectopic gestation occurs in the fallopian tube, when it is called **tubal pregnancy**. In rare cases, it may occur in the ovary, the rudimentary horn of a bicornuate uterus, cervix and peritoneal cavity. Lately, ectopic pregnancy at the site of previous caesarean scar has been reported. Primary abdominal pregnancy is indeed a very rare phenomenon, but secondary abdominal pregnancies have been reported.

TYPES OF ECTOPIC GESTATION

Extrauterine

- Tubal (90%–95%)
- Ovarian (1%)
- Abdominal (1%–2%) – rare

Uterine but ectopic location in the uterus

- Interstitial (2%)
- Rudimentary horn of a bicornuate uterus
- Cervical (0.5%)
- Caesarean scar
- Heterotopic pregnancy: Coexistence of ectopic pregnancy with intrauterine pregnancy.

EPIDEMIOLOGY

1. Ectopic pregnancy may occur at a rate of 1:80 pregnancies or more often. The significance of ectopic pregnancy lies in the fact that it often goes undiagnosed and patient may have massive intraperitoneal bleeding risking her life. It constitutes one of the leading causes of pregnancy-related maternal deaths and accounts for about 10% of maternal mortality.
2. In last 30 years, the incidence has increased six times, related to increase incidence of sexually transmitted diseases and induced abortions
3. Increasing incidence of pelvic inflammatory disease (PID) in the community, the use of intrauterine contraceptive devices (IUCD) and the wider use of assisted reproductive technology (ART), increase in the detection and diagnosis due to more sensitive ultrasound technology have contributed significantly to this rising incidence.

INCIDENCE

The incidence of ectopic pregnancy has been increasing over the past three decades, but the number of hospitalizations is decreasing because of increasing outpatient management. It has risen from 1:150 pregnancies to about

1:40–1:25 pregnancies in present times. TE Goldner et al. (1993) reported a fivefold increase in its incidence in the USA. Racial, genetic and environmental factors have been implicated. Promiscuity, rising incidence of sexually transmitted infections and the practice of resorting to induced abortions have contributed to this increased incidence. Social and lifestyle changes such as late marriage and older age at the time of childbearing amongst career women have become a common practice. Those women who seek postponement of pregnancy may have used contraceptives in an irregular pattern. Modern technology today offers hope to many infertile couples in the form of ART procedures. However, their widespread use in clinical practice has been accompanied by a 5% increase in the incidence of ectopic pregnancies. The important risk factors for ectopic pregnancy are a history of tubal surgery, including tubal ligation, prior ectopic pregnancy. A few early ectopic pregnancies resolve spontaneously and are not recognized. Therefore, the exact prevalence of ectopic pregnancy is difficult to estimate. Repeat ectopic pregnancies are reported in 13%–15% of cases.

AETIOLOGY (Table 17.1)

Tubal pregnancy occurs either because the fallopian tube offers the fertilized egg a congenial environment for implantation or because a delay in the ovum transport across the fallopian tube causes the fertilized egg to implant in the tube itself. The risk factors predisposing to ectopic tubal implantation include – previous salpingitis, previous ectopic pregnancy, tubal damage following genital tuberculosis, previous tubal surgery such as tubectomy (especially Madlener) or tubal reanastomosis, the presence of IUCD, prolong infertility and following ART procedures in infertile women.

The commonest cause is PID including sexually transmitted infections such as *Chlamydia trachomatis* and gonorrhoea. Other leading causes of salpingitis are septic abortion, postabortal sepsis and puerperal sepsis commonly seen in developing countries. With reduction in the incidence of gonococcal infection, chlamydial infection predominates and causes extensive and a subclinical damage to the fallopian tube than that caused by gonococcal infection. RE Barlow et al. evidenced the presence of chlamydial infection in 50% of women presenting with ectopic pregnancy. By treating chlamydial infection in women, a Swedish study showed a drop in the incidence of ectopic pregnancy by 45%.

Table 17.1 Aetiology of Tubal Ectopic Pregnancy

- Previous pelvic inflammatory diseases
- Genital tuberculosis
- Endometriosis in the pelvis causing distortion of the fallopian tube
- Previous ectopic pregnancy
- Pelvic adhesions
- Congenital elongation, accessory ostia, diverticula
- Transmigration
- Previous tubal surgery, tubectomy
- IVF programme
- IUCD, progesterone containing IUCD
- Progestogen-only pills (POP)

Almost 40% of women suffering from ectopic pregnancy have evidence of PID. Westrom reported that following one episode of salpingitis, 12.8% of the affected women showed a partial or complete tubal blockage; this figure rose to 30% following two episodes of salpingitis and 75% after three episodes. He reported a sevenfold increase in the incidence of ectopic pregnancy among women found to have stigmata of PID at laparoscopy. The incidence of ectopic pregnancy following one episode of PID rises from 1:150 pregnancies to about 1:25. The incidence also increases in women who have undergone induced abortion and who have suffered genital tuberculosis. The pelvic adhesions following appendicitis and endometriosis may kink or distort the fallopian tube so as to interfere with ovum transport. Acute salpingitis leads to congestion and oedema of the tubal wall and exfoliation of tubal epithelium during the healing process. Often the tubal musculature is also involved in fibrosis following PID, thus causing a partial blockage of its lumen, an impaired tubal peristaltic activity and a delay in the transport of the fertilized egg.

AETIOPATHOGENESIS

Situations favouring delay in tubal transport of the fertilized egg, or those contributing to its tubal implantation, are discussed below:

- Congenital defects in the fallopian tubes such as accessory ostia, diverticula, partial stenosis and polyp may entrap the fertilized egg and prevent it from reaching the uterine cavity. A cornual fibroid, by narrowing the tubal lumen, can predispose to tubal pregnancy.
- Transperitoneal migration of the ovum from one ovary to the opposite fallopian tube has been reported on the basis of the presence of the corpus luteum in one ovary and an ectopic pregnancy in the opposite fallopian tube. Berlind observed this migration in 8% of cases of ectopic pregnancies.
- Delayed transport of the fertilized ovum along the tubal lumen may result from impaired ciliary and peristaltic activity in the fallopian tube as a consequence of injury or inflammation.
- Hormonal contraceptives, especially progestogen-only pills (POP), are known to reduce tubal motility and thereby favour an ectopic pregnancy.
- Pelvic adhesions and endometriosis may distort the tube and cause kinking. Following the surgical procedure of ventrosuspension, kinking at the isthmic portion of the tube may contribute to ectopic pregnancy.
- Surgical procedures such as tubectomy (especially Madlener), by virtue of spontaneous reanastomosis, and tuboplasty may end up in partial stenosis at the anastomosis site favouring ectopic pregnancy. Conservative surgery for an ectopic pregnancy is reported to cause repeat tubal pregnancy in 15% of cases.
- Laparoscopic cauterization in sterilization operation may lead to the formation of a fistulous opening in its medial end of ligated portion of tube permitting the sperms to reach the ovary. The fertilized egg however is large and

gets entrapped in the distal segment causing ectopic pregnancy. GC Wolf et al. reported that 7.4% of ectopic pregnancies occurred in previously sterilized women. With the use of rings and clips for tubal sterilization the incidence is now reduced. In vitro fertilization (IVF) favours occurrence of ectopic pregnancy on account of fundal insertion of two or more eggs during embryo transfer. The number of eggs and the quantity of fluid medium used during embryo transfer may push an egg into the tubal lumen. This also explains the occurrence of heterotopic pregnancy in 1%–2% of IVF cases.
- In some cases, it is probable that the ovum itself is at fault. The rapid development of trophoblast may favour premature implantation in the fallopian tube. In contrast, delayed trophoblastic development may end up as a cervical pregnancy.
- Extraneous causes such as appendicitis and pelvic endometriosis may involve the fallopian tubes in adhesions, impair its mobility or cause kinking. This partly explains a higher incidence of ectopic pregnancy on the right side.
- About 4% of pregnancies with IUCD are ectopic pregnancies. The presence of IUCD is effective in preventing intrauterine pregnancies, but not ectopic pregnancies. If proper asepsis is not followed at the time of insertion of IUCD, it can predispose to subsequent ectopic pregnancy.
- Progestogen-containing IUCDs and progestogen-only contraceptive pills decrease tubal peristalsis and thereby contribute to the occurrence of an ectopic pregnancy.
- Induction of ovulation with gonadotropins may increase the risk of ectopic pregnancy because of multiple ovulation and multiple pregnancy.

PATHOLOGY

TUBAL PREGNANCY

Tubal pregnancy accounts for 90%–95% of all ectopic pregnancies. In a tubal pregnancy, the most frequent site of implantation is the ampullary portion of tube (80%) because the plicae are most numerous in this part and previous salpingitis is more likely to produce crypts here than elsewhere in the fallopian tube. If the fertilized ovum implants on the antimesenteric border, the trophoblast eventually erodes through the peritoneal surface of the tube and leads to intraperitoneal haemorrhage. If attached caudally, erosion of the trophoblast leads to formation of a broad ligament haematoma.

In favourable cases, the haemorrhage is slow and slight blood clot around the trophoblast dislodges the ovum and produces a tubal mole. The size of the mole depends partly on the extent of the haemorrhage and partly upon the stage of pregnancy. This mole may remain within the tube and gradually gets absorbed. More often, it gets expelled through the abdominal ostium into the peritoneal cavity – tubal abortion. The blood may form a clot around the rupture site or near the fimbrial end – peritubal haematocele. A profuse haemorrhage causes blood to collect in the pouch of Douglas to form a pelvic haematocele (Fig. 17.1). The worst form of haemorrhage results when the trophoblast erodes through all the layers of the tube causing tubal rupture (Figs 17.2–17.7). A rare rupture into the broad ligament forms a broad ligament haematoma (Figs 17.8 and 17.9).

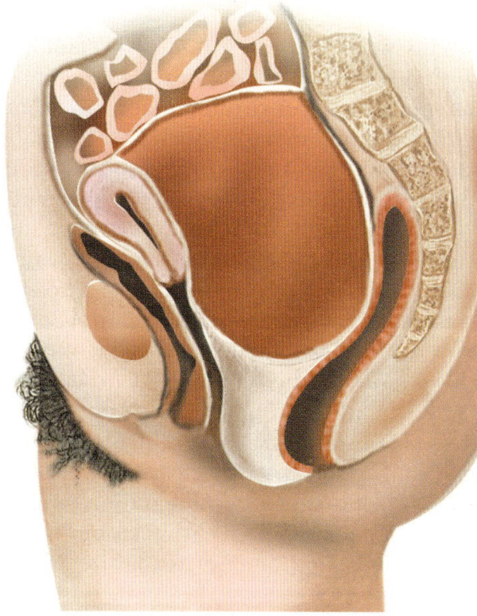

Figure 17.1 A large pelvic haematocele from a case of a ruptured tubal gestation. Note how the swelling pushes the uterus forwards, and how retention of urine may develop from elongation of the urethra. Note the close relation to the rectum.

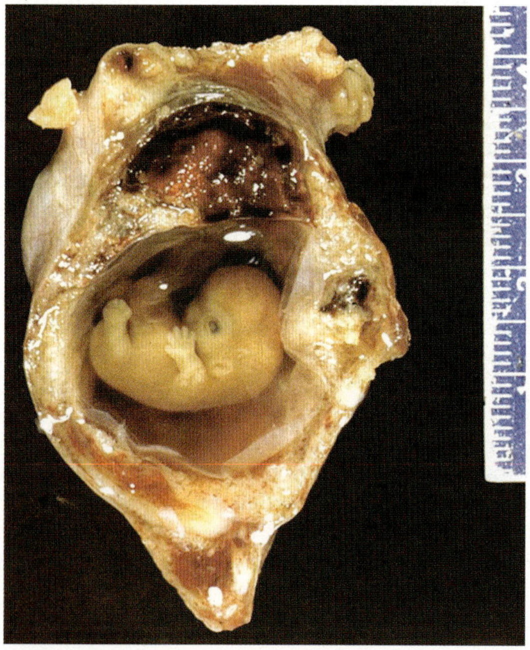

Figure 17.2 Tubal rupture with intact gestational sac – a rare event. (*Source*: C Crum, K Lee, C Crum, Marisa Nucci, K Lee. Diagnostic Gynecologic and Obstetric Pathology. Complications of Previable Pregnancy. Saunders, 2011.)

The ampullary portion is the most frequent site of ectopic pregnancy in 80%, fimbrial ends in 6%, isthmus in 12% and interstitial portion of tube in 2%.

OVARIAN PREGNANCY

Ovarian pregnancy is relatively an uncommon site of ectopic pregnancy seen in 1%–2% of cases however, because of the increase use of IUCDs is being seen more often.

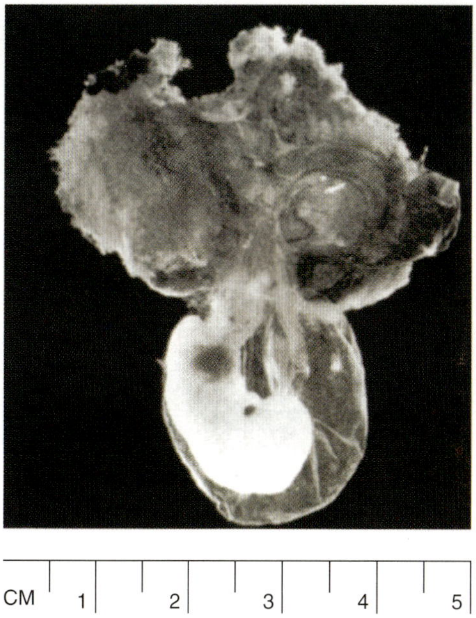

Figure 17.3 Actual specimen removed at operation.

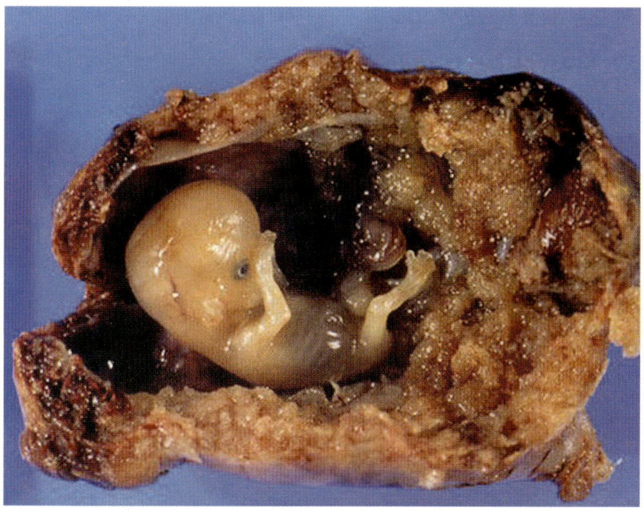

Figure 17.4 The fallopian tube containing ectopic gestation on the point of rupture, removed intact at operation. In the lower half of the picture, the point of erosion is shown by a blood clot. (*Source*: Sciencephoto library.)

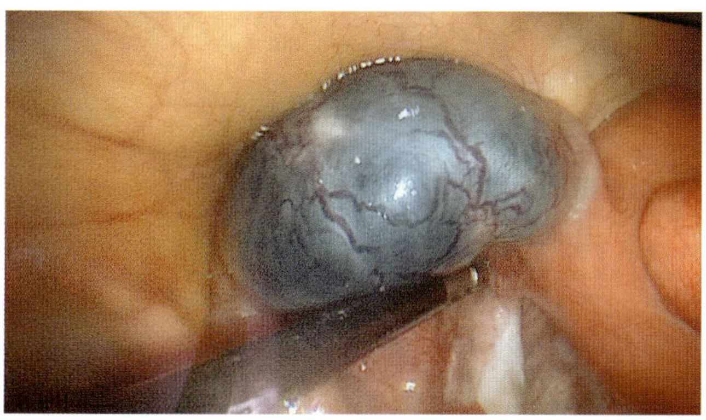

Figure 17.5 Laparoscopic view of left ampullary unruptured ectopic pregnancy. The uterus has a subserosal fundal fibroid.

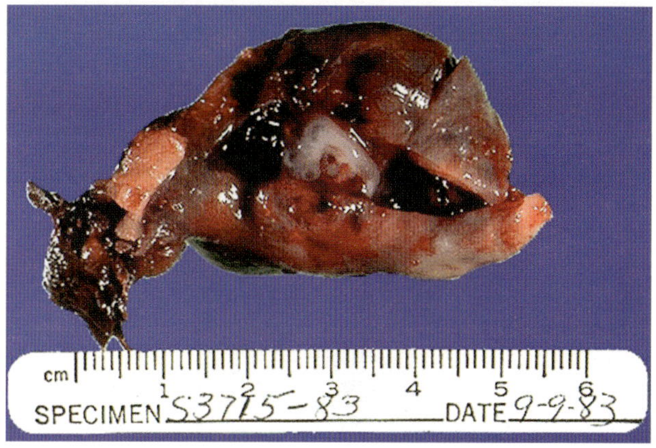

Figure 17.6 Ruptured tubal pregnancy. Note the fetus surrounded by a haematoma being extruded through the wall of the distended tube. (*Source*: Robbins & Cotran Atlas of Pathology. Chapter 13: Figure 13–104. Elsevier.)

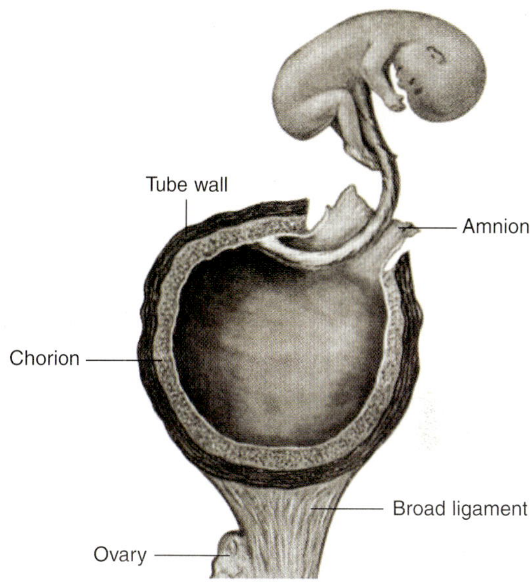

Figure 17.7 Tubal rupture with rupture of gestational sac – the more common event.

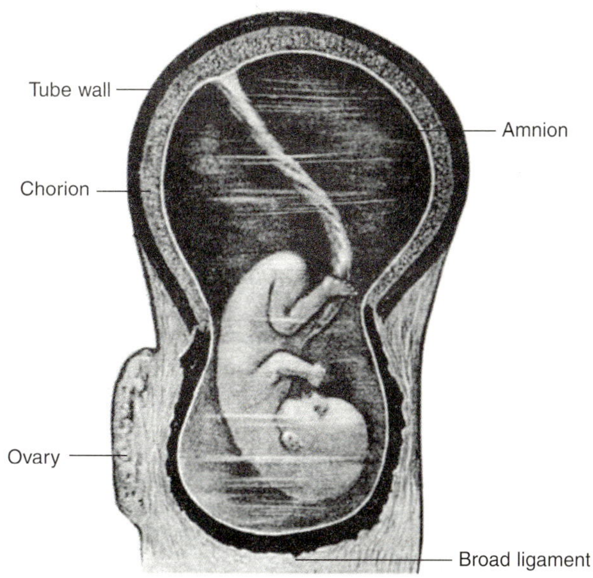

Figure 17.8 Intraligamentary rupture of tube. Gestational sac intact.

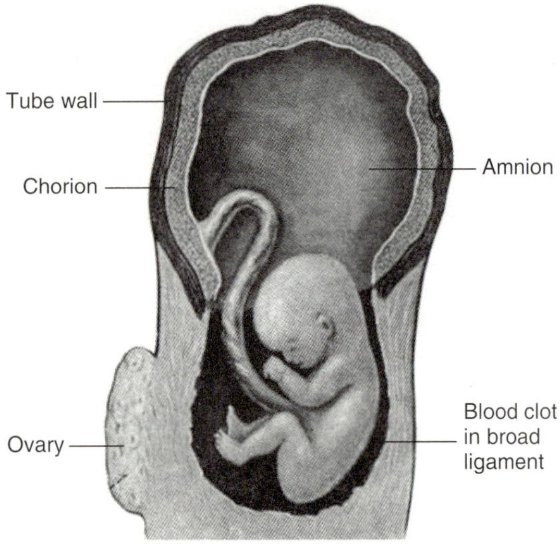

Figure 17.9 Same as Fig. 17.8, but with the gestational sac ruptured.

Although IUCD prevents implantation of pregnancy in the uterus, it has no protective effect on the tubal pregnancy and on ovarian pregnancy. As the fertilized egg lodges in the corpus luteum, ovarian pregnancy gives the appearance of a corpus luteal haematoma. Histological examination will establish the diagnosis. Ovarian pregnancy accounts for 20%–30% of all ectopic pregnancy in IUCD users and 0.5%–3% of all ectopic pregnancies.

ABDOMINAL PREGNANCY

PRIMARY ABDOMINAL PREGNANCY

This condition is extremely rare where a pregnancy implants anywhere in the abdomen without any connection with uterus or tubes. It is possible that the ovum is implanted in areas of ectopic decidua.

SECONDARY ABDOMINAL PREGNANCY

Although rare, a secondary abdominal pregnancy results when a ruptured tubal pregnancy implants anywhere on pelvic or abdominal viscera and a communication with the tube or uterus can be identified during surgical management. In most cases, this condition gets diagnosed in second trimester on the basis of clinical examination and ultrasound. On rare occasions, an abdominal pregnancy continues till term when during laparotomy for a suspected ruptured uterus, this condition comes to lime light. In most cases, fetus dies in abdomen or soon after laparotomy, profuse haemorrhage may occur at surgery trying to remove placenta implanted on the surface of bowel loops or some other structure.

A woman may suffer mild abdominal pain and threatened abortion in the early weeks, but pregnancy proceeds with abdominal discomfort throughout pregnancy. At term, the woman goes into spurious labour but fails to deliver spontaneously or with a Syntocinon drip.

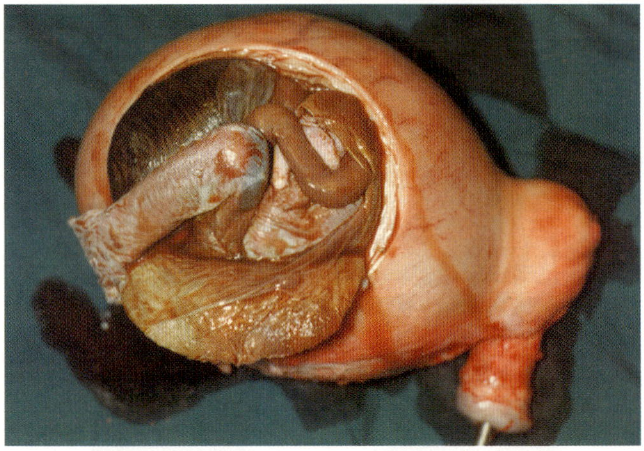

Figure 17.10 Heterotopic pregnancy with ectopic pregnancy in rudimentary horn.

Ultrasound or radiograph reveals an abnormal and a high position of a malformed or a dead fetus outside the uterus. Rarely, a normal live fetus is seen. The uterus is normal in size. Long-standing abdominal pregnancy causes calcification and shrinkage of the fetus which is then called a lithopaedion.

INTERSTITIAL PREGNANCY

Interstitial pregnancy is a very rare form of ectopic gestation, when the ovum is implanted in the interstitial portion of the tube (2%). Usually a muscular septum intervenes between the gestational sac and the cavity of the uterus. Interstitial pregnancy usually terminates by rupture into the peritoneal cavity during the 3rd month of pregnancy (Fig. 17.10).

PREGNANCY IN AN ACCESSORY HORN OF UTERUS (CORNUAL PREGNANCY) (Fig. 17.11)

Rarely, a pregnancy may implant and grow in the accessory horn of a bicornual uterus. The pregnancy may continue up

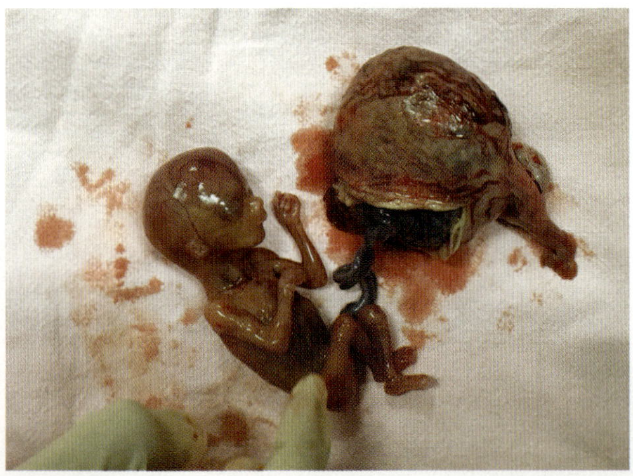

Figure 17.11 Ectopic tubal pregnancy – fetus expelled from the fallopian tube.

Scan to play Ectopic pregnancy

to 12–16 weeks. The condition may get diagnosed by a routine ultrasound done in early pregnancy of patients and may present rupture of accessory horn with resultant intraperitoneal bleeding. The fate of pregnancy in a duplicated uterus depends upon the degree of development of the horn. In uterus didelphys or when both horns are well developed, pregnancy usually proceeds to term or near-term, and parturition may be normal. If one horn is ill-developed, the muscle wall becomes thinned out and may rupture during pregnancy. This complication usually develops during the 4th month and causes severe internal bleeding. At operation, the condition is recognized by its attachment to the round ligament and body of uterus. Pregnancy in an accessory horn has been seen when the corpus luteum was present in the opposite ovary indicating transperitoneal migration of fertilized ovum.

CO-EXISTING INTRAUTERINE PREGNANCY AND ECTOPIC PREGNANCY (HETEROTOPIC PREGNANCY)

This combination of ectopic pregnancy with intrauterine pregnancy is uncommon; however, in recent years because of widespread use of assisted reproduction techniques this combination has become somewhat frequent. Combined uterine and extrauterine pregnancy is reported in 1%–3% of successful IVFs. In a spontaneous pregnancy, the incidence of combined pregnancies is very low (1:4000 to 1:30,000). Ultrasound done to diagnose early pregnancy in IVF cycle may help to discover a heterotopic pregnancy. *The importance of examining both tubes when operating on a case of ectopic gestation must be emphasized.*

Caesarean scar ectopic pregnancy is relatively a newer type of ectopic pregnancy recognized recently. In this rare variety of an ectopic pregnancy, the gestational sac is seen embedded and surrounded by myometrium and fibrosis of the caesarean scar.

SYMPTOMS, SIGNS AND DIAGNOSIS

SYMPTOMS

Accurate diagnosis of ectopic pregnancy is based on symptoms and clinical signs. To begin with patients have signs and symptoms of normal pregnancy; however, soon symptoms such as pain in the lower abdomen, spotting PV and fainting spell set in. *One should consider the possibility of an ectopic pregnancy when a woman in early pregnancy presents with bizarre clinical features.*

The key to a successful outcome is an early diagnosis of ectopic pregnancy.

The clinical picture in ectopic gestation is related to the pathological anatomy. A tubal rupture is an acute emergency associated with internal bleeding and shock. A tubal mole, with peritubal and paratubal haematocele, causes abdominal pain and irregular vaginal bleeding. This is a less urgent condition and is called the subacute or chronic ectopic gestation. The subacute ectopic pregnancy may eventually rupture and become an acute emergency.

Occasionally, with routine ultrasonic scanning in early pregnancy, unruptured ectopic pregnancy can be detected before the clinical features develop.

AMENORRHOEA

About 75% of patients present with a history of amenorrhoea of less than 6 weeks duration. Rarely, an ectopic pregnancy may rupture even before patient misses her periods, this is more likely to happen with isthmic tubal pregnancy. In a rare case of abdominal pregnancy, amenorrhoea may proceed into the third trimester or even beyond 9 months. Duration of amenorrhoea may be 3–4 months in cases of interstitial and cornual pregnancies. Early bleeding simulating uterine abortion is seen in caesarean scar ectopic pregnancy.

PAIN

Abdominal pain, generally severe, is a consistent feature of ectopic pregnancy in 95% of cases. Sudden acute pain in the abdomen is caused by tubal rupture resulting in haemoperitoneum. Occasionally, internal haemorrhage in peritoneal cavity can irritate the undersurface of the diaphragm and phrenic nerve leading to the complaints of shoulder tip and epigastric pain. In a young patient brought in a condition of shock complaining of abdominal as well as shoulder pain, the diagnosis of ectopic pregnancy is almost certain. In subacute variety, the patient complains of vague abdominal pain but signs of shock are absent hence, the diagnosis often gets missed. Pain is often absent in early unruptured ectopic pregnancy.

VAGINAL BLEEDING

Vaginal bleeding is usually little in amount in the form of either dark altered blood or blood-stained fluid. The bleeding is usually as a result of separation of decidua in the endometrial cavity. Rarely, it may come as a trickle from the fallopian tube. Under the hormonal effects the endometrium shows decidual changes, however, there is the absence of chorionic villi. When tubal pregnancy is disturbed, withdrawal of the hormonal support results in shedding of the deciduas. Sometimes, the whole of the uterine decidua separates from the endometrium and is expelled as a decidual cast (Fig. 17.12). Decidual cast has a smooth glistening inner surface and shaggy maternal surface. The chorionic villi are conspicuously absent. The passage of a decidual cast is pathognomonic of ectopic gestation. If a young woman with a short period of amenorrhoea complains of continuous or intermittent but slight vaginal bleeding, ectopic pregnancy should be considered even if the abdominal pain may be slight or might have been short-lived and almost forgotten. Vaginal bleeding and pain are absent in early unruptured ectopic pregnancy. Bleeding may occur very early in cervical and caesarean scar ectopic pregnancies.

ACUTE RETENTION OF URINE

In a subacute variety of ectopic pregnancy, the blood collects in the pouch of Douglas to form a pelvic haematocele. This haematocele forms an irregular mass of differing consistency due to a mixture of clot and blood, and bulges forwards displacing the cervix against the bladder neck leading to retention of urine.

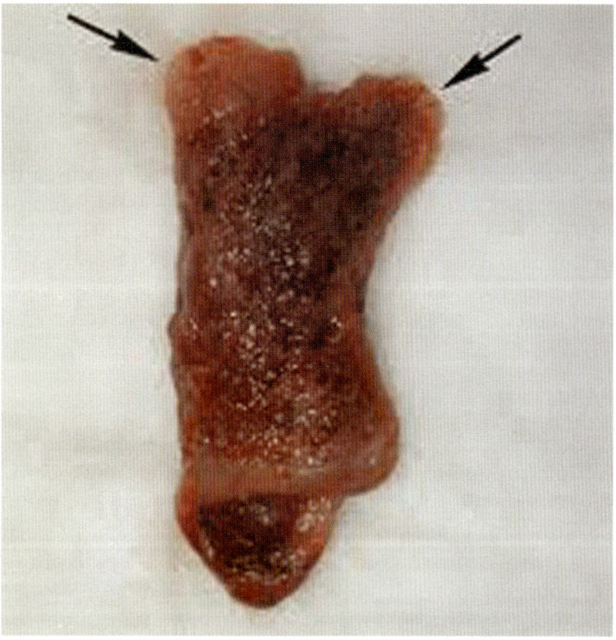

Figure 17.12 Complete decidual cast extruded from the uterus in a patient operated for ectopic gestation.

Table 17.2 Clinical Features of Ectopic Pregnancy

Acute ectopic pregnancy	Haemorrhagic shock
	Acute pain in the abdomen
	Amenorrhoea
	Vaginal bleed
	Abdominal tenderness
Subacute ectopic pregnancy and chronic ectopic pregnancy	Amenorrhoea
	Abdominal pain
	Vaginal bleeding
	Retention of urine
	Abdominal mass and tenderness
	Ultrasound
	β-hCG level
Abdominal pregnancy	Amenorrhoea
	Colicky pain
	Postmaturity
	Failed induction
	Ultrasound: Abdominal fetal position – Malformed, dead

FEVER

If the pelvic haematocele gets secondarily infected, the patient develops slight fever. It is rare to find high-grade fever in a case of ectopic pregnancy.

PHYSICAL SIGNS

The physical signs may vary in acute tubal rupture, subacute or chronic variety of ectopic pregnancy.

ACUTE ECTOPIC PREGNANCY

A patient with sudden tubal rupture with acute intraperitoneal haemorrhage presents in a state of shock with marked pallor, tachycardia and hypotension. The patient is cold, the skin is clammy, the temperature subnormal and the pulse thready with marked tachycardia. Blood pressure will be low. Breast changes of pregnancy may or may not be present depending upon the duration of pregnancy and parity. The abdomen is usually slightly distended and markedly tender with restricted movements. The distension is partly due to ileus of intestine due to the presence of blood in the peritoneal cavity. Rebound tenderness can be elicited in the lower abdomen, rigidity may or may not be present. Signs of free fluid in the abdomen are present in a case with profuse internal haemorrhage. Cervical movements during vaginal examination causes severe pain. Due to abdominal tenderness, it becomes difficult to make out exact size of uterus during bimanual examination. In a case of pelvic haematocele, a bulge may be felt in the posterior fornix during pelvic examination.

Clinical features of various types of ectopic pregnancies are explained in Table 17.2.

DIFFERENTIAL DIAGNOSIS

- Acute PID: Acute PID remains the most common differential diagnosis in a suspected case of ectopic pregnancy. The absence of amenorrhoea, fever, tachycardia and raised TLC and the presence of bilateral tender masses in lateral fornices in a young patient following a recent sexual encounter should raise a possibility of acute PID.
- Corpus luteal haematoma simulates ectopic gestation both in the history and clinical findings. With a history of short period amenorrhoea, pain, vaginal bleeding and a tender mass with internal haemorrhage, it is difficult to rule out this condition. Ultrasound gives an identical finding in both conditions. However, a negative urine pregnancy test and negative serum hCG go in favour of corpus luteum haematoma. Rupture of intraabdominal organs: Splenic rupture though uncommon in gynae practice can produce a similar clinical picture; however, history of blunt trauma to abdomen and the absence of amenorrhoea go in favour of diagnosis of splenic rupture.
- Perforated gastric and duodenal ulcer produce acute abdominal pain, but signs of internal haemorrhage are absent. Abdominal palpation reveals board-like rigidity which is absent in ectopic pregnancy. Air may be seen under the diaphragm in gastric perforation.
- Perforated appendix and acute pancreatitis will demonstrate high fever and signs of peritonitis. Raised TLC and serum amylase level will help in making diagnosis of these conditions.
- Myocardial infarct has occasionally been considered when the patient complains of epigastric pain and

collapses. Normal ECG and the gynaecological history will lead to accurate diagnosis.
- The diagnosis may be much more difficult with ruptured secondary abdominal pregnancy as the differential diagnosis of ruptured uterus and concealed accidental haemorrhage have to be considered.

SUBACUTE AND CHRONIC VARIETY OF ECTOPIC PREGNANCY

In this condition, there may be some degree of constitutional disturbance as a result of the localized intraperitoneal bleeding, but the predominant features are recurrent abdominal pain and vaginal bleeding. Retention of urine may occur due to pelvic haematocele.

The pulse rate is raised in proportion to the severity of the bleeding. It is exceptional for the temperature to be raised to more than 99.48°F. The absence of pyrexia may be of help in distinguishing ectopic gestation from pyosalpinx. The breasts may show signs of early pregnancy. On examination of the abdomen, tenderness in one or other iliac fossa is noted. Distension of abdomen and rigidity may be rarely noted in cases with localized pelvic haematocele.

The characteristics physical signs are found on vaginal examination. The peculiar brownish uterine bleeding can be noted, the cervix is found to be soft and the uterus slightly enlarged. The other physical signs may vary with the type of case. With pelvic haematocele, an irregular swelling can be felt through the posterior fornix or in the pouch of Douglas during rectal examination. It has a peculiar consistency which is almost pathognomonic, as it has no definite outline, is neither fluid nor solid and its consistency varies in different areas. Occasionally, the haematocele may be extremely tender. It pushes the uterus forwards and upwards, and on occasions produces retention of urine. Occasionally, it may extend upwards into the abdomen and is palpable during abdominal examination. A tubal mole and the haematosalpinx form a retort-shaped swelling which is tense, firm but smooth, and which pushes the uterus to the opposite side of the pelvis. Peritubal haematocele forms a firm swelling which may be mistaken for subserous myoma. Firmness, tenderness and smoothness are characteristics of the localized haematomas of ectopic gestation. One danger of vaginal examination is that it may possibly disturb a quiescent ectopic. For this reason, if an ectopic gestation is strongly suspected, vaginal examination should be performed gently. Ultrasound diagnosis may help in arriving at a diagnosis in difficult cases.

Diagnosis of ectopic gestation is often difficult and get missed as it is not suspected. In a young patient and during the childbearing period of life, whenever a woman complains of pain in the lower abdomen associated with continuous/irregular vaginal bleeding, a diagnosis of ectopic pregnancy should be kept in mind.

DIFFERENTIAL DIAGNOSIS OF CHRONIC ECTOPIC PREGNANCY

Clinical diagnosis remains a challenge as the condition may simulate other conditions. *Think of ectopic pregnancy when the woman presents with atypical features in early pregnancy.*

PYOSALPINX

In acute pyosalpinx, patient runs high-grade fever, patient may complain of a vaginal discharge. The signs of internal haemorrhage are absent; so also the history of amenorrhoea, though slight irregular vaginal bleeding may be present in a pyosalpinx. In chronic pyosalpinx, the patient may be afebrile, pain and tenderness are mild and the pelvic mass is often bilateral. In tubercular pyosalpinx, a history of amenorrhoea, pain and a pelvic mass may resemble chronic ectopic pregnancy. Investigations such as laparoscopy and endometrial biopsy may help to establish a diagnosis of pelvic tuberculosis.

SEPTIC ABORTION

A history of amenorrhoea, pain and bleeding per vaginum with a history interference by a trained or untrained person for termination of pregnancy helps in making a diagnosis of septic abortion. Fever usually is high with marked leucocytosis in septic abortion. An offensive vaginal discharge goes in favour of septic abortion.

PELVIC ABSCESS

Pelvic haematocele may be mistaken for pelvic abscess, especially if the patient has fever. Culdocentesis reveals the true nature of the swelling.

TWISTED OVARIAN CYST

Twisted ovarian cyst causes acute abdominal pain and sometimes slight vaginal bleeding, but amenorrhoea is absent; so also signs of internal haemorrhage. Ultrasound examination is of immense help in such a situation.

RUPTURE OF A CHOCOLATE CYST

Although an extremely rare condition, the rupture of a chocolate cyst can mimic ectopic pregnancy. It causes shock and collapse, with acute abdominal pain. The absence of amenorrhoea and negative β-hCG and ultrasound help in making a correct diagnosis.

UTERINE FIBROID

Uterine fibroids can cause acute pain in the abdomen and a palpable abdominal mass if a subserous fibroid undergoes torsion or if red degeneration develops in a fibroid uterus. In such cases, history is more reliable than the pelvic findings. Ultrasound can make a correct diagnosis.

CORPUS LUTEAL HAEMATOMA

Corpus luteal haematoma usually presents with a short period of amenorrhoea, acute abdominal pain, vaginal bleeding and rarely shock due to haemorrhage. The pelvic findings resemble that of an ectopic gestation. A negative urine pregnancy test/negative serum β-hCG and carefully done transvaginal ultrasound (TVS) help to make a correct diagnosis. At times, a laparoscopy will clinch the diagnosis.

ACUTE APPENDICITIS

Patients usually have fever with leucocytosis and vomiting, the absence of amenorrhoea and vaginal bleeding helps to differentiate it from ectopic pregnancy. Tenderness is felt high up in the right fornix.

Risk Factors for Ectopic Pregnancy

- Previous PID
- Pelvic tuberculosis
- IUCD and POP users
- Previous tubal surgery
- IVF – gamete intrafallopian transfer (GIFT) technique
- Previous ectopic pregnancy

DIAGNOSTIC INVESTIGATIONS (Table 17.3)

In the management of acute ectopic gestation, when a patient presents with acute abdomen and in shock due to severe internal bleeding, there is no need and no time for any investigation other than haemoglobin, blood grouping, cross-matching and immediate laparotomy. However, in the subacute/chronic variety, investigations may be required to confirm the diagnosis.

URINARY/SERUM hCG

A positive urine pregnancy test along with ultrasound findings and clinical suspicion helps in making a diagnosis; however, a negative urine pregnancy test cannot be relied upon to rule out ectopic pregnancy. Serum β-hCG level less than 6500 mIU/L is seen in ectopic pregnancy and missed abortion. A slow rise in serum hCG level is seen in a case of ectopic pregnancy.

β-hCG

β-hCG is detected in the serum 9 days (5–10 mIU/mL) and in the urine 13 days after ovulation, around the time of implantation and before the missed period. The level doubles every 48 hours in a normal pregnancy. However, in ectopic pregnancy this doubling of β-hCG is absent rather the increase in β-hCG may be marginal or absent. Therefore, in case of doubt and if the condition of the woman remains stable, serial study and doubling time study are useful. If the level does not rise or rises by less than 66% from the previous reading, ectopic pregnancy or missed abortion should be suspected (N Kadar et al.). When hCG level is more than 6500 mIU/L, intrauterine sac is visible on abdominal ultrasound. Similarly, with a serum hCG value of 1500 mIU/L an intrauterine gestation sac should be visible on TVS.

Table 17.3 Investigations

- Pregnancy test
- Serum β-hCG level; repeat every 2 days
- Ultrasound – MRI
- Culdocentesis
- Laparoscopy

Failure of rise in hCG by two folds in 48 hrs is suggestive of an ectopic pregnancy (Fig. 17.20). In ectopic pregnancy, the doubling rate of β-hCG is slow with less than 66% increase over 48 hours.

Rapid bedside qualitative hCG test with a sensitivity of 25–50 mIU/L should be used, if available, in an acute emergency case (takes 1 hour). Progesterone level less than 20 ng/mL also suggests abnormal pregnancy, but this hormone test has a limited value and takes time (24 hours). It is not used in a routine work-up of a suspected case of ectopic pregnancy. It has a sensitivity of only 80%.

ULTRASOUND

Ultrasound has come to occupy the place of most important investigation in a case of ectopic pregnancy. At ultrasound, the uterine cavity appears empty and a mass can be seen in the region of adnexal. A gestational sac in the adnexal is however identified only in 5%–15% cases of early ectopic pregnancy. β-hCG in the urine and serum, an empty uterine cavity, an adnexal mass with free fluid in the peritoneal cavity is pathognomonic of an ectopic pregnancy. The ultrasonic findings at times may resemble that of PID and endometriosis (Figs 17.13 and 17.14). The main advantage

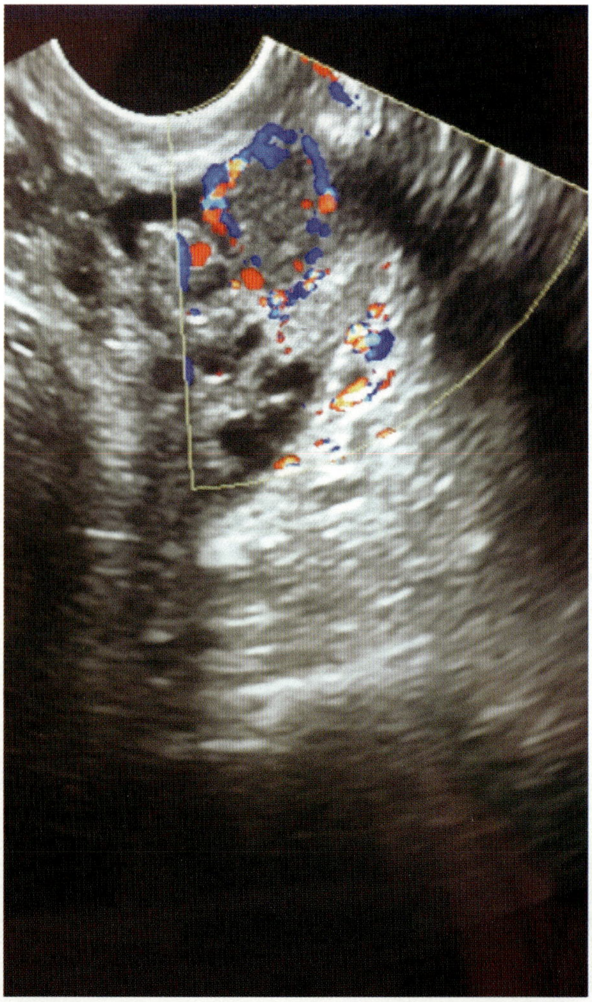

Figure 17.13 Ultrasonographic view of adnexal ectopic pregnancy with a ring of fire appearance on Doppler.

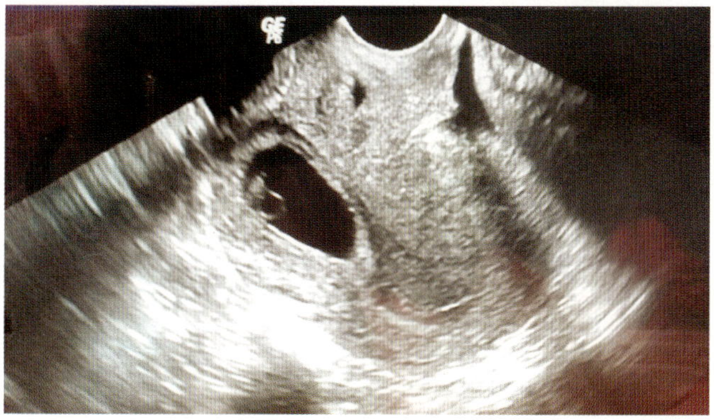

Figure 17.14 Ultrasound showing an empty uterine cavity with live tubal ectopic pregnancy.

of transvaginal sonography lies in making an early diagnosis of an intrauterine pregnancy. At 5 weeks of gestation when the serum β-hCG reaches 1000 mIU/L, a gestational sac with a yolk sac is visible. In an ectopic pregnancy, a pseudosac or an empty sac without yolk is formed by decidual thickening and is centrally placed in uterus.

Other ultrasonic features are 'blob' sign and 'bagel sign'. A blood clot with a trophoblastic tissue is known as blob sign. An empty gestational sac in the fallopian tube is known as bagel sign. Corpus luteal haemorrhage shows spider-web like contents with haemorrhagic areas. Doppler ultrasound reveals increased vascularity and a sign called fireball appearance has been described in cases of ectopic pregnancy.

TVS detects uterine gestational sac 1 week earlier than transabdominal probe (TAS) and gives a clearer image because of its proximity to the pelvic organs. Pregnancy can be detected by TVS approximately 14 days after pregnancy detection by serum hCG at 1000 mIU/L level (5th week of gestation). Pulsed Doppler ultrasound can add further information regarding the vascularity of the peritrophoblastic structure and reduce false-positive findings (Fig. 17.15). In a cervical pregnancy, the uterus is empty but a gestational sac occupies the cervical canal. In a caesarean scar site pregnancy, the uterus as well as the cervix are empty; however, the sac is located over the isthmus.

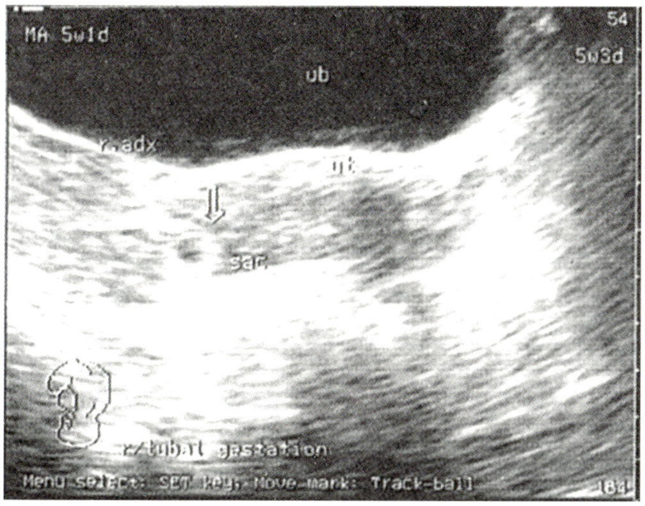

Figure 17.15 Ultrasonography showing ectopic pregnancy with free fluid in the pouch of Douglas.

CULDOCENTESIS OR ASPIRATION OF THE POUCH OF DOUGLAS

In the past aspiration from the pouch of Douglas by placing patient in a lithotomy position was a commonly done test to make a diagnosis of ectopic pregnancy. Aspiration of 2–5 mL of nonclotting blood was taken as a diagnostic of ectopic pregnancy. A needle with its tip in a wrong place or the presence of adhesions in the pouch of Douglas could lead to false-negative results. Currently with the availability of TVS and sensitive β-hCG measurement culdocentesis is not a preferred test.

OTHER HORMONAL STUDIES

Placental proteins, especially PP14 (placental protein 14), are reduced in ectopic pregnancy and their diagnostic value appears to be useful. Schwangerschafts protein-1 (SP1) and pregnancy-associated plasma protein-A (PAPP-A 1) appear late, after 6 weeks of gestation; therefore, their value in the early diagnosis of ectopic pregnancy remains doubtful. Normal progesterone level in early pregnancy is 25 ng/mL. Less than 2 ng/mL is seen in ectopic pregnancy but its use in clinical practice is limited at present as it takes 24 hours to perform.

LAPAROSCOPY

When an ectopic pregnancy is suspected, but the diagnosis is in doubt in spite of equivocal findings of hormonal tests, ultrasound, one should proceed with laparoscopic visualization of the pelvic organs. Not only laparoscopy helps to confirm the diagnosis, most cases can be surgically managed by laparoscopy

TREATMENT

For long, surgery (laparotomy) was the only management for ectopic pregnancy. It is a life-saving measure for acute tubal rupture with massive intraperitoneal haemorrhage. However, now there are options such as expectant management, medical management and a conservative surgical treatment in early diagnosed cases of ectopic pregnancy who are haemodynamically stable. With a diagnosis of very early, unruptured ectopic pregnancy made by ultrasound, a medical treatment can give equally good results.

MEDICAL MANAGEMENT

METHOTREXATE THERAPY

The principle for its use is based on the fact that methotrexate (mTX) is a folate antagonist that inactivates dihydrofolate reductase enzyme, leading to a fall in tetrahydrofolate (essential cofactor in the synthesis of DNA and RNA during cell division). A single dose of mTX therapy given in a dose of 50 mg/m^2 i.m. can help in a slow decline of β-hCG and ultimately dissolution of ectopic pregnancy.

This form of therapy has a 90% success rate (Tanaka), although about 4% may require one more dose of mTX as recognized by a slow decline in hCG value or the failure of a treatment, which is defined as a failure of hCG to fall below 15% in the 1st week (4–7 days). A higher failure rate (18.6%, Lipscomb 2004) has been reported in women with previous ectopic pregnancy. About 80% conceive but repeat ectopic pregnancy is observed in 15% of cases. About 85% of these cases reveal patent fallopian tubes during the follow-up. Five per cent patients still require surgery because of a failed medical treatment.

- Injection mTX 25–50 mg injected into the gestation sac under ultrasound/laparoscopic guidance has also shown a similar success rate. It is an invasive procedure, so it is not a commonly used method of treatment.

Prerequisites for mTX therapy in ectopic pregnancy for consideration of suitability of a patient with ectopic pregnancy for mTX therapy, the following criteria should be met:

- The women should be haemodynamically stable.
- Ectopic pregnancy should be unruptured.
- Serum β-hCG level should not exceed 6500–10,000 mIU/mL.
- The size of the gestation sac should not exceed 3–5 cm in its longest diameter.
- Fetal cardiac activity should be absent.
- The patient should be willing to come for follow-up.
- There should be no contra-indication to mTX (liver disease, anaemia).
- The patient should be desirous of future fertility.
- Hb%, WBC and liver function test should be normal

Side Effects of Methotrexate

- Anaemia: Hb% should be at least 9 g%
- Leucopenia: WCC should be at least 4000 mm^3
- Agranulocytosis: Platelet count 100,000 mm^3
- Thrombocytopenia: Platelet count <100,000 mm^3
- Hepatorenal toxicity
- Nausea, vomiting, gastric haemorrhage
- Alopecia

Contraindications

- Serum creatinine level > 1.3 mg%
- Liver function tests, serum SGOT and SGPT > 50 IU/L
- Low Hb and platelet count
- Preexisting blood dyscrasias
- Acute pulmonary disease
- Peptic ulcer
- Immunodeficiency disease
- Breast feeding
- Known drug sensitivity or the presence of drug allergy
- Gestational sac > 3.5 cm
- The presence of fetal cardiac activity
- Cervical caesarean scar and interstitial pregnancy.

Other Surgically Administered Medical (SAM) Drugs

- Mifepristone (RU486)
- Prostaglandins
- 20% KCl solution
- Glucose solution – all injected into the gestation sac under ultrasound/laparoscopic control
- Of all these, mTX has proved the most effective.

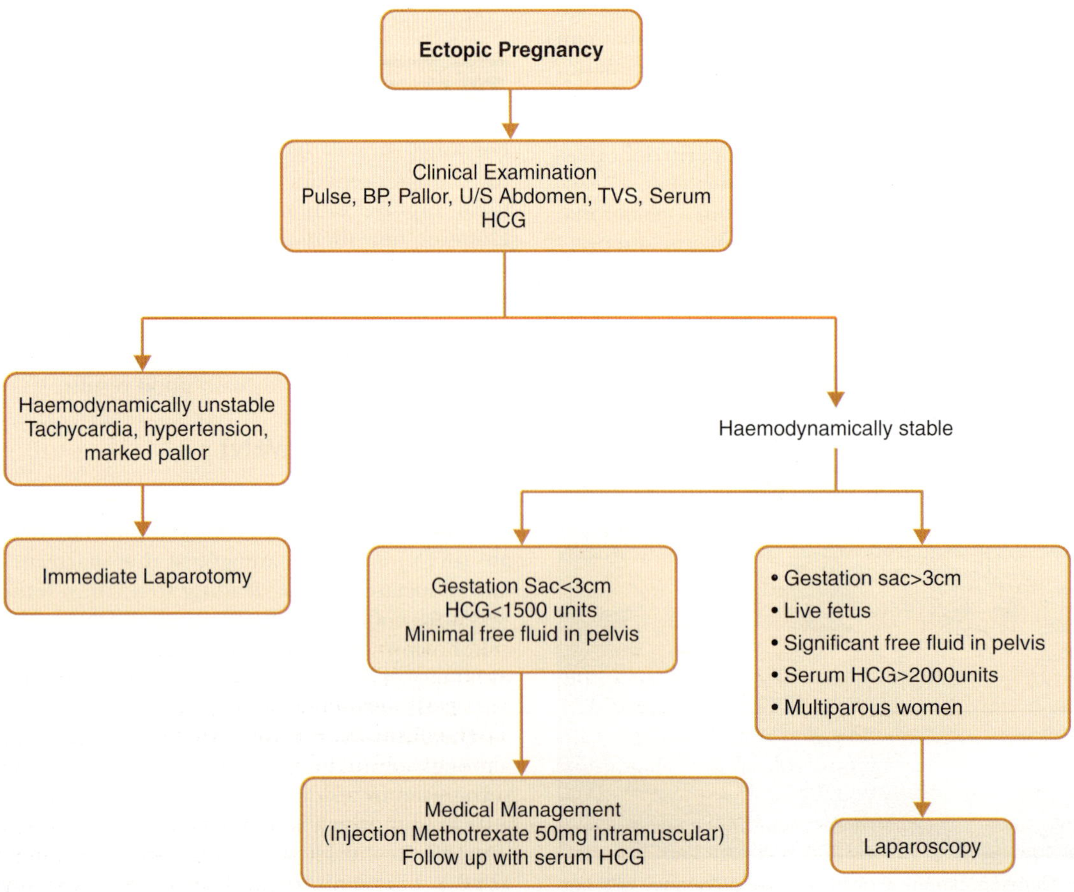

Postmedication Management

Postmedication management comprises following:

- Avoid use of alcohol
- Avoid pregnancy until ectopic pregnancy resolves and serum hCG becomes undetectable. Use of barrier methods of contraception is advocated during the follow-up.

Response to mTX therapy: Following mTX, a fall in the level of hCG to 15% or below the initial level is considered a satisfactory resolution of a trophoblastic tissue. It is important however to note that there may be an initial rise in serum hCG level in the first 4–7 days before the decline, increase in the size of the gestation sac and abdominal pain due to release of hCG and slight bleeding during resolution. Ultrasound scanning therefore should be delayed until after a week. Follow-up with hCG and ultrasound is mandatory. Serum hCG should be done every 48–72 hours initially and then weekly until the levels become undetectable.

SURGICAL TREATMENT

All patients with acute ectopic pregnancy should be operated upon at the earliest once the diagnosis is made. The operation essentially consists of open laparotomy, identifying the affected tube, clamping the mesosalpinx and performing salpingectomy as described by Lawson Tait in 1884. The pedicles are transfixed and the blood present in abdominal cavity and pelvis is removed. Before removing the affected fallopian tube always look at the contralateral fallopian tube. This is important in case the patient has infertility and it is desired to preserve the fallopian tube for subsequent fertility. Most patients show immediate improvement in their condition following surgical management.

It is very important to inspect the contralateral tube for two reasons.

1. Rarely bilateral tubal pregnancy may be encountered or the other fallopian tube is diseased/damaged.
2. Condition of the tube needs to be assessed to check the prognosis of future pregnancy.

In most cases it is possible to preserve the ovary as it is separate from the gestation sac in the tube. Rarely, if ovary is buried in a tubo-ovarian mass, salpingo-oophorectomy is performed. In the past the blood in the peritoneal cavity was used for autotransfusion. The advantages of autotransfusion are that blood is available immediately without any need for a cross-match. Also, there is no fear of transmission of HIV, malaria and hepatitis B.

TYPES OF SURGERY ON THE FALLOPIAN TUBE

The surgical treatment may comprise salpingectomy, partial salpingectomy, salpingostomy and milking of the tube (Fig. 17.16).

- Salpingectomy if the gestation sac is >4 cm, most of the tube is damaged and the other tube is healthy (Fig. 17.17).
- Partial salpingectomy if more than 6 cm of the tube can be preserved. Later, tubal anastomosis can be performed (Figs 17.18 and 17.19).

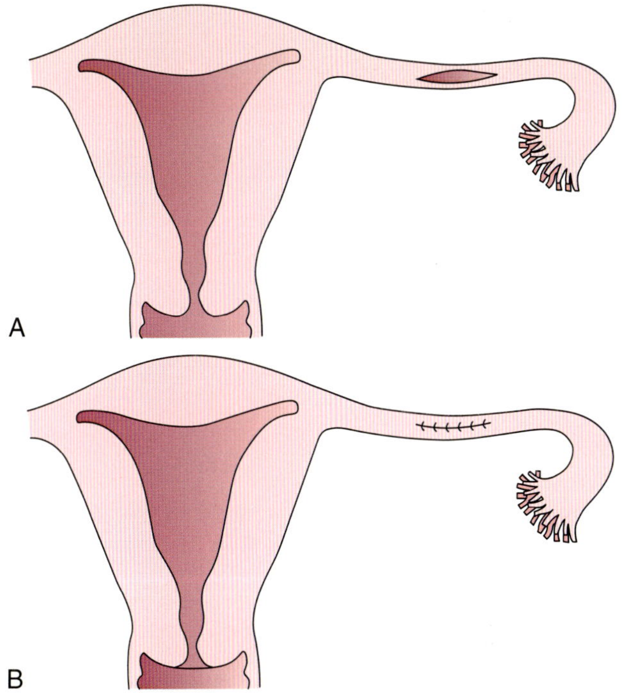

Figure 17.16 **(A)** Salpingostomy. **(B)** Salpingotomy.

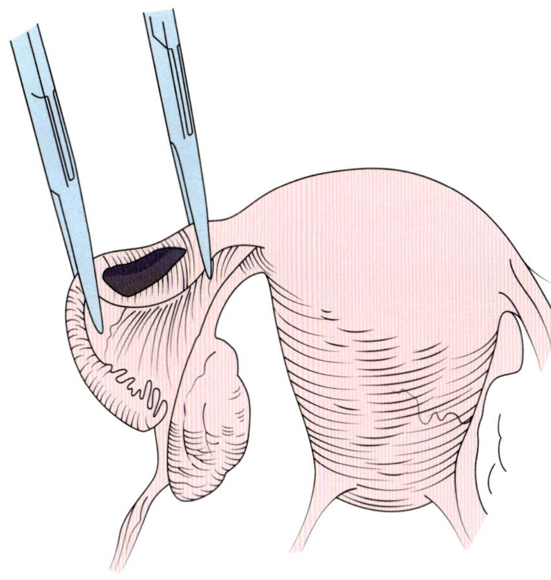

Figure 17.17 Total salpingectomy for a tubal pregnancy.

- Salpingostomy – Antimesenteric border is incised, conceptus removed, haemostasis secured and the wound left open for secondary healing. The pregnancy rate is better than with salpingotomy (Fig. 17.16) and repeat ectopic pregnancy is low. Salpingotomy – The wound is closed with fine Vicryl sutures.
- Milking of the tube is possible with fimbrial pregnancy, but because of a risk of persistent intratubal bleeding and a persistent trophoblastic tissue and an increased risk of recurrent ectopic pregnancy this technique is not

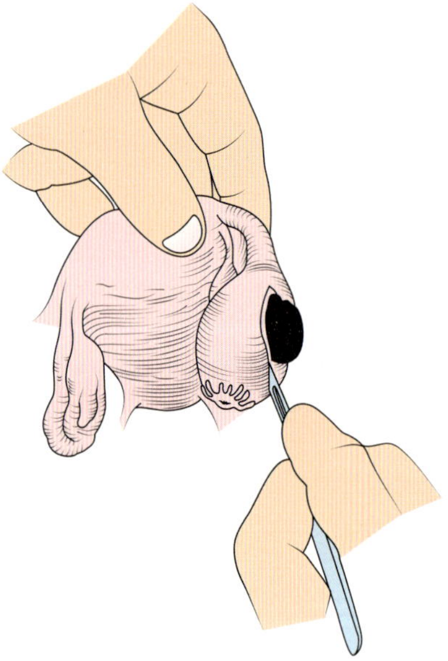

Figure 17.18 Partial salpingectomy for a tubal pregnancy.

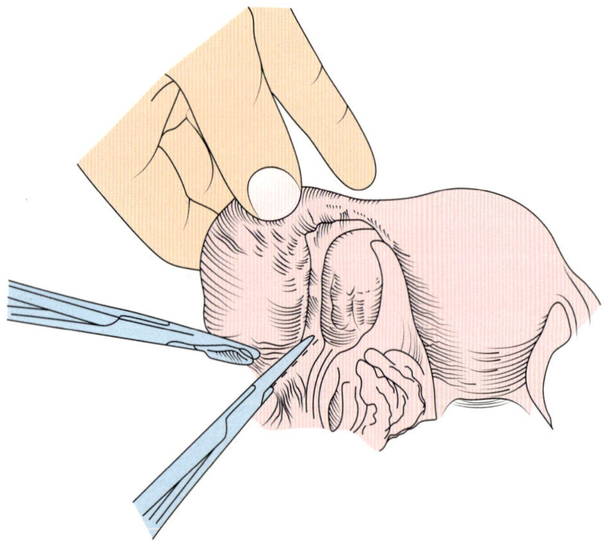

Figure 17.19 Removing an ampullary tubal pregnancy with conservation of tube.

popularly used. With improved technique, laparoscopically performed above-mentioned procedures have become the gold standard in the treatment, with early recovery, less pain and a short hospital stay. The future outcome is similar to that of laparotomy. Most cases can be managed by laparoscopy.

CONSERVATIVE TUBAL SURGERY

Conservative tubal surgery is justifiable only if the contralateral tube has already been removed or is diseased, because this type of surgery exposes the woman to a recurrent ectopic pregnancy.

Fifty per cent women undergoing conservative surgery conceive and have uterine pregnancy.

With improved awareness and screening procedures, life-threatening ectopic pregnancy has changed to a benign condition, especially in the case of an asymptomatic woman in stable condition at the time of diagnosis (unruptured ectopic). Conservative medical treatment then applied is safe and cost effective. It also improves the subsequent pregnancy outcome.

The treatment of secondary abdominal pregnancy includes performing a laparotomy and removing the fetus and placenta. If the placenta is adherent to a vascular organ, it may be safer to clamp the cord close to the placenta, leave the latter in situ and close the abdomen without a drainage. Hreschchyshyn et al. (1965) proposed administration of mTX to resolve the placental tissue. Ultrasonic monitoring and estimating serum β-hCG level are mandatory in such a situation.

INTERSTITIAL PREGNANCY

TREATMENT

Although an extremely rare variety of ectopic pregnancy, interstitial pregnancy can be associated with massive intraperitoneal haemorrhage, rarely a hysterectomy is indicated in ruptured interstitial pregnancy. In unruptured pregnancy, conservative management may be possible. Incision and emptying the gestational sac following ligation of the ipsilateral uterine artery, ovarian and round ligament is followed by suturing the muscular layer. The risk of uterine rupture in subsequent pregnancy mandates careful antenatal monitoring and caesarean delivery. Recently, hysteroscopic removal of the sac has been attempted. Early interstitial pregnancy has been managed with local or intramuscular mTX injection and a follow-up until serum β-hCG disappears. In all ectopic pregnancies if woman is Rh-negative, it is advisable to administer 100 mcg anti-D gamma globulin to the Rh-negative patient to safeguard against isoimmunization.

PROGNOSIS

Due to a delay in diagnosis or a failure to diagnose ectopic pregnancy still remains a cause of maternal deaths. Ten per cent deaths in ectopic gestation are primarily due to haemorrhage. Following treatment, 50%–80% of the women conceive and of these 50% have intrauterine pregnancies, 15% will have repeat ectopic pregnancy. The rest remain infertile, due to tubal damage.

UNRUPTURED ECTOPIC GESTATION

Recent advances in immunoassays for hCG and high-resolution ultrasound have made significant progress in the diagnosis and management of early unruptured ectopic pregnancy. In these cases, there has been a shift from ablative surgery to conservative fertility-preserving therapy/ medical management. Schenker observed that 15% of ectopic cases will have recurrent ectopic pregnancies and 60%–70% have fertility problems. To improve future fertility, and to avoid catastrophic haemorrhage, it is necessary to make a

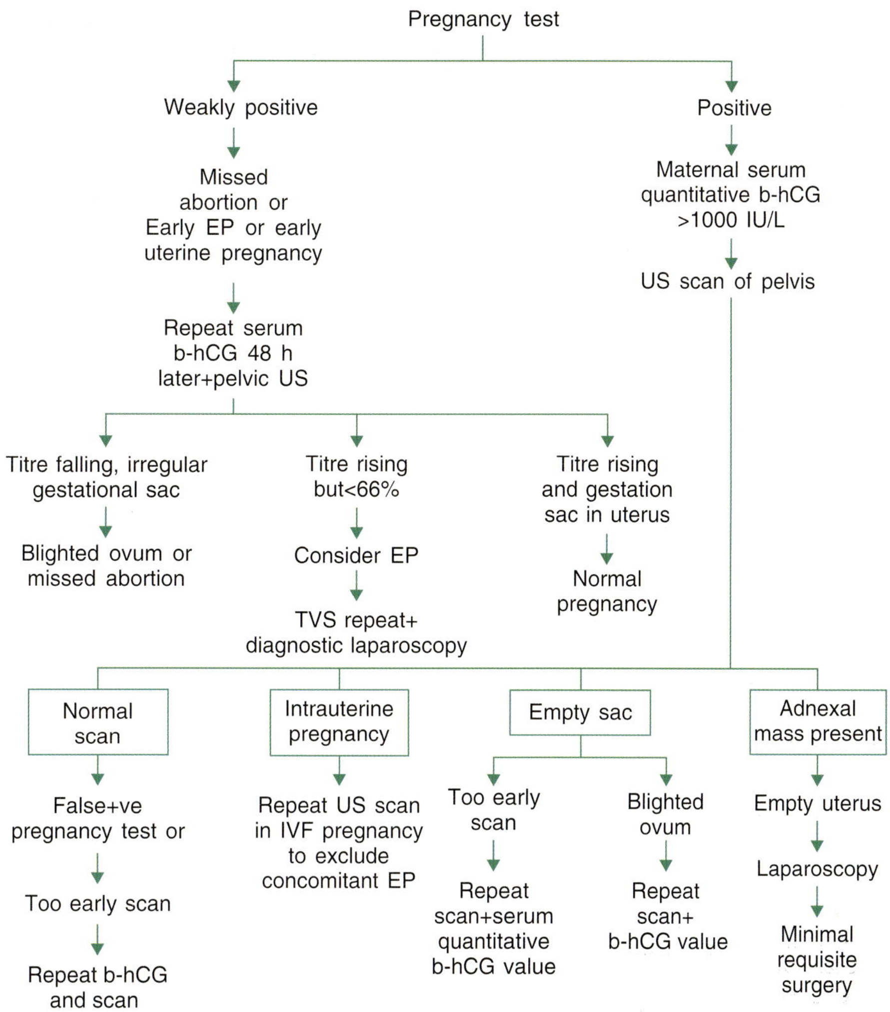

Figure 17.20 Positive pregnancy test: Features suggestive of ectopic pregnancy (EP).

diagnosis before the ectopic sac ruptures. *This is possible with routine ultrasonic scanning in early pregnancy. Early diagnosis is the key to conservative management.*

If a woman in the reproductive age complains of amenorrhoea, mild abdominal pain and abnormal uterine bleeding, she should be suspected of ectopic pregnancy. Early diagnosis of ectopic pregnancy allows laparoscopic conservative surgery or medical therapy. This not only reduces mortality and morbidity due to haemorrhage but also improves subsequent fertility.

EXPECTANT TREATMENT (Fig. 17.21)

The expectant treatment comprises follow-up with serial hCG levels and ultrasound scanning. It is applicable only if the gestational sac is less than 2 cm and hCG levels are not very high (< 500 mIU/mL) and the absence of haemoperitoneum. In most cases pregnancies resolve without any surgical or medical management. However, due to the uncertainty and a prolonged follow-up, it is not practical in large number of cases.

Table 17.4 Spiegelberg Criteria to Diagnose Ovarian Pregnancy

- Pregnancy is in close relation to ovary.
- Fallopian tube on affected side is normal.
- Mass is attached to uterus by ovarian ligament.
- Histologically chorionic tissue is in intimate contact with ovarian tissues.

OVARIAN PREGNANCY

Ovarian pregnancy constitute 0.5%–1% of all ectopic pregnancies. The criteria for diagnosis of ovarian pregnancy were described by Spiegelberg (Table 17.4) In most cases condition comes to notice at the time of surgery for suspected tubal pregnancy. The treatment comprises either oophorectomy or partial resection of ovary with the reconstruction of remaining ovarian tissues.

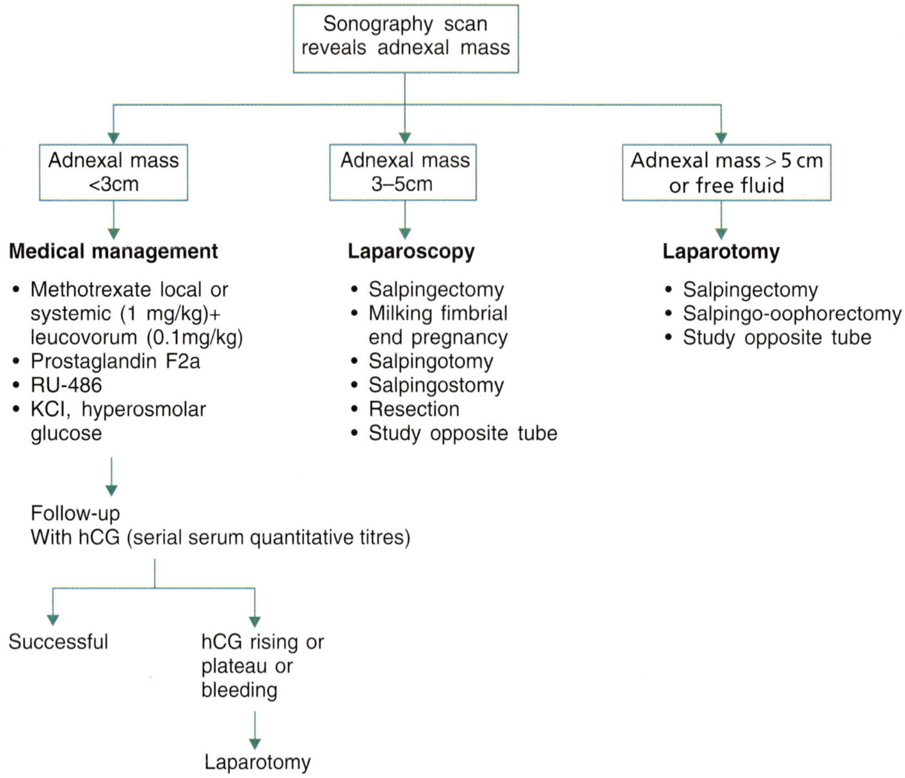

In laparoscopic salpingectomy, the ectopic tube is removed using a tissue removal bag. Before removal, endo-loop is slipped into the mesosalpinx and tightened.

Diathermy knife or laser can be used in salpingotomy and salpingostomy to cut and secure haemostasis.

Figure 17.21 A treatment of ectopic tubal pregnancy (ETP).

CERVICAL PREGNANCY

Cervical pregnancy is extremely rare (0.5%–1%), though in Japan, the incidence is 1/1000 pregnancies and it is the second most common variety of ectopic pregnancy. The woman presents with profuse painless bleeding following a short period of amenorrhoea. Pelvic examination reveals a patulous external os and products of conception in the cervical canal; the internal os is closed and the uterus is firm and normal in size. Ultrasound helps in a correct diagnosis; clinically, the diagnosis of inevitable abortion is initially made. Doppler blood flow mapping and MRI improve the diagnostic accuracy.

The risk factors are previous endocervical curettage and Asherman syndrome.

ULTRASOUND

Rubin's criteria for diagnosis of cervical pregnancy.

- There should be no fetal tissue in uterine cavity.
- There should be cervical glands opposite the placental tissue.
- The sac and fetal tissue present in cervical canal should be below the level of reflection of peritoneum in the pelvis.

Ultrasound criteria are as follows:

- Empty uterus
- Ballooned cervix
- Gestational sac and fetal tissue below the level of internal os.
- Internal os is closed
- The blood flow in the cervix is increased
- The absence of sliding sign – the pressure over the cervix causes sliding down of the gestational sac in a miscarriage, whereas the cervical pregnancy remains static, because it is attached to the cervix.

TREATMENT OF CERVICAL PREGNANCY

Because of a risk of profused bleeding during any surgical procedure, the treatment consists of ligating the uterine vessel vaginally, suction evacuation and tamponade by inserting a Foley catheter in the cervical canal for 24 hours. In case of profuse haemorrhage occasionally hysterectomy may be needed. Hysteroscopic resection of the cervical pregnancy using resectoscope has been described by Ash and Farroll in the USA. mTX has also been injected locally, followed if necessary a week later with suction evacuation. Unlike in tubal pregnancy, i.m. mTX injection 50 mg may have to be repeated weekly until β-hCG level disappears.

Uterine artery embolization has been attempted to reduce blood loss, prior to evacuation of cervical and caesarean scar pregnancy.

CORNUAL PREGNANCY

Cornual pregnancy is a pregnancy in the accessory horn or bicornuate uterus. Pregnancy may continue up to

14–16 weeks when a sudden rupture into the peritoneal cavity results in features of acute abdomen. In most cases diagnosis becomes obvious at the time of surgical management for suspected ectopic pregnancy. Excision of rudimentary horn at laparotomy or laparoscopy is the treatment. Most cases in subsequent pregnancy should be managed by an elective caesarean section as a site of excision of rudimentary horn remains a weak area in the uterine musculature.

HETEROTOPIC PREGNANCY

Heterotopic pregnancy, i.e. combined uterine and ectopic tubal pregnancy, is very rare in spontaneous conception cycles; the incidence is not more than 1:4000 to 1:7000 pregnancies. The incidence is however higher in IVF programmes because of the higher number of embryos transferred, with a possibility of one embryo migrating to the tube. The possibility is also related to the amount of fluid injected with the embryo. At present, IVF centres have reported an incidence of 1%–3% for heterotopic pregnancy.

The diagnosis is not easy. The serum β-hCG may not be proportionately high. Ultrasound can visualize multiple pregnancy in early pregnancy. A carefully done TVS in early pregnancy may help to diagnose this condition.

TREATMENT

Medical treatment in the form of mTX, mifepristone and prostaglandin is contraindicated because of their adverse effects on the normal uterine pregnancy. Glucose and KCl have been injected in the tubal pregnancy with the aim of continuation of intrauterine pregnancy. A surgical approach in the form of laparoscopic salpingectomy may help to manage condition successfully allowing uterine pregnancy to grow.

In IVF programme, the following prophylactic measures have been suggested:

- Bilateral tubectomy prior to IVF.
- Transfer of not more than two embryos.
- A small amount of fluid medium to be transferred.
- A routine ultrasound scanning in early pregnancy, in case conception follows.

CAESAREAN SCAR ECTOPIC PREGNANCY

Caesarean scar ectopic pregnancy is recently reported in 6% of ectopic pregnancies. The ultrasound shows an empty uterus and cervix and the gestational sac is attached low to the lower segment caesarean scar. Doppler imaging confirms the diagnosis. The woman presents with clinical features of threatened or inevitable abortion.

The gestation sac is embedded in the myometrium and fibrosis of the caesarean scar. MRI is a diagnostic test.

ULTRASOUND

Ultrasound shows following:

- Gestational sac located over the lower anterior uterine segment.
- The absence of sliding sign.
- Increased blood flow over the lower uterine segment.

TREATMENT

- mTX injection.
- Surgery – Suction curettage may be risky even under ultrasonic guidance and the risk of caesarean scar rupture remains. A surgical removal of an ectopic site bearing area in the regional isthmus with reconstruction of uterus is the preferred treatment.
- In a young woman desirous of childbearing, resection and suturing of scar can be done but the risk of scar rupture in subsequent pregnancy is considerable. There is an increased risk of repeat scar ectopic pregnancy as well as placenta accreta. Hysterectomy is recommended in a multiparous woman.

PERSISTENT ECTOPIC PREGNANCY (PEP)

PEP complicates conservative therapy, especially milking of the tube, when a portion of the conception products is left behind. Following laparoscopic salpingostomy, PEP is reported in 16% against 1% following laparotomy.

Persistent elevation of serum β-hCG is a diagnostic. A repeat injection of mTX may help resolution of PEP.

RECURRENT ECTOPIC PREGNANCY

Recurrent ectopic pregnancy is seen in about 15% of cases, irrespective of the method of previous treatment for ectopic pregnancy. Such an event is more likely in cases with previous PID.

When a woman suffers from a recurrent ectopic pregnancy, it may be prudent to perform salpingectomy and offer IVF as a treatment for subsequent fertility.

MORTALITY AND MORBIDITY

Ectopic pregnancy is responsible for 11.5% maternal mortality mainly due to a delay in diagnosis or a failure of diagnosis. Early diagnosis and management can avoid maternal death.

Morbidity includes following:

- Infertility
- Recurrent ectopic pregnancy
- Pelvic adhesions and chronic pelvic pain
- Psychological morbidity and fear of future pregnancy outcome

KEY POINTS

- Of all the ectopics, tubal pregnancy is the most common. PID, previous tubal surgery and IUCD are the common predisposing factors for ectopic pregnancy.
- Although an acute ectopic pregnancy is life-threatening condition and requires an emergency surgery, subacute and chronic ectopic pregnancy may be managed medically or surgically after careful confirmation of diagnosis.

- It is now possible to detect an early unruptured ectopic pregnancy by ultrasound, aided by serum β-hCG level, and at times by laparoscopy.
- Conservative surgery and medical therapy can preserve the fallopian tube for future fertility. However, 15% are at a risk of recurrent ectopic pregnancy.
- Cervical pregnancy, pregnancy in a rudimentary horn, caesarean scar pregnancy and abdominal pregnancy are rare.
- Heterotopic pregnancy is becoming commoner due to ART. Management requires continuation of intrauterine pregnancy with an appropriate treatment for tubal pregnancy. Recurrent pregnancy remains a threat to a woman with one ectopic pregnancy, and she needs good monitoring in the subsequent pregnancies.
- Early diagnosis is the key to successful medical and minimally invasive conservative surgery; it reduces mortality.
- TVS and serial β-hCG help in early diagnosis of ectopic pregnancy in a suspected case.

SELF-ASSESSMENT

1. What are the causes of ectopic pregnancy?
2. Discuss the symptoms and signs of chronic ectopic pregnancy. How will you manage a case of chronic ectopic pregnancy?
3. A 24-year-old woman presents with 2 months amenorrhoea. Pregnancy test is positive, but ultrasound shows an empty uterus. How will you manage this case?
4. A young primigravida presents with 2 months amenorrhoea, slight abdominal pain and vaginal bleeding. Discuss the management.
5. A woman is brought to emergency with amenorrhoea 2 months and features of shock. Discuss the management of such a case.

SUGGESTED READING

ACOG practice bulletin. Tubal ectopic pregnancy. Feb 2018.

Duncan Jeffrey S, Shulman Lee P Duncan, Schuman. Year Book of Obstetrics, Gynaecology, and Women's Health. Page 295, John Wiley & Sons, 2010.

Maya Chetty, Janine Elson. Treating non-tubal ectopic pregnancy. Best Practice & Research. Clinical Obstetrics & Gynaecology, Vol 23(4): 529–538, Elsevier, 2009.

Sengupta, Chattopadhyay, Varrma. Textbook of Gynaecology for Postgraduates and Practitioners, Elsevier, 2007.

Acute and Chronic Pelvic Pain

18

CHAPTER OUTLINE

Pelvic pain is a fairly common complaint amongst women resulting in disruption of their day-to-day activity, personal life and sexual life. It is one of the common conditions for which women attend gynaecological OPD. Often managing these cases is difficult and taxing for gynaecologist.

Acute pelvic pain is mostly due to some significant pathology such as acute pelvic inflammatory disease (PID), ectopic pregnancy or torsion of an ovarian cyst, and requires prompt attention. Urgent investigations may help in clinching the diagnosis. In most cases, a prompt treatment either medical or surgical is indicated.

Chronic pelvic pain (CPP) mostly a condition with significant alteration in day-to-day activities of a woman. Before coming to hospital she may have visited several doctors and may have undergone large number of investigations and at times surgical interventions without much relief. Although some gynaecological conditions such as endometriosis, pelvic congestion syndrome or chronic PID can be the cause, in most cases no obvious pathology is identified.

ACUTE PELVIC PAIN

Causes of acute pelvic pain may vary in different age groups. Following are the common causes of acute pelvic pain:

PREMENARCHE

- **Congenital** causes: Haematocolpos and haematometra (Chapter 5)
- Ovarian cyst: Torsion, rupture haemorrhage and malignancy (Chapter 32).
- Abdominal tuberculosis
- Nongynaecological causes: UTI, acute appendicitis, gastrointestinal problems, acute porphyria.

In young adolescents, mostly acute pain is of a nongynaecological origin. They may be related to urinary tract, gastrointestinal tract or abdominal tuberculosis.

TWISTED OVARIAN CYST

Dermoid cyst is the commonest ovarian cyst seen in young girls, because of long pedicle this cyst has a tendency to undergo torsion resulting in acute abdominal pain. Less commonly other germ cell tumours of ovary can be the cause of acute abdominal pain due to torsion, rupture or infection.

REPRODUCTIVE AGE GROUP

Acute pain may be due to obstetrical, gynaecological and nongynaecological conditions.

OBSTETRICAL CAUSES

- *Abortions.* Pain may be due to inevitable, incomplete or septic abortion. Inevitable abortion is associated with severe vaginal bleeding and the diagnosis is obvious.
- *Septic abortion.* In septic abortion, the woman suffers from high fever, severe abdominal pain and vomiting. Foul-smelling vaginal discharge may be present.
- *Ectopic pregnancy.* Acute ectopic pregnancy is associated with severe abdominal pain and short period of amenorrhoea with or without vaginal bleeding. Ultrasound reveals free fluid in the abdominal cavity and a pelvic mass. It requires immediate surgery.
- *Red degeneration of fibroid.* A woman in pregnancy may develop acute abdominal pain and often vomiting, uterus is enlarged and tender. Ultrasound is of help in differentiating this condition from other causes. In most cases, a conservative treatment in the form of rest and analgesics helps.
- *Twisted ovarian cyst.* This requires immediate surgery.
- *Acute hydramnios.* More common in a multiple pregnancy, acute hydramnios presents with unduly enlarged uterus in mid-pregnancy and abdominal pain and respiratory distress. Ultrasound shows multiple pregnancy and hydramnios. Invariably, patient goes into preterm labour and delivers.
- *Molar pregnancy.* Pain is due to sudden enlargement of the uterus filled with molar tissue. Occasionally excessive bleeding may occur. Evacuation of the mole is required.
- *Retention of urine.* Retention of urine may occur due to acute UTI, retroverted gravid uterus or pelvic haematocele of ectopic pregnancy. Fibroid or ovarian cyst impacted in the pouch of Douglas can also cause retention of urine. Catheterization of bladder and treatment of underlying course is warranted.

- *Abruptio placentae.* Bleeding in retroplacental space in a case of abruption placentae can cause acute abdomen. It is accompanied by features of shock and marked abdominal tenderness. Immediate treatment in the form of induction of labour/delivery is indicated to prevent severe complications such as Disseminated Intravascular Coagulation (DIC), renal failure and shock.

GYNAECOLOGICAL CAUSES (Figs 18.1 and 18.2)

- *Dysmenorrhoea* due to pelvic pathology such as endometriosis, fibroids or a primary dysmenorrhoea can cause acute abdominal pain. Although primary dysmenorrhoea is present since menarche, dysmenorrhoea due to conditions such as fibroids, endometriosis or adenomyosis begins later in reproductive life.
- *Mittelschmerz* is a mid-cycle pain, not lasting more than 12–24 hours, is noted around time of ovulation. Pain is located in one of the iliac fossa and may be accompanied with slight vaginal bleeding. Analgesics may be required for severe pain.
- *PID.* Acute pain felt in the lower abdomen accompanied by fever, urinary symptoms may be due to acute PID. Often patient correlates onset of pain to a recent sexual relation or some procedure on uterus. Pain is mostly bilateral in lower abdomen.

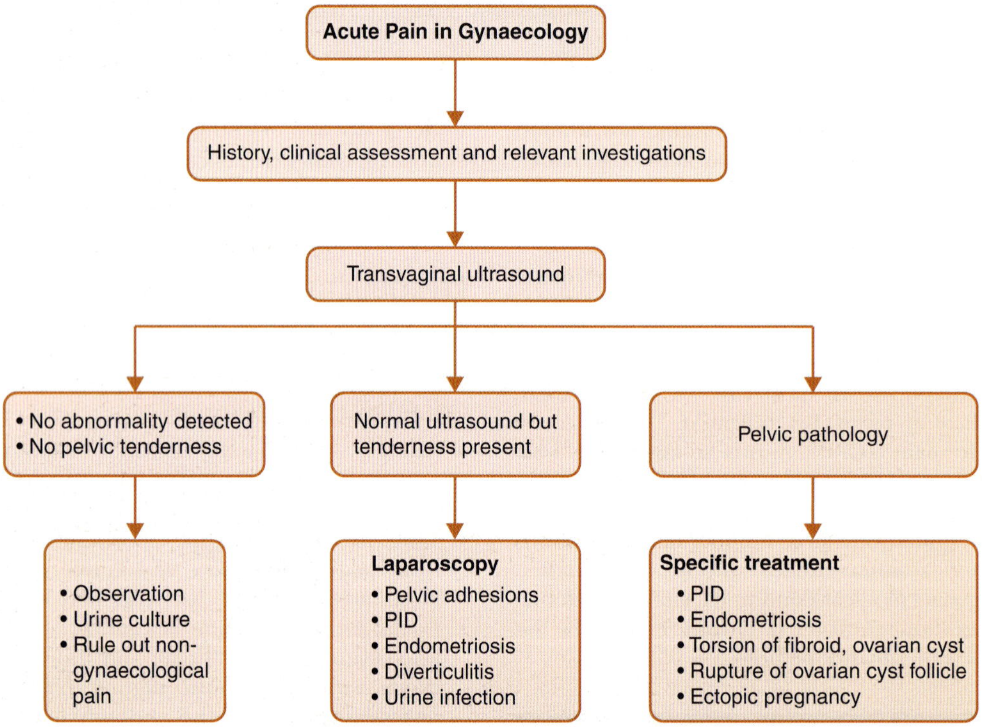

Figure 18.1 Acute pain in gynaecology.

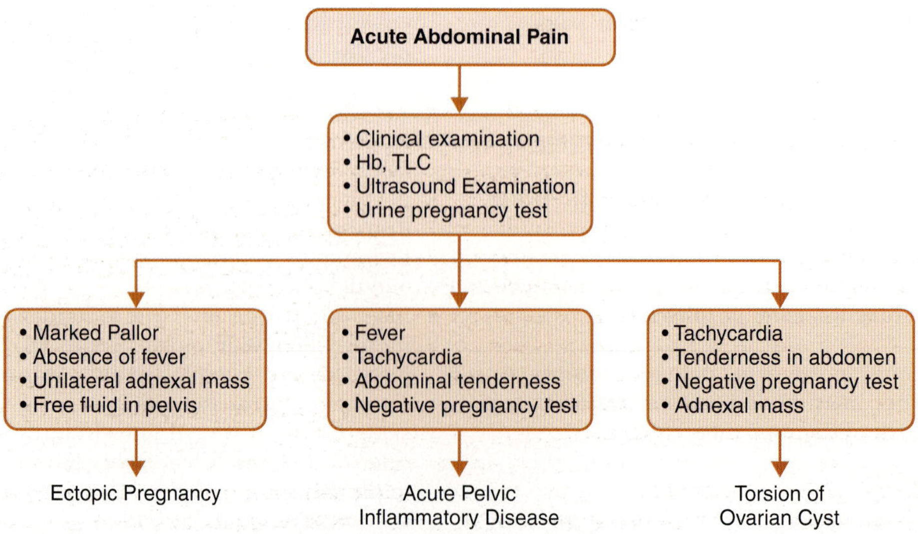

Figure 18.2 Acute abdominal pain.

- *Endometriosis.* Acute pain in endometriosis is either due to rupture of a chocolate cyst or due to leakage of blood into the peritoneal cavity. Ultrasound helps to detect the cause. Laparoscopy or laparotomy is required.
- *Ovarian hyperstimulation syndrome.* In a woman with infertility who is undergoing induction of ovulation, acute abdominal pain may be due to ovarian hyperstimulation. In most cases, hyperstimulation begins with the injection of Human Chorionic Gonadotropin (hCG) for release of mature ovum from the ovary. It may be noted that severe case requires hospitalization, intravenous fluid and close observation (see Chapter 15).
- *Uterine fibroids.* Normally, a fibroid does not cause acute pain unless a pedunculated fibroid undergoes torsion or the vessels on the capsule ruptures causing intraperitoneal haemorrhage. Treatment is *prompt diagnosis and surgical intervention.*
- *Ovarian tumours.* Torsion, infection of haemorrhage in a cyst and rupture cause acute pain in the abdomen. Malignant tumours mostly do not produce acute pain and remain 'silent' until in an advanced stage (Chapter 32).

NONGYNAECOLOGICAL CAUSES

- *Retention of urine* in women can occur due to an ovarian tumour or fibroid impacted in the pouch of Douglas. Acute cystitis and bladder stone cause severe pain in the suprapubic region. In a ureteric colic, pain is felt along the course of ureter.
- *Gastrointestinal pain* is often colicky and associated with gastrointestinal symptoms. Appendicitis can confuse the diagnosis, but the pain is localized in the right iliac fossa.
- Abdominal tuberculosis.

MENOPAUSAL AND POSTMENOPAUSAL WOMEN

- *Pyometra, collection of pus in the uterine cavity,* can occur in endometrial carcinoma or following radiotherapy or when the cervix gets stenosed due to tubercular and senile endometritis. The pain is localized in the central portion of the lower abdomen and may or may not be accompanied with fever. Ultrasound reveals an enlarged uterus with fluid in the cavity. Treatment comprises cervical dilation for drainage of pus and antibiotics. A subsequent endometrial curettage will help to rule out underlying malignancy or tuberculosis.
- *Ovarian tumours in elderly, postmenopausal woman are mostly malignant.* They can present with acute abdominal pain.
- *Sarcoma of uterus. Although rare, sarcoma can develop in a uterus with fibroids. A diagnosis is made when the fibroid starts growing rapidly causing pain,* postmenopausal bleeding or low grade fever (Chapter 13).
- *Retention of urine* can occur in a postmenopausal woman due *to bladder neck ob*struction, prolapse uterus or urinary infection and requires drainage and appropriate management.

CHRONIC PELVIC PAIN

Chronic pelvic pain (CPP) refers to acyclical pelvic pain of more than 6-month duration. This type of pain has been a recognized as a symptom of organic conditions such as endometriosis, adenomyosis, chronic PID, uterine fibroids and due to postoperative adhesion formations. It needs appropriate medical and surgical management.

However, a CPP in the absence of any palpable or demonstrable pelvic pathology is more difficult to manage. It is easy to attribute this to neurosis, as many of these women present with neurotic personality. However, it is now confirmed that neurosis is the result and not the cause of this CPP. Chronic pelvic pain syndrome (CPPS) does exist. It is important therefore to elucidate the cause of CPPS by detailed investigations such as transabdominal and transvaginal ultrasound and a diagnostic laparoscopy.

Laparoscopy may reveal small foci of endometriosis and pelvic adhesions which are invariably missed on pelvic examination. The absence of pelvic pathology and findings of normal pelvic organs is reassuring to the woman as well as the doctor that no serious disease such as cancer exists. At times, the congestion and dilatation of pelvic veins is the only abnormal finding noted.

INCIDENCE

About 15% of women complain CPP. About 10% women visit the gynaecologists. In some centres, as many as 30%–40% diagnostic laparoscopies are performed for CPP.

AETIOLOGY (Table 18.1)

The causes of CPP are diverse. They may be gynaecological and nongynaecological.

1. *Gynaecological causes* are mostly organic but can be functional at times.
   The well-recognized organic causes are as follows:
   - Pelvic endometriosis, chocolate cyst of the ovary (30%–35%)
   - Ovaries – ovarian adhesions, residual ovarian syndrome, ovarian tumours (benign and malignant)
   - Tubal – chronic PID, tubal adhesions, postoperative adhesions, parametritis due to infection or malignancy (24%)
   - Pelvic tuberculosis and adhesions
   - Uterine – uterine fibroids and adenomyosis, pyometra in menopausal women, fixed retroverted uterus
2. *Functional causes* include the following:
   - Congestive dysmenorrhoea, Mittelschmerz and postcoital pain
   - CPPS, pelvic varicose or dilated veins (30%)
3. *Nongynaecological causes are as follows:*
   - Intestinal tuberculosis, diverticulitis, colitis, appendicitis, irritable bowel syndrome which account for 20% cases
   - Carcinoma rectum
   - Chronic intestinal obstruction
   - Renal – ureteric colic, bladder stone, urinary tract infection, cystitis, chronic retention of urine.
   - Skeletomuscular – joint pains (referred pain).
   - Hernias
   - Sickle cell disease, porphyria
   - Neurological – herpes zoster, nerve entrapment, nerve compression, referred pain
   - Scar – scar site pain, scar endometriosis

Table 18.1 Correlation of History of Pelvic Findings and the Possible Diagnosis

History	Physical Finding	Diagnosis
Progressive worsening of dysmenorrhoea and dyspareunia	Tenderness and nodules in the posterior fornix and uterosacral ligaments	Pelvic endometriosis
Pelvic pain (postoperative)	Restricted mobility of pelvic viscera	Pelvic adhesions
Menorrhagia, dysmenorrhoea	Bulky uterus	Uterine fibroid or adenomyosis
Shifting pain on body movement	Normal pelvic findings	Pelvic venous congestion
Dyspareunia, postcoital pain following surgery	Tender ovaries at the vault	Residual ovarian syndrome
Pain and bulge over the abdomen or scar	Hernia	Hernia scar endometriosis
Urinary frequency, dysuria urgency, pain suprapubic	Bladder distension or empty bladder	Cystitis
Pain left iliac fossa	Tender colon	Colitis
Pain right iliac fossa	Tender McBurney point	Chronic appendicitis
Referred pain, localized pain on trigger points	Trigger points	Nerve and muscle pain

NO OBVIOUS CAUSE FOUND FOR CHRONIC PELVIC PAIN

In quite a few cases, no cause of CPP can be detected in spite of detailed work up (35%). Even laparoscopic findings appear normal, and investigations undertaken do not reveal a definite cause. It is also observed that even when a lesion is detected, it may not be the cause of the CPP, i.e. loose peritoneal adhesions, mainly postoperative adhesions do not cause chronic pain, and adhesiolysis does not cure the symptom.

ORGANIC CAUSES

ENDOMETRIOSIS, CHOCOLATE CYST OF OVARY

Endometriosis presents as dull lower abdominal pain associated with dysmenorrhoea, menorrhagia and dyspareunia. It is important to note that small lesions with fibrosis may cause only dull chronic pain. Tender nodules felt in the posterior fornix and tender pelvic masses with the above history may help to recognize the clinical condition of endometriosis. Ultrasound confirms the presence and extent of the pelvic mass. Laparoscopic examination is useful not only to confirm the unsuspected clinical diagnosis but also to surgically manage by coagulation on the lesion. If a chocolate cyst is noted in the ovary, it can be laparoscopically managed.

Surgical removal of chocolate cyst by laparotomy may be necessary if the cyst is huge.

A correlation of macroscopic findings with histological and clinical findings is rather poor. Severity of endometriosis does not always correlate with severity of pain. Small lesions near uterosacral ligaments may cause more severe pain than caused by large chocolate cyst.

OVARIAN ADHESIONS AND POLYCYSTIC OVARIAN DISEASE

Polycystic ovarian diseases usually do not cause any pelvic pain, however, following surgical management in the form of ovarian drilling and subsequent ovarian adhesions can cause chronic pelvic pain.

CHRONIC PELVIC INFLAMMATORY DISEASE

Chronic PID causes chronic persistent lower abdominal pain, dyspareunia, dysmenorrhoea, menorrhagia and infertility. The uterus is retroverted and fixed. Thickened and slightly tender fornices or a tubo-ovarian mass is noted. If medical treatment fails, the removal of adnexa or hysterectomy may be needed.

PERITONEAL AND POSTOPERATIVE PELVIC ADHESIONS

Not all adhesions cause pain. Loose adhesions which do not restrict mobility of abdominal viscera remain asymptomatic and do not require adhesiolysis. Rather, breaking these adhesions may result in reformation of denser adhesions which may cause persistent chronic pain later. Dense adhesions and adhesions which restrict visceral mobility will lead to CPP. If these adhesions entrap the ovaries, pelvic pain can result. It is observed that some adhesion tissue contains nerve fibres, and these adhesions when stretched during movement of viscera can cause pain.

PELVIC TUBERCULOSIS

Pelvic tuberculosis is a common condition in India affecting women of reproductive age. Apart from chronic pain, the woman often suffers from amenorrhoea, oligomenorrhoea and infertility. Endometrial curettings may in some cases reveal the tubercular nature of the infection. Laparoscopy may be necessary to confirm the diagnosis. Anti-TB treatment is needed. Polymerase Chain Reaction (PCR) on endometrial tissue and biopsies from pelvic structures helps to diagnose tuberculosis when histology fails to do so.

UTERINE FIBROIDS AND ADENOMYOSIS

Uterine fibroids and adenomyosis cause dysmenorrhoea and menorrhagia. Dull abdominal pain is due to heaviness and pelvic congestion, and at times due to associated PID. Submucous fibroid can cause colicky pain in the form of spasmodic dysmenorrhoea. Interstitial fibroids can cause dysmenorrhoea more often than subserous fibroids which cause more of heaviness and dull pain. Bimanual examination and ultrasound will help to establish the cause of the pelvic pain.

OVARIAN CYST OR TUMOUR

In most cases ovarian cyst or tumour causes dull aching pain or a sensation of heaviness in lower abdomen. However, rapid increase in size of the tumour or changes such as haemorrhage, infection or torsion can cause pain. A dermoid cyst may cause dull pain due to infection and gradual torsion of its pedicle. Malignant tumour is a silent tumour causing pain only in the advanced stage.

RESIDUAL OVARIAN SYNDROME

Residual ovarian syndrome is seen when one or both ovaries are saved at the time of hysterectomy. These ovaries develop adhesions with surrounding structures causing CPP and dyspareunia. Extensive and dense adhesion may require surgical removal of the ovaries. With the availability of hormone replacement therapy (HRT), some believe in removing both ovaries at the time of hysterectomy to avoid occurrence of residual ovarian syndrome and the remote possibility of ovarian cancer.

DYSMENORRHOEA

Congestive dysmenorrhoea is present in endometriosis, PID and uterine fibroids. It is felt as a dull ache in the lower abdomen starting a few days before menstruation and is relieved following the onset of menses. The woman may also complain of backache and heaviness, in the lower abdomen. Dysmenorrhoea is related to menstrual cycles.

OVULATION PAIN (MITTELSCHMERZ)

Ovulation pain occurs in mid-cycle, is often acute, but at times a sharp pain is followed by a dull pain lasting for several hours. It may be due to rupture of a Graafian follicle, timing corresponds to time of LH peak and generally noted 24 hours before ovulation. It is postulated to be due to contractility of ovarian perifollicular smooth muscle mediated through PGF2α. In such cases, anti-inflammatory drugs (nonsteroidal anti-inflammatory drugs, NSAIDs) are effective.

CHRONIC PELVIC PAIN SYNDROME

CPPS is a condition characterized by CPP not associated with any clinical evidence of pelvic pathology. At laparoscopy, pelvic veins are seen dilated and some are associated with venous stasis. The woman is generally in reproductive age and complains of dull aching pain in the lower abdomen; in rare cases, severe pain which responds to postural adjustment. Lying flat relieves or reduces pain, whereas standing, walking or bending worsens it. Other associated symptoms are congestive dysmenorrhoea (60%–70%), dyspareunia and postcoital ache. Polycystic ovary syndrome (PCOS) is seen in 50% of the cases and menorrhagia is present in same number of cases. Shifting location of pain with body movements is characteristic of this syndrome. Doppler ultrasound and venography help in the diagnosis.

INTESTINAL CAUSES

Chronic lower abdominal pain related to intestines and sigmoid colon is seen in irritable bowel syndrome and bowel symptoms such as constipation, chronic diarrhoea and colicky pain. Sigmoid colon pain is felt in the left iliac fossa, lasts for a few minutes to a few hours. Intestinal colic is often related to food and accompanied by flatulence. Appendicitis may present with chronic pain in the right iliac fossa. Irritable bowel syndrome and inflammatory bowel diseases are not uncommon in women in age group of 30–40 years, and may be associated with pelvic venous congestion (20%).

Stool examination for amoebiasis, sigmoidoscopy, colonoscopy and barium enema may reveal the cause of abdominal pain. Irritable bowel syndrome responds to drotaverine and mebeverine.

URINARY TRACT

Infection, cystitis and bladder stones cause CPP, but are associated with urinary symptoms. Chronic retention of urine caused by bladder neck obstruction or a pelvic tumour causes chronic pain in the suprapubic region and difficulty in passing urine. A full bladder is palpable in the suprapubic region. Catheterization will empty the bladder and relieve the discomfort. Chronic retention of urine with over flow is not uncommon in postmenopausal woman due to narrowing of urethra or senile urethritis. Urine culture, cystoscopy, radiography of pelvis for stone and ultrasound are useful diagnostic procedures.

PSYCHOLOGICAL FACTORS

Some women with CPP appear neurotic and this was considered to be the cause in women with CPP. As mentioned before, now it is proved, that in many cases neurosis is the result of CPP and not vice versa. Some elements of neurosis may eventually contribute to exaggeration of symptoms. Antidepressants do not relieve pain in majority of these women, though when given along with medications do alleviate neurosis. Psychotherapy may also help.

SKELETOMUSCULAR PAIN

Diseases of bone and joints can cause CPP. Ilioinguinal nerve may be trapped in a wide Pfannenstiel incision. Postoperative muscle pain is also possible. Trigger points can be located by pressing a finger where the woman complains of pain. Pain following surgery and accidents are the obvious causes of chronic pain. Referred pain from the spine is an identifiable cause of chronic pain (Table 18.1).

WORKUP OF A CASE OF CHRONIC PELVIC PAIN

HISTORY

CPP is common in reproductive years. The onset, type, duration and location of pain will provide guidance to the probable cause of the pain. Radiation of pain and its relation to menstruation is important. Obstetric and sexual history is important. History of use of intrauterine contraceptive device suggests possibility of pelvic infection. Associated urinary and bowel symptoms should be enquired into. Some women with CPP also complain of dysmenorrhoea and dyspareunia.

A history of tuberculosis and psychiatric problem will help. History of cancer in the family will suggest probable cancer phobia in the woman.

General examination may reveal lymphadenopathy (tuberculosis), anaemia and swelling of feet. Abdominal mass, ascites and tenderness suggest organic cause.

Vaginal discharge is seen in PID. Bimanual pelvic examination is necessary to rule out organic pelvic pathology. A full bladder is felt anterior to the uterus and is tender on palpation. Rectal examination may reveal a mass in the pouch of Douglas or a stricture in rectum. Pain and restriction of joint movements, especially hip joint or lumbosacral spine, suggest referred pain to the pelvis. Tenderness in the pelvis is caused by endometriosis, adenomyosis, pelvic adhesion, PID diverticulitis and urinary infection.

Ovarian pain is located at the junction of the middle and inner two-third of a line between the anterior superior iliac spine to the umbilicus, and tenderness can be elicited here.

INVESTIGATIONS

A firm diagnosis and cause of pain cannot always be elicited clinically. Ultrasound, diagnostic laparoscopy, Doppler ultrasound for pelvic congestion, urine tests, barium enema, colonoscopy, sigmoidoscopy, radiography of joints and intravenous pyelography (IVP) will be needed in accordance with the patient's history and examination. CT and MRI may be helpful in some cases. MRI can miss a small nodule, but it picks up rectovaginal endometriosis.

Laparoscopy detects small foci in the pelvis suggestive of endometriosis which are undetected clinically. It can detect pelvic adhesions and small inflammatory masses apart from obvious pelvic pathology. Therapeutic treatment can be applied in the same sitting such as adhesiolysis and cauterization of endometriosis. Pelvic venous congestion and dilated vessels are not always revealed because of a head low position and pressure of pneumoperitoneum.

A poor correlation between macroscopic view and histological evidence exists at laparoscopy and the diagnosis can be missed if peritoneal biopsies are not taken. The burnt-out healed areas of endometriosis can also cause CPP due to fibrosis and entrapment of nerve fibres.

Even if a pelvic pathology is detected at laparoscopy, i.e. fibroid or a small ovarian cyst, adhesions, it may not be the real cause of CPP; it could be just a coincidental finding. '*Conscious pain mapping' at diagnostic laparoscopy under local anaesthesia is useful in deciding the cause and location of chronic pain.*

When laparoscopy fails to reveal any pathology and pelvic venous congestion is suspected to be the cause of pelvic pain, transuterine pelvic venography is performed by injecting the dye myometrially or pelvic venography using contrast medium. In pelvic congestion syndrome, dilated ovarian and uterine vessels more than 10 mm with delayed clearance of dye are observed. Hysteroscopy picks up intrauterine lesions.

MANAGEMENT

The detection of pelvic pathology or cause for pain determines the therapy appropriate for the case. Negative investigations at least assure the woman that no serious pathology exists; this way, cancer phobia can be eliminated. *Diagnostic laparoscopy remains the gold standard when a woman fails to respond to hormones.*

The problem however remains when no cause is found. Doppler ultrasound or pelvic venography will demonstrate the dilated veins. Treatment comprises progestogen therapy or hysterectomy. NSAIDs are effective in mild cases. Gonadotropin-releasing hormone (GnRH) can shrink the endometriosis and the pelvic veins.

The rationale behind progestogen treatment is that oestrogen causes dilatation of pelvic vessels and progestogens, by their antioestrogenic effect, constrict the veins, reduce the blood flow and suppress ovulation. Medroxyprogesterone acetate (MDPA) up to 30 mg daily (Provera) given for 9–12 months relieves pelvic pain. Unfortunately, pain may recur after stoppage of the drug and a prolonged therapy can produce side effects such as increase in body weight, pain, bloating and menstrual irregularity; thus, it is not desirable. Micronized progesterone is a natural progesterone available in India as utrogestan 100 mg oral and vaginal tablet. In a patient with liver disease, a vaginal route may be preferred. It causes dizziness in a few cases, so one tablet daily is advocated at bedtime for 10 days in the premenstrual phase. For premenstrual tension, one tablet twice daily is recommended for 10 days premenstrually.

Mirena IUCD which releases MDPA at a rate of 20 mcg has emerged as an alternative to prolonged oral progestogen therapy. Mirena is very effective in relieving pain and effective for 5 years. Besides, it acts as a contraceptive when the woman is not desirous of pregnancy.

Selective serotonin reuptake inhibitor (SSI) fluoxetine 10–60 mg daily, or sertraline 50–200 mg daily are drugs useful in some cases.

In the past, people have tried diethyl ergotamine in tablet and injection forms to reduce pelvic pain caused by dilatation of vessels. Diethyl ergotamine causes vasoconstriction of veins and reduces pelvic congestion. Long-term use of this drug is not recommended because of serious side effects. Ligation of ovarian veins has been attempted with variable results.

Surgery in the form of hysterectomy and bilateral salpingo-oophorectomy may be resorted to if drug therapy fails in elderly women. Psychotherapy alone or combined with drugs will be useful in pelvic pain syndrome and irritable bowel syndrome.

Acupuncture and short-wave diathermy are adjuvants, and are effective in some women. Presacral neurectomy and laparoscopic uterosacral nerve ablation (LUNA) are recommended in intractable pain in young women.

LUNA may lead to prolapse and bladder dysfunction. Ureteric damage can also occur. Presacral neurectomy causes bleeding and haematoma in presacral space.

Static magnetic therapy for 4 weeks or transcutaneous nerve stimulation helps in some cases.

Varicosity of pelvic veins have been treated with embolization of ovarian vessels or laparoscopic injection of sclerosing agents (sclerotherapy) using 5% ethanolamine maleate. Gel foams and coils are also used.

Conscious pain mapping. Conscious pain mapping involves laparoscopy under local anaesthesia and interaction with the woman on touching individual organs to localize the organ of pain. This method helps in improving diagnostic accuracy.

Backache is one of the symptoms often accompanying CPP and is due to following gynaecological diseases:

- Pelvic endometriosis
- Pelvic adhesions
- PID and fixed retroverted uterus
- Prolapse of uterus
- Uterine fibroids

- In orthopaedic conditions, pain is limited to below the fourth lumbar spine; it is diffuse and cannot be pinpointed to a spot

KEY POINTS

- Acute pelvic pain is an emergency, and requires immediate attention and treatment.
- CPP is a well-recognized entity in clinical practice often due to obscure causes.
- The pain may be of functional origin without any recognizable evident pathology.
- Common underlying causes of CPP are PID, pelvic adhesions, endometriosis and adenomyosis, uterine fibroids, fixed retroverted uterus, ovarian enlargements due to benign causes and neoplasia, genital tuberculosis and residual ovarian syndrome following hysterectomy.
- Blood investigations, ESR, pelvic ultrasonography with colour Doppler, CT/MRI scan, laparoscopy, hysteroscopy may be necessary to establish a diagnosis.
- Conscious pain mapping at laparoscopy is emerging as most important diagnostic tool.
- Treatment consists of proper counselling, antibiotics, and anti-inflammatory drugs such as NSAIDs, analgesics, hormones, short-wave diathermy and surgery in selected cases.
- Presacral neurectomy and LUNA are reserved for intractable pain in young women.

SELF-ASSESSMENT

1. Discuss the causes of chronic pelvic pain in a young nulliparous woman.
2. A 30-year-old woman, para 1+0, presents with chronic pelvic pain for 6 months. How will you manage?
3. A 28-year-old woman, nulliparous, complains of dysmenorrhoea, menorrhagia and chronic pelvic pain. Discuss the differential diagnosis.
4. A 32-year-old woman presents with acute abdominal pain and vomiting. A lump is felt per abdomen. Discuss the differential diagnosis and management.

SUGGESTED READING

Arulkumaran S. Clinics in Obstetrics and Gynaecology 2006;20:5.

Studd J. Acute abdominal pain. Progress in Obstetrics and Gynaecology 1998;13:311.

Studd J. Chronic pelvic pain. Progress in Obstetrics and Gynaecology 1991;9:245.

19 Temporary and Permanent Methods of Contraception

CHAPTER OUTLINE

BIRTH CONTROL

There has always been a need felt for avoiding unwanted pregnancies and restricting family size among the married couples. Such a desire and need has always been higher among women than men. The risks associated with repeated and unwanted pregnancies have serious long-term effects on the health of women and at times the entire family. Nowadays, there is a pressing need for limiting the family size at a personal level and for the control of population at the national level. The need of birth control at a personal level has arisen through an increased cost of living, scarcity of accommodation, a desire for better education of children in the present competitive world and an overall desire for an improved standard of living.

The population in India has been growing rapidly. The socioeconomic problems of overpopulation are felt all around. The world population is also a major problem with more than 6.3 billion living on this earth and 26 children born every second.

Reproductive health and medical grounds are other considerations for choosing a birth control. A woman younger than 18–20 years is not physically grown up to have a child. If she does reproduce, she becomes a high-risk case during pregnancy and labour, and is likely to deliver a low birthweight (LBW) baby. Spacing births, 3 years apart, is considered beneficial for both the mother and the child. *Birth control is thus seen as a health measure for these young women.* Multiparous women from low-income group are generally anaemic and malnourished and are predisposed to prolapse, stress incontinence, chronic cervicitis and cancer of the cervix. The spacing of childbirth and limiting the number of pregnancies are strongly desirable for this reason.

There are following three approaches to limiting family size:

- Contraceptives – prevent fertilization
- Emergency contraception – prevents implantation
- Medical termination of pregnancy (MTP) – abortion

However, use of effective contraception remains the best choice.

DEFINITION OF CONTRACEPTION

A method or a system which allows intercourse and yet prevents conception is called a contraceptive method. This contraception may be temporary when the effect of preventing pregnancy lasts, while the couple uses the method but the fertility returns immediately or within a few months of discontinuation of its use. The permanent contraceptive methods are surgical approaches such as tubectomy in a woman and vasectomy in a man with permanent contraception.

In spite of great advances in technology, all methods of contraceptions have a small undesirable risk of failure. Unfortunately, no contraception has proved perfect and its effectiveness, safety and techniques vary. This therefore requires counselling, screening of the couple and offering the best method suited to the couple. It also requires monitoring while the woman uses any contraception.

Choice of contraception depends upon the following:

- Age and parity of the couple.
- Availability, cost.
- Reliability (failure rate).
- Side effects, contraindications to a particular method.
- Advantages and disadvantages.
- Need for follow-up.
- Counselling and allowing the couple to make a suitable choice. The couple may need to change from one contraception to another from time to time during the reproductive period. Personal, medical and social factors should also be taken into consideration during counselling.

METHODS OF CONTRACEPTION

1. **Natural methods:**
   - Abstinence during the fertile phase.
   - Withdrawal method (coitus interruptus).
   - Breastfeeding (lactational amenorrhoea method [LAM]).
2. **Barrier contraceptives:**
   - Condoms by male and females.
   - Spermicidal agents

- Diaphragm, or the cervical cap in the vagina, use of a female condom.
- Hormones which alter the cervical mucous and prevent entry of sperms into the cervical canal.

3. **Intrauterine contraceptive devices (IUCDs).**
4. **Suppression of ovulation with hormones – hormonal contraceptives.**
5. **Interceptive agents (postcoital contraception).**
6. **Immunological methods.**
7. **Suppression of spermatogenesis in males.**
8. **Surgical sterilization.**

Failure rate of any contraceptive method is described in terms of pregnancy rate per 100 woman-years (Pearl index).

Ideal contraceptive methods should be effective, long acting, safe, coital-independent and reversible. Besides, they should be easily available and affordable with minimal side effects.

Refer to Fig. 19.1 for various sites of action of contraceptive techniques.

1. NATURAL METHODS OF CONTRACEPTION

Abstinence during the Fertile Phase

'Fertility awareness' means the woman learns to know when the fertile time starts and when it ends. The fertile phase of the menstrual cycle can be predicted in various ways.

The Calendar Method or the Rhythm Method. This depends upon the avoidance of sexual intercourse around ovulation. In a 28-day cycle, ovulation generally occurs on the 14th day of the cycle, but may occur anytime between the 12th and 16th day. Spermatozoa deposited in the female genital tract may survive for 24 hours. The ovum itself may live for 12–24 hours so that intercourse between the 11th and 17th day may result in a pregnancy. The safe period is, therefore, calculated from the first day of the menstrual period until the 10th day of the cycle and from the 18th to the 28th day. An alternative method is to calculate the risk period, which is from 3 days before ovulation to 3 days after ovulation. In a 35-day menstrual cycle, therefore, ovulation will occur on the 21st day (i.e. 14 days before the next period) so that the risk period is from day 18 to day 24. Various methods are available to help a woman know about the approaching unsafe period. However, cost, privacy and low sensitivity limit use of these methods.

Persona. This is a microcomputer attached to a microlaboratory. It measures the levels of oestrone-3 glucuronide and luteinizing hormone (LH) in the morning urine by dipping a test stick in the urine 'green light' shows conception unlikely and 'red light' shows fertile period and warns the probable ovulation and conception. The failure rate with this technique is approximately 6 per 100 woman-year.

Calendar Method. In Knaus–Ogino method, the fertile period is determined by subtracting 18 days from the shortest cycle and 10 days from the longest cycle which gives the first and the last day of fertile period, respectively.

This method will result in approximately 25 pregnancies per 100 woman-years. The failure results from irregular ovulation or from irregular menstrual cycles. Some couples prefer this method on religious grounds or because they find other methods unacceptable. The methods of predicting ovulation have been described in chapter 16.

Mucus Method (Billings or Ovulation Method). The properties of the cervical mucus change under the influence of the ovarian hormones on different days of the menstrual cycle. The woman attempts to predict the fertile period by feeling the cervical mucus. Under oestrogen influence, the

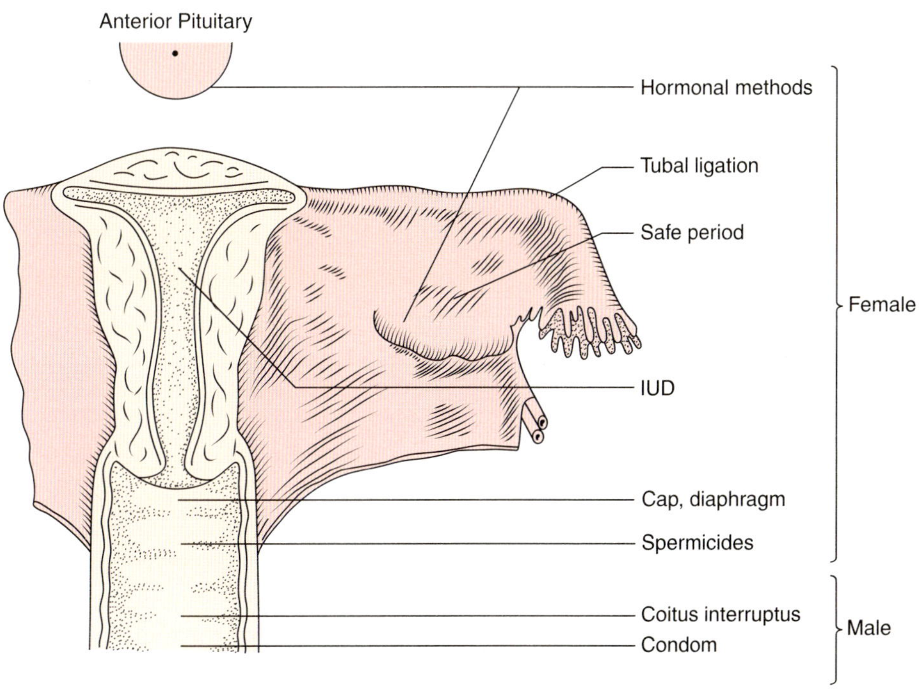

Figure 19.1 Sites of action of modern contraceptive techniques.

mucus increases in quantity and becomes progressively more slippery and elastic until a peak is reached. Thereafter, the mucus becomes thicker, scanty and dry under the influence of progesterone until the onset of menses. Intercourse is considered safe during the 'dry days' immediately after the menses until mucus is detected. Thereafter, the couple must abstain until the 4th day after the 'peak day' (Fig. 19.2).

Temperature Method. Progesterone is known to exert a thermogenic effect on the body. Therefore, if the woman records her basal body temperature (BBT) daily after waking up in the morning and plots the readings graphically, the BBT chart will be biphasic in an ovulatory cycle (Fig. 19.2). The day of temperature shift indicates the time of ovulation. Avoidance of intercourse during the fertile days can prevent an unwanted pregnancy. This method is cumbersome method, hardly practised.

Symptothermal Method. This combination method is more effective. The first day of abstinence is predicted either from the calendar, by subtracting 21 from the length of the shortest menstrual cycle in the preceding 6 months, or the first day mucus is detected, whichever comes first. The end of the fertile period is predicted by use of the 'BBT' chart. The woman resumes intercourse 3 days after the thermal shift. Apart from the long periods of abstinence required, this method is not reliable if the woman is lactating or has irregular cycles or develops fever.

Withdrawal Method (Coitus Interruptus)

Coitus interruptus is a common practice among married couples. Coitus takes place in a normal manner but the penis is withdrawn immediately before ejaculation. The unreliability of this method is obvious, but it has the advantage that it costs nothing and it requires no device. Nevertheless, it has a failure rate of approximately 25 pregnancies per 100 woman-years. The main cause of the failure is not that ejaculation occurs inside the vagina but that prostatic fluid secreted prior to ejaculation, frequently contains active spermatozoa. This practice at times imposes a great mental strain upon the husband and can cause considerable anxiety. It is also a cause of failure in the wife to enjoy intercourse fully. Some couples seem to prefer this method and make no complaints of suffering from strain or anxiety.

Advantages. *Advantages* of fertility awareness methods are (i) no cost, (ii) no contraindications, (iii) no systemic side effects, (iv) no effect on lactation and (v) no need to visit a health personnel.

Disadvantages. *Disadvantages* are (i) failure rate is high, (ii) requires motivation and (iii) no protection against human immunodeficiency virus (HIV) and sexually transmitted disease (STD).

Breastfeeding (Lactational Amenorrhoea Method)

Regular breastfeeding with at least one feed at night is shown to prevent pregnancy for initial 6 months after delivery, with a failure rate of only 0.5%–1.5%. This occurs due to prolactin preventing LH surge and ovulation. Thereafter, the protective effect wears off. Apart from the beneficial effects of lactation on the newborn, it is advocated as the natural method of family planning in the first 6 months after childbirth. Beyond 6 months of breastfeeding, prolactin level falls and ovulation can occur. It is the frequency rather than the duration of feed that decides an ovulation in a nursing mother.

2. BARRIER METHODS

Condoms

In this method, the erectile penis is completely covered by a very thin rubber (condom) which is used only once. It is desirable to use a condom with a water-based spermicidal agent to improve the efficacy of the method (Fig. 19.3).

Condoms are made of latex which can be damaged by oil-based spermicidal agents; therefore, water-based spermicides

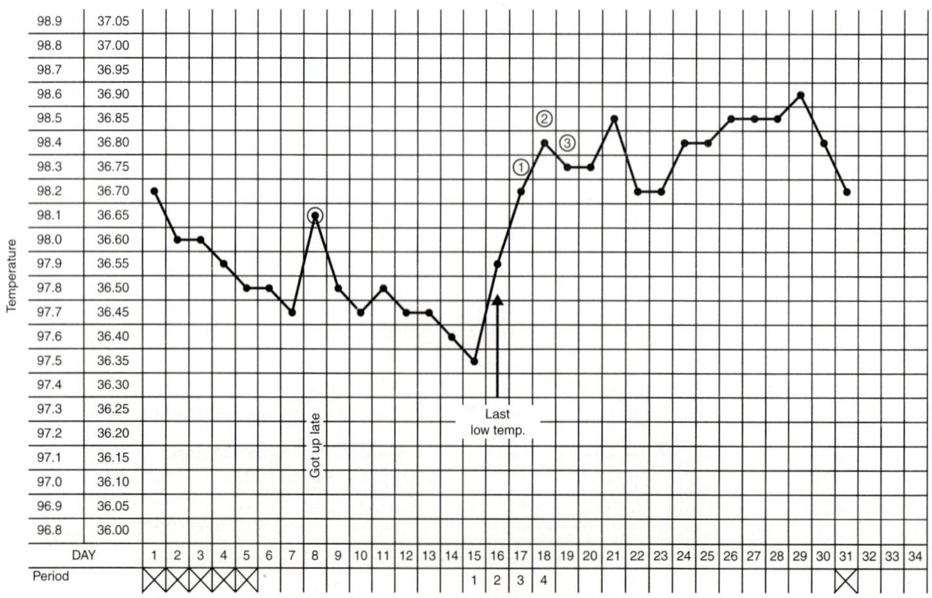

Figure 19.2 Basal body temperature chart.

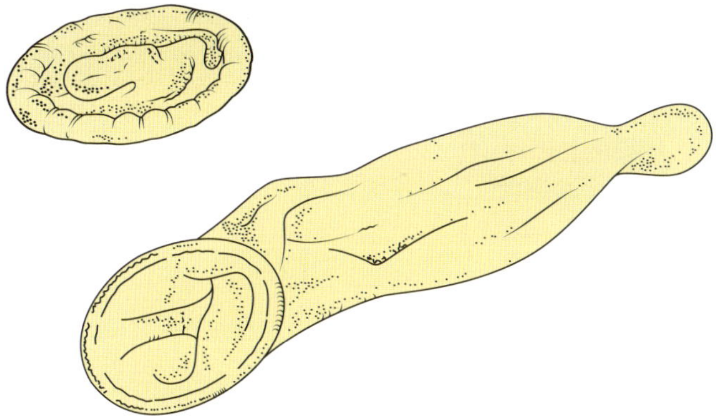

Figure 19.3 Condoms rolled and unrolled.

should be used. Because of irritation by latex in some women, nonlatex polyurethane condoms are available. They, however, slip and break easily and are more costly than the latex condoms.

Advantages

- It is easily available, cheap, easy to carry, free from side effects and requires no instruction.
- Male involvement in contraceptive effort and is immediately effective.
- It has no adverse effect on pregnancy, should the method fail. *Nirodh* brand is distributed free of cost in the government hospitals in India.
- Prevent transmission of STDs from one partner to the other.
- Decreased incidence of cervical cancer: In women whose partners use condom, sexual transmission of the viral infection causing this disease is prevented. Condom has also a place in checking the spread of the dreaded AIDS infection.

Disadvantages

- High failure rate, pregnancy rate of 10–14 per 100 woman-years. This is partly due to bursting of the condom or slipping and partly due to noncompliance.
- Vaginal irritation or allergy to the latex. To avoid allergy to latex rubber, polyurethane condoms and Tactylon material are used; however, these are slightly more expensive.
- Inability to obtain full sexual satisfaction.
- Method is coitus-dependent.

Other indications for use of condoms:

- Following vasectomy: For 12 ejaculation following vasectomy, as these ejaculations may contain sperms from the ejaculatory duct.
- In the past use of condoms for 3 months was advocated, if sperm antibodies are the cause of infertility. The antibodies clear by end of this period. However, with intrauterine insemination need for such a therapy is reduced.
- To prevent transmission of gonococcal, *chlamydia*, syphilis, trichomonas and fungal infection. Use of condoms has an important role in preventing transmission of HIV from one partner to the other.

Spermicidal Agents

The spermicidal agents kill the sperms before the latter gain access to the cervical canal. These chemical contraceptive agents contain surfactants, such as nonoxynol-9, octoxynol and menfegol and enzyme-inhibiting agents, and are available as foam tablets, soluble pessaries, creams, jellies or as films along with other contraceptives such as the diaphragm, occlusive cervical cap and condom. Used alone, failure rate is high, approximately 30 per 100 woman-years. When used in conjunction with a mechanical barrier, they give a reliable contraceptive effect. The spermicidal agent remains effective for 1–2 hours after the application.

By causing irritation and abrasions with chronic use, they can cause vaginal ulceration and perhaps increase the risk of HIV spread rather than preventing it. Therefore, the spermicidal agents should not be recommended to HIV couples. A new spermicidal cream, Tenofovir, prevents viral attachment to the vaginal mucosa and is nonirritant and is under development.

The use of condoms with spermicidal agents and postcoital agents as back-up technique is effective in avoiding pregnancy.

Praneem from neem is spermicidal and prevents transmission of sexually transmitted infections. This is under trial in India.

Occlusive Diaphragms

These provide a barrier in the vagina against direct insemination. The diaphragm is effective when used in conjunction with a chemical spermicide in the form of a jelly or cream, and when sufficient time is allowed for complete destruction of the sperms before the diaphragm is removed. In practice, the diaphragm liberally smeared with spermicide can be inserted at any convenient time and is left in place for a minimum of 8 hours after coitus. It causes no discomfort and no douching is required when these precautions are observed.

Alterations in the size and type of diaphragm may be required as a result of changes in weight, illness, delivery. Initially a visit to a doctor or trained nurse is required to choose a suitable size of diaphragm and to learn how to insert it. Subsequently, repeat visit at 6 months and 1 year is desirable. A refitting of the diaphragm is always required after childbirth, and this can be done about 6–8 weeks after childbirth.

The woman needs initial training in insertion and removal of diaphragm.

Types

1. *The Dutch cap or diaphragm.* This consists of a dome-shaped diaphragm of thin rubber, with a rubber-covered metal rim which may be either a watch spring or spiral spring. The diaphragm is made in a wide range of sizes varying from 50 to 95 mm diameter (the ones in common use range between 65 and 80 mm) and fit obliquely in the vagina, stretching from just behind the pubic ramus into the posterior fornix, thus covering the cervix. It is held in position by the tension of the spring rim. It is the easiest type of cap for the patient to use, fits in the majority of cases, causes no discomfort to either partner when correctly fitted (Fig. 19.4). Contraindications to use of diaphragm are (i) prolapse, cystocele, rectocele because accurate fitting is not possible; (ii) recurrent urinary tract infection; and (iii) allergy to rubber or spermicidal agent. Toxic shock syndrome (TSS) may occur if the diaphragm is left in the vagina for a long period. TSS is caused by staphylococcal pyogenic infection.

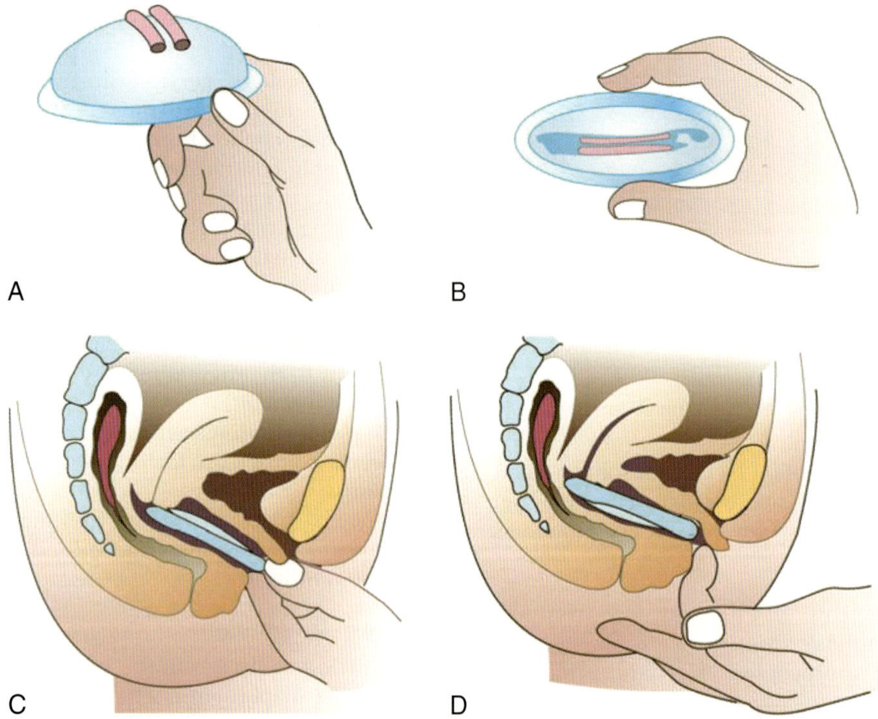

Figure 19.4 **(A)** Two strips of contraceptive paste are placed over the dome of the cap. **(B)** The rim is squeezed together so as to enclose the paste. **(C)** Insertion of Dutch cap – first stage. **(D)** Insertion of Dutch cap – second stage. The anterior rim is pushed up well behind the symphysis pubis.

The failure rate with the use of the Dutch cap is about 4–6 per 100 woman-years and is nearly always associated with poor fitting and noncompliance.

2. *The cervical cap.* This is a cup-shaped rubber somewhat like a thimble, with a solid rolled rubber rim. It fits closely to the cervix and is suitable where the cervix is long and firm. When a woman has a prolapse of uterus and vagina, a cervical cap is preferred to the vaginal diaphragm. Chronic cervicitis, erosion and cervical laceration contraindicate its use. The cervical caps are available in four sizes, varying from 22 to 31 mm (Fig. 19.5).
3. *Dumas cap.* It is a cup-shaped rubber with a thickened rim which fits well into the vault of the vagina so that it encloses the cervix. The size varies from 55 to 75 mm diameter.
4. *Femshield (female condom).* It is known as 'FEM' or Femidom. It is a newly developed female barrier contraceptive and is woman oriented. It is a loose-fitting 15–17 cm long sheath made of polyurethane prelubricated. It has a polyurethane ring at the closed end of the sheath, serving as an insertion and anchoring device, and the second end is open and lies outside the vagina after insertion. It has the combined features of a diaphragm and a condom (Fig. 19.6). It covers the entire vagina, cervix as well as the external genitalia. It is highly protective against spread of STDs, and AIDS in particular. It can be removed immediately after intercourse. The advantages of the Femshield are (i) it is coital-independent and can be worn well in advance of the sexual act; (ii) it does not slip off easily, and the failure rate is expected to be low; (iii) it is stronger than the condom and does not burst easily; and (iv) it can be worn during the puerperal period unlike the diaphragm. Failure rate is 5–15 per 100 woman-years. The Femshield is expensive, costing $2–3 per piece. Besides, its reuse more than once has not yet been recommended. It was initially developed as a safety method for women from contracting HIV infection. Only those female condoms which cover not only vagina but also skin vulva and perineum can prevent HIV infection.

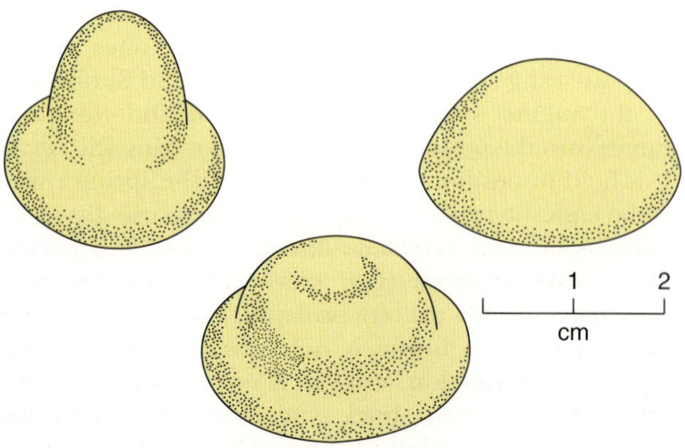

Figure 19.5 Types of cervical caps.

5. *Today.* It is a mushroom-shaped polyurethane disposal sponge, 2 inches in diameter, 1.25 inches thick and contains 1 g of nonoxynol-9 (Fig. 19.7). It is provided with a loop for its easy removal. It should be placed high up in the vagina with the concave side covering the cervix. It can remain effective for 24 hours. It is used only once. It acts as a mechanical barrier and prevents entry of sperms into the cervical canal, absorbs semen and contains a spermicidal agent.

Failure rate is similar to those of other barrier methods and spermicidal agents (9–30 per 100 woman-years). It is

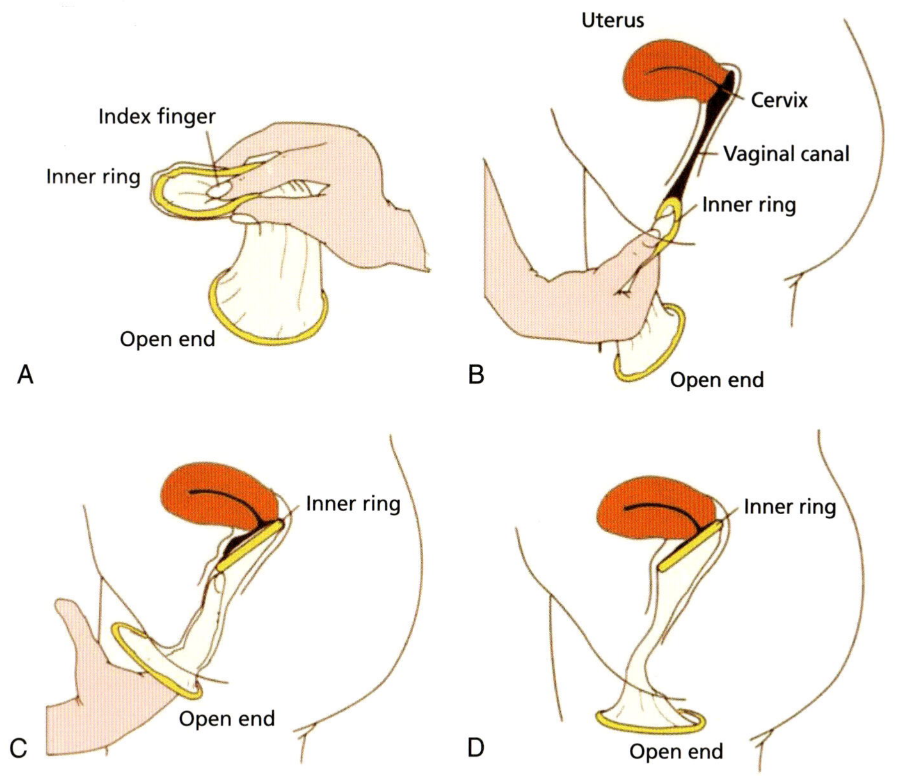

Figure 19.6 Femshield or female condom.

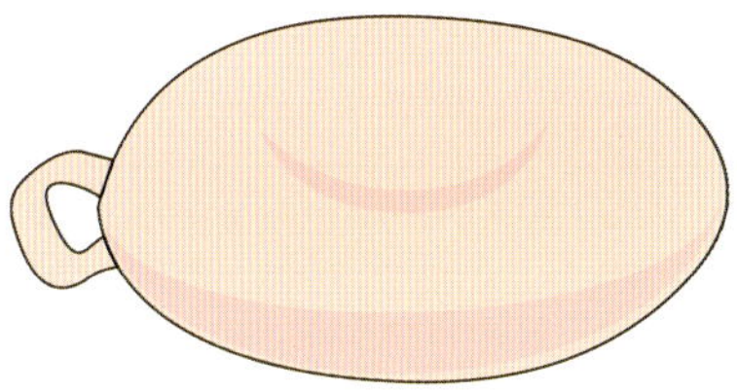

Figure 19.7 'Today' vaginal sponge.

however expensive, coital-dependent, and may cause Toxic Shock Syndrome if left over a long period.

Occlusive diaphragms are cheap and easy to use. One diaphragm can be used for over a year if it is washed, dried and kept properly after each use. Like the condom, the diaphragm prevents transmission of STDs from one partner to another and the incidence of cancer of the cervix is low in women using this contraceptive. It does not, however, prevent transmission of HIV, because it allows vaginal secretion to mix with semen. The lack of bathroom facilities and of privacy in low socioeconomic groups prevents its wider use in India. An occasional woman develops vaginal irritation to latex.

Advantages

- Instant contraception. Reversible in 2–4 months
- No toxicity
- No decreased libido

Disadvantage. Scrotal swelling is sometimes reported.

INTRAUTERINE CONTRACEPTIVE DEVICES

IUCD is an effective, reversible and long-term method of contraception, which does not require replacement for a long period and does not interfere with sexual activity. The device is commonly made of polyethylene which is impregnated with barium sulphate to render it radiopaque so that the presence or absence of the device in the pelvis can be easily detected by radiograph or ultrasound. Initial intrauterine devices contained only polyethylene (Lippe's Loop). Subsequently, medicated devices which contain copper, progesterone hormone and other pharmacologic agents have been introduced. The plastic devices are flexible so that they can be straightened and loaded into an introducer by which they are passed through the cervical canal and gently released within the uterine cavity to take up their original shape. Each device has a nylon thread attached to its lower end and this thread protrudes through the cervical canal into the vagina, where it can be felt by the patient and doctor, and can be removed by pulling it with the forceps.

Types of Commonly Used IUCDs (Fig. 19.8)

Inert IUCDs (first-generation IUCD): Lippe's loop is still commonly used in China. In India, this was the first IUCD introduced in National Family Planning Programme. Other inert devices such as Saf-T-coil, Mahua ring (Chinese double-coiled ring) and Ota ring are no longer in use.

1. **Copper-carrying devices**. In these, copper wire with a surface area of 200/220/250/375/380 mm is wrapped round the vertical stem of a polypropylene frame. Among these devices are Copper-T 200, Copper 7, Multiload Copper 250, Copper-T 380, Copper-T 220 and Nova T. The copper devices are more expensive than inert devices but are reported to have a better contraceptive efficacy, with fewer side

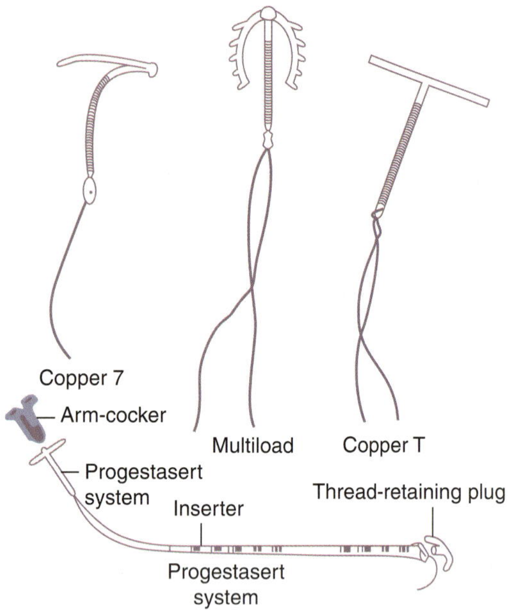

Figure 19.8 IUCDs in common use.

effects. They have an effective life of about 3–5 years. It is estimated that about 50 mcg of copper is released daily in the uterus. Copper-T 380A, known as ParaGard, has a lifespan of 10 years. Nova T has silver added to the copper wire, thereby increasing its lifespan to 5 years.

2. **Hormone-releasing IUCDs: Progestasert and Mirena.** Progestasert is a T-shaped device carrying 38 mg of progesterone in oil reservoir in the vertical stem. It releases 65 mcg of the hormone per day. The hormone released in the uterus forms a thick plug of mucus at the cervical os which prevents penetration by the sperms and thus exerts an added contraceptive effect. Menstrual problems such as menorrhagia and dysmenorrhoea noticed with Copper-T are less with this device (40% reduction). It is expensive and requires yearly replacement. A new device, Mirena, containing 52 mg of levonorgestrel (LNG) and releases the hormone in very low doses (20 mcg/day). It acts for a period of 5 years and has a low pregnancy rate of 0–3 per 100 woman-years. However, the incidence of ectopic pregnancy is higher with the use of progesterone-containing devices in comparison to copper devices. It can be safely recommended for nursing mothers.

Frameless IUCD and **fibroplant** releasing 14 mcg progestogen daily for 3 years is under trial. GyneFlex is 3–4 cm long, 1.2 mm in width and adapts to the shape of the uterine cavity. Because it is small in size, complications such as pain, bleeding, ectopic pregnancy and expulsion are less reported. It contains six copper beads on a monofilament polypropylene thread. The thread is knotted at one end which is fixed to the fundus. Frameless IUCD contains several copper cylinders tied together on a string, and it is anchored 1 cm deep into fundus (Fig. 19.9). Essure device placed within the intramural portion of the fallopian tube is being tried (Fig. 19.10).

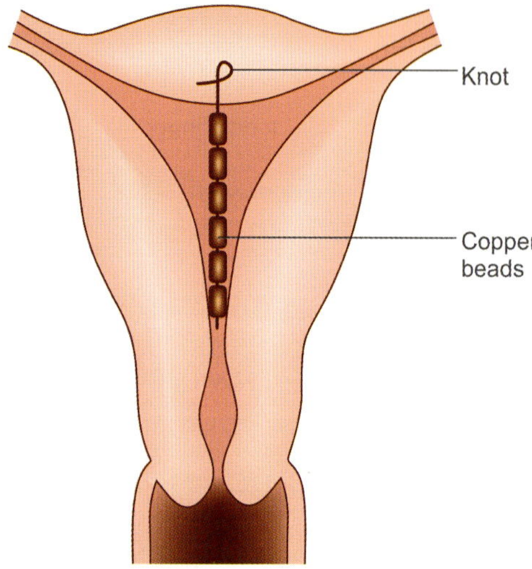

Figure 19.9 Frameless IUCD.

All IUCDs fall in category 1 or 2 when choosing their use in any associated medical or surgical conditions. For a full detail, please see WHO contraceptive wheel (Fig. 19.10).

SELECTION OF A CONTRACEPTIVE METHOD

WHO has given a MEC for contraceptive use revised in 2015, in which the safety of each contraceptive method is determined by several considerations in the context of the medical condition or medically relevant characteristics; primarily, whether the contraceptive method worsens the medical condition or creates additional health risks, and secondarily, whether the medical circumstance makes the contraceptive method less effective. The safety of the method should be weighed along with the benefits of preventing unintended pregnancy.

WHO Medical Eligibility Criteria for a Contraceptive Use

1. A condition for which there is no restriction for the use of the contraceptive method
2. A condition where the advantages of using the method generally outweigh the theoretical or proven risks
3. A condition where the theoretical or proven risks usually outweigh the advantages of using the method
4. A condition which represents an unacceptable health risk if the contraceptive method is used.

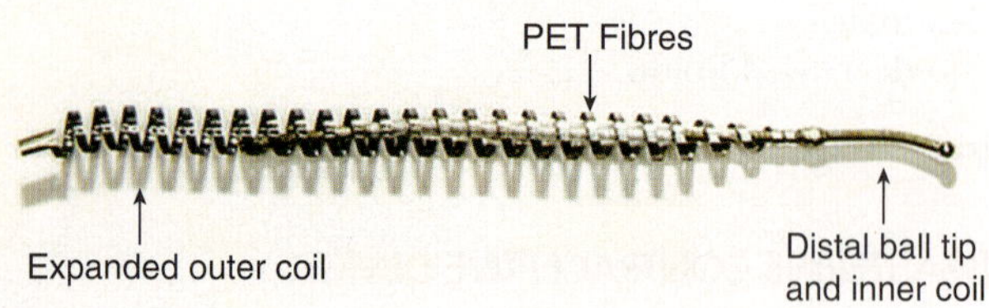

Figure 19.10 Essure Device

A new MEC contraceptive wheel was launched in 2015, making the method of choosing contraceptive method easier (Fig. 19.11).

Patient Selection. IUCDs are a good contraceptive choice for the following groups of women:

- Low risk of STD
- Multiparous woman
- Monogamous relationship
- Desirous of long-term reversible method of contraception, but not yet desirous of permanent sterilization
- Unhappy or unreliable users of oral contraception or barrier contraception

Uses of IUCD

- As a contraceptive
- Postcoital contraception (emergency contraception)
- Following intrauterine procedure such as adhesiolysis and septal resection prevents development of Asherman syndrome (to be used after removing the copper)
- Hormonal IUCD (Mirena) in menorrhagia and dysmenorrhoea, and hormonal replacement therapy in menopausal women

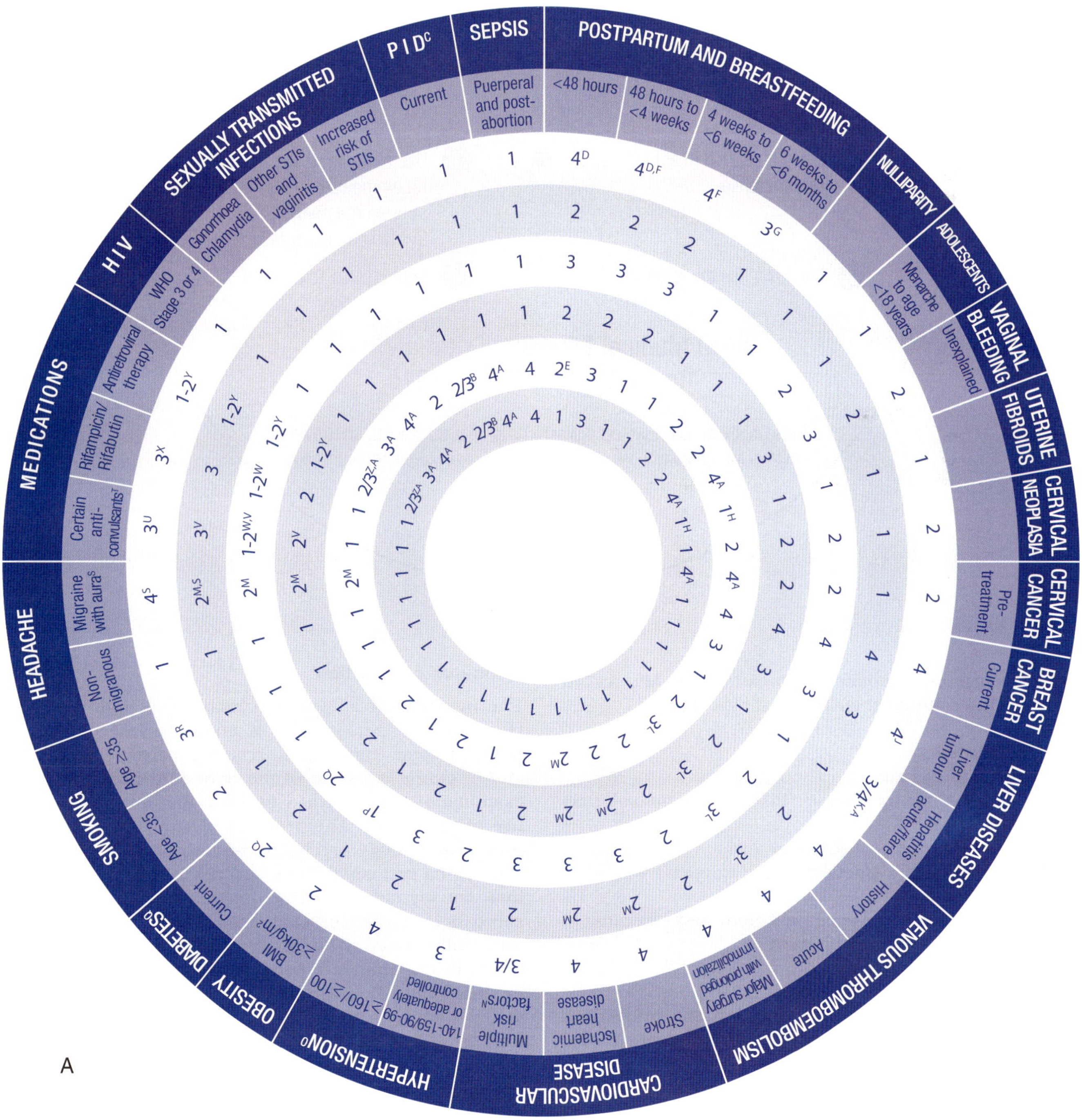

A

Figure 19.11 (A and B) MEC contraceptive wheel, the method of choosing contraceptive method. (*Source*: WHO Medical council.)

Continued

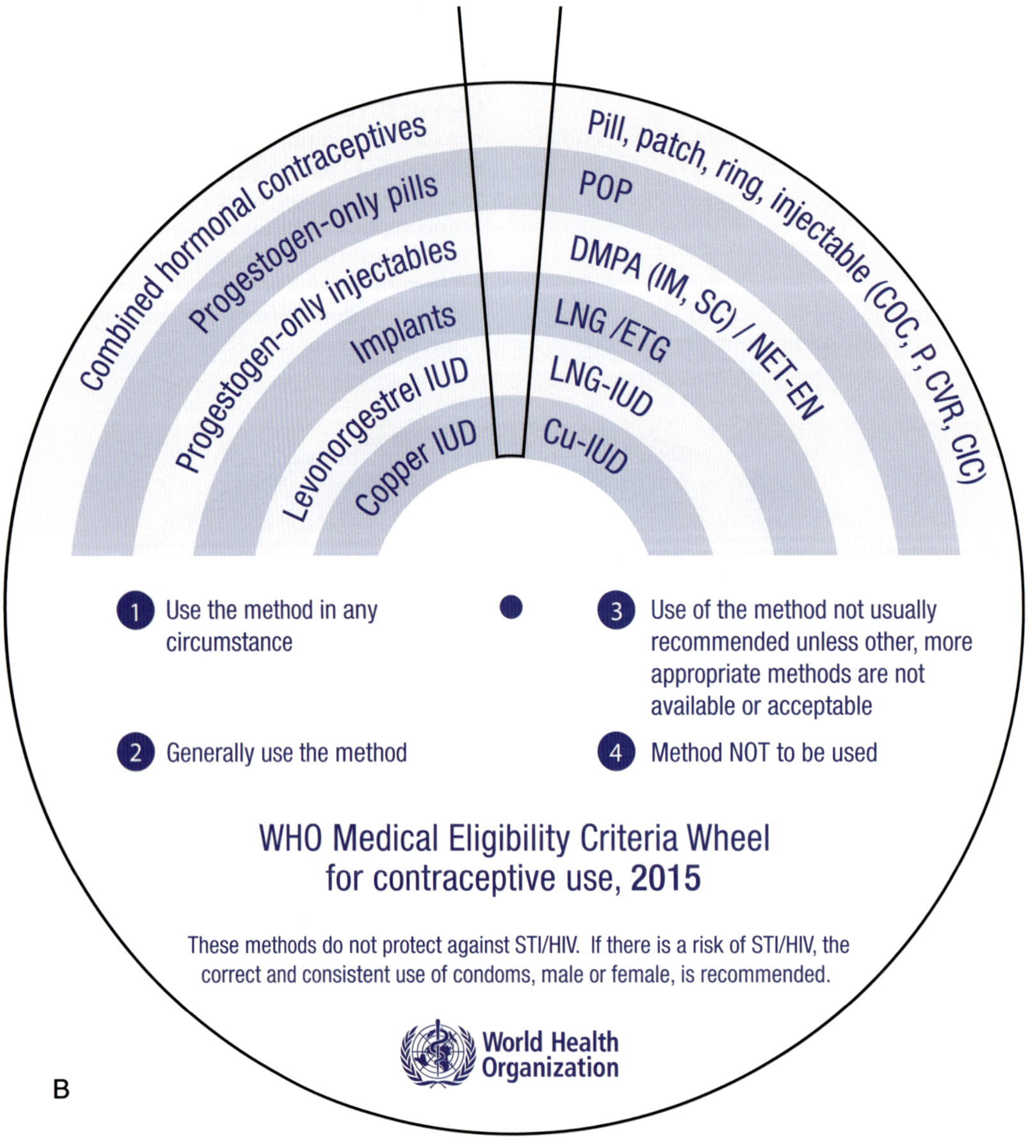

Figure 19.11, cont'd

- In a woman on Tamoxifen for breast cancer, Mirena can be used to counteract endometrial hyperplasia

Contraindications

- Suspected pregnancy
- Pelvic inflammatory disease (PID), lower genital tract infection
- Presence of fibroids – because of misfit
- Menorrhagia and dysmenorrhoea, if Copper-T is used
- Severe anaemia
- Diabetic women who are not well controlled – because of slight increase in pelvic infection
- Previous ectopic pregnancy
- Scarred uterus
- Preferably avoid its use in unmarried and nulliparous patients because of the risk of PID and subsequent tubal infertility
- LNG IUCD in breast cancer
- Uterine anomalies such as bicornuate uterus, septate uterus

Technique of Insertion

The insertion of an IUCD is relatively simple and easy. However, the person who is going to insert a device requires some training in accurate pelvic examination and in gentle insertion of the device. A thorough pelvic examination is performed to determine the position and size of the uterus. The presence of any uterine, tubal or ovarian pathology precludes the insertion of the device. The vagina and cervix are inspected by means of a speculum. Any vaginal or cervical infection must be treated and cured before a device is inserted. The cervix is grasped with a vulsellum or Allis forceps. The device with the introducer is available in a presterilized pack. The device is mounted into the introducer, and the stop on the introducer is adjusted to the length of the uterine cavity. The introducer is then passed through the cervical canal and the plunger is pressed home. This is known as 'push-in technique'. The better method is 'withdrawal technique' with less chance of uterine perforation. In this, the rod containing IUCD is inserted up to the fundus. The outer

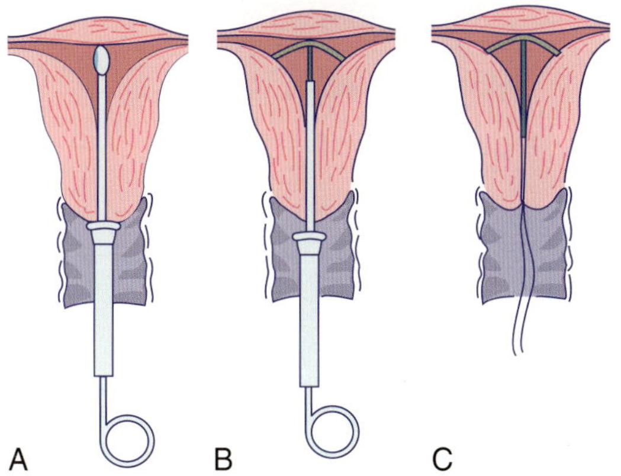

Figure 19.12 **(A)** IUCD inserted. **(B)** Inserter withdrawn. **(C)** IUCD released.

rod is withdrawn followed by inner rod (multiload). The device uncoils within the uterine cavity (Fig. 19.12). The nylon thread is cut to the required length. The forceps and the speculum are removed and the patient is then instructed to examine herself and feel for the thread every week. The acceptance rate of the IUCDs varies. The removal rate at the end of 1 year, because of pain, discomfort, continuous or heavy bleeding or vaginal discharge, is reported to be about 15%–20%. The pregnancy rate varies from 2 to 6 per 100 woman-years. It is advisable to insert IUCD during or soon after menstruation and after abortion or MTP. *Lately, immediate postpartum insertion within 10 minutes of placental expulsion or within 24 hours of delivery is practiced and is found effective.* This saves the woman second visit to the clinic. There is no clinical evidence of increase in perforation, expulsion. The failure rate is less than 1%. Progestogen-containing IUCDs having a thicker vertical stem require cervical dilatation in a few cases.

Mechanism of Action

Several mechanisms are responsible for the contraceptive effect of an IUCD.

- The presence of a foreign body in the uterine cavity renders the migration of spermatozoa difficult.
- A foreign body within the uterus provokes uterine contractility through prostaglandin release and increases the tubal peristalsis so that the fertilized egg is propelled down the fallopian tube more rapidly than in normal and it reaches the uterine cavity before the development of chorionic villi and thus is unable to implant.
- The device in situ causes leucocytic infiltration in the endometrium. The macrophages engulf the fertilized egg if it enters the endometrial tissue.
- Copper-T elutes copper which brings about certain enzymatic and metabolic changes in the endometrial tissue which are inimical to the implantation of the fertilized ovum.
- Progestogen-carrying device causes alteration in the cervical mucus which prevents penetration of sperm, in addition to its local action. It also causes endometrial atrophy. It prevents ovulation in about 40%.

Complications

With improvements in the new devices, the acceptability and compliance have improved. The complications of an IUCD are as follows:

Immediate
- Difficulty in insertion
- Vasovagal attack
- Uterine cramps

Early
- Expulsion (2%–5%)
- Perforation (1%–2%)
- Spotting, menorrhagia (2%–10%)
- Dysmenorrhoea (2%–10%)
- Vaginal infection
- Actinomycosis

Late
- PID – 2%–5%. IUCD does not prevent transmission of HIV
- Pregnancy – 1–3 per 100 woman-years (failure rate)
- Ectopic pregnancy
- Perforation
- Menorrhagia
- Dysmenorrhoea

IUCD can be inserted in HIV-positive woman on medication.

Long-term follow-up of women wearing IUCD has shown no ill effects on systemic diseases. There is no evidence that the device predisposes to either cervical or endometrial cancer.

Perforation can occur at the time of insertion, particularly during puerperium. Its incidence is 1–3 per 100 insertions, lately reduced with improved devices. Perforation is rare with withdrawal than push-in technique. Menorrhagia can be controlled with NSAID drugs.

Expulsion may occur in 5%–15% and is due to small size of IUCD. It is common during the puerperal period or following MTP of a large gestation size.

PID occurs usually within 4 weeks of insertion and may be due to existing unrecognized vaginal infection, or the tail of IUCD causing ascending infection. Actinomycosis is an infection commonly associated with IUCD.

IUCD is removed by grasping the thread with an artery forceps and gently pulling it out.

Misplaced IUCD

It is defined as the condition when the tail of the IUCD is not seen through the os. The causes are (i) uterus has enlarged through pregnancy, (ii) thread has curled inside the uterus, (iii) perforation has occurred or the IUCD is buried in the myometrium and (iv) it has been expelled (Fig. 19.13).

A plain radiograph or pelvic ultrasound will show whether the IUCD is still inside or has been expelled. If it is inside, the uterine sound or another IUCD inserted in the uterine cavity will show on radiograph its proximity to the misplaced IUCD and perforation can be diagnosed (Fig. 19.13). An abnormal shape or location of IUCD on radiograph indicates likely perforation. Hysteroscopy is useful not only to locate it but also for its retrieval. If the IUCD is in the uterine cavity, it can be retrieved with Shirodkar's hook, a curette or through a hysteroscope and ultrasonic guidance. In case of perforation, a laparotomy is needed,

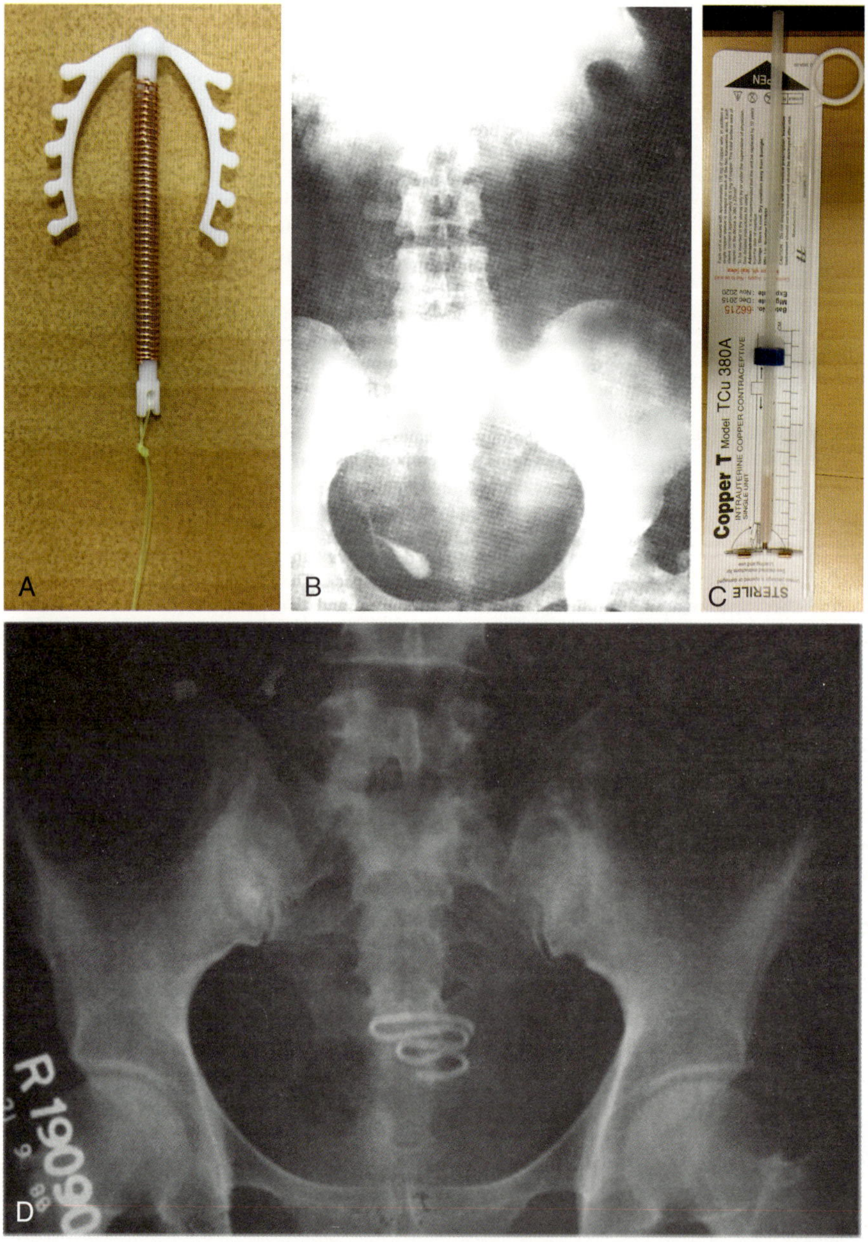

Figure 19.13 **(A)** Multiload Copper-T 375. **(B)** Displaced Copper-T with calcium deposition at tip of T. **(C)** Copper-T 380A. **(D)** Pelvic radiograph showing Lipple's loop in the pelvic cavity. (*Courtesy* **(B):** Dr K.K. Saxena, New Delhi.)

because Copper-T causes adhesions to the omentum or a gut and cannot be retrieved easily through a laparoscope.

Pregnancy. *Pregnancy* occurs with IUCD in situ in 1–3 per 100 woman-years. If this happens, it is important to do ultrasound and rule out ectopic pregnancy. The uterine pregnancy can be associated with complications such as infection; therefore, it is mandatory to remove the IUCD if the tail is visible. While doing so, the risk of abortion should be explained to the woman. If the thread of the IUCD is not seen, termination of pregnancy is offered, not because IUCD has any teratogenic effect but because the risk of uterine infection is considerable. Alternatively, if woman decides to continue pregnancy she may be allowed to continue after counselling and explaining the risk.

Ectopic Pregnancy. It occurs in 1:30 pregnancies in woman wearing IUCD. This is because IUCD has a local contraceptive action on the uterus and prevents a uterine pregnancy but does not protect against tubal or ovarian pregnancy. Progestasert has the highest incidence of ectopic pregnancy (six to nine times more than Copper-T). PID caused by IUCD also contributes to the occurrence of an ectopic pregnancy.

Advantages of IUCD

- It is coital-independent.
- One-time insertion gives continuous protection for a long period. It is cost-effective.
- It is highly effective, newer IUCDs being as effective as oral contraceptives. Three per cent failure rate at the end

of 1 year is reduced to less than 1% at the end of 5 years. There is no user failure.

- There is no evidence of reduced fertility following its removal. About 75% women conceive within 6 months of its removal and almost 90% conceive within a year.
- There are no systemic ill effects, unlike oral contraceptives. No adverse effect on lactation is observed.

Copper-T 380A (Fig. 19.12C) is provided free in the National Family Planning Programme.

Disadvantages of IUCD

- A trained medical or paramedical personnel is required to screen and insert an IUCD.
- Certain complications such as menstrual irregularities, dysmenorrhoea, pelvic pain make woman gets it removed.

Mirena IUCD

It is 32 × 32 mm IUCD with the vertical rod containing 52 mg LNG progestogen in a silastic reservoir in its vertical arm: 20 mcg hormone is eluted in 15 minutes after its insertion, and the peak level reaches in a few hours. The hormone does not get absorbed into the general circulation (or minimal amount) so the side effects of systemic administrations are not seen. It does not suppress ovulation, and its effect is mainly on the endometrium and cervical mucus. Because of this, Mirena is also used in abnormal uterine bleeding (AUB), endometrial hyperplasia, in HRT and in a woman on Tamoxifen for breast cancer to combat hyperplasia of endometrium caused by oestrogen. It may cause irregular bleeding during the first 3–6 months. The pregnancy rate is 0.5 per 100 woman-years (equal to that of tubectomy).

- Teratogenic, if pregnancy occurs with Mirena in situ due to progestogen.
- Incidence of ectopic pregnancy 0.02%.
- 20 mcg hormone is daily eluted.

Compared to tubectomy, Mirena is an effective contraceptive, reversible and reduces dysmenorrhoea and menorrhagia unlike tubectomy. Mirena, because it cures menorrhagia and is as effective as tubectomy, is expected to reduce the number of hysterectomies. It is safe. Continuation rate of 80% is reported at the end of 1 year.

Advantages of Mirena

1. One-time insertion
2. Effective for 5 years
3. Compliance
4. Reduces menorrhagia and dysmenorrhoea

Fibroplant: Is a frameless LNG IUCD; releases 14 mcg LNG daily, and is under clinical development.

MALE HORMONAL CONTRACEPTIVE

There have been several attempts at finding out an effective male contraceptive. However, due to a number of reasons till date there is no effective male contraceptive other than condoms which may be advocated for mass use. A number of approaches have been utilized to develop a reliable and effective male contraceptive, most of these are based upon suppression of spermatogenesis.

HORMONAL CONTRACEPTION

Hormonal contraception comprising use of oestrogen and progesterone combination in the form of oral tablets, injectables, vaginal rings, dermal patches has come to occupy most prominent place in the field of female contraception. In western countries, this has become the most commonly used method among women. In India, popularity of oral pills is not very high rather tubectomy remains most often used method by the women. Progesterone alone in the form of depot injections, implants, vaginal rings and IUCD has also become popular because of lesser side effects yet giving as reliable contraception as with combination of oestrogen and progesterone.

Following sections describe various types of hormonal contraceptives which are in use nowadays.

SUPPRESSION OF OVULATION (HORMONAL CONTRACEPTIVE AGENTS) (Table 19.1)

Hormonal contraception is one of the most effective contraceptive methods available nowadays. Since 1956, when Pincus came out with an oral contraceptive drug, more than 30 millions of women have used this method in one form or the other. A wide variety of hormonal preparations are now available for contraceptive use. The mode of action depends upon the hormone used, the mode of delivery and the time of administration. The hormones can be delivered orally, by intramuscular route, subcutaneous implants, vaginal rings, intrauterine devices or by dermal patches.

Oral Contraceptives

There are three types of hormonal oral contraceptives, i.e. monophasic combined oral pills (Table 19.2), triphasic combined pills and minipills.

Combined Oral Pills (OCP). Combined oral pills contain a combination of ethinyloestradiol (EE_2) in a dose of 20–30 mcg

Table 19.1 Hormonal Contraceptives

Oral	Insertions	Injections
	• Vaginal ring • IUCD Mirena	• Monthly • 2 monthly, 3 monthly • Combined
COC, POP Progest/ Combined Pills • Once daily for 21 days	• Implants	E_2 + P injection monthly
3 weeks cyclically • 2 monthly, 3 monthly • Yearly • Triphasic • Emergency pills	• Testosterone implants in male	Progestogen patch • Subdermal self-administration injection of DMPA on trial in males • Testosterone injections in males

Table 19.2 Types of Monophasic Combined Oral Pills

First generation	Ethinyloestradiol	Norethindrone
Second generation	Ethinyloestradiol	Norgestrel, LNG
Third generation	Ethinyloestradiol	Desogestrel, gestodene norgestimate
Fourth generation (Yasmin)	Ethinyloestradiol	Drospirenone

and an orally active progestogen such as norgestrel or Novelon. Mala-D and Mala-N both have same composition containing LNG 0.15 mg and ethinyloestradiol (EE) 30 mcg the latter is available free of cost in Family Planning Clinics in India. The tablets are taken starting on the first day of the cycle for 21 days. A new course of tablets should be commenced 7 days after the completion of the previous course. Tablet should be taken at a fixed time of the day, preferably after a meal.

Mechanism of Action. The combined oral pill suppresses pituitary hormones, FSH and LH peak and through this suppression prevents ovulation. At the same time, progestogen causes atrophic changes in the endometrium and prevents nidation. Progestogen also acts on the cervical mucus making it thick and tenacious and impenetrable by sperms.

OCP also increases the tubal motility, so the fertilized egg reaches the uterine cavity before the endometrium is receptive for implantation.

Pregnancy rate with combined oral pill is 0.3 per 100 woman-years (with perfect use) and 5–8 per 100 woman-years (with typical use) is the lowest of all contraceptives in use nowadays. During the first cycle of use, ovulation is not always suppressed and as a precaution patient may be advised to use an additional method. Lately, starting the pill on the first day of the cycle has reduced such a failure rate and the need to take the additional precaution in the first cycle. If she forgets to take a tablet pill, she should take two tablets the following day. If she forgets to take the tablet more than twice in a cycle, she is no longer adequately protected and must use a barrier method for remaining part of the cycle. The majority of failures with oral combined pills are due to the failure to take the pills regularly. With proper compliance, most women have regular 28-day menstrual cycles. The bleeding is less in amount and shorter in duration than a normal menstrual period. In a nonlactating woman, OCP can be started after 3 weeks of delivery, but can be given soon after an abortion, MTP or an ectopic pregnancy. Following vesicular mole, one should start OCP only after serum β-hCG is negative. Antiretroviral drugs (ART) reduce effectiveness of OCP but when combined with condoms, OCP are effective in protecting against pregnancy.

Noncontraceptive Benefits of Combined Pills. Oral contraceptive pills offer a number of short-term and long-term benefits when used as contraceptives.

1. Use of OCP results in regular cycles and average blood loss during menstruation. It is helpful in women with menorrhagia and polymenorrhoea. It also relieves dysmenorrhoea and premenstrual tension.
2. It prevents anaemia by reducing the menstrual blood loss.
3. It lowers the incidence of benign breast conditions such as fibrocystic disease.
4. It reduces the incidence of functional ovarian cyst (50%).
5. Reduce incidence of malignancies. Both ovarian and endometrial malignancies are less common among regular users of OCP. The incidence of ovarian malignancy is reduced by 40% and uterine malignancy by 50% if taken for 1 year, this protective effect lasts as long as 10 years after stoppage of use of OCPs. The incidence of PID is reduced, though it does not reach the same low level as seen with the barrier method. This protective effect is due to the thick cervical mucus caused by progestogen, preventing the microorganisms entering into the uterine cavity.
6. **Reduced incidence of ectopic pregnancy** is due to suppression of ovulation and reduction in PID.
7. It protects against rheumatoid arthritis.
8. Reduces the risk of anorectal cancer by 30%–40%.
9. It is useful in acne, Polycystic Ovarian Disease (PCOD) and endometriosis.

Side Effects with the Use of OCPs and Contraindications

- Intermenstrual spotting is common in the first 3 months of use of the pills, subsequently it gradually disappears. Frequent spotting can be stopped by choosing a pill containing higher dose of oestrogen or other combination of hormones. Often menstrual bleeding becomes scanty and occasionally a woman may become amenorrhoeic causing a fear of pregnancy. Amenorrhoea lasting more than 6 months requires investigations. Postpill amenorrhoea is not related to the type, dose or duration of pill intake. Those with previous menstrual irregularity (oligomenorrhoea) are more likely to suffer from amenorrhoea.
- Genital tract candidiasis. Oral pills are associated with monilial (candidial) vaginitis.
- No documented association is seen with carcinoma of cervix; however, dysplasia is more frequent. Recently an increase incidence of cervical adenocarcinoma and glandular abnormalities has been reported with long-term use of OCPs.
- No adverse effect has been noted on uterine fibroids, and it is oestrogen singly that increases their size.
- Breast. The combined pills should not be offered to a woman suffering from cancer of the breast. Some have reported the breast cancer in a nulliparous woman (25%) who has taken oral contraceptive pills before the age of 24 years for over a period of 4 years. This should be considered while prescribing oral pills to a young nulliparous woman. There are some reports indicating higher incidence of breast cancer among users of OCPs. Periodic breast examination and necessary investigations in a user of OCPs will help to detect breast cancer at an early stage. Progestogen component also contributes to the potential of development of breast cancer. However, if breast cancer develops, it is well differentiated with good prognosis. The risk of malignancy disappears after 10 years of stoppage.
- Pituitary adenoma was attributed to the use of the pill but its exact role in its development is not clear and doubtful.

- Breast milk amount in lactating woman who chooses to use OCPs is reduced. The combined pills may preferable be avoided during the first 6 months after delivery if a woman is lactating. However, progesterone only pills (POP) do not suffer this disadvantage and can be safely used during the first 6 months of lactation. Nausea and vomiting are common initially mainly due to oestrogen and subsequently disappears. It can be avoided by taking the pills at bedtime. If vomiting occurs within 1 hour of taking pill, repeat dose.
- Liver. Adenomas have been reported and though they are benign rarely a rupture of a hepatoma can be fatal. Because the hormones are metabolized in the liver, chronic liver diseases and recent jaundice contraindicate the use of pills.
- Gall bladder function may be adversely affected.
- Carbohydrate metabolism. Carbohydrate tolerance may be reduced. Therefore, combined oral pills are contraindicated or given cautiously to a diabetic woman.
- Lipid metabolism. Oestrogen increases the high-density lipoprotein (HDL) and lowers low-density lipoprotein (LDL). Some progestogens have a reverse effect and the overall effect on the myocardial function and lipid metabolism depends upon the combined effect of both hormones. Rifampicin, an antibiotic prescribed for a tubercular infection, reduces the absorption of drugs in the pill; hence, OCPs are contraindicated in a tubercular patient on rifampicin. Other drugs interfering with OCPs are tetracycline, anticonvulsants, antifungal, cephalosporin and phenobarb. Ritonavir for HIV also interferes with absorption of OCPs.
- Headache, migraine, depression, irritability, increased weight and lethargy can occur due to progestogen.
- Thromboembolic disorders. Pulmonary embolism and cerebral thrombosis, both venous and arterial, are 7–10 times more frequent in the pill users than in the nonusers in the first year of use. This is due to an increased clotting mechanism (platelet aggregation and increased fibrinogen factor VII, VIII and decreased fibrinolysis) caused by the oestrogen component of the pill. The effect is dose-dependent, and the reduction of the oestrogen content of the pill from the original 100–30 mcg in currently used pills and of late a newer oral pill (Femilon) which contains 20 mcg EE_2 reveal an improved safety and tolerance profile, and at the same time retain its contraceptive efficacy. The incidence of thromboembolic disorders has thus dropped without diminishing the efficacy of the pill. A woman older than 40 years, a woman with stroke, heavy smoker, a cardiac and hypertensive patient, a woman with familial hyperlipoproteinaemia are all high-risk cases for this complication. The pills containing desogestrel and gestodene (third generation) also carry a higher risk of venous thromboembolism than the pills containing LNG.
- Sickle cell anaemia patients can develop thrombosis and crisis.
- A woman who wears contact lenses should be warned of oedema and irritation of eyes (thrombosis of optic vessels) – it is a relative contraindication. Combined oral contraceptive (COC) pill do not protect a woman against HIV and sexually transmitted infections. This is important while counselling a woman at a high risk for these infections. Barrier methods reduce the risk of transmission of HIV and other infections. In HIV patients a dual method of barrier contraceptive with OCPs are recommended.
- Pills have no adverse effects on thyroid functions.

Contraindications to the Use of OCPs

1. Cardiac disease, hypertension, smoker older than 35 years.
2. Diabetes.
3. History of thrombosis, myocardial infarction, sickle cell anaemia, severe migraine.
4. Chronic liver diseases such as cholestatic jaundice of pregnancy, cirrhosis of liver, adenoma, porphyrias.
5. Breast cancer, gall bladder disease.
6. Gross obesity.
7. Patient on enzyme-inducing drugs such as rifampicin, and antiepileptics except sodium valproate.
8. 4–6 weeks prior to a planned surgery.
9. Lactating woman.

A woman can take OCPs regularly up to the age of 35 years, and thereafter until 45 years if she is healthy, nonobese and nonsmoker. However, she should remain under the supervision of the doctor and have Pap smear done regularly to check on cervical dysplasia.

Return of Menstruation and Fertility. Ninety-nine per cent of women will have normal menstrual cycles within 6 months after stopping use of OCPs but return of fertility may be slightly delayed due to delayed return of ovulation. Ninety per cent ovulate within 3 months of stopping the drug. There is no evidence of increased fetal malformations or increased rate of abortion in those who conceive while on pills.

Triphasic Pills. With the aim of further reducing the amount of hormones during OCP use, the biphasic and triphasic pills were introduced. The composition of pills in initial part of menstrual cycle is different from the pills given in the last 10 days, this way the total amount of oestrogen and progesterone in a month is reduced. The triphasic preparations currently in use contains EE_2 and LNG in an amount 30 mcg EE_2 plus 50 mcg LNG during the first 6 days of the cycle, for the next 5 days 40 mcg EE_2 plus 75 mcg LNG, and during the last 10 days 30 mcg EE_2 and 125 mcg LNG. Next pack of triphasic pills is started after 1 week. These pills have no adverse effect on carbohydrate and lipid metabolism; therefore, they can be prescribed to diabetic women and without expecting any increased risk of myocardial infarct. They are as effective as the monophasic oral pills but not recommended in woman with menorrhagia and for other indications.

How to Maintain Compliance with the Use of Oral Pill?

- Three-monthly course of pills. 'Seasonale' which contains EE_2 plus LNG is available as a packet containing 84 tablets (with a gap of 7 days), which means only four menstrual cycles in a year, and has been attractive to many working women especially in the USA. However, some may face the problem of prolonged breakthrough bleeding. Yearly continuous pills are under trial (one period a year) – Lybrel is effective for 1 year.

- OCPs containing only 10 mcg EE_2 (ultra low dose pills).
- Once-a-month pill containing 3 mg quinestrol and 12 mg megestrol acetate, popular in China and Latin America. Two tablets in the first month are followed by one tablet monthly.
- EE_2 + drospirenone (Yasmin, Tarana, Janya) contain 21 tablets in a packet. Janya contains 24 tablets (gap of four tablets in a cycle), and contains 20 mcg EE_2.
- EE_2 + cyproterone acetate (Dianette) 35 mcg EE_2 is more useful in women with PCOD, hirsutism.
- Quadriphasic pills containing E_2 + dienogest, daily – no pill-free days, better tolerated and a good control of menses.
- Chewable tablets containing 35 mcg EE_2 and 0.4 mg norethindrone.
- Lybrel-continuous daily use for 1 year contains 20 mcg EE_2 + 90 mcg LNG in a tablet.

Newer Pills with Antiandrogenic Properties. Drospirenone reduces fluid retention and has no adverse effect of spironolactone, has antimineralocorticoid (3 mg drospirenone is equivalent to 25 mg of spironolactone, cures acne and hirsutism. It reduces fluid and sodium retention, and has no adverse effect mg of latter), has antimineralocorticoid and with antiandrogenic activity. It inhibits ovulation, and has no effect on bone mineral density. It also prevents obesity and maintains good lipid profile. Because of this property and relief from acne, it is also been called 'beauty pill'.

Main side effect is potassium retention because of which it is contraindicated in renal and liver disease and in a woman with previous thromboembolism.

Different Generations of Oral Pills. Depending on the progesterone content in an OCP, oral pills have been called the first generation, second generation, third generation and fourth generation.

- **First generation** – contains norethindrone progesterone and 50 mcg or more of EE
- **Second generation** – contains LNG, norgestimate, norethindrone progesterone formulation and 20, 30 or 35 mcg EE.
- **Third generation** – contains gestodene, desogestrel progesterone formulation and 20, 30 or 35 mcg EE
- **Fourth generation** – contains spironolactone, dienogest or cyproterone acetate.

Progestogens. Progestogens alone have also being successfully used as hormone contraceptives. Besides being devoid of oestrogenic side effect these contraceptives can be used during lactation, during menses and in woman where oestrogen are contraindicated.

Progestogens are available as oral pills (minipills), intramuscular injections, implants, patches, vaginal ring and Mirena IUCD.

Progestogen-Only Pill (POP – Minipill). The low-dose POP (norethisterone 350 mcg, norgestrel 75 mcg or LNG 30 mcg) has been introduced to avoid the side effects of oestrogen in the combined pills. The tablet is taken daily without a break. The pill should be started within 5–7 days of the menstruation and taken at the same time with a leeway of 3 hours on either side of the fixed time each day. If this regime is not observed any day, the woman continues with POP but observes extra precaution for next 48 hours. The mode of action of progestogen has already been discussed earlier.

POP is started 21 days postpartum and soon after abortion. The woman needs to take precaution in the first 48 hours in the first cycle.

Minipill does not have some of the major side effects of the combined pill and *it is well suited for lactating women*; some progestogens, in fact, increase milk secretion. However, it has a higher pregnancy rate of 2–3 per 100 woman-years which is higher than that of the combined pill though comparable to an IUCD and is higher in obese women. Strict daily compliance is a drawback. Other drawbacks are irregular bleeding (20%), amenorrhoea, depression, headache, migraine and weight gain, ectopic pregnancy, functional ovarian cysts besides a higher failure rate.

The use of newer generation of synthetic progestogen, namely desogestrel in POP. It has no androgenic effect, no adverse effect on carbohydrate and lipid metabolism, and is considered to be safe, especially for lactating women. *However, the incidence of thromboembolism is higher with this progestogen.*

Contraindications. Contraindications to POP are previous ectopic pregnancy, ovarian cyst, breast and genital cancers, abnormal vaginal bleeding, active liver and arterial disease, porphyria, liver tumour, valproate, spironolactone and meprobamate. *Because of osteopenia, it is contraindicated in adolescents and young women.*

Advantages of Progestogen-Only Pill. Advantages of POP are that they can be recommended to:

- Lactating women.
- Women older than 35 years.
- Those with focal migraine.
- Those intolerant to oestrogen or oestrogen contraindicated.
- Diabetic, hypertensive woman, sickle cell anaemia. As regards to return of fertility, it is faster than in COC users because ovulation is not suppressed in all cases (suppressed in 40%)

Mode of Action of Minipills

- Cerazette which contains desogestrel in a dose of 75 mcg suppresses ovulation in 97%–100%, whereas other POPs suppress ovulation in only 40%.
- It forms a thick plug of mucus in the cervical canal and acts as a barrier to sperms.
- It alters tubal peristalsis and fertilized egg reaches the uterine cavity too early for implantation.

Cerazette containing 75 mcg desogestrel has the following advantages over other POPs:

- Stringent time compliance not necessary, as it suppresses ovulation in 97%, through pituitary hormone suppression.
- No androgenic effects such as acne.
- No ectopic pregnancy, no effect on carbohydrate or lipid metabolism.
- Failure rate only 0.21 per 100 woman-years. It acts through metabolite etonogestrel which binds to progesterone receptors

Side effects: (1) weight gain, (2) irregular menstrual bleeding, (3) depression, (4) breast cancer and (5) thromboembolism.

Depot Injections of Progesterone. Although not very popular in India depot injections of progesterone (Depot medroxyprogesterone acetate, DMPA; norethisterone enanthate NET-EN) are two commonly used intramuscular injections of progesterone. In fact, in more than 125 countries these are available in the Family Planning Programs. Ease of administration, repeating action at 2–3 monthly intervals and high efficacy have made this mode of administration of contraceptives very popular. To overcome the inconvenience of daily compliance, depot injections of progestogens have been developed. DMPA is given in a microcrystalline aqueous suspension and NET-EN in a castor oil solution, both by deep intramuscular injection (subcutaneous preparation of DMPA is also available in 104 mg). Lately a monthly DMPA combined with 25–50 mg of medroxyprogesterone acetate combined with 5 mg oestradiol is available and is considered to be more effective with lesser menstrual disturbances. Other preparations in use are the DMPA 150 mg 3-monthly, DMPA 300 mg 6-monthly and NET-EN 200 mg 2-monthly. After stoppage, the contraceptive effect of DMPA lasts longer than that of NET-EN. Menstrual irregularity though common is accepted by puerperal woman as physiological. The injection should be started within a month of delivery in a non-lactating woman and during the third month in a lactating woman because ovulation is delayed up to at least 10 weeks in lactating mothers. Pregnancy rate is 0.4 per 100 woman-years for DMPA and 0.6 per 100 woman-years for NET-EN.

Injection DMPA has recently been introduced free of cost in the National Family Planning Programme of India with the name of 'Antara'.

The injection should be administered within 7 days of menstruation with a grace period of 2 weeks for DMPA and 1 week for NET-EN for a repeat injection. Action lasts 12–14 weeks of the first injection for DMPA and 8–9 weeks for NET-EN.

Advantages

- Injections are easy to administer and there is no worry over 'missing pill'. They are long-acting and reversible.
- The compliance is good and the woman remains under regular medical supervision.
- The side effects on lipid and carbohydrate metabolism are avoided. DMPA is least androgenic.
- It is suited to lactating women.
- The incidence of PID, ectopic pregnancy and functional ovarian cysts is low, so also endometrial cancer.
- Avoids oestrogenic side effects.
- Can be given to a woman with sickle cell anaemia.
- Return of fertility is slightly delayed in DMPA group compared to NET, but 80% conceive within a year (5 months for DMPA and 3–4 months for NET-EN).
- Independent of coitus.
- They turn out to be more cost-effective for mass usages.

Disadvantages

- Once administered, the side effects, if any, need to be tolerated until the progestogenic effect of the injection is over.
- Menstrual irregularities are common in the form of amenorrhoea or irregular bleeding. Amenorrhoea is reported in 20%–50% users of DMPA at the end of 1 year and are more common with DMPA than NET. Heavy and irregular bleeding is reported in 1%–2% users and is more common with the use of NET.
- Do not prevent STD and HIV.
- There is a delay in return of fertility but 80% are expected to conceive by end of 1 year. With DMPA, ovulation returns in 5 months, and with NET within 3 months of the last injection.
- The side effects in the form of weight gain, depression, bloated feeling and mastalgia can occur with injectable progestogen.
- Prolonged DMPA use, by virtue of antioestrogenic action, may reduce bone density mass and induce osteopenia.
- Contraindicated in breast cancer.
- It does increase LDL but does not adversely affect the blood pressure.
- It may decrease libido, cause dry vagina.

Because of risk of osteopenia, this contraceptive is contraindicated in adolescents, and should not be used for more than 2 years in others. Lately, subcutaneous injections are under development to enable self-administration by the woman.

Once-a-Month Injections. Once-a-month intramuscular injections of combined oestrogen and progestogen are available in some countries.

These are as follows:

- **Mesigyna** – (1/2 mL containing NET 50 mg with oestradiol valerate 5 mg) is given by deep intramuscular injection once a month with ± 3 days. The low failure rate of 0.4% at the end of 1 year is encouraging.
- **Cyclofem and Lunelle** – 1/2 mL contains 25 mg DMPA and oestradiol cypionate 5 mg. The failure rate is 0.2% at the end of 1 year. The menstrual irregularity is less than with progestogen-alone injections.
- **Marvelon** – Desogestrel 150 mcg with EE_2 30 mcg.
- **Femovan** – Gestodene 75 mcg with EE_2 30 mcg.
- **Anafertin** – Dihydroxyprogesterone acetophenide 75 mg + estradiol enanthate 5 mg.

It should be remembered that the first menstrual period comes 10–15 days after the first injection but thereafter every 30 days and lasts for 5 days. Failure rate of 0.1%–0.4% is reported. Ovulation returns in 6 months.

Subdermal Implants

In the quest to find alternative routes of giving hormonal contraceptives, subdermal implants were discovered. With this method, the progestogens are delivered into general circulation with a slow and sustained release manner with lesser side effects. There are two types of subdermal implants, biodegradable and nondegradable. Once implanted they release drug slowly over a period of 1–5 years depending upon the implant.

The subdermal implant has no 'nuisance value' of continuous compliance which often adversely affects motivation. Besides, being nonoral it avoids 'hepatic first-pass effect and thus, reduces systemic side effects'.

Norplant I. Norplant I (Figs 19.14–19.16) was the first subdermal implant introduced for contraception containing six silastic capsules, it has now been withdrawn from the market and replaced by a single rod implant.

Norplant II (Jadelle) was the second implant system introduced for contraception. It consisted of two rods each

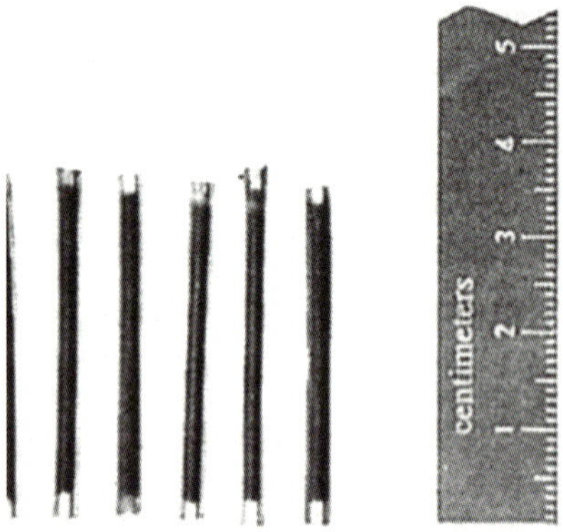

Figure 19.14 Norplant I and Norplant II.

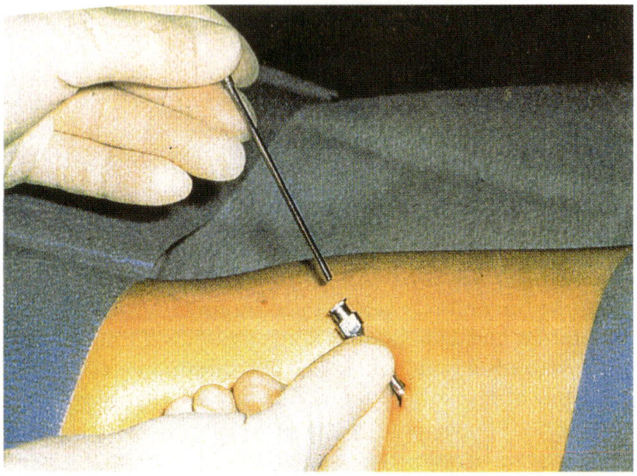

Figure 19.15 Insertion of Norplant.

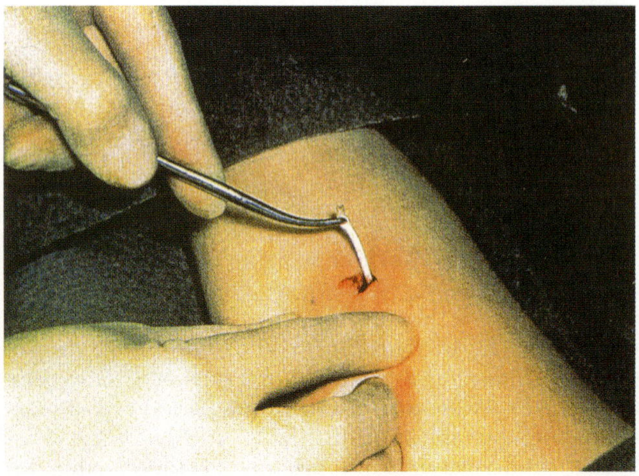

Figure 19.16 Removal of Norplant.

containing 70 mg LNG with a daily release of 50 mcg and provides contraception for 3–5 years.

The implants suppress ovulation in 50% of the cycles but the main mechanism of action is suppression of endometrium.

Insertion of Implants. The implants are inserted on the first day of the menstrual cycle or within 5 days of abortion, and 3 weeks after the delivery. The woman needs to use barrier contraception or abstain in the first 7 days after insertion.

It takes 5–10 minutes to insert under local anaesthesia. It is best inserted on the medial aspect of the upper arm. The capsules are nonbiodegradable, so they need removal at the end of its use or earlier, if side effects are intolerable.

The insertion and removal is made easier using a single rod system called Implanon (40 × 2 mm), which contains 68 mg etonogestrel and does not require an incision to insert. It releases 30 mcg of the hormone daily and is effective for 3 years. There has been no failure to date. It prevents ovulation and is reversible within 1 month of removal.

With the use of Implanon, amenorrhoea is common at the end of 1 year. Acne is reduced and it has no effect on bone density.

Advantages. The advantages of implants are as follows:

- They are long-acting with sustained effect – compliance is good.
- Coital-independent with no 'nuisance' of daily oral or frequent injections.
- Pregnancy rate varies between 0.2 and 1.3 per 100 woman-years. The failure rate is higher in obese women weighing more than 70 kg.
- Systemic side effects are few and the first-pass effect on the liver avoided.
- Return of fertility is prompt (within 4–12 weeks).
- Can be used by lactating mothers and women older than 40 years.

Disadvantages

- Breakthrough bleeding, irregular cycles, amenorrhoea occur as seen with other progesterone only contraceptives.
- Other side effects of progestogens are seen.
- Ectopic pregnancy is reported in 1.3%.
- Local infection at the site of insertion may occur.
- Requires insertion and removal with nonbiodegradable implants; however, it is a minor surgical procedure.
- The implants are expensive.
- Infertility may be seen in a few cases after the removal of implant.

Contraceptive Vaginal Rings (CVR)

Another route which has been tested and found suitable for delivery of hormonal contraceptive is in the form of contraceptive vaginal rings. In an attempt to reduce the side effects of systemic hormonal contraception and the surgical method of insertion of implants, silastic vaginal rings carrying progestogens in different doses have been tried. The ring is 50–75 mm in diameter and 5–9 mm thick. The ring currently available contains LNG released at a rate of 20 mcg of hormone daily. The ring needs a change after

3 months. Another ring which contains both oestrogen and progesterone is available in the market by the name of NuvaRing containing 11.7 mg etonogestrel and 2.7 mg ethinyloestradiol. NuvaRing is effective for 1 month. Advantage of NuvaRing is that incidence of breakthrough bleeding and spotting is less compared to vaginal ring containing only progesterone. Failure rate is 1.8 per 100 woman-years.

Recently, a lot of research is going on in this field, some progestin-containing rings (3-keto desogestrel 10 mg) have been left in for 3 months at a time. The pregnancy rate with this is reported to be 3.5 per 100 woman-years (WHO, 1985). A ring releasing 30 mcg EE_2 with either 120 mcg desogestrel or 650 mcg norethisterone is under trial.

Other rings are as follows:

1. **NuvaRing** – 120 mcg etonogestrel + 15 mcg EE_2 daily release can be removed during intercourse but not for more than 3 hours at a time.
2. **Nestorone** – 150 mcg progesterone +15 mcg EE_2, effective for 1 year; failure rate is 1.2 per 100 woman-years.

Advantages of Contraceptive Vaginal Rings
- Self-insertion and removal, good compliance.
- Other advantages of progestogen contraceptives.
- Quick reversibility.

Disadvantages
- Expensive; Rs 700 per ring per cycle.
- Local irritation is felt by few, vaginitis 5%.
- Expulsion can occur especially in woman with vaginal prolapse.
- Systemic side effects of progestogens have been noted in some women.

IUCDs Containing Progestogen. Another route of delivering hormonal contraceptives which has been successfully employed is in the form of IUCD impregnated with progestogens. Progestasert and Mirena are two such devices which have been extensively used. Mirena contains 52 mg LNG in the vertical arm of T device and elutes 20 mcg daily. The effect lasts for 5 years.

The failure rate is 0.1% similar to oral combined pills.

Though primarily used in AUB, its contraceptive benefit is also appreciated.

The menstrual irregularity in the first 3 months settles down to normal cycles and dysmenorrhoea is also cured. The incidence of PID and ectopic pregnancy is reduced.

The insertion is however difficult due to the thick vertical stem. Amenorrhoea is reported in about 20% at the end of 1 year. Mirena costs Rs 7000.

Skin Patches

Hormonal Patch (Ortho-Evra). Another route of hormonal contraceptives which has been tested in clinical practice is a skin patch impregnated in hormone. A Ortho Evra Hormonal patch releases 6.00 mg norelgestromin (NGMN) and 0.75 mg EE. A patch lasts 7 days. Three patches are required in each cycle followed by 1-week patch-free interval. The patch should be applied within 5 days of menses over the buttocks or abdomen but not over the breasts.

The failure rate is 1–2.8 per 100 woman-years. Compliance of 90% is reported. The breakthrough bleeding (18%), skin reaction (20%) and breast discomfort are the side effects. The other symptoms are headache, nausea and mastalgia. The site of patch should be changed often and is contraindicated in obese women.

Although found popular among women in rich countries, its popularity is low in India. Because of sweating, excessive heat the patch may get displaced decreasing its effectiveness.

Percutaneous Gel. Three grams daily of percutaneous gel of oestradiol with cyclical progestogen is easy to apply. One should wait for 1 hour for the gel to dry up and not to be in contact with other members. It should not be applied over the breasts.

Centchroman (Ormeloxifen)

Centchroman is a nonsteroidal contraceptive developed in India at Central Drug Research Institute, Lucknow. Centchroman is a synthetic nonsteroidal contraceptive to be taken as 60 mg tablet twice a week for initial 3 months followed by a weekly dose. It is started on the first day of menses and taken twice weekly for 12 weeks and weekly thereafter (half-life is 170 hours). It does not prevent ovulation. It prevents implantation through endometrial changes. It exhibits a strong antioestrogenic and a weak oestrogenic action peripherally at the receptor level. The return of fertility occurs soon after stoppage of the drug (within 6 months).

Centchroman is not teratogenic or carcinogenic, exerts no pharmacological effect on other organs. The only side effect noted is prolonged cycles and oligomenorrhoea in 8% of cases. This is due to a prolonged proliferative phase. Pregnancy rate is 1.83 per 100 woman-years. The drug can also be used as a postcoital pill, given in 60 mg dose within 24 hours of coitus (two tablets repeated 12 hours later with failure rate of 1%). It has been developed by Central Drug Research Institute, Lucknow, and has been released in India under the name of *Saheli. It was introduced free of cost in India under family planning with the name of 'Chhaya'.*

Side Effects
- Headache, nausea, vomiting.
- Gain in weight.
- Does not protect against HIV and STD.
- Some delay in return of fertility (up to 6 months).
- Prolonged use causes – hyperplasia of endometrium.

Contraindications
- During 6 months of lactation.
- PCOD, hepatic dysfunction, cervical dysplasia, allergy to the drug.

EMERGENCY CONTRACEPTION (POSTCOITAL CONTRACEPTION)

Postcoital contraceptive agents are the methods used after unsafe coitus which prevent pregnancy by interfering with fertilization or implantation. They interfere with postovulatory events which normally result in pregnancy and are therefore known as **interceptives**. Recently, there is lot of emphasis on emergency contraception as it has been seen that most pregnancies result because of unexpected, unprotected intercourse or as a result of failure of contraceptives.

Emergency contraception is used following rape, unprotected intercourse or accidental rupture of a condom during coitus taking place around ovulation. It can also be used as backup method if woman has forgotten to take oral pills. These postcoital methods should be used mainly as 'backup' methods in these conditions and not as a regular contraceptive technique. If used frequently Emergency Contraception (EC) can cause menstrual irregularities, EC are also less effective than regular contraceptives.

The preparations available include following:

Two tablets of relatively high doses of a combined pill (ovral/Eugynon 50), containing 100 mcg EE_2 and 1 mg norethisterone, or 500 mcg LNG, taken within 72 hours of intercourse followed by two tablets taken 12 hours later (Yuzpe and Lancee, 1977). Failure rate is 3.2 per 100 woman-years.

Mode of action. The hormones may delay ovulation if taken soon after intercourse, cause corpus luteolysis and bring about cervical mucus changes and endometrial atrophy.

1. LNG Tablets

Prostinar tablet contains 0.75 mg LNG. One tablet should be taken within 72 hours of unprotected intercourse and another 12 hours later. Alternately, two tablets can be taken as a single dose. The failure rate is 1.1%. The tablets can be offered up to 120 hours; however, sooner the tablets taken after unprotected intercourse more effective they are but its efficacy decreases with the longer coital-drug interval. LNG prevents ovulation and causes desynchronization of endometrium through its receptors (luteal phase deficiency). The next menses may come earlier or delayed.

Side effects are those of progestogens. The hormone is not teratogenic in case pregnancy does occur but risk of ectopic pregnancy remains.

Advantages

- It has no oestrogen and its associated side effects.
- It can be offered to hypertensive, cardiac and diabetic woman.
- It can be offered to a lactating woman.
- It can be given as late as 120 hours after the unprotected intercourse.
- Single-dose therapy is an advantage.

Contraindicated in liver disease, contains lactate, so allergy to galactose. The drug is also contraindicated in a woman with history of thrombophlebitis and migraine.

2. RU486 (Mifepristone)

RU486 is a steroid with an affinity for progesterone receptors. It does not prevent fertilization but by blocking the action of progesterone on the endometrium, it causes sloughing and shedding of decidua and prevents implantation. It is not teratogenic.

A single dose of 25–50 mg is effective in preventing pregnancy in 99.1% cases (failure rate 0.9%). It causes delayed menstruation. Ectopic pregnancy is not avoided. The drug is expensive compared to LNG.

3. Ulipristal

Ulipristal is a synthetic progesterone hormone receptor modulator, it attaches to progesterone receptor and prevents/delays ovulation and suppresses endometrium, prevents implantation. A 30 mg tablet should be taken within 5 days. Two per cent pregnancy rate has been reported. Side effects are headache and mood changes.

4. Centchroman

Two tablets (60 mg) taken twice in 24 hours within 24 hours of intercourse can prevent implantation in 99% of women.

5. Prostaglandins

Self-administered vaginal suppository containing prostaglandin following an unprotected intercourse, by virtue of its luteolytic effect on the ovary and its increased motility effect on fallopian tubes and the uterus, prevents implantation and brings about menstruation. Its specific role as emergency contraceptive is however yet to be established.

6. Copper-T IUCD

Inserted within 5 days of unprotected intercourse can prevent implantation of a fertilized ovum. Advantages of Copper-T as emergency contraception are as follows:

- It can be inserted as late as 5 days after the unprotected intercourse.
- It is cheap.
- Failure rate is 0.1%.
- It can remain as on-going contraceptive method for 3–5 years.

The contraindications and complications of IUCD have already been mentioned.

IMMUNOLOGICAL METHODS OF CONTRACEPTION

Immunological approach to family planning is still in a developmental stage. Should immunology prove successful, family planning efforts will be simplified and will be more acceptable to the couples. The antigens which are being experimented upon are as follows:

- β-hCG subunit (300 mcg) i.m. 6-weekly × 3 doses evokes specific antibodies and thereby produces temporary sterility for 1 year.
- Zona pellucida plays an important role in fertility. The zona pellucida antibodies can either prevent penetration of ovum by the sperm or prevent shedding of zona after fertilization so that implantation is impossible.
- Antibodies to sperm antigens. These trials have not yet proved successful in human beings.
- Anti-FSH vaccine (inhibin) is also under trial.

PERMANENT METHODS OF CONTRACEPTION

Surgical Sterilization

The sterilization operation is undertaken with the primary objective of preventing further pregnancy permanently. Sterilization is suited to those couples who have completed their families and do not want to bear the inconvenience or cost of the other methods of contraception, and when the other methods are contraindicated.

An ideal method of sterilization should have the following characteristics:

- It should be an outpatient procedure.
- The anaesthesia should be local or short general anaesthesia, so that the woman or man can return home in a few hours.
- The surgical technique should be simple and quick.
- The instruments should be inexpensive.
- Minimal scar is desirable.
- The method should be 100% effective.
- Cost effective.
- The complications and sequelae of surgery should be minimal.
- The technique should be surgically reversible in case of unexpected disaster such as death of children.

MALE STERILIZATION

VASECTOMY

Vasectomy consists of dividing the vas deferens and disrupting the passage of sperms. It is done through a small incision in the scrotum, under local anaesthesia. The sterility is not immediate. The sperms are stored in the reproductive tract for up to 3 months. The couple must therefore abstain from intercourse during this period or use some other methods of contraception such as condoms. Approximately, 20 ejaculates clear the semen of all sperms. Two semen analysis reports must confirm the absence of sperms before the man can be declared sterile. No-scalpel technique has been now adopted. One single incision is made with a special forceps and skin stitch is not required. Clips and plugs can be applied over the vas instead of cutting. Vasectomy is cheaper than tubectomy (Fig. 19.17).

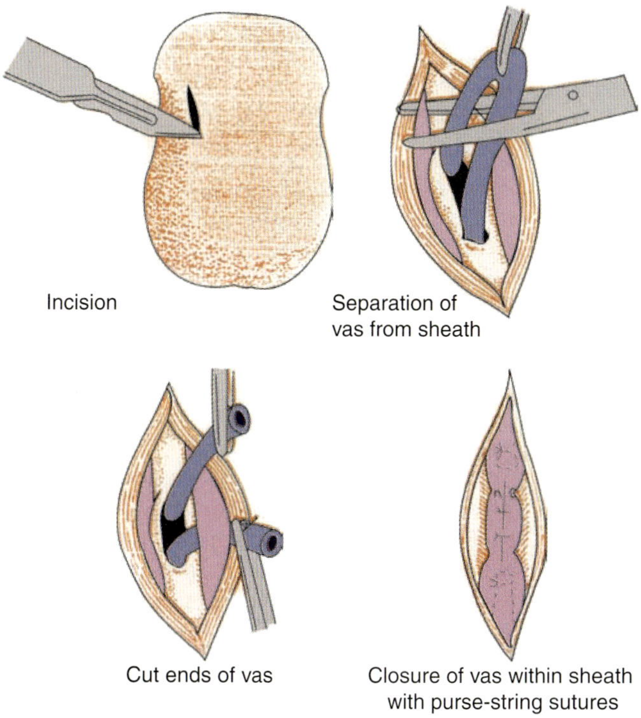

Figure 19.17 Vasectomy operation.

Reversible inhibition of sperm under guidance (RISUG) has been experimented by All India Institute of Medical Sciences and Indian Institute of Technology in India. A polymer gel is injected into the vas. Reversibility is possible by flushing the vas with sodium bicarbonate. This technique is under trial.

Complications of Vasectomy

- Local pain, skin discolouration, bleeding, haematoma formation (1%–2%).
- Infection (1%), trauma to the testicular artery causing gangrene, rare.
- Antibody formation and autoimmune disease (40%).
- Failure rate of 0.15 per 100 woman-years at the end of 1 year.
- Granuloma formation in 0.1%–3% cases.
- Spontaneous recanalization.
- Formation of spermatocele.
- Decreased libido or impotency are mainly psychological in origin and occur in men who were not properly motivated.
- Does not prevent HIV, STD.

Advantages

- It is an outpatient procedure.
- Local anaesthesia is adequate.
- It is a minor surgical procedure and the man can resume duty after rest of 1 or 2 days.
- Libido not affected. No evidence of prostate cancer.

REVERSIBLE INHIBITION OF SPERM UNDER GUIDANCE (RISUG)

NEWER TECHNIQUES

New nonsclerotic occlusive copolymer of styrene maleic anhydride (SMA) – lowers pH of semen and alters sperm transportation and morphological changes in the sperms. This copolymer is injected in the lumen of vas deferens under ultrasound guidance with the help of a fine hypodermic needle. Its action begins immediately and action can be reversed subsequently by injection of another copolymer which neutralizes its action.

Chemical sclerosing agents such as 90% ethanol, 3.6% formaldehyde, silver nitrate, hydrogen peroxide, acetic acid can eliminate the need of surgery, are effective and easily administered. However, the consequence of intravascular injection and excessive destruction of the vas by even a slight increase of instillation can be disastrous and the procedure is irreversible.

Occlusive plugs and intravasal devices are still in the experimental stage.

Plugs

A device called 'SHUG' consists of two flexible silicon plugs connected by a nylon thread which lies outside the vas. This thread prevents migration of plugs and allows easy removal through a small incision.

Contraindications to vasectomy are as follows:

- Local skin infection
- Varicocele, hernia
- Undescended testis

FEMALE STERILIZATION (TUBECTOMY, TUBAL STERILIZATION)

Tubal ligation can be done at any time convenient to the patient (Fig. 19.18 ▶). Postpartum sterilization is done within the first week of delivery when the patient is already hospitalized. Interval sterilization is done when the woman is not pregnant or any time after 6 weeks of delivery. Tubectomy can also be combined with caesarean section.

INDICATIONS

Apart from multiparity and the need of permanent method of family planning, sterilization may be advisable in women with medical diseases. Indications are as follows:

- Multiparity
- Three caesarean deliveries
- Medical diseases making a subsequent pregnancy high risk.
- Psychiatric problems
- Breast cancer

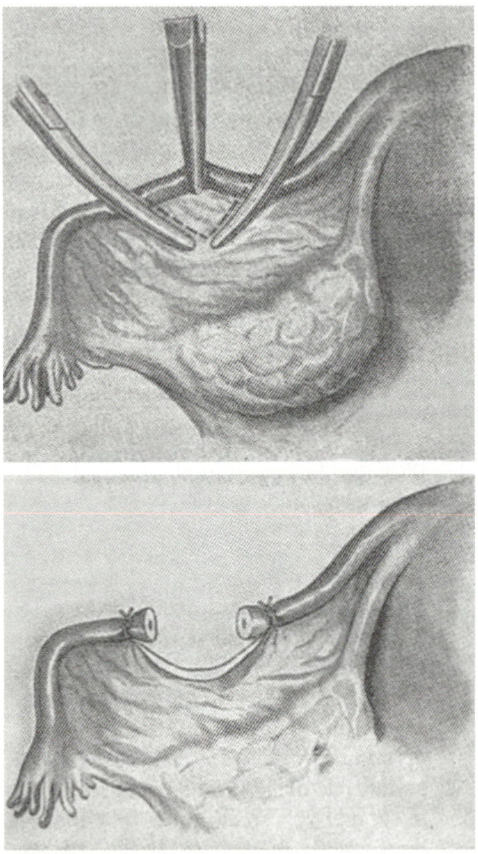

Figure 19.18 Operation for sterilization. The fallopian tube is drawn up with dissecting forceps in a position where the broad ligament is relatively bloodless and curved clamps are placed in position on each side. The tissue enclosed by the two clamps is then excised with a scalpel. Subsequently, the tissue enclosed in the clamps is ligatured. No effort is made to bury the cut ends of the fallopian tube. Although the operation is simple, it gives excellent results and subsequent adhesions have been shown to cause no trouble. (*Source:* From: Shaw's Textbook of Operative Gynaecology, Elsevier.)
▶ Scan to play Laparoscopic tubal sterilization

- Eugenic – repeat fetal malformations, haemophilia, Rh incompatibility, Wilson disease, Tay–Sachs disease and Marfan syndrome.

The interval surgery should preferably be done soon after menses to avoid the potential risk of pregnancy in the postovulatory period.

CONTRAINDICATIONS

1. Woman younger than 25 years (as directed by the Government of India).
2. Parity less than two children (as per the Government rule).
3. Local infection.

METHODS OF STERILIZATION (Figs 19.18–19.20)

1. Laparotomy
   - Pomeroy method
   - Madlener method
   - Irving method
   - Aldridge method
   - Cornual resection
   - Uchida method
   - Fimbriectomy
2. Minilaparotomy
   - Pomeroy
   - Madlener
   - Aldridge
   - Uchida
   - Fimbriectomy
3. Vaginal route
4. Laparoscopy – Silastic ring, bipolar cautery, Filshie clip.
5. Hysteroscopy – Chemical agents, Essure

Laparotomy

Laparotomy sterilization is performed during caesarean section and during gynaecological surgery.

Minilaparotomy

The operation is performed through a small incision less than 2.5 cm in length (Fig. 19.18). Because of its simplicity and ease of doing operation this procedure is advocated for routine sterilization especially in a smaller set up.

Pomeroy Method. The most popular technique of tubal ligation is the Pomeroy operation. The fallopian tube is identified on each side, brought out through the incision, the middle portion is held with a Babcock forceps and a small loop of fallopian tube is tied at the base with catgut suture and the portion between tied points is excised. The failure rate is 0.4% and it is mainly due to spontaneous canalization. The operation is simple, requires short hospitalization, does not require sophisticated and expensive equipment such as a laparoscope and can be performed in a primary health centre by a doctor trained in this procedure. If desired reversal of sterilization is possible.

Madlener Operation. A loop of the tube is crushed and ligated with a nonabsorbable suture. Failure rate of 7% and occurrence of ectopic pregnancy are unacceptable, though it is a simple procedure to perform.

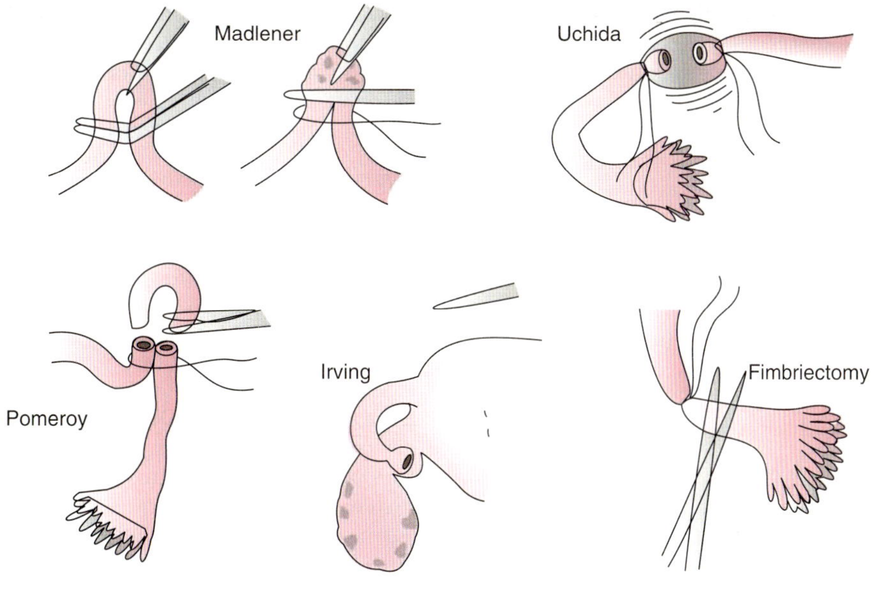

Figure 19.19 Different surgical techniques of sterilization.
Scan to play Minilap Tubal sterilization

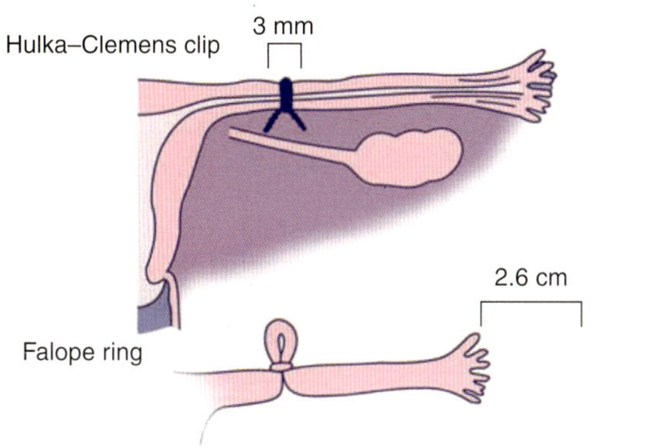

Figure 19.20 Application of Hulka–Clemens clip and Falope ring.

Irving Method. The mid-portion of the tube is ligated and the intervening portion excised. The proximal end is buried in the myometrium and the distal end is buried in the broad ligament. It is a reliable method but irreversible and may require a laparotomy incision.

Aldridge Method. A hole is made in the anterior leaf of the broad ligament and the fimbrial end is buried into this. The high failure rate is due to the fimbrial end popping out and restoring the patency of the tube.

Cornual Resection. The cornual portion of the tube is resected near its uterine attachment. The technique is complicated and the uterine end tends to bleed heavily. This may also require a laparotomy incision.

Uchida Method. The tubal serosa is stripped off the muscular layer in the mid-segment of the tube, which is then excised. The proximal end is ligated and buried in the broad ligament. The minimal excision of the tube preserves the potential for tuboplasty.

Fimbriectomy. Excision of fimbria results in permanent sterilization and leaves no potential for reversibility.

Vaginal Tubal Ligation

Vaginal tubal ligation is not popular because of higher morbidity and because of relatively more difficulty in performing the procedure. The pouch of Douglas is opened after placing patient in a lithotomy position, the fallopian tube is hooked out with finger or Babcock and tubectomy performed. It is associated with risk of pelvic infection, higher failure rate and it is more difficult to perform. It is mainly combined with the Manchester repair operation for prolapse of uterus.

Laparoscopic Sterilization

This technique has become the most commonly used technique of tubal sterilization. Laparoscopic sterilization is carried out under local or general anaesthesia. A small subumbilical incision is made and pneumoperitoneum created by inserting a Veress needle and introducing CO_2. CO_2 is safer than air and nitrous oxide which can cause air embolism and accidental explosion, respectively. With the patient in the head low position, the trocar and cannula are inserted through the incision and an operating laparoscope introduced after removing the trocar. The illumination of the pelvic organs for visualization is by fibreoptic light. The uterus is manipulated from below by an assistant so that the fallopian tubes are moved to the centre of the operating field. Each fallopian tube is picked up near the isthmic end (2–3 cm away) and it clipped/banded (silastic bands) (Filshie, Hulka band, silastic ring) or cauterization of a segment of the tube done with a bipolar cautery. The gas is allowed to escape at the end of the procedure and the instruments are removed. A subcuticular skin stitch completes the operation. The failure rate with this technique is 0.6 per 100 woman-years.

The earlier cauterization technique has now been replaced by the silastic Falope ring, Hulka clip and Filshie clip, which are safer (Fig. 19.19). Monopolar cauterization is liable to cause accidental intestinal burns and destroy a considerable part of the tubal structure with a disadvantage if recanalization is required at a later date. The Falope silastic ring destroys 2–3 cm of the fallopian tube. The Hulka and

Filshie clips destroy a smaller segment (3–4 mm), thus preserving the potential for successful reversal of sterilization if needed later. The failure rate varies between 0.2% and 1.5%.

Falope ring, introduced by Yoon in 1974, is a silastic band with 3.6 mm and 1 mm outer and inner ring diameter, respectively, and is 2.2 mm thick. It is impregnated with barium sulphate for radiological visualization.

Advantages. Laparoscopic sterilization has gained popularity all over the world as it has a number of advantages:

- Subumbilical scar is small and nearly invisible.
- It can be done under local anaesthesia in the out-patient department.
- It is highly reversible, with a success rate of 70% or more.

Disadvantages.
- The equipment is expensive and maintenance is not easy.
- Experienced personnel are required to perform this operation.
- Mortality of 1–2 per 100,000 and is now very low with experience.

Complications. Complications are uncommon but when they do occur, they are serious in nature. Seen usually in the hands of inexperienced personnel:

- Abdominal wall emphysema due to a wrong placement of the needle.
- Bleeding from superior epigastric vessel by trocar injury.
- Tearing of the mesosalpinx and bleeding.
- Uterine perforation.
- A wrong application of the ring, e.g. putting the ring on round ligament/mesosalpinx/utero-ovarian ligament, will cause operation failure.
- Failure rate varies between 0.4% and 2.5%. Although cauterization carries a failure of 0.8%, Hulka clip has a failure rate of 2.3% and Falope ring 0.8%. Most failures occur within 2 years of operation. At the end of 10 years, failure is reported in 1.8% of cases.
- Spontaneous recanalization occurs if cauterization is incomplete.
- Ectopic pregnancy is reported in 0.2%–0.3%.
- Hydrosalpinx formation if the tube is occluded at two places some distance apart.

Contraindications. The laparoscopic sterilization is contraindicated in following situations:

- In a patient with a cardiac or pulmonary disease, head low position and CO_2 are contraindicated.
- Previous abdominal surgery exposes the patient to the risk of intestinal trauma in case parietal adhesions are present.
- Puerperal cases. The fallopian tubes are oedematous and vascular and may easily get torn. The uterus is soft and can get easily perforated with the uterine manipulator.
- Extreme obesity, diaphragmatic or umbilical hernia. The increased risk of interstitial injury in these cases.
- In PID, the fallopian tubes may not be easily visible amongst the adhesions.

Due to associated morbidity, the Government of India has forbidden laparoscopic sterilization combined with MTP or in the puerperal period.

- Skin infection, anaemia, thrombophlebitis.

Hysteroscopic Sterilization

In this technique during hysteroscopy either a chemical agent or some plug is introduced in the cornual of the fallopian tube. The technique of using sclerosing agents and quinacrine has been abandoned because of high failure rate, and other complications such as uterine perforation, burn injury and infection.

Essure Contraceptive Device (Fig. 19.10). Recently, a new device called Essure has become available in developed countries, which is inserted in the cornual of the tube during hysteroscopy. The technique of 'Essure permanent device' is a dynamically expanding microinserter consisting of a flexible inner coil made of stainless steel and a dynamic outer coil made of nickel titanium alloy (Nitinol). The device is 4 cm long with inner 0.8 mm diameter. Running along and through the inner coil is a layer of polyethylene terephthalate (PET) fibres, which initiate a benign local fibrous tissue growth responsible for the occlusion of the fallopian tube. The guide wire guides the device into the fallopian tube.

During the insertion, the outer coil is wound down to keep it in a low-profile position. Upon release, the outer coil expands to 1.5–2 mm from 0.8 mm and anchors tissue device firmly in the fallopian tube. It takes 3 months to occlude the tube, during which other contraceptive is required to protect against pregnancy. This is an irreversible and permanent technique. Hysterosalpingography 3 months later should confirm tubal blockage.

Kerin devised this technique. PET fibres are effective and unlike liquid sclerosing agents, do not cause chemical peritonitis.

Buscopan and NSAID are required to prevent tubal spasm and facilitate proper insertion via hysteroscope. Failure rate of 3.5% is reported.

Optimal placement of Essure device at the proximal fallopian tube allows the device to span the utero-tubal junction. The device is placed far enough to allow the tubal block, while a portion of the device trails into the uterine cavity (4–8 coils).

Disadvantages
- Hysteroscopy is required.
- Cost and expertise required.
- Permanent method.
- hCG to confirm blockage.
- 3 months waiting.
- Bilateral insertion difficult due to spasm in 15% of cases.
- Tuboplasty for reversal not possible.
- Perforation of the tube

Advantage. No abdominal scar and can be done under local anaesthesia.

Complications and Sequelae of Female Sterilization
- Anaesthetic complications.
- Mortality of 4 per 100,000 procedures is due to haemorrhage, sepsis and embolism, and anaesthetic risks.

- Morbidity is due to postoperative lung infection, abdominal wound sepsis, peritonitis.
- Trauma to the bladder, bowel may occur with a laparoscopic technique.
- Thrombophlebitis and embolism is rare, but may complicate puerperal sterilization.
- Pelvic adhesions.
- Failure rate of sterilization varies from 0.4% in Pomeroy technique, 0.3%–0.6% by laparoscopic method to 7% by Madlener method. Pregnancy occurs either because of undiagnosed corpus luteal phase pregnancy, faulty technique or due to spontaneous recanalization.
- Ectopic pregnancy. Partial spontaneous recanalization may result in ectopic pregnancy, and estimated rate is 0.6 per 1000 sterilized women.
- AUB following sterilization is seen in 15% of cases but the exact aetiology is not known.
- Regret and depression may ensue especially when death of a child follows sterilization. Request for tuboplasty is made when a child dies or a change of partner occurs as in remarriage. The success of tuboplasty is 70%–80%. Libido is not usually affected.

MIRENA VERSUS TUBECTOMY (Table 19.3)

Lately, Mirena is emerging as an alternative to tubectomy especially in young women who may want to retain fertility and avoid a permanent method.

Mirena may be a better choice in the presence of following conditions:

1. Heavy menstrual bleeding.
2. Dysmenorrhoea.
3. Pelvic endometriosis, adenomyosis and myoma.

CONTRACEPTION FOR ADOLESCENTS

In India, many girls get married at an early age and become mothers. They need counselling regarding spacing and delaying the birth of the next child. Unmarried adolescents are exposed to the risk of unwanted pregnancy and unsafe abortion, as well as the possibility of acquiring AIDS and sexually transmitted infections.

Family planning and contraception become important health care issues amongst adolescents. Although sex education will provide benefit, many will require contraceptive guidance and provision of a suitable contraception.

Table 19.3 Comparison of Mirena and Tubectomy

Mirena	Tubectomy
• Effective	Effective
• Reversible	Surgically reversible – success 70%
• Bleeding, dysmenorrhoea less	Menstrual Bleeding may increase in 15%
• Cheaper than surgery	Costly
• No Surgery, anaesthesia complications avoided	Surgery, anaesthesia required
• Ectopic pregnancy (0.2/1000)	Risk of ectopic pregnancy slightly increased
• Ovarian function not compromised	May be compromised

BARRIER METHOD

It is the best method in young girls. Apart from providing contraceptive method, it can prevent transmission of infections from one partner to the other.

If the man refuses to use condoms, a married woman can use *Today* sponge with spermicidal cream. A recently married woman may find barrier method cumbersome in the initial stages.

The adolescent should receive informed knowledge on 'unsafe period' when ovulation occurs, and be provided with emergency contraception such as LNG, two tablets. This is because periodic abstinence is difficult amongst the young couples.

IUCD

While IUCD may not be a suitable contraceptive device in the unmarried and recently married nulliparous women, it is a long-term coital-independent method suited to young parous women, provided no contraindication exists for its use. It is one of the best methods for spacing childbirth. Progesterone copper device is recommended if the woman has heavy periods with dysmenorrhoea.

HORMONAL CONTRACEPTIVES

COC pills can be safely prescribed to adolescents. One must remember the possibility of breast cancer at a later date if the young nulliparous woman younger than 24 years of age takes COC for more than 4 years.

POPs are not preferred over COC, because of the irregular bleeding, amenorrhoea, a higher failure rate and osteopenia.

Three-monthly injections or implants, skin patches and vaginal rings may be acceptable to young married adolescents, and side effects tolerated. Occasional failure may be backed up with MTP facilities.

Sterilization should not be offered to young couples. The Government of India has passed a law that the surgical procedure should not be performed in a woman younger than 25 years with two or less children and the youngest child less than 2 years old.

MTP and emergency contraception should form the backup procedures in these girls.

PERMANENT STERILIZATION AFTER CHILD BIRTH

A multiparous woman may be counselled on sterilization or vasectomy. This is done any time after 24 hours of delivery, so the woman need not return to the hospital for tubectomy later, and this is cost-effective and convenient. Minilaparotomy is a simple and a quick procedure done under local or a short general anaesthesia.

CONTRACEPTION FOR A LACTATING WOMAN

LACTATING WOMAN

Regular lactation with one feed at night delays ovulation and pregnancy for up to 6 months, provided she remains amenorrhoeic. After 6 months, lactation has no bearing on ovulation and pregnancy can occur, despite amenorrhoea. Thereafter, the woman needs some form of contraceptive precaution.

POP does not suppress lactation or alter the quantity and quality of milk. It can be started after 6 weeks of delivery. Irregular periods during this period is taken as a puerperal event and accepted by the woman. Instead of oral pills, implants and injection are other alternatives.

Oral combined pill in a lactating woman is contraindicated because of following reasons:

- It reduces the quality and quantity of milk.
- Hormone secreted in the milk may be harmful to the infant.
- There is increased risk of thromboembolism.

IUCD can be inserted immediately after the delivery.

- Male condoms are safe and effective.

CONTRACEPTION FOR A WOMAN WITH HIV INFECTION

Condoms are the best in prevention of transmission of infection from one partner to the other. Female barrier methods are not as effective as male condoms, except Femshield.

The failure rate with condom is high, so dual method of using hormonal contraceptives (COC) or IUCD is desirable. IUCD can be inserted provided the woman has not suffered from PID and is on medication. The screening for other STD becomes part of screening procedures before inserting an IUCD. Surgical procedures are not contraindicated in these women.

CONTRACEPTION FOR WOMEN OLDER THAN 35 YEARS

Women older than 35 years constitute 20% of the contraceptive users, and selection of the proper contraception is an essential component of family planning counselling. A woman after the age of 35 years may become obese, hypertensive and diabetic. She is likely to suffer AUB. The choice depends upon the suitability, contraindication and side effects.

STERILIZATION

When considering a permanent method of sterilization, one should weigh the risk of surgical procedure against the number of years a woman needs contraceptive protection. In a woman nearer the menopause with a fewer years of fertility, surgical procedure may not be a wise proposition, and temporary methods will be cost-effective as well as safe, with emergency contraception and MTP as a back-up method.

LOW-DOSE COC PILLS

They are safe, if the woman is thin, nonsmoker without any medical disease up to the age of 45 years.

Although POPs may be safer than COC, its adverse effect on bone density and occurrence of osteoporosis must be borne in mind if given over a prolonged period. Besides, they cause irregular bleeding, and the risk of breast cancer increases.

IUCD may be suitable and effective. If the woman suffers from menorrhagia, Mirena may be inserted and is effective for 5 years.

Desogestrel and gestodene cause thromboembolism and are contraindicated in elderly women.

CONTRACEPTION FOR A WOMAN WITH MEDICAL DISEASE

The risk of pregnancy should be weighed against the risk of any contraception in a woman with medical disorder. While prescribing a family planning method, *due consideration and counselling related to side effects is necessary*.

If the risk is negligible, sterilization provides the permanent method to prevent a pregnancy. Vasectomy would be ideal, with no risk to the woman.

IUCD is carefully considered in cardiac and diabetic women, because of the possibility of pelvic infection.

COC is contraindicated in a hypertensive, cardiac and diabetic women, as well as a woman with breast cancer, liver disease and previous thromboembolism. An epileptic woman and a woman on antitubercular drugs such as rifamycin may face a higher failure rate due to interaction with rifamycin and antiepileptic drugs except sodium valproate.

Similarly POP is contraindicated in liver diseases, vascular disorders and breast cancer. It is safe in sickle cell anaemia.

Emergency contraception (LNT tablets) is safe in a woman with medical disorders.

Contraception for a Woman with Psychiatric Disorder.

If a woman is considered unfit to bear children, and permanent method considered, a written opinion regarding psychiatric problem should be obtained. The written consent should be obtained from the husband or guardian, as the psychiatric patient may not be mentally aware of the nature of sterilization.

Emergency contraception is no bar to a woman with a medical disorder, as only two tablets are given in 24 hours.

WHO CONTRACEPTIVE WHEEL

WHO has introduced a small wheel-like device which can help doctor to decide whether a particular method of contraception is safe for a woman who has some associated disease. Recently WHO has come out with an easy to use disc like device called Contraceptive Wheel. It helps clinician to choose a safe method of contraception in the presence of a significant medical/surgical condition. Each contraceptive has been categorized into four categories with a range where category I means safe to use without any health risk, whereas category II indicates use of a method is more advantageous than risk, category III indicates risks are more than usual, however, method of contraception can be used with caution whereas category IV means that use of contraceptive method is absolutely contraindicated in a given health condition which women might be suffering. This contraceptive wheel is user friendly and makes clinician decide the best contraceptive for a woman.

MALE CONTRACEPTION

There have been attempts to find out a safe method of contraception for males other than vasectomy. Till now there is no proven method of male contraception because of several reasons such as high count of sperms in ejaculate, a long period of 72 days for spermatogenesis and high incidence of side effects.

Following approaches are being tested for male contraception.

METHODS BASED ON SUPPRESSION OF SPERMATOGENESIS

GOSSYPOL

Its use as a male contraceptive was discovered in China. Gossypol is a yellow pigment isolated from cottonseed oil. It is administered orally 10–20 mg daily for 3 months and thereafter 20 mg twice weekly. The action is directly on the seminiferous tubules inhibiting spermatogenesis without altering FSH and LH levels. The side effects such as weakness, hypokalaemia and permanent sterility in 20% of cases limit its use.

TESTOSTERONE ENANTHATE

- Testosterone enanthate 200 mg injection weekly causes azoospermia in 6–12 months. Testosterone buciclate 600 mg 3-monthly is also effective through negative feedback mechanism without loss of libido.
- Instead of weekly injection, testosterone decanoate 1000 mg i.m. followed by 500 mg 4-weekly is more convenient.
- Four implants of 200 mg each of testosterone every 4–6 months with 300 mg medroxyprogesterone 3-monthly is successful in 96% of cases with count less than 1 million/mL.

Side effects – osteopenia, liver and lipid metabolism dysfunction, prostate enlargement.

GNRH

The continuous administration of analogues of gonadotropin-releasing hormone (GnRH) causes a fall in the sperm count and sperm motility. The level of testosterone also falls. The loss of libido and osteoporosis make this regime unacceptable over a long period. Besides, it is very expensive and needs to be given subcutaneously.

MEDROXYPROGESTERONE ACETATE

Medroxyprogesterone acetate 250 mg i.m. with 200 mg norethisterone given as weekly injections is reported to suppress spermatogenesis with 97% success.

DESOGESTREL

It has androgenic property. 75–300 mcg daily with subcutaneous pellets of testosterone 300 mcg causes oligospermia, without altering the level of HDL.

The hormonal suppression of spermatogenesis causes loss of libido and is toxic in high doses. Besides, the injection of hormones is inconvenient to administer regularly. The acne, weight gain and decreased HDL are other side effects. Immunological methods of suppressing spermatogenesis have not yet been successful.

Synthetic hormone – 7 alpha-methyl-nortestosterone (MENT) used as substitute of testosterone–no side effects.

KEY POINTS

- Family planning and contraception has gained momentum world over with an urgent need to control the world population as well as to promote woman's health.
- This has resulted in continuous effort to discover newer methods and new modes of delivery with optimal effectiveness but with minimal side effects.
- Barrier methods, both male and female, apart from their contraceptive effect, have the advantages of preventing transmission of STDs, HIV and reducing the incidence of cancer of the cervix. A high failure rate of 10–14 per 100 per woman-year users with barrier methods can be improved by a backup method such as use of emergency contraception if unprotected intercourse occurs around ovulation. These advantages along with the low cost and excellent reversibility can enhance the use of this method in preventing an unwanted pregnancy.
- Newer formulations containing extremely small dose of oestrogens and an effective progestogen has reduced the failure rate and side effects of oral contraceptive pills.
- IUCD is an established method of female contraception in India on account of one-time insertion, low cost and long efficacy. Progesterone-impregnated IUCD has an added advantage of reducing menstrual bleeding, but it is expensive. The removal rate of 5%–10% on account of side effects is acceptable.
- Newer drug delivery systems are continuously on trial, and their advantages, disadvantages, effectiveness and reversibility are being studied. This has resulted in availability of implants, vaginal rings and contraceptives skin patches.
- OCPs offer a number of health benefits in addition to contraception.
- POP are particularly useful when oestrogen is contraindicated or its side effects are intolerable. POP is as effective as IUCD but less effective than COC. It can be used by the lactating woman, unlike COC.
- Centchroman as an oral contraceptive pill is available in India. It is cheap and needs to be taken once a week.
- Vasectomy and tubectomy are the surgical methods offered only when a permanent method is desired by the couple.
- Emergency contraceptive also known as postcoital contraception is an innovative technique of preventing conception if rape or unprotected intercourse occurs around ovulation. This method has a 95%–98% success rate and thus avoids MTP.
- A wide range of contraceptives allow a wider selection of choice to the couples and improves the acceptability of one or more methods.

SELF-ASSESSMENT

1. Discuss the advantages and disadvantages of oral combined contraceptive pills.
2. What are the contraindications to oral combined pills?
3. What is the role of minipills in contraception?
4. Discuss the complications and contraindications of intrauterine device.
5. Write short notes on:
   - Hormonal implants
   - Vasectomy
   - Barrier contraceptives
6. Discuss the uses of Mirena and Copper-T.

SUGGESTED READING

Alison Scott, Anna Glasier: Evidence based contraceptive choices. Best Practice and Research Clinical Obstetrics and Gynaecology. Vol 20:5,665–680, Elsevier, 2006.

Duncan Jeffrey S, Shulman Lee P Duncan, Schuman. Year Book of Obstetrics, Gynaecology, and Women's Health. Page 295, John Wiley & Sons, 2010.

Panay N, Studd J: Noncontraceptive uses of the hormone releasing intrauterine system. Studd J: Progress in Obstetrics and Gynaecology. Vol 13:379–395, Churchill Livingstone: Elsevier, 1998.

Medical Termination of Pregnancy

20

CHAPTER OUTLINE

MEDICAL TERMINATION OF PREGNANCY

Voluntary termination of pregnancy before 20 weeks of pregnancy has been legalized in India by a law passed by the Parliament in the year 1972. This legislation was adopted with an aim of reducing incidence of unsafe abortion by an untrained person. There has always been a need for termination of pregnancy if it is associated with risk to the life of women, pregnancy resulted because of sexual abuse or where pregnancy was undesirable or as a result of contraceptive failure. Before this Act, a pregnant woman sought help of untrained persons to get rid of unwanted pregnancy risking her physical health and her life. A number of other countries in the world also have legalized abortions as a safety measure for pregnant woman. Although law is called as medical Termination of Pregnancy (MTP), both medical and occasionally surgical methods are employed for termination of pregnancy. However, many governments in the world over have liberalized 'Abortion Laws' in keeping with changing times, accepting the recognition of the right of the individual to bear a child at her chosen time and helping to curb the malpractices accompanying illegal abortions. In India, the MTP Act was adopted as a health measure way back in 1972 to avoid death due to criminal abortions.

DEFINITION

The MTP Act permits the wilful termination of pregnancy before the age of fetal viability (20 weeks' gestation) for well-defined indications. It has to be performed by recognized medical practitioners in a recognized place approved by the competent authority under the Act.

INCIDENCE

It has been estimated that the total number of abortions performed globally is approximately 46 million annually; of these, 26 million take place in countries where abortions are legalized. In India, 6.7 million MTPs take place annually. However, exact incidence remains unknown. In women undergoing MTP, 40% pregnancies are unplanned and 25% are unwanted. Despite the law, 40%–50% of abortions are unsafe terminations of pregnancy done by unqualified persons under unhygienic conditions.

GROUNDS FOR PERFORMING MTP

The MTP Act has permitted termination of pregnancy for following indications:

MEDICAL GROUNDS

When the continuation of pregnancy is likely to (i) endanger the life of the pregnant women or (ii) cause grievous injury to her physical and/or mental health, as in cases of severe hypertension, cardiac disease, diabetes, psychiatric illnesses, genital and breast cancer.

EUGENIC GROUNDS

When ultrasound shows a malformed embryo or fetus or there is a substantial risk of the child being born with serious physical or mental abnormalities. For example, hereditary disorders, congenital malformation in previous offspring with a high risk of recurrence in subsequent childbirth/Rh-isoimmunization, teratogenic drugs and maternal rubella posing risk of anomalies in the fetus. Chorion villus biopsy, cordocentesis and sonographic evaluation of the fetus have contributed significantly in identifying the fetuses at risk.

HUMANITARIAN GROUNDS

In cases when the pregnancy is caused by rape or incest.

SOCIAL GROUNDS

When: (i) in the actual or reasonably foreseeable future, her environment (social or economic) might lead to risk of injury to her mental or physical health. (ii) pregnancy resulting from failure of contraceptive device or method.

The written consent of the patient on a specially prescribed form is necessary before undertaking the procedure. The written consent of the legal guardian must be obtained in case the woman is younger than 18 years or she is mentally ill, even if she is older than 18 years.

Indications of MTP are as follows:

- Maternal medical disorders
- Fetal conditions
- Rape, incest
- Failure of contraceptives
- Social grounds

WHO CAN PERFORM MTP?

Only doctors who have been registered and authorized by the District Health Authorities for the purpose of carrying out MTP can carry out MTP. Generally for carrying out the first-trimester MTP, opinion and signature of one doctor is sufficient. However, for the termination of pregnancy between 12 and 20 weeks, opinion of two certified doctors is must.

THE PLACE FOR PERFORMING MTP

The Act stipulates that MTP can be performed only at: (i) a hospital established and maintained by the government, (ii) a place recognized and approved by the government, under this Act.

- Abortion services are provided under this Act at these centres under strict confidentiality.
- The identity of the person is treated as a statutory personal matter.
- Ultrasonic scanning plays an important role in confirming uterine pregnancy, estimating gestational age, detecting malformed embryo and sometimes in performing MTP under ultrasonic guidance.

HOW TO COMPLY WITH THE INDIAN MTP ACT AND ENSURE QUALITY CARE

- Ensure proper case selection: Document meticulously the patient' age, gestational maturity and indication for MTP.
- Essential investigations performed such as haemoglobin, urine routine, blood group and Rh factor and sonography whenever necessary.
- Opinion of one medical practitioner for the first-trimester MTP, and opinions of two medical practitioners for the second-trimester MTP.
- MTP to be performed by a registered medical practitioner approved for undertaking MTP in a place recognized under the MTP Act.
- Documents to be maintained: Form I, Form II and admission register.

IMPLICATIONS OF THE MTP ACT

In countries with liberal abortion laws, maternal morbidity and mortality have declined, and women have been motivated to accept birth control measures. Deaths due to illegal abortions (500 per 100,000) are mostly due to haemorrhage (20%), sepsis, embolism (20%–25%), anaemia and gut injury. Mortality and morbidity increases with each week of gestation, and is fivefold to tenfold higher in the second trimester compared to the first-trimester MTP.

Table 20.1 Methods of the First-Trimester MTP

6–8 weeks pregnancy	Medical abortion, menstrual regulation
8–12 weeks pregnancy	Suction evacuation, medical methods
12–14 weeks pregnancy	Extra amniotic drugs, intramuscular prostaglandins, vaginal misoprostol

Repeated abortions are not conducive to a woman's health; hence, MTP should not be considered as a birth control measure and should not replace prevailing methods of contraception. Even in the best of circumstances, there is a small inherent risk in the procedure of MTP. This should serve as a warning that MTP can never be as safe as efficient contraception. The woman undergoing MTP should be counselled to accept a safe method of contraception.

When properly counselled, MTP can indirectly promote family planning and population control.

METHODS OF MTP

There are different methods adopted for termination of the first- and second-trimester pregnancies.

Methods of MTP can be broadly classified as follows (also refer Table 20.1):

Methods of the first-trimester MTP

- Menstrual regulation
- Dilatation and suction evacuation
- Cervical softening before dilatation and suction evacuation
- Medical methods

Methods of the second-trimester MTP

- Prostaglandins given vaginally, intraamniotic, extra amniotic or intramuscular
- Surgical evacuation
- Extraovular instillation of drugs such as ethacridine lactate
- Extrauterine methods

The above methods are used singly or in combination. The oxytocic drugs stimulate myometrial activity and shorten the induction–abortion interval in the second trimester. Similarly, the use of prostaglandins (gel, suppository) a few hours before the procedure helps to attain a gradual softening and atraumatic dilatation of the cervix, facilitating further dilatation and evacuation procedures.

FIRST-TRIMESTER MTP

SURGICAL METHODS

Menstrual Regulation

Menstrual regulation consists of aspiration of the contents of the uterine cavity by means of a disposable plastic cannula (Karman's cannula). It has an attached plastic 50 mL syringe capable of creating a vacuum of 65 cm Hg (Fig. 20.1). It has a simple thumb-operated pressure control valve and a

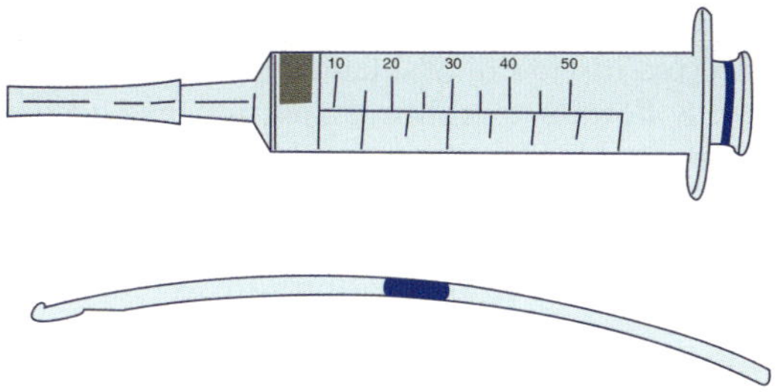

Figure 20.1 Menstrual regulation syringe with Karman cannula.

piston-locking handle. It is independent of electricity, is portable and washable. It is effective when carried out on pregnancy within 42 days of the last menstrual period (LMP). A paracervical local anaesthetic block or preoperative sedative alone usually suffices but sometimes in an apprehensive patient, general anaesthesia may be necessary. This procedure can be performed in an office set-up, outpatient clinic or day-care centre. Since 1972, this method has been extensively evaluated and found to be efficient, safe and easy to use in terminating early pregnancy. It is a good practice to examine the products of conception following the procedure. The occasional complications encountered include failure to evacuate leading to continuation of pregnancy, incomplete evacuation, haemorrhage, cervical laceration, perforation, infection and anaesthetic complications. If pregnancy was not confirmed by ultrasound, an ectopic pregnancy may be missed.

A failure to evacuate is due to following reasons:

1. Too early a pregnancy.
2. Ectopic pregnancy.
3. Uterus bicornuate, aspiration being carried out in a non-pregnant horn.

Rh anti-D globulin 50 mcg i.m. should be given to an Rh-negative nonimmunized woman with pregnancy less than 12 weeks.

Medical Abortion

Of late termination of early pregnancy (less than 49–63 days) is being carried out with the use of mifepristone (RU486) and misoprostol. This method avoids need for a surgical method such as menstrual regulation. In India termination of pregnancy up to 49 days has been permitted for the use of a medical method. In a confirmed pregnancy, the woman is initially given a tablet of mifepristone containing 200 mg of drug, followed by vaginal administration of 800 mcg of misoprostol. In most cases, abortion is successful within few hours after administration of misoprostol. Most women experience continuation of bleeding for a period of 7–14 days. A repeat ultrasound after 14 days is carried out to check for any retained products or possible continuation of pregnancy. Some patients may require suction evacuation for heavy bleeding after medical abortion. Prophylactic antibiotics are given for a period of 48 hours to 5 days. Rh-negative woman should receive anti-D injection. World over this method has taken over the surgical evacuation for termination of early pregnancy. To avoid complications on a rare occasion, it will be good idea to visit a doctor and avoid self-administration of drugs. In India, regulations advise registration of cases in an MTP clinic and drugs to be dispensed on the prescription of a certified doctor.

TERMINATION OF PREGNANCY BETWEEN 8 AND 12 WEEKS

Vacuum Evacuation (Suction Evacuation)

Vacuum evacuation is the most efficient method of terminating pregnancy up to 12 weeks of gestation. It has gained rapid acceptance worldwide. The operation can be generally undertaken under local anaesthetic, paracervical block, coupled with some sedation if necessary. Apprehensive patients may need general anaesthesia. The procedure involves examination of the patient in the operation theatre observing full aseptic precautions. The gestation size and the position of the uterus are carefully assessed. After administering a paracervical block, the cervix is held with an Allis/vulsellum forceps and dilated by means of Hegar's or some other metal dilators until adequate dilation is achieved to permit introduction of the suction cannula of the appropriate size (diameter corresponding to the weeks of gestation) into the uterine cavity (Fig. 20.2). A standard negative suction of 650 mm (65 cm) of Hg is created and the products are aspirated. When the procedure is completed, a grating sensation is felt all around the uterine cavity, no further tissue is aspirated and the internal os begins to grip the Karman cannula which may also reveal a blood-stained froth. There is no need to follow this up with a check curettage with a sharp curette, as this step can be traumatic and lead to complications such as perforation, synechiae (Asherman syndrome), and predispose to placenta accreta in a future pregnancy. In case the pregnancy exceeds 8-week gestation size, the patient is nulliparous or there is presence of a uterine scar, general anaesthesia may be preferred.

In case of large uterus of 10- to 12-week gestation size, or nulliparous cervix, priming the cervix with prostaglandin gel or suppository, at least 4 hours earlier helps to soften the cervix so that it yields more easily and undue force is avoided during cervical dilatation. This precaution safeguards against complications such as cervical tear, lacerations and injury to the internal os leading to incompetent cervix; 200–400 mcg misoprostol pessary is inserted in the vagina (prostaglandin E_1).

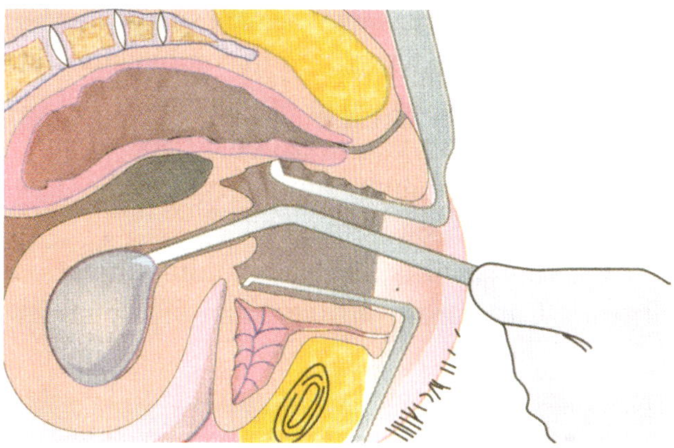

Figure 20.2 Suction evacuation - aspiration of the products of conception.

Vacuum aspiration as a method of MTP has a very low failure rate (<1%). Complications such as incomplete evacuation, infection, uterine perforation and excessive bleeding occur in less than 2% of cases. The mortality is less than 2 per 100,000 procedures. Nonimmunized Rh-negative mothers must receive 100 mcg of anti-D immunoglobulin after undergoing MTP. Failure to end pregnancy is due to a very early pregnancy, unrecognized ectopic pregnancy and pregnancy in a rudimentary horn. Preoperative ultrasound is useful in preventing these complications.

MEDICAL METHODS

Prostaglandins and RU486 have been extensively used as medical methods of MTP in early pregnancy. Acting singly, they are not as effective as when used in combination. The medical method avoids hospitalization but the prolonged observation, occasional need of surgical termination (failure) and the cost of the drugs are some of the disadvantages.

Prostaglandins

Prostaglandin Injections (Prostin, Carboprost-prostaglandin $F_2\alpha$) 250 mcg given i.m. every 3 hours up to a maximum of 10 doses has been found to be effective in initiating the process of abortion. It has not been popular in the first trimester because of an unacceptably high incidence of incomplete abortion (20%) requiring surgical intervention to complete the procedure, and the high rate of unpleasant side effects such as nausea, vomiting, diarrhoea, cramping abdominal pain, bronchospasm and mild fever at times.

Mifepristone (Mifegest – RU486)

First invented in France, in 1980, RU486 stands for Roussel Uclaf 486 (laboratory number).

It is a synthetic steroid, a derivative of 19-nortestosterone, with antiprogestogenic effect. It also has antiglucocorticoid and weak antiandrogenic action. By competing with progesterone receptors, it reduces the endometrial glandular activity, accelerates degenerative changes and increases stromal action, thereby causing sloughing of endometrium. It thus prevents or disturbs implantation of the fertilized ovum through luteolysis.

It also causes uterine contractions, softens and slightly dilates the cervix.

Used singly, it is effective in 83% cases, and causes incomplete abortion in 10%–20% cases. Adding prostaglandin yields a success rate of 95% in pregnancies less than 63 days duration, with 4% incomplete abortion and continuation of pregnancy in 1% cases.

The protocol is as follows:

- Written consent for MTP is required.
- Blood group Rh, Hb%, urine albumin
- Ultrasound is done to confirm uterine pregnancy and duration, and exclude ectopic pregnancy.

  Day 1: 200 mg of mifepristone given as a single dose – the woman is observed for half an hour and then allowed to go home. Anti-D globulin given to an Rh-negative woman.

  Day 3: 800 mcg of oral misoprostol (prostaglandin) is administered unless abortion has occurred. Sublingual or vaginal misoprostol is also used but a stronger action of a sublingual route can cause uterine rupture in a scarred uterus. Pulse and BP are observed for 2 hours, if all is well patient is allowed to go home.

  Nowadays, misoprostol (PGE_1) vaginal tablet of 400 mcg is inserted instead of oral tablet.

  Day 14: Follow-up to confirm abortion has occurred; if not, surgical MTP is done.

  The bleeding usually starts within few hours of taking mifepristone, and abortion occurs in about a week.

Contraindications to mifepristone are as follows:

- IUCD in situ – IUCD should be removed before medical termination to avoid the risk of perforation.
- Suspected ectopic pregnancy – ultrasound should be done before termination.
- Hypertension, anaemia, glaucoma, cardiovascular disease, smoker, asthmatic.
- A woman on anticoagulant (coagulopathy) and glucocorticoid therapy.
- Allergy, porphyria, seizures (adrenal failure).
- Previous uterine scar – scar rupture can occur with misoprostol.
- Fibroid uterus.
- Lactating woman – Since the drugs are secreted in the milk, leading to diarrhoea in infants. Lactation may be stopped temporarily.
- Gestation period should not exceed 63 days (preferably 49 days).

Advantages of misoprostol are as follows:

- Easily stored in room temperature
- Shelf life: 3 years
- Cheap
- Easy administration

Not contraindicated in patients with asthma.

Complications

- Adrenal failure
- Headache, malaise, skin rash, fever, nausea vomiting, diarrhoea
- Failure to abort, 1%
- Misoprostol causes Möbius syndrome in the fetus (congenital facial palsy, limb defects, bladder extrophy, hydrocephalus). Therefore, termination of pregnancy is strongly recommended if medical termination fails.
- It takes longer time for termination compared to surgical termination and longer follow-up of 2 weeks is necessary.
- Surgery is required in case of failure or is incomplete. In case the woman starts bleeding profusely, emergency surgical evacuation is required. Therefore, emergency surgical backup is a must for medical termination of pregnancy.
- The subsequent menstruation may be delayed by 10–14 days.
- Sublingual misoprostol is as effective as vaginal pessary, but side effects are more severe than with oral tablets and vaginal pessaries.
- If vomiting occurs soon after oral misoprostol, repeat the dose. Vaginal pessary is safe.

  Alternative protocols used are as follows:
- 200 mg of oral mifepristone followed by 800 mcg vaginal misoprostol on the third day.
- 200 mg mifepristone and 1 mg tablet of prostaglandin E_1 analogue, gemeprost vaginally – pregnancy failure is reported in 0.2%–2.3% cases.
- Methotrexate 50 mg intramuscular or oral followed 5–7 days later by 800 mcg vaginal misoprostol (repeat misoprostol 24 hours later, if required).

- Epostane – A progesterone-blocking agent is administered in doses of 200 mcg every 6 hours for 7 days.

Misoprostol alone for termination of pregnancy between 8 and 12 weeks:

For termination of pregnancies between 8 and 12 weeks, misoprostol alone has been used extensively. Several dosages regime have been employed with a variable success rate. In most cases induction–abortion interval may last 24 hours or longer with a risk of incomplete abortion or excessive bleeding.

Medical versus Surgical Methods for Termination of Early Pregnancy

While choosing between medical and surgical methods for termination of early pregnancy, there is not much difference in terms of safety and efficacy of two methods. However, surgical method has inherent risk of complications such as perforation of uterus, infection and excessive bleeding during the procedure.

SECOND-TRIMESTER MTP

The MTP Act 1972 permits termination of pregnancies up to 20 weeks. Opinion of two certified doctors is needed and such a termination should be carried out in a place fully equipped with anaesthesia and an operation theatre to handle any complication. The second-trimester MTP is associated with higher complication rates and risk of serious complications. The incidence of the second-trimester MTP has dropped with the passage of time, from about 30% of all MTPs performed two decades ago to about 10% in the present times and is mostly performed for fetal malformations.

SURGICAL METHODS

Dilatation and Evacuation

In some western countries, MTP up to 16 weeks is carried out by a slow and deliberate dilatation of the cervix with the use of laminaria tents, prostaglandin gel or pessary, before evacuation of the uterine contents using either vacuum aspiration or aspirotomy with ovum forceps. Complications such as cervical trauma, uterine perforation or tear, incomplete evacuation, haemorrhage and infection are more common with the second-trimester MTP than the first-trimester MTP. In India, surgical method for the termination of the second-trimester MTP is not commonly used.

MEDICAL METHODS OF MTP

Medical methods employ use of abortifacient drugs given by vaginal, extramniotic, intra-amniotic or intramuscular route to accomplish pregnancy termination.

Extraovular Instillation of Drugs

Several drugs such as ethacridine lactate, hypertonic saline and prostaglandins have been successfully used in the past, but the drug of choice has been ethacridine lactate.

Ethacridine Lactate. Ethacridine lactate is available as Emcredil. The advantage is that extraovular instillation can be easily performed in the second trimester with a low failure rate.

The procedure should be undertaken in an operation theatre. After steadying the anterior lip of the cervix, a Foley catheter is introduced transcervically into the extraovular space. The bulb of the Foley catheter is inflated with 10–20 mL of distilled water to seal off the internal os. Ethacridine lactate 0.1% pre-prepared solution is instilled into the extraovular space in a dose of 10 mL/week of gestation up to a maximum of 150 mL. The catheter is left in place for 6 hours, whereupon it gets gradually expelled spontaneously. Alternatively, the Foley catheter bulb is deflated and the catheter removed. Uterine activity usually begins within 12–18 hours. The mean induction–abortion interval varies between 24 and 36 hours. About 30% of the abortions are incomplete and require oxytocin infusion and occasionally blunt curettage to remove the retained placental tissue. In the event of failure to initiate uterine activity within 24 hours, an augmenting oxytocin drip is desirable. In case of failure in 72 hours, reinstillation of ethacridine may be tried or some other method of MTP should be resorted to.

To increase the success rate with ethacridine lactate, most gynaecologists prefer starting a drip containing 10–20 units of oxytocin till abortion is complete. Alternatively, supplementation with prostaglandins helps to hasten the process of abortion. Amongst the methods tried, the following methods merit mention: (i) instillation of 1 mL of carboprost or Prostodin injection diluted in 10 mL of distilled water into the extraovular space just before removing the Foley catheter, (ii) instillation of 0.5 mg prostaglandin E_2 gel (Cerviprime gel, Prostodin tablet) 4–6 hours before instillation of Emcredil solution in the extraovular space, (iii) Inj. prostaglandin $F_2\alpha$250 mcg i.m. every 3 hours, commencing from the time of removal of the catheter. In all such cases, the induction–abortion interval may be reduced to 12–18 hours with a higher success rate of 75%–80%.

Intracervical or Extraovular Instillation of Cerviprime (PGE_2)

Contraindications to the use of prostaglandins are cardiac disease, renal disease, hypertension, bronchial asthma and previous caesarean scar.

Mifepristone and Misoprostol

Oral mifepristone (200 mg) followed 36–48 hours later by 600 mcg of vaginal misoprostol and then 400 mcg of vaginal misoprostol every 3 hourly with a maximum of five doses or 200–600 mcg of vaginal misoprostol every 12 hourly for a maximum of five doses has also been used. A combination of mifepristone and misoprostol gives a higher success rate for the second-trimester MTPs compared to misoprostol alone.

Postoperatively all women should receive antibiotics, analgesics and Rh anti-D globin in an Rh-negative nonimmunized woman.

Prostaglandins

Before the availability of misoprostol, Prostaglandin $F_2\alpha$ was widely used. It is available as Inj. prostodin 1 mL ampoule (Astra-IDL) containing 0.25 mg of the drug, for parenteral use. It has been used in doses of 250 mcg (1 mL) i.m. every 3 hours, for a maximum of 10 doses. Prostaglandins have also been used instead of laminaria tents to soften the cervix before undertaking dilatation and evacuation.

Combined Methods. These involve the use of several methods in combination to take advantage of their synergistic effects on myometrial activity, thereby hasten the abortion process and minimize complications. Amongst the popular combinations in use are: (i) Emcredil plus PG, (ii) PG and laminaria tent and (iii) Emcredil and oxytocin.

In a nulliparous woman, prior ripening of cervix before using any medical method increases success rate. This can be achieved by local application of prostaglandins or by use of devices such as laminaria tent.

LATE SEQUELAE OF MTP

Late sequelae of MTP include following:

- Pelvic Inflammatory Disease (PID) – chronic pelvic pain.
- Infertility caused by tubal infection and blockage.
- Incompetent os following trauma to the cervix; this may lead to preterm births and recurrent mid-trimester abortions.
- Adherent placenta in the subsequent pregnancy.
- Asherman syndrome.
- Ectopic pregnancy as a result of PID.
- Cervical ectopic pregnancy caused by trauma.
- Intrauterine Growth Restriction (IUGR).
- Rh-isoimmunization if anti-D has not been administered after the MTP to nonimmunized Rh-negative mothers.
- Psychological problems, if MTP was done without proper counselling, and there is a feeling of regret, especially if infertility follows the procedure.

INDIAN EXPERIENCE WITH MTP

- Nearly 15 million MTPs are taking place in India; of these, 10 million are performed by unrecognized providers. Nearly 15,000–20,000 or more women die annually as a result of complications of unsafe illegal abortions.
- Vacuum aspiration for the first-trimester MTP has proved to be effective in 98.6% cases and it can be accomplished in 94.8% cases under paracervical block anaesthesia with or without sedation. Slowly, there is a trend for adopting medical methods for termination of early pregnancy, thus avoiding complications associated with surgical procedure.
- The Indian Council of Medical Research while investigating the sequelae of induced abortions reported an incidence of minor complications in 3.13% procedures and major complications in 0.21%.
- Administration of tablet of 200–400 mcg of misoprostol inserted into the posterior fornix of the vagina 3–4 hours before suction evacuation brings about softening of the cervix and dilation, thus facilitating cervical dilatation and reducing the time of surgery as well as its accompanying blood loss.
- The second-trimester MTP with ethacridine lactate remains widely used method because of its simplicity, lack of serious side effects and low cost. Success rate can be increased with the addition of prostaglandins to the instillation fluid or setting up oxytocin drip.
- Termination of pregnancy in India is permitted up to 20 weeks.

KEY POINTS

- MTP service is available in India as a health measure to avoid criminal abortion and not as a contraceptive technique. Its indications are clearly defined by the government and should be abided by the gynaecologists.
- The first-trimester MTP by suction evacuation is safer than the second-trimester termination.
- Medical method of using mifepristone and misoprostol has proved successful, but the drugs are expensive and requires 2-week follow-up. The surgical method may still be required in failed cases.
- The choice between medical and surgical methods of termination of pregnancy depends on the choice of the woman and contraindications of a method.
- Newer prostaglandins have fewer side effects
- Availability of short-acting and long-acting contraceptives allows the couple to choose a method of their need and convenience.

SELF-ASSESSMENT

1. Describe MTP Law prevailing in India.
2. Describe medical and surgical methods of the first-trimester MTP.
3. Describe commonly used methods of the second-trimester MTP.
4. Describe complications of the second-trimester MTP.

SECTION 4

BENIGN CONDITIONS IN GYNAECOLOGY

SECTION OUTLINE

21 Genital Prolapse

CHAPTER OUTLINE

Uterine prolapse is a fairly common condition especially among elderly women. Downward displacement of uterus from its normal position is called prolapse of uterus. Uterus is held in its normal position by its supports. Damage to muscles and ligamentous supports of uterus results in prolapse of uterus. Because of a close relationship with vaginal walls, prolapse of uterus is associated with prolapse of anterior and posterior walls of vagina.

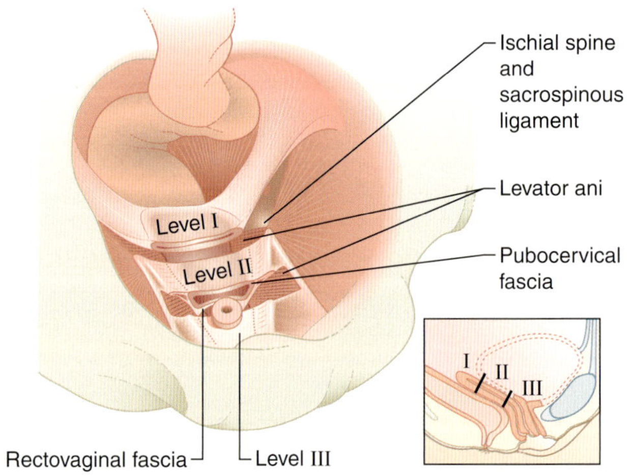

Figure 21.1 Supports of the genital tract. (*Source:* From Figure 21-5. Ian Symonds and Sabaratnam Arulkumaran: Essential Obstetrics and Gynaecology, 5th Ed., Elsevier, 2013.)

SUPPORTS OF THE UTERUS

Knowledge of supports of uterus is helpful in understanding aetiopathogenesis of prolapse of uterus. Three levels of supports of uterus have been identified in the pelvis.

DeLancey described three levels of supports of pelvic organs.

- Level I – Uterosacral and cardinal ligaments support the uterus and vaginal vault. The cervix remains at or just above the level of ischial spines.
- Level II – Pelvic fascia and paracolpos which connect the vagina to the white line on the lateral pelvic wall through the arcus tendineus fascia pelvis. This includes the pubocervical fascia anteriorly and the rectovaginal fascia and septum posteriorly.
- Level III – Levator ani muscle supports the lower one-third of the vagina. The levator muscle forms a platform against which the pelvic organs (uterus and upper vagina) get compressed during straining.
- Damage to Level I supports causes uterine descent, enterocele and vault descent.
- Damage to Level II supports causes cystocele, rectocele.
- Damage to Level III supports causes urethrocele, gaping introitus and deficient perineum.

For diagrammatic representations of DeLancey's three levels of support to the genital tract, refer to Figs 21.1 and 21.2.

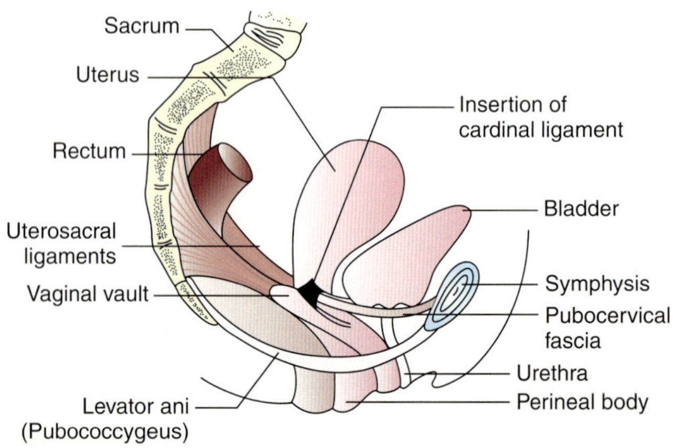

Figure 21.2 Various supports of the uterus.

To view the lecture notes scan the symbol or log in to your account on www.MedEnact.com

Clinically unrecognized damages and breaks in these supports can be detected by ultrasound and MRI.

AETIOLOGY OF PROLAPSE UTERUS (Table 21.1)

Weakness or injury to normal supports of uterus results in uterovaginal prolapse. In most cases, damage to supports occurs as a result of a mismanaged childbirth. However, a congenital defect or weakness of supports of uterus can result in prolapse of uterus and vagina. Withdrawal of hormonal support, especially oestrogen, following menopause is an important factor for the onset of symptoms of prolapse. Rarely pelvic trauma or nerve damage to pelvis can result in prolapse uterus. Raised intraabdominal pressure, chronic constipation, chronic obstructive airway diseases also play a role in the development of pelvic organ prolapse.

Mismanaged childbirth: Unsupervised or wrong practices during labour or puerperium can predispose a woman to subsequent development of uterine prolapse. Prolonged bearing down efforts in the first stage of labour before the full dilatation of cervix result in undue stretching or tears in Mackenrodt and uterosacral ligaments. Similarly, application of forceps before the full dilation of cervix results in tears in cervix and Mackenrodt ligaments with subsequent risk of uterine prolapse. Birth of a big-size baby can also predispose to prolapse uterus by damaging cervix and supporting ligaments. Following a childbirth, poor rehabilitation in puerperium, early resumption of physical activity, lifting heavy weights can predispose woman to prolapse uterus.

As discussed later, prolapse of uterus due to a mismanaged childbirth is mostly seen in women in reproductive age. This type has been called uterovaginal prolapse and has elongation of supravaginal portion of cervix, vaginal mucosa is well epithelialized and associated with good tone of levator muscles.

Menopause: Menopause is characterized by declining levels of oestrogens. All the supports of uterus are under the effect of oestrogen during reproductive years. Declining levels of oestrogen after menopause result in loss of tone of muscular supports and relaxation of ligamentous supports of uterus. These changes predispose a woman to uterine prolapse in the presence of preexisting weakness in supports of uterus.

Table 21.1 Aetiology of Prolapse

Atonicity	• Menopause • Congenital weakness
Birth injuries	• Prolonged labour • Perineal tear • Pudendal nerve injury • Operative delivery • Multiparity • Big baby
Other causes	• Raised intraabdominal pressure • Chronic bronchitis

Prolapse uterus seen after menopause is clinically characterized by atrophy of vaginal mucosa, the presence of enterocele, poor tone of levator muscles and the absence of cervix elongation.

CLASSIFICATION OF PROLAPSE (Figs 21.3 and 21.4)

Uterine prolapse has been classified in a number of ways. However, recently for the purpose of a uniform reporting and comparison of results, a new classification has been proposed by International Society for Study of Vulvovaginal Disorders.

Following section describes two commonly used classification systems of prolapse, namely Uterovaginal Prolapse System and Pelvic Organ Prolapse Quantification System (POP-Q).

Uterovaginal Prolapse System

A. *Anterior vaginal wall* (Fig. 21.5)
   Upper two-thirds—Cystocele }
   Lower one-third—Urethrocele } Cystourethrocele

B. *Posterior vaginal wall*
   Upper one-third – Enterocele (the pouch of Douglas hernia) (Fig. 21.6)
   Lower two-thirds – Rectocele

C. *Uterine descent*
   - Descent of the cervix into the vagina
   - Descent of the cervix up to the introitus
   - Descent of the cervix outside the introitus

Procidentia – Entire uterus is outside the introitus (Figs 21.7–21.9).

CYSTOCELE

Prolapse of upper two-thirds of anterior vaginal wall is called cystocele. The bladder is supported by pubocervical fascia which extends laterally to the arcus tendineus and

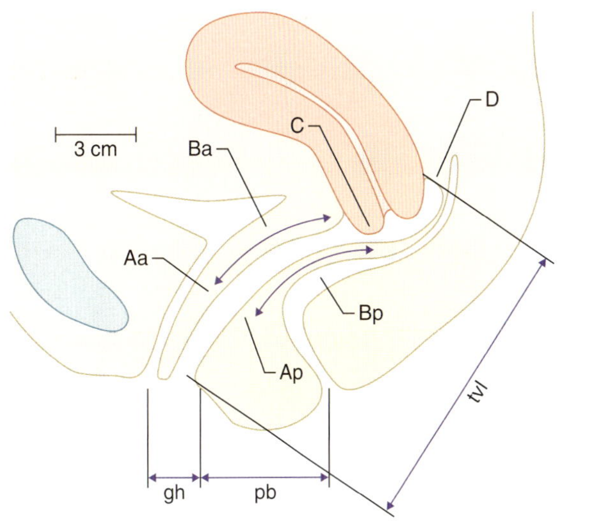

Figure 21.3 Pelvic organ prolapse quantification system (POP-Q). (*Source:* From Figure 21-9. Ian Symonds and Sabaratnam Arulkumaran: Essential Obstetrics and Gynaecology, 5th Ed., Elsevier, 2013.)

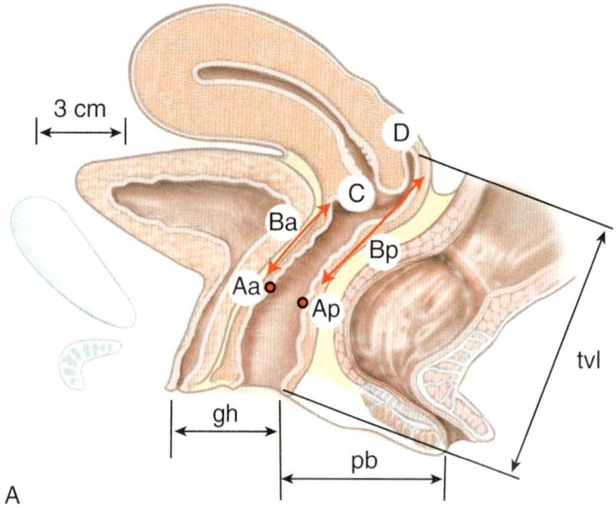

A

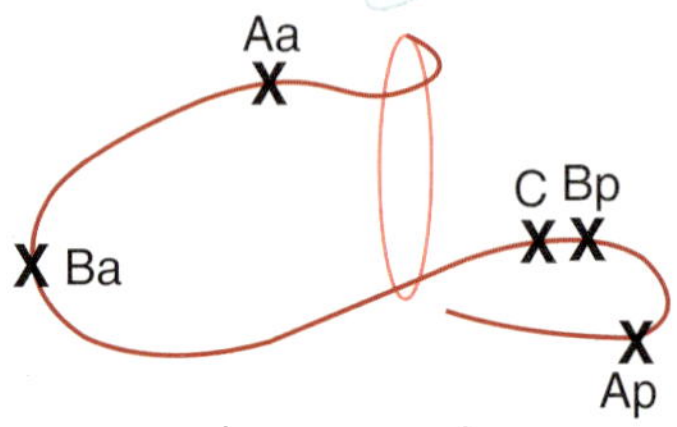

$+3_{Aa}$	$+6_{Ba}$	$+2_{C}$
4.5_{gh}	1.5_{pb}	6_{tvl}
-3^{Ap}	-2^{Bp}	–

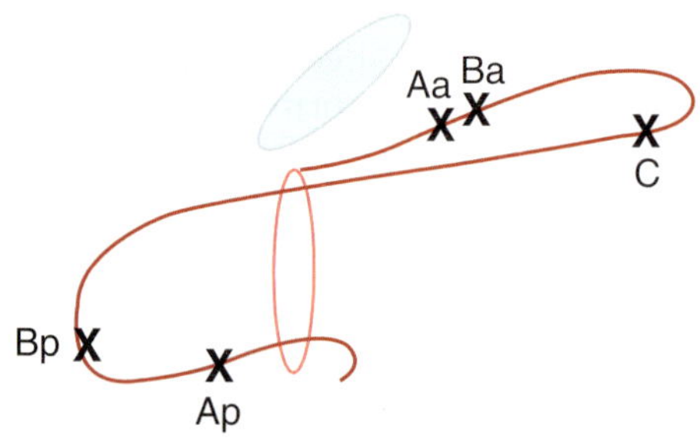

-3_{Aa}	-3_{Ba}	-6_{C}
4.5_{gh}	1_{pb}	8_{tvl}
$+3^{Ap}$	$+5^{Bp}$	–

B Profile A Profile B

Figure 21.4 Pelvic organ prolapse quantification (POP-Q) system for staging pelvic organ prolapse. Aa, Point A anterior; Ap, Point A posterior, Ba, Point B anterior; Bp, Point B posterior; C, Cervix or vaginal cuff; D, Posterior fornix (if cervix is present); gh, Genital hiatus; pb, Perineal body; tvl, Total vaginal length. (*Source:* From Figure 1.11. Victor Nitti: Vaginal Surgery for the Urologist. Saunders: Elsevier, 2012.)

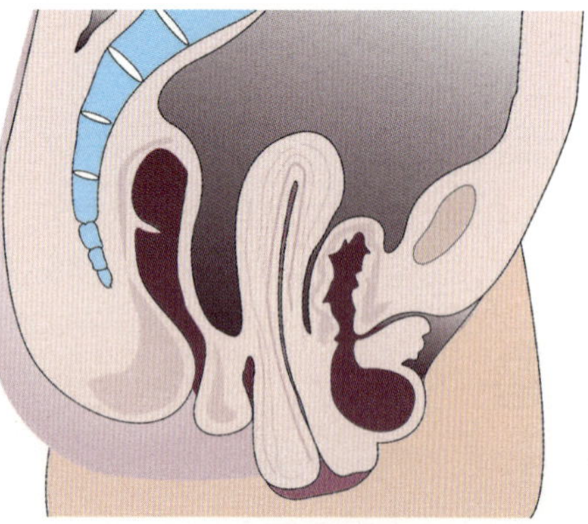

Figure 21.5 Prolapse of the cervix, anterior vaginal wall and bladder. The cervix is elongated and hypertrophied. The anterior vaginal wall and bladder have prolapsed outside the vaginal orifice. The cervix is also prolapsed. In this case, the ligamentary supports hold up the body of the uterus. Note that the almost vertical direction of the uterosacral ligament from the cervix to the junction of the second and third sacral vertebrae. Compare this figure with Fig. 21.8.

fuses with the levator ani muscle below. The urethra is supported by the posterior urethral ligament which is fixed to the pubic bone.

In prolapse of the anterior vaginal wall, the upper part of the anterior vaginal wall descends and in advanced cases it may protrude outside the vaginal orifice. In these cases, the vesicle and vaginal fasciae are thinned out and fail to support the bladder, so that the bladder prolapses with the anterior vaginal wall. This condition is termed as cystocele. In mild cases, the lower portion of the anterior vaginal wall does not prolapse, and the urethra is well supported by the posterior urethral ligament. When the urethra along with the **lower one-third of the anterior wall prolapses, it is termed urethrocele,** and the patient invariably complains of stress incontinence. When the cystocele protrudes outside the vulva, owing to friction, the vaginal epithelium becomes thickened, hypertrophied and keratinized. Ulceration can occur over the vaginal wall. Senile vaginitis in menopausal women shows a thin reddened vagina. The breaks in the

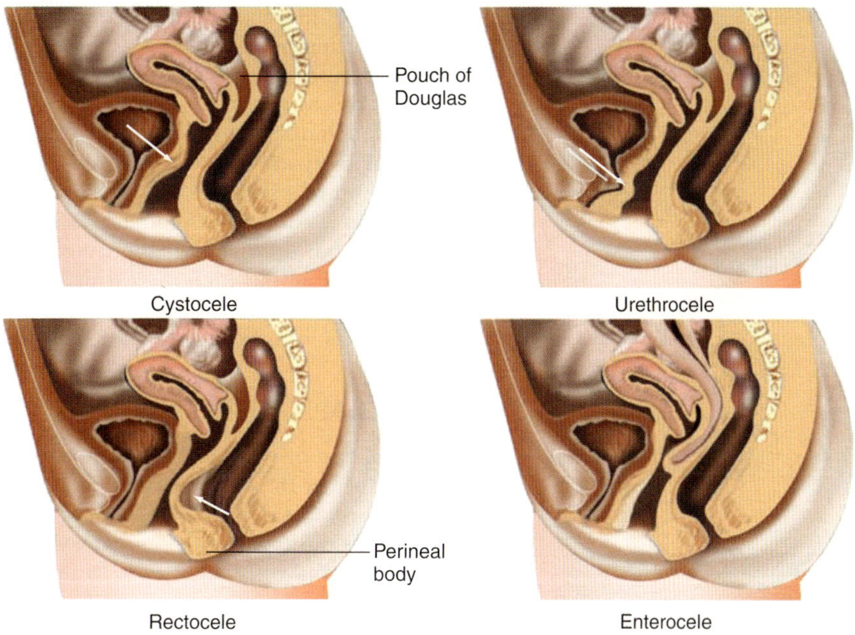

Figure 21.6 The anatomy of prolapse.

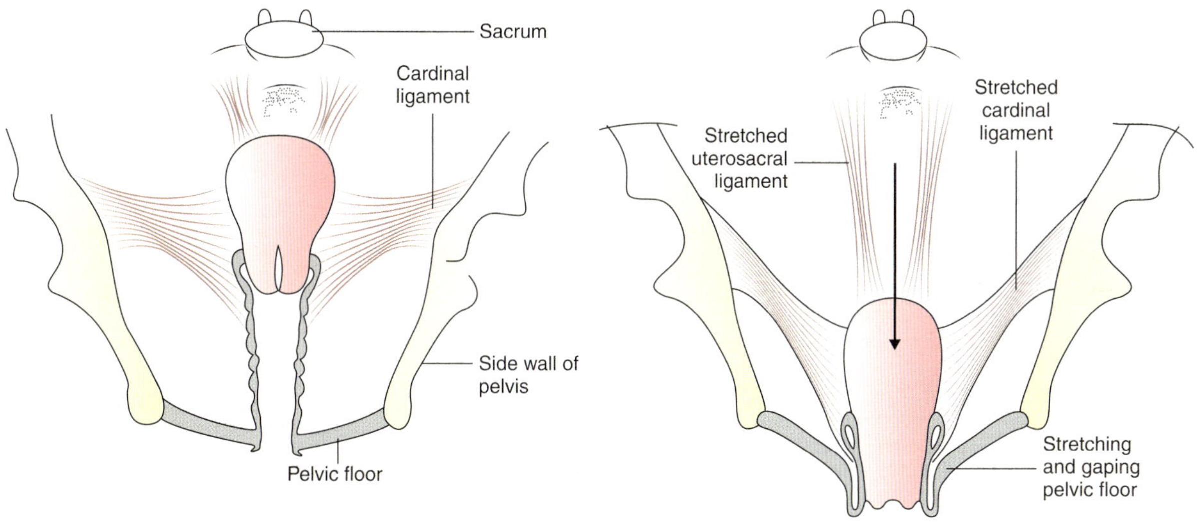

Figure 21.7 Lateral supports of the uterus showing cardinal ligaments.

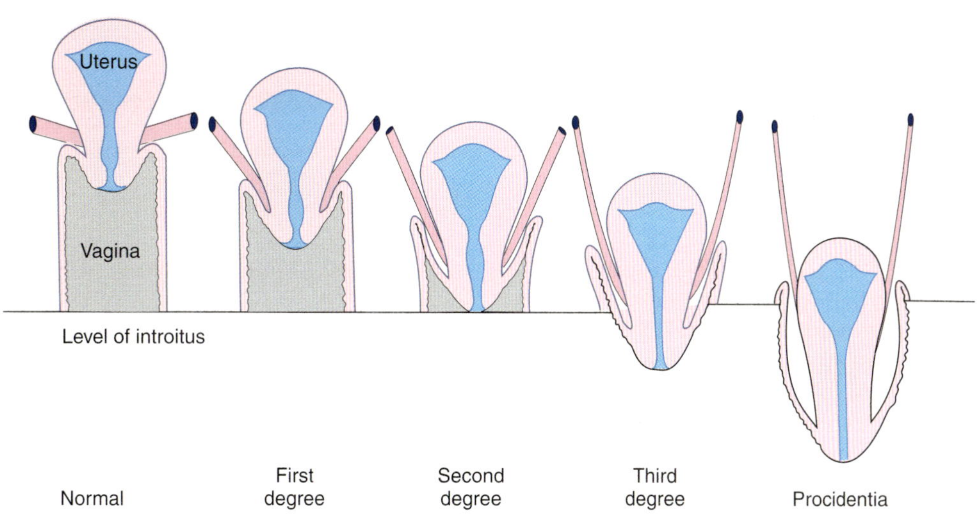

Figure 21.8 Note the descent of the cervix which is accompanied by stretching of the ligaments and by supravaginal elongation of the cervix.

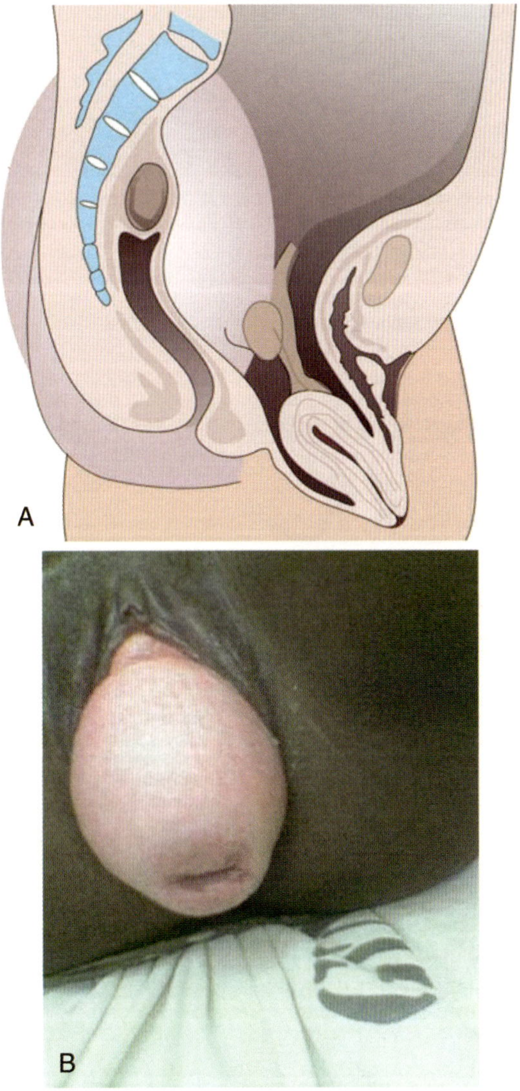

Figure 21.9 (A) Complete procidentia. Note that the whole of both vaginal walls lie outside the vaginal orifice. The whole of the uterus also lies below this level. Clearly the ligamentary supports of the uterus must be greatly stretched to allow such a degree of prolapse. Compare this figure with Fig. 21.8. (B) Procidentia with cystocele, enterocele. (*Source* **(B)**: From Figure 2. Cyril C Dim, Uchenna A Umeh, Hyginus U Ezegwui, et al. Uterine Procidentia in an African Adolescent: An Uncommon Gynecological Challenge. Journal of Pediatric and Adolescent Gynecology, Vol 2(1): 37–39, 2008.)

lateral attachment cause the vaginal sulci to disappear and the lateral portion of the bladder prolapses.

PROLAPSE OF THE UTERUS

If the uterus prolapses, there is always some associated descent of the anterior vaginal wall. It is customary to describe three degrees of prolapse of the uterus. In the first degree, the cervix descends into the vagina; in the second degree, the cervix descends to the level of the introitus; while in the third degree, the cervix protrudes outside the vaginal orifice. In **procidentia** (Fig. 21.9A), the whole of uterus protrudes outside the vagina, bringing with it both the anterior and posterior vaginal walls, and it may be possible to feel the loops of the small intestine in the pouch of Douglas. In most cases, the vaginal portion of the cervix is hypertrophied and in uterine prolapse of the third degree, the epithelium covering the cervix is often thickened – keratinization. It is not uncommon for trophic ulcers to form both on the cervix and prolapsed anterior wall – these are called decubitus ulcers.

In prolapse of the uterus, the supravaginal portion of the cervix is sometimes elongated. Supravaginal elongation of the cervix must be distinguished from congenital cervical elongation, in which the fornices are deep and the elongation is restricted only to that portion of the cervix which projects into the vagina (Figs 21.5, 21.8, 21.10 and 21.11).

PROLAPSE OF THE POSTERIOR VAGINAL WALL

Prolapse of middle third of posterior vaginal wall is called rectocele. In rectocele, the rectum protrudes with the posterior vaginal wall. The tissues which normally intervene between the posterior vaginal wall and the rectum may have been damaged by obstetric injury, and the vagina and rectum may become adhered by scar tissue. Prolapse of upper one-third of posterior vaginal wall is called enterocele. This portion lies in relation to the pouch of Douglas; it is not uncommon for the upper part of the posterior vaginal wall to protrude outside the vulva and loops of the intestine to be palpable in the prolapsed part. The term 'enterocele' is used to describe this type of prolapse (Fig. 21.6). Enterocele is herniation of the pouch of Douglas into the rectovaginal septum. It is often associated with uterine prolapse.

If a woman with prolapse is examined and asked to strain, the usual sequence of events is for the anterior wall to protrude first, followed by the cervix and then the posterior vaginal wall.

DECUBITUS ULCER

Keratinization and pigmentation of the vaginal mucosa as well as ulceration of the prolapsed tissue are caused by

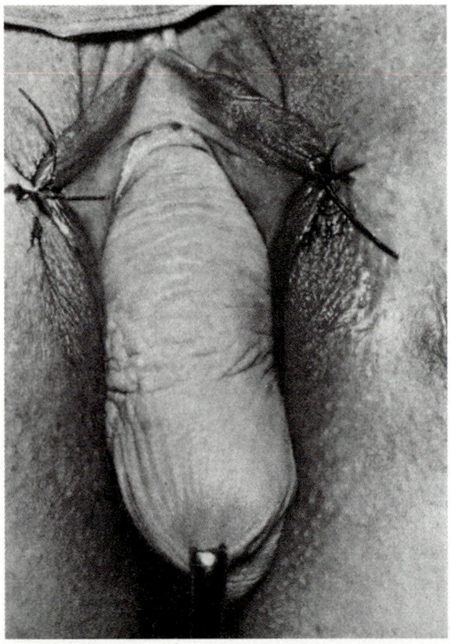

Figure 21.10 Prolapse of the uterus at operation. The cervix has been drawn down, and the whole of the uterus can be pulled outside the vaginal orifice.

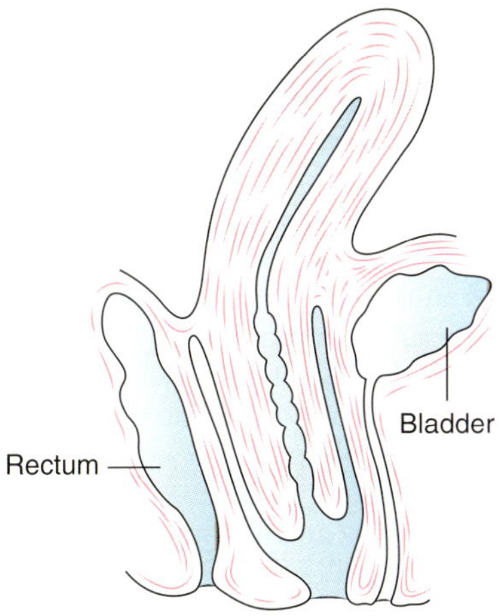

Figure 21.11 Congenital elongation of cervix.

friction, congestion and circulatory changes in the dependent part of the prolapse. Reduction of the prolapse with daily packing of tampons soaked in glycerine and Acriflavine solution or Betadine in the vagina helps in healing of the ulcer within a week or two. Decubitus ulcer needs to be differentiated from cancer of the cervix. Apart from cytology and biopsy, the other distinguishing features are that the decubitus ulcer shows a clean edge and heals on reposition with vaginal packing. In rare cases, carcinoma develops at the site of decubitus ulcer or when a ring pessary is left in situ for a long period.

ELONGATION OF THE CERVIX

As the supravaginal portion of the cervix is well supported by Mackenrodt ligaments but the vaginal portion of the cervix prolapses with the vagina, the supravaginal portion gets stretched and elongated. This usually happens with the second-degree and third-degree prolapse of the uterus. In procidentia, the entire uterus slides with the vagina and hence the cervix retains its normal length. It is not uncommon for the cervix to elongate to as much as 10 cm in a case of uterovaginal prolapse. The cervix may show hypertrophy and congestion. The uterus is invariably retroverted.

OBSTRUCTION OF THE URINARY TRACT

A large cystocele may cause kinking of urethra leading to hypertrophy of the bladder wall and trabeculations. The kinking of the distal ureters in procidentia can lead to hydroureter and hydronephrosis, if prolapse is not surgically corrected. Urinary tract infection is not uncommon as residual urine remains in the bladder in a large cystocele.

Incarceration of the prolapse is encountered in rare cases when, due to oedema and congestion, the prolapse becomes irreducible. Head low position, ice packing or packing with magnesium sulphate reduces the oedema, enabling the prolapse to be reduced.

POP-Q SYSTEM (Table 21.2, Fig. 21.3)

Quantification of prolapse has lately been described by the International Continence Society, and it is objective and site specific. The hymen is taken as a fixed point (O). Six reference points are measured, using a scaled spatula, and tabulated in a grid (Fig. 21.4). The points above the hymen are described as "minus" and points below as "plus".

Table 21.2 Staging of POP

Stage 0	No demonstrable prolapse
Stage 1	All points <–1
Stage 2	Lowest point within 1 cm of hymen (between –1 and + 1)
Stage 3	Lowest point > 1 cm below hymen but not complete prolapse
Stage 4	Complete prolapse with lowest point equal to TVL-2

SYMPTOMS OF PROLAPSE

The patients mostly complain of something descending in the vagina or of *something protruding outside vagina.* The prolapse is aggravated by straining and coughing, and by heavy work, whereas on rising from the bed in the morning, the physical signs of prolapse are least. Often the patient states that the prolapse reduces by itself when she lies down. If there is a large prolapse, the external swelling may cause inconvenience to her during walking or carrying out her day-to-day routine activities. Even in mild degree, patients are conscious of a sense of weakness and of a lack of support around the perineum.

Towards the end of the day, the patient may complain of a vague mid-sacral discomfort and backache, which are relieved by rest. This symptom is most logically explained as a strain on uterosacral ligaments. Some women suffer from a 'bearing-down' feeling above the pubes.

In most cases of prolapse, there is some degree of vaginal discharge. The discharge may emanate from a chronically inflamed lacerated cervix, but may also be caused by the relaxation of the vaginal orifice which allows bacteria to invade the vagina and produce a mild degree of vaginitis. A friction or decubitus ulcer is an obvious cause of discharge and bleeding. Menstrual cycles are usually normal.

One of the important symptoms associated with prolapse of uterus is urinary complaint in the form of incomplete evacuation of bladder or frequency of micturition; however, the most frequent is stress incontinence of urine. In this condition, there is involuntary escape of little amount of urine during any act associated with raised intraabdominal pressure such as coughing, sneezing, change of posture or lifting heavy weight. This imperfect control of micturition is caused by lack of support to the sphincter mechanism of the urethra. Frequency of micturition is also a common symptom, caused in some, by chronic cystitis and in others, by incomplete emptying of the bladder. In the presence of large cystocele, patients frequently complain that they have difficulty in micturition, and that the more they strain, the more difficult it becomes to pass urine. The explanation of this symptom is that when the intraabdominal pressure is raised during straining, the urine is pushed down into the cystocele below the level of the internal meatus. Patients often mention that they are able to pass urine by repositioning prolapse in vagina with the help of a finger. This is termed as "splinting". Stress incontinence of urine occurs when the neck of the bladder and internal urinary meatus descend below the level of the pelvic floor muscles. Urinary symptoms develop when pubocervical fascia is damaged and breaks occur at level III support.

Rectal symptoms are less remarkable, and constipation is rare (level III damage).

Coital difficulties with the third-degree uterine prolapse and procidentia are obvious. A major degree of prolapse prevents penetration and orgasm due to a lax outlet. However, digital reposition of prolapse before coitus can help these women in having intercourse.

INVESTIGATIONS

Patients with prolapse should be carefully examined, because the treatment is based on the physical signs observed. Although most patients are examined in the supine position, examination in a squatting position or standing position will help to assess degree of prolapse. During examination she is made to cough and strain, and the nature and degree of prolapse noted. In a patient with symptom of stress incontinence, examination is done with a partially full bladder. The vulva is examined for evidence of any perineal laceration. Inspection will show whether the vaginal orifice is relaxed. The perineal body and levator muscles are palpated to determine the muscle tone and the dimensions of the hiatus urogenitalis. Stress incontinence should be looked for by asking the patient to strain.

Speculum examination determines the degree of uterine descent and associated prolapse of anterior and posterior vaginal walls. Cervical cytology may be obtained, but it is important to remember that in the third-degree uterine prolapse and procidentia, a satisfactory smear might not be obtained as cervix lying outside the vagina may be dry. Enterocele should be looked for carefully. If missed, vault prolapse can occur subsequently. The per vaginal examination should include measuring the length of the cervix, position and mobility of uterus. Any adnexal mass present should be noted. The general condition of the patient should be evaluated to decide on her fitness for surgery. On the whole, there is not much difficulty in arriving at a correct diagnosis.

The laboratory investigations include: (i) haemogram, (ii) urine examination, urine culture, (iii) blood urea, (iv) blood sugar, (v) X-ray of the chest, (vi) ECG and other investigations necessary before major gynaecological surgery.

IVP is rarely indicated and may reveal ureteric obstruction in a major degree of prolapse. Ultrasound and MRI may help in localizing the defects in the supporting structures.

Transperineal and vaginal ultrasound may reveal defects in the levator ani muscles and lateral supports, whereas transrectal ultrasound is useful to confirm the presence of enterocele.

DIFFERENTIAL DIAGNOSIS

- *Vulval cyst* and Gartner cyst can be easily differentiated from prolapse.
- The *cyst of the anterior vaginal* wall is usually tense with well-defined margins and cannot be reduced on pressure.
- *Urethral diverticula* are rare, always small and are situated low down in the anterior vaginal wall. Urethroscopy helps in the diagnosis.
- *Congenital elongation of the cervix* can be differentiated from prolapse as it is the vaginal portion of the cervix that is elongated and there is no accompanying vaginal wall prolapse. The fornices are deep.
- *Cervical fibroid polyps* can be easily identified as the cervix is high up and a rim of cervix can be felt above the pedicle of cervical polyp.
- *Chronic inversion* of uterus can be recognized because the cervix is further up, and the uterus cannot be defined. The uterine sound will confirm the diagnosis. Ultrasound and laparoscopy will identify the fundal depression with an absence of uterine fundus in the pelvis.
- In rare cases, the patient may complain of vaginal prolapse, but, in fact, a rectal prolapse is evident.

COMPLICATIONS OF PELVIC ORGAN PROLAPSE

1. Kinking of ureter with a resultant renal damage can occur in procidentia. During surgery sometimes, the ureters can get included in the sutures at the vaginal vault.
2. Urinary tract infection; In a large cystocele with residual urine there can be frequent Urinary Tract Infection (UTI) leading to upper renal tract infection and renal damage.
3. In rare cases, cancer of the vagina can develop at the site of decubitus ulcer or if a ring pessary is left in over a long period.

PREVENTION OF PROLAPSE

Careful attention during childbirth can do much to prevent prolapse.

- Antenatal physiotherapy; relaxation exercises and due attention to weight gain and anaemia are important.
- Proper supervision and management of the second stage of labour.
- An episiotomy if indicated as in primigravidae, breech delivery, instrument delivery should be performed. Recently, however, the usefulness and the role of episiotomy in prolapse have been questioned, and complications of episiotomy are listed.
- Forceps delivery/ventouse should be resorted to if there is delay in the second stage of labour.
- A perineal tear must be immediately and meticulously repaired after delivery.
- Postnatal exercises and physiotherapy are beneficial.
- Early ambulation in postpartum period.
- Provision of adequate rest for the first 6 weeks after delivery and the availability of home help for heavy domestic duties.
- A reasonable interval between pregnancies allows recovery of muscle tone and ligamentous support in pelvis. Using a family planning method so that family size can be limited avoids strain on the ligamentary supports of uterus.

TREATMENT (Table 21.3)

Surgery remains the main mode of treatment of prolapse uterus; however, before resorting to any surgical treatment, the most important decision to consider is the appropriate treatment for prolapse in a young woman following childbirth. It is a great mistake to advise immediate operative treatment in such a case. If the operation is performed within 6 months of delivery, there is always a possibility of recurrence of prolapse following the subsequent childbirth. Besides, these women rapidly improve if well-directed conservative measures are adopted. Abdominal exercises, massage and perineal exercises practised regularly, will prevent or reduce the prolapse. *Conservative measures should be advised following delivery for initial 4–6 months.*

Surgery is advised in women older than 40 years, unless it is contraindicated on account of some medical disorders. Surgery for prolapse is contraindicated during pregnancy.

PESSARY TREATMENT OF PROLAPSE

The ring pessary for prolapse is nearly a thing of the past in elderly women and very young women desirous of further childbearing. With modern anaesthesia and good preoperative care, advanced age is no longer a contraindication to a surgical procedure for prolapse.

The pessary treatment of prolapse has certain following limitations:

- It can cause vaginitis, ulcerations in vagina.
- Pessary needs to be changed every 3 months.
- The wearing of a pessary is not comfortable to some women and may cause dyspareunia.
- If the vaginal orifice is patulous, the pessary often gets expelled especially in a squatting position as during defecation or urination.
- A forgotten pessary can be the cause of ulcers in vagina, and in rare cases can produce carcinoma of the vagina and a vesicovaginal fistula.
- A ring pessary is not helpful for symptom of stress urinary incontinence.

Table 21.3 Management of Genital Prolapse

Nulliparous	Abdominal sling operations
Pregnancy	Ring pessary up to 16 weeks
Postnatal	• Ring pessary and pelvic floor exercises for 3–6 months • Surgery if required thereafter
Young woman < 40 years	Conservative vaginal surgery (fertility sparing surgery) • Cystocele, rectocele repair • Manchester repair • Sling operation
Woman older than 40 years and multipara	Vaginal hysterectomy and pelvic floor repair

Current indications for use of pessary are as follows:

- In a young woman who wants to have subsequent children; prolapse during early pregnancy.
- Puerperium.
- Temporary use while treating infection and decubitus ulcer.
- A woman unfit for surgery.
- In a woman who declines surgery.

The ring pessary is made of a soft plastic polyvinyl chloride material and available in different sizes. A pregnant woman with prolapse may need a ring pessary limited to the first trimester of pregnancy as subsequently the uterus becomes an intra-abdominal organ and the prolapse spontaneously gets reduced. Pessary treatment may be again needed during puerperium in a woman with a severe degree of prolapse and distressing symptoms.

OPERATIVE TREATMENT OF PROLAPSE

Surgery remains the main treatment of cure for prolapse. The type of surgery depends upon her desire to retain uterus for the subsequent fertility. However, for women older than 40 years, a vaginal hysterectomy with repair of anterior and posterior vaginal walls prolapse is the desired treatment. In younger women desirous of retaining uterus, a conservative surgical procedure such as Manchester operation (Fothergill's operation) is the surgical procedure of choice.

The aims of surgery are as follows:

- Relieve symptoms
- Restore anatomy
- Restore sexual function
- Prevent recurrence

PREOPERATIVE PREPARATION

Oestrogen cream applied locally for senile vaginitis will help in improving condition of vaginal mucosa, but should be stopped a few days before surgery. The patient should receive a course of urinary antibiotics if urinary infection is present. Decubitus ulcer may heal by daily insertion of vaginal tampon soaked in Acriflavine or Betadine solution for 2 weeks.

SURGERY

A number of surgical procedures with minor variations in techniques have been described for surgical repair of prolapse.

- Surgery for anterior vaginal wall prolapse – Anterior colporrhaphy
- Surgery for posterior vaginal wall prolapse – Posterior colporrhaphy
- Surgery for prolapse of uterus – Manchester operation in young women
- Vaginal hysterectomy in women older than 40 years
- Surgical procedures for nulliparous prolapse – Sling operation
- Surgical procedure for vault prolapse – Abdominal or vaginal surgical procedures

ANTERIOR COLPORRHAPHY

Anterior colporrhaphy operation is performed to repair a cystocele and cystourethrocele. Traction is given on the cervix to expose the anterior vaginal wall. An inverted T-shaped incision is made in the anterior vaginal wall, starting with a transverse incision in the bladder sulcus. Through its midpoint, a vertical incision is extended up to the urethral opening (Fig. 21.12). The vaginal walls are reflected on the either side to expose the bladder and vesicovaginal fascia (Fig. 21.13). The overlying vesicovaginal fascia is tightened, and the excess vaginal wall excised to correct the laxity. Then the vaginal is wall sutured. In women suffering from stress incontinence, in addition a Kelly suture is placed in the region of bladder neck to correct stress incontinence. The breaks or defects in the lateral supports require further suturing of the pubocervical tissue to the arcus tendineus. This also elevates the vaginal wall. In repeat surgery for recurrence or failed surgery, a mesh may be supplemented to strengthen the support to the bladder.

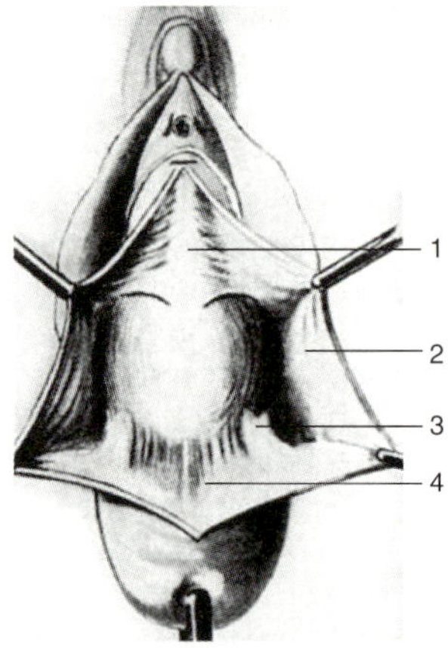

Figure 21.13 The appearance after the dissection of the vaginal flaps: (1) posterior urethral ligament – the well-defined cranial border is emphasized. In the illustration, the vesicovaginal space has been opened up, and the vaginal fascia (2) remains attached to the vaginal wall. (3) Bladder septum. (4) Vesicocervical ligament.

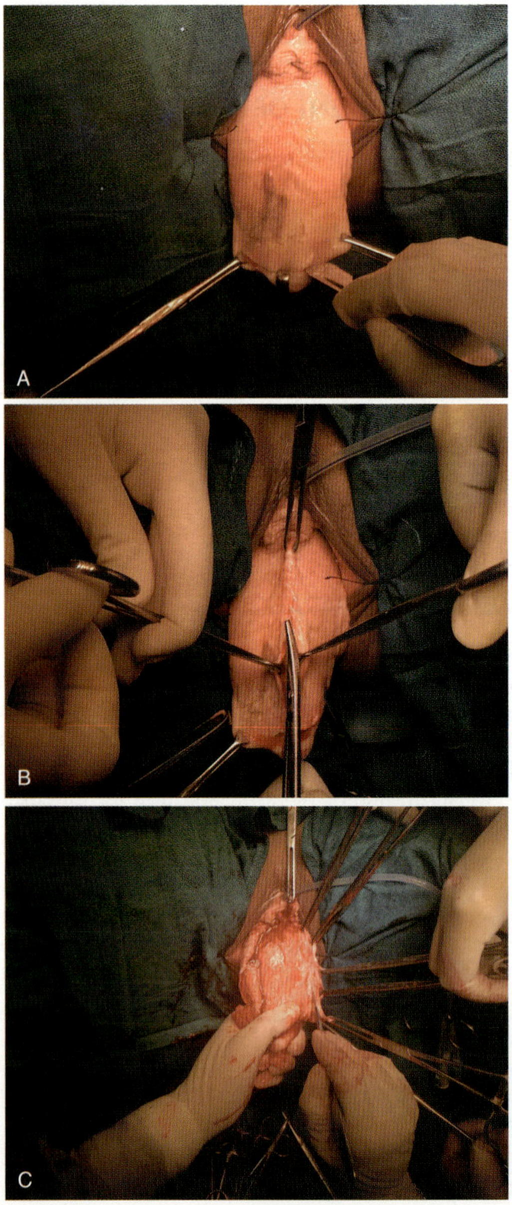

Figure 21.12 (A) Anterior colporrhaphy. A Transverse incision is given in the bladder sulcus. (B) Mid line vertical incision is given extending up to urethral opening. (C) Vesico vaginal space is opened up. The vesicle fascia is recognized because of the dilated veins which ramify in its layer. The anterior vaginal wall is reflected away from the bladder on either.

POSTERIOR COLPORRHAPHY AND COLPOPERINEORRHAPHY

Posterior colporrhaphy operation is done to correct a rectocele and repair a deficient perineum.

The lax vagina over the rectocele is excised, and the rectovaginal fascia repaired after reducing the rectocele. The approximation of the medial fibres of the levator ani helps to restore the calibre of the hiatus urogenitalis, restore the perineal body and provide an adequate perineum separating the hiatus urogenitalis from the anal canal (Fig. 21.14).

It is commonly combined with an anterior colporrhaphy, or vaginal hysterectomy. To avoid recurrence and to reinforce the weak supportive fascia, some use mesh in the fascial layer. However, dyspareunia, erosion of mesh or infection requiring its removal and sinus formation are the disadvantages, in addition to the high cost.

FOTHERGILL'S REPAIR (MANCHESTER OPERATION)

In this operation, the surgeon combines an anterior colporrhaphy with amputation of the cervix. The cut ends of the Mackenrodt ligaments are sutured in front of the cervix, and the raw area on the amputated cervix is covered with vaginal mucosa. A special technique of covering cervix with vaginal mucosa has been described and is called as sturmdorff sutures. It is followed up with a colpoperineorrhaphy.

The operation preserves uterus for menstrual and childbearing functions. However, subsequent pregnancies may be associated with a mid-trimester abortion or preterm delivery. In some cases, there may be failure of dilatation of cervix during labour requiring a caesarian section. It is a suitable procedure for women younger than 40 years who are desirous of retaining their menstrual and reproductive

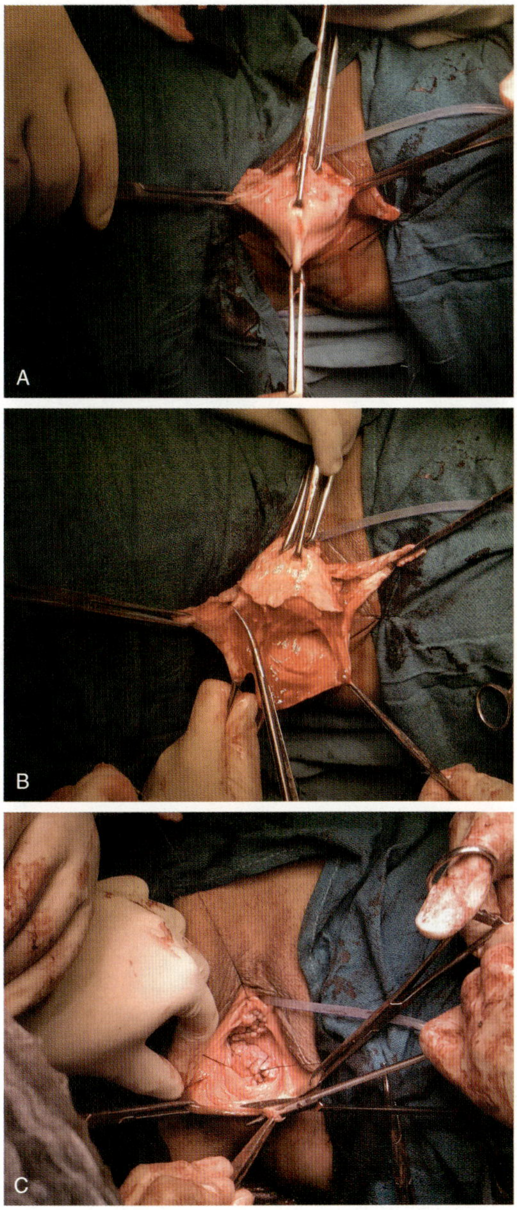

Figure 21.14 (A) Colpoperineorrhaphy. The posterior vaginal wall is caught by an allis clamp and traction provided. (B) The posterior vaginal wall is reflected away from the cervix. (C) A triangular piece of vagina has been removed and the free edges of the wound are drawn apart. The perineal fascia has been divided and the levator ani muscles have been sutured together in the midline.

functions. In younger women, the procedure can be combined with tubal sterilization if family is complete.

To avoid complications such as stenosis of cervix some include dilatation of cervix and endometrial curettage as a preliminary step in Fothergill's repair. This is optional, but desirable in a woman complaining of menstrual disorder associated with prolapse.

Cervical amputation may lead to incompetent cervical os, habitual abortions or preterm deliveries. Excessive fibrosis may lead to cervical stenosis and dystocia during labour. In rare cases, it may cause haematometra. Recurrence of prolapse may occur following vaginal delivery in some cases.

To avoid the obstetric complications of Fothergill's operation, Shirodkar modified this operation as follows.

SHIRODKAR'S PROCEDURE

In this procedure, amputation of cervix is avoided. Anterior colporrhaphy is performed as usual, and attachment of Mackenrodt ligaments to the cervix on each side is exposed. The vaginal incision is then extended posteriorly round the cervix. The pouch of Douglas is opened, uterosacral ligaments identified and divided close to the cervix. The stumps of these ligaments are crossed and stitched together in front of the cervix. A high closure of the peritoneum of the pouch of Douglas is carried out. As cervix is not amputated, subsequent pregnancy complications are avoided. The rest of the operation is similar to Fothergill's operation.

Other conservative surgeries used are as follows:

- Vaginal sacrospinous hysteropexy.
- Abdominal/laparoscopic sacrohysteropexy.

These can be combined with cystocele, rectocele repair. The advantages are as follows:

- Vaginal length is maintained.
- Cervix is preserved for sexual function.

VAGINAL HYSTERECTOMY WITH PELVIC FLOOR REPAIR

Vaginal hysterectomy with pelvic floor repair is suitable for women older than 40 years, those who have completed their families and are no longer keen on retaining their child-bearing and menstrual functions.

The operation alleviates the women of her prolapse symptoms, in addition to any associated menstrual problems. A Kelly stitch is needed while doing anterior colporrhaphy in case she has associated stress incontinence.

The Steps of Vaginal Hysterectomy (Figs 21.15–21.18)

A circular incision is made over the cervix below the bladder sulcus, and the vaginal mucosa dissected off the cervix all around. The pouch of Douglas is identified posteriorly and peritoneum incised and opened. The bladder is now pushed upwards until the uterovesical peritoneum is visible, and is similarly incised. The uterus is now free in the front and behind. The pedicles containing Mackenrodt's and uterosacral ligaments are clamped on the either side close to the cervix, cut on the uterine side and the pedicles transfixed. Next, the uterine vessels are identified, clamped, cut and ligated. The upper portion of the broad ligament holding the uterus contains round, ovarian ligaments and the fallopian tube. These are similarly dealt with on both sides, and the uterus removed. The peritoneal cavity is closed with a purse-string suture, using chromic catgut 0. Anterior colporrhaphy and posterior colpoperineorrhaphy are performed as required.

The vagina is packed with Betadine or Acriflavine pack for 24 hours, a Foley catheter left in place for continuous drainage of urine for 48 hours. In case Kelly's stitches were placed for SUI the catheter is kept for 5–7 days.

Complications of surgery.

1. Haemorrhage
2. Sepsis

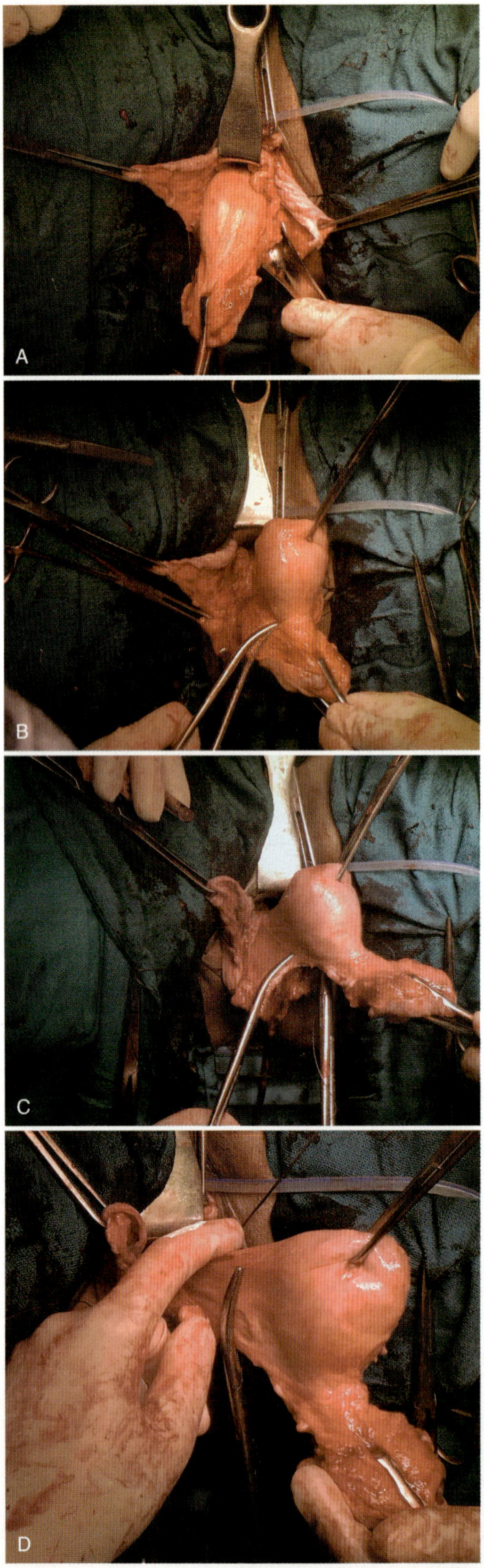

Figure 21.15 (A) The vaginal skin has been excised and pulled down over the cervix. (B) Mackenrodt's ligaments have been clamped and cut, and a suture ligature has been inserted in the left of Mackenrodt's ligament. Note that the bladder has been freely mobilized and pushed well up out of danger. (C) Clamp is being applied over the cornuo fundal structures.

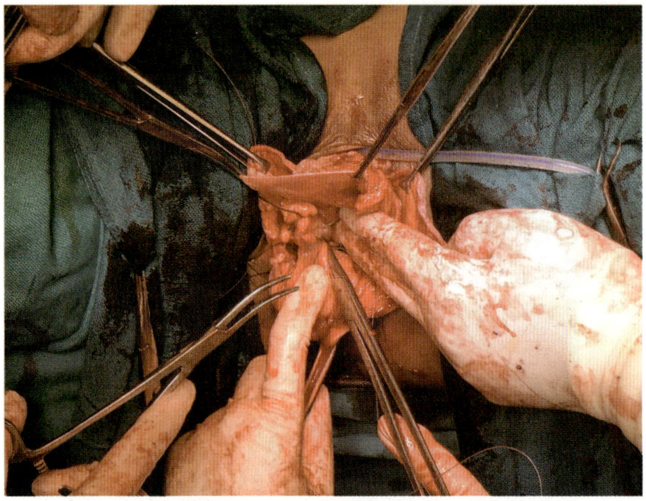

Figure 21.16 Cystocoele repair is being done with buttressing sutures.

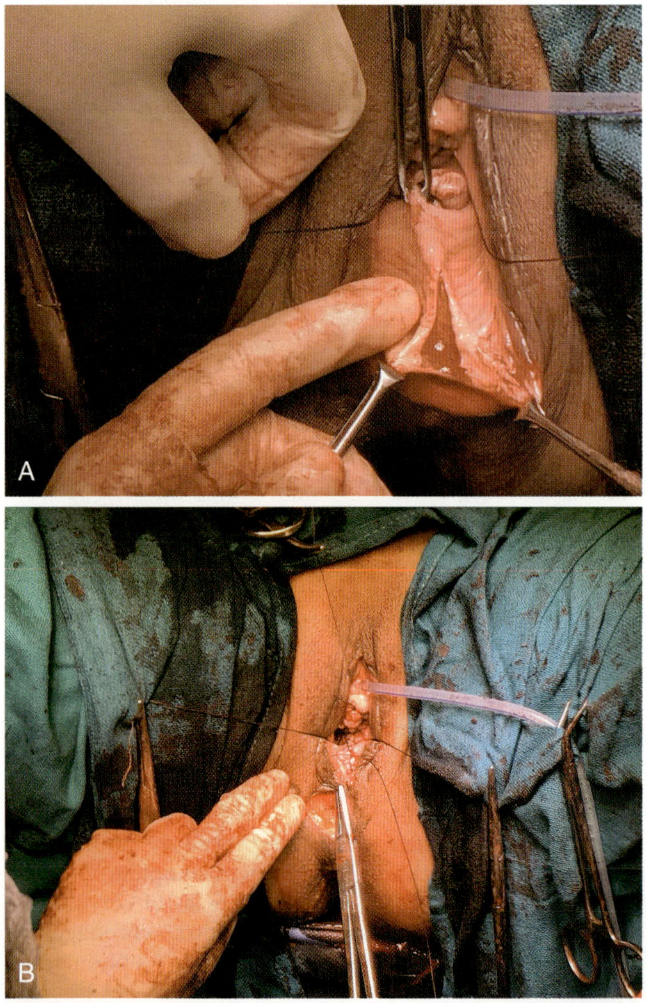

Figure 21.17 (A) Rectocoele repair. An incision given over posterior vaginal wall (B) Lax vagina is excised and the rectovaginal fascia repaired.

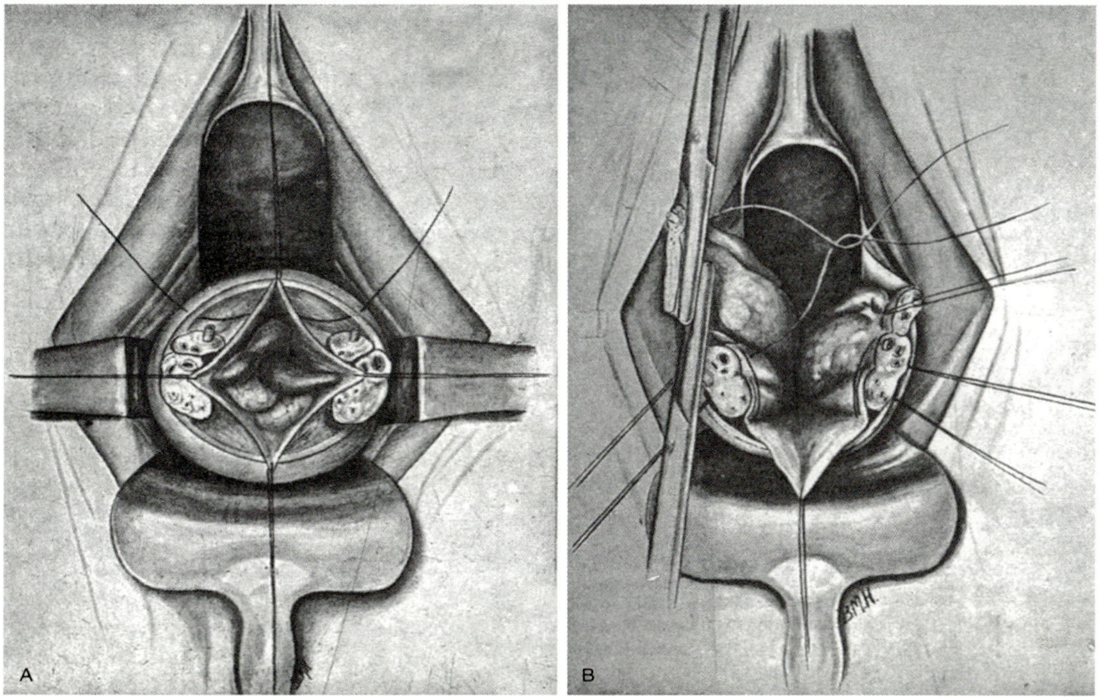

Figure 21.18 **(A)** Peritoneal opening closed in vaginal hysterectomy. **(B)** Pedicles clamped and ligated in vaginal hysterectomy.

3. Urinary tract infection
4. Complications related to anaesthesia
5. Subsequent vault prolapse
6. Dyspareunia due to narrow/short vagina

Alternative Methods of Tying Pedicles during Surgery

LigaSure. LigaSure vessel sealing system is lately used to secure the pedicles in vaginal hysterectomy. The device consists of a bipolar radiofrequency generator, reusable hand piece and disposable electrodes. The electrodes melt the collagen and elastin in the vessel wall to form a seal zone. Quick surgery with LigaSure is an advantage.

While choosing the vaginal route for performing hysterectomy in a uterus without prolapse, the following points should be observed.

Vaginal hysterectomy is contraindicated if

- Uterus is very bulky (more than 12–14 weeks).
- The uterus is fixed by abdominal adhesions and inflammatory disease. Abdominal adhesions are likely to be present if the woman had previous abdominal surgery or caesarean section.
- Other pelvic pathology exists such as endometriosis and ovarian tumour. In such cases, proper laparotomy is indicated.

Some experts are also able to remove the ovaries by the vaginal route.

LE FORT'S REPAIR

Le Fort's repair is reserved for the very elderly menopausal woman unfit for major surgery. In this procedure, anterior and posterior vaginal walls are approximated below the level of cervix.

Before the procedure, a Pap smear and pelvic sonography should be obtained to exclude possible pelvic pathology.

The procedure can be performed under sedation and local anaesthesia, or epidural anaesthesia. The flaps of the vagina from the anterior and posterior vaginal walls are excised, the raw areas apposed with catgut sutures. Thus, a wide area of adhesion is created in the midline which prevents the uterus from prolapsing, the small tunnels on either side permitting drainage of discharge.

This operation limits marital functions; hence, it should not be advised in women who are leading an active sexual life. Some women may develop stress incontinence. Other contraindications are menstruating women and women with diseased cervix and uterus.

ABDOMINAL SLING OPERATIONS

A number of abdominal sling operations have been described for young women suffering from nulliparous prolapse or the second- or third-degree uterine prolapse, who are desirous of retaining their childbearing and menstrual functions. The objective of these operations is to buttress the weak supports of uterus (Mackenrodt's and uterosacral ligaments) by reinforcing these with a nylon mesh or Dacron tapes used as slings. The advantage of these synthetic tapes/mesh is that they are strong and non-tissue reactive.

Sling operations are best suited for nulliparous prolapse.

The operations in common use are as follows:

- Abdominal wall cervicopexy.
- Shirodkar's abdominal sling operation.
- Khanna's abdominal sling operation.

Abdominal Wall Cervicopexy

The operation entails opening of the abdominal wall through a low transverse suprapubic incision deepened down, up to the rectus sheath. By means of transverse incisions made in the rectus sheath, two musculofascial slings are elevated from the midline outwards and laterally up to the lateral border of the rectus abdominis muscles on the either side. The peritoneum is opened in the midline, and the uterus brought up into view. The uterovesical fold is incised, and the bladder mobilized from the front of the uterine isthmus. The medial ends of the fascial sling are now directed retroperitoneally between the two leaves of the broad ligaments up to the space created in front of the uterine isthmus; the slings are pulled through and anchored there with stout nonabsorbable ligatures after ensuring an adequate correction in the position of the uterus in the pelvis. The uterovesical fold is next sutured, followed by closure of the abdomen in layers. Presently, the surgeon uses a 12-inch-long Mersilene/nylon tape to provide the new artificial supports for the uterus. The tape is fixed at its midpoint to the uterine isthmus anteriorly, and its lateral ends brought out retroperitoneally between the two leaves of the broad ligament, so as to emerge at the lateral border of the rectus abdominis muscle on the either side. The ends of the tape are now fixed to the aponeurosis of the external oblique muscle of the abdominal wall either by weaving it through the aponeurosis on the either side from the medial to the lateral side or by fixing it to the undersurface of the aponeurosis with interrupted nonabsorbable sutures.

Purandare and Mhatre have improved on the original operation by attaching the tape posteriorly on the cervix close to the attachments of the uterosacral ligaments. The ends of the tape are then brought forward retroperitoneally as described above, and are attached to the external oblique aponeurosis.

The sling operations can be combined with a Moschcowitz repair to treat associated enterocele. Anterior colporrhaphy and colpoperineorrhaphy can be combined to correct additional genital laxity of the vagina.

Many Indian gynaecologists have contributed significantly to the operative repair of genital prolapse. Amongst thse, the important modifications worth noting are Virkud's sling operation, Mangeshkar's laparoscopic technique and Neeta Warty's laparoscopic modification of Shirodkar's operation.

Shirodkar's Abdominal Sling Operation for Uterine Prolapse

This operation was designed to meet the special needs of the case of a nulliparous prolapse having inherently weak supports. It is a technically a difficult operation to perform but it is based on sound anatomical principles and gives excellent results. Using Mersilene tape, the cervix is fixed to the lumbosacral fascia by passing the tape extraperitoneally.

Khanna's Sling Operation

In this operation, the Mersilene tape is fixed to the isthmus posteriorly, and the two free ends brought out retroperitoneally to emerge out at the lateral margin of the rectus abdominis muscle on the either side. They are anchored to the anterosuperior iliac spine on the either side. The sling supports Mackenrodt's ligaments.

ENTEROCELE

Whenever an enterocele is encountered during prolapse operation, it should be repaired.

During vaginal hysterectomy, the enterocele is repaired after the uterus is removed. The redundant peritoneum of the pouch of Douglas is dissected, the peritoneal sac excised and the neck of the enterocele is ligated. The enterocele aperture is closed and strengthened by approximating the two uterosacral ligaments and the levator ani muscles. Failure to recognize and repair the enterocele can lead to vault prolapse later.

Enterocele can also be repaired during an abdominal operation. The cul-de-sac of the pouch of Douglas is obliterated by several purse-string sutures starting from below. This operation is known as Moschcowitz repair. One should take care not to include the ureter in the stitch.

VAULT PROLAPSE

Vault prolapse is a delayed complication of abdominal and vaginal hysterectomy. It results because of poor attention paid to anchoring the supporting structures to the apex of vagina. It also results from failure to identify and repair an enterocele during hysterectomy. A technical error in previous surgery, age, oestrogen deficiency in a menopausal woman, parity, obesity and chronic cough may all contribute to its occurrence. Sling operations for urine stress incontinence leave a defect in the posterior fornix, leading to enterocele in 15% of cases. The vault prolapse follows soon after the technical error in surgery, but within 2 years in remaining 50% due to weakness in the supporting structures. Vault prolapse occurs equally, commonly following vaginal and abdominal hysterectomies.

The current incidence of vault prolapse is 3–6 per 1000, but is increasing due to increase in longevity and desire for sexual life beyond menopause that brings the woman to the gynaecologist.

The woman with vault prolapse complains of coital difficulty and difficulty in walking. Backache, urinary and rectal symptoms may exist.

DEGREES OF VAULT PROLAPSE

First degree – The vaginal apex is visible at the introitus.
Second degree – The vault protrudes through the introitus.
Third degree – The entire vagina is outside the introitus.
Vault prolapse is often associated with cystocele and enterocele.

PREVENTION

- Enterocele should be recognized and repaired during the primary surgery (vaginal/abdominal hysterectomy).
- Attachment of the uterosacral and cardinal ligaments to the vaginal vault during hysterectomy reduces the incidence of vault prolapse.

TREATMENT (Table 21.4)

- *Right transvaginal sacrospinous colpopexy* in obese and elderly women not fit for abdominal surgery was first described by Ritcher in 1968. Bilateral fixation is rarely required. It is now the preferred surgery in most cases.

The vaginal vault is fixed to the sacrospinous ligament, so that in the upright position, the vagina lies in the

Table 21.4 Vault Prolapse

Vault prolapse	
Young woman	**Old woman**
Abdominal sling surgery	Vaginal sling surgery
Sacropexy	• Right transvaginal sacrospinous colpopexy
Colpopexy	• Transabdominal (laparoscopy) sacropexy
Laparoscopy	• Colpocleisis
Colpopexy	• Le Fort's operation
	• Abdominoperineal surgery
	• Ring pessary
	• Posterior intravaginal slingoplasty

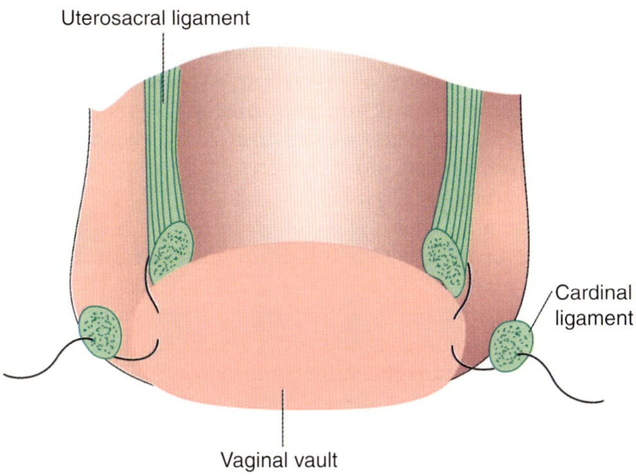

Figure 21.19 McCall's culdoplasty.

horizontal position and gets compressed against the levator ani muscles. McCall culdoplasty comprises fixing the uterosacral and Mackenrodt's ligaments to the vaginal vault and the peritoneum of the pouch of Douglas. Ureteric obstruction and kinking are reported in 10% of cases(Fig. 21.19). Vaginal route is safer for elderly women. A choice of an abdominal surgery to treat vault prolapse especially in young women avoids dyspareunia.

Complications of surgery for vault prolapse:

Early complications

- Haemorrhage – primary, reactionary, secondary haemorrhage.
- Sepsis
- Trauma to the bladder, urethra rectum mainly in repeat surgery.
- Urinary infection.
- Thromboembolism

Late sequelae

- Narrow scarred vagina causing dyspareunia.
- Granulation tissue.
- Recurrence of vault prolapse
- Fistula

VAGINAL SACROSPINOUS COLPOPEXY

Following opening of the posterior vaginal wall vertically, a window space is created between the vagina and the rectum towards the right sacrospinous ligament. A synthetic sling such as the Mersilene mesh fixes the vault to the sacrospinous ligament with a Miya hook 2 cm away from the ischial spine using a nonabsorbable suture. During surgery, care is taken not to injure the rectum, pudendal vessels and nerves at the ischial spine, sciatic nerve and sacral plexus which lie above the ligament. Ninety per cent success has been reported. Previous rectal surgery and drainage of pelvic abscess contraindicate this surgery. Buttock pain (15%) following this operation resolves gradually. It is caused by a nerve injury. Cystocele may develop at a later date. Recurrence of vault prolapse (20%–30%) and detrusor overactivity are reported (Fig. 21.20). Enterocele should be repaired before closing the vagina.

Abdominal sacrocolpopexy: In this procedure, the vault is fixed to the sacral promontory by interposing a mesh between apex of vagina and sacral promontory. The mesh is covered with pelvic peritoneum to make it retroperitoneal. The same procedure can also be done laparoscopically. A careful dissection can avoid injuries to bladder, ureters and presacral vessels. It is best suited for younger women, because coital difficulty following vaginal surgery is avoided (Fig. 21.21).

- *Colpocleisis* as a treatment for vault prolapse is used only in selected very old women unfit for a major surgical procedure due to underlying medical conditions. This procedure precludes any sexual activity hence is not suitable in younger women. In this treatment, vaginal mucosa is denuded all around and the cavity is obliterated with a series of purse-string sutures starting from the apex downwards. Stress incontinence of urine may follow this operation.
- *Le Fort's* operation is another alternative. It is a kind of partial colpocleisis. A small rectangular portion of the anterior and posterior vaginal wall is denuded and

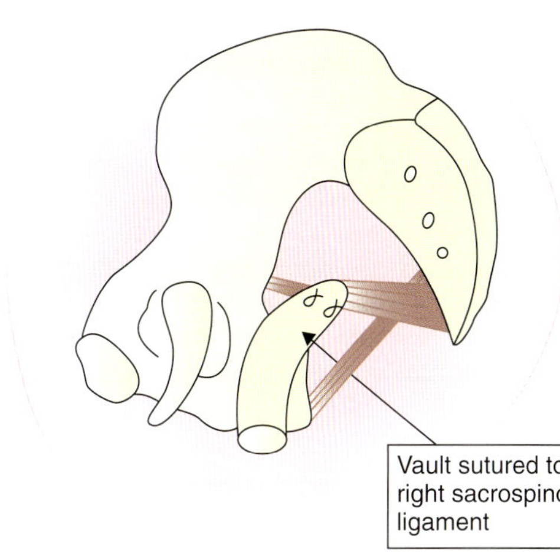

Figure 21.20 Sacrospinous fixation.

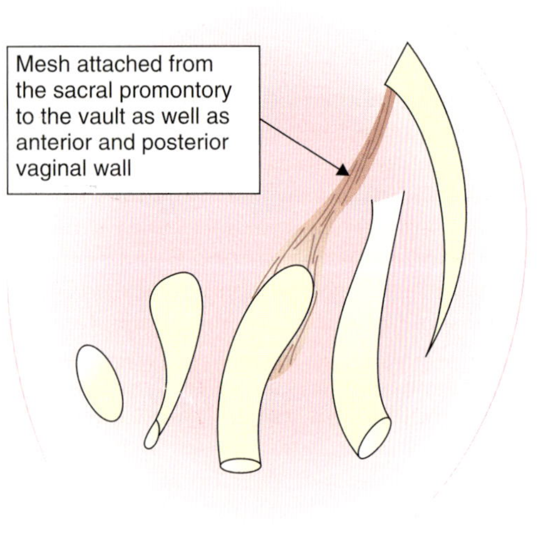

Figure 21.21 Sacrocolpopexy.

sutured to each other with several Vicryl sutures, thus obliterating the vagina in the middle. It is suited for old women not interested in sexual function.

- *Abdominoperineal surgery as* described by Zacharin is a difficult surgery required in complicated cases, especially if rectal prolapse is also present.
- Ring pessary is recommended in a woman not fit for surgery.
- Anterior and posterior colporrhaphy may be required for cystocele and rectocele in addition.

Posterior intravaginal slingoplasty; Petros described this operation in 1997. Posterior intravaginal sling plasty with a monofilament polypropylene tape (8-mm wide, 40-cm long) is used to support uterosacral ligaments by creating neo-uterosacral ligaments and by relocating the vault. Although associated with less morbidity, this surgery can cause ureteric and rectal injury, and postoperative coital difficulties and pain. Recurrence of prolapse in 10% of cases is also a disadvantage. Mesh erosion can also occur.

Abdominal surgery is preferable in young women with vault prolapse as it avoids coital difficulties, and also in women who develop recurrence following vaginal repair.

POSTOPERATIVE CARE

Postoperative care is important and comprises following:

- Parental fluids until bowel sounds return. Early oral fluids are now advocated.
- Antibiotics, sedatives, metronidazole i.v. for 24 hours.
- Indwelling catheter for 48 hours.
- Vaginal pack for 24 hours.
- Early ambulation.

RECURRENT PROLAPSE AND PROSTHETICS

About 30% of women who have undergone previous surgery for genital prolapse suffer from recurrence. They often need repeat surgical interventions. The high failure rate of primary surgery is attributed to poor collagen tissue strength of the patient's damaged tissues. Further stress and menopausal changes predispose to recurrence.

The introduction of synthetic and biological prosthesis has been utilized extensively to reduce recurrence in high-risk cases. Use of synthetic meshes as a primary surgical tool is debatable.

Classification:

1. Synthetic materials
   A. Macro porous, nonabsorbable (Marlex, Prolene): The pore size is more than 75 micrometer to allow infiltration by macrophages, fibroblasts, new vessels and collagen fibres. The long-term problem is mesh erosion, infection and dyspareunia caused by hard mesh; it may require its removal surgically.
   B. Absorbable polyglactin (Vicryl): It is free of mesh complications, but long-term results need further evaluation.
2. Biological materials
   A. Autologous material (rectus fascia, fascia lata): This requires two sites of operation, vaginal and in fascia lata, and hence results in a prolonged surgery. The poor quality of tissues can also cause recurrence of prolapse and wound infection.
   B. Xenografts of porcine.
3. New system
   A. A polypropylene tape is used in posterior intravaginal sling plasty.
   B. Apogee and perigee, used in a sling operation. The mesh is secured to the arcus tendineus pelvic fascia through a transobturator approach.

KEY POINTS

- Pelvic organ prolapse is a common problem encountered in clinical practice.
- Genital organ descent results from congenital weakness of the pelvic connective tissues, acquired tissue damage following prolonged or difficult childbirth or vaginal instrumental delivery. Conditions causing raised intraabdominal pressure and menopause with a resultant oestrogen deficiency predispose to prolapse.
- Cystocele, urethrocele, rectocele and uterine descent are manifestations of the same pathology.
- These women suffer from symptoms such as protruding of cervix outside vagina, urinary symptoms such as frequency, incomplete voiding, stress incontinence, repeated urinary infections and in rare cases, retention of urine. Difficulty during defecation, infertility, coital problems, backache and difficulty in walking around are also encountered.
- In younger women desirous of retaining childbearing functions, conservative surgical repair operations are indicated, whereas in perimenopausal and menopausal women, vaginal hysterectomy with repair of the pelvic floor is the operation of choice.
- In a younger woman desirous of further child bearing, Manchester operation (Fothergill's operation) is the

procedure of choice. However, amputation of cervix as a part of this operation may lead to repeated mid-trimester abortions/preterm deliveries. Vault prolapse is a sequelae of abdominal as well as vaginal hysterectomy which requires surgical repair. Both abdominal and vaginal operations can be undertaken to repair vault prolapse. A ring pessary is applicable only in a woman unfit for surgery.
- Recent introduction of prosthetic materials to supplement weakened tissues has resulted in long-term benefits in the management of recurrent prolapse, but the cost and complications should be borne in mind.
- A patient with vault prolapse may also have other vaginal defects. These need additional corrective procedures along with repair for vault prolapse.
- By fixing the uterosacral and cardinal ligaments to the vaginal vault at the time of hysterectomy, vault prolapse can be prevented.
- Sacrocolpopexy is considered the gold standard surgical procedure for vault prolapse.

SELF-ASSESSMENT

1. Describe the normal supports of the uterus.
2. How would you classify genital prolapse?
3. Describe the symptomatology of genital prolapse.
4. Discuss the prophylaxis of genital prolapse.
5. Describe the surgical procedures for repair of genital prolapse.
6. A 50-year-old woman presents with third-degree uterine prolapse. How will you manage this case?
7. A 30-year-old woman, para 2, complains of something coming out per vagina. Discuss the investigations and management of this case.
8. Discuss the management of nulliparous prolapse.
9. A 60-year-old woman presents with something coming out per vagina following abdominal hysterectomy 2 years ago. How will you manage the case?

SUGGESTED READING

Beecham CT. In: Classification of vaginal relaxation. Am J Obstet Gynecol 136(7):957,1980.

Clifford L, Regan L. In: Recurrent pregnancy loss.In: John Studd. Progr Obstet Gynaecol Vol 11:387,1994.

Nichols DH. Transvaginal sacrospinous fixation. Pelvic Surgery 1:10,1981.

Richter K. Massive eversion of the vagina: Pathogenesis, diagnosis and therapy of the 'true' prolapse of the vaginal stump. Clinical Obstetrics and Gynecology 25:897,1982.

Ridley JH. Evaluation of the colpocleisis operation: A report of 58 cases. Am J Obstet Gynecol 113:1114,1972.

Seigworth GR. Vaginal vault prolapse with eversion. Obstet Gynecol 54:255,1979.

Studd J (ed). Progress in Obstetrics and Gynaecology 17:381. Churchill Livingstone, Elsevier

Sturdee D. Year Book of Obstetrics and Gynaecology Year Book of Obstetrics and Gynaecology. 61–70,2001.

22 Displacements of the Uterus

CHAPTER OUTLINE

INTRODUCTION

The uterus is kept in place by a cross-formation of four ligaments (pubocervical ligaments, uterosacral ligaments and a pair of cardinal or Mackenrodt's or transverse cervical ligaments, and by the pelvic floor muscles and a sheet of connective tissue enveloping the hollow pelvic viscera providing them support.

The uterus is normally maintained in an anteverted, anteflexed position. However, the uterus is a mobile organ and its position may vary depending on the status of bladder, parity of the person, the position she is lying down in and by the presence of fibroids and other condition in the uterus. For different reasons, uterine displacement may occur; the displacement may happen sideways but more commonly backwards, or downwards.

Pelvic inflammatory disease and endometriosis may leave behind adhesions that may bind the uterus to other structures, thus leading to uterine displacements – commonly presenting as a fixed retroversion or a lateral tilting following adhesions with adnexal structures. Uterine tumours may push or drag the uterus into various abnormal positions. Similarly, tumours in surrounding structures may move the uterus out of its normal position. A faulty development of the structures supporting the uterus may also cause uterine displacement.

There are **two common types of uterine displacements** which are often the cause of physical distress – **retroversion and prolapse**.

In retroversion, the uterus tips backwards and also possibly sags downward. In prolapse, the uterus settles downward; sometimes, the displacement is so extreme that the cervix protrudes out from the vulva, and may even drag down with it part of the rectum and bladder. In other cases, the entire uterus and vagina prolapse out of the introitus causing procidentia. Prolapse is more common after menopause. Prolapse has been discussed in chapter 21.

Mostly displacement of the uterus has no bearing on the reproductive function or menstrual functions; however, in an uncommon situation a uterine displacement may prevent a woman from conceiving; if she does become pregnant under such a condition, it may lead to retention of urine in early pregnancy and vary rarely may end in abortion. With the backward position of the uterus, as in retroversion, the ligaments which support the organ may be stretched which can result in kinking of the fallopian tubes, and congestion of the ovaries and the uterus itself. The same condition can likewise cause backache, dyspareunia, dysmenorrhoea, infertility, abortion, menstrual irregularities, leucorrhoea and constipation. Most patients with mobile retroversion, however, are symptomless.

RETROVERSION

The usual position of the uterus is one of anteversion and anteflexion, in which the uterine body is bent forwards at its junction with the cervix. Version refers to the direction of the cervical canal, whereas flexion refers to the inclination of the body of the uterus at the cervix. The normal uterus is not a static organ; its position is altered by the state of the bladder which, when full, displaces the uterus backwards. In most cases of retroversion, the uterus is also retroflexed, so that the body of the uterus is flexed backwards (Fig. 22.1).

AETIOLOGY

It is difficult to explain why the uterus is normally anteverted and anteflexed. The round ligaments do not maintain this position on their own, although they are used to correct the retroversion during surgery. It appears that the position of the uterus in relation to the cervix is largely inherent in the uterine myometrium.

MOBILE RETROVERSION

The uterus is retroverted in 20%–50% of patients, with no obvious gynaecological symptoms.

The uterus is usually retroverted in case of prolapse, but it is difficult to say if it precedes prolapse or if prolapse causes retroversion. Sometimes, the displacement of the uterus is caused by tumours such as anterior wall myomas and ovarian cysts in the pelvis, which push the uterus backwards.

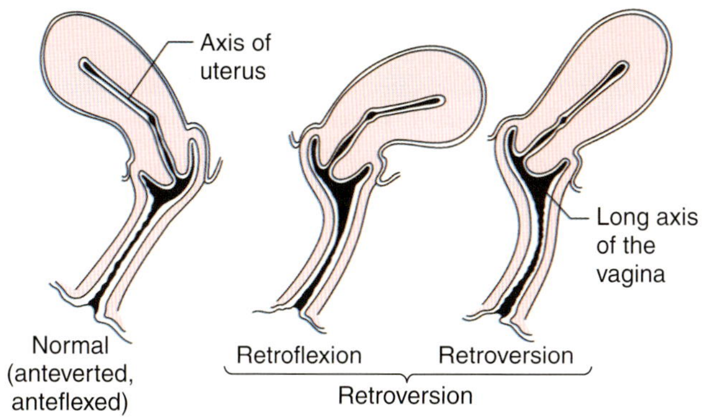

Figure 22.1 Normal and retroverted uterus.

Retroversion is commonly noted in women after childbirth. Such displacements often correct themselves spontaneously once the patient's muscle tone improves.

FIXED RETROVERSION

Fixed retroversion means that the uterus is bound down by adhesions or tumours in the retroverted position. Most fixed retroversions result from pelvic inflammatory diseases (PID) such as salpingo-oophoritis and pelvic tumours. In salpingo-oophoritis, the oedematous, the distended fallopian tubes prolapse behind the uterus and, partly by their weight and partly through formation of adhesions to the posterior surface of the uterus, pull back the uterus. In the process of healing, adhesions form which bind the uterus firmly in its retroverted position. Fixed retroversion is also caused by chocolate cysts of the ovary and pelvic endometriosis.

SYMPTOMS

The significance of retroversion per se in clinical practice has declined during the last few decades. This is due to the appreciation of the fact that the symptoms earlier attributed to this displacement are not to it, rather they are related to the aetiological factors causing retroversion. Therefore, asymptomatic retroversion does not need treatment, and treatment of symptomatic fixed retroversion is directed towards the disease that causes it.

DYSMENORRHOEA

Both congestive and spasmodic dysmenorrhoea have been wrongly attributed to mobile retroversion. The incidence of dysmenorrhoea is the same in women with the retroverted uterus as it is in women with an anteverted uterus. The fixed retroverted uterus can cause dysmenorrhoea.

MENORRHAGIA

Menorrhagia associated with mobile retroversion is either due to myohyperplasia or abnormal uterine bleeding (AUB). A manual or surgical correction of retroversion will not relieve the menstrual symptoms. In fixed retroversion, menorrhagia is due to pelvic congestion caused by pelvic pathology.

PRESSURE

A normal-sized retroverted uterus does not cause pressure on the rectum or on the bladder.

BACKACHE

More likely, the backache is due to an orthopaedic cause and not due to the retroverted uterus.

DYSPAREUNIA

Of all the symptoms of retroversion, dyspareunia may be one which is genuine and attributable to retroversion. During vaginal examination, the body of the retroverted uterus is tender and the patient may wince when it is touched. Besides, the ovary may prolapse in the pouch of Douglas and thus cause dyspareunia during coitus. Following coitus, she may complain of a dull ache in the pelvis that persists for 12–24 hours. This may lead to frigidity and marital disharmony.

INFERTILITY

To implicate retroversion as a cause of infertility, it is necessary to perform all other investigations for infertility. In the past a lot of emphasis has been given to retroversion in a woman with unexplained infertility. Sims–Huhner test (postcoital test) with abundant motile sperms seen in the vaginal pool and cervical mucous rules out retroversion as a cause of infertility. On the contrary, failure to detect sperms in the cervical canal indicates that the cervical canal is away from the seminal pool and is not accessible to the motile sperms. In such a case, retroversion may be the cause of infertility. A surgical correction of the retroversion may result in conception in such a rare situation. Fixed retroversion due to salpingo-oophoritis causes infertility because of associated tubal blockage.

ABORTION

Retroversion as a cause of abortion has been greatly exaggerated. Fixed retroversion would more often lead to infertility rather than abortion, because of the associated tubal block.

RETROVERTED GRAVID UTERUS CAUSING RETENTION OF URINE

Retroverted gravid uterus especially in a multigravida may cause retention of urine around 12–14 weeks of pregnancy. This is as a result of failure of the retroverted uterus to correct its position thus causing overstretching of anterior vaginal wall and lumen of urethra. In most cases, the uterus tends to rise out of pelvis at 12–14 weeks; however, in an acutely retroverted uterus this may not happen thus resulting in retention of urine. The management of such a case comprises placing an indwelling Foley's catheter for 48 hours and allowing urine to escape slowly after the initial placement of the catheter. Subsequently, woman may be asked to lie in an extreme lateral position or prone position to prevent recurrence of such an event.

DIAGNOSIS

There should be no problem in the diagnosis of the retroverted uterus on bimanual vaginal examination. In rare cases, the uterus felt in the pouch of Douglas may be mistaken for an ovarian tumour or a fibroid. The fact that the mass in the pouch of Douglas moves with the cervix confirms that this is the uterine body.

TREATMENT

If the retroversion is mobile and the patient is free of symptoms, no treatment is required.

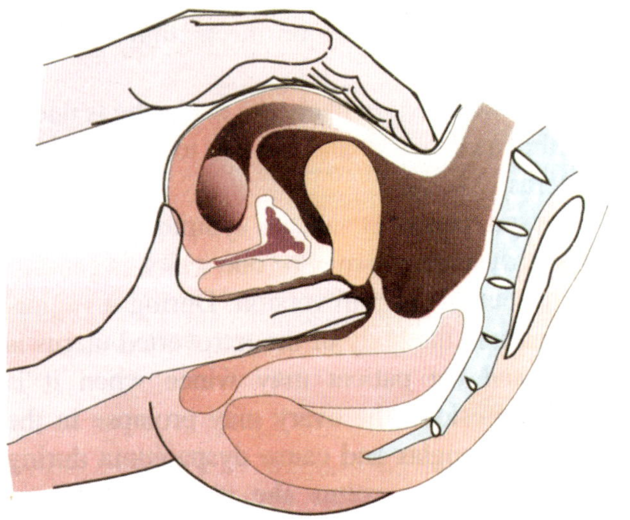

Figure 22.2 Digital replacement of a retroverted uterus. The fingers placed on the abdomen, by pressing the body of the uterus downwards, together with help from the internal fingers which push the cervix upwards, correct the displacement.

PESSARY TREATMENT

If the patient complains of dyspareunia or backache and the uterus is found to be retroverted, the uterus is bimanually replaced (Fig. 22.2) and kept in the anteverted position by inserting a Hodge pessary into the vagina (Fig. 22.3). The pessary is made up of plastic.

The pessary is retained in position for 3 months and then removed. If the symptoms persist in spite of the uterus being in anteversion, one should look for other causes of the underlying symptoms and no operative treatment for the retroversion should be undertaken. This is known as the pessary test. Recurrence of symptoms as soon as the pessary is removed strongly suggests retroversion as the cause the underlying symptom.

SURGERY

INDICATIONS

1. Fixed retroversion requires surgery for the primary organic lesion such as the pelvic inflammatory mass and tumour. At the end of the surgery, the uterus is brought forward by shortening the round ligaments, as mentioned below, and maintained in an anteverted position.

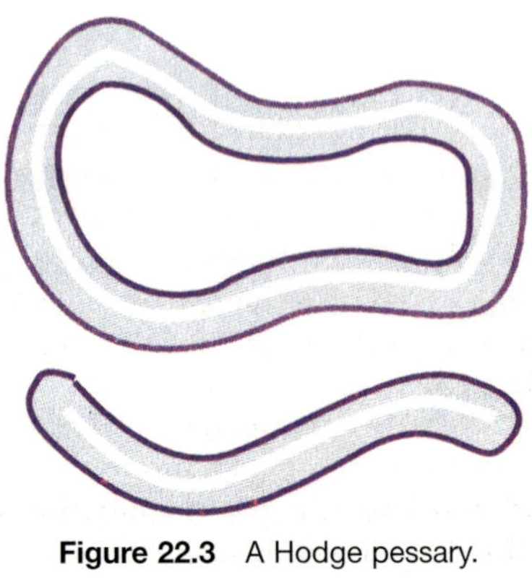

Figure 22.3 A Hodge pessary.

2. In patients for whom the pessary test proves that the symptoms and infertility are caused by retroversion.
3. Following tuboplasty and myomectomy operation, uterus is ventrosuspended to prevent or minimize the formation of tubal and pelvic adhesions.

VENTROSUSPENSION

One of the most popular surgical procedures to correct the retroversion is the **modified Gilliam's operation** in which the round ligament is first held by nonabsorbable suture, close (1 cm) to the uterine cornua. The ends of this suture are left long. A long, curved forceps is now passed between the anterior rectus sheath and the muscle at the level of the anterior superior iliac spine. It is now directed close to the internal abdominal ring into the space between the two layers of the broad ligament towards the uterine cornua. The forceps point is then pushed through the peritoneum of the broad ligament and the ends of the ligature around the round ligament withdrawn along the tract of the forceps. These ends are now anchored to the anterior rectus sheath. The round ligament is thus drawn up against the anterior abdominal wall. This operation was frequently undertaken in the past with a mistaken impression that it will improve fertility; however, it is of historical significance in the modern times.

PLICATION OF ROUND LIGAMENTS

Shortening of round ligaments by plication using a nonabsorbable suture is a simple form of ventrosuspension operation for fixed retroversion associated with organic pelvic disease and fibroids.

BALDY–WEBSTER OPERATION

The round ligaments are passed through the anterior and posterior leaves of the broad ligament and are sutured to the posterior surface of the uterus, thus shortening the round ligaments and ventrosuspending the uterus.

INVERSION OF THE UTERUS

In inversion, the uterus is turned inside out. At first, the fundus is pushed down into the cavity of the uterus leaving a cup-shaped depression on the peritoneal surface. As a result of contractions of the uterus, the invagination is pushed further and further down, until finally the whole uterus is turned inside out and hangs in the vagina. If the peritoneal surface of the uterus is inspected, the fallopian tubes, the ovarian and the round ligaments can be seen to pass down into a deep hollow in the position where the body of the uterus should have been. Inversion of the uterus is classified as **complete or partial** according to the degree to which the uterus is turned inside out (Figs 22.4 and 22.5).

ACUTE INVERSION

In most cases an inversion of the uterus occurs as a result of mismanagement of the third stage of labour. Attempt to pull the umbilical cord before the separation of placenta predisposes to acute inversion of the uterus. Certain practices during labour, such as Crede's manoeuvre, are well-known predisposing factors for acute inversion of the uterus.

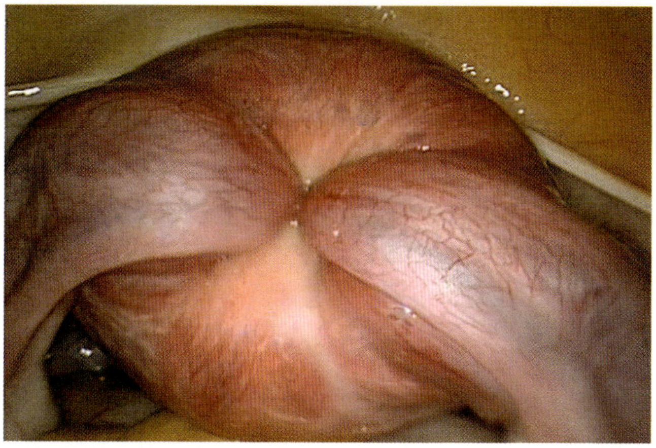

Figure 22.4 Inversion of the uterus. (*Source*: LJ Shephard, H Shenassa, SS Singh. The Journal of Minimally Invasive Gynecology. Laparoscopic Management of Uterine Inversion, 2010.)

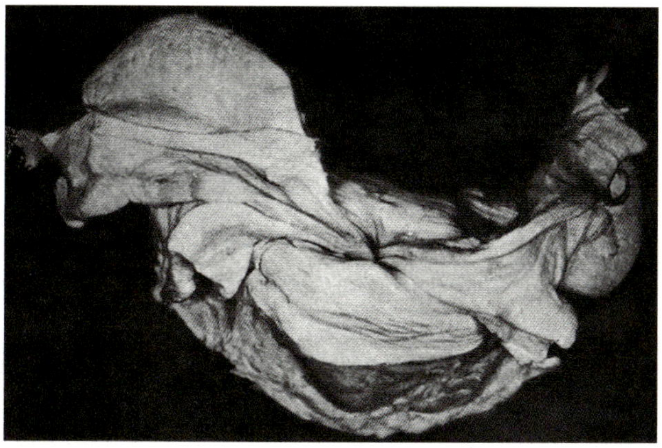

Figure 22.5 The fallopian tubes, broad ligaments and ovarian ligaments pass into a cup-shaped depression at the fundus of the uterus.

In some cases it may be due to traction being applied to the umbilical cord when the placenta is morbidly adherent, whereas others are due to squeezing a relaxed uterus immediately after delivery. Nevertheless, most puerperal inversions are probably spontaneous, although the exact aetiology is unknown. It has been suggested that the puerperal contractions of the body tend to invaginate the fundus into the uterine cavity. The presence of muscle defects in the region of the uterine fundus may also allow a dimple to occur and progressive invagination to follow. Puerperal inversion of the uterus is complete when the whole uterus lies outside the vagina. The condition is associated with a severe degree of shock, and the inverted uterus may bleed profusely. Shock may be neurogenic or hemorrhagic.

PREVENTION

Proper management of the third stage of labour can prevent acute inversion.

TREATMENT

The treatment of acute puerperal inversion depends on how soon after delivery it is recognized. The ideal treatment is an immediate replacement. If the inversion occurs in the presence of a doctor or nurse, it should be promptly reposited by exerting a firm and constant pressure on the inverted uterine fundus. If the placenta is attached to the uterus, it should not be removed until after the replacement of the uterus has been effected. In all instances, the shock should be treated simultaneously by transfusion with blood or plasma substitute. In domiciliary midwifery, resuscitation must be continued until woman is shifted to a facility with a proper arrangement for replacement of the uterus and management of shock.

The best method of performing this has been described by **O'Sullivan.** The patient is anaesthetized with the least possible delay. One gallon of warm sterile water is prepared for instillation into the vagina, using an irrigating can, raised 3–4 feet above the level of the patient. After gently pushing the inverted uterine fundus back into the vagina, the nozzle of the irrigating cannula is inserted into the vagina, and the vaginal orifice is closed manually by the operator and an assistant. As much as 3 L of fluid may be needed. The inversion usually corrects under the hydrostatic pressure. If this method fails, manual reposition may be attempted under deep anaesthesia. As a last resort, the abdomen should be opened and, if the inverted fundus cannot easily and without damage be pulled back into position with a simultaneous pressure from the vagina, the tight cervical ring may be divided following which the uterus is restored to it's original position and then its cut edges are repaired. Antibiotic cover should be given.

CHRONIC INVERSION

Chronic inversion of the uterus occurs as a result of the late presentation of puerperal cases in which the diagnosis was missed at the initial stages of the inversion. Chronic inversion of the uterus can also occur along with extrusion of a submucous fundal fibroid. Clinically, chronic inversion associated with fundal myoma is suspected if the woman complains intermittent lower abdominal pain and irregular vaginal bleeding. Over the period, the myoma becomes infected and causes offensive blood-stained discharge. In a longstanding fibroma associated with inversion, sarcoma may often exist, which by softening the uterine wall is responsible for the inversion. A diagnosis of chronic inversion is often difficult to make. A cup-shaped depression must be identified in the fundus. In complete inversion, the cervix is drawn up and the vaginal portion of the cervix will not be palpable. In partial inversion, the uterine sound can be passed only for a short distance along the uterine cavity, and this will help to distinguish the partial inversion from a myomatous polyp arising from body of the uterus. When the tumour which protrudes through the cervix is pulled down with a vulsellum forceps, if the cervix moves upwards, then it is most suggestive of an inverted uterus. If the tumour is a polypus, traction brings down the cervix and the tumour may be pulled further through the external os without the cervix being drawn up. In chronic inversion, the inverted fundus is likely to be ulcerated and infected, and may resemble an infected fibroid polyp or a malignancy.

Ultrasound and laparoscopic examination of the pelvis will confirm the diagnosis of inversion.

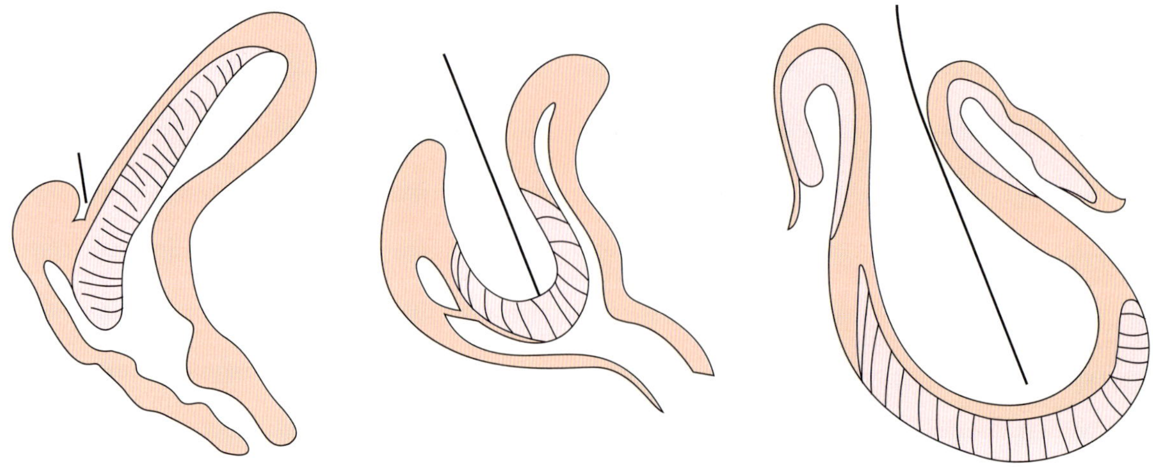

Figure 22.6 Inversion of the uterus. (A) First degree. (B) Second degree. (C) Third degree.

DEGREES OF INVERSION (Fig. 22.6)

- In first-degree inversion, the fundus of the uterus inverts into the uterine cavity.
- In second-degree inversion, the uterine fundus protrudes through the cervix and lies in the vagina.
- In third-degree inversion, the whole uterus is inverted and protrudes through the introitus.

TREATMENT

Before attempting any surgical correction of chronic inversion, the patient should be treated with antibiotics and local antiseptic packing.

- If it is desirable to conserve the uterus in young patients, the inversion can be corrected either by vaginal or by an abdominal approach. In the either instance, the important step in the operation is the division of the constricting ring of the cervix after which it is easy to restore the fundus to its correct position. The transected cervix is then repaired by suturing. In vaginal Spinelli's operation, the cervical ring is cut anteriorly and the inversion is corrected followed by repair of the cut edges of cervix. In some cases the rim of cervix may have to be divided posteriorly (Kustner's operation) followed by reposition of the uterus and repair of the cut edges of cervix. In abdominal repair of chronic inversion of the uterus after dilatation of constriction band through which tubes and ovaries are prolapsing an attempt is to restore the normal position of the uterus; in difficult cases the rim of cervix may have to be divided to reposit the inversion followed by repair of incision (Haultain's operation).
- If it is not desired to conserve the uterus in a multiparous woman, vaginal or abdominal hysterectomy is performed.
- Inversion caused by extrusion of fundal myoma with underlying sarcomatous changes will mandate radical hysterectomy followed by radiotherapy.

In a young woman, vaginal myomectomy under laparoscopic guidance will safeguard against uterine perforation.

KEY POINTS

- The uterus is a mobile organ; however, in most cases its usual position is that of anteversion and anteflexion.
- The uterus is retroverted in about 20%–50% of women; mobile retroversion is often asymptomatic and requires no treatment. It is more likely in multiparous women.
- Fixed retroversion is a result of pelvic inflammatory disease or a result of endometriosis; these women may complain of chronic backache and deep dyspareunia which may contribute to infrequent coitus and infertility.
- Pessaries to correct retroversion were in vogue some years ago. A surgical correction is indicated in women with symptomatic retroversion. The operation of choice is ventrosuspension. This procedure is carried out concomitantly with laparotomy performed for other gynaecological operations such as myomectomy or tuboplasty.
- Acute inversion is always due to mismanaged third stage of labour. If not recognized immediately it may result in severe shock and at times, demise of the patient. An immediate reposition of the uterus can prevent such a serious complication.
- Chronic inversion of the uterus is a rare clinical entity. It is likely to be mistaken for a submucous polyp or cervical cancer. A careful pelvic examination, pelvic ultrasound examination and laparoscopy will help to establish the diagnosis. Treatment of the condition is surgical.

SELF-ASSESSMENT

1. Describe the varieties of displacement in the pelvis observed in clinical practice
2. Describe uterine retroversion. When would it require a surgical correction?

3. Describe the role of pessary in the treatment of the retroverted uterus.
4. Describe the clinical features of an acute inversion of the uterus. How would you manage such a case?
5. Describe the clinical features of chronic inversion of the uterus and its management.
6. Enumerate the various causes of the uterine inversion.
7. What is the place of the operation of ventrosuspension? Describe the various surgical operations for the same.

SUGGESTED READING

Allen WM, Masters WM. Traumatic lacerations of uterine support. Am J Obstet Gynecol 70:500,1955.

Kresch A, Seifer DB, Sachs LD, et al. Laparoscopy in 100 women with chronic pelvic pain. Obstet Gynecol 64:672,1984.

Lawson JO. Pelvic anatomy I. Pelvic muscles. Ann R Coll Surg Engl 54:244–52,1974.

Sternbach RA, Wolf SR, Murphy RW, et al. Aspects of chronic low back pain. Psychosomatics 14:75,1973.

Wall DP, Melzack R (eds): Textbook of Pain. Churchill Livingstone: New York, 1984.

Zdeblick TA. In: The treatment of degenerative lumbar disorders: A critical review of literature. Spine 20(suppl 24):126S–137S,1995.

23 Diseases of the Broad Ligament, Fallopian Tubes and Parametrium

CHAPTER OUTLINE

DISEASES OF BROAD LIGAMENT

Diseases of broad ligament are mostly benign and are seen in association with other conditions affecting ovaries or uterus. These conditions may be in the form of cysts, tumour masses or infections. Following section describes these conditions which are seen in clinical practice.

BROAD LIGAMENT CYSTS

Broad ligament cysts are fairly common. However, they are small and are of no clinical importance except the paraovarian cyst which may attain a large size and undergo torsion.

ANATOMICAL CONSIDERATIONS

Vestigial remnants of the Wolffian duct (mesonephric duct) are seen in the broad ligament, lying between the fallopian tube and the hilum of the ovary. The mesonephric duct extends from the outer aspect of the ovary, parallel to the fallopian tube in an inward and downward direction until it enters the myometrium in the region of the cervix. Its lowermost limit is the region of the hymen. It should be rememebered that wolffian dust is same as mesonephric duct or gartners duct.

Associated with the mesonephric duct and opening into it are the tubules of the upper part of the Wolffian body, the epoophoron or parovarium (sometimes called the organ of Rosenmüller). They are situated in the broad ligament adjacent to the hilum of the ovary. These mesonephric tubules are sometimes called Kobelt's tubules. Besides these, a number of blind isolated tubular remnants are seen near the inner border of the ovary and are known as paroophoron.

The lining of the mesonephric duct is a nonciliated, low columnar epithelium. Although the lining of the mesonephric tubules is low columnar or cuboidal, both ciliated and nonciliated cells are present in it.

Cysts may arise in the broad ligament from either the mesonephric duct or its tubules. These cysts are usually small, pedunculated or intraligamentary, lying between the layers of the broad ligament where they may attain a considerable size. Mesonephric duct cysts are never lined with ciliated epithelium, whereas cysts of the mesonephric tubules may be. These cysts of mesonephric origin lie between the ovary and the fallopian tube, but are always separate and easily identified being separate from the ovary.

PARAOVARIAN CYSTS

Paraovarian cysts are extraperitoneal cysts lying in the broad ligament adjacent to the ovary, below the fallopian tube. The tube is stretched and flattened over the top of the cyst which tends to enlarge in a lateral direction so that it may lie to the side of ovary. Small paraovarian cysts are extremely common and are often found at operation without their presence having previously been suspected. They sometimes form a cyst as large as 15–30 cm in diameter. The cyst is usually unilocular, and contains clear fluid. Its wall is smooth, thin and translucent. Sometimes, a few loculi are present, and papilloma, similar to the stationary papillomas of papillary cystadenomas of the ovary, may be scattered over the inner surface of the cyst. Unlike the ovarian cyst, the wall of a paraovarian cyst frequently contains smooth muscle as do the mesonephric tubules. It is therefore possible to establish the origin of these cysts by histological examination.

Paraovarian cyst is clinically diagnosed as an ovarian cyst, and at laparotomy, it can be identified as a broad ligament

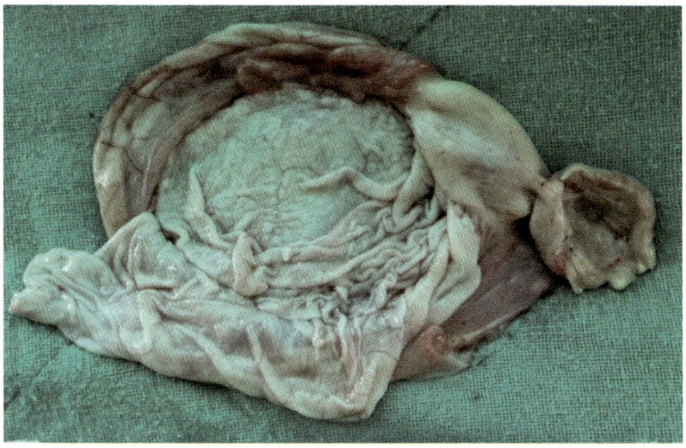

Figure 23.1 A paraovarian cyst which had undergone torsion involving also the appendages.

cyst with a normal looking ovary being present. Although an ovarian cyst can also burrow into the broad ligament but in such a case, the normal ovary is not identifiable unlike in a paraovarian cyst. Histological identification of the muscle in a cyst establishes the correct diagnosis.

The paraovarian cyst is usually seen in young women. It displaces the uterus to the opposite side, and may be fixed in between the two layers of the broad ligament. As these cysts can undergo torsion, they are sometimes misdiagnosed as twisted ovarian cysts (Fig. 23.1).

TREATMENT

Surgical removal of the paraovarian cyst becomes necessary when it attains a large size. A delicate incision is made in the peritoneum over the cyst from which it is reflected by a blunt dissection. A finger is then swept around the cyst, between it and its bed until it is sufficiently free to be enucleated. Only a few small vessels will need ligation in the cyst bed. The ureter is found very close to the cyst and may be at a risk of injury. It is mandatory therefore to identify it or trace it down from the pelvic brim before any structure is cut or clamped. Paraovarian cyst can also be removed by laparoscopy after initial decompression of the cyst followed by its removal. In most cases, it is possible to save the ovary on the same side.

TUMOURS OF THE FALLOPIAN TUBES

Neoplasms of the fallopian tubes are extremely rare and often malignant. See chapter 36.

CONDITIONS AFFECTING THE BROAD LIGAMENT AND PARAMETRIUM

HAEMATOMA

Haematoma of the broad ligament and parametrium may result from ectopic gestation which ruptures extraperitoneally into the broad ligament. A large haematoma may develop following rupture of the uterus or cervical laceration during childbirth. Haematoma may follow dilatation of the cervix, if the cervix gets split and uterine vessels get torn. The condition may also develop in cases of concealed accidental haemorrhage. A broad ligament haematoma tends to spread extraperitoneally. It may extend upwards and cause a swelling above the Poupart's ligament and may even spread to the perinephric region. A haematoma may sometimes be encountered following abdominal and vaginal hysterectomy when a vascular pedicle slips and retracts into the cellular tissue. Pain, tachycardia and haemorrhagic shock ensue. A painful lump is felt in the lower abdomen. Prophylactic or therapeutic anticoagulants in the postoperative period can also at times produce a haematoma. A small haematoma usually resolves with conservative treatment, but a large haematoma requires laparotomy, drainage and ligation of the bleeding vessel in broad ligament.

PARAMETRITIS

Parametritis, first described by Matthews Duncan, is a cellulitis of the soft tissues of the parametrium. Well-marked parametritis almost invariably follows childbirth or abortion, when the parametrium is infected from lacerations of the vaginal portion of the cervix, the vaginal vault or from lacerations of the lower uterine segment. Some degree of parametritis is present in all acute infections of the uterus and fallopian tubes and in advance carcinoma of the cervix. The cases which are of clinical importance are those complicating childbirth and abortion. The condition causes symptoms at the beginning of the second week when the patient complains of pain in the hypogastrium and back. The temperature rises to about 102°F; the pulse rate is raised in the same proportion. The inflammation of the pelvic cellular tissue leads to the development of a large indurated swelling in the pelvis. In the early stages, the uterus is pushed to the opposite side and the indurated swelling of the parametrium extends from the uterus to the lateral wall of the pelvis, and fixes the uterus in the pelvis. It is impossible to separate the uterus from the swelling, because the parametrium extends to the wall of the uterus. The effusions in parametrium may spread backwards along the uterosacral ligaments, and it may also extend upwards and point above Poupart's ligament. On rare occasions, the effusion may point in the perinephric region, in the ischiorectal fossa and even in the buttock, having tracked through the greater sciatic foramen. Suppuration in parametric effusion is uncommon. It is rare for frank pus to form, needing evacuation. As the effusion is extraperitoneal, symptoms of peritoneal irritation are absent, but rectal symptoms may arise as the result of inflammation involving the rectum.

Most parametrial effusions subside with antimicrobial treatment, but they are followed by scarring of the parametrium and this causes chronic pelvic pain. The scarred tissue draws the uterus over to the affected side and the thick scar tissue is readily palpated on bimanual examination. Ureteric kinking may occur resulting in hydronephrosis.

Parametritis is often complicated by some degree of pelvic thrombophlebitis with its risk of pyaemia, pulmonary infarction and extension to the lower extremities to produce a 'white leg'. This clinical syndrome is especially common if the responsible organism is the anaerobic *Streptococcus.* Almost all effusions in parametrial space are lateral to the uterus and vagina, where the parametrium is most plentiful. However, on rare occasions, an anteroposterior parametritis develops situated between the cervix and the rectal wall posteriorly, and the bladder and urethra anteriorly. The *treatment* of parametritis consists of bed rest, local heat and a full course of the appropriate antibiotic – similar to that described in the treatment of acute salpingo-oophoritis.

TUMOURS OF THE BROAD LIGAMENT AND PARAMETRIUM

MYOMA

The most common tumour found in a broad ligament is myoma. It may be primary (true broad ligament fibroid), when it arises from the uterosacral or round ligament, and tissues in the broad ligament, or secondary (false broad ligament fibroid), when it arises from the lateral wall of the uterus or the cervix and grows laterally between the two layers of the broad ligament. In the latter, the myoma retains its attachment to the uterus, and the uterine vessels as well as the ureter are pushed laterally. In case of a primary myoma, the uterine vessel is medial to the fibroid, but the ureter may lie anywhere in relation to it though usually it is beneath the tumour. Primary myoma is also known as true broad ligament myoma and secondary myoma as false broad ligament fibroid.

SARCOMA

Sarcoma in broad ligament is very rare. It presents with clinical features of a myoma. In the early stages, surgery is feasible, but in advanced stages, it can be treated only by radiation.

LIPOMA

Lipoma is rare and can be enucleated without much difficulty during surgery. However, all precautions should be exercised to avoid injury to ureter and major vessels.

RETROPERITONEAL TUMOURS

Retroperitoneal tumours are included here because they are often mistaken for an ovarian tumour or a broad ligament tumour, and their exact nature is revealed only at laparotomy. These tumours are classified as follows:

- Congenital: Ectopic pelvic kidney should be suspected when a fixed pelvic mass is associated with the absence or malformation of the genital tract. Ultrasound and intravenous pyelography reveals its true condition.
- Dermoid cyst: Rarely dermoid cyst can be retroperitoneal in location.
- Tumours of neurogenic origin: Neurofibromas and tumours arising from the spinal meninges can be present in the retroperitoneal space.
- Solid tumours arising from the bony pelvis, i.e., osteoma, chondroma and sarcoma can also be present in retroperitoneal space.

When faced with a retroperitoneal tumour, a thorough preoperative investigations, i.e., IVP and barium enema, CT and MRI are indicated. Diagnostic laparoscopy and biopsy are helpful. The ultrasound will indicate its location. Two dangers are encountered during removal of the retroperitoneal tumour, injuries to ureter and injury to major pelvic vessels.

- The ureter may be close to the tumour and be cut or ligated unless it is identified at the start of the surgery.
- Large vessels of the hypogastric system may obtrude into the operative fields and these must be secured.

In case of inoperable fixed growth, radiotherapy is an alternative.

The different types of abdomen lumps encountered in gynaecology are illustrated in Table 23.1

Table 23.1 Differential Diagnosis of Lumps in the Lower Abdomen

Adolescents	Reproductive Age	Menopause
• Haematocolpos • Haematometra • Ovarian tumour • Uterine fibroids (rare) • Tubercular mass • Pelvic kidney	• Pregnancy • Ectopic pregnancy • Full bladder – gravid uterus • Fibroid or ovarian tumour associated with pregnancy • Uterine fibroid • Pelvic Inflammatory Disease (PID) • Ovarian tumour	• Pyometra • Endometrial carcinoma • Ovarian tumour • Fallopian tube cancer • Uterine sarcoma • Chronic retention of urine

KEY POINTS

- Remnants of the Wolffian body and the mesonephric duct are present in the broad ligament between the fallopian tube and the ovary; these can enlarge and cause cystic neoplasms. The paraovarian cyst can grow to a large size. It can undergo torsion or rupture.
- The parametrium can be the site of a haematoma formation or infection causing parametritis.
- The connective tissue in the broad ligament can be the site of a true broad ligament fibroid. However, more common is a fibroid arising from lateral wall of uterus extending into broad ligament.
- Retroperitoneal tumours may mimic broad ligament neoplasms.
- The nature of the abdominal tumours varies according to the age.

SELF-ASSESSMENT

1. Describe the different abdominal tumours encountered in gynaecology.
2. Write short notes on following:
   a. Haematoma of the broad ligament
   b. Retroperitoneal tumours

SUGGESTED READING

American College of Obstetricians and Gynecologists Committee on Gynecologic Practice. Committee Opinion No. 477: the role of the obstetrician-gynecologist in the early detection of epithelial ovarian cancer. Obstet Gynecol 2011; 117:742.

American College of Obstetricians and Gynecologists. ACOG Practice Bulletin. Management of adnexal masses. Obstet Gynecol 2007; 110:201.

Givens V, Mitchell GE, Harraway-Smith C, et al. Diagnosis and management of adnexal masses. Am Fam Physician 2009; 80:815.

Grab D, Flock F, Stohr I, et al.: Classification of asymptomatic adnexal masses by ultrasound, magnetic resonance imaging, and position emission tomography. Gynecol Oncol. Vol 77:454–459, 2000.

National Institutes of Health Consensus Development Conference Statement. Ovarian cancer: screening, treatment, and follow-up. Gynecol Oncol 1994; 55:S4.

Studd, J, et al. Progress in Obstetrics and Gynaecology 17:306, Elsevier, 2006.

Studd, J, et al. Progress in Obstetrics and Gynaecology 18:299–313, Elsevier, 2008.

24 Benign Diseases of the Ovary

CHAPTER OUTLINE

Ovaries can be site of a variety of diseases. These diseases include functional cysts, ovarian endometriosis, polycystic ovaries and neoplastic diseases. In this chapter, functional cysts and polycystic ovaries are described.

Ovarian enlargements, cystic or solid, may occur at any age. Functional and inflammatory enlargements of the ovary develop almost exclusively during the childbearing years. They may be asymptomatic or produce local discomfort, menstrual disturbances, infertility or in rare cases cause acute symptoms due to complications such as haemorrhage, rupture or torsion.

The ovary is complex in its embryology, histology, steroidogenesis and has the potential to develop malignancy. Therefore, ovarian neoplasms exhibit a wide variation in structure and biological behaviour. Unlike the cervix and uterus, the ovaries are not clinically accessible, and therefore, suitable screening methods for detecting ovarian neoplasms are not available. The ovary, after the cervix, is the second most common site for development of gynaecological malignancy, with a dismal prognosis.

Ovarian tumours may occur at any age.

In adolescents, the ovarian tumours are mostly malignant and are of germ cell origin. In perimenopausal and postmenopausal women they tend to be epithelial in origin. During the childbearing age, these ovarian enlargements are functional in 70% of cases, neoplastic (mostly benign) in 20% of cases and due to ovarian endometriomas in 10% of cases.

NONNEOPLASTIC ENLARGEMENTS OF THE OVARY (Table 24.1)

Enlargement of ovaries can be as a result of pelvic congestion as seen in a pelvic inflammatory disease, ovarian endometriosis causing a chocolate cyst or persistence and enlargement of physiological structures in the ovary such as the Graafian follicle or corpus luteum. The lesions due to inflammatory conditions are discussed in the chapter on a pelvic inflammatory disease, and endometriosis affecting the ovary is dealt in Chapter 27. In this chapter, nonneoplastic enlargement of the ovaries, and polycystic ovarian syndrome (PCOS) are described in detail.

Table 24.1 Varieties of Cystic/neoplastic Enlargements of the Ovaries

1. Functional cysts	• Follicular cysts • Lutein cysts • Multiple functional cysts • Corpus luteal cyst • (PCOS)
2. Inflammatory	• Salpingo-oophoritis • Puerperal, abortal, IUCD related
3. Metaplastic	• Endometrioma
4. Neoplastic benign and malignant	• Benign • Borderline tumor • Malignant

FUNCTIONAL CYSTS IN OVARY

Ovaries can be the site of functional cysts such as follicular cyst, theca lutein cyst or corpus luteum cyst. These cysts usually form because of nonregression of functional cysts in ovary.

To define a functional cyst, its size must be at least 3 cm, but not more than 7 cm.

FOLLICULAR CYSTS

Follicular cysts are not uncommon. They may be single or multiple, may be bilateral and vary in size from small blebs to cysts of large size but generally do not exceed 5.0 cm in diameter (Fig. 24.1). They form as a result of failure of absorption of the fluid in an incompletely developed follicle or anovulation. They are usually asymptomatic unless haemorrhage, rupture or torsion supervenes, in which case symptoms and signs of an acute abdomen develop.

Large and multiple cysts may cause pelvic pain, dyspareunia and irregular bleeding. The enlarged ovary may be recognizable clinically or documented on sonography.

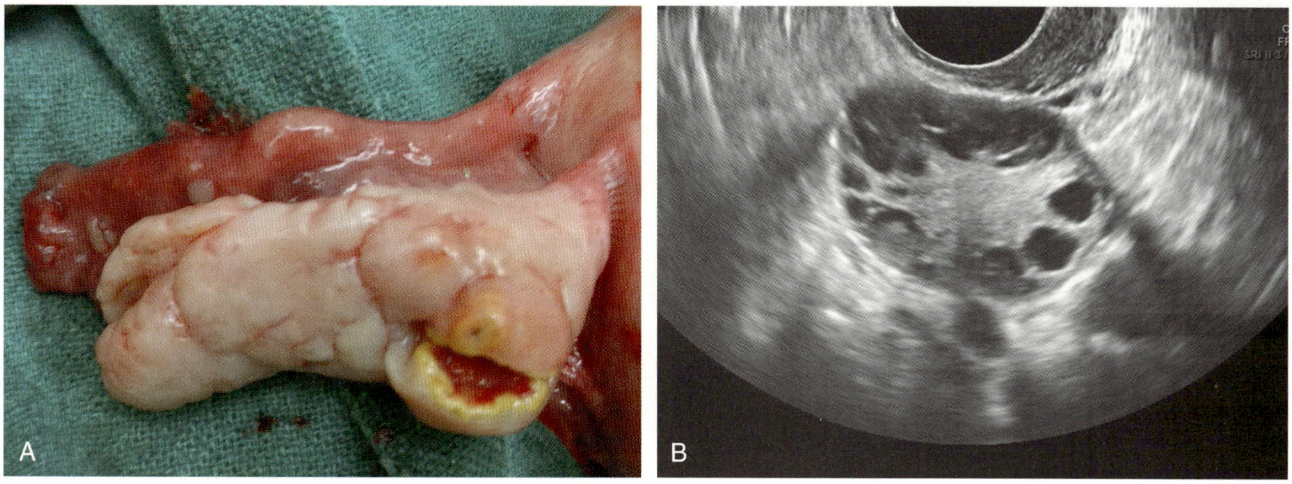

Figure 24.1 (A) Corpus luteum cyst. **(B)** Transvaginal ultrasound showing polycystic ovary.

Ovarian neoplasms, inflammatory adnexal enlargement and endometriosis must be considered in the differential diagnosis.

Most follicular cysts disappear spontaneously within 4–8 weeks. In the presence of symptoms such as amenorrhoea administering oral medroxyprogesterone 10 mg twice a day over a period of 5 days will generally bring on menstruation. Norethisterone tablet (Primolut N) 5 mg t.i.d. for 5 days also induces menstruation. Oral combined pills administered for 3 months help resolve the persistent cyst in most cases.

If any cyst persists for longer than 3 months, or size increases to > 7 cm, the possibility of a neoplastic cyst must be kept in mind, and the patient investigated.

FOLLICULAR HAEMATOMAS (FOLLICULAR CYST WITH HAEMORRHAGE)

Small follicular haematomas are common. To the naked eye, the ovary contains haemorrhagic cysts. Old cysts appear to contain tarry material and are likely to be mistaken for endometriosis. Many of these are asymptomatic and of no clinical significance except for the rare case, when the cyst ruptures into the peritoneal cavity causing acute abdomen, and is mistaken for an ectopic pregnancy.

LUTEIN CYSTS OF THE OVARY

Two types of lutein cysts are recognized:

- Granulosa lutein cysts found within the corpus luteum.
- Theca lutein cysts associated with a trophoblastic disease and chorionic gonadotropin therapy.

CORPUS LUTEUM (GRANULOSA LUTEIN) CYSTS

Corpus luteum cysts are functional, nonneoplastic enlargements of the ovary. Persistent corpus luteum cysts may cause local pain, tenderness or delayed menstruation. These cysts are often palpable clinically. Unless complications such as torsion or rupture lead to an acute abdomen requiring surgical treatment, most cysts will resolve in due course of time. Hence observation is recommended whenever this condition is suspected. As it resembles unruptured ectopic pregnancy sonography and serum quantitative estimations of β-hCG can help to make a correct diagnosis.

Ultrasound reveals a spider web–like structure with or without a clot. Doppler shows increased vascularization with a high blood flow velocity.

THECA LUTEIN CYSTS

These cysts can sometimes enlarge to several centimetres in diameter. They are usually bilateral and filled with straw-coloured fluid. Theca lutein cysts are often noted in cases of hydatidiform moles, choriocarcinoma. Induction of ovulation with gonadotropin (hCG) and clomiphene can also result in the formation of theca lutein cyst. The cysts spontaneously regress after evacuation of the mole, therapeutic curettage and treatment of choriocarcinoma. In a case undergoing induction of ovulation with gonadotropin or clomiphene one should avoid giving hCG injection to prevent further enlargement of ovary.

Functional cysts are distinguished from neoplastic cysts by *the fact that they never grow more than 7 cm in size, are unilocular with clear fluid and regress after some time.* The hyperstimulation syndrome by clomiphene therapy has been described in the chapter on Infertility: Male and Female.

MULTIPLE FUNCTIONAL CYSTS

Multiple functional cysts are usually caused by following conditions:

- Follicle-stimulating hormone (FSH)-secreting pituitary adenoma.
- Ovarian hyperstimulation syndrome (OHSS)
- PCOS

PITUITARY ADENOMA

In pituitary adenoma, ovarian cysts measure more than 1 cm; FSH and oestrogen levels are raised, but luteinizing hormone (LH) level is low. Other signs of hyperstimulation such as haemoconcentration and coagulation profile are not present. Amenorrhoea, oligomenorrhoea and infertility are the clinical features. Pituitary adenoma may require transsphenoidal excision of the adenoma, but no surgery is required for the ovarian cysts. These eventually resolve.

OVARIAN HYPERSTIMULATION SYNDROME

OHSS is caused mainly by administration of human chorionic gonadotropin injection in a woman undergoing control ovarian stimulation with gonadotropin or clomiphene. The follicular size is usually more than 3 cm.

POLYCYSTIC OVARIAN SYNDROME

PCOS is characterized by multiple small cysts less than 1 cm; LH is raised and LH/FSH ratio is ≥2. This condition is fairly common affecting 5%–15% of adolescent girls. It may also be seen among women in reproductive age suffering from infertility, menstrual irregularities or hirsutism. Following section describes in detail about aetiopathogenesis, diagnosis and management of this condition.

POLYCYSTIC OVARIAN SYNDROME OR DISEASE PCO, PCOS, PCOD

PCOD is a heterogeneous, multisystem endocrinopathy in women of reproductive age with the ovarian expression of various metabolic disturbances and a wide spectrum of clinical features such as obesity, menstrual abnormalities and hyperandrogenism. This disease was described by and named as Stein–Leventhal syndrome in 1935. To diagnose PCOS, adrenal and androgen-producing ovarian tumour should be excluded.

INCIDENCE

Current incidence of PCOS (5%–15%) is increasing fast lately due to change in lifestyle and stress. It is also becoming a common problem amongst adolescents, developing soon after puberty. Amongst infertile women, about 15%–20% of infertility cases are due to anovulation caused by PCOS. Some of the women who develop a cardiovascular disease, hypertension, endometrial cancer and type 2 diabetes later in life appear to have suffered from PCOS in earlier years.

AETIOLOGY AND PATHOGENESIS

The exact aetiology of PCOS remains unknown. A number of theories have been postulated in the genesis of PCOS. Some of the well-known factors which may influence the onset of PCOS are lifestyle changes, sedentary life, diet and stress. Initially, the ovaries were thought to be the primary sight which sets the series of changes in the endocrine pattern resulting in PCOS. Genetic, familial and environmental factors (autosomal dominant inherited factors) were later added as aetiological factors in the development of PCOS. The environmental factors may function in utero or in early adolescent life, manifesting clinically a few years later as PCOS. CYP_{21} gene mutation has been identified in this connection. Familial occurrence has also been reported where a sex-linked mode of inheritance has been postulated.

Another view held for the development of PCOS is an enhanced serine phosphorylation unification activity in the ovary (hyperandrogen) and a reduced insulin receptor activity peripherally (insulin resistance).

Obesity is related to PCOS. At least 50%–70% of patients with PCOS tend to be obese or overweight. The adipose tissue (fat) is considered an endocrine and immunomodulatory organ; it secretes leptin, adiponectin and cytokines which interfere with the *insulin signalling* pathways in the liver and muscles resulting in *insulin resistance*, and *hyperinsulinaemia*. Increased birth weight in obese and PCOS mothers can also cause PCOS in their adolescent daughters.

Raised LH secretion by insulin can cause infertility or miscarriage through improper oocyte maturation.

Obesity is characterized as the condition when body mass index > 30 kg/m^2 and waist line >88 cm; waist/hip ratio > 0.85.

Endogenous β-endorphin also stimulates insulin release and may contribute to insulin resistance.

Hyperandrogenism and resulting anovulation were initially thought to arise primarily in the ovaries. It has now being proved that insulin resistance with resultant hyperinsulinaemia initiates PCOS in 50%–70% cases, though hypothalamic–pituitary–ovarian axis, adrenal glands also play a role in the genesis of PCOS to some extent.

OVARIAN STEROIDOGENESIS IN PCOS

Insulin induces LH to cause theca-cell hyperplasia and secrete androgens, testosterone and epi-androstenedione which are converted to oestrogen in the granulosa cells. Epi-androstenedione is converted in the peripheral fat to oestrone. This leads to rise in the oestrogen and inhibin level. These in turn cause high LH surge.

While oestrone level increases, oestradiol level remains normal with the result that the oestrone/oestradiol ratio rises.

Hyperandrogenism lowers the level of hepatic sex hormone–binding globulin (SHBG), as a result levels of free testosterone in serum rises leading to hirsutism. *Androgen also suppresses the growth of the dominant follicle and prevents apoptosis of smaller follicles which are normally destined to disappear in the late follicular phase.*

PCOS may set in early adolescent life, but clinically manifest in the reproductive age with long-term complications such as diabetes, hypertension, hyperlipidaemia and a cardiovascular disease; this cluster of disorders is known as the 'X syndrome' or 'metabolic syndrome'.

Endocrinological changes in PCOS are as follows:

1. Oestrone/E_2 level rises.
2. LH level is raised over 10 IU/mL.
   FSH level remains normal, but FSH/LH ratio falls.
3. SHBG levels fall due to hyperandrogenism.
4. Testosterone and epi-androstenedione levels rise.
5. Fasting blood glucose/fasting insulin < 4.5 suggests insulin resistance.
6. Triglyceride level > 150 mg/dL-hyperlipidaemia High Density Lipoproteins (HDL) < 50 mg/dL.
   Testosterone > 2 ng/mL, free T > 2.2 pg/mL (Normal level 0.2–0.8 ng/mL)
   Normal androstenedione.
   Raised Dehydroepiandrosterone Acetate Sulfate (DHEA-S) level
7. Prolactin is mildly raised in 15% of cases.
8. Fasting insulin levels are raised (>10mIU/L in 50-70% cases of PCOS).

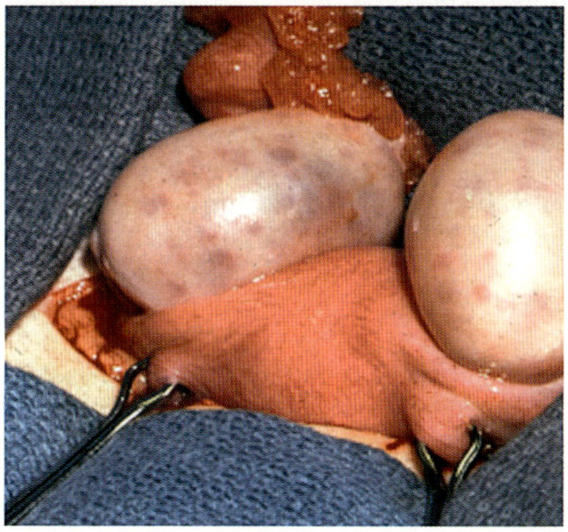

Figure 24.2 Bilateral enlarged ovaries with a smooth and thickened capsule. (*Source:* From Figure 22.3A. R. Jeffrey Chang: Polycystic Ovary Syndrome and Hyperandrogenic States. Jerome F Strauss and Robert L Barbieri: In: Yen & Jaffe's Reproductive Endocrinology: Physiology, Pathophysiology, and Clinical Management, 7th Edition. Saunders: Elsevier, 2014.)

9. Thyroid function tests may be abnormal (hypothyroidism).
10. Urinary cortisol < 50 mcg/24 hours.

PATHOLOGY

Macroscopically, both ovaries are enlarged. The ovary shows a thick white capsule of tunica albuginea. The ovarian surface may be lobulated but the peritoneal surface is free of adhesions.

Multiple cysts (12 or more) of 2–9 mm size are located peripherally along the surface of the ovary giving it a 'necklace' appearance on ultrasound. These are persistent atretic follicles. Theca-cell hyperplasia and stromal hyperplasia account for the increase in the size of the ovary which amounts to more than 10 cm^3 in volume. The laparoscopic view of the polycystic ovarian disease is shown in Fig. 24.2.

CLINICAL FEATURES (Table 24.2)

The pathogenesis appears to be initiated either in utero or in early adolescent life. Early adrenarche in the form of early pubertal hair and early menarche is observed in some of these girls. Menstruation for the initial few years may be normal, but as clinical features of PCOS develop the cycles become oligomenorrheic (87%) or they develop a short period of amenorrhoea (26%) followed by prolonged or heavy periods (a common complaint in a majority of cases). Dysmenorrhoea is absent.

In the reproductive years, infertility is seen in a number of these women. This is due to anovulatory cycles. If a woman with PCOS conceives, she develops carbohydrate intolerance, diabetes and hypertension. Pregnancy loss occurs in 20%–30% cases due to abortions.

Hyperandrogenism appears in the form of acne (30%) and hirsutism. Facial hair appears over the upper lip, chin, breasts and thighs. Baldness is sometimes noted, but virilism does not develop.

History of lifestyle, diet and smoking and exogenous hormone administration should be enquired. Family history of diabetes and hypertension should also be asked.

EXAMINATION OF A GIRL WITH PCOS

Look for

- Obesity, especially waistline. Waist to hip ratio > 0.85 is abnormal; 50% of women are obese.
- Body mass index between 25 and 30 – overweight; and above 30 – obesity.
- Thyroid enlargement.
- Hirsutism and acne.
- Hyperinsulinaemia which may manifest as acanthosis nigricans (5%) over the nape of the neck, axilla and below the breasts; 75% of obese PCOS women have hyperinsulinaemia.
- Blood pressure in obese women.

Pelvic findings are usually normal, and it is not easy to palpate the enlarged ovaries.

DIAGNOSTIC CRITERIA FOR MAKING A DIAGNOSIS OF PCOS

For the diagnosis of PCOS, the Rotterdam criteria (2003) are generally followed. It states that at least two of three criteria should be present. These criteria are as follows:

- Oligo/amenorrhoea, anovulation, infertility
- Hirsutism/acne
- Ultrasound findings (see section 'Investigations')

Table 24.2 Clinical Features of PCOS

Clinical Features	Hormonal	Sequelae

• Young woman
• Central obesity
  ◦ BMI > 30 kg/cm^2
  ◦ Waist line > 88 cm
• Oligomenorrhoea, amenorrhoea
• Infertility (20%)
• Hirsutism
• Acanthosis nigricans due to insulin resistance; thick pigmented skin over the nape of neck, inner thigh and axilla
• Most androgen come from ovary
• ↑fasting insulin > 10 mIU/L
	• ↑E_2 level
	• ↑ LH levels
	• ↑ FSH/LH ratio
	• ↑Androgens
	• Testosterone, epi-androstenedione, ↑ dehydro-epiandrosterone
	• 17-α-hydroxyprogesterone > 300 ng/dL
	• Testosterone > 2 ng/mL
	• Prolactin ↑
	• Sex hormone–binding globulin (SHBG) ↓
	• ↓E_2/oestrone (E_1) ratio
	• F. glucose/insulin ratio < 4.5
		• Diabetes (15%)
		• Cardiovascular Disease (CVO)
		• Lipidaemias
		• Hypertension
		• Endometrial cancer
		• Breast cancer
		• Premature ovarian failure following surgery

DIFFERENTIAL DIAGNOSIS

Although the diagnosis is easy in most cases, congenital or adult adrenal hyperplasia, Cushing disease and ovarian masculinizing tumours should be considered in differential diagnosis especially, if a woman is extremely obese or had features of virilism. With irregular cycles in young girls, hormonal assays will identify a hypothalamic–pituitary–ovarian dysfunction. Thyroid function tests may be called in for a few cases.

INVESTIGATIONS

Ultrasound is diagnostic of PCOS.

- It confirms the enlarged ovaries, their size and increased stroma. Ovarian volume will be more than 10 mm^3.
- It shows 12 or more small follicles each of 2–9 mm in size placed peripherally.
- It helps to rule out ovarian tumour.
- It can also show endometrial hyperplasia, if present.

In a case with suspicious adrenal tumour/adrenal hyperplasia, abdominal scan, estimation of DHEA, 17-OH hydroxyprogesterone level will help in diagnosis of these conditions. To make a diagnosis of PCOS, ultrasound should preferably be performed in the early follicular phase. An increased blood flow is sometimes revealed on Doppler ultrasound. Ultrasound is also used to watch the response of medication and to decide when to stop the drug therapy. Sometimes, only one ovary may show features of PCOS. These ovarian changes cannot be relied upon if a woman is on combined oral pills, as these pills change the ovarian morphology.

- Hormonal study mentioned earlier is not performed routinely, but specific hormonal studies are undertaken in a woman as and when required. All hormonal studies are not needed as a routine.
- Thyroid function tests in an obese woman.
- Laparoscopy is reserved for a therapeutic purpose. In most cases diagnosis can be confirmed on ultrasound. Laparoscopy reveals enlarged bilateral ovarian cysts.

TREATMENT

The aims of treatment are as follows:

- To cure a woman with menstrual disorders
- To treat hirsutism
- To treat infertility
- To prevent long-term effects in the form of X syndrome in later life.

The treatment should be tailored to the requirement of the woman.

- **Weight loss.** Weight loss of more than 5% of previous weight alone is beneficial in mild hirsutism; it restores the hormonal milieu considerably. Weight loss increases the secretion of the SHBG, reduces insulin level and testosterone level.
- **Lifestyle changes.** Cigarette smoking should be stopped. It lowers E_2 level and raises DHEA and androgen level.
- Hormones to regulate menstruation are as follows:
  - Oral combined pills (OC)
  - OC containing cyproterone acetate or drospirenone
  - Spironolactone and OCs
- Ketoconazole 200 mg daily reduces testosterone secretion.

Oestrogen suppresses androgens and adrenal hormones (DHEA). It raises the secretion of SHBG in the liver, which binds with testosterone, thus reducing free testosterone. It also suppresses LH. It is best given as low-dose combined pills, having progestogen with lesser androgenic effect. Fourth generation of combined pills which contains 30 mcg E_2 and 2–3 mg drospirenone (progestogen with anti-androgenic action) are best for PCOS (Yasmin, Janya, Tarana). It helps to reduce acne and further development of hirsutism. It prevents water retention and reduces weight; it maintains a lipid profile.

- Progestogen may be required to induce menstruation in an amenorrhoeic woman prior to initiating a hormonal cyclical therapy.
- Oral Contraceptive Pills (OCP) containing cyproterone is prescribed, if the woman has hirsutism (see Chapter 9).
- Eflorinthine cream topically prevents hair growth.

Hirsutism. Anti-androgens used are described in detail in chapter on Hormone Therapy in Gynaecology. Acne can be managed by a clindamycin lotion 1% or erythromycin gel 2%, if pustules form. For severe acne, isotretinoin is used, but it is teratogenic and pregnancy should be avoided while on this medication. *The drugs take 3–6 months before improvement in hirsutism is noted.*

Dexamethasone (0.5 mg) at bedtime reduces androgen production, and is used in some infertile women if DHEA-S is raised above 5 ng/mL.

Infertility. For managing infertility in a PCOS woman *Clomiphene is the first line of treatment.* It induces ovulation in 80% and 40%–50% conceive. A 25%–40% abortion rate has been reported in a PCOS woman who conceives after ovulation induction, it may be due to a corpus luteal phase defect. There is an increased risk of ovarian hyperstimulation in a woman with PCOS when ovulation is induced. Clomiphene with dexamethasone improves fertility rate. In a resistant case, tamoxifen 20–40 mg daily for 5 days or letrozole (2.5 mg daily for 5 days or 20 mg single dose on day 3) can be tried. Failure after the above therapy calls for FSH, LH or GnRH analogues therapy. A woman with insulin resistance requires, in addition, metformin.

These women also have raised level of homocysteine in which case *N*-acetyl-cysteine (NAC) 1.2 g may be added to clomiphene therapy. NAC is a mucolytic drug and an insulin sensitizer.

Metformin. Metformin treats the root cause of PCOS, rectifies endocrine and metabolic functions and improves fertility rate. It is used as an insulin sensitizer. It reduces insulin level, delays glucose absorption and production of glucose in liver (liver neoglycolysis). It also improves peripheral utilization of glucose; Liver and renal function tests should be performed prior to metformin administration.

Besides reducing the level of insulin, metformin also reduces the level of total and free testosterone and increases the SHBG. Ovulation occurs in 70%–80%, and pregnancy in 30%–40%. It does not cause hypoglycaemia and does not reduce weight. It is contraindicated in a hepatic and renal disease, and causes gastrointestinal disturbances and lactic acidosis. Therefore, starting with 500 mg daily, the dose is gradually increased to 500 mg three times a day. Metformin should not be administered for more than 6 months. If metformin is contraindicated, acarbose 300 mg daily can be used. Octequitide peptide hormone secreted by hypothalamus which inhibits the growth hormone and insulin has also been used to treat these cases. It enhances ovulation in clomiphene-resistant infertility.

Lately, to improve the pregnancy rate in PCOS, instead of metformin, some gynaecologists have started using *N*-acetyl cysteine with micronutrients. This reduces the homocysteine level. The micronutrients include vitamin D, minerals, chromium, selenium, inositol and folic acid (Ovacare, one tablet twice daily).

It is important to inform the patient that PCOD can recur.

SURGERY

Surgery is reserved for those in whom

- Medical therapy fails
- Hyperstimulation occurs
- Infertile women
- Previous pregnancy losses

Surgery comprises laparoscopic drilling or puncture of not more than four cysts in each ovary either by laser or by unipolar electrocautery (Fig. 24.3).

Surgery restores endocrine milieu and improves fertility for a period of 6–12 months. Pelvic adhesions caused by surgery may reduce fertility rate. Hydroflotation reduces adhesion formation.

Advantages of surgery are as follows:

- Tubal testing with chromotubation can be performed simultaneously.
- Other causes of infertility, i.e. endometriosis looked for.
- One-time treatment.
- Intense and prolonged monitoring not required.
- Cost-effective compared to In-vitro Fertilization (IVF).
- Reduces androgen and LH production
- Following surgery, single ovulation occurs with drugs, and hyperstimulation and multiple pregnancy are avoided.
- Ovulation occurs in 80%–90% and pregnancy in 60%–70%.

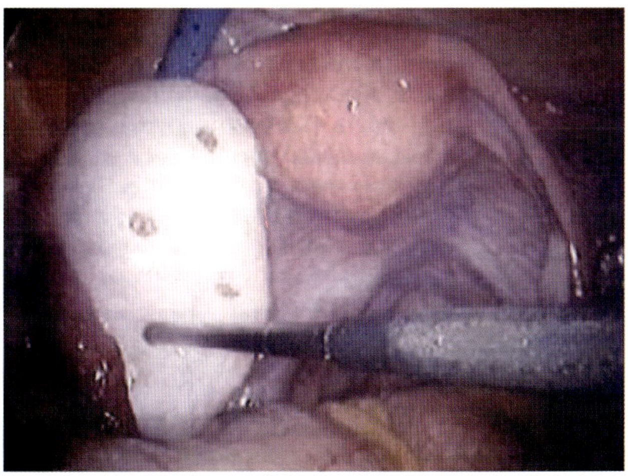

Figure 24.3 Laparoscopic ovarian drilling. (*Source*: From Figure 2. Suresh Kini: In: Polycystic ovary syndrome: diagnosis and management of related infertility practice points. Obstetrics, Gynaecology and Reproductive Medicine. Vol 22(12): 347–353, 2012.)

Disadvantages of surgery are as follows:

- Surgery involves anaesthesia and laparoscopy.
- Adhesions may form postoperatively.
- Premature ovarian failure due to destruction of ovarian tissue if cautery is used. For this reason, many now prefer a simple puncture of the cysts.

Surgery is not a preferred treatment for management of PCOS as it may result in a decrease in ovarian reserve and adhesions might form around ovaries.

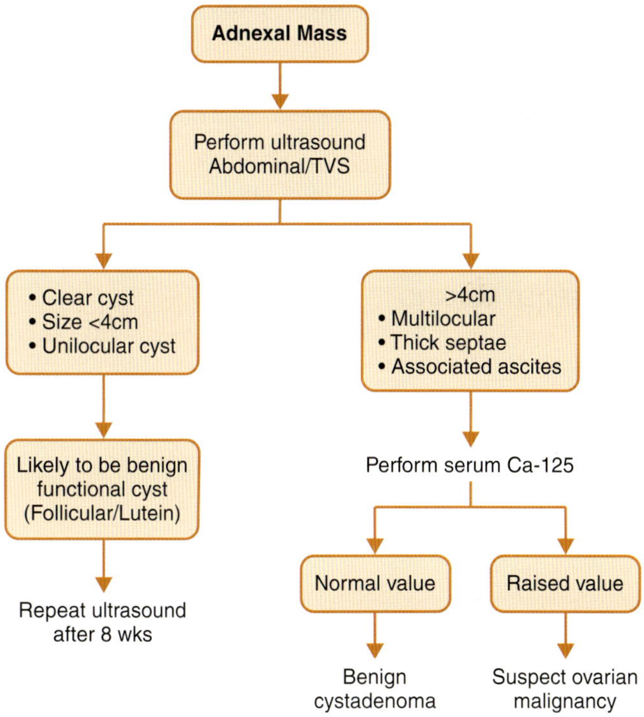

PREVENTION

With the knowledge that PCOS has long-term adverse effects (threefold) on the health of the woman, such as development of diabetes, hypertension, a cardiovascular disease and hyperlipidaemia, endometrial cancer, it is now suggested that PCOS should be adequately treated at the earliest. These women should be observed for these ailments in later life. Obesity in adolescents needs to be avoided and corrected. Lifestyle changes should be recommended.

KEY POINTS

- Polycystic ovary is a multisystem endocrine disorder with features of oligomenorrhoea, anovulation, obesity and hirsutism. It is a disease of young women.
- PCOS originates from insulin resistance; hyperinsulinaemia and obesity are linked.
- PCOS causes oligomenorrhoea, hirsutism and infertility.
- Ultrasound is the gold standard investigation in the diagnosis of PCOS. Hormonal study is performed only if required.

- Decrease in weight and change of lifestyle improves the condition considerably.
- Surgery is performed if medical therapy fails and to improve fertility rate.
- Follow-up should be ensured to avoid late sequel such as diabetes, hypertension, a cardiovascular disease and hyperlipidaemia.
- Raised E_2 level, LH level and androgens with low or normal FSH characterize this syndrome.
- Clomiphene remains the first line of treatment for infertility in PCOS. Resistant cases require laparoscopic puncture or gonadotropins and metformin.

SELF-ASSESSMENT

1. Describe the clinical features of PCOS.
2. Discuss the management of PCOS.
3. Discuss long-term sequelae of PCOS.

SUGGESTED READING

ACOG Committee on Practice Bulletins–Gynecology. ACOG Practice Bulletin No. 108: Polycystic ovary syndrome. Obstet Gynecol 2009; 114:936.

American College of Obstetricians and Gynecologists Committee on Gynecologic Practice. Committee Opinion No. 477: the role of the obstetrician-gynecologist in the early detection of epithelial ovarian cancer. Obstet Gynecol 2011; 117:742.

American College of Obstetricians and Gynecologists. ACOG Practice Bulletin. Management of adnexal masses. Obstet Gynecol 2007; 110:201.

Bonnar J. Recent Advances in Obstetrics and Gynaecology Vol 19:121, 1995.

Bonnar J. Recent Advances in Obstetrics and Gynaecology 21:111, 2001.

Fauser BC, Tarlatzis BC, Rebar RW, et al. Consensus on women's health aspects of polycystic ovary syndrome (PCOS): the Amsterdam ESHRE/ASRM-Sponsored 3rd PCOS Consensus Workshop Group. Fertil Steril 2012; 97:28.

Goodman NF, Cobin RH, Futterweit W, et al. American association of clinical endocrinologists, american college of endocrinology, and androgen excess and pcos society disease state clinical review: Guide to the best practices in the evaluation and treatment of polycystic ovary syndrome–Part 1. Endocr Pract 2015; 21:1291.

Rotterdam ESHRE/ASRM-Sponsored PCOS Consensus Workshop Group. Revised 2003 consensus on diagnostic criteria and long-term health risks related to polycystic ovary syndrome. Fertil Steril 2004; 81:19.

Studd J. Progress in Obstetrics and Gynaecology 11:851, 1994.

Studd J. Progress in Obstetrics and Gynaecology Vol 16:227, 2005

Benign Diseases of the Vulva

25

CHAPTER OUTLINE

INTRODUCTION

A variety of developmental, trophic, inflammatory, allergic and neoplastic diseases can occur in the vulvar skin and its appendages. The common vulvar diseases affecting the vulva are as follows:

1. *Epidermis and dermis.* Common dermatological disorders, allergies, infections, naevi, dystrophies, ulcers and new growths.
2. *Skin appendages.* Folliculitis, sebaceous cysts, hidradenomas, Bartholin's cyst or abscess and Paget disease.
3. *Adjacent structures.* Lipomas, fibromas, haemangiomas, varicosities, carcinomas, sarcomas and endometriosis.
4. *Developmental.* Vulvovaginal cysts, imperforate hymen, vulval anus and intersex problems.
5. *Hormonal.* Vulval atrophy in menopausal women.
   - Despite the fact that vulvar diseases are not uncommon, and the vulva is easily accessible to clinical examination, there is often a delay in arriving at diagnosis due to delay in seeking medical advice out of a sense of modesty which prevails and prevents the patient from seeking early advice.
   - The symptoms most commonly produced by vulvar lesions are excoriation, swelling, ulceration or altered pigmentation which may be accompanied by itching, pain or bleeding. An accurate diagnosis can usually be made by inspection, palpation, smear and culture examination and biopsy.

BENIGN DISEASES OF THE VULVA

Benign conditions of the vulva may be classified as follows:

- *Inflammatory lesions.* (a) Skin diseases, (b) sexually transmitted diseases, (c) contact vulvitis and (d) vulvar infections associated with vaginitis.
- *Ulcers.* (a) Simple acute ulcers, (b) tubercular, (c) traumatic ulcers and (d) malignant ulcers.
- Atrophy.
- Dystrophies.
- Cysts and neoplasms.

INFLAMMATORY LESIONS

SKIN INFECTIONS

INTERTRIGO AND FOLLICULITIS

Intertrigo and folliculitis are commonly seen in obese women, using tight garments which prevent evaporation of the moisture from these parts leading to chaffing followed by bacterial and fungal infection. Pyogenic bacteria, staphylococcus can cause folliculitis. The treatment involves weight reduction, use of loose undergarments, advice regarding personal hygiene, use of a bland soap and an unmedicated protective dusting powder. Antimicrobial ointments may be used initially to control secondary bacterial infection. Occasionally, oral antibiotics may be needed. Local application of 0.5% hydrocortisone ointment three to four times daily helps to relieve itching in intertrigo.

TINEA CRURIS

Tinea cruris or ringworm of the thigh, vulva and groin is not infrequently encountered in the tropics. The causative organism is *Trichophyton rubrum.* It tends to be chronic and frequently relapses after treatment. The characteristic erythematous circumscribed areas are found in the skin flexures of the thighs and outer aspect of the labia. A fine papular rash is usually seen sharply demarcated from the adjacent healthy skin. Patients experience intense itching; scratching leads to superimposed infection. Treatment consists of meticulous hygiene, the use of frequently changed light underclothes, dusting with a fungicidal powder or application of a fungicidal ointment containing benzoic and salicylic acids. Oral administration of griseofulvin is also highly effective.

THREADWORMS

Enterobius vermicularis may secondarily infect the vulva from the anorectal area, particularly in children. The diagnosis is easily established on stool examination. The treatment is with anthelmintic drugs such as piperazine or mebendazole.

VULVOVAGINITIS

Vulvovaginitis in children may be nonspecific due to a foreign body accidentally introduced in the vagina or due to threadworm infection. Gonococcal and fungal infection may rarely be due to sexual abuse or contamination. Bartholinitis is mostly gonococcal but other cocci may also be responsible, and present with a painful and tender swelling over the labia majora (Fig. 25.1). Recurrent bartholinitis is not uncommon. Bartholinitis needs antibiotics.

BARTHOLIN'S ABSCESS

Bartholin's gland is mainly infected by gonococci, though other nonspecific organisms may be involved. The woman presents with a painful vulval swelling and purulent discharge. The swelling is inflamed and painful. It requires drainage under anaesthesia. The pus should be cultured and appropriate antibiotics instituted. After drainage, the area heals by granulation. It has a propensity for frequent recurrences.

PSORIASIS

Psoriasis (Fig. 25.2) affects the vulval skin causing plaques of scaly well-defined patches. The silvery scale can be easily scraped off to reveal a red papular underlying surface. The aetiology is not known but the condition responds satisfactorily to treatment with local steroids. Psoriasis is also seen characteristically on the elbows and knees. A search for lesions at these sites helps in establishing the diagnosis.

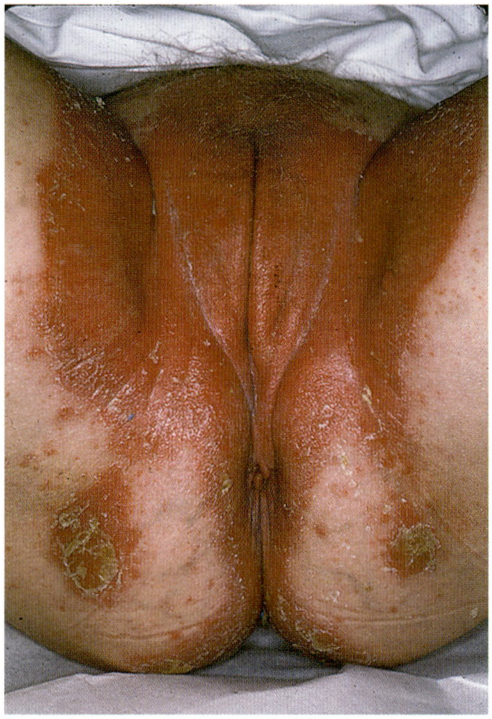

Figure 25.2 Psoriasis of the vulva. Note the extent of the lesion extending laterally to the inner thighs and posteriorly to involve the perianal skin and cleft. (*Source*: Danielle Mazza. Women's Health in General Practice. Genital tract disorders. Churchill Livingstone, 2011.)

FILARIASIS

This is caused by the worm *Wuchereria bancrofti* which is spread by mosquitoes. The parasite reproduces in the lymphatics and causes lymphatic oedema of the legs and elephantiasis of the legs and vulva. It is prevalent in tropical countries.

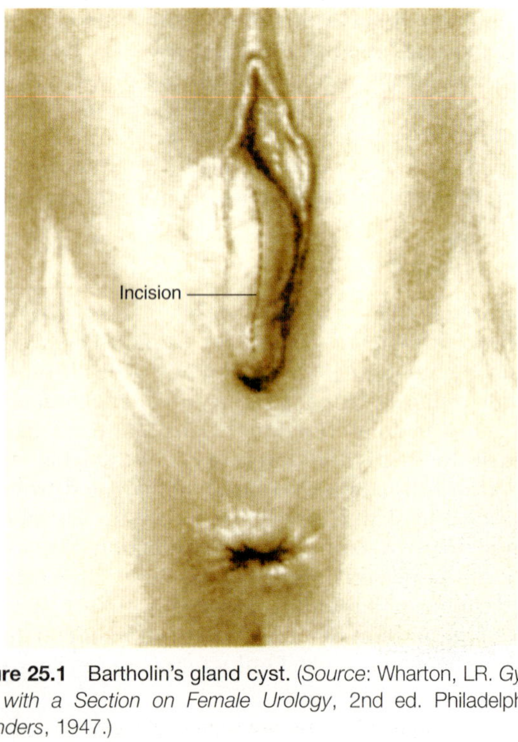

Figure 25.1 Bartholin's gland cyst. (*Source*: Wharton, LR. *Gynaecology with a Section on Female Urology*, 2nd ed. Philadelphia: WB Saunders, 1947.)

CONTACT VULVITIS

Contact vulvitis often represents a local reaction to undergarments made from synthetic materials, to soaps and detergents, to chemicals (deodorants) and occasionally to medicaments and industrial pollutants. Examination reveals oedema and reddening of the vulvar skin and vestibule without accompanying vaginitis. The acute symptoms can be controlled by administering oral antihistamines, application of local steroidal ointments or creams, using cotton underwear, advocating the use of bland soaps and scrupulously avoiding offending drugs.

PRURITUS VULVA

Pruritus vulva is an itching sensation with an intense desire to scratch the vulva. Vulvar irritation is not the same as pruritus, but it is a painful condition associated with burning sensation. Prolonged or severe pruritus can eventually lead to vulval irritation through scratching and abrasions.

Causes of Pruritus Vulvae

There are several causes, though often it may be difficult to elucidate the cause, and the treatment becomes empirical. Some of the known aetiological factors in pruritus vulva are as follows:

- *Vaginal discharge* due to *Trichomonas vaginalis* or fungal monilial infection accounts for 80% of all cases of pruritus vulva. The vaginal discharge may be slight but causes intense pruritus within the introitus as well as on the vulva. Purulent discharge on the other hand, produces irritation rather than pruritus.

- *General* disease. For example, diabetes, jaundice, uraemia, cirrhosis, haemochromatosis.
- *Nutritional.* Iron deficiency anaemia, vitamin A and B_{12} deficiency, achlorhydria.
- *Generalized or* localized dermatitis, such as psoriasis, eczema.
- *Allergy* to drugs, contact dermatitis, allergy to soap, detergents, antiseptics, phenol, dusting powder, deodorants, wearing tight synthetic undergarments, imperfectly rinsed underclothes.
- *Cervical* conditions such as cervicitis; erosion produces excessive mucoid secretion which causes vulval itching.
- *Vulval parasitic infections* such as pediculosis, scabies.
- *Vulval diseases* such as condyloma acuminata, granulomas, Behcet syndrome, Paget disease and vulval cancer.
- *Anal.* Threadworm infestation.
- *Urinary.* Bacilluria, acidic urine, incontinence and glycosuria, bladder fistula.
- *Allergy* to condoms or diaphragms, spermicidal agents.
- *Psychological.* Psychoneurosis due to stress. The scratching habit may develop following sexual frustration, feeling of guilt, overmasturbation or other sexual practices.
- *Chronic vulval dystrophies* of vulval skin such as leukoplakia, lichen sclerosis, kraurosis vulva and Paget disease.
- Radiation vulvitis.
- Clinically, the woman develops an itching sensation and begins to scratch the vulva. Persistent and prolonged scratching can lead to abrasions, inflammation and irritation with soreness. The patient may lose sleep because of itching and becomes irritable.

Treatment

The cause of pruritus should be investigated systematically and treated with antihistamines and sedation may allay the symptoms. Hydrocortisone ointment/steroid ointment locally or Eurax ointment often helps. Oestrogen cream is useful in kraurosis vulva due to menopausal changes. Fungal infection is treated with nystatin cream or one of the imidazole group of antifungal drugs such as miconazole, econazole, clotrimazole, terconazole or oral antifungal drugs such as fluconazole/ketoconazole or itraconazole. Oral metronidazole is specific for *Trichomonas* infection. If the skin is hard and tends to crack, a cream made of zinc oxide (40 parts) and olive oil (60 parts) or cod liver oil helps to soften the skin. Injection of absolute alcohol subcutaneously 0.5–1 mL breaks the scratch habit, but if given very superficially or in deep tissues or in excessive amount, it may cause sloughing of the tissues. Ball's operation, now rarely performed, comprises division of cutaneous nerves by a circular incision around the vulva. The effect lasts for 3–6 months. Lately, *interferon* is used as an ointment (human leucocyte *interferon*) with 90% regression in symptoms; Applying 4000 units/g ointment four times a day for 5 weeks is recommended. Systemic intramuscular *interferon* 2,000,000 units daily for 10 days has yielded 90% cure rate. Fever, myalgia, headache are the side effects with the systemic use of *interferon.*

ULCERS

Traumatic ulcers are easily recognized by their appearance, contused edges and history of hurt. Treatment comprises local applications of antibiotic ointment to prevent infection and administration of oral analgesics to relieve pain.

- Tuberculous ulcers appear as thin serpiginous ulcers with undermined edges and a thin yellowish discharge at the base. Biopsy from the edge reveals the typical, tuberculous granulomatous lesions showing the presence of Langhans type of giant cells.
- Venereal diseases such as syphilis, chancroid and granuloma inguinale present with ulcers on the vulva.
- Vulval cancers present as nonhealing ulcers with raised everted edges or as growths which breakdown and ulcerate.
- Vulval ulcers are classified as follows:
  - Primary disease
    - Fungal infection, streptococcal infection, syphilis, TB.
    - Chancroid, Behcet disease, traumatic ulcer, amoebiasis, lymphogranuloma venereum, granuloma inguinale.
  - Dermatitis
    - Lichen sclerosus, lichen planus, Crohn disease, allergy to drugs.
    - Viral infection, herpes simplex (Fig. 25.3)
    - Immunological.
    - Vulvar intraepithelial neoplasia (VIN), Paget disease, malignant ulcer.

CLINICAL FEATURES

Most ulcers are painful except malignant ulcers. Pruritus if present suggests infective condition. General and systemic examination will reveal general or primary skin lesion. Serological tests, culture and biopsy confirm the nature of the ulcer.

BEHCET DISEASE

Behcet disease is associated with oral and ocular ulcers. It is a chronic inflammatory multisystem disorder of unknown aetiology, so the treatment is nonspecific. Corticosteroid cream helps.

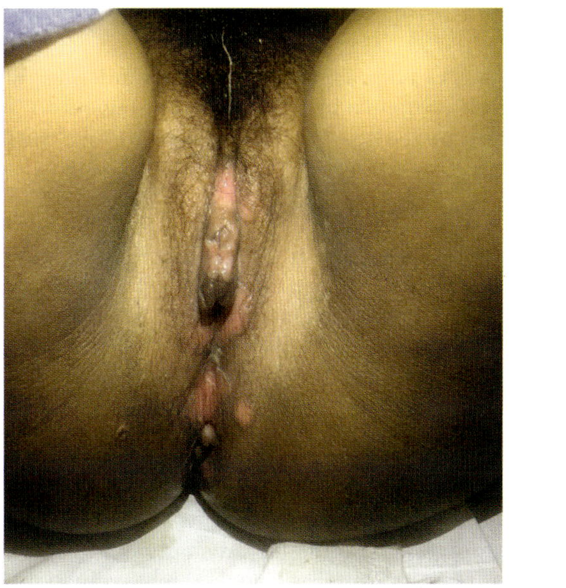

Figure 25.3 Herpes simplex of vulva

ATROPHY

Atrophy occurs as a normal consequence of decreased oestrogen levels after menopause. The labia become flatter and the skin hangs loosely due to loss of subcutaneous fat. The epithelium is pale, smooth and thin. The introitus narrows down. Atrophic changes can be prevented by timely administration of oestrogens in the form of local creams or at times by systemic administration. However, once the tissues undergo atrophy, these changes cannot be reversed by the use of hormones. Women who undergo menopause after radiation therapy or following surgical castration appear to be more prone to this change. The condition is akin to lichen sclerosus.

VULVAL PAIN SYNDROME

Lynch introduced this term in 1991 to describe women with unprovoked 'chronic vulval discomfort of burning, stinging and irritation' in the absence of any visible abnormality in the vulva, or raw area around the vulva.

- Several causes have been implicated and it is at times difficult to elucidate and treat the cause. Urinary oxalate excretion and deficient immune system are the probable causes. The treatment remains empirical. Some of the known causes are as follows:
  - Skin infection – Human papilloma virus and fungal infection, herpes simplex infection.
  - Organic disease
  - Autoimmune disease
  - Iatrogenic – Topical agents, deodorants
  - Irritants and allergy
  - Tense levator ani muscles
  - Psychological
  - Urinary oxalate causing vulval burning
  - Hormonal – Low oestrogen levels in body and use of oral contraceptives
  - Pelvic floor muscle tension
  - Vulval vestibulitis.
  - The woman with chronic vulval pain is usually 20–40 years of age.

VESTIBULITIS

Vestibulitis causes pain on touch, local tenderness on pressure and erythema in the vestibular region. A woman of childbearing age may complain superficial dyspareunia. Intensity of pain varies from mild to severe discomfort.

DYSAESTHETIC VULVODYNIA

Dysaesthetic vulvodynia is a cutaneous dysaesthesia which causes nonlocalized vulval pain, unprovoked constant neurologic pain in the vulva and perianal region. A burning ache similar to postherpetic pain occurs usually in perimenopausal and postmenopausal woman; therefore, history of dyspareunia is rarely reported. A woman is often psychologically disturbed and anxious. This affects normal activity, walking, social life and sexual function.

MANAGEMENT

- Eliminate and treat the underlying cause.
- Thirty per cent have spontaneous remission in a year's time.
- Medical – Topical lignocaine 1%–2% may help, so also steroid creams.
- *Interferon* gel cures only 20% of the cases. Amitriptyline, tricyclic antidepressant for neuralgic pain in a dose of 10 mg daily is given, gradually increasing to 60 mg daily as required. The drug causes dry mouth, weight gain and has a sedative effect. The woman should not conceive or breastfeed while on these drugs. Other drugs are Tegretol (carbamazepine), in severe cases, gabapentin 300 mg orally. In a severe case, a woman may need vestibulectomy. It consists of excision of the horseshoe-shaped vestibule and inner labial fold and covering the raw area with vaginal mucosa dissected from the posterior vaginal wall.

VULVAL DYSTROPHIES

Now known as **nonneoplastic epithelial disorders**, vulvar dystrophies represent a spectrum of atrophic and hypertrophic lesions caused by a variety of conditions resulting in circumscribed or diffuse 'white lesions'. These lesions also often show differing microscopic patterns varying from mild dysplasia to frank malignancy in different parts of the same lesion. Multiple biopsies are therefore necessary, and the toluidine blue test helps in identifying areas of maximum epithelial hyperactivity that are most suitable for biopsy. A variety of causes are implicated in the development of vulval dystrophies, such as trauma of scratching, allergy, folic acid and B_{12} deficiency, chronic infection, metabolic disorders such as diabetes and thyroid, immunosuppression and autoimmune diseases such as systemic lupus erythematosus (SLE).

- Currently used histological classification of vulvar dystrophy (Table 25.1) is based on the recommendations of the International Society for the Study of Vulvar Diseases. The histological classification is more meaningful in the management than relying on the gross morphology which may not be helpful in the diagnosis.

HYPERPLASTIC DYSTROPHY (SQUAMOUS CELL HYPERPLASIA), PREVIOUSLY KNOWN AS LEUKOPLAKIA

Chronic irritation or chronic vulvovaginal infection often leads to benign epithelial thickening and hyperkeratosis. Some of these women suffer from autoimmune diseases such as diabetes, thyroiditis, achlorhydria. During the acute phase, the lesions may appear red and moist due to secondary infection. As epithelial thickening develops, vulval skin appears as raised white lesion which may be circumscribed or diffuse; it looks rubbery. It may involve any part of the vulva, perianal area, perineum or skin of the adjacent thighs. These lesions have also been designated as lichen simplex chronicus or neurodermatitis. Patients suffer from pruritis, soreness, discharge and dyspareunia (Fig. 25.4). The woman is often premenopausal. The lesion begins as white polygonal papules which coalesce to form plaques giving the appearance of being **'splashed with white wash'** – fissures may develop due to scratching.

- Microscopic examination reveals irregular down growth of the rete pegs deep into the dermis. The cells of the

Table 25.1 Vulvar Dystrophies

Type of Dystrophy	Hyperplastic Lesions	Lichen Sclerosis	Mixed Dystrophy
Gross appearance	White/greyish white, focal or diffuse	Small bluish-white papules that coalesce into white papules	Combination of both
Symptoms	Pruritus	Pruritus, dyspareunia, dysuria	Combination of both
Feel on palpation	Firm, cartilage like	Thin, parchment-like	Combination of both
Histology	Thickened keratin with proliferative epithelium – Acanthosis	Moderate hyperkeratosis with epithelial thinning. Loss of rete hyalinization in dermis	
Pathophysiology	Reactive phenomenon from irritation	Unknown	
Method of diagnosis	Biopsy	Biopsy	
Treatment	Fluorinated corticosteroids	Testosterone cream	

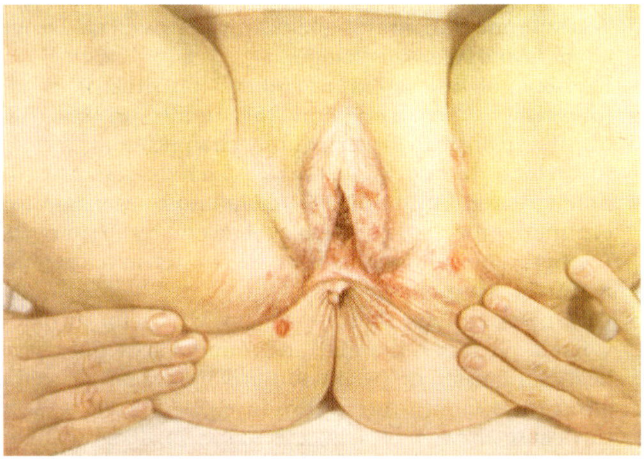

Figure 25.4 Leucoplakia of the vulva showing scratch marks and ulcerations. (*Source:* Novak Emil and Novak Edmund, *Gynaecologic and Obstetric Pathology*, 4th ed., Philadelphia and London: WB Saunders, 1958.)

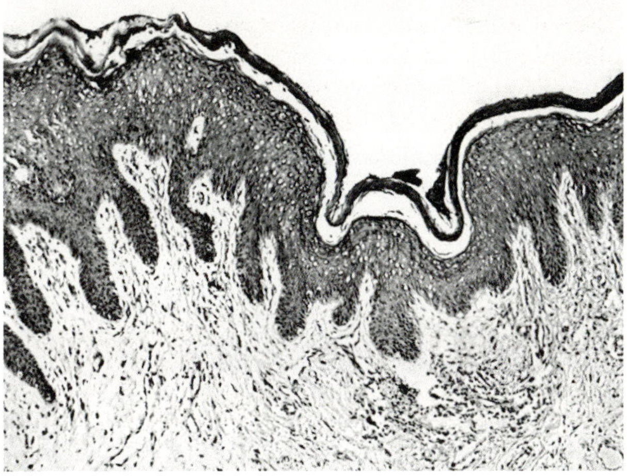

Figure 25.5 Hypertrophic leucoplakia of vulva showing irregular down growth of papillae, abnormal basal cells and superficial keratinization.

basal layers show active mitosis, the prickle cell layer is increased in thickness, and there is a heavy accumulation of keratin on the surface. The dermis reveals infiltration with inflammatory cells (Fig. 25.5). About 10%–30% of these cases develop malignant change. Initial treatment with oestrogens is worthwhile. Oral administration of 0.625 mg of conjugated equine oestrogen (Premarin) helps to control vulval pruritus. Bland local medicaments such as Calamine lotion, crotamine or zinc oxide paste are soothing. In case of suspected superadded inflammation, steroid ointment containing 1% hydrocortisone, betamethasone, fluocinolone with or without antimicrobial agents such as neomycin, Soframycin (antibiotic), miconazole or chiniofon (antifungal) are useful. A prescription for a mild sedative at bedtime ensures adequate rest, helps recovery and prevents patients from scratching. Two per cent lignocaine ointment also relieves pain. Clobetasol 0.05% cream is most useful.

- In case malignancy is suspected, multiple biopsies from suspicious areas are mandatory. Lesser degrees of dysplasia require observation, but in more advanced lesions, surgical excision is indicated to relieve pruritus as well as to remove the potential site of malignancy. Colposcopic inspection using acetic acid and toluidine blue is desirable. One per cent aqueous toluidine blue is applied and washed off after 1 minute with 1% acetic acid. Blue areas are biopsied.

LICHEN SCLEROSUS (ATROPHIC DYSTROPHY)

With ageing, endogenous oestrogen decreases and atrophic changes in the vulvar skin and subdermal tissues appear some years after advanced atrophy of the vaginal mucous membrane. There is contracture of the vaginal introitus, and the vaginal mucous membrane becomes thin and is easily traumatized (Figs 25.6 and 25.7).

- Goolamal et al. showed that this lesion is linked to autoimmune diseases in 40% of cases and is seen

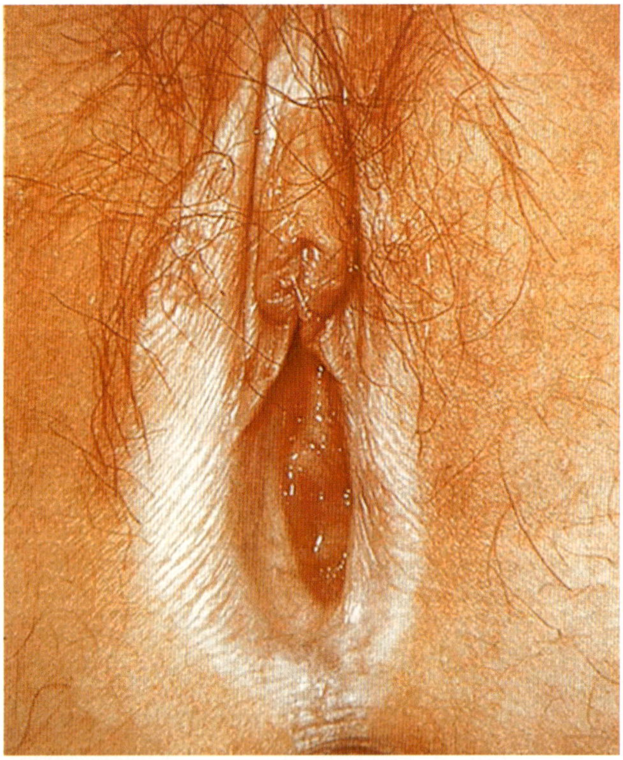

Figure 25.6 Lichen sclerosus et atrophicus of the vulva. (*Source*: Juan Rosai. Rosai and Ackerman's Surgical Pathology. Female reproductive system. Mosby, 2011.)

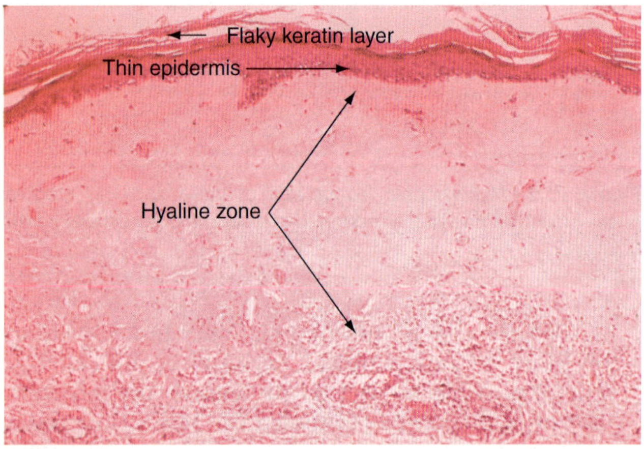

Figure 25.7 Lichen sclerosis. Histology shows hyperkeratosis, but the epidermis is thinner than normal. The most striking feature of lichen sclerosis is the presence of a hyaline zone in the superficial dermis. This is the result of oedema and degeneration of the collagen and elastic fibres of the dermis. (*Source:* Hacker NF, Gambone JC, Hobel CJ, *Hacker and Moore's Essentials of Obstetrics and Gynecology*, 5th ed. Philadelphia: Elsevier, 2010.)

in diabetes, thyroid disorders, SLE syndrome and pernicious anaemia. Antithyroid antibodies are often detected.

- It is usually a disease of elderly women older than 65 years of age; genetic and familial tendency is also noted. During the acute phase, the lesion may appear dusky involving the vulva, perineum and perianal area in an hour-glass pattern (figure-of-eight). The skin is papery thin and wrinkled. As the disease progresses, the labia minora blend into the labia majora thus causing a narrow introitus. Although the lesion is essentially atrophic in longstanding lesions areas of dysplasia and malignancy may occur in 1%–5% of cases. Longstanding Lichen sclerosus is a well-recognized predisposing factor for development of carcinoma vulva. All suspicious areas must be biopsied. The chief symptoms are intense pruritus, dysuria, dyspareunia and local discomfort. Biopsy reveals hyperkeratosis, thinning of the epidermal epithelium, flattening of the rete pegs and hyalinization of the tissue beneath the epidermis. Treatment with bland creams is recommended. The condition responds well to local application of steroids, such as oestrogen cream and testosterone propionate.
- Two per cent testosterone ointment in a white petroleum jelly resolves pruritus in 6–8 weeks. Andractim gel (5 g) dose can be gradually reduced because of the risk of virilization and acne. About 80% response is reported. Testosterone by converting to dihydrotestosterone brings about favourable skin changes.
- Excision of the areas to relieve pruritus is often followed by recurrence of the lesion around the excised margins. Hypertrophic changes may follow, for which biopsy is advisable. Lichen sclerosus is now treated with 0.05% clobetasol (Dermovate) ointment for 8–12 weeks followed by Trimovate (clobetasone plus nystatin and oxytetracycline) to maintain symptomatic relief.
- Oestrogen and testosterone creams are useful in older women. Vitamin A is useful, and retinoid analogues have been administered. Twenty to thirty milligrams acitretin given for 4 months is effective in 60%–70% of cases. It can cause dryness of skin, eye irritation, hair loss and myalgia. Its teratogenic effect prevents its use during pregnancy, and young women should use contraceptives to prevent pregnancy. Intralesional *interferon* is successful in some cases.
- It must be emphasized that before medical treatment, multiple or selective biopsy is mandatory to rule out malignancy or preinvasive lesion, as 5%–10% of these lesions show concomitant malignancy or develop these changes in due course of time. Pap smear is also desirable to check on the cervical histology.
- *Surgery is rarely employed and is not curable.* Fresh lesion may appear in the vicinity of the excised area. Skinning vulvectomy, cryoablation and laser ablation and vulvectomy in older women have been employed.
- The treatment therefore, is directed towards symptomatic relief, preventing cancer by regular follow-up and improving the appearance of the vulval skin. This indicates the need for prolonged and continuous follow-up.
- Mixed variety shows histological changes of hypertrophied as well as atrophic dystrophy at different sites in the same lesion. The treatment is also based on predominance of type of lesion seen.
- Denervation of vulva by 'Mering' procedure with a curved incision around the vulva up to the subcutaneous tissue is sometimes recommended.

CYSTS AND NEOPLASMS

VULVAL CYSTS

SEBACEOUS CYST

Sebaceous cyst results from blockage of the duct of the sebaceous gland and contains cheesy material. It is commonly seen between the labia majora and labia minora and can get infected.

BARTHOLIN'S CYST

Bartholin's cyst is formed when its duct is blocked either by inflammation or by inspissated secretion. It appears as a swelling on the inner side of the junction of the anterior two-thirds with the posterior one-third of the labium majus. A small cyst remains asymptomatic, but a larger one bulges across the vaginal introitus and causes dyspareunia, discomfort – it may get infected, thus needing excision or marsupialization. The latter is easy to perform, causes less bleeding and retains the function of the gland. The incision runs along the long axis of the labia majora away from the introitus to avoid a painful scar and dyspareunia. The cavity is scraped, haemostasis secured and the edge sutured to the skin. The cavity shrinks and heals by granulation tissue.

CYST OF THE CANAL OF NUCK

Cyst of the canal of Nuck is a remnant of the processus vaginalis beneath the anterior part of the labia minora.

VULVAL NEOPLASMS

FIBROMA AND LIPOMA

Fibroma and lipoma are occasionally seen in vulva. They present as pedunculated benign swelling that can be easily excised.

HIDRADENOMA

Hidradenoma arises in the apocrine glands, rarely exceeding 1 cm in size. Histologically, it shows cystic spaces enclosing a papillary adenomatous mass. In rare cases, it may undergo malignant change, therefore requiring excision.

PIGMENTED MOLE OR NAEVI

Pigmented mole or naevi are not uncommon over the vulva and may develop into melanoma. A growing mole should be excised and subjected to histology.

ENDOMETRIOSIS

Endometriosis of vulva is a purplish swelling seen over the labia majora or episiotomy scar over the perineum. It grows during menstruation and becomes painful but recedes in between menstruation. It requires excision. It does not respond to drugs.

ELEPHANTIASIS OF VULVA (Fig. 25.8)

Elephantiasis of vulva is a filarial disease of the tropics and is caused by *Wuchereria bancrofti*. It causes elephantiasis vulva and inguinal lymphadenitis. By the time chronic lymphatic obstruction occurs, filariae are not detected. If diethylcarbamazine fails to cure the condition, surgical excision is needed. Tuberculosis is a rare cause of elephantiasis vulva.

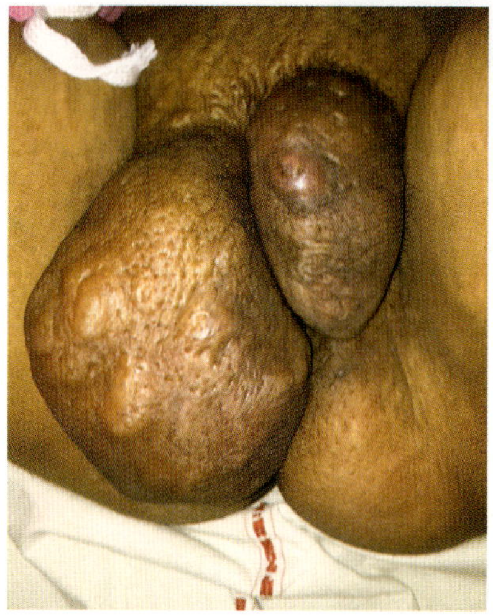

Figure 25.8 Elephantiasis of vulva.

KEY POINTS

- Vulva is a common site of sexually transmitted diseases such as syphilis, herpes, condyloma acuminata.
- Pruritus vulva has several aetiological factors which need evaluation. Some are idiopathic and respond to empirical treatment.
- Vulval dystrophies represent a spectrum of atrophic and hypertrophic lesions which may be localized or diffuse. About 10%–30% develop malignancy, and malignancy may exist in the same lesion. It is therefore important to rule out cancer by toluidine blue test, colposcopy and biopsy.
- Vulvodynia is a painful vulval condition without an obvious clinical lesion. It is difficult to elucidate the cause. Symptomatic relief with drugs is the first line of treatment.

SELF-ASSESSMENT

1. Describe the benign lesions of the vulva encountered in clinical practice.
2. How would you manage a case of vulval pruritus?
3. How would you manage a complaint of vulvodynia?
4. What are the types of vulval dystrophies? Discuss their management.

SUGGESTED READING

ACOG Practice Bulletin No. 93: diagnosis and management of vulvar skin disorders. Obstet Gynecol 2008; 111:1243.

Bracco GL, Carli P, Somni L, et al. Clinical and histological effects of topical treatments of vulval lichen sclerosus: A clinical evaluation. J Reprod Med 38:37–40, 1993.

Elchalal U, Gilead L, Vardy DA, et al. Treatment of lichen sclerosus in the elderly: An update. Obsetet Gynecol Surv 50:155–62, 1998.

Faber MT, Sand FL, Albieri V, et al. Prevalence and type distribution of human papillomavirus in squamous cell carcinoma and intraepithelial neoplasia of the vulva. Int J Cancer 2017; 141:1161.

Hood AF, Lumadue J. In: Benign vulvar tumours. Dermatologic Clinics 10:371–385, 1992.

Lawson JO. In: Pelvic anatomy I, Pelvic floor muscles. Ann R Coll Surg Eng 154:244–252, 1974.

26 Benign Diseases of the Vagina

CHAPTER OUTLINE

The vagina is usually a site of benign conditions such as infections, ulceration and other changes related to age of the patient; however, rarely the vagina can be a site of malignancy. Nature has provided a number of protections in the form of high acidic pH, thick squamous cell epithelium in the vagina which prevents occurrence of common diseases, whenever these normal defences of vagina are altered there is an increased risk of diseases of the vagina.

BIOLOGY OF THE VAGINA

In a healthy adult woman of childbearing age, the vaginal secretions consist of white coagulated material comprising squamous cells, Döderlein's bacilli and coagulated secretion. Döderlein's bacilli are large Gram-positive bacteria which are sugar fermenting. This ability to convert glycogen into lactic acid is responsible for the high acidity (pH) of the normal healthy adult vagina. The vaginal contents are mostly derived from the squamous cells of the vaginal mucosa. Some contribution comes from endometrial and cervical secretion. In a healthy woman, cervical secretions are small in amount and there is little secretion from the endometrium of the body of the uterus even during the secretory phase of the menstrual cycle. Pathological conditions such as erosions and ectropion of the cervix cause increased mucus secretion and the patient complains of mucous discharge at the vaginal orifice.

The superficial cornified cells of the vaginal mucosa produce glycogen under oestrogen stimulation and are continuously desquamated. Subsequently, as a result of the breaking down of the cells, glycogen is liberated and ultimately converted into lactic acid. In the newborn, before the appearance of Döderlein's bacilli, glycogen is broken down into lactic acid and there is some evidence that the process is brought about by enzyme action. After the appearance of Döderlein's bacilli, the production of the lactic acid is augmented by the action of bacilli on glycogen.

The amount of normal vaginal secretion varies with age, in health and in disease. During pregnancy, it increases and it is maximal in the early puerperium and in women following an abortion. It varies at different times in the menstrual cycle increasing at ovulation and just before menstruation. In health, it is dependent on the vascular state of the genitalia, and this itself is largely oestrogen dependent. Congestive conditions of the genitalia and adjacent pelvic organs increase vaginal transudation such as in prolapse with hypertrophied cervix and cervicitis and in retroversion of the uterus with a congested and myohyperplastic uterus. The pelvic congestion of chronic constipation also aggravates vaginal discharge.

1. The normal moistness of the vagina is sufficient to lubricate the vagina and labia minora without staining or moistening the underclothes except at ovulation, in immediate premenstrual phase, during pregnancy and under the stimulus of sexual excitation.
2. With a moderate increase in vaginal secretion, the underclothes are undeniably soiled and require changing and washing frequently.
3. An excessive amount of vaginal secretion requires the wearing of some extra absorbent pad, diaper or internal tampon and is genuinely pathological. It is to be stressed, however, that this excessive discharge is not necessarily pathological.

The components of vaginal secretion are from the following:

- The sweat and sebaceous glands of the vulva and the specialized racemose glands of Bartholin's. The characteristic odour of vaginal secretion is provided by the apocrine glands of the vulva.
- The transudate of the vaginal epithelium and the desquamated cells of the cornified layer. This is strongly acidic.
- The mucous secretions of the endocervical glands which is alkaline.
- The endometrial glandular secretion.

All these play a varying part at different times of the menstrual cycle, the last two being most active just before menstruation.

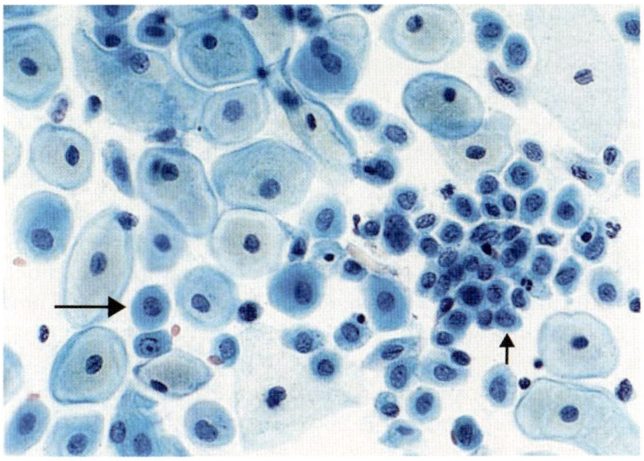

Figure 26.1 Parabasal and basal cells (postpartum smear). Parabasal cells (large arrow) are oval and typically have dense cytoplasm. Basal cells (small arrow) are similar but have less cytoplasm. Many cells have abundant pale-yellow staining glycogen, a characteristic but nonspecific feature of squamous cells of pregnancy and the postpartum period. (*Source*: From Figure 1-5. Edmund S Cibas and Barbara S Ducatman. Cytology: Diagnostic Principles and Clinical Correlates, 4th ed. Saunders: Elsevier, 2014.)

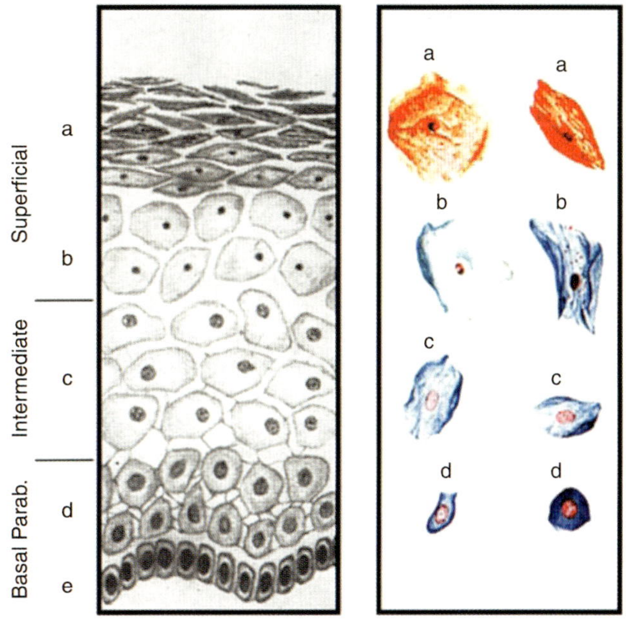

Figure 26.2 The layers of vaginal epithelium of the well-oestrogenized adult. The superficial layer contains surface cells that are cornified (squamous) with eosinophilic cytoplasm and pyknotic nuclei (a) as well as large intraepithelial cells that are also karyopyknotic but basophilic (b). The intermediate zone contains basophilic cells that have less cytoplasm and intermediate-size nuclei (c). Parabasal and basal cells have successively smaller amounts of basophilic cytoplasm and more vesicular nuclei (d, e). (*Source*: From Figure 15-29. Mark A Sperling: Pediatric Endocrinology, 4th Ed. Saunders: Elsevier, 2014.)

STRUCTURE OF VAGINAL EPITHELIUM

The squamous cells of vagina are divided into three layers: superficial, intermediate and deep. The deep layer consists of two types of cells, basal and parabasal. **The basal cells** are the less mature, smaller and more basophilic cell. It is a small round cell with a basophilic cytoplasm and a relatively large central nucleus which is uniform in shape and size. Vaginal smears where this cell predominates are typical of low oestrogen content, for example, menopausal, lactating or postpartum smears (Fig. 26.1). The parabasal cell is similar to the basal cell but slightly more mature. The intermediate cell type is represented by a cell intermediate between the basal and the superficial or fully cornified cell. It is three times larger than the basal cell and ellipsoid or quadrilateral in shape. The cytoplasm stains light and the nucleus is smaller and has less deep staining than in the basal cell. The nucleus is vesicular. The presence of parabasal cells in a vaginal smear indicates a low but not absent oestrogenic influence as seen in normal menopause. Its presence in large numbers is also characteristic of rapid desquamation of the vaginal epithelium which may result from vaginal infection or basal cell hyperplasia. **The superficial cells** are of two types: precornified and cornified. The precornified cell is larger than the intermediate cell, being a hexagonal or octagonal flat wafer. Its main point of distinction from the fully cornified cell is that its cytoplasm is still fairly basophilic. Its nucleus is small and pyknotic. The cornified or fully mature cell represents the final phase of complete oestrogenic maturity. It has a pink eosinophilic cytoplasm, the largest cytoplasm of any vaginal cell (Fig. 26.2). The nucleus is pyknotic. The maximum level of cornification is usually seen in the late proliferative phase of a normally menstruating woman when oestrogen production is maximum near the time of ovulation.

PHYSIOLOGICAL CHANGES IN THE VAGINAL EPITHELIUM

It is possible to demonstrate cyclical variations in the vaginal epithelium during the menstrual cycle by cytological examination. This technique has become so well authenticated that a competent cytologist can diagnose the date of the menstrual calendar from an examination of the vaginal smear with nearly the same accuracy as can be accessed from the study of the endometrium. The cornification index (the percentage of the cornified cells) is one simple method of assessing oestrogen activity. The vaginal cytology during the different phases of menstrual cycle is as follows:

1. **Menstruation**. Endometrial debris, red and white blood corpuscles and histiocytes are present. The vaginal squames are immature in that they have basophilic cytoplasm; they are adherent or conglomerate and their nuclei are larger than those of mature cells.
2. **Early proliferative phase**. Polymorphs are few and the squames tend to be discrete and more mature, their cytoplasm more acidophilic and their nuclei more pyknotic and smaller; the cornification index rises.
3. **Late proliferative phase**. As the oestrogen activity reaches its maximum, the squames become uniform and mature, and the nuclei are small and pyknotic. The cells are separate, and the cornification index is the highest.
4. **Early secretory phase**. The squames become clumped together in clusters. They are less mature, the cytoplasm is now largely basophilic, and the nuclei are bigger, less

dark-staining and vesicular. The cells are no longer flat but appear to be folded with a crinkled or crumpled appearance. Some are pointed and characteristically spear shaped. The cornification index falls.

5. **Late secretory phase**. Intermediate precornified cells predominate. There is lack of cornification. Cytoplasm is basophilic – the cells are crumpled and folded. The nuclei are large, pale staining and vesicular. Pyknosis and concentration of nuclear substance are absent. Polymorphs are on the increase. The background is mucky (dirty).

The cyclical changes in the vaginal epithelium show that the activity is at its maximum during the week before the onset of menstruation. Brown staining of the vagina, when the walls are painted with Lugol's iodine, gives a rough indication of the glycogen content of the cells lining the vaginal epithelium, and thereby the oestrogenic titre of the patient's blood. The maximum glycogen content in the vaginal epithelium is found in the vaginal fornices, where it is present to the extent of 2.5–3.0 mg%, and it is at its lowest in the lower third, where its value is 0.6–0.9 mg%.

CYTOLOGY OF THE VAGINA

Cornification of the vagina is well marked in the vagina of the newborn because of the high oestrogen level which has been transferred from the mother. After about 10 days, the vaginal epithelium becomes thinner and remains in this state until the approach of puberty. At puberty, the functional layer increases in thickness. In the first half of a normal pregnancy, the cornification index is low and should not exceed 10%. In the presence of progesterone deficiency there is a rise in the cornification index, and if the index rises over 25%, the patient is likely to abort. In late pregnancy, the cornification index falls even lower and at term, it may fall below 10%. After menopause, although the ovaries have ceased to function, some degree of cornification is usually present, the oestrogens probably being derived from the adrenal cortex and from conversion of androstenedione (from ovary) to oestrone in the peripheral adipose tissue.

After menopause, the vaginal epithelium atrophies with withdrawal of the oestrogen support. The epithelium becomes thin and parchment-like and is prone to infection (senile vaginitis). The vaginal smear shows mainly the basal basophilic rounded cells with large nuclei. The background shows leucocytic infiltration. The superficial squames are absent and the intermediate cells are few and far between.

VAGINAL ACIDITY

The vaginal acidity is due to lactic acid, which may be present in a variable amount. The pH value is 5.7 in the newborn and reaches 6–8 in children, and falls to 4 at puberty. During pregnancy, the pH value is usually 4. After menopause, the pH rises to 7. The normal pH in healthy women during the childbearing period is about 4.5.

It is important to understand that Döderlein's bacillus is the only organism which will grow at a pH of 4–4.5. As the acidity of the vagina falls and the pH rises, nonresident pathogens are able to thrive.

NATURAL DEFENCE MECHANISM OF THE VAGINA

The skin of the vagina is a tough stratified squamous epithelium devoid of glands. It presents a smooth unbroken surface to the attack of pathogenic organisms. There are no crypts where organisms could multiply unlike in the endocervix. The pH is low and the high acidity mitigates against bacterial growth. The thickness of the epithelium and the hostile pH depend upon oestrogen, and therefore, it is only in extreme young girls, before puberty, and in senescence, i.e. after menopause, that bacterial inroads are likely. There are following certain phases when the pH is raised:

- During menstruation, when the cervical and the endometrial discharge, which is alkaline, tends to neutralize the vaginal acidity.
- After abortion and childbirth, when the alkaline lochia has a similar effect.
- An excessive cervical discharge, such as occurs in endocervicitis, has the same effect.

Apart from these exceptions, the vagina is naturally self-sterilizing under the action of Döderlein's bacilli.

FLORA OF THE FEMALE GENITAL TRACT

In healthy women, the fallopian tubes, the cavity of the uterus and the upper third of the cervical canal are free of microorganisms. The lower third of the cervical canal always contains microorganisms, as does the vagina.

a. **Lactobacilli (Döderlein's bacilli)** – mainly responsible for the production of hydrogen peroxide which is toxic to anaerobes. They also protect against bacteria and candida.
b. **Facultative organisms** (low, nonpathogenic numbers)
   (1) Diphtheroids
   (2) Coagulase negative staphylococci
   (3) Streptococci (groups B and D)
   (4) *Escherichia coli*
   (5) *Ureaplasma urealyticum*
   (6) *Mycoplasma hominis*
c. **Anaerobic organisms** (poor concentration)
   (1) Peptostreptococci
   (2) *Bacteroides*
   (3) *Fusobacterium* species

In healthy women, Döderlein's bacillus is the only organism found in the upper two-thirds of the vagina; but in the neighbourhood of the vulva, both saprophytic and parasitic organisms can be demonstrated. Döderlein's bacilli have been found in the vagina of the newborn within 9 hours after delivery, although the usual time for them to appear is 15 hours. The vagina of the newborn is probably inoculated during parturition.

During the puerperium, acidity of the vagina is reduced and foreign organisms such as coliform bacilli and other pathogens can grow.

Vaginal discharge increases around ovulation, during pregnancy and intercourse. Antibiotics and barrier contraceptives also make vaginal secretion more alkaline.

During the climacteric and after menopause, the number of Döderlein's bacillus is reduced and sometimes, this organism cannot be demonstrated in the vagina. The importance of Döderlein's bacillus is that its presence is associated with the production of lactic acid contained in the vagina and this acidity inhibits the growth of other organisms. In multiparous women, when the vaginal orifice is patulous as a result of childbirth, foreign organisms may be found in the lower part of the vagina which by producing a low-grade vaginitis give rise to discharge.

LEUCORRHOEA

The term *leucorrhoea* should be restricted to those conditions when the normal vaginal secretions are increased in amount. In such patients, there will be no excess of leucocytes present when the discharge is examined under the microscope, and the discharge is macroscopically and microscopically nonpurulent. Purulent discharges due to specific infections such as gonorrhoea, trichomoniasis and moniliasis. Ulcerated growths of the cervix and the vagina and discharges caused by urinary fistulae are of a different type and should be excluded from the term 'leucorrhoea'. Some clinicians use the term to describe any white or yellowish-white discharge from the vagina. An increase in the normal vaginal secretions is physiological at puberty, during pregnancy, at ovulation and, in some women, during the premenstrual phase of the menstrual cycle. During pregnancy, the normal discharge is increased in amount because of increased vascularity of the female genital tract. During the latter part of the menstrual cycle, the hypertrophied premenstrual glands of the endometrium secrete mucous which is discharged through the cervix into the vagina. The leucorrhoea of puberty is probably caused by the increased vascularity of the uterus, cervix and vagina at that time. It is of short duration and needs no treatment. This secretion contains proteins, polysaccharides, amino acids, enzymes and immunoglobulins.

Nonpathogenic leucorrhoea, therefore, can be classified into: (i) cervical and (ii) vaginal.

EXCESSIVE CERVICAL SECRETIONS (CERVICAL LEUCORRHOEA)

Mucous discharge from the endocervical glands increases in such conditions as chronic cervicitis, cervical erosion, mucous polypi and ectropion. When the mucous secretions of the cervix are produced in excess, it undergoes little change in the vagina and appears as mucoid discharge at the vulva.

EXCESSIVE VAGINAL SECRETIONS (NONPATHOGENIC VAGINAL LEUCORRHOEA)

This form of leucorrhoea is seen when the discharge originates in the vagina itself as a transudation through the vaginal walls. Normally lactic acid of the healthy vagina is formed from the glycogen contained in the keratinized cells of the vaginal mucosa and the vaginal portion of the cervix. These cells are constantly being desquamated when their glycogen liberated is fermented by Döderlein's bacilli, which produces lactic acid. This process is under the control of oestrogen, the level of which determines the pH of the vagina.

Local conditions in pelvis with an increase in blood flow to the pelvic organs as seen in pregnancy, acquired retroversion and prolapsed congested ovaries, chronic pelvic inflammatory disease (PID) and chronic constipation are causes of an increased vaginal secretions.

Leucorrhoea must be distinguished from specific vaginitis by performing bacteriological examination and care must be taken to differentiate between the cervical discharge of chronic cervicitis and excessive vaginal secretion. A speculum examination of the vagina usually helps to decide the source of leucorrhoea. If cervical, an excessive mucoid discharge will be obvious at the external os.

PATHOLOGICAL VAGINAL INFECTIONS

- Gonococcal
- Trichomonal 15%–20%
- Monilial 20%–25%
- Chlamydial
- Bacterial vaginosis 50%

Except bacterial vaginosis, the other infections are mostly sexually transmitted and therefore described in chapter on Sexually Transmitted Diseases.

VAGINITIS

Vaginitis causes significant inflammatory response seen in the vaginal wall. There is evidence of increase in WBCs in the vaginal fluid. This is commonly seen in infections caused by trichomoniasis, candidiasis and herpes, STDs including HIV infections.

General Features

1. **Symptoms** – Pruritus, burning in vagina
   a. Malodourous discharge and dyspareunia.
2. **Physical findings:**
   a. Congestion of vaginal walls, microhaemorrhages, the presence of abnormal vaginal discharge – It may be copious in amount and frequently foul smelling.
   b. Increase in vaginal pH.
   c. Tenderness/discomfort during pelvic examination.
3. **Investigations**
   a. **Hanging drop examination** – Reveals the presence of motile *Trichomonas* organisms in a case of *Trichomonas* vaginitis.
   b. **KOH treated preparation of vaginal discharge** – This reveals the presence of pseudomycelia and spores in a case of Candida vaginitis.
   c. **Whiff test** – The fishy odour on adding a drop of 10% KOH to the vaginal secretion is suggestive of the presence of bacterial vaginosis.
   d. **Gram's stain** – This may reveal presence of Gram-negative intracellular and extracellular diplococci suggestive of gonococci. The presence of *Clue cells* is suggestive of bacterial vaginosis.
   e. **Culture:**
      Chocolate Agar – Gonococci
      Sabouraud's medium or Nickerson's medium – Candida
      Special enriched medium – Trichomonas
      Trichomonas infection

CANDIDAL VAGINITIS

Candida albicans is the next common cause of vaginitis. It is not a sexually transmitted infection. It is commonly seen whenever there is increase in content of glycogen in vagina in conditions such as pregnancy, diabetics, woman taking oral pills or in the immunocompromised woman. Often infection may occur following a course of oral antibiotics for some conditions.

1. **Risk factors altering the immune response include**
   a. Pregnancy
   b. Medications – Oral contraceptives, antibiotics, corticosteroids, cancer chemotherapy
   c. HIV and other STDs
   d. Diabetes mellitus
2. **Poor personal hygiene**
3. **Run down condition of health in general**.

Diagnosis

1. **Clinical**
   - Complaints of pruritus, burning, dysuria
   - Evidence of vulvar erythema, oedema, scratch marks
   - Discharge: whitish, flaky or curd-like
   - Vaginal pH 4.5

Investigations

- **A KOH wet mount** preparation of the vaginal discharge helps to dissolve all cellular debris, leaving behind the resistant hyphae and spores of candida thus making diagnosis easy.
- **Culture**: Though not routinely advocated, vaginal discharge can be cultured on Sabouraud's agar – The presence of discrete creamy rounded colonies appears in 48–72 hours, giving a typical yeast-like odour.
- Nickerson's Medium is a special medium, on which candida colonies appear in 48–72 hours as brown-black discrete round colonies.

Treatment

Preventive measures – These include the following:
   a. Improve personal hygiene
   b. Discontinue offending medications
   c. Control diabetes

The treatment of candida vaginitis comprises of use of antifungal creams or pessaries for a duration of 7–14 days. Some of the commonly used antifungal pessaries contain clotrimazole, miconazole, terconazole or butoconazole.

Oral antifungal agents – Rarely oral antifungal agents may have to be used especially in young unmarried girls or in women who have frequent recurrences with vaginal antifungal agents. Fluconazole can be given as a single oral dose of 150 mg. Itraconazole and newer antifungal agents which are active against candida can be given orally.

TRICHOMONAS VAGINITIS

Diagnosis: This is based on clinical suspicion followed by confirmatory tests to establish the diagnosis.

(1) **Clinical Findings:** These include
Vulvar erythema and oedema
Copious frothy yellowish-green foul smelling discharge
Punctate lesions of cervix (strawberry cervix)
Vaginal pH > 4.5

(2) **Hanging drop test:** Reveals presence of actively motile pear-shaped flagellate organisms.

(3) **Culture:** Requires use of special media, these are not routinely used.

Treatment

Being a protozoal infection *Trichomonas* vaginitis response well to Metronidazole or one of the drugs belonging to Imidazole group. Metronidazole is given in a dose of 400 mg three times a day for a period of 5 days. Alternatively, same drug can be given in a single dose of 2 gm. Both the partners need to be given treatment at the same time to prevent risk of recurrence. Tinidazole 2 g as a single dose or secnidazole in a single dose of 2 g has also been used for the treatment of *Trichomonas* vaginitis. There may be a bitter metallic taste in case patient or husband is alcoholic. Single dose therapy ensures better compliance.

VAGINOSIS (BACTERIAL)

Vaginosis (also known earlier as nonspecific vaginitis/ *Gardnerella vaginalis*/Corynebacterium vaginitis and anaerobic vaginitis) is associated with minimal inflammatory response; the vaginal fluid reveals few leucocytes.

Bacterial vaginosis is termed *vaginosis* rather than *vaginitis*, because it is associated with alteration in the normal vaginal flora rather than due to any specific infection. There is a considerable decrease in the number of lactobacilli in the vaginal discharge with 100-fold increase in growth of other anaerobic bacteria. Lactobacilli reduce pH and release hydrogen peroxide toxic to other bacteria, so reduction in their number allows other bacteria, i.e. aerobic and anaerobic bacteria, to grow. These are *Haemophilus vaginalis, G. vaginalis, Mobiluncus* and *M. hominis. Mobiluncus* is a Gram-positive rod-shaped bacterium with a characteristic corkscrew spinning anaerobe. Bacterial vaginosis is therefore a polymicrobial condition (Fig. 26.3).

It is not sexually transmitted and has a variable incubation period. About 50% women are asymptomatic carriers of infection, but majority complain vaginal discharge without itching.

The characteristics of vaginal discharge in bacterial vaginosis are as follows (Amsel's criteria):

- White, milky, nonviscous discharge adherent to the vaginal wall.
- pH of the discharge is more than 4.5. (pH 5–7).
- Fishy odour when mixed with 10% KOH is due to amino-metabolites from various organisms (amine or whiff test).
- Presence of clue cells – the epithelial cells have a fuzzy border due to adherence of bacteria (Fig. 26.4A and B).
- Increased number of *G. vaginalis* and other microorganisms and reduced number of lactobacilli and leucocytes.

The woman has minimal vulval irritation. The diagnosis is based on wet smear and culture. The smear reveals clean background with few inflammatory cells and other organisms, but scanty lactobacilli. Many epithelial cells present a granular cytoplasm caused by small Gram-negative bacilli adhering on their surface, the so-called ***clue cells***. Free floating clumps of *Gardnerella* are seen. Gram stain is 90% sensitive and 83% specific. DNA probe for *G. vaginalis* is now available. Gas liquid chromatography is useful.

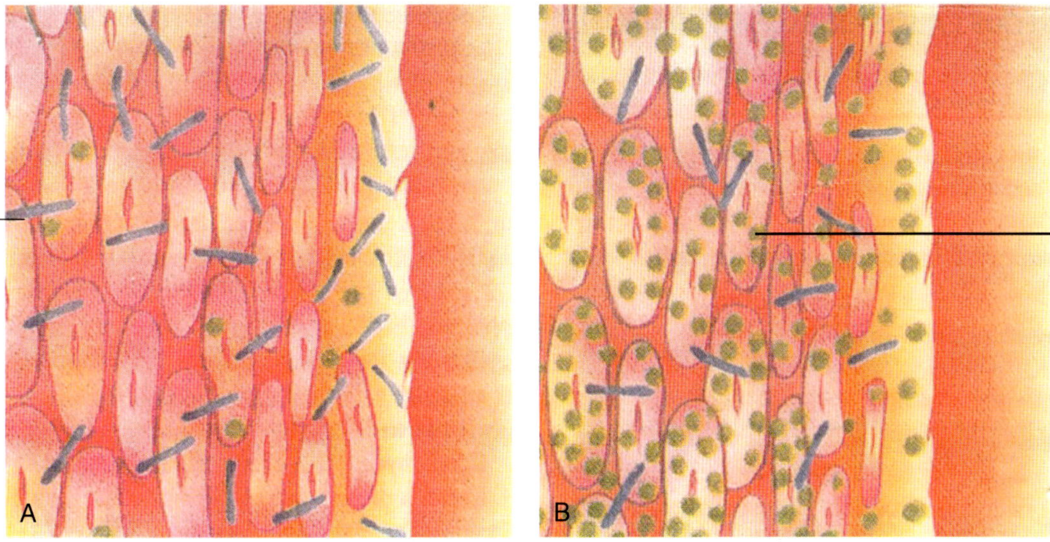

Figure 26.3 **(A)** Normal mature vaginal cells with Döderlein's lactobacilli. **(B)** Clue cells with very few Döderlein's bacilli.

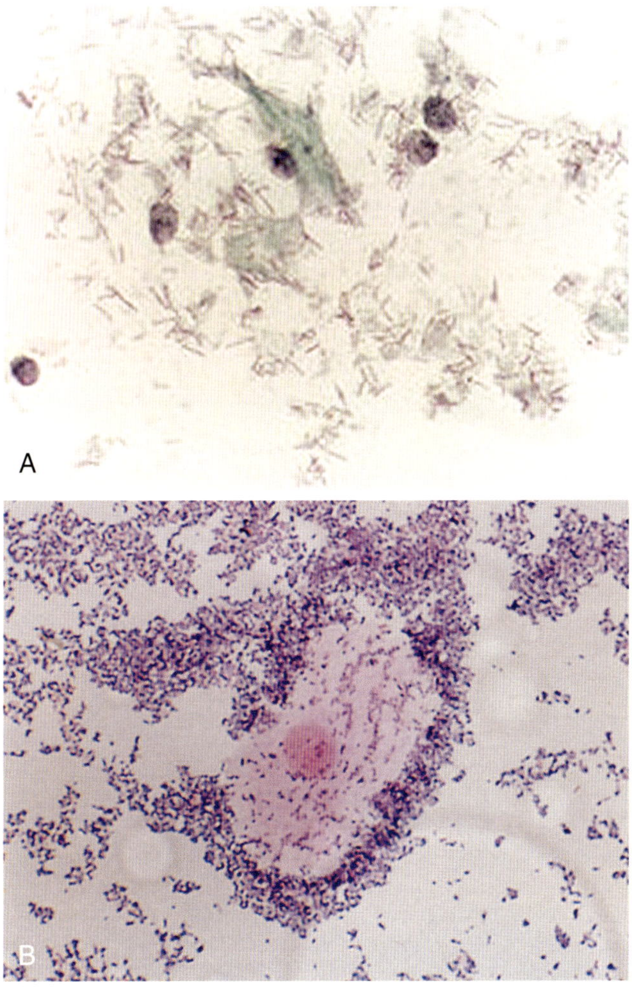

Figure 26.4 Bacterial vaginosis. **(A)** Vaginal smear showing Döderlein's bacilli. **(B)** Clue cells suggestive of bacterial vaginosis.

Bacterial vaginosis can cause PID, chorioamnionitis, premature rupture of membrane (PROM) and preterm labour.

TREATMENT

The 7-day course of metronidazole 400 mg twice daily is effective in 85% of cases, whereas a single dose of 2 g cures only 45% of cases. Ampicillin 500 mg or cephalosporin 500 mg b.i.d. for 7 days is also effective. Tetracycline 500 mg four times a day, doxycycline 100 mg twice a day and sulphafurazole for 10–14 days are the alternative antibiotics in nonpregnant women.

Clindamycin 2% cream locally is effective in 85% of cases. Oral clindamycin 300 mg daily for 7 days is also effective. Ornidazole 500 mg vaginal tablet daily for 7 days is also effective, use of vaginal tablets avoid the first-pass effect in liver seen with oral route.

Lacteal is a protein-free acidifying lactate gel which neutralizes the vaginal pH (lactic acid 5% W/V, 0.1% glycogen) – 5 mL is applied daily for 7 days. Recurrence rate is 30%.

Metronidazole does not reduce the number of lactobacilli unlike clindamycin and may be considered superior to the latter. Metronidazole to treat bacterial vaginosis may be avoided in first trimester.

PROBIOTICS

Ecoflora

Ecoflora capsule contains *Lactobacillus rhamnosus GR-I* and *Lactobacillus reuteri Rc-14*. These are probiotic agents, effective against Gram-negative pathogens and resistant to spermicides. They also have anti-inflammatory activity. They secrete collagen-binding proteins that prevent pathogen adhesions. The ecoflora adheres to the epithelial cells, prevent adhesion of other pathogens and produce H_2O_2, thus maintaining pH in the vagina. One to two capsules daily for 30 days are followed by one capsule daily for another 30 days. The drug is, however, contraindicated during pregnancy.

MISCELLANEOUS CAUSES OF EXCESSIVE VAGINAL DISCHARGE

a. **Excessive physiological discharge**
  (1) **Common causes**
    Sexual excitement
    Cervical erosion
    Ovulation time
    Psychological factors
  (2) **Management**
    Clinical evaluation to exclude pathology
    Counselling and education
    Electrocautery of erosion cervix
b. **Other infections**
  (1) **Common microorganisms suspected include**
    Chlamydia trachomatis
    Gonorrhoea
    Herpes
    Foreign body
    Chemical irritation
    Senile vaginitis
c. **Management options**
  Advice about personal hygiene.
  Avoid use of irritants such as douches, vaginal contraceptives (chemical creams, foam tablets) if they are the cause.
  Remove foreign body – retained condom, tampon, pessaries)
  Chlamydia – treat with tetracycline/doxycycline/erythromycin.
  Gonorrhoea – treat with penicillin/ceftriaxone/ciprofloxacin, cefixime.
  Herpes – treat with acyclovir and allied derivatives.

INFLAMMATION OF THE VAGINA

In this important group of disorders, a variety of mixed pathogens are recoverable on smear and culture, i.e. *Staphylococcus, Streptococcus*, both haemolytic and anaerobic, and *E. coli*.

AETIOLOGY

Chemicals, drugs, douches, pessaries, tampons, trauma, foreign bodies such as rubber ring pessaries, contraceptives and even vaginal and cervical operations are all causative. Alteration in the pH towards alkalinity always favours non-specific infection; hence, it is common in the puerperium. Often present infection with trichomoniasis is important, because the isolation of the secondary organism may mask the presence of the *Trichomonas*, which is really responsible for the discharge. Hence, it is important to use selective culture media in all cases where response to treatment is disappointing.

SYMPTOMS AND SIGNS

A red, swollen, tender vagina with irritation, burning and often dysuria with frequency of micturition is present. The vaginitis is mild or severe and acute or chronic, and the colour, consistency and amount of discharge are variable. The infection is more common following menstruation or following intercourse.

DIAGNOSIS

Diagnosis is established by smear and culture of vaginal discharge.

TREATMENT

Treatment varies according to the infecting organism and is general as well as local.

GENERAL

All measures are designed to improve the general health of the patient.

LOCAL

The correction of the vaginal pH to 4.5 by a water-dispersible, buffered vaginal jelly which can be inserted in graduated amounts with a special disposable applicator (Fig. 26.5).

A locally applied bactericidal cream such as triple sulpha (sulphathiazole 3.42%, N-acetyl sulphanilamide 2.86% and N-benzoyl sulphanilamide 3.70%, excipient to 100%) (Fig. 26.6) or antibiotic pessaries when the organism and sensitivity are known.

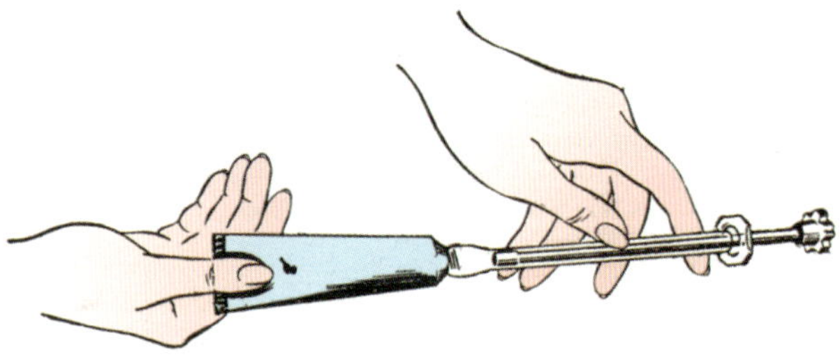

Figure 26.5 pH corrected using a special disposable applicator.

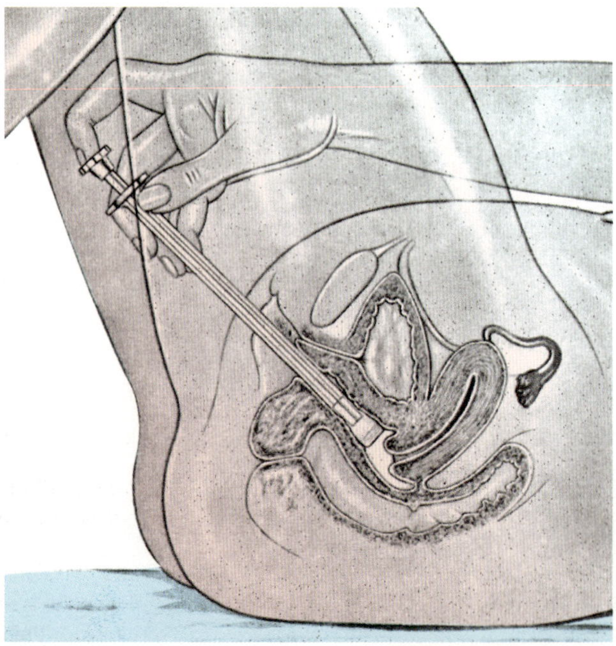

Figure 26.6 Applicator inserted in the vagina and the cream injected (local application).

The elimination of infection in the genital tract such as chronic endocervicitis by diathermy cauterization and conization. A woman with nonspecific vaginitis can be conveniently treated without extensive laboratory investigations with 1-day therapy using the kits containing combination of fluconazole 150 mg, azithromycin 1 g and secnidazole. Instead of azithromycin, doxycycline can be used for 10–14 days. Same way cefixime can be used for gonorrhoea and chlamydia, and 1 g of secnidazole with 45% cure rate. Advantage of using such a combination is that it avoids detail diagnostic work up. This is repeated a week later if required.

OESTROGEN DEFICIENCY–RELATED VAGINITIS

Oestrogen deficiency vaginitis is seen as vulvovaginitis in children and as senile vaginitis in postmenopausal women. In both these age groups, the vaginal epithelium is thin and ill-protected against infection; glycogen content is low. Döderlein's bacillus is thinly populated and the vaginal pH is higher than normal, approaching or exceeding 7.4. Cytology reveals predominantly basal and parabasal cells.

VULVOVAGINITIS IN CHILDREN

The commonly affected age group is in the first 5 years of life, but other prepubertal girls can be affected. The infecting organism may be any pyogenic coccus or *E. coli*, *Trichomonas vaginalis* and *Monilia* are uncommon except in a case of sexual abuse. Infection is transmitted from adults or another child by hands, toilet, utensils or clothes. Threadworms which encourage scratching are a fairly common causative factor in this age group. In children, always think about a possibility of a foreign body inserted in the vagina, the variety of which baffles enumeration, must not be forgotten. This primitive Freudian urge accounts for many otherwise inexplicable vaginal discharge in young children. Occasionally, vulvovaginitis in children may be due to sexual abuse.

SYMPTOMS AND SIGNS

A reddened, oedematous vulva bathed in a profuse purulent discharge, with soreness and irritation. The child is fidgety and constantly handling or scratching the external genitalia. Labial adhesions may sometimes form.

DIAGNOSIS

Examination under anaesthesia is probably the most effective method of excluding a foreign body, obtaining an adequate smear and inspecting the upper vagina.

TREATMENT

Local and systemic antibiotics will provide prompt relief from the symptoms.

Ethinyloestradiol 0.01 mg increases the vaginal epithelial resistance and improves the vaginal acidity and is often all that is needed to affect a cure.

- Specific antibiotics such as ampicillin or cephalosporins are effective to which the infecting organism is sensitive. This is best given systemically and not locally.
- No local treatment is desirable in young girls.
- Isolation from other children to prevent cross-infection is desirable.
- If not adequately treated and speedily eradicated, the infection can become chronic and resistant.

SENILE VAGINITIS

In many aspects, senile vaginitis is comparable to vulvovaginitis in children. As a result of oestrogen deficiency, the vaginal epithelium becomes thin and atrophic, the glycogen content and acidity of the vagina are lowered and the ever present mixed pathogens obtain a footing.

AETIOLOGY

Apart from women with natural menopause, prolonged lactation or premature menopause, women who have undergone oophorectomy are prone to develop senile vaginitis.

SYMPTOMS AND SIGNS

Dry vagina, dyspareunia and a purulent, often slightly blood tinged, discharge are evident. The vagina is inflamed and tender and the mucosa is excoriated. Urinary symptoms in the form of increased frequency and dysuria are common. On examination, the urethral meatus is pouting and shows a low-grade chronic urethritis often misdiagnosed as a urethral caruncle. There is patchy granular vaginitis, the spots of which are red and bleed easily when swabbed. These raw and inflamed areas may become adherent and cause an obliteration of the canal in the region of the fornices or vault. The infection may spread upwards to involve the endometrium and produce a senile endometritis, and later a pyometra.

DIAGNOSIS

The clinical features outlined above are easy to interpret, but certain reservations are of great importance.

- Senile vaginitis does produce a blood-stained discharge, but this does not exclude the coincident cancer of the endometrium or endocervix.
- Senile vaginitis and senile endometritis may coexist.

It is therefore obligatory to examine women with postmenopausal bleeding under anaesthesia and perform a diagnostic curettage to exclude cancer of the endometrium, endocervix and a pyometra.

TREATMENT

Oestrogen therapy is given to improve the resistance of the vaginal epithelium, raise the glycogen content and lower the vaginal pH. Ethinyloestradiol 0.01 mg daily for 3 weeks should suffice.

Local treatment by pessary/ointment containing oestrogen can be employed.

As an alternative to pessaries which may be difficult for the patient to insert, a vaginal cream containing the same ingredients may be instilled by patient with the help of special applicator illustrated in Figs 26.5 and 26.6. This treatment is usually effective and can be repeated if the symptoms recur.

SECONDARY VAGINITIS

All varieties of vaginitis in which the primary cause is not vaginal are included in this section.

- *Foreign body.* The presence of a vaginal pessary to manage prolapse or retroversion invariably causes vaginitis. Contraceptives and vaginal tampons operate in a similar way, especially if forgotten and left inside for a long period.
- *Infective conditions of the cervix.* Vaginitis is frequently secondary to chronic infection of the cervix, usually an endocervicitis, the effective eradication of which is sufficient to clear up the vaginal infection. Childbirth injuries of the genital tract, such as cervical tear are other causes
- *Vesicovaginal, ureterovaginal urinary fistulae and rectovaginal fistulae.* These are causes of secondary vaginal infection, and cause persistent discharge.

GROWTH ON CERVIX

A growth on cervix especially carcinoma cervix or a cervical polyp is always infected and may cause secondary vaginitis.

VAGINITIS MEDICAMENTOSA

It is a special type of vaginitis usually caused by chemicals, douches, arsenic pessaries and occasionally contraceptives.

RARE FORMS OF VAGINITIS

EMPHYSEMATOUS VAGINITIS

In this extremely rare condition, the vaginal walls are distended with gas-containing vesicles. The subepithelial tissues are indurated and oedematous, and the clinical picture suggests a malignant infiltration. There is, however, no ulceration. The main symptom apart from a swollen vagina is profuse vaginal discharge. The aetiology is unknown except that the patients are usually pregnant. Treatment is expectant as the condition resolves spontaneously. Less-severe varieties of this emphysema have been described in which the gas-containing vesicles are found on a routine inspection of the vagina, and these cause minimal symptoms.

TREATMENT

In case of vaginal discharge in which there is some local cause, such as a retained pessary, the cause must be removed. In vaginitis due to prolapse and secondary vaginitis caused by the fistulae, it is usually waste of efforts to treat vaginitis without dealing with the primary cause. Specific infections of the vagina are treated by appropriate antibiotics as soon as the causative organism has been identified. There are various methods of treating vaginal discharge.

Vaginal Irrigations

Vaginal irrigation is rarely employed nowadays. In cases of prolapse, Betadine is the best antiseptic cleansing agent, but occasionally acriflavine pack has been used.

Vaginal Pessaries

The pessaries may contain the following:

- Oestrogen to promote keratinization of the epithelium and to increase glycogen content and vaginal acidity. The pessaries contain 0.1 mg (1000 international units) or 1 mg (10,000 international units) oestrone.
- Antibiotics.
- Cortisone or bacteriostatic agents, Betadine.
- Specific fungicidal drugs, nystatin (100,000 units), imidazole derivatives, ketoconazole or the more recent terconazole; antiprotozoal and other bactericidal drugs.

Bactericidal Creams

Bactericidal creams such as triple sulpha cream, Betadine. Swabs should be taken for culture from the cervix, vagina and the urethra and the appropriate antibiotic given systemically or locally as soon as the organisms and their sensitivities are known.

TOXIC SHOCK SYNDROME

Toxic shock syndrome is a septicaemic shock, reported first by Todd in 1978, which follows the use of vaginal tampons during menstruation, and at times during the puerperium.

It is caused by *Staphylococcus aureus* and rarely by β-haemolytic streptococci, both organisms release the endotoxin which causes sudden pyrexia over 39.9°C, myalgia, diffuse skin rash and oedematous erythema. The patient may suffer from vomiting, diarrhoea and hypotension. Leucocytosis, thrombocytopenia and increased serum bilirubin and liver enzymes are noted. The blood culture, however, is sterile. Toxin and release of bradykinin account for the syndrome.

Treatment

The treatment comprises correction of hypovolaemia with intravenous fluid, β-lactamase-resistant penicillin, cephalosporin and gentamicin. Unless correctly diagnosed and promptly treated. The mortality may be around 15%.

Prevention

Vaginal tampons or contraceptive sponge (Today Sponge) should never be left in the vagina for more than 24 hours at a time.

ULCERATIONS OF THE VAGINA

Ulcerations of the vagina are rare. Foreign bodies such as a retained pessary usually cause ulceration high up in the posterior vaginal fornix, and the presence of granulation tissue and unhealthy offensive vaginal discharge are other manifestations. Following longstanding irritation, an ulcer may undergo malignant transformation; hence, a biopsy is mandatory in suspicious cases. Removal of the ring pessary, local douche and oral antibiotics can heal the ulcer.

VENEREAL ULCERS

These are commonly seen on the vulva, but occasionally the vagina may also be involved.

TUBERCULOUS ULCERS

Tuberculous ulcers are rare and if they do occur, concomitant lesions are commonly present on the cervix or the vulva.

CHEMICAL ULCERS

Introduction of potassium permanganate pessaries to induce abortion has been a practice in some communities. The chemical irritation can cause ulceration, occasionally followed by widespread cicatrization and stenosis of the vagina.

RADIATION ULCERS

Ulceration of the vagina may develop following radiotherapy particularly in cancer of the cervix. Ulcers of this kind do not heal readily; they may cause adhesion and distortion of the vaginal vault.

TROPHIC ULCERS

These are observed in women suffering from procidentia.

VAGINAL GRANULATION TISSUE

These are seen in scars/vault following surgical procedures such as vaginal hysterectomy or abdominal hysterectomy. The most common site is the vaginal vault. Patients complain of an offensive, occasionally blood-stained discharge which may persist for a few weeks to months after surgery. Cauterization of the granulation tissue gives relief.

SCARS, STENOSIS AND ATRESIA OF THE VAGINA

Scarring of the vaginal and the paravaginal tissues is not uncommon. The possible causes are injuries during childbirth, extensive repair operations for genital prolapse, radiotherapy for genital malignancy or chemical burns. Severe fulminant vulvovaginal infections in young girls and puerperal or menopausal women may also lead to such sequelae.

AMOEBIASIS OF VAGINA

Amoebiasis of vagina appears as a fungating subcutaneous ulcer causing foul smelling discharge and postmenopausal bleeding. The biopsy confirms the diagnosis. Oral Metronidazole 400 mg twice daily for 7 days cures the ulcer.

CYSTS AND NEOPLASMS OF THE VAGINA

VAGINAL CYSTS

The vaginal cyst is rare, and is most commonly located in the anterior vaginal wall. This is usually small, but may attain a size of 7.5 cm in diameter.

Gartner's duct cyst arises from the remnants of the mesonephric duct and lies in the anterolateral aspect of the vaginal wall. A small cyst remains asymptomatic. A large cyst if causing dyspareunia requires excision.

Inclusion cyst is mainly seen at the lower end of the vagina on its posterior surface and is caused by tags of mucosa embedded inside the scar that later forms a cyst.

Bartholin cyst at times extends into the vagina and causes dyspareunia.

Endometriotic cyst appears as a bluish bulge in the posterior fornix. It behaves similar to endometriotic cyst of the vulva. It is treated by surgical excision.

VAGINAL NEOPLASMS

Tumours of the vagina are rare. In rare cases, a benign tumour such as a fibromyoma can occur.

Malignant tumours are described in chapter on Malignant Lesions of Vulva and Vagina.

KEY POINTS

- Leucorrhoea is a common complaint in women of childbearing age. Apart from cervical lesions and nonspecific causes, specific vaginitis is caused by gonococci *Trichomonas, Chlamydia* and *Monilia* and bacterial vaginosis.
- Vulvovaginitis in children is not uncommon. It is mostly due to foreign body or pinworm infections in anal canal.
- Senile vaginitis due to oestrogen deficiency in menopausal women causes dry vagina, dyspareunia and urinary symptoms, and needs to be treated with vaginal oestrogen.
- Bacterial vaginosis is the most common vaginal infection caused by reduction in the number of lactobacilli. This allows *Gardnerella,* aerobic and anaerobic organisms to over grow and produce typical discharge with fishy odour. The clue cells in the smear are pathognomic of this infection. During pregnancy, it can cause of chorioamnionitis, premature rupture of membrane and preterm labour.

SELF-ASSESSMENT

1. Describe normal commensals of vagina.
2. What are the common causes of leucorrhoea? Discuss its management
3. Enumerate and briefly describe the causes of ulcers in the vagina.
4. Describe the microscopic appearance of the normal vaginal epithelium in an adult woman. Describe the cytological changes observed during the normal menstrual cycle. What alterations in structure occur after onset of menopause?
5. Describe the management of senile vaginitis.
6. What are the causes of bacterial vaginosis? How will you treat it?
7. Write a short note on vulvovaginitis in a child.

SUGGESTED READING

Hamill HA. In: Normal vaginal flora in relation to vaginitis. Obstet Gynecol Clin N Am 16:329–336, 1989.

MacCue JD. Evaluation and management of vaginitis. An update for primary care practitioners. Arch Int Med 149:565–568, 1989.

Mardh PA. The vaginal ecosystem. Am J Obstet Gynecol 165: 1163–1168, 1991.

O'Connor MI, Sobel JD. Epidemiology of recurrent vulvo vaginal Candidiasis: Identification and strain differentiation of *Candida albicans.* J Infect Dis 154:358–363, 1986.

Peeters M, Piot P. Adhesion of *Gardnerella vaginalis* to vaginal epithelial cells: Variables affecting adhesion and inhibition of Metronidazole. Genitourin Med 61:391–395, 1985.

SECTION 5 INFECTIONS IN GYNAECOLOGY

SECTION OUTLINE

Pelvic Inflammatory Disease

27

CHAPTER OUTLINE

PELVIC INFLAMMATORY DISEASE

Pelvic inflammatory disease (PID) implies inflammation of the upper genital tract involving the uterus, fallopian tubes as well as the ovaries. Because most cases of the PIDs are due to ascending or blood-borne infection, the lesion is often bilateral, though one tube may be more affected than the other. The ovaries are so closely linked to the fallopian tubes anatomically that they are incidentally involved in all infections, and it is therefore customary to consider inflammations of the two organs together. The only exception to this is involvement of only ovaries in mumps where the fallopian tubes are not affected.

AETIOLOGY

Normally there exist several natural barriers to the ascent of pathogenic organisms from the vagina to the fallopian tubes. Intact hymen prevents ascending infection. When a young, unmarried girl presents with PID, it is more likely to be tubercular in nature.

The acidic pH of the vaginal secretion inhibits the growth of bacteria; the cervical canal has a relatively small lumen and is normally filled with a plug of alkaline mucus. The ciliary movement of endometrial lining in the uterus and the cervical canal is directed downwards and discourages the upward spread of nonmotile organisms to the cavity of the uterus. This natural protective mechanism is impaired during menstruation, after abortion and delivery, as the cervical canal becomes dilated, the protecting epithelium of the endometrium is shed, and raw surfaces are present in the cavity of the uterus. The vaginal pH is increased, rendering the genital tract more vulnerable to infection. In addition to these factors, intrauterine manipulations such as curettage for evacuation in abortion and manual removal of placenta favour entry and spread of pathogenic organisms. Intrauterine contraceptive device (IUCD) is also a source of infection, particularly when it is not introduced under aseptic conditions, or introduced in the presence of a vaginal infection.

The most common cause of PID is *sexually transmitted diseases* (STD), the incidence of which has risen in the past 20 years. Gonococcal and chlamydial infections are two most common causes of acute PID; the incidence of these two causes varies in different communities. About 60%–75% of PIDs are caused by STD, of which gonorrhoea accounts for about 30% in the developed countries. The importance and high incidence of chlamydial infection has been recognized with availability of culture facilities and enzyme-linked immunosorbent assay (ELISA) kits. Penicillinase-producing gonococci resistant to penicillin have also been identified recently in cultures in 2%–10% of the cases.

Gonococci and *Chlamydia* travel up the genital tract along the mucous membrane to reach the fallopian tubes and cause salpingo-oophoritis. The organisms probably ride up the tract along with the motile sperms in a piggy-back fashion. Sperms also help in transportation of *Trichomonas* similarly. Other organisms directly ascend along the lining of the genital tract. This partly explains the absence of gonococcal inflammatory disease in a woman whose husband is azoospermic. *Chlamydia* infection (obligate Gram-negative intracellular organisms) remains asymptomatic in the endocervix or produces minimum symptoms, and therefore the infection goes unnoticed and untreated, but the damage it causes to the tube is more devastating than with gonorrhoea (fivefold). The cervix and the urethra are the common sites where *Chlamydia* lodge and ascend upwards. The incidence of this infection is not easy to find out in many countries because of the lack of culture facilities. The development of immunological tests has now made it possible to detect the antibodies in the sera of infected patients. Gonococci and *Chlamydia* create an environment for secondary invasion by other organisms normally residing in the lower genital tract. Other organisms which can cause PID include (i) mycoplasma (*Mycoplasma hominis* and *M. ureolyticus*), (ii) tubercle bacillus, (iii) viruses and (iv) *Escherichia coli* (30%) (Table 27.1).

Mycoplasma hominis is isolated in 50% of sexually active women, but detected in only 7% of PID cases. *Mycoplasma genitalium* is now a new organism that is seen to cause PID. Bacterial vaginosis can also cause upper genital tract infection. These organisms reach the tube via the lymphatics bypassing the endometrium.

Table 27.1 Organisms Responsible for Pelvic Inflammatory Disease

- Sexually transmitted
  - *Gonococcus*
  - *Chlamydia*
  - *Mycoplasma*
- *Trichomonas*
- Pyogenic
  - Aerobes
  - Staphylococci
  - Streptococci
  - *E. coli*
- Anaerobes
  - *Bacteroides fragilis, Peptococcus, Clostridium*
  - *Actinomyces*
- Tubercular salpingitis

The polymicrobial nature of this infection has been observed and some 40 microorganisms, both aerobes and anaerobes, have been implicated in causation of PID:

Aerobes. Both Gram positive and Gram negative.

Anaerobes. Bacteroides fragilis (20%), fusobacteria, *B. melaninogenicus*, anaerobic cocci such as peptococci and peptostreptococci, clostridia, facultative anaerobes, *Actinomyces* (Gram positive) and *E. coli* (30%–40%).

The infection by anaerobic organisms is greatly favoured by blood loss, anaemia and tissue damage such as infection occurring in septic abortion. A polymicrobial infection in PID mandates the administration of more than one antibiotic covering Gram-positive, Gram-negative and an aerobic bacteria.

- In India like many other developing countries, many deliveries are conducted at home by *dais* (untrained midwives). Criminal abortions continue to take place despite the Government of India's liberal policy on induced abortions. *Postabortal and puerperal sepses* are therefore common occurrences. It is estimated that about 40%–50% of all PID cases in the developing countries are caused in this manner and the rest by STDs.
- Minor *operative procedures* such as Dilatation and Curettage and hysterosalpingogram and other procedures can cause ascending infection. Manual removal of placenta and evacuation of products of conception are other important sources of infection in the upper genital tract.
- The use of IUCDs has increased the incidence of PID threefold. Most infections occur at the time of insertion of IUCD. By observing proper asepsis at the time of insertion of IUCD, PIDs can be avoided. This is not to condemn this method of family planning, but to emphasize the need for strict asepsis during insertion of the device and careful follow-up of the women wearing these devices. *Actinomyces* Gram-positive anaerobes is reported in 7% of IUCD users, if the device is worn for more than 2 years as against 1% in nonusers. *It is important to note that barrier contraceptives prevent STD and pelvic infection.*
- *Tuberculosis* of the fallopian tubes is blood borne in most cases and rarely ascending in nature.
- *Pelvic peritonitis* due to appendicitis and diverticulitis may spread to involve the fallopian tube of that side.

The PID is a disease of young women, who are sexually and reproductively active. The promiscuity and frequent change of sex partners are mainly responsible for PID in the developed countries, and amongst sex workers. About 75% cases of PID are due to STDs in the developed countries. Septic abortions and puerperal sepsis are the important aetiological factors in the developing countries (Fig. 27.1). Sterilization operation prevents PID by blockage of the tubes. Apart from barrier contraceptives, progestogen-containing pills produce a thick plug of mucous in the cervical canal and prevent ascent of microorganisms.

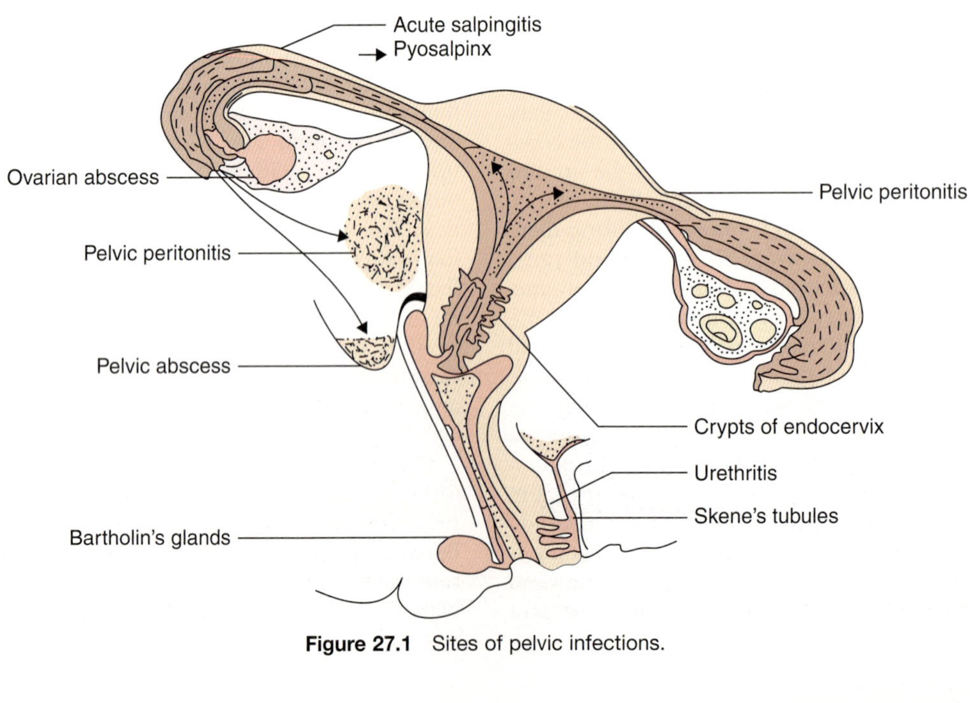

Figure 27.1 Sites of pelvic infections.

Westrom (1975) reported that women with one previous attack of PID are predisposed to another attack in 12% of the cases. Two attacks of PID increase the risk to 35% and three attacks to as much as 75%. Golden (2003) reported 8% recurrence in a woman with previous PID versus 1% occurrence with no history of PID previously.

PATHOLOGICAL ANATOMY

ACUTE SALPINGITIS

In acute salpingitis, the fallopian tubes are swollen, oedematous and hyperaemic with visible dilated vessels on the peritoneal surface. Some degree of serous exudation is seen around the fallopian tube. The sure sign of salpingitis is the discharge of seropurulent fluid from the fimbrial end of the tube at the time of laparoscopy or laparotomy.

The mucous membrane is oedematous, infiltrated with leucocytes and plasma cells. In ascending infection, as seen in gonorrhoea, the mucous membrane is first affected. The inflammatory exudate is discharged into the lumen of the tube which now distends, mainly at the ampullary end. The ulceration of the mucous membrane that follows leads to adhesions and tubal blockage or narrowing of the lumen which may subsequently be the cause of infertility or ectopic pregnancy (Fig. 27.2), compared with the normal pregnancy (Fig. 27.3).

In early stages, when the fimbrial end is not closed by adhesions, pus pours out into the pelvic cavity causing pelvic abscess. Eventually, with the sealing of the fimbrial end by fibrinous adhesion, pus accumulates in the tubal lumen. The ovaries are involved and a tubo-ovarian abscess (TOA) or tubo-ovarian mass results, both getting surrounded by adhesions. The ampullary portion of the tube distends more than the isthmic portion, resulting in a retort-shaped pyosalpinx. An acute pyosalpinx is surrounded by adhesions which fix it to the back of the broad ligament, the ovary, the sigmoid colon, adjacent coils of intestine and posterior surface of the uterus. The wall of the tube is thickened and the tube is tense with pent-up fluid (Figs 27.4 and 27.5). On a rare occasion, the infection may spread upwards to cause generalized peritonitis, paralytic ileus and pelvic or even subdiaphragmatic and perinephric abscess. Septic thrombophlebitis, bacteraemia and metastatic abscess are rare nowadays, because of a prompt and effective antibiotic therapy.

In PID following postabortal and puerperal infection, the pathogenesis is different. The infection spreads through the cervix via lymphatics to the cellular tissue in the broad ligament, causing cellulitis. The fallopian tube is affected from the outside and the mucosa last of all. The wall of the tube is thickened considerably with hardly any distension of the lumen. Eventual involvement of mucosa ends up in blockage of the fallopian tube by multiple intraluminal adhesions.

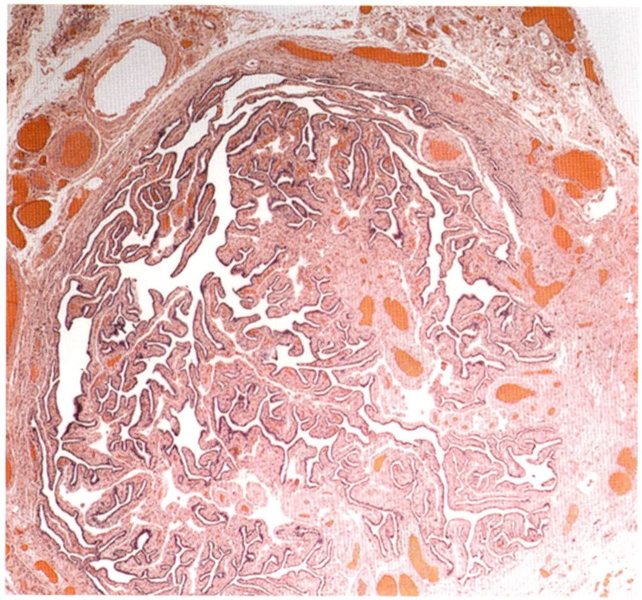

Figure 27.3 Normal fallopian tube between isthmus and ampulla. Note the convolutions of the plicae.

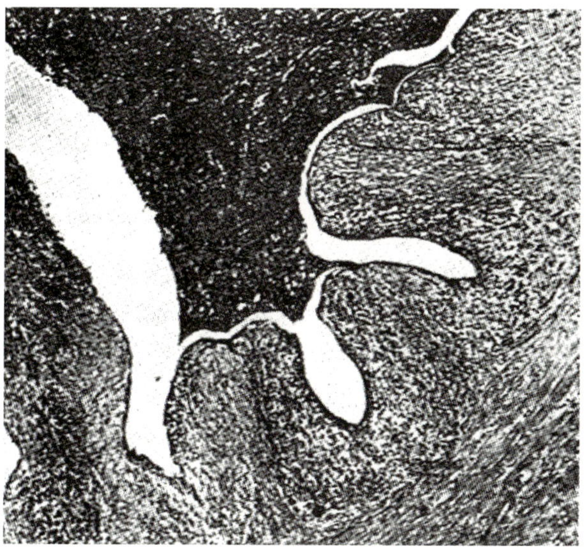

Figure 27.2 Acute suppurative salpingitis showing the tubal plicae infiltrated with inflammatory cells, with desquamation of the surface epithelium and a transudation of inflammatory cells into the lumen of the tube (×48).

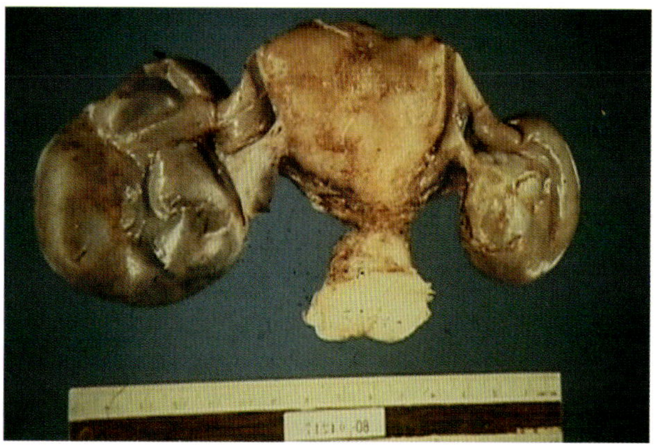

Figure 27.4 Bilateral tubo-ovarian abscess. It was impossible at operation to define or separate the ovaries from the tubes. (*Source*: Public domain-Brookside Press, http://www.brooksidepress.org/Products/Military_OBGYN/Textbook/Problems/Hydrosalpinx640.jpg.)

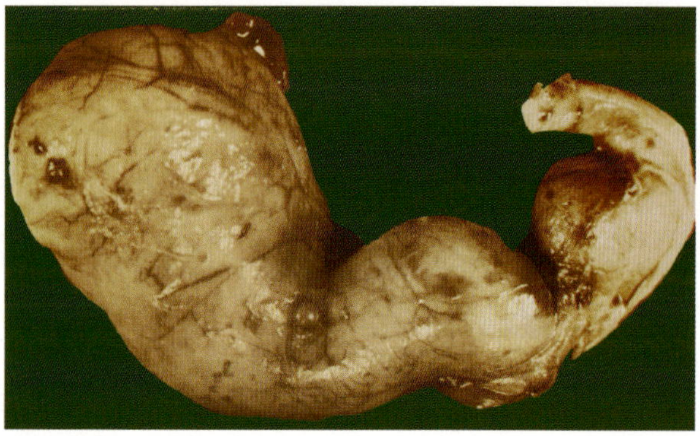

Figure 27.5 A retort-shaped pyosalpinx. (*Source*: H. Fox (editor), Haines and Taylor Obstetrical and Gynaecological Pathology, 3rd ed., London: Churchill Livingstone, 1987, pp. 411–456.)

Subacute PID results from inadequate treatment or from reinfection by the infected partner. Tuberculosis also manifests in the form of recurrent pelvic infection due to secondary infection.

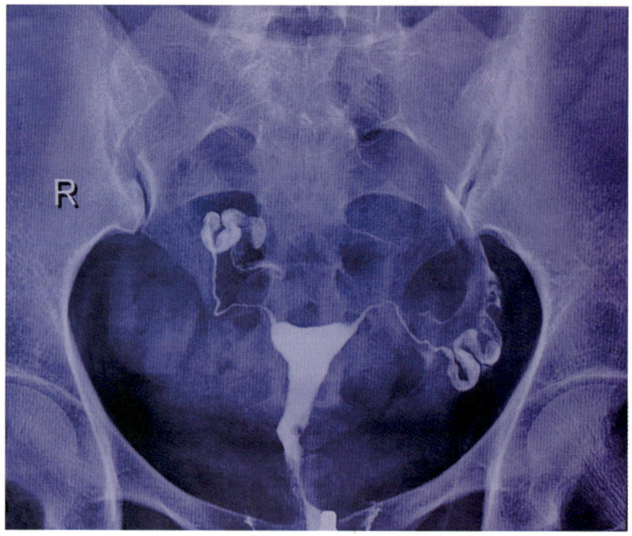

Figure 27.7 Hysterosalpingography showing bilateral hydrosalpinx.

CHRONIC PID

Failure of acute pelvic infection to resolve or end result of acute infection results in chronic tubo-ovarian masses. These masses manifest in the following forms:

- Hydrosalpinx
- Chronic pyosalpinx
- Chronic interstitial salpingitis
- Tubo-ovarian cyst and TOA
- Tubercular tubal-ovarian masses

Hydrosalpinx (Figs 27.6 and 27.7)

Hydrosalpinx is the distension of the fallopian tubes by collection of fluid in the lumen. If a pyosalpinx or TOA responds to antibiotics, the pus contained therein becomes sterile within 6 weeks of the initial attack, but the damage to the tube persists presenting as chronic pyosalpinx or hydrosalpinx.

A hydrosalpinx represents the end result of a previous acute salpingitis, and is often bilateral. It is retort-shaped swelling of the tube due to enormous dilatation of the ampullary region filled with a clear fluid and may be as large as 15 cm. The fimbrial end of the fallopian tube is usually closed; fimbriae are indrawn so that the outer surface of the hydrosalpinx is smooth and rounded. The interstitial end of the tube is curiously patent, as the dye can be visualized in the lumen during hysterosalpingogram (Fig. 27.7). The wall of the hydrosalpinx is thin and translucent. At times, the hydrosalpinx is mobile and can undergo torsion. Quite often, however, the outer surface is covered with adhesions which fix the hydrosalpinx to the back of the broad ligament and the pouch of Douglas (POD). Histology reveals flattening of the tubal plicae and exfoliation of the lining epithelium (Fig. 27.8).

Chronic Pyosalpinx (Figs 27.4 and 27.5)

A chronic pyosalpinx is thick-walled swelling of the fallopian tube, surrounded by dense adhesions and filled with pus. The inner wall is replaced by a granulation tissue. A pyosalpinx is often fixed to the POD, posterior surface of the broad ligament and the uterus by dense adhesions.

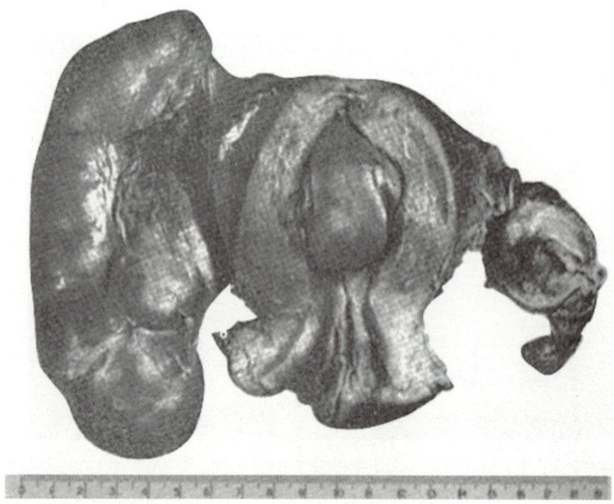

Figure 27.6 Right-sided hydrosalpinx. The left appendage shows less obvious but well-marked chronic salpingitis.

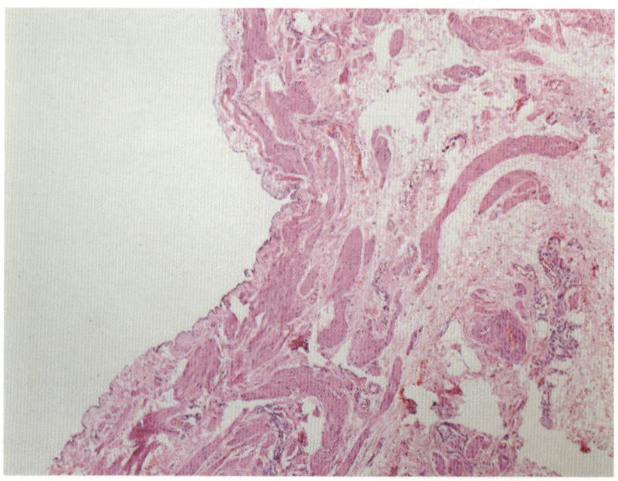

Figure 27.8 The wall of a hydrosalpinx. Note the flattening of the plicae (×360).

Table 27.2 Stages of PID

Stage I – Acute salpingitis without peritonitis – no adhesions
Stage II – Acute salpingitis with peritonitis – purulent discharge from tubal ostia
Stage III – Acute salpingitis with superimposed tubal occlusion or tubo-ovarian complex
Stage IV – Ruptured tubo-ovarian abscess
Stage V – Tubercular salpingitis

Chronic Interstitial Salpingitis

In chronic interstitial salpingitis, the wall of the fallopian tube is thickened and fibrotic, but there is no accumulation of pus in the lumen. Involvement of the ovary in adhesions results in chronic salpingo-oophoritis.

Tubo-Ovarian Cyst

In tubo-ovarian cyst, a hydrosalpinx communicates with a follicular cyst of the ovary, while in TOA, pyosalpinx communicate with an ovarian abscess. It is difficult to identify a normal ovarian tissue in these pathological conditions.

Tuberculous Form

Pelvic tuberculosis is described in Chapter 28.

STAGING

The spectrum ranges from mild-to-moderate and severe PID. Depending upon the severity of tubal damage, Gainesville has described five stages of PID (Table 27.2).

SYMPTOMS AND SIGNS OF PID

ACUTE PELVIC INFECTION

A young, sexually active woman is prone to PID. The most common symptom of acute PID is abdominal pain. It is bilateral and restricted to the lower abdomen. Pain spreads upwards if generalized peritonitis ensues. It is severe in the acute stages and is accompanied with high-grade fever. Vomiting may also follow. The sexually transmitted organisms may cause dysuria and vaginal discharge. Menstrual irregularity, if any, is due to preceding endometritis in a case of ascending infection or due to the antecedent abortion or delivery. The patient may develop abnormal uterine bleeding at a time when menstruation is not expected and the bleeding is often profuse and prolonged. In criminal abortion, the patient may deliberately conceal the history of amenorrhoea, making the diagnosis more difficult. In case of a pelvic abscess (Fig. 27.9), in addition to the above symptoms, the patient develops severe diarrhoea and passes small and frequent loose motions due to rectal irritation. In *chlamydial infection, symptoms are less pronounced and often an asymptomatic course.*

The patient with acute PID looks ill with high temperature (103–104°F). Tachycardia is present, and the tongue shows dehydration and is coated. Abdominal examination shows distension combined with tenderness and rigidity in the lower abdomen. It is rare for an abdominal swelling to be palpated in acute salpingo-oophoritis. Later, as the tenderness becomes less with treatment, a tender fixed mass

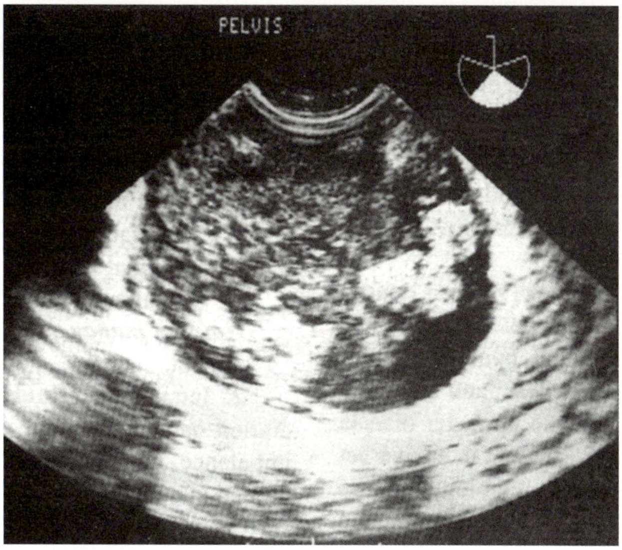

Figure 27.9 Ultrasound showing pelvic abscess.

arising from the pelvis may be palpable. Speculum examination shows purulent discharge from the cervical canal. A torn cervix or damaged tissue is evident in postabortal sepsis and criminal abortion. Swabs should be taken from the cervix and high vagina for culture. In an acute stage, cervical movement tenderness and tenderness in the fornices are the only evidence of pelvic infection. Later (Fig. 27.10), tender pelvic masses are felt in the lateral fornices. These masses are fixed and at times palpable behind the uterus in POD. A pelvic abscess produces a fluctuating tender swelling in the POD, bulging into the posterior fornix. TOA formation occurs in 30% of the cases of PID and is a frequent reason for hospitalization.

DIFFERENTIAL DIAGNOSIS

ACUTE APPENDICITIS

In appendicitis, the pain is initially central, around the umbilicus and then localizes to the right iliac fossa. Vomiting is severe, but temperature is not as high as in PID. The

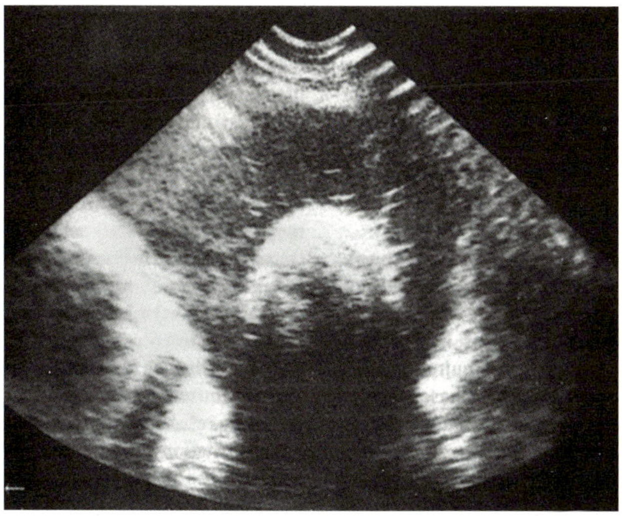

Figure 27.10 Ultrasound showing a pelvic mass.

lower margin of the appendicular mass can be reached, but this is not so in case of PID. Vaginal discharge and menstrual irregularities are absent in acute appendicitis.

ECTOPIC GESTATION

Amenorrhoea followed by irregular uterine bleeding and abdominal pain are the characteristic features seen in ectopic pregnancy. Cervical movement pain and a tender mass during per vaginal examination are the features of ectopic pregnancy. Criminal abortion with history of amenorrhoea may mimic ectopic pregnancy. Mostly temperature is normal or only slightly raised in ectopic pregnancy. The signs of internal bleeding are absent in PID. Vaginal discharge, leucocytosis and raised erythrocyte sedimentation rate (ESR) go in favour of a diagnosis of PID. Ultrasound may reveal bilateral tubo-ovarian masses.

DIVERTICULITIS

Diverticulitis may simulate the clinical picture of PID, but it usually seen after the age of 50 years, whereas PID is a disease of the young, sexually active females. The signs of infection are confined to the left iliac fossa in diverticulitis.

A TWISTED OVARIAN CYST

A twisted ovarian or paraovarian cyst (fimbrial cyst) causes sudden pain in the abdomen with vomiting, but pyrexia is usually absent or of very low grade (Fig. 27.11). Menstrual irregularity and vaginal discharge are absent, and an abdominal lump is felt distinctly, which is usually tender. The normal-sized uterus is felt separate from the lump. Ultrasound is helpful in making a diagnosis.

Inflammatory bowel diseases and urinary tract infection are associated with bowel and urinary symptoms, and do not usually have high fever or vaginal discharge.

RUPTURED ENDOMETRIOTIC CYST

Rupture of an endometriotic cyst is not a common event; however, in rare situation a ruptured endometriotic cyst can be mistaken for PID. The patient with endometriosis will have suffered dysmenorrhoea, menorrhagia and pelvic pain before this acute episode. Besides, the patient is afebrile and has no vaginal discharge.

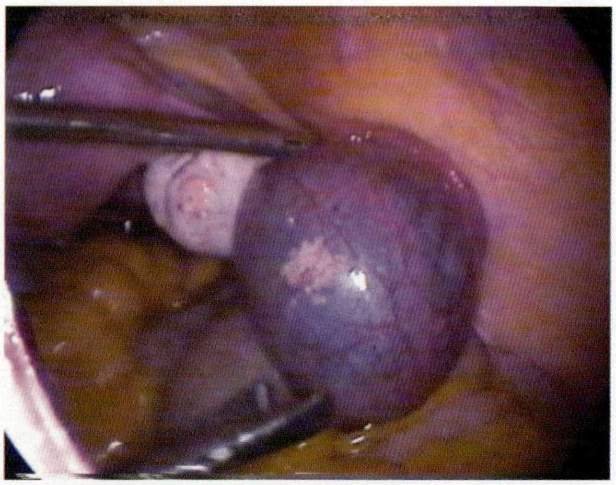

Figure 27.11 Laparoscopy revealed torsion of fimbrial cyst (paraovarian cyst) to be the cause of acute abdominal pain.

SEPTIC ABORTION

Septic abortion may mimic the clinical features of PID; amenorrhoea preceding the abdominal pain is present in septic abortion. A detailed clinical evaluation will help in establishing a diagnosis of septic abortion. The treatment with antibiotics is similar in both these conditions.

CHOLECYSTITIS

Occasionally, a woman with PID complains of acute right-sided upper abdominal pain simulating cholecystitis. This is due to a fibrous band extending from the right adnexa to the under surface of the liver in PID caused by gonococcal and chlamydial infection. This goes by the name of Fitz-Hugh–Curtis syndrome.

INVESTIGATIONS

Clinical diagnosis of PID is accurate in only 65%–70% cases, and specific investigations are required to confirm the diagnosis as well as to identify the offending organisms.

- Haemoglobin.
- Blood counts reveal rise in total leucocyte count.
- ESR is also raised.
- *Cervical and high vaginal swab culture* for both aerobic and anaerobic organisms is necessary. Urethral swab culture should be done, if gonorrhoea is suspected. For chlamydial infection, a long-wire swab tipped with calcium alginate is used to collect the specimen from the tube, urethra and endocervix, and this is inoculated on cycloheximide-treated McCoy cells for culture. Serological microfluorescence test for detection of IgM and IgG antibodies is useful. Polymerase chain reaction (PCR) test is now available for *chlamydia*. Actinomycosis is difficult to culture and is diagnosed histologically.
- To diagnose *chlamydia*, a culture from the endocervix is necessary. Direct chlamydial enzyme immunoassay and direct immunofluorescence examination of the smear are also useful. In case of IUCD, vaginal smear should be studied for the presence of *Actinomyces*.
- *Blood culture* is needed if there are features of septicaemia.
- Blood urea and serum electrolytes.
- *Urine* can be tested by PCR for chlamydial infection.

One must be aware, however, that a high vaginal swab culture does not always indicate or represent the bacterial flora present in the upper genital tract infection. Attempts to culture laparoscopically aspirated material or culdocentesis aspirate have been unsatisfactory. Moreover, gonococci and *chlamydia*, which are the primary organisms involved, are difficult to culture once invasion by other pathogens occurs.

- *Culdocentesis* in the past was used frequently to rule out an ectopic pregnancy and to establish the diagnosis of a pelvic abscess.
- *Laparoscopic* examination though recommended and practiced by some should not be used in routine practice. This investigation is limited to cases in which diagnosis is uncertain and it is not easy to aspirate pus for culture. **The pus extruding from the fimbrial end and peritubal**

adhesions is a sure sign of PID. Other signs of pelvic infection besides exudates are hyperaemia of the fallopian tubes, oedema and fibrinous band of adhesions in perihepatic space (Fitz-Hugh–Curtis syndrome) mentioned above, seen in 15% of cases.

- *C-reactive protein,* an acute-phase reactant protein generated in response to inflammation, is increased to 20–30 mg/dL or more, and it helps to distinguish between infective and noninfective mass.
- *Ultrasound, computed tomography (CT) and magnetic resonance imaging (MRI).* TOA appears on ultrasound as a complex cystic adnexal or cul-de-sac mass with thick irregular walls and septations. It often contains internal debris and echoes (Figs 27.9 and 27.10). This is safer and noninvasive compared to laparoscopy. 3D and 4D ultrasonography is used nowadays to define tubo-ovarian masses.

CT shows a spherical or tubular structure, with a low attenuation centre, in addition to thick walls and septations, but it is difficult to differentiate it from endometriosis. Internal gas bubbles, if seen, are pathognomonic of inflammatory mass.

MRI does not provide more specific information than ultrasound, and is much more expensive.

It is important to test the all cases of PID for HIV and other sexually transmitted infections. The partner should also undergo investigations for sexually transmitted infections. In a menopausal woman, tubo-ovarian mass indicates probable malignancy and should be investigated accordingly.

CHRONIC PELVIC INFLAMMATORY DISEASE

The history of previous pelvic infection helps in the diagnosis, but often this history is not forthcoming and not recalled by the patient. The patient complains of constant lower abdominal pain which gets worse before menstruation. Low backache and deep dyspareunia caused by pelvic masses prolapsed in the POD are common complaints. Vaginal discharge may be absent and if present, may be due to chronic cervicitis. Menorrhagia, polymenorrhagia, and congestive dysmenorrhoea are attributed to chronic pelvic congestion. Infertility results from blockage of the fallopian tubes. Rectal irritation may be complained of by few patients. These debilitating symptoms act upon the general health of these patients. Abdominal pain is due to pelvic adhesions or superimposed infections.

Pelvic examination in chronic PID is less painful than in the acute stage of the disease. The appendages are found to be tender, thickened and fixed, and an associated fixed retroversion of uterus is a very common finding. At times the uterus and appendages are densely adherent to each other, so the uterus cannot be defined separately from the pelvic masses, thus forming a fixed hard mass. A 'frozen pelvis' is the descriptive term used in these cases.

DIFFERENTIAL DIAGNOSIS

Ectopic Gestation

Chronic ectopic pregnancy may be easily mistaken for PID. Pregnancy test, ultrasound and laparoscopic examination will confirm the diagnosis of ectopic pregnancy.

Uterine Fibroids

The symptoms are very similar, so also the pelvic findings if appendages are adherent to the uterus, giving the impression of an irregular enlarged uterus. Fixity and tenderness however go more in favour of chronic PID.

Pelvic Endometriosis

Pelvic endometriosis produces similar clinical features as chronic PID. Laparoscopic examination will confirm the diagnosis.

Ovarian Tumour

A benign ovarian tumour is often unilateral and causes neither menstrual problem nor dyspareunia. A malignant ovarian tumour usually occurs in elderly women and is rapidly growing; hence, symptoms come up faster than in chronic PID. The tenderness is absent in an ovarian tumour. Ultrasound examination, CA-125 and fine-needle aspiration cytology (FNAC) can be useful.

Tubercular Tubo-Ovarian Masses

Tubercular tubo-ovarian masses may present as recurrent or chronic PID. It is sometimes unilateral. Laparoscopic examination, endometrial biopsy and culture help in establishing the diagnosis. PCR testing of endometrial tissue can also be done.

TREATMENT

Aim is to treat infection, minimize tubal damage and prevent adhesions, thus avoiding sequel of tubal damage.

TREATMENT OF ACUTE PID

The mild cases of acute PID are treated at home with antibiotics. Moderate and severe cases of acute PID need hospitalization.

Treatment modalities comprise following:

- Medical treatment, antimicrobial
- Minimal invasive surgery
- Major surgery

Syndromic management – laboratory tests take time and may delay the treatment. To avoid sequelae such as blocked tubes, chronic pelvic pain and infertility or ectopic pregnancy, the modern management is to initiate antibiotics while waiting for the final reports. This has a small risk of unnecessary treatment or overtreatment, but is worthy.

Hospital management consists of following:

- Rest.
- Intravenous fluids in the presence of dehydration or vomiting and correction of electrolyte imbalance. Ryle's tube aspiration may be needed in peritonitis or distension of abdomen, in which case correct intake–output chart should be maintained.
- Analgesics, once the diagnosis is confirmed.
- *Antibiotics.* Because of the damaging effect of gonococci and *chlamydia* on the fallopian tubes and polymicrobial nature of the infection, it is mandatory to institute antibiotic therapy at the earliest and not wait for the culture results.

In most cases of PID, both aerobes and anaerobes form the bacterial flora, hence it is essential to administer combination of antibiotics to cure the disease and prevent permanent damage to the fallopian tubes. Initially, intravenous route is resorted to, but as the infection settles down, oral therapy may be started. When the culture report is available or if the patient fails to respond to the antibiotics, an appropriate change in the antibiotic therapy will be needed.

Antibiotics effective are as follows:

- Azithromycin 500 mg for 14 days.
- Doxycycline 100 mg b.i.d. for 14 days.
- Clindamycin 450 mg q.i.d. for 10 days.
- Gentamycin 80 mg IM 8 hourly for 5 days.

For managing a case of PID, the guidelines given by CDC are extremely useful and help in better management of a case (Table 27.3).

Table 27. 3 CDC Guidelines for Treatment of PID (2015)

Recommended Parenteral Regimens
- ***Cefotetan*** *2 g i.v. every 12 hours*
  PLUS
- ***Doxycycline*** *100 mg orally or i.v. every 12 hours*
  OR
- ***Cefoxitin*** *2 g i.v. every 6 hours*
  PLUS
- ***Doxycycline*** *100 mg orally or i.v. every 12 hours*
  OR
- ***Clindamycin*** *900 mg i.v. every 8 hours*
  PLUS
- ***Gentamicin*** *loading dose i.v. or i.m. (2 mg/kg), followed by a maintenance dose (1.5 mg/kg) every 8 hours. Single daily dosing (3–5 mg/kg) can be substituted.*

Alternative Parenteral Regimen
- **Ampicillin/Sulbactam** 3 g i.v. every 6 hours
  PLUS
- **Doxycycline** 100 mg orally or i.v. every 12 hours

However, for subacute cases or those who can take antibiotics orally, a regimen has been suggested by CDC as given in Table 27.4.

The *side effects* of clindamycin are skin reaction, nausea and vomiting. Other antibiotics useful are cephalosporins, and penicillin with beta-lactamase inhibitors.

The following are the newer antibiotic regimens:

1. Cefoxitin 2 g i.v. 6-hourly + Doxycycline, 100 mg i.v. followed by oral route.
2. Azithromycin 500 mg i.v. 6-hourly for 2 days, then orally for *chlamydia*.
3. Ofloxacin 400 mg orally b.i.d. for 14 days. Cefotetan 2 g i.v. 12-hourly plus doxycycline 100 mg b.i.d. orally/ i.v.. Drugs are continued for at least 48 hours after the clinical improvement. After the discharge from the hospital, doxycycline is continued 100 mg for 10–14 days.
4. Levofloxacin 500 mg b.i.d. for 14 days with or without metronidazole.

Table 27.4 Subacute Cases Who Can Take Antibiotics Orally (the following regimen have been suggested by CDC)

Recommended Intramuscular/Oral Regimens
- **Ceftriaxone** 250 mg i.m. in a single dose
  PLUS
- **Doxycycline** 100 mg orally twice a day for 14 days
  WITH or WITHOUT
- **Metronidazole** 500 mg orally twice a day for 14 days
  OR
- **Cefoxitin** 2 g i.m. in a single dose and **Probenecid**, 1 g orally administered concurrently in a single dose
  PLUS
- **Doxycycline** 100 mg orally twice a day for 14 days
  WITH or WITHOUT
- **Metronidazole** 500 mg orally twice a day for 14 days
  OR
- Other parenteral third-generation **cephalosporin** (e.g. ceftizoxime or cefotaxime)
  PLUS
- **Doxycycline** 100 mg orally twice a day for 14 days
  WITH or WITHOUT
- **Metronidazole** 500 mg orally twice a day for 14 days

5. Clindamycin 900 mg i.v. every 8-hourly plus gentamicin in a loading dose i.v. or i.m.(2 mg/kg) followed by maintenance dose (1.5 mg/kg) 8 hourly (regimen continued for at least 48 hours after the clinical improvement). After discharge from the hospital, doxycycline is given 100 mg b.i.d. orally for 10–14 days or clindamycin 450 mg orally 4 times a day for 10–14 days.

Newer cephalosporins, i.e. ceftizoxime, cephalotaxine and ceftriaxone, may be given. In penicillin-resistant gonococci, amoxicillin 3 g orally, metronidazole 500 mg i.v. 8-hourly, and azithromycin 1 g single dose for gonorrhoea and *chlamydia* are the alternatives.

Royal College of Obstetricians and Gynaecologists (RCOG) green top guideline now recommends a single dose of i.m. Ceftriaxone 250 mg followed by oral doxycycline 100 mg twice daily with metronidazole 400 mg twice daily for 14 days as outpatient treatment or ceftriaxone i.m. followed by Azithromycin 1 g per week for 2 weeks.

Partner should be investigated and treated. There is no need to remove IUCD if the woman responds to antibiotics. A failed response calls for its removal. Barrier contraceptives should be recommended thereafter.

Surgical Treatment

Surgery may be needed for the following:

- Drainage of a pelvic abscess by colpotomy (Fig. 27.12).
- Dilatation and evacuation of septic products of conception or for haemorrhage in postabortal sepsis.
- Acute spreading peritonitis not responding to a full course of chemotherapy. The presence of pockets of pus in peritoneum mandates laparotomy. Laparotomy, drainage of pus and insertion of drainage may be lifesaving.
- Intestinal obstruction.

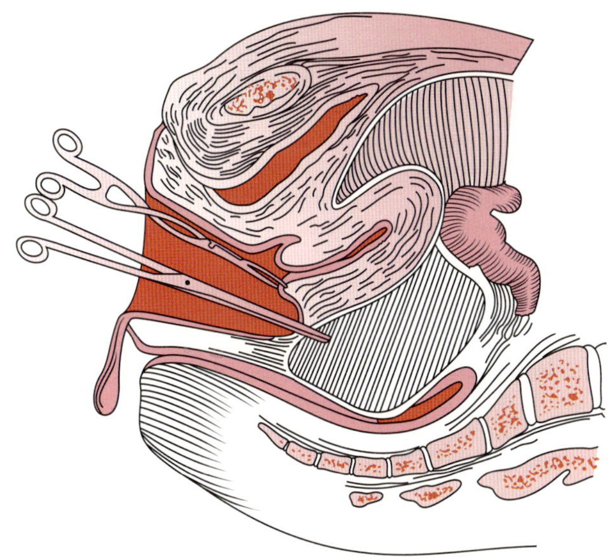

Figure 27.12 Posterior colpotomy for pelvic abscess.

- Suspected intestinal injury in a criminal abortion.
- Ruptured TOA.

Minimal Invasive Surgery

Minimal invasive surgery may be possible in selected cases for following conditions:

- The size of the abscess is more than 10 cm.
- The abscess fails to respond to antibiotics in 48–72 hours.
- Abscess collection in POD.
- Pockets of pus collection in abdomen or pelvis.

Ultrasound-guided vaginal aspiration of pelvic abscess with or without drainage yields 70% success. Sequelae include rupture of abscess during aspiration, pelvic vein thrombosis and chronic infection.

Percutaneous abscess drainage (PAD) under CT/ultrasound guidance of abdominal mass and pyoperitoneum yields 50% success and reduces the need for major surgery, with its associated morbidity and mortality. It also preserves the ovarian function and shortens the hospital stay. However, bowel injury is a risk in abdominal drainage.

Disadvantages of PAD are septicaemia, bladder and bowel injury, haemorrhage and recurrence.

Minimal invasive surgery may result in late *complications* of recurrence, chronic PID, tubal blockage and chronic pelvic pain. The minimal surgery has the advantage of minimal ovarian tissue damage in young women.

SURGICAL TREATMENT OF CHRONIC PID

Chronic PID needs a surgical treatment as the condition indicates the end result of acute infection and that some form of pelvic pathology has ensued. Surgery depends on the age and parity of the patient, the symptoms and pelvic pathology.

In a young woman, conservative surgery in the form of salpingectomy and salpingo-oophorectomy is performed. When extensive damage precludes conservative management or when the patient is multiparous, total abdominal hysterectomy with bilateral salpingo-oophorectomy is needed.

In a mild case of PID adequately treated, the tubal damage may be minimal but the infection may lead to infertility. Such patients need some form of tuboplasty/in-vitro fertilization depending on the site of tubal blockage.

Tuboplasty is required if the tubal lumen is blocked. Hysteroscopic falloposcopy or laparoscopic salpingoscopy should assess the extent of damage and decide the success rate of tuboplasty.

Laparoscopic breaking of external adhesions either by electrocautery is indicated if the tubal blockage is due to external adhesions.

If IVF is considered necessary, removal of hydrosalpinx or clipping of both tubes should be undertaken before IVF. This helps to improve the success rate and prevent ectopic pregnancy with IVF.

Hysteroscopic balloon plasty or cannulation is successful if the tubal block is due to luminal debris or a mild stricture.

PROGNOSIS

Boer–Meisel system of prognostic evaluation has been described and depends on following:

- Extent of adhesions.
- Nature of adhesions, such as flimsy or dense adhesions.
- Size of hydrosalpinx.
- Macroscopic condition of hydrosalpinx.
- Thickness of the tubal wall.

END RESULTS

PID remains the source of considerable morbidity in the form of chronic pelvic pain, menorrhagia, ectopic pregnancy (tenfold) and infertility, which would in turn require further surgical procedures, both investigatory and therapeutic. Other symptoms are backache, dyspareunia and vaginal discharge, recurrent PID.

It has been stated that despite adequate treatment, 15% of patients fail to respond to antibiotics, 20%–25% have at least one recurrence and 20% develop chronic pelvic pain (Te Linde). About 15% of patients suffer from infertility and 8% of those who conceive will have an ectopic pregnancy.

PREVENTION OF PID (Table 27.5)

- Safe and Clean Birth Practices: Hospital delivery is ideal. Realizing that the country cannot provide enough beds and that it is not easy for the rural women to come to the urban centres for delivery, the Government of India has started training programme for *dais* in aseptic techniques. This may help reduce the incidence of puerperal infection.
- Safe Abortion Practices: Induced abortions are carried out free of cost in government institutions to avoid criminal abortions in India. Though one continues to see such postabortal septic cases admitted to the hospitals, the number has definitely come down during the last two decades or so.
- Contraception. Barrier methods prevent STD. Oral contraceptives, especially minipills, are also effective.

Table 27.5 Antimicrobial Prophylaxis for Gynaecological Procedures

Procedure	Antibiotics	Dose
Hysterectomy	Cefazolin	1–2 g single dose i.v.
	Cefoxitin	
	Cefotetan	
	Metronidazole	500 mg i.v. 8 hourly for 24 hours
Hysterosalpingogram	Doxycycline	100 mg b.i.d. for 5 days
MTP/D&C	Doxycycline	100 mg orally 1 hour before and 200 mg after the procedure

IUCD causes PID in 5%. To avoid PID, it is necessary to see that only trained personnel introduce the device under aseptic conditions. Vaginal infection should be treated before insertion of the device.

- Sex education. Young women should be educated regarding the risk of STD. The awareness of AIDS and its related complications should promote safe sex practices and use of barrier methods of contraception.
- Female condom known as Femshield has been recently introduced, which covers the cervix, entire vagina and the external genitalia, and is highly effective not only as a barrier method, but is also protective against AIDS and STD. Femshield may have a better compliance than the male condom.
- Contact tracing and treatment of partner is also necessary.

RARE VARIETY OF PID DUE TO ACTINOMYCES

Actinomyces are anaerobic Gram-positive filamentous, nonsporing bacteria causing infection often associated with IUCD use. The incidence is 7% with IUCD worn for more than 2 years against 1% in nonusers. The woman develops fever, abdominal pain, abnormal bleeding and discharge. Sulphur granules can be recognized. The infection is treated with 250,000 units/kg daily of penicillin i.v. in four divided doses for 2–6 weeks. Thereafter, oral 100 mg/kg daily in divided doses is administered for 3–12 months. Other antibiotics are tetracycline, erythromycin, clindamycin and chloramphenicol.

KEY POINTS

- PID implies inflammation of the upper genital tract involving the uterus and the adnexa.
- Natural barriers exist to protect the ascent of organisms from the vagina to the upper genital tract; these include the ciliary movement of the endosalpinx downwards, the periodic shedding of the endometrium, the thick cervical mucous plug in the endocervical canal and the acidic pH of the vagina.
- The natural protective barrier may get breached during menstruation, abortion and the puerperium; uterine instrumentation or the insertion of an IUCD may initiate infection.
- Both aerobes and anaerobes may be implicated; however, amongst the common causes of infection are STDs caused by *Chlamydia* and gonococci. Septic abortions are often the result of pregnancy termination carried out under unhygienic conditions. Bleeding, anaemia, tissue damage and lack of proper asepsis predispose to this life-threatening condition.
- Tuberculous infection usually causes chronic PID. It is a blood-borne infection which affects both the adnexae.
- In PID the patient suffers from manifestations such as abdominal pain, leucorrhoea, menorrhagia, congestive dysmenorrhoea, dyspareunia, backache and infertility. The uterus is often retroverted with restricted mobility and there may be thickening of the appendages which are painful on palpation.
- Use of barrier contraceptives, observance of proper asepsis during instrumental manipulations and a prompt treatment of suspected infection are the best approaches to safeguard the patient from infections.
- Prophylactic antibiotics during surgery can reduce incidence of PID.
- Sex education, using barrier contraceptives, can reduce sexually transmitted infections and thereby avoid PID.

SELF-ASSESSMENT

1. What are the causes of PIDs?
2. Discuss the clinical features and management of acute PID.
3. What are the complications and sequelae of PIDs?

SUGGESTED READING

Arulkumaran S. Clin Obstet Gynaecol 2009, Elsevier, UK.

Drugs for sexually transmitted infections. Treat Guidel Med Lett 2004; 2:67.

Jeffrey S Dungan, Lee P Shulman. Year Book of Obstetrics, Gynecology, and Women's Health. 301, 2013.

John Bonnar, J, Ed. Recent Advances in Obstetrics and Gynaecology 16:165, RCOG Press, London 2010.

Soper DE. Pelvic inflammatory disease. Obstet Gynecol 2010; 116:419.

Studd J. Progr Obstet Gynaecol. 9:259, Churchill Livingstone, Edinburgh, 1991.

Thompson SE, Brooks C, Eschenbach DA, et al. High failure rates in outpatient treatment of salpingitis with either tetracycline alone or penicillin/ampicillin combination. Am J Obstet Gynecol 1985; 152:635.

Tuberculosis of the Female Genital Tract

28

CHAPTER OUTLINE

INTRODUCTION

Tuberculosis (TB) has been recognized as a debilitating disease since ancient times. But the credit for the first authentic description of genital tuberculosis is attributed to NA Morgagni (1744) who first described the autopsy findings of genital tuberculosis in a young woman aged 20 years who died of tuberculosis. In his report, he clearly mentioned that the uterus and tubes were filled with caseous material. Robert Koch discovered the organism *Mycobacterium tuberculosis* in 1882. Since the early part of the twentieth century, the incidence of general tuberculosis and its consequence, pelvic tuberculosis have progressively declined in the developed countries, so much that the disease has become rare in many industrialized countries of Europe and America. However, it still continues to be seen amongst the destitute, immigrants of Asian and African descent in the UK and in the inner city communities of the USA. The disease continues to be rampant in developing countries of Latin America and Asia. It is endemic in India. The actual incidence of pelvic tuberculosis is difficult to assess as many patients are asymptomatic and the disease often comes to light only incidentally during the course of investigation for a gynaecological complaint. G Schaefer (1970) reported that 4%–12% of women dying from pulmonary tuberculosis have evidence of genital involvement. He further mentioned that 5%–10% of infertile women suffer from tuberculosis. In India, PK Malkani (1975) reported an incidence of 9.3% in infertility patients in New Delhi. Padubidri V. from New Delhi reported tuberculosis in 4% of all endometrial aspirations examined. Usha Krishna et al. (1979) from Mumbai reported an incidence of genital tuberculosis in 13% of infertile women. Chitra Kumar et al. (2000) from Darbhanga (Bihar) reported an incidence of genital tuberculosis in 18.6% of infertile women. Surveys from Mumbai about the prevalence of tuberculosis amongst infertile women reported by several authors have been mentioned here – R Merchant (1989) reported an incidence of 14.7%, FR Parikh et al. (1995) reported genital TB as the cause of infertility in 15.3% and BM Desai et al. (1995) reported a high incidence of 39% in patients referred for assisted reproduction procedures. Classically, female genital tuberculosis (FGT) has been described as a disease of young women with 80% diagnosed between the ages of 20 and 40 years, although the disease has also been reported in older women around menopause and occasionally even thereafter. V Falks (1980) reported that 46% of his patients of genital tuberculosis from Sweden were aged more than 50 years.

PATHOGENESIS

The causative agent is mostly *M. tuberculosis* (95%), but in a few cases it is caused by the *M. bovis* (5%), particularly in underdeveloped countries where effective tuberculosis control programs for cattle are not in place and pasteurization of milk is not routinely practiced. These organisms are identified on routine staining of infected material with Ziehl–Neelson's acid-fast stain. Genital tuberculosis occurs almost always secondary to a primary focus elsewhere, the commonest site being the lungs (50%), followed by other sites such as lymph nodes (40%), the kidneys, joints, gastrointestinal tract or as part of a generalized miliary infection. The mode of spread is generally haematogenous or via lymphatics, and rarely from direct contiguity with an intraabdominal organ or affected peritoneum (G Schaefer, 1976; AM Siegler, 1979). Once the genital tract has been colonized, the granulomata containing viable tubercle bacilli form within the various pelvic organs. Following the development of tubercular hypersensitivity, these foci become generally silent for many years, before reactivation of the focus takes place. The active growth and increase in blood supply to the genital organs around menarche constitutes the event leading to its reactivation and establishment of the disease process.

The genital infection thus acquired in childhood may remain dormant until puberty. As a rule, *the fallopian tubes are always the first to be involved*; hence the disease is commonly bilateral in distribution, with subsequent dissemination to other genital organs and the peritoneum. Bilateral pelvic lymph nodes involvement often follows. Vulvovaginal involvement is usually secondary to uterine involvement.

Primary genital tuberculosis is rare; there are reports in the literature of cases of primary genital tuberculosis affecting the vulva and cervix, in which the male sexual partner has been suspected to be the source of the disease (1%). The presence of *M. tuberculosis* organisms in the semen of men suffering from urogenital tuberculosis has been well documented. Apart from semen being a source of infection, the practice of using saliva for lubrication before intercourse by some men may also be a source of infection in cases of open pulmonary tuberculosis.

Pathology of genital tuberculosis:

The general distribution of involvement of reproductive organs in cases of genital tuberculosis has been stated by Schaefer as follows:

1. Fallopian tubes: 90%–100%
2. Endometrium: 50%–60%
3. Ovaries: 20%–30%
4. Cervix: 5%–15%
5. Vulva and vagina: <1%

In a more recent survey of more than 1400 cases of genital tuberculosis by Nogales-Ortiz et al., they found involvement of the fallopian tubes in 100% of their cases, endometrium in 79%, myometrium in 20%, cervix in approximately 25% and the ovaries in only 11% of cases.

When the tubercle bacilli infect a susceptible host, the initial reaction is a polymorphonuclear inflammatory exudate. Within 48 hours this is replaced by mononuclear cells which become the primary site for intracellular tubercle replication. As cellular immunity develops, destruction of the tubercle bacilli begins, leading to caseation necrosis. Later, reactivation of the lesion leads to the classical granulomatous lesion characterized by central caseation and necrosis surrounded by concentric layers of epithelioid cells and giant cells with peripheral distribution of lymphocytes, monocytes and fibroblasts.

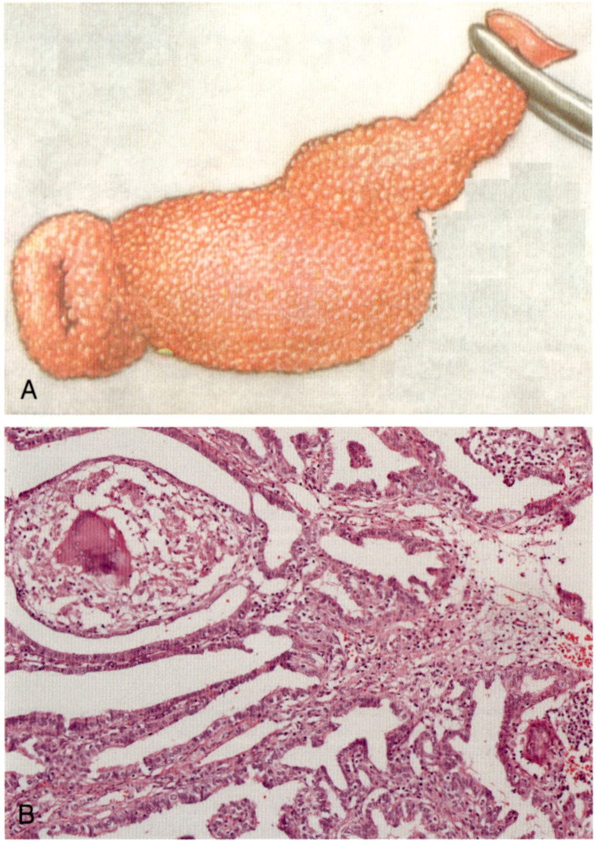

Figure 28.1 **(A)** Tuberculous salpingitis. **(B)** Tubercular salpingitis: Fallopian tube showing epithelioid cell granulomas and giant cells. (*Courtesy*: Dr Sandeep Mathur, AIIMS.)

GENITAL TRACT LESIONS

Detailed description of lesions is as follows:

Fallopian tubes: Involvement of the tubes is almost 100%, and is bilateral. It is secondary to haematogenous spread from a primary focus usually in the lungs, and less commonly from lymphatic spread from the bowel or direct transperitoneal extension from a nearby focus such as the appendix or the large bowel. The tubal mucosa is the most favourable nidus for blood-borne spread of the disease resulting in endosalpingitis – usually bilateral. It is the earliest lesion with a propensity for transluminal spread to the ovary and endometrium. Thus, the fallopian tubes play the central role in the initiation and dissemination of pelvic tuberculosis, although occasionally the cervix and endometrium can be infected primarily from the bloodstream. The fallopian tubes may appear normal initially but in minimal disease, they may be thickened with a whip-like consistency. There may be evidence of tubercles on the surface (tuberculous exosalpingitis). At times, following a direct extension of tuberculosis from adjacent organs, the exosalpingitis manifests in the form of diffusely spread miliary tubercles on the serosal surface of the fallopian tube, the ampullary part of the tube appears dilated with the fimbrial end open and pouting. This lesion has been described as the *tobacco-pouch appearance* (Fig. 28.1).

In more than 50% of cases, the tubes are dilated, with their external surfaces appearing roughened due to adhesions or may show the presence of greyish tubercles, these may be discrete or confluent. On cut section, the lumen reveals the presence of yellowish grey caseous material or fluid along with blood (tuberculous haematosalpinx) and pyosalpinx. At times, violin string adhesions are noted between the right fallopian tube and the undersurface of the liver, known as Fitz-Hugh–Curtis syndrome. Leakage of infected material into the peritoneal cavity causes peritubal abscess, tuberculosis peritonitis and ascites.

In 20% of cases, the tubes assume an elongated **retort-shaped structure.** The tubes remain patent in almost 25%–50% cases of genital tuberculosis with a minimal disease, but as the disease advances, reactive fibrosis sets in and the tubes get occluded. However, even in the advanced form of the disease presenting with bilateral tubal masses the fimbriae are often spared, giving the tubes the typical tobacco-pouch appearance (Figs 28.2 and 28.3).

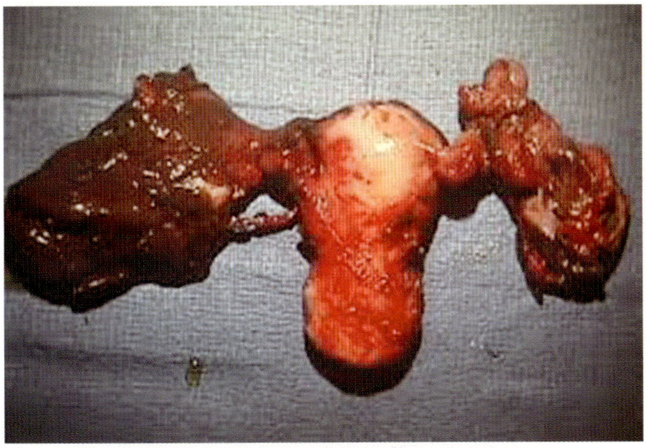

Figure 28.2 Bilateral tuberculous pyosalpinx. Note the retort-shaped tubes, absence of surface tubercles and adhesions.

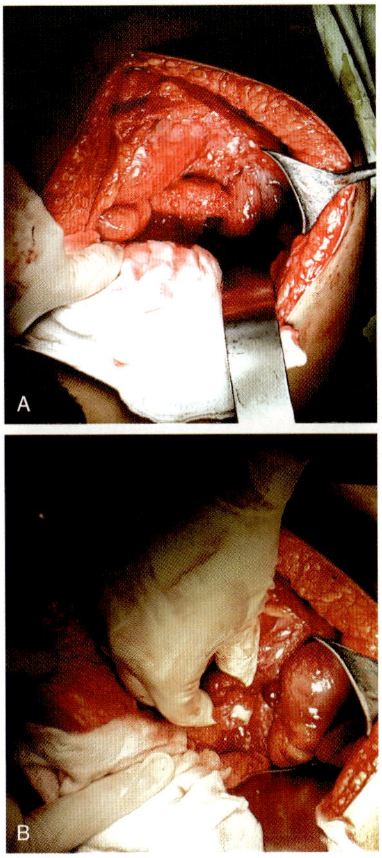

Figure 28.3 **(A)** laparotomy picture of a patient having mutliple miliary tubercular deposits all over the bowel, peritoneum and uterus. **(B)** Pus extruding through the fimbrial end of fallopian tube- a sure sign of genital tuberculosis.

Microscopically, granulomas and chronic inflammatory infiltrate may involve the full thickness of the tubal wall; on occasions these telltale granulomas are difficult to find. The ampullary part is the most common to be affected, the fimbriae and interstitial parts of the tubes are often spared. The brunt of the attack is borne by the endosalpinx, it often exhibits focal or widespread reactive adenomatous hyperplasia which may be severe enough to be mistaken for carcinoma. The diagnosis of tubal tuberculosis is based on the demonstration of acid-fast bacilli in the tissues, or by positive cultures or by guinea pig inoculation. It is a well-known fact that the tubercle bacilli are difficult to demonstrate even with fluorescent techniques. Hence, the onus of initial suspicion lies squarely on the pathologist reporting the slide. Presently, with availability of the polymerase chain reaction (PCR) technique based test, the diagnosis of tuberculosis can be established with greater certainty in samples of suspicious tissue. The granulomas may be single or confluent with a variable tendency to frank caseation with the surrounding muscular layers showing a dense lymphocytic infiltration and patchy areas of fibrosis. Caseation necrosis is not uncommon in advanced cases. The mucosa often exhibits a hyperplastic adenomatous pattern with a complex network of fused papillae, and has been associated with a higher incidence of *ectopic pregnancy* (F Novak and JD Woodruff, 1979). Whether this predisposes to the occurrence of future adenocarcinoma is debatable (Novak and Woodruff, 1979). The differential diagnosis includes foreign body granulomas usually related to previous hysterosalpingography or surgery, sarcoidosis, Crohn disease or associated with *Enterobius vermicularis*.

Uterus – tuberculosis of the endometrium: The endometrium is involved in about 50%–60% of cases of genital tuberculosis. Grossly the endometrium appears unremarkable in the majority of cases because of cyclic menstrual shedding. Endometrial histology reveals the characteristic lesion showing central caseation, surrounded by epithelioid cells and stroma infiltrated with giant cells (Fig. 28.4A and B). Tuberculosis is a descending infection from the fallopian tube, and the cornual ends are the first to be involved.

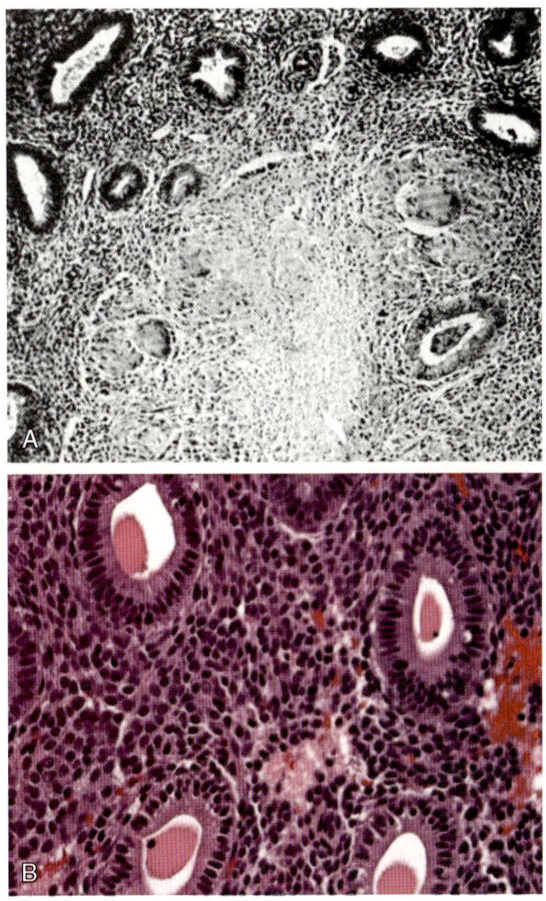

Figure 28.4 **(A)** and **(B)** Tuberculous endometritis depicting typical giant cells in the stroma (×115). (*Source:* Textbook of Gynaecology, India: Elsevier, 2008.)

Occasionally there may be ulcerative, granular or fungating lesions. On other occasions, the uterine cavity may appear smooth and devoid of endometrium, attempts at curettage yielding scanty or no material. The cavity may appear shrunken due to underlying fibrosis. The tubal ostia may appear recessed and narrowed, like golf holes. In 2%–5% of cases, total destruction of the endometrium with resulting amenorrhoea secondary to end organ failure may lead to pyometra formation, in case the internal os gets occluded. At times the cavity may be partially or extensively obliterated with intrauterine adhesions appearing as strands, ridges or thick bands (Asherman syndrome).

Endometrial lesions are frequently focal and typically immature because they tend to shed monthly except in cases of amenorrhoea or pyometra. It is believed that the endometrium is regularly reinfected from the tubes or from the basal layer of the endometrium which is not shed monthly. Granulomas are best identified on endometrial sampling on day 24–26 of the cycle or within a few hours of the onset of menses (Fig. 28.4).

Ovaries: These are involved in 20%–30% of cases of genital tuberculosis. Most frequently this is perioophoritis resulting from spread from the adjacent fallopian tubes, when the ovary seems to be encased within adhesions. However, it may sometimes follow a haematogenous spread and cause caseating granulomas within the parenchyma of the ovary.

Cervix: In most cases, there are no gross changes in the cervix. Ulcerative lesions are uncommon. Occasionally a polypoidal hypertrophic lesion mimicking cancer of the cervix may be seen. Microscopy may reveal scarce granulomatous lesions surrounded by large numbers of lymphocytes. Reactive hyperplasia of the glandular epithelium may lead to papilla formation, sometimes there may be evidence of epithelial atypia. On examination, the patient reveals presence of an ulcer on the cervix covered with yellowish-brown offensive discharge which it may bleed on touch. Cervical biopsy helps in establishing a diagnosis of tuberculosis. As a result of involvement of the endocervical mucosa, there is increase in secretion of mucin. The cervical involvement is mostly due to descending spread from the infected uterine cavity, though occassionally, it may be primarily from transmission of infection from the husband suffering from genital tuberculosis through sexual intercourse.

Vulva and vagina: Tuberculosis of the vulva is rare compared to rest of the female genital tract (1%). Vulval lesions arise by a direct extension from lesions in the upper genital tract, or as an exogenous infection. Children as well as adults may be affected. Exogenous infection may arise from sputum or through sexual intercourse with a partner suffering from either tubercular epididymitis or renal tuberculosis. Bartholin's gland may be affected at times, often unilaterally with a focus of tuberculosis elsewhere in the body. In all cases, lymph nodes would be involved. Bartholin's gland may reveal induration or abscess formation. With the recent epidemic of HIV sweeping through many countries globally, the reduced body resistance has favoured an upsurge in tuberculosis. Clinically a vulval lesion may appear as a discharging ulcer, sinus or a nodular hypertrophic lesion (Fig. 28.5). A vaginal nodule may ulcerate and cause a discharging sinus. Microscopy reveals the typical tubercular granuloma.

Ulcerative vaginal lesions whenever present are always found to co-exist with cervical disease. Tubercular vaginitis has also been reported. The diagnosis has been made on cervico-vaginal smears. Ulcerative lesions often heal by fibrosis causing vaginal stenosis. *Recto-vaginal fistula* is a rare complication of genital tuberculosis.

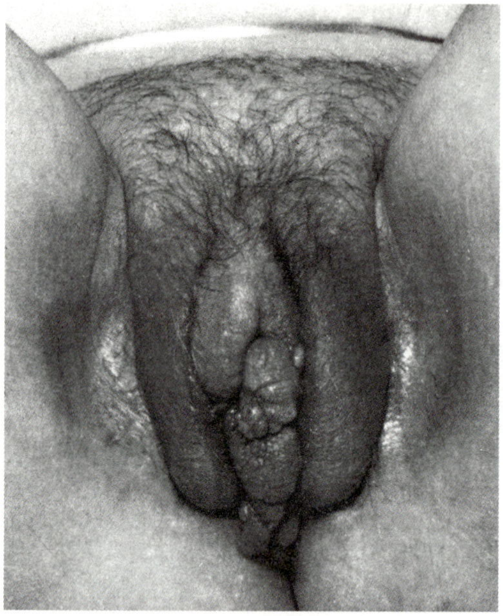

Figure 28.5 Hypertrophic tuberculosis of vulva. Note considerable oedema of labia majora and elephantiasis-like appearance of labia minora. (*Source:* From: Macleod and Read, Gynaecology, 5th ed. Churchill, 1955.)

CLINICAL FEATURES OF GENITAL TUBERCULOSIS

It is an important observation that about 10%–15% of women suffering from genital tuberculosis are asymptomatic and 15% of them may have successfully conceived earlier. However, the leading presenting complaints in women suffering from genital tuberculosis include **infertility, menstrual irregularities, abdominal pain, vaginal discharge and suspicion of neoplasm.** Fistula formation is a rare occurrence. Sometimes general symptoms of low-grade fever, weight loss, fatigue and a feeling of listlessness may raise the suspicion of hitherto unsuspected diagnosis of genital tuberculosis. Pelvic examination often reveals nothing significant; in 20% of cases the adnexae may feel thickened or cord-like, tubo-ovarian masses may be palpable. These may be tender if secondarily infected. In cases of nonhealing scars following surgery, always suspect the possibility of tuberculosis and biopsy from the scar tissue will reveal the diagnosis.

Clinical features of female genital tuberculosis are as follows:

- Infertility
- Menstrual irregularity
- Abdominal pain
- Vaginal discharge
- Abdominal mass
- Fistula formation
- Ectopic pregnancy
- Asymptomatic in 10%–20% cases

Infertility (primary or secondary): This is an important presenting symptom. In fact, in 35%–60% cases infertility may be the only complaint for which the patient seeks medical attention. Of these women, about 75% present with primary infertility and 25% give history of previous conceptions. In almost half of these cases, there may be a history of a past infection or contact with a person suffering from tuberculosis. In any suspicious case, it may be wise to obtain a histological report on the endometrium early in the course of the work up for infertility. Infertility is attributed to tubal damage and endometrial adhesions (Asherman syndrome), and at times ovarian damage.

Menstrual irregularity(amenorrhoea, hypomenorrhoea, menorrhagia): It has been observed in 10%–40% of cases. The menstrual disturbances reported include menorrhagia, menometrorrhagia, intermenstrual bleeding, oligomenorrhoea, hypomenorrhoea, amenorrhoea and even postmenopausal bleeding. In the West, dysfunctional bleeding is more frequently encountered, whereas in India oligomenorrhoea and hypomenorrhoea are seen more frequently associated with genital tuberculosis. This has been attributed to the higher association with pulmonary disease in our country. Tuberculosis should be suspected if puberty menorrhagia does not respond to medical therapy.

Chronic pelvic pain: This pain may be dull aching in type, sometimes aggravated premenstrually, or it might be intermittent in nature.

Vaginal discharge: Blood-stained vaginal discharge, postcoital bleeding, leucorrhoea and serosanguinous/seropurulent discharge from ulcers are occasionally encountered from lower genital tract tubercular lesions.

Abdominal mass: Some women may present with a mass in the abdomen, which consists of rolled-up omentum, with dense adhesions to the uterus and adnexae. The history of associated menstrual disturbances accompanying the presence of fixed abdomino-pelvic mass should raise the suspicion of genital tuberculosis. Encysted ascites, matted intestinal loops, uterine pyometra and adnexal masses may present as lumps. A doughy feel on palpation of the abdomen is suggestive of tuberculous peritonitis. Other symptoms include dysmenorrhoea, dyspareunia and repeated episodes of pelvic inflammatory disease (PID). In a young, unmarried girl presenting with a pelvic inflammatory mass, it is almost always of a tubercular origin. PID which fails to respond to the standard treatment and recurrent PID is often due to tuberculosis.

Fistula formation: This complication generally follows surgical interventions such as draining of an abscess, or abdominal hysterectomy.

Ectopic pregnancy: Women with genital tuberculosis rarely conceive. However, patients successfully treated for the disease have a high risk of ectopic pregnancy. The high risk is attributed to residual tubal scarring causing narrowing and distortion of the tube.

Prospects of future childbearing: Treatment of patients with genital tuberculosis for infertility has generally yielded poor results. In case pregnancy occurs, the risk of ectopic pregnancy and abortions is substantially high. However, live pregnancies have been reported. In women with a tubal disease but having receptive endometrium and a normal uterus, cases of successful pregnancy outcomes have been reported with assisted reproductive techniques. However, in case of the endometrium being unfavourable and nonreceptive, surrogate pregnancy may need to be considered.

INVESTIGATIONS

General: Routine investigations may reveal nothing significant.

1. **Complete blood count:** A differential leucocyte count often shows the presence of *lymphocytosis*.
2. **Erythrocyte sedimentation rate (ESR):** This is frequently raised. However, ESR is a nonspecific investigation.
3. **Mantoux test:** A positive test is indicative of exposure to tubercle bacilli in the past. It has been reported to be positive in more than 90% of cases. A negative test goes against tuberculosis. QuantiFERON test is superior to Mantoux test.
4. **Hysterosalpingography** reveals features suggestive of genital tuberculosis in many patients, where endometrial biopsy has failed to reveal the diagnosis. Hysterosalpingography should not be performed if genital tuberculosis is suspected because of risk of spread of infection. If performed in an asymptomatic woman, it may show the following patterns(Figs 28.6–28.8):
   - A rigid nonperistaltic pipe-like tube (lead pipe appearance)
   - Beading and variation in the filling
   - Calcification of the tube
   - Cornual block
   - A jagged fluffiness of the tubal outline
   - Tobacco-pouch appearance of hydrosalpinx and pyosalpinx
5. **The enzyme-linked immunoabsorbent assay (ELISA) tests – IgG and IgM:** In recent times, mycobacterial purified protein antigens used in ELISA have been favourably evaluated.
6. **Ultrasound examination:** It can reveal an abdominal mass, but cannot identify its nature. However, ultrasound guided fine-needle aspiration cytology (FNAC) from the adnexal mass is feasible, as is USG-guided transvaginal

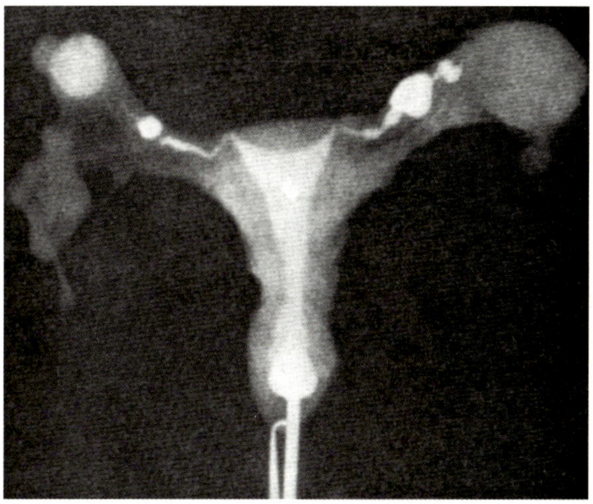

Figure 28.6 Tuberculous tubes and uterus injected after removal. (*Source:* From: Stallworthy, 1952, J Obst Gynaecol Br Emp.)

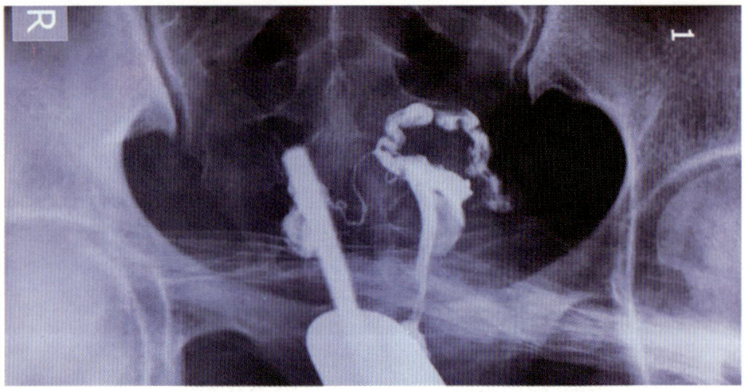

Figure 28.7 Beaded appearance of the fallopian tube and extravasation of the dye in pelvic tuberculosis.

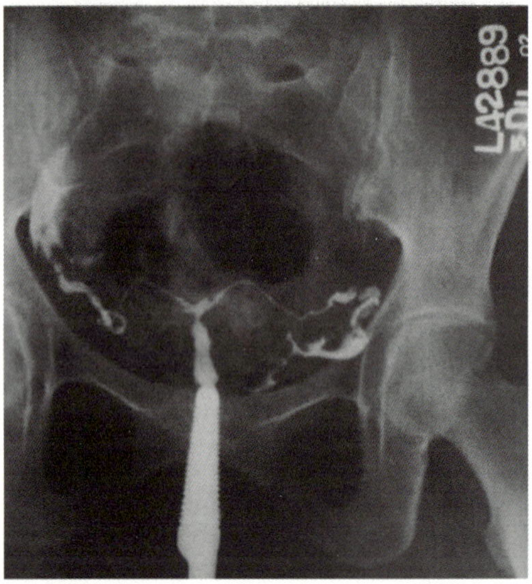

Figure 28.8 HSG showing a reduced size of the uterine cavity with irregularity of lumen outline and adhesions suggestive of Asherman syndrome. (*Courtesy*: Dr K.K. Saxena, New Delhi.)

tri-cut biopsy of the peritoneum as an alternative to laparoscopic biopsy of the peritoneal tissue.

7. **Endometrial histology and PCR testing:** Endometrium tissue is obtained by D&C/hysteroscopy-directed biopsy. The ideal time for planning this procedure is the late premenstrual phase, the reason being that the tubercles are present near the superficial layers of the endometrium and are shed during menstruation. The endometrial scrapings are divided into three portions: (i) for *histopathology*, (ii) for *PCR testing* and (iii) *for AFB smear and culture*. This test has been used successfully for detecting tuberculosis in endometrial biopsy taken from affected tissues. PCR is a rapid, sensitive and specific method of detecting mycobacterial DNA, and report is available within 24 hours. False negative results are reported in 8% cases and false positive results in 10-20% cases.

   Guinea pig inoculation and tissue culture; In case of positive culture, the bacteriologist should further attempt to type the bacillus and test its sensitivity. Acid-fast staining of endometrial tissues to detect *M. tuberculosis* is not accurate.
8. **Hysteroscopy:** This often reveals the presence of synechiae, partial obliteration of the cavity, recessed golf-hole appearance of tubal ostia or rarely the presence of ulcers.
9. **Laparoscopy:** Diagnostic laparoscopy is widely used to establish the diagnosis of genital tuberculosis/abdomino-pelvic tuberculosis. Tuberculous lesions can be seen on the parietal peritoneum, intestinal serosa, omentum, surface of the uterus and fallopian tubes (thickened rigid tubes/hydrosalpinx, pyosalpinx, tubo-ovarian adnexal masses) and perihepatic adhesions may be present. Histology and PCR testing from selected tissue biopsies often help to settle the diagnosis.
10. **Tissue biopsy:** Local excision tissue biopsies from suspected lesions from the lower genital tract (vulva and vagina) submitted for histology help to establish the diagnosis.
11. **Chest X-ray (CXR):** To detect site of primary lesion.
12. **Radiography of bones:** In case of suspected tuberculous pathology.
13. **Nucleic acid amplification technique (NAAT)** detects tuberculosis within a few hours compared to culture.
14. CA 125 is at times raised, but is nonspecific.

Other tests to be considered in selective situations include:

15. **Gas chromatography:** A direct demonstration of compounds characteristic of mycobacteria shows great promise (90% sensitive) to provide rapid diagnosis.
16. **SAFA** (soluble antigen fluorescence antibody) test has been evaluated, the drawback being a false positive reporting of 11%. It is no longer used.
17. **BACTEC:** This is a rapid culture method where radioactive carbon labelled substrate such as palmitic acid or formic acid is used as a marker for bacterial growth. It takes 5–7 days to culture.
18. **Gene expert**: It is a new test introduced for diagnosis of drug-resistant tuberculosis. It is based on PCR. Initially this test was introduced for tubercular meningitis cases, but is being explored for diagnosing drug resistance in other forms of tuberculosis.
19. **Semen culture:** Advised in patients with vulvovaginal tuberculous lesions.
20. **Biochemical markers:** Ascitic fluid is tested for the presence of markers such as adenosine deaminase activity. The test is highly specific sensitive.

DIFFERENTIAL DIAGNOSIS

The clinician has to consider several other possibilities before settling on the diagnosis of FGT:

1. ***Ovarian cyst, broad ligament cyst, encysted fluid:*** These cysts are fixed and immobile. However, the menstrual history is usually normal unlike in women with tubercular encysted lesion. Any history of previous extragenital tuberculosis goes in favour of genital tuberculosis.
2. ***PID:*** Infertility and menstrual disturbances are common to both PID and FGT. However, history of frequent recurrences or a failure of response to treatment should raise the suspicion of genital tuberculosis.
3. ***Ectopic pregnancy:*** History of amenorrhoea, abdominal pain and the presence of a unilateral adnexal mass should raise the suspicion of ectopic pregnancy. Urine pregnancy test, transvaginal sonography with colour Doppler blood flow studies and diagnostic

laparoscopy should help in the diagnosis and management of the case.

4. *Carcinoma cervix:* In women presenting with local cervical lesions (ulcer, polypoidal growth) clinical findings such as lack of induration, lack of friability should raise suspicion of alternative pathology. Tissue biopsy and histological examination will help to settle the issue.
5. *Elephantiasis of the vulva:* Filariasis of the vulva can mimic hypertrophic tuberculosis of the vulva. Biopsy helps to establish the diagnosis.
6. *Pregnancy:* Amenorrhoea and abdominal mass may raise the suspicion of pregnancy.
7. *Puberty menorrhagia and postmenopausal bleeding* due to other causes need to be excluded.
8. ***Fungal infections and sarcoidosis*** cause granulomatous lesions – histologically resembling tubercular granulomas.

TREATMENT

Most patients are in good health and there is no need for hospitalization. Only those who have fever and abdominal pain are admitted to the hospital in the initial stages of the treatment.

CHEMOTHERAPY

The first line of treatment is with antitubercular drugs (Category I drugs) (Table 28.1). WHO recommends **rifampicin** (450–600 mg daily depending upon the body weight) combined with 300 mg of **isoniazid** daily in a single oral dose before breakfast. Rifampicin is hepatotoxic and liver function tests (LFTs) should be undertaken before instituting this drug. **Pyrazinamide** is a new oral drug (1.5–2.0 g daily in two divided doses) which is very effective against slow multiplying organisms and enhances the effect of rifampicin, but causes hyperuricaemia. **The modern therapy consists of rifampicin, isoniazid, ethambutol and pyrazinamide for initial 2 months, followed by rifampicin and isoniazid biweekly for another 4 months.** This short course gives quick and successful results and prevents emergence of drug-resistant bacilli. Some prefer to add ethambutol, 15 mg per kg body weight in a single dose after breakfast or 50 mg per kg/body weight twice weekly during the first 2–3 months. Ethambutol should not be administered for a longer period as it may affect the vision (optic neuritis) and cause skin rash. Ophthalmic examination is mandatory before starting the drug. Oral contraceptives should not be combined with rifampicin. Pyridoxine (B_6) 10 mg daily prevents peripheral neuritis. The oral contraceptives are less effective in the presence of rifampicin, as the latter interferes with their absorption.

Resistant cases associated with HIV need extended treatment for a year.

The new drugs introduced in resistant cases are (Table 28.2) as follows:

- Capreomycin
- Kanamycin
- Ethionamide
- *para*-Aminosalicylic acid
- Cycloserine

The main reasons for a failure of treatment are due to noncompliance and incomplete treatment.

For good compliance, Revised National TB Control Programme (RNTCP) of India in 2004 incorporated DOT strategy (direct observed treatment). It covered 87% of the population with 72% detection rate and 86% treatment success, with a sevenfold decline in death rate from 29% to 4%.

DOTs – a short course therapy of 6 months.

First 2 months

- Isoniazid – 15 mg/kg body weight
- Rifampicin – 450–600 mg
- Pyrazinamide – 30 mg/body weight
- Ethambutol – 30 mg/kg body weight

Three times a week.

Next 4 months – continue with Rifampicin and Isoniazid (same dose) three times a week.

Table 28.1 Chemotherapeutic Drugs for Tuberculosis

Drug	Action	Side Effects
Rifampicin 10 mg/kg o.d. daily	Bactericidal	Hepatotoxic, fever, purpuric rash, orange urine
Isoniazid 5–10 mg/kg o.d. daily	Bactericidal	Hepatotoxic, peripheral neuritis, hypersensitivity
Pyrazinamide 25–30 mg/kg o.d.	Bactericidal	Hepatitis, hyperuricaemia
Ethambutol 15 mg/kg o.d.	Bacteriostatic	Optic neuritis, skin rash

Table 28.2 Drugs Used in Resistant Cases

Drug	Dose	Side Effects
1. Capreomycin	15–30 mg/kg i.m.	Auditory, vestibular and renal toxicity
2. Kanamycin	15–30 mg/kg i.m.	Auditory, vestibular and renal toxicity
3. Ethionamide	15–30 mg/kg i.m.	Hepatitis hypersensitivity
4. *para*-Aminosalicylic acid	150 mg/kg	Hepatitis, GI tract
5. Cycloserine	15–20 mg (1 g maximum)	Psychosis, convulsions, skin rash

Resistant cases (8-month course)

First 2 months – streptomycin three times a week + four drugs as above

Third month – Four drugs as above

Next 3 months – Isoniazid, rifampicin, ethambutol (same dose) three times a week.

HIV–TB patients should also receive Highly Active Antiretroviral Therapy (HAART) therapy.

PLACE OF SURGERY IN TREATMENT OF FEMALE GENITAL TUBERCULOSIS

Surgery is generally avoided; however, may be needed if *there are signs of* progression of the disease, persistent active lesion, persistence of large inflammatory masses, i.e. pyosalpinx and pyometra; persistence of symptoms, i.e. pain, menorrhagia and persistence of fistula, despite the chemotherapy.

Contraindications to surgery are active lesions elsewhere in the body and plastic adhesions of bowels. Any attempt to separate the adhesions would result in injury to bowel and fistula formation. Surgery should be preceded by several weeks of chemotherapy, followed by a full course of chemotherapy.

TYPES OF SURGERY

- Total hysterectomy with removal of ovaries and the fallopian tubes. It is very rarely required nowadays.
- Vulvectomy in cases of hypertrophied vulva.
- Tuboplasty is contraindicated. Any surgery on the tube to improve fertility would cause reactivation of the disease. Moreover, fertility cannot be restored when the tubal walls are damaged.
- Removal of adnexal mass in a young woman.
- Drainage of pyometra.
- Fistula repair.

FOLLOW-UP

The patient needs to be followed up for at least 5 years, as reactivation of the lesion during this period has been reported. A yearly, or when indicated earlier, endometrial biopsy should be carried out to check for any reactivation. Hysterosalpingogram is however not advisable, as it may reactivate the dormant infection.

PROGNOSIS

Nearly 90% of the cases get cured with chemotherapy. However, prospects of fertility are extremely low in the region of 10% only. Of those who conceive, 50% have a tubal pregnancy, 20%–30% abort. Only 2% of women with genital tuberculosis will have live births.

IN VITRO FERTILIZATION (IVF)

Women successfully treated for genital tuberculosis are now offered assisted reproduction by in vitro fertilization. RS Marcus et al. have reported 40% success, provided the endometrium is normal. However, pregnancy rates following IVF-ET are lower in treated cases of genital tuberculosis.

KEY POINTS

- Tuberculosis of the genital tract is common in India, and is secondary to primary focus in the lungs (50%), lymph nodes (40%), urinary tract (5%) and bones and joints (5%).
- The infection primarily attacks the fallopian tubes causing PID. Later it spreads downwards, causing uterine synechiae and Asherman syndrome. Cervical and vulval lesions are very rare.
- Very often, genital tuberculosis remains silent and goes unnoticed. Infertility, amenorrhoea, abdominal mass and pain develop in an advanced stage.
- Endometrial biopsy, laparoscopy and blood tests help to discover its existence.
- Newer techniques such as PCR, NAAT and BACTEC rapid culture methods which offer results in 24 hours and 5–7 days, respectively, are now being employed. NAAT detects tuberculosis in a few hours.
- Treatment is essentially medical. Category I drugs given for a period of 6 months is the standard of treatment. In drug-resistant cases and HIV-positive cases, a longer duration of treatment with Category II may be needed.
- Surgery may be required if the disease persists and does not respond to drugs, and the treatment is hysterectomy and bilateral salpingo-oophorectomy, and removal of tubo-ovarian mass in a young woman.
- Reactivation may occur within 5 years; therefore, follow-up becomes necessary.
- Pregnancy rate following treatment is only 10%, of which one-third abort and another 50% develop ectopic pregnancy.
- High degree of suspicion is required in an asymptomatic woman, especially in an infertile woman.

SELF-ASSESSMENT

1. Describe the pathogenesis of female genital tuberculosis.
2. Describe the lesions of the female genital tract caused by tubercular infection.
3. How would you investigate a case of suspected genital tuberculosis?
4. Describe the common clinical manifestations of genital tuberculosis.
5. How would you treat a patient of genital tuberculosis?

SUGGESTED READING

Alwani CM, Arun HN, Ranjana B, Shirish B. Genital tuberculosis. J Obstet Gynaecol Family Welfare 1995;1:14.

Bhattacharya N, Banerji AK, Roy S, et al. Endometrial tuberculosis (A ten year study of 525 cases).

Bhattacharya P. Hypertrophic tuberculosis of the vulva. Obstet Gynecol 1978; 51:225.

Chhabra S. Genital tuberculosis a baffling disease. J Obstet Gynaecol India 1990; 40:569.

Coetzee LF. Tuberculous vaginitis. S Afr Med J 1972; 46:1225.

Czernobilsky B. Endometritis and infertility. Fertil Steril 1978; 30:119.

Dalal AR, Venkatesan R. Management of genital tuberculosis. In Tank DK, Saraiya UB, Patel MK (eds). Postgraduate Frontiers in Obstetrics and Gynaecology. 2nd Ed. New Delhi, FOGSI Publications, J. P. Brothers, 1999.

Daly JW, Monif GRG. Infectious diseases in Obstetrics and Gynecology. In Monif (ed). Mycobacteria. 2nd Ed. Philadelphia, Harper & Row, 1982.

Das S, Chaudhari P. Cervical tuberculosis in suspected carcinoma cervix. J Obstet Gynaecol India 1993; 43:453.

Desai SK, Allahabadia GN (eds). Infertility and Tuberculosis–Current Concepts. New Delhi, Jaypee Brothers Medical Publishers, 1995.

Desai SK. Endometrial receptivity in genital tuberculosis. J Obstet Gynaecol India 2002; 52:23.

Deshmukh K, Lopez J, Naidu AK. Genital tuberculosis. J Obstet Gynaecol India 1987; 37:289.

Dodhwal V, Kumar S, Mittal S. Sonohysterography in evaluating intrauterine pathology. J Obstet Gynaecol India 2001; 51:113.

Falk V, Ludviksson K, Agren G. Genital tuberculosis in women. Analysis of 187 newly diagnosed cases from 47 Swedish hospitals during the ten year period 1968–1977. Am J Obstet Gynecol 1980; 138:933.

Frydman R, Eibschitz I, Belaesch-Allart JC. Genital tuberculosis-infertility treated with IVF-ET. J In Vitro Fert Embryo Transf 1985; 4:184.

Gupta N, Arora HL, Gupta A. Tuberculosis of the female genital tract. J Obstet Gynaecol India 1991; 41:238.

Gurgan T Urman B, Yarali H. Genital tuberculosis. Fertil Steril 1996; 65:367.

Halbrecht HV. Healed genital tuberculosis. Obstet Gynecol 1957; 10:73.

Jedberg H. A study on genital tuberculosis on women. Acta Obstetric Gynecol Scand 1950; 31(Suppl):117

Kherdekar M, Kher A, Sharma AD. Tuberculosis of the endometrium: A histopathological study of 355 cases. Indian J Pathol Microbiol 1977; 20:39.

Krishna UK, Sathe AV, Mehta H, et al. Tuberculosis in infertility. J Obstet Gynaecol India 1979; 29:663.

Kumar C, Sinha S. Laparoscopic evaluation of tubal factor in cases of infertility. J Obstet Gynaecol India 2000; 50:67.

Lattimer JK, Colmore HP, Sanger G, et al. Transmission of genital tuberculosis from husband and wife via the semen. Am Rev Tuberculosis 1954; 69:618.

Manjari Mridu, Khanna S, Kahlan SK. Genital tuberculosis. Indian J Pathol Microbiol 1995; 42:227.

Meisels A, Fortin R. Genital tuberculosis Acta Cytol 1975; 19:79.

Merchant RJ. Genital tuberculosis and infertility. J Reprod Med 1989; 34(7):468.

Millar JW, Holt S Gilmour HM, et al. Vulvar tuberculosis. Tubercle 1979; 60:173.

Munshi MM, Chiddarwar S, Patel A. Tuberculosis in gynaecology. Indian J Pathol Microbiol 1993; 36:356.

Nagpal M, Pal D. Genital tuberculosis: A diagnostic dilemma in OPD patients. J Obstet Gynaecol India 2001; 51:127.

Nogales-Ortiz F, Tarancion I, Nogales FF. The Pathology of female genital tuberculosis: A 31 year study of 1436 cases. Obstet Gynecol 1979; 53:422.

Novak ER, Woodruff JD. Novak's Gynaecologic and Obstetric Pathology, 8th Ed. Philadelphia, WB Saunders, 1979.

Parikh FR, Nadkarni SG, Kamat SA, et al. Genital tuberculosis in infertility. Fertil Steril 1995; 67:497.

Premi HK, Kumar A, Kumar S. Cervical tuberculosis. J Obstet Gynaecol India 1990; 40:826.

Ridley CM. Recent Advances in Vulval Disease. Churchill Livingstone, Edinburgh, 1985.

29 Sexually Transmitted Diseases Including HIV Infection

CHAPTER OUTLINE

The term 'sexually transmitted diseases (STDs)' refers to a variety of clinical syndromes and infections caused by pathogens that can be acquired and transmitted through sexual activity.

It has become a global threat to the health of the population, and its increasing incidence is due to promiscuity and frequent change of partners. Symptoms caused by infections of the lower genital tract are amongst the most common complaints in gynaecologic patients. Genital tract infection can lead to pelvic inflammatory disease (PID), infertility and ectopic pregnancy if the fallopian tubes are involved. Viral infections are liable to cause vulval and cervical cancers. Obstetric complications include repeated pregnancy losses, intrauterine fetal death, neonatal eye and throat infections, and septicaemia. Vertical transmission to the fetus and neonate is known to occur in women with syphilis and human immunodeficiency virus (HIV) infection. Antenatal routine testing and treatment can avoid or reduce risk of their transmission.

Of all the vaginal infections known, bacterial vaginosis (BV) accounts for 40%–50% of cases, monilial infection 20%–25% of cases and *Trichomonas* infection 15%–20% of cases. The others are rare, though the incidence of chlamydial infection is increasing.

Types of vaginal infections:

- **Bacterial** – Syphilis, gonorrhoea, chlamydial infection, lymphogranuloma, *Mycoplasma genitalium* infection, chancroid
- **Viral** – Human papillomavirus (HPV), herpes simplex virus (HSV), HIV infection
- **Protozoal** – *Trichomonas vaginalis* infection
- **Fungal** – Candidal infection
- **Infestations** – Scabies, pediculosis

Most of the genital tract infections are sexually transmitted. However, unscreened blood transfusions can also spread syphilis, HIV infection and hepatitis B. Other rare causes are use of infected needles and sharing of toilets or towels.

VULVAR INFECTIONS

The normal vulva is composed of the skin consisting of stratified squamous epithelium. It contains sebaceous, sweat and apocrine glands, underlying subcutaneous tissue and the specialized Bartholin's glands. Vulvar pruritus and burning account for approximately 10%–15% of presenting complaints. Following infections can affect vulva:

PARASITIC INFECTION (PEDICULOSIS PUBIS)

Pediculosis pubis is one of the most contagious STDs caused by crab louse or *Phthirus pubis.* It is also transmitted through intimate contact and shared towels or sheets. The parasites deposit their eggs at the base of hair follicles. The louse feeds on human blood (Fig. 29.1).

CLINICAL FEATURES

The patient complains of intense itching in the pubic area; there may be the presence of a vulvar rash. The intense itching can cause insomnia, irritation and social embarrassment.

DIAGNOSIS

Diagnosis is established on inspection – finding of eggs/lice in the pubic hair. The louse can be identified under the microscope.

TREATMENT

Local application of permethrin cream 5% – two applications 10 days apart – to kill newly hatched eggs or local application of gamma-benzene hexachloride 1% as lotion/cream or shampoo after showering so that the drug effects last for 12 hours on 2 successive days. This treatment is

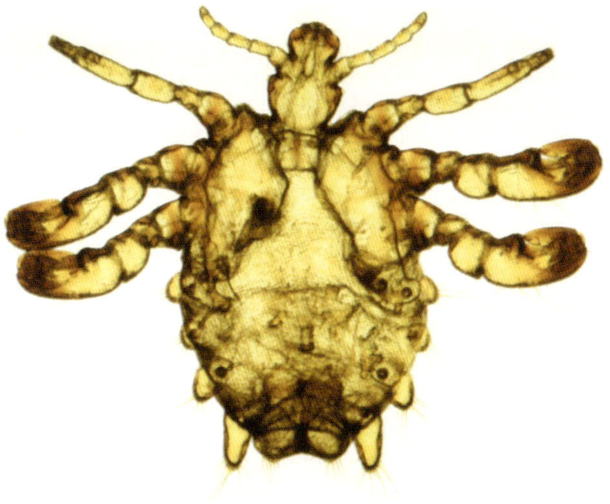

Figure 29.1 Crab louse (*Phthirus pubis*). (*Source:* Robert S. Dill, Associate Professor, Biological Sciences, Bergen Community College.)

contraindicated in pregnant and nursing mothers. All clothes should be properly laundered.

SCABIES

It is transmitted through close contact/fomites and caused by *itch mite.*

CLINICAL FEATURES

It generally affects the flexure aspects of the elbows and wrists, buttocks and the external genitalia. The adult female burrows beneath the skin to lay its eggs. The patients suffer from intense burning along with intermittent episodes of intense itching/burning. Itching is more severe at night. It may present as papules, vesicles or burrows.

DIAGNOSIS

It is established on microscopic examination of skin scrapings under oil.

TREATMENT

It consists of local application of permethrin cream 5% twice a day for 2 successive days or application of 30 mL of lotion over the entire skin surface, leaving it on for 12 hours. Pruritus may persist for a while; this should be controlled with antihistamines. Treatment should be withheld during pregnancy and lactation. Clothes should be properly laundered.

MOLLUSCUM CONTAGIOSUM

It is a benign viral infection caused by the *poxvirus.* It is spread by close sexual or nonsexual contact and by autoinoculation. The incubation period ranges from several weeks to months.

CLINICAL FEATURES

The patient presents with a crops of small domed vesicles, with central umbilication measuring 1–5 mm in size. White waxy material can be expressed out of it.

DIAGNOSIS

Giemsa staining of the discharge (white waxy material) reveals intracytoplasmic molluscum bodies confirmatory of the diagnosis.

TREATMENT

It consists of evacuation of the white material, excision of the nodule with a dermal curet and treatment of the base with Monsel's solution (ferric subsulphate) or 85% trichloracetic acid. Cryotherapy and electrocoagulation may be considered as an alternative therapy.

CONDYLOMATA ACUMINATA (Figs 29.2 and 29.3)

Also called **venereal warts,** these are caused by the HPV, which is a small DNA double-stranded virus. These warts spread diffusely over the whole of the vulval area. The verrucous growths may appear discrete or coalesce to form large cauliflower-like growths. They affect the skin of the labia majora, perineum, perianal region and vagina. The growths are seen in women of the childbearing age and are mainly sexually transmitted. Vaginal discharge, use of oral contraceptives and pregnancy favour their growth. There are several varieties of the HPV of which HPV 6, 11, 16 and 18 as well as 31, 32 and 33 are of significance to the gynaecologist. HPV 6 and 11 are implicated in the development of condyloma acuminatum, and HPV 16 and 18 are implicated in the development of cancers of the cervix and vulva. The presence of **koilocytes** constitutes the histological marker for the virus. Apart from koilocytes, other histological features are perinuclear halo, multinucleation, organophilic cytoplasm, acanthosis and chronic inflammatory infiltrate. Dysplasia may be seen in warts in elderly women. The typing of virus is based on DNA, DNA hybridization and polymerase chain reaction (PCR). HPV is a small DNA virus, 55 nm in diameter, is epitheliotropic and contributes to 15% of all cancers. In young women, the infection is transient; it disappears in 90% of cases without

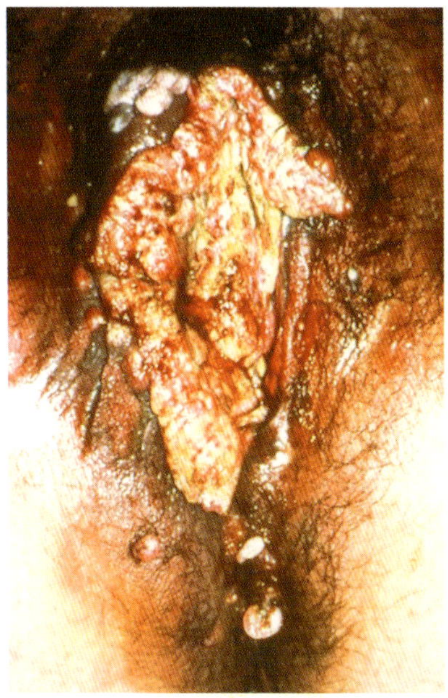

Figure 29.2 Condyloma acuminatum of the vulva. (From Russell AH: Cancer of the vulva. In Leibel SA, Phillips TL, eds: Textbook of radiation oncology, ed 2, Philadelphia, 2004, Saunders, p 1180.)

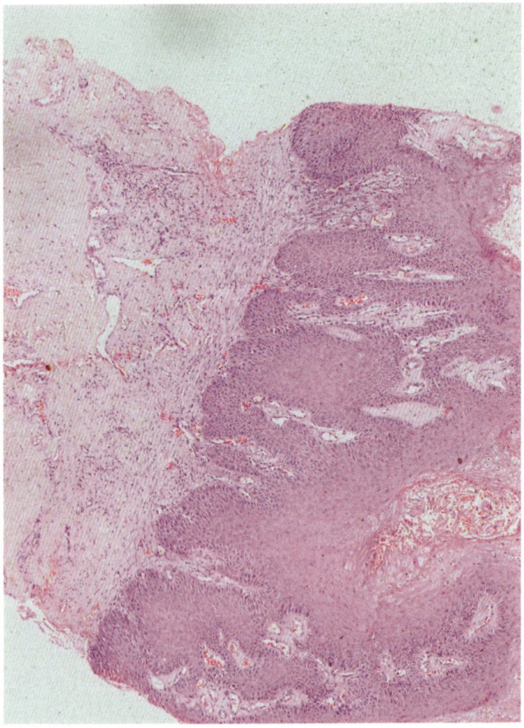

Figure 29.3 Condyloma accuminata: Hypertrophic stratified squamous epithelium arranged in knuckle-like fronds. The epithelium shows acanthosis and papillomatosis. (*Courtesy*: Dr Sandeep Mathur, AIIMS.)

any alteration in DNA. In older women and immunocompromised persons, it often persists and progresses to carcinoma in situ in 30% of cases in 1–3 years and cancer of the cervix. Both squamous cell carcinoma and adenocarcinoma can occur.

Condyloma is associated with vulval, vaginal and cervical cancers in 20% of cases. Cervical cancer accounts for about 80% of HPV-related cancers.

DIAGNOSIS

Colposcopic study of this lesion aided by acetic acid application is important in the diagnosis of lesions on the cervix and 1% toluidine blue staining for the vulval lesions. Toluidine blue dye is washed off with 3% acetic acid 1 minute after application on the vulva. The abnormal vulval skin with the abnormal nuclei retains the blue dye, whereas the normal skin allows the dye to be washed off. Acetic acid can cause burning in the vulva, and it should be diluted to 50% before use. Vulval skin is first smeared with water-soluble K-Y jelly and then treated with dilute acetic acid. The vascular pattern is studied. The abnormal areas stained with toluidine blue are biopsied.

COLPOSCOPIC FINDINGS

Meisels described colposcopic appearance of condylomas as patches of raised projection of acetowhite epithelium with speckled appearance. Immunochemical technique can demonstrate viral antigen in the tissue sections.

TREATMENT

Young women with flat condyloma may be observed for 6 months, especially when it develops during pregnancy, because the lesions often disappear spontaneously. Local application of podophyllin 25% in alcohol or podophyllin 20% in tincture benzoin for 6 hours daily or 25% trichloracetic acid plus 5% fluorouracil causes sloughing off of small warts in 3–4 days in 70%–80% of cases. The treatment may need to be repeated weekly as the warts recur at 3–6 weeks' interval. Local podophyllin cream (podofilox) is also available. This treatment is, however, contraindicated in the first trimester of pregnancy because the drug is absorbed into the circulation and is cytotoxic, causing abortion and peripheral neuropathy. This treatment is also contraindicated in vaginal and cervical lesions because of severe inflammatory reaction provoked at these sites. The larger lesions are best removed by diathermy loop or laser ablation. The surgical excision of a localized growth is another alternative. Associated syphilis and malignancy need to be excluded. The husband of the infected woman should be treated simultaneously or protected from infection by advising the use of condoms.

Vulval and vaginal warts during pregnancy mandate caesarean section to avoid papillomatous laryngitis in the neonate.

Lately, Ikic et al. advocated the use of interferon in the form of local ointment or cream or intralesional injection. The cream is applied four to five times daily 1 g each time (1 g contains 2 × 106 IU), with total daily dose of 6 g for 8 weeks. Ninety per cent of lesions regress by this application. Intramuscular injection of 2 × 106 IU of interferon daily for 10 days yields 90% success. Side effects are fever, myalgia and headache. *Cream is preferred to injection, as the latter is painful. Interferon inhibits the viral and cellular growth.* Interferon therapy is avoided during pregnancy. Apart from surgery, the warts can be removed by cryosurgery, diathermy or laser. *Needless to say, biopsy is mandatory to rule out malignancy. Pap smear of the cervix is also required to rule out cervical malignancy.*

Other measures include the following:

- Improve body immunity with antioxidants such as vitamin C and folic acid.
- Avoid smoking.
- Vaccines at 0, 1 and 6 months before exposure to sexual activity in adolescent girls and boys are available, though they are expensive. Bivalent vaccine against HPV 16 and 18 is known as Cervarix. Quadrivalent vaccine against HPV 6, 11, 16 and 18 is known as Gardasil or Silgard. The high cost of vaccine precludes the prophylactic use in general population. Cervarix is given at 0, 1 and 6 months. Gardasil is given at 0, 2 and 6 months. Recently, two doses of HPV vaccine given at 0 and 6 months have been found to be effective. Inosiplex is an immunomodulator which is used as an adjunct to conventional therapy. Orally, it is given 5 mg/kg daily for 12 weeks. About 20% complete response and 40% partial response are reported.
- Imiquimod cream applied three times a week for 4 months cures 75% of cases of condylomata accuminata but recurs in 15% of cases. Some develop local erythematous reaction to the cream.

GENITAL ULCERS

Sexually transmitted infections (STIs) such as genital herpes, granuloma inguinale (donovanosis), lymphogranuloma venereum (LGV), chancroid and syphilis often present with ulcerative lesions of the vulva.

GENITAL HERPES

It is a recurrent STD caused by the double-stranded DNA virus of *HSV group (almost 80% are type II infections)*. The prevalence of the disease has reached epidemic proportions in the developed countries of the world. The *incubation period* is 3–7 days. HSV type I accounts for only 30% of vulval lesions.

It mostly affects women between 20 and 30 years of age.

CLINICAL FEATURES

Primary Infection

The patient often complains of constitutional symptoms such as malaise, fever and vulval paraesthesia, followed by appearance of vesicles on the vulva resulting in ulcers which are shallow and painful. These often coalesce. Multiple crops of vesicles and ulcers tend to occur in 2–6 weeks. The lesions peak in 7 days and last for approximately 2 weeks. The outbreak is self-limited. The lesions heal without scarring. Viral shedding, however, tends to continue for weeks after the appearance of lesions.

Recurrent Herpetic Lesions (Fig. 29.4)

These are generally of shorter duration and milder in severity of symptoms. Prodromal symptoms of burning or itching in the affected area often precede the attacks. Systemic symptoms are generally absent. About 50% of the affected women experience their first recurrence within 6 months and have on an average of about four recurrences within the first year; thereafter, the episodes of recurrences tend to occur at variable intervals. Latent herpes virus residing in the dorsal root ganglia of S_2, S_3 and S_4 may get reactivated whenever the immune system gets compromised as seen during pregnancy or any other immunocompromised states.

COMPLICATIONS

Known rare complications include encephalitis and urinary tract involvement causing retention of urine, severe pain or both.

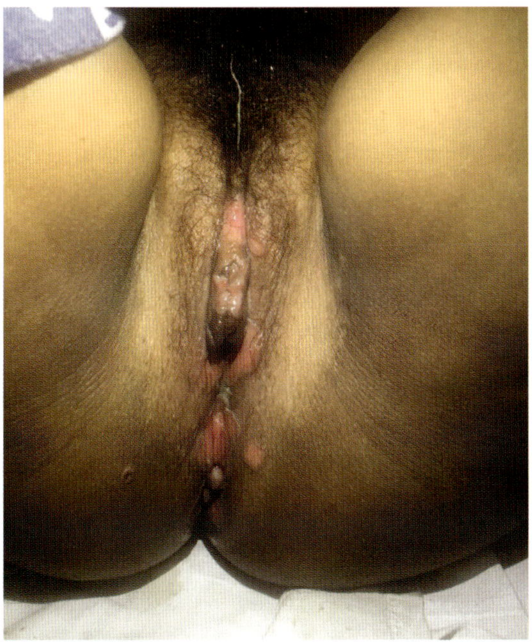

Figure 29.4 Recurrent herpes genitalis. (*Source:* Wikimedia commons.)

Table 29.1 Recommended Regimens for Treatment of Herpes Simplex (CDC, 2015)

- Acyclovir 400 mg orally three times a day for 7–10 days
  OR
- Acyclovir 200 mg orally five times a day for 7–10 days
  OR
- Valaciclovir 1 g orally twice a day for 7–10 days
  OR
- Famciclovir 250 mg orally three times a day for 7–10 days

[a]Treatment can be extended if healing is incomplete after 10 days of therapy.

DIAGNOSIS

Diagnosis is essentially based on clinical inspection of the lesions; immunologic or cytologic tests are not very sensitive; viral cultures from swabs taken from the base of the vesicles are positive in 90% of cases. In 6 weeks, nucleic acid amplification test (NAAT) offers greater sensitivity than the culture. Biopsy reveals characteristic 'ground glass appearance' of the cellular nuclei and numerous small intracellular basophilic particles and acidophilic inclusion bodies. Cytology shows multinucleated giant cells. The antibody detection in serum and PCR staining is also diagnostic. Antibodies can be detected 2 weeks after the infection.

TREATMENT (Table 29.1)

- **Aims of the treatment include the following:**
  - To shorten the duration of the attack.
  - Prevent complications.
  - Prevent recurrences.
  - Diminish risks of transmission.
- The virus cannot be effectively eradicated.
- In severe cases, administer acyclovir 5 mg/kg body weight intravenously every 8 hours for 5 days.
- Treat primary outbreaks.
- Prescribe 200 mg acyclovir five times daily orally for 5 days. Local application of acyclovir cream provides relief and accelerates healing of local lesions. Thus, *treatment reduces the duration and severity of the attack but does not prevent latency of the disease or episodes of recurrence.* Valaciclovir 500 mg b.d. or famciclovir 125–250 mg b.d. is also effective, given for 7 days.
- Centers for Disease Control and Prevention (CDC) has given guidelines for the effective treatment of herpes simplex infection (Table 29).
- Counselling: The couple is advised to abstain from intercourse from the time of experiencing prodromal symptoms until total re-epithelialization of the lesions takes place. These patients are more susceptible to HIV infection and other STDs.
- Caesarean section is recommended in the presence of active infection to avoid neonatal infection.

Vaccine against genital herpes is not yet available, but immune enhancers reduces the frequency of recurrences. Imiquimod is being tried, but clinical trial is lacking.

GRANULOMA INGUINALE (DONOVANOSIS) (Fig. 29.5)

The causative organism for granuloma inguinale is *Calymmatobacterium granulomatis*. It is a Gram-negative bacillus

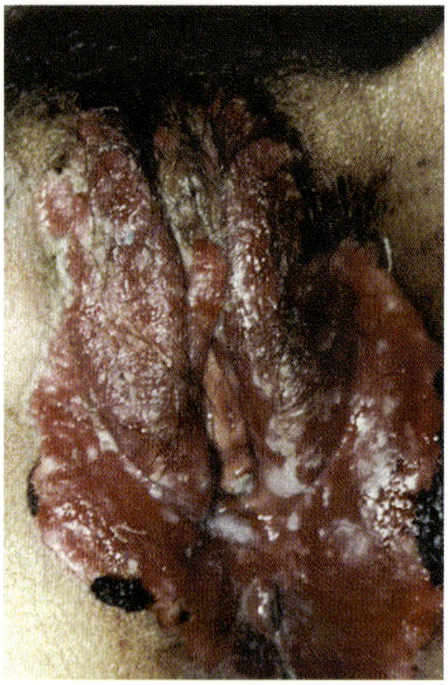

Figure 29.5 Granuloma inguinale. (*Source*: OmarLupi, Vandana Madkan, Stephen K.Tyring. Journal of the American Academy of Dermatology, Tropical dermatology: Bacterial tropical diseases, 54(4) 2006.)

causing chronic ulcerative infection of the vulva. It is prevalent in the tropics. It is not only highly contagious but also transmitted through repeated sexual or nonsexual contacts. The *incubation period* is 1–12 weeks.

CLINICAL FEATURES

It begins as a painless nodule which later ulcerates to form multiple beefy red painless ulcers that tend to coalesce; the vulva is progressively destroyed, and minimal adenopathy may occur.

DIAGNOSIS

Microscopic examination of smears from the lesion/biopsy specimens reveals pathognomonic **intracytoplasmic Donovan bodies** and clusters of bacteria with a bipolar (safety pin) appearance (Gram negative). Blue–black stained organisms are seen in the cytoplasm of mononuclear cells.

TREATMENT (Table 29.2)

Table 29.2 Recommended Regimen for Granuloma Inguinale (donovanosis) CDC 2015

Azithromycin 1 g orally once per week or 500 mg daily for at least 3 weeks and until all lesions have completely healed

Alternative regimens

- Doxycycline 100 mg orally twice a day for at least 3 weeks and until all lesions have completely healed
  OR
- Ciprofloxacin 750 mg orally twice a day for at least 3 weeks and until all lesions have completely healed
  OR
- Erythromycin base 500 mg orally four times a day for at least 3 weeks and until all lesions have completely healed
  OR
- Trimethoprim-sulfamethoxazole one double-strength (160 mg/800 mg) tablet orally twice a day for at least 3 weeks and until all lesions have completely healed

LYMPHOGRANULOMA VENEREUM

It is an uncommon STD that affects men more commonly than women. It is generally prevalent in Africa and Asia.

RISK FACTORS

- Sexually active before the age of 20 years
- Multiple sexual partners
- Low socioeconomic status
- History of having suffered from other STDs

The incubation period is 7–21 days.

PATHOPHYSIOLOGY

The causative organism is *Chlamydia trachomatis* (any one of the 'L' serotypes 1, 2 and 3), an intracellular Gram-negative bacteria. *Sexual transmission*: In women, the organism is carried by lymphatic drainage from the genital lesion to the perirectal node, both inguinal and pelvic lymph nodes. Rectal involvement is common in females and occurs by contiguous spread from the perirectal nodes, leading to proctocolitis and rectal stricture formation. The drainage is primarily to the inguinal nodes, leading to **bubo** formation; this may burst, ulcerate or cause sinus. It can also affect the urethra, perineum and cervix.

CLINICAL FEATURES

The lesion starts as painless vesicopustular eruption that heals spontaneously. After some weeks, the sequelae of lymphatic spread begins with hardly any clinical manifestations. The general features are fever, headache, malaise and arthralgia.

DIAGNOSIS

It is essentially a clinical diagnosis. Determination of LGV is extremely difficult until the late stage of the disease.

INVESTIGATIONS

The *Frei test* based on delayed skin hypersensitivity to the antigen becomes positive 2–8 weeks after primary infection. The *complement fixation test* is more sensitive than the Frei test. Culture can be grown, and inclusion bodies in the smear can be detected. DNA probing is specific.

COMPLICATIONS

Complications are as a result of scar tissue formation. It includes the following: (a) proctitis, (b) severe stricture formation leading to intestinal obstruction, (c) rectovaginal fistulae following stricture formation and (d) vulvar cancer.

TREATMENT (Table 29.3)

Table 29.3 Treatment of Lymphogranuloma Venereum (CDC- 2015)

Recommended regimen

- Doxycycline 100 mg orally twice a day for 21 days

Alternative regimen

- Erythromycin base 500 mg orally four times a day for 21 days

MYCOPLASMA GENITALIUM

Mycoplasma genitalium, first discovered in 1983, is an intracellular organism which lacks cell wall and is not stained by Gram stain. It is difficult to culture and takes weeks or months. NAAT and PCR are the detection tests. No commercial test is available. The infection causes urethritis, endocervicitis and PID.

TREATMENT

- Moxifloxacine 400 mg o.d. × 7 days

  or
- Azithromycin 500 mg stat and 250 mg every 6 hour × 4 days

CHANCROID (SOFT SORE)

It is an acute STD caused by small Gram-negative bacilli *Haemophilus ducreyi (anaerobe)*. It is common in the underdeveloped countries of the world. It affects males five to ten times more often than females. It may facilitate the spread of HIV infection. It is highly contagious, but it requires the presence of broken/traumatized skin for entry. The *incubation period is* 3–6 days.

CLINICAL FEATURES

Initially, there appears a small papule that develops into a painful pustule that ulcerates. Multiple lesions at various stages of development may be evident at one and the same time. The ulcers are shallow, ragged and painful. Often, a unilateral inguinal lymphadenopathy may be evident in 50% of cases. Recurrence rate at the same site has been observed in 10% of cases. The ulcers are sharply demarcated without induration. Distal spread is rare. In 10% of cases, soft sore is associated with syphilis or herpes.

DIAGNOSIS

This is based on investigation of the purulent discharge from the lesion or aspirate from the lymph node showing the typical extracellular 'school of fish' appearance on Gram staining. Culture, enzyme-linked immunosorbent assay (ELISA) and PCR staining can also be used as diagnostic tests.

TREATMENT

Recommendations include the following options:

- Azithromycin 1.0 g orally as a single dose with 98% effectiveness.
- Erythromycin 500 mg orally every 6 hours for 7 days.
- Alternatives include ceftriaxone 250 mg i.m. as a single dose or oral trimethoprim and sulphamethoxazole (Bactrim DS) b.i.d. for 7 days or oral ciprofloxacin 500 mg b.i.d. for 3 days.
- Spectinomycin 2 g i.m. as a single dose.
- The woman should be screened for other STDs.

SYPHILIS (Fig. 29.6)

It is an STI caused by the motile spirochete *Treponema pallidum*. Humans are natural hosts. It also spreads by contact with broken skin/intact mucous membrane. The most frequent entry sites in the female include the vulva, vagina and cervix.

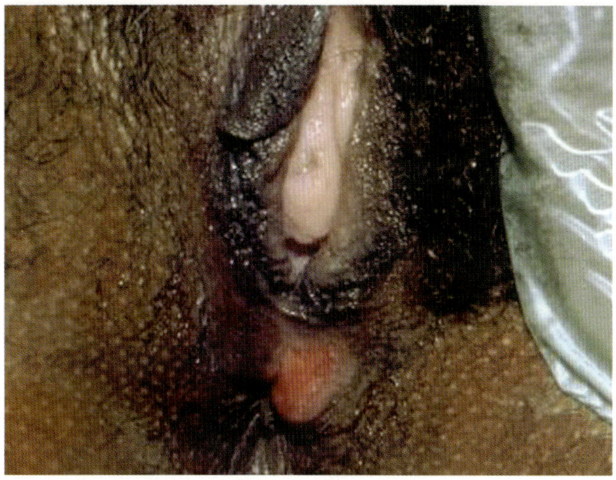

Figure 29.6 Hard chancre of syphilis. (*Source:* Logical images, www.logicalimages.com)

CLINICAL FEATURES

When the disease is untreated, its natural evolution is as follows.

Primary Syphilis

The classic lesion designated as the chancre appears within 9–90 days from the first exposure. The macular lesion becomes papular and then ulcerates. The ulcer(s) is painless and firm, with a punched out base and rolled out edges. Left unattended, these heal within 3–9 weeks. There occurs an accompanying painless inguinal, discrete lymphadenopathy. The latent period is 8 weeks after inoculation and 3–6 weeks after chancre. The serological test becomes positive 1–4 weeks after chancre.

Secondary Syphilis

This is evidence of widespread dissemination of the spirochetes.

Onset of systemic manifestations includes symptoms such as malaise, headache, loss of appetite, sore throat and the appearance of a generalized symmetric, asymptomatic maculopapular rash on the palms and soles of the feet. It is not uncommon to find a generalized adenopathy in 50% of cases. *Condylomata lata* are a classic finding; these are highly contagious exophytic broad excrescences that ulcerate. These are commonly seen on the vulva, perianal area and upper thighs. After 2–6 weeks, it passes into the phase of latent syphilis. No clinical manifestations are present; however, the serologic test for syphilis is positive. This stage lasts for 2–10 weeks (Fig. 29.7).

Tertiary Syphilis

Syphilis left untreated may develop into tertiary syphilis in about a third of the affected patients 5–20 years after the chancre has disappeared. The disease remains latent in the remaining persons. Manifestations of diffuse organ system involvement include the following:

- *Neurosyphilis:* Manifests as meningitis, tabes dorsalis or paresis and mental disease.
- *Cardiosyphilis:* Manifests as valvular disease, aortitis and aneurysm.
- *Skin manifestations* such as gummas.

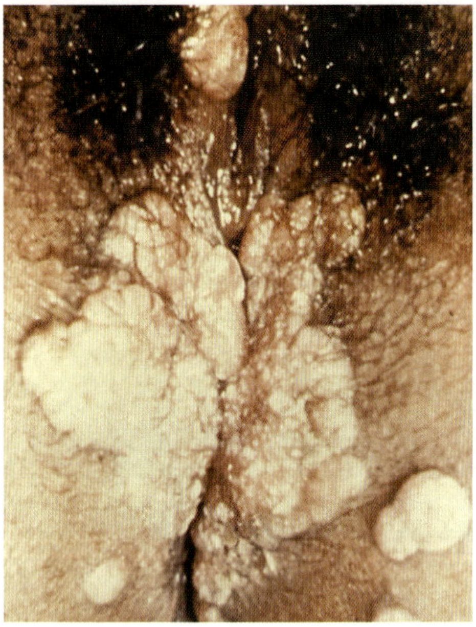

Figure 29.7 Early condylomas of secondary syphilis.

During pregnancy, syphilis can cause late abortion and stillbirth. Congenital syphilis in newborns manifests few weeks after birth.

LABORATORY INVESTIGATIONS

These include the following:

- Primary syphilis: Dark-field microscopy of chancre scrapings reveals spirochetes. Serological test (VDRL test) at this stage is negative.
- Secondary syphilis: Dark-field microscopy of scrapings from condylomata lata reveals spirochetes. Serological test (VDRL test) is positive. Immunofluorescent technique is also available.
- Tertiary syphilis: Serological test (VDRL test) is positive. Lumbar puncture and examination of cerebrospinal fluid are recommended in cases of suspected neurosyphilis.
- Confirmatory tests such as the fluorescent titre antibody (FTA) absorption test and the microhaemagglutination assay for antibodies to *Treponema pallidum* (MHA-TP) are advocated. The important point to remember is that a *false-positive VDRL is seen in women with systemic lupus erythematosus and other conditions.*
- Biopsy may be needed to differentiate it from tubercular and cancerous ulcers.
- PCR testing is now available.

TREATMENT

The following are recommended:

- Screen for other STDs and HIV infection.
- Counselling about treatment, expected course of the disease, risk of fetal transmission and its sequelae in the case of pregnancy.
- Treating all sexual partners of the infected individual.
- Specific treatment: (a) Intramuscular injection of 2.4 million units of benzathine penicillin after a test dose. Male partner should receive the same dose preferably on the same day. (b) If latent disease is present for over a year, the dose of penicillin is repeated weekly for 3 weeks. Patients who are allergic to penicillin should undergo desensitization or they should be prescribed erythromycin, doxycycline or azithromycin as an alternative drug.

Alternative drugs for person sensitive to benzathine penicillin

- Doxycycline 100 mg b.d. × 14 days.
- Erythromycin 500 mg q.i.d. × 14 days.
- Azithromycin 500 mg o.d. × 10 days.
- Amoxicillin 500 mg q.i.d. × 14 days.
- During follow-up, serology titres should show a decrease by fourfolds after 3–6 months.
- Recommend use of barrier contraceptives to prevent spread of the disease.
- Seek joint consultation with a specialist in STDs.
- All newborns to a mother who was found to be VDRL positive should receive neonatal prophylaxis in the form of procaine penicillin for 14 days.

VAGINITIS

GONOCOCCAL VULVOVAGINITIS

This is an STD that can lead to sequelae adversely affecting subsequent reproductive functions.

EPIDEMIOLOGY

The causative organism is a Gram-negative intracellular diplococcus called *Neisseria gonorrhoeae*. The incubation period is 2–10 days. The vaginal squamous epithelium is resistant to gonococcal infection. The gonococci attack the columnar epithelium of glands of Skene and Bartholin, urethra, cervix and fallopian tubes. It ascends in a piggyback fashion attached to the sperms to reach the fallopian tubes. It is destroyed easily by drying, heat, sunlight and disinfectants.

Sites for bacterial recovery: These include the urethra, cervix, anal canal and pharynx. *Principal sites of invasion:* These include columnar epithelium of the genital tract, transitional epithelium of the urethra and Bartholin's gland. *Infection rates:* The likelihood of contracting infection is 35% for men from women and 75% for women from men. Childhood infection occurs due to contamination with infected material.

DIAGNOSIS

Early clinical findings: Gonorrhoea causes an asymptomatic infection of the pharynx, cervix and anal canal/rectum. *Complaints*: These include urinary frequency and dysuria, dyspareunia, rectal discomfort and vaginal discharge. Vulvovaginal/perineal infection often results in inflammation, discharge, irritation causing pruritus and dysuria. Examination reveals swollen, painful external genitalia, purulent vaginal discharge, erythema surrounding external urinary meatus, opening of Bartholin's ducts, vaginitis and endocervicitis.

Late clinical findings: Bartholinitis, Bartholin's abscess, Bartholin's cyst, tubo-ovarian abscess, pyosalpinx, hydrosalpinx and blocked tubes. The disseminated infection may lead to polyarthralgia, tenosynovitis, dermatitis, pericarditis, endocarditis, meningitis and ophthalmologic manifestations causing conjunctivitis and uveitis. End result of chronic pelvic infection causes chronic pelvic pain, dysmenorrhoea, menorrhagia, infertility with fixed retroversion and at times dyspareunia. In the past, it was the cause of neonatal ophthalmitis occurring in newborns born to infected mothers. The routine practice of instilling in all neonates sulphacetamide/antibiotic eye drops has helped control this problem.

As much as 50%–80% of women may remain asymptomatic.

LABORATORY INVESTIGATIONS

These include Gram staining of smear prepared from any suspicious discharge. The terminal urethra and endocervix are favoured sites for obtaining the discharge. Culture from urethra and cervix on Thayer–Martin medium or blood agar, and McLeod chocolate agar in 5% CO_2 moist atmosphere is performed.

Complement fixation tests and PCR staining are also possible.

NAAT from urine, endocervical discharge: though 90% sensitive, is now in vogue. If NAAT is positive, there is no need of culture.

Self-collected samples yield similar results to that prepared by the physician.

Laparoscopy reveals, apart from tubal disease, a band of fibrous tissue on the right side stretching from the fallopian tube to the undersurface of the liver (Fitz–Hugh–Curtis syndrome) (Fig. 29.8).

COMPLICATIONS

PID, pyosalpinx formation, tubo-ovarian abscess, pelvic abscess, followed later on by hydrosalpinx formation, infertility, menstrual disturbances, chronic pelvic pain, dysmenorrhoea and dyspareunia.

TREATMENT

Treatment options include the following (Table 29.4):

- Injecting cefoxitin 2.0 g i.m. plus probenecid 1.0 g orally, followed by 14 days of treatment with oral. Doxycycline 100 mg b.i.d. for 14 days or oral. Tetracycline 250 mg q.i.d. for 14 days.
- Ceftriaxone 250 mg i.m. + 1.0 g probenecid orally, followed by oral. doxycycline 100 mg b.i.d. for 14 days or oral tetracycline 500 mg q.i.d. for 14 days.
- Oral ciprofloxacin, levofloxacin or ofloxacin 400 mg b.i.d., followed by 14 days of clindamycin 450 mg orally q.i.d. or metronidazole 500 mg b.i.d. for 14 days.
- Injection spectinomycin 2 g i.m. single dose.
- Surgery includes drainage of abscess, excision of the cyst, tuboplasty for tubal infertility.
- Treat the male partner as well and look for chlamydial infection and syphilis.

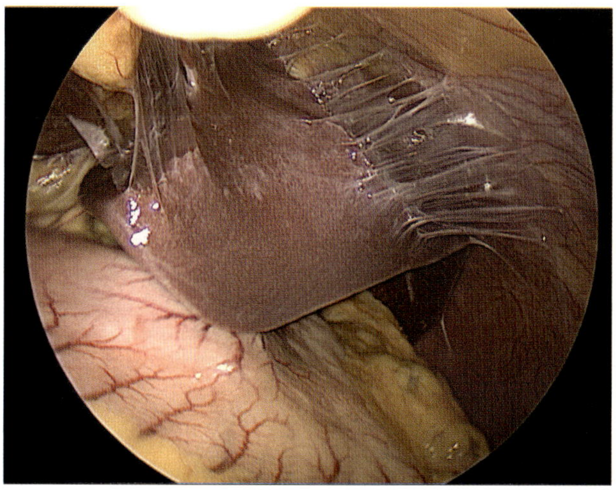

Figure 29.8 Laparoscopic view of gonococcal and chlamydial infection showing Fitz–Hugh–Curtis syndrome. (*Courtesy*: Dr Vivek Marwah, New Delhi.)

Table 29.4 Treatment of Gonorrhoea (CDC-2015)

Recommended Regimen
- Ceftriaxone 250 mg i.m. in a single dose PLUS azithromycin 1 g orally in a single dose

Alternative Regimens
If ceftriaxone is not available:
- Cefixime 400 mg orally in a single dose PLUS azithromycin 1 g orally in a single dose

CHLAMYDIAL INFECTION

Chlamydial infection is common in young, sexually active women but rare after the age of 40 years. About 2%–10% of pregnant women are found to have this infection during the antenatal period and it accounts for 1% of all abortions. The incubation period is 6–14 days. It is sexually transmitted during vaginal and rectal intercourse.

Chlamydia trachomatis is a small Gram-negative bacterium, an obligate intracellular parasite that appears as intracytoplasmic inclusion body, and is of two varieties, one that causes LGV and the other non-LGV, which causes nonspecific lower genital tract infection. Often, the infection is silent and the woman is asymptomatic but may develop vaginal discharge, dysuria and frequency of micturition, and at times cervicitis. Sometimes, chlamydial infection may cause Reiter syndrome with arthritis, skin lesions, conjunctivitis and genital infection. It also causes perihepatitis and Fitz–Hugh–Curtis syndrome similar to that caused by gonorrhoea. During pregnancy, abortion, preterm labour and intrauterine growth retardation (IUGR) may occur. Newborn may suffer from conjunctivitis, nasopharyngitis, otitis media and pneumonia. Pneumonia may develop in 6 weeks to 3 months after vaginal delivery. The cervix is the first site of infection but the disease may spread upwards to develop PID and spread to the partner and neonate. It can cause chorioamnionitis and preterm labour if infection occurs during pregnancy.

By ascending upwards, it may cause salpingitis and infertility, though the symptoms of salpingitis may go unnoticed. The tubal damage is, however, more severe than that caused by gonococci.

In the endocervix, chlamydial infection alters sperm parameters. Fragmentation of DNA causes loss of motility or dead sperms – this results in infertility.

DIAGNOSIS

The use of fluorescein-conjugated monoclonal antibody in immunofluorescence tests on smears prepared from urethral and cervical secretion allows a direct diagnosis of the infection. IgM antibodies can be detected in 30% of cases of recent infection. Cervical smear shows leucocytes but no organisms. ELISA can also detect the antigen. *Chlamydia* is cultured from the cervical tissue in 5%–15% of asymptomatic women. Polymerase and ligase chain reactions are fast, highly sensitive and specific tests (96%) and now considered 'gold standard' in the laboratory diagnosis. Uripath-UK (clear view) is a simple, rapid and bedside test.

Cervical ectopy with bleeding on touch and mucopurulent discharge is seen when the cervix is infected.

Chlamydial infection and gonococcal infection often coexist and both attack the columnar epithelium of the genital tract and urethra. Urine can be cultured in suspected chlamydial infection. Urine for PCR is simple and accurate to perform. NAAT is also possible.

TREATMENT (Table 29.5)

During pregnancy, erythromycin or amoxicillin t.i.d. or q.i.d. is given for 7 days. Contact tracing, avoidance of sex or barrier contraceptive is necessary to avoid recurrence.

TRICHOMONIASIS

In clinical practice, this is amongst the most common STDs. Nearly half of the patients who complain of pruritus vulvae harbour this organism. It is almost entirely a disease of the child-bearing age, though young girls and postmenopausal women are not all immune. There is no doubt that this infection is sexually transmissible, but in some instances, it can be acquired by inadequate hygiene or the use of an infected person's towels, bath or clothes. Its ingress to the vagina is favoured by a low general resistance particularly when the pH is raised such as during a menstrual period (pH 5–6). It is not uncommon during pregnancy and is often associated with gonococcal infection.

Trichomonas vaginalis is a protozoan, actively motile and slightly larger than a leucocyte and is anaerobic. Three types of *Trichomonas* are known. Men may harbour *Trichomonas vaginalis* in the urethra and prostate. A trichomonad has four anterior flagella and one posterior flagellum, and they move along the mucous membrane (Fig. 29.9). The posterior flagellum is responsible for motility.

Table 29.5 Treatment of Chlamydial Infection (CDC-2015)

Recommended regimens
- Azithromycin 1 g orally in a single dose
  OR
- Doxycycline 100 mg orally twice a day for 7 days

Alternative regimens
- Erythromycin base 500 mg orally four times a day for 7 days
  OR
- Erythromycin ethylsuccinate 800 mg orally four times a day for 7 days
  OR
- Levofloxacin 500 mg orally once daily for 7 days
  OR
- Ofloxacin 300 mg orally twice a day for 7 days

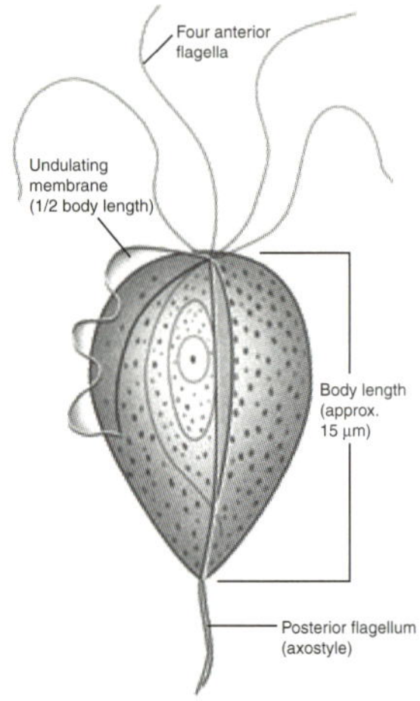

Figure 29.9 *Trichomonas vaginalis*. The protozoa are seen only in a wet film and are of varying shapes. They may be adherent to a squamous cell, or they may be attached to pus cells (diagram after Glen Liston).

SYMPTOMS

About 20% of cases remain asymptomatic – others develop symptoms 4–28 days following sexual contact with an infected partner or contact with an infected material. About 70% of cases show typical discharge, which is profuse, thin, creamy or slightly green in colour, irritating and frothy. The vaginal walls are tender and angry looking, and the discharge causes pruritus and inflammation of the vulva. There are often multiple small **punctate strawberry spots** on the vaginal vault and portio vaginalis of the cervix (strawberry vagina). The characteristic frothy discharge is almost diagnostic, but the presence of secondary infection may alter and mask this initial sign. The patient may also complain of urinary symptoms such as dysuria and frequency, and a low-grade urethritis may be discovered on examination. Abdominal pain, low backache and dyspareunia may also be complained of, if pelvic infection occurs.

DIAGNOSIS

In all suspected cases, it is necessary to examine a wet film preparation under the microscope. The preparation should be fresh, and the temperature should be at least 35°C. *Trichomonas* is in constant motion, which distinguishes it from pus cells (leucocytes) (Fig. 29.9). *Trichomonas* is usually accompanied by a mixed group of secondary infecting organisms such as *Escherichia coli* and pathogenic cocci. If the wet film stained with Gram stain or Leishman stain is negative, the parasite can be cultured. The culture is 98% reliable. *Trichomonas* may also be diagnosed on a smear stained for cytology. The other sensitive techniques include PCR and antigen testing. Pap smear shows greyish-blue pear-shaped structure without the flagella. PCR and NAAT are more sensitive tests but are hardly needed in routine clinical practice.

TREATMENT (Table 29.6)

Male partner should be treated at the same time with one of the aforementioned drugs.

Table 29.6 Treatment of Trichomonas Vaginitis (CDC-2015)

Recommended regimen
- Metronidazole 2 g orally in a single dose
  OR
- Tinidazole 2 g orally in a single dose
  Or
- Secnidazole 2 g orally in a single dose

Alternative regimen
- Metronidazole 500 mg orally twice a day for 7 days

Metronidazole and related drugs are best avoided in the first trimester of pregnancy. Recurrent infection is treated with tinidazole 500 mg q.i.d. and vaginal pessary 500 mg b.d. for 14 days. Prolonged use causes pancreatitis, neutropenia and neuropathy. Breastfeeding is contraindicated during therapy.

CANDIDAL (MONILIAL) VAGINITIS

It is a fungal infection caused by yeast-like microorganisms called *Candida or Monilia*. The commonest species causing human disease is *Candida albicans*, which is Gram positive and grows in acidic medium. It may be sexually transmitted. Almost 25% of women harbour *Candida* in the vagina.

RISK FACTORS

These include promiscuity, immunosuppression, HIV infection, pregnancy, steroid therapy, following long-term broad-spectrum antibiotic therapy, use of oral contraception pills, diabetes mellitus, poor personal hygiene and obesity.

CLINICAL FEATURES

Pruritus vulva is the cardinal symptom. It is often accompanied by vaginal irritation, dysuria, or both, and passage of thick curdy or flaky discharge. Speculum examination reveals vaginal wall congestion, with curdy discharge often visible at the vulval mucocutaneous junction and in the posterior fornix.

DIAGNOSIS

It is essentially based on clinical findings. The diagnosis can be confirmed on microscopic examination of a smear of the vaginal discharge treated with 10% KOH solution, which dissolves all other cellular debris, leaving the mycelia and spores of the *Candida* (Fig. 29.10). Gram staining of the discharge or Pap smears may also reveal the presence of *Candida*. Culture on Sabouraud's agar or Nickerson's medium helps identify *Candida*.

Pap smear shows thick red-stained hyphae and dark red spores. The colonies on culture appear as black rounded colonies, 1-2 mm in diameter with yeast-like odour.

TREATMENT

Local intravaginal application of antifungal agents such as imidazole, miconazole, clotrimazole, butoconazole or terconazole vaginal pessaries or creams used for 3–6 days is effective. A single oral dose of fluconazole 150 mg has been found to be very effective. Ideally, both partners should be treated and the underlying predisposing factor corrected to give long-term

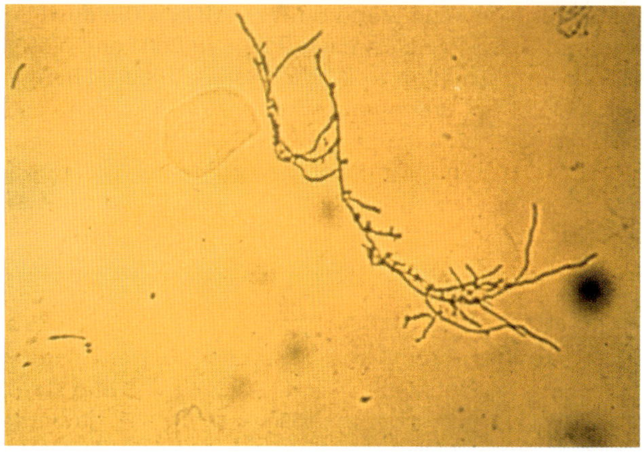

Figure 29.10 Mycelial tangles of yeast pseudohyphae in KOH wet-mount preparation. (*Source:* Hacker NF, Gambone JC, Hobel CJ. Hacker and Moore's Essentials of Obstetrics and Gynecology. 5th ed. Philadelphia: Elsevier, 2010.)

relief. Recurrent infections require fluconazole orally 150 mg every 72 hours for three doses and then weekly dose for a few weeks.

- Nystatin pessary b.d. × 10 days
- Miconazole cream 2% × 7 days
- Clotrimazole 100 mg vaginal tablet × 7 days or 1% cream for 7–10 days
- Ketoconazole 400 mg daily × 5 days

HUMAN IMMUNODEFICIENCY VIRUS INFECTION

HIV infection made its first appearance in 1981, and the virus was discovered in 1983. Since then, it has spread very rapidly and reached epidemic proportions (Fig. 29.11).

Acquired immunodeficiency syndrome (AIDS) is the clinical end stage of HIV infection, resulting in severe irreversible immunosuppression and acquisition of various

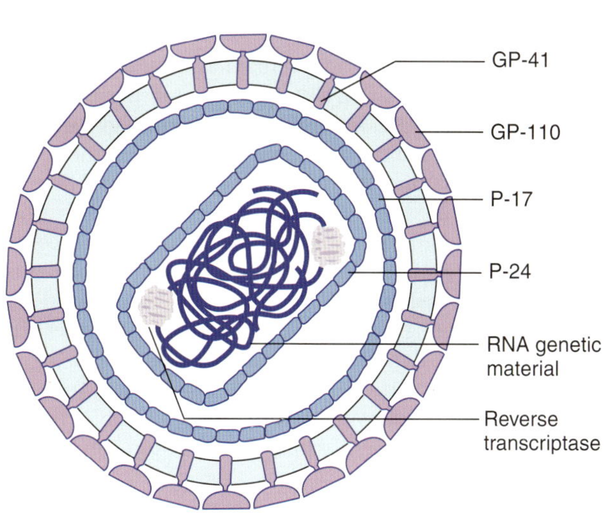

Figure 29.11 HIV virus.

opportunistic infections and cancers. AIDS is the third generation of STDs. Prevalence was 0.39% in 2004 and 0.3% in 2009 (from 2.6 million to 2.39 million in 2009). There are worldwide efforts to contain further spread of this deadly infection. Most affected people are young below the age of 25 years. It is common among homosexuals and intravenous drug users, as well as results from blood transfusion and perinatal transmission from infected mothers.

MICROBIOLOGY

HIV is a small RNA retrovirus. HIV-1 and HIV-2 are members of the Lentivirus subfamily. The virus gains entry into the cell through CD_4 receptor on the surface of T cells, transcribes genomic RNA into DNA and then integrates into the DNA of the host cell. It remains as provirus until the life of the cell. It replicates within the host cells at the expense of the host cell resources. When cell death occurs, the HIV viral load is released in large numbers. HIV cells show preference for human T cells, where it can lie dormant for many years. HIV-1 is a more severe virus, and HIV-2 is a slowly progressive virus.

EPIDEMIOLOGY

High-risk group includes sex workers, with other associated STDs, smokers, cocaine users who are immunocompromised and also those who have received infected blood transfusion. The majority of HIV-infected patients belong to the childbearing age. Spread of the disease occurs through sexual contact (homosexual and heterosexual), through shared use of infected needles among intravenous drug users, and through contact with infected body fluids such as blood, semen, vaginal secretions, saliva, tears and breast milk. In the past, many people got inadvertently infected through administration of HIV-contaminated blood transfusions. Health care workers handling infected subjects are vulnerable to the infection. The virus infects macrophages, white cells and T-helper lymphocytes (T_4 cells).

Following initial infection, antibodies develop in 2–3 weeks' time and the person becomes seropositive. At times, it may take as long as 6 months. This period is known as 'window period'.

NATURAL COURSE OF THE DISEASE

After infection, the person may remain asymptomatic or manifest symptoms within 3–6 weeks; there are nonspecific features such as fever, headache, malaise, myalgia, arthralgia, rash and gastrointestinal upset. Thereafter, the patient enters the 'asymptomatic phase', lasting for 8–10 years. Evidences of compromised immune-like generalized enlargement of lymph nodes may become evident within 3 years, with a drop in CD_4 counts. The symptoms of AIDS complex begin to manifest such as unexplained fever, rashes, thrush, weight loss, fatigue and diarrhoea. AIDS-defining disease includes opportunistic infections, tuberculosis (TB), Kaposi sarcoma and cervical cancer.

Retrovirus has a core protein with an envelope of glycoprotein. It can be destroyed by sterilization at 56°C for half an hour or with the use of hypochlorite, lipid solvents and glutaraldehyde.

Horizontal transmission from male to female is higher than that from female to male. This is because of the larger vaginal area exposed to infection and small abrasion that occurs during intercourse. Male-to-female transmission per intercourse is 0.2%–0.5% but only 0.1% from female to male. In a man, this infection does not interfere with fertility in the initial stages. With advancing infection, it can cause orchitis with oligospermia and aspermia and viscous semen. In a woman, infertility is unlikely, but vertical transmission to the neonate is a big risk. Seminal wash in intrauterine insemination and in vitro fertilization (IVF) removes the virus and is employed if the man alone is infected.

CLINICAL HIV INFECTION

The median time from acquiring infection to full-blown AIDS is about 10 years. The clinical features of the disease include the following:

- Generalized lymphadenopathy
- Unexplained fever
- Malaise, fatigue, arthralgia, weight loss and cachexia
- Oral lesions – aphthous ulcers not responding to usual treatment, thrush and leucoplakia
- Reactivation of herpes zoster
- Recurrent oral and genital herpes, candidiasis skin infection
- Thrombocytopenia
- Molluscum contagiosum, condylomata acuminata and basal cell carcinoma
- Opportunistic infections such as *Pneumocystis carinii* pneumonia (PCP), toxoplasmosis and cytomegalovirus infection
- Tuberculosis
- Peripheral neuropathy, encephalopathy, meningitis, myopathy, meningitis and dementia
- Kaposi sarcoma and cancer of the cervix
- Perinatal transmission

The WHO estimates that by the turn of the last century (AD 2000), about 3 million women worldwide had died of AIDS. About 10 million children were the victims of perinatal infection, and many of these were orphaned. The incidence of HIV-positive cases in antenatal clinics has risen from 2% to almost 4%–5% over the last 15 years. Many HIV-infected women choose to become pregnant, continue their pregnancies in spite of counselling and availability of medical termination of pregnancy (MTP) services.

PERINATAL HIV TRANSMISSION

The rate of perinatal transmission without drugs is estimated to be 20%–30%. It may occur as transplacental transmission, intrapartum spread of disease or postpartum transmission through lactation. The highest risk of vertical transmission of the disease is during labour. Administration of antiviral drugs to the mother during pregnancy and delivery has brought down the incidence of vertical transmission of HIV significantly to 1%. Neonatal administration of antiviral drugs and avoiding lactation have further made a downward dent into the incidence of neonatal disease.

DIAGNOSIS

Diagnosis of HIV infection is based on the initial screening test for specific antibodies using ELISA, usually against the core antigen or envelope antigen. All positive tests are confirmed by western blot. The median time between acquiring infection and AIDS is about 10 years. Clinical progress of the disease is monitored on the basis of CD_4 counts. It provides the basis for therapeutic intervention.

- At CD_4 counts of >500/mL, patients do not demonstrate evidence of immunosuppression.
- At CD_4 counts of 200–500/mL, patients are likely to develop symptoms and in need of intervention.
- At CD_4 counts of <200/mL, patients often present with oral thrush, unexplained fever and increasing lassitude.

The 'window period' mentioned earlier mandates repeat test for antibodies in 6 months in a suspected case because of false-negative result in the first sample. Testing for virus becomes positive earlier than testing for antibodies (window period).

TREATMENT

- Screening for HIV should be offered to all pregnant women and all those at risk.
- Pregnant women suffering from HIV infection are at an increased risk of infections such as TB, bacterial pneumonitis and PCP. Prophylaxis against PCP includes aerosolized pentamidine. It appears to be safe during pregnancy. Cotrimoxazole (TMP/SMX-DS) is prescribed to prevent opportunistic infections; Pap smear is done periodically.

NACO

With a view to control HIV infection, the National AIDS Control Organization (NACO) was established in India.

Along with other voluntary and foreign collaborations, this organization works towards:

1. Mapping and screening high-risk cases of HIV infection, i.e. sex workers, single migrants, lorry drivers, homosexuals and injectable drug abusers.
2. Treating HIV-infected cases free of cost and follow-up.
3. Avoiding spread of infection from husband to wife, and vice versa, through adoption of barrier contraception and preventing spread to offspring through adoption of proper hygienic practices.
4. Taking care of affected children and orphans.
5. Educating the public, particularly the adolescents, regarding sex education and contraceptives.

STRATEGIES TO PREVENT PERINATAL TRANSMISSION

- Decreased fetal viral exposure by preventing chorioamnionitis and decreasing the duration of labour. Decrease the contact of the fetus from infected maternal fluids by preventing rupture of membranes and mucosal inflammation. This practice has led to increase in rates of elective caesarean section.
- Initiate zidovudine (Retrovir) therapy. If the maternal CD_4 count is less than 500/mL and the viral load by DNA-PCR is 10,000 copies/mL, then it is advised to initiate zidovudine at 14–16 weeks of gestation. The recommended dosage is 600 mg per day in two to three divided doses. The drug is teratogenic in the first trimester (neural tube defect) and causes maternal anaemia and neutropenia.
- *A larger viral* load *with a low CD_4 count mandates triple-drug therapy after proper counselling.*
- Intrapartum therapy consists of administration of zidovudine 2.0 mg/kg i.v. during the first hour of labour, followed by 1.0 mg/kg per hour throughout the rest of labour. Avoid amniotomy, fetal scalp electrodes and intrauterine pressure catheters. Later, advise on safe sex practices (barrier contraception) and postpartum contraception. It is preferable to avoid lactation. However, in poor countries, this advice may not be practical where exclusive breastfeeding (not even water) is advised.

Fetal therapy: Maternal administration of zidovudine is associated with decreased risk of vertical transmission by as much as two-thirds in mildly affected asymptomatic women. Maternal zidovudine therapy is followed by 6 weeks of neonatal zidovudine therapy in oral doses of 2.0 mg/kg i.v. every 6 hours for 6 weeks.

In the latest revised guidelines for treating HIV infection during pregnancy, WHO recommends use of triple-drug regimen throughout pregnancy comprising lamivudine, tenofovir and efavirenz irrespective of the CD4 counts.

ANTIRETROVIRAL THERAPY (ART)

Options for directly treating HIV-infected women have greatly increased since the introduction of zidovudine, a retroviral drug that inhibits reverse transcriptase. Early trials with zidovudine monotherapy demonstrated a survival advantage and delay in the progression of AIDS-defining illnesses. More recent studies have focused on combination therapies such as zidovudine with didanosine or zalcitabine. Zidovudine with lamivudine may be a superior choice (Fig. 29.12). Protease inhibitors such as ritonavir and indinavir appear more efficacious, possibly because of better bioavailability. Data from short-term clinical trials suggest that combinations of zidovudine with ritonavir or indinavir demonstrated dramatically improved viral burdens and CD_4 counts. The combined therapy is popularly known as highly active antiretroviral therapy (HAART). Three or more drugs in combination with different modes of action are used in HAART.

Lately, WHO has come out with revised guidelines for the treatment of HIV infection in 2016.

In HIV-positive women, the main gynaecological problems to deal with are as follows:

1. To detect other associated STDs and treat them.
2. Prevent further viral load (horizontal transmission) by using barrier contraceptives.
3. To avoid pregnancy and vertical transmission to the offspring by using contraceptives. Barrier methods are not effective, so 'dual contraceptives' are recommended by adding hormonal contraceptives or emergency contraceptives.

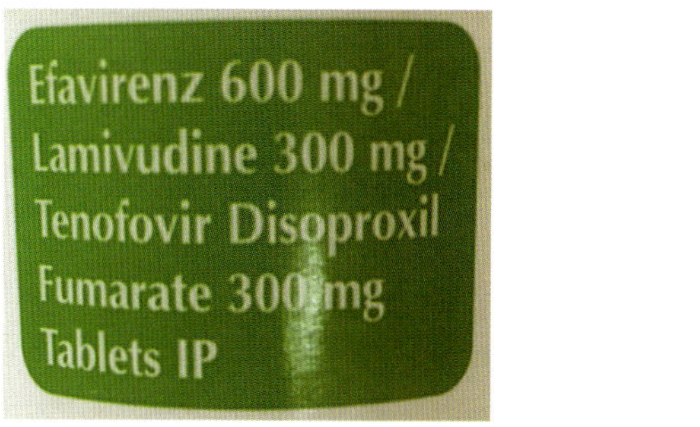

Figure 29.12 ART in pregnancy.

4. Regular Pap smear to detect cervical intraepithelial neoplasia (CIN). Excisional therapy is superior to ablation to avoid recurrence if CIN exists.
5. Vitamin A improves immunity. Avoid smoking and drug abuse.
6. Hepatitis B: Hepatitis B virus (HBV), a DNA virus, can be transmitted sexually, though the partner may remain an asymptomatic carrier, more so in HIV infected patients. The transmission is avoided by prophylactic vaccine 1 mL at zero, first and sixth months.

A single dose of nevirapine during labour and to the newborn reduces the risk by 50%.

PROPHYLAXIS

The medical and other personnel exposed to the viral infection should receive combined drugs within 2–4 hours of exposure but definitely not later than 72 hours. Needless to say, it is important to screen the women for other STDs and treat them.

CONTRACEPTION

Barrier methods in the form of condom help prevent horizontal transmission between the partners. Though female condom is also effective, diaphragm use does not protect the woman, as considerable portion of the vagina is exposed to infection. Spermicidal agents also are not effective. Circumcision in males has proved to reduce the horizontal transmission by 70%.

If the woman is taking antiviral drugs, intrauterine contraceptive device (IUCD) can be inserted. If not on therapy or if she is suffering from other STDs, IUCD is not suitable for contraception, as it increases the risk of PID.

Oral combined pills are excellent contraceptives against pregnancy but do not protect against viral infection. Rather, the antiviral drugs reduce the bioavailability of the contraceptive hormones, making them less effective than in HIV-negative women. They, however, will improve the contraceptive effect of the condoms.

Surgical methods are not contraindicated but require additional condom use to also prevent horizontal transmission.

Dual contraception, one to stop transmission of infection (barrier) and one to prevent pregnancy, is strongly recommended.

Oral pills are contraindicated if the woman is taking anti-TB drugs. Cerazette (progestogen-only pill) is permissible as a contraceptive pill or 3-monthly progestogens such as DMPA is effective.

DRUGS

Several drugs are now available, but HAART (combination of drugs) is the best choice.

- Zidovudine 300 mg b.d.
- Lamivudine 150 mg b.d.

One of the aforementioned drugs plus one of the following:

- Tenofovir 300 mg daily
- Nelfinavir 1250 mg b.d.
- Lopinavir/ritonavir three capsules b.d. or indinavir 800 mg daily

Instead of zidovudine, stavudine 30–40 mg b.d. depending upon the body weight can be given.

Instead of lamivudine, didanosine 400 mg daily (250 mg in a thin woman) may be added.

During therapy, haemoglobin, total leucocyte count (TLC), differential leucocyte count (DLC) and liver function tests should be performed periodically. These drugs cause lactic acidosis, which can cause pregnancy-induced hypertension. The drugs contraindicated during pregnancy are amprenavir and a combination of stavudine and didanosine.

The successful treatment does not prevent transmission. It definitely reduces the viral load and reduces the risk of transmission.

If an HIV-negative woman insists on pregnancy, intrauterine insemination with washed semen is safe. The virus does not attach to the sperm, and semen wash helps get rid of the virus. Unprotected intercourse only around ovulation is an option, though it may expose the woman to a slight risk of infection. An HIV-positive woman should use a barrier method but may be offered intrauterine insemination at ovulation so that the man is protected.

Breastfeeding: Either exclusive breastfeeding or total artificial feed is the mode of nutrition to the neonate. Mixed feeding with breast milk and formula feeds increases the risk of viral transmission and hence, contra-indicated.

All newborns to HIV-positive mothers are given nevirapine for a duration of 6 weeks. They can receive all immunizations except the BCG vaccine if they are HIV positive.

PROPHYLAXIS

An attempt to develop vaginal microbicides has failed, but it is hoped that tenofovir may prove more specific in preventing infection in future.

Tenofovir vaginal gel is expected to reduce transmission by 40%. No toxicity (renal) has been reported so far.

SCREENING (Table 29.7)

Table 29.7 Screening Recommendations for STDS (CDC, 2015)

Routine laboratory screening for common STDs is indicated for sexually active adolescents.

- Routine screening for *C. trachomatis* on an annual basis is recommended for all sexually active females younger than 25 years.
- Routine screening for *Neisseria gonorrhoeae* on an annual basis is recommended for all sexually active females younger than 25 years.
- HIV screening should be discussed and offered to all adolescents. Frequency of repeat screenings of those who are at risk for HIV infection should be based on the level of risk.
- The routine screening of adolescents who are asymptomatic for certain STDs (e.g. syphilis, trichomoniasis, and BV, and HSV, HPV, hepatitis A virus [HAV] and HBV infection) is not generally recommended.
- Cervical cancer screening begins at the age of 21 years.

SEXUALLY TRANSMITTED INFECTIONS AND INFERTILITY

A link between STIs and infertility is well recognized. According to the WHO report, almost 90 million STI-related infertility cases are recorded annually. The highest prevalence is reported in sub-Saharan Africa. The risk factors for acquiring an STI are young age when indulging in sexual activity (younger than 30 years), multiple sex partners, no use of barrier contraceptives and sex workers.

STIs cause infertility both in men and in women by several mechanisms.

Gonococci and *C. trachomatis* are mainly responsible for infertility, with other organisms playing a minor role. Recently, *M. genitalium* was discovered to be one of the causal agent of infertility. With decreased prevalence of *N. gonorrhoea, C. trachomatis* is now the commonest organism causing infertility.

In a male, gonorrhoea causes urethritis initially, but chronic infection can ascend to cause epididymitis and orchitis and damage the upper genital tract. It is reported that unilateral epididymo-orchitis results in infertility in 25% of cases, but bilateral infection is responsible for as much as 40% of cases of infertility. In women, it causes PID and tubal damage.

Chlamydia trachomatis is often a silent infection in both sexes (75% in females, 50% in males), but it causes extensive damage in the fallopian tube and impairs sperm morphology and sperm function by causing fragmentation of sperm nuclei, reducing motility and apoptosis (sperm death) via lipopolysaccharide component of *Chlamydia* and intracellular changes in the tyrosine phosphorylation in the sperm. With azithromycin or doxycycline, infection can be eradicated, but recurrence is not uncommon. Therefore, it is suggested that a vaccine such as that developed for HPV is the best option to prevent chlamydial infection and is under research.

Mycoplasma genitalium is sexually transmitted. It colonizes in the cervix, ascends upwards and causes PID in the female. It is difficult to culture because it takes months to cultivate and other mycoplasmas overgrow in the meantime. Now with PCR, it is possible to detect this organism.

PRACTICAL APPROACH TO COMMON VAGINAL INFECTIONS

A woman is liable to several infections in the lower genital tract, most common of which are gonorrhoea, chlamydial infection, *Trichomonas* infection, monilial infection and BV. The tests and cultures take time, are costly and invite more visits to the clinic.

Lately, therefore, 'syndromic management' approach is implemented. This consists of giving multiple-drug therapy in one sitting and comprises 1 g azithromycin, 2 g metronidazole and 150 mg fluconazole. Only those who fail to respond or those who are resistant are subjected to detailed investigations.

The following are the advantages of this approach:

1. One visit
2. Cost-effective in most cases
3. Quicker treatment

Disadvantage is perhaps the woman will receive unnecessary multiple therapies if only one organism is involved.

HEPATITIS B VIRUS

HBV is a DNA virus that can be transmitted sexually, though the partner may remain the asymptomatic carrier. This infection can be avoided by prophylactic vaccination with 1 mL of hepatitis B vaccine at 0, 1 and 6 months.

STDS IN ADOLESCENTS

There has been an upsurge in the incidence of STDs amongst the younger generation in present times. Economic and social liberalization, widespread education, increase in social networking opportunities, migration for work, greater opportunities for interaction and intermingling between the sexes, and changing moral values in society have contributed to this increase in the prevalence of STDs.

The incidence of STDs is higher in homeless people, runaway adolescents and those in detention facilities. There has been a noticeable rise in the incidence of chlamydial infections and veneral warts. The practice of HBV vaccination has reduced the prevalence of hepatitis B infections. HIV infections are more common amongst drug users and alcoholics. Adolescents are often tempted to respond to their physical and emotional changes by indulging in high-risk sexual behaviours to gain peer group approval; they are often ignorant of the consequences that may follow or wilfully choose to ignore them. It is not unusual to find them in relationship with multiple partners and failing to use barrier contraceptives. Clinicians treating adolescents should bear in mind to use on-site single-dose antibiotics whenever possible because of the unreliability of adolescents to return for treatment. This opportunity should be utilized to educate them about the use of condoms and to recommend immunizations whenever available. An attempt should be made to treat the partner as well.

KEY POINTS

- STIs mostly affect young people and young women in reproductive years. Syphilis, gonorrhoea, chlamydial infection and, lately, HIV infection are recognized as major STIs.
- Condyloma acuminatum is caused by HPV infection (HPV 6, 11). High-risk HPV infection (HPV 16 and 18) is closely associated with development of intraepithelial neoplasia and subsequent invasive carcinoma of the vulva and cervix. It requires adequate treatment and follow-up.
- HPV vaccine is now available as prophylactic vaccine against HPV and needs to be given ideally before the start of sexual activity.
- Herpes virus II accounts for recurrent painful vulval ulcers. Acyclovir ointment or oral drug is the treatment of choice.
- Syphilis is a systemic disease which starts as genital infection, posing health problem in cardiovascular

(CVS) and central nervous systems (CNS) in long-standing cases. It can cause late abortions, stillbirth and congenital syphilis.
- Gonococcal and chlamydial infections often attack the urethra and cause vaginal infection. Ascending infection is responsible for tubal damage, PID and infertility.
- Chlamydia is a silent infection but inflicts more tubal damage than gonorrhoea.
- Trichomonal and monilial infections can be easily recognized clinically and treated. Recurrent infection needs prolonged therapy.
- AIDS is a life-threatening health problem. HAART is a promising therapy both for the woman and for her offspring, and vertical transmission can be reduced from 30% to 2%.
- HIV-positive women need regular follow-up with Pap smear, dual contraceptives and screening for other STDs.
- BV accounts for 40%–50% of cases of vaginal discharge, 20%–25% for monilial infection and 10%–15% for *Trichomonas* infection.

SELF-ASSESSMENT

1. Enumerate the STDs encountered in clinical practice.
2. Discuss the management of chlamydial infection.
3. How would you manage a patient with gonorrhoea?
4. Discuss the management of HIV infections.
5. Discuss the problems of STDs in adolescents.

SUGGESTED READING

American College of Obstetricians and Gynecologists. Healthcare for Adolescents. Washington, DC: ACOG, 2003.

Burstein GR, Gaydos CA, Diener-West M, et al. Incidental chlamydial trachomatis infections in inner-city adolescent females. JAMA 1998; 280: 521–26.

Holmes KK, Mardh PA, Sparlin PF, et al. Sexually Transmitted Diseases. 3rd Ed. New York, McGraw-Hill, 1999.

Revised guidelines for HIV counseling, testing, and referral and revised recommendations for HIV screening of pregnant women. Centers for Disease Control and Prevention. MMWR Recomm Rep 2001; 50(RR-19): 1–86

Sexually transmitted diseases, treatment guidelines. Centers for Disease control and Prevention. MMWR Recomm Rep 2002; 51(RR-6): 1–78.

SECTION 6

URINARY AND INTESTINAL TRACT IN GYNAECOLOGY

SECTION OUTLINE

30 Diseases of the Urinary Tract

CHAPTER OUTLINE

Urinary symptoms are frequently complained by the gynaecological patients. Gynaecological disorders and pelvic operations often contribute towards their occurrence or aggravation. On occasions, the underlying disease may be neurological and has no gynaecological bearing. Hence, it is important for the gynaecologist to identify urinary problems attributable to gynaecological causes in order to institute rational therapy. The establishment of a proper diagnosis will call for a detailed history, meticulous examination and often a full urological workup including laboratory tests, cystoscopy, radiological evaluation, cystometry and ultrasound scanning.

Often a sole kidney may be located in the pelvis and mistaken for a tumour. The dire consequence of its removal in a mistaken identity is very obvious.

Because of the close association between the urinary and genital organs embryologically, malformation of one organ may also reveal malformation of the other and it should be searched for.

COMMON URINARY SYMPTOMS

Common urinary symptoms include difficulty in micturition, retention and incontinence of urine (Fig. 30.1).

Acute urinary retention follows sudden inability to void urine. The condition causes discomfort and pain. Catheterization yields a large volume of urine. Detailed interrogation often reveals the underlying cause. An attempt should be made to exclude the neurological causes (especially in patients who experience inability to void urine but experience no painful sensation). Most patients with disorders of bladder sensation experience pain rather than lack of bladder sensation. Elderly women, smokers and those with chemical exposure are vulnerable to bladder cancer; accompanying haematuria must raise the suspicion of underlying cancer.

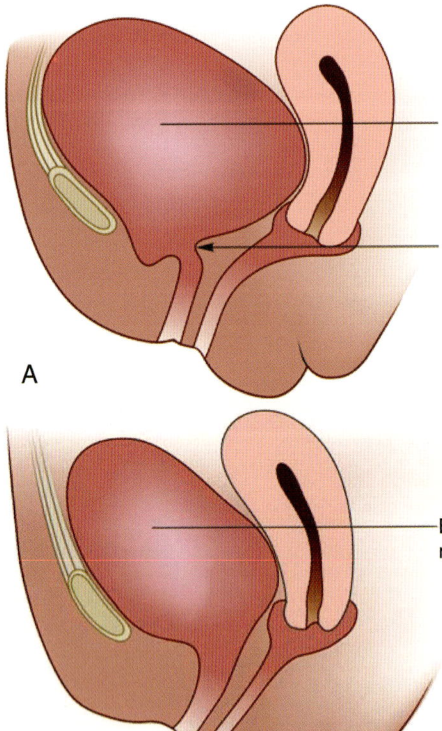

Figure 30.1 A tracing of the urethra and the bladder: **(A)** At rest and **(B)** during micturition.

ACUTE RETENTION OF URINE (Table 30.1)

CAUSES

Several conditions may lead to the occurrence of retention of urine.

POSTOPERATIVE RETENTION

Urinary retention is common after surgical operations of the vagina and perineum. Postoperative oedema may cause

Table 30.1 Causes of Acute Retention of Urine in Gynaecology

1. Postoperative retention
2. Retroverted gravid uterus
3. Urinary infection
4. Prolapse of the uterus with cystocele
5. Tumours impacted in the pouch of Douglas
6. Ectopic pregnancy
7. Advanced cancers of cervix, vagina and vulva
8. Imperforate hymen

obstruction to the flow of urine, and pain in the pelvic region may lead to a reflex spasm of the bladder sphincter. Radical operations such as Wertheim's hysterectomy involves extensive dissection causing denervation of the bladder, leaving the patient with an insensitive bladder resulting in retention of urine with overflow. The treatment of postoperative retention consists of timely and continuous catheterization until the residual urine volume comes down to less than 100 mL. Urinary antiseptics and analgesics should be concomitantly administered. Spinal and epidural anaesthesia accounts for retention of urine in the first 12–24 hours of the postoperative period. Surgery for stress urinary incontinence and the vagina also can cause retention of urine.

PUERPERAL RETENTION OF URINE

After delivery, the patient is often unable to appreciate the filling of the bladder as a result of bruising of the vagina and painful perineal wound.

OBSTRUCTIVE CONDITIONS

Obstructive conditions intrinsic to the urethra are rare. Cicatricial stenosis may follow surgery of the bladder neck for a fistula or lower down in the urethra for a caruncle. Inflammatory stenosis following gonorrhoea is rare in women. Sling operations for stress incontinence performed with undue enthusiasm may occlude the bladder neck and cause retention of urine, which can only be relieved by cutting the sling. Cancers of the cervix, vagina, bladder or urethra may lead to extensive tissue infiltration and obstruction to the flow of urine.

SPACE-OCCUPYING LESIONS IN THE PELVIS

Space-occupying lesions in the pelvis may obstruct the urethra or bladder neck region. Some of the lesions encountered are as follows:

- Haematocolpos in adolescent girls
- Retroverted gravid uterus at about 14 weeks of gestation
- Haematocele complicating an ectopic gestation
- Cervical myomas or a posterior uterine wall myoma impacted in the pouch of Douglas
- Ovarian neoplasm impacted in the pelvis

NEUROLOGICAL CAUSES

Spinal cord lesions, disseminated sclerosis, tabes dorsalis and denervation of the bladder during extensive surgery for a malignant disease in the pelvis are recognized causes.

Anticholinergic and antidepressant drugs may also cause retention.

CHRONIC RETENTION WITH OVERFLOW

Chronic retention of urine in old women is due to bladder neck narrowing owing to senile changes in urethra.

Treatment of Urinary Retention

In the presence of an organic lesion, attend to the removal of the primary cause.

Retention of urine due to a retroverted gravid uterus is encountered relatively frequently. This occurs between the 12th and 14th weeks of pregnancy when the retroverted gravid uterus fails to grow out of the pelvis into the abdomen. The anterior vaginal wall and the attached urethra get unduly stretched as the retroverted gravid uterus sinks low into the pelvic cavity. Sometimes, the urethral meatus may be drawn upwards into the vagina. A soft rubber catheter can usually be passed into the bladder without difficulty, suggesting that rather than occlusion of the urethra, it is the disturbance of the reflex mechanism of voiding which causes the retention.

On examination, the full bladder is palpable as an abdominal mass. On pelvic examination, the cervix is lifted up high behind the symphysis pubis and the gravid uterus is palpable as a large mass filling up the pouch of Douglas.

The treatment consists of slow emptying of the bladder by an indwelling catheter draining into a sterile drainage bag over 12–14 hours. The patient is encouraged to lie down on her face so that posture and gravity assist the gravid uterus to assume the anteverted position. Digital reposition of the gravid uterus is neither safe nor successful, hence not recommended.

URETHRAL SYNDROME

A patient with urethral syndrome is usually a postmenopausal woman with complaints of dysuria, frequency of micturition and occasional stress incontinence. Urine is sterile. The cause of urethral syndrome is oestrogen deficiency at menopause causing weakening of the internal urethral sphincter and urethral mucosal changes. Oestrogen cream applied vaginally improves the blood supply to the urethral sphincter and urethral mucosa and improves the symptoms in about 3 months.

In a young woman, urethral syndrome is associated with sterile urine, but the presence of pus cells indicates probable infection with tubercle bacilli or Chlamydia.

DIFFICULT MICTURITION

Difficulty in emptying the bladder is a symptom present with those conditions which eventually produce retention of urine. It also occurs in growth of the bladder and urinary calculi. One of the most common gynaecological causes of difficulty in micturition is a severe degree of prolapse of the anterior vaginal wall and procidentia. When such patients strain to micturate, the anterior vaginal wall prolapses further and the bladder descends so that a large sacculation of the bladder comes to lie below the level of the internal urinary meatus. The more the patient strains, the less likely is she to empty her bladder, as the urine is forced down into the cystocele instead of the urethra. The only way the act of micturition can be started by the patient is by her own digital manipulation by pushing back the prolapsed anterior vaginal wall and the uterus this is termed "splinting". Treatment consists of anterior colporrhaphy, combined with a pelvic floor repair, and vaginal hysterectomy if indicated.

PAINFUL MICTURITION

Pain may be experienced either during or immediately following the act of micturition. Pain during micturition is usually of vesical origin due to infection but may be of urethral origin and referred to the urethra itself, whereas an intrinsic lesion of the bladder gives rise to bladder spasm felt in the mid-hypogastrium so that, as soon as the patient has voided urine, she has an urge to pass urine again, though the bladder is empty. Gonococcal urethritis causes scalding pain, as urine passes over the inflamed mucous membrane. Other causes of painful micturition are tender caruncles at the meatus, prolapse of the urethral mucous membrane and disease of the vulva such as kraurosis and carcinoma of the urethral meatus. The recently consummated marriage somewhat traumatizes the urethra and leads to pain and frequency of micturition. This has been called **honeymoon cystitis**. All operations performed upon or near the urethra and instrumentation of the canal, even with a soft catheter, cause some degree of dysuria. Painful micturition is a prominent symptom in cystitis; the pain is experienced at the end of micturition when the inflamed surfaces of the bladder come into apposition. Other conditions which cause painful micturition are papilloma, carcinoma, tuberculosis and stone. One important cause of dysuria and pain is radiation cystitis, which in severe degrees can cause a small-capacity irritable bladder. This is seen after a radium treatment of carcinoma of the cervix and can be very distressing. The urine should be examined in all cases where the symptom is present and the presence of infection excluded or confirmed by culture. Cystourethroscopy must be performed to exclude the presence of the more serious causes of dysuria. The postradiation bladder often shows telangiectasia of the vessels in the region of the trigone.

INCREASED FREQUENCY OF MICTURITION

Voiding urine more than eight times during day and more than once during night is considered frequency of micturition. Frequency of micturition is one of the most common symptoms complained of by gynaecological patients, and although many causes of frequency lie in the urinary tract, a large number are gynaecological in origin. The nongynaecological causes are diabetes mellitus, diabetes insipidus or polyuric phase of renal failure when urinary output increases. Frequency of micturition is present when the patient passes small amount of urine at short intervals, and it is often associated with other symptoms of bladder irritability such as urgency of micturition and incontinence. Common causes of cystitis include *Escherichia coli* infection, tuberculous infection, stone or growth. Frequency of micturition is a normal symptom of early pregnancy and develops again during the last few weeks when the presenting part enters the pelvis. Pressure upon the bladder by pelvic tumours such as myomas of the uterus and ovarian cysts can also cause frequency. Patients with cystocele often complain of the symptom because chronic cystitis results from incomplete emptying of the bladder. Inflammatory swellings around the bladder such as parametritis and inflamed appendages can also lead to frequency of micturition. Infiltration of the bladder by carcinoma of the cervix or of the vagina can cause frequency of micturition. Apart from the urological causes, this symptom also develops in retention overflow when the bladder is overdistended. One very important cause of frequency is bladder neurosis. In the fully established bladder neurosis, the patient's life is ultimately dominated by her bladder—though this at first happens only in the day time. The condition is readily misdiagnosed as stress incontinence. The urine is sterile, with normal cystoscopy, and no local cause is discoverable.

The investigation of frequency of micturition requires, in addition to the usual gynaecological examination, a complete examination of the urine, urine culture test, cystoscopy and intravenous pyelography, and ultrasound scanning.

Treatment is by simple applied psychotherapy, bladder discipline and sedatives. Increased frequency due to an organic lesion, usually cystitis, occurs equally at night as during the day, and the nocturia score gives a rough indication of the severity of the condition.

Other causes of frequency need prompt treatment.

INCONTINENCE OF URINE

In true incontinence of urine which is due to a vesicovaginal or ureterovaginal fistula, the urine is discharged involuntarily and continuously so that the patient is constantly wet; the bladder is always empty without residual urine in the case of a vesicovaginal fistula and contains only half the expected normal in the case of an ureterovaginal fistula. True or complete incontinence of urine is present besides urinary fistulae in malformations such as ectopia vesicae, ectopic ureter opening into the vagina and in some diseases of the spinal cord.

False or partial incontinence is much more common. It is exemplified by the nocturnal enuresis in young girls when the urine is voided during sleep and when local reflex caused by threadworms may be found. One of the most common types of partial incontinence is the stress urinary incontinence with prolapse of the anterior vaginal wall. In this condition, the patient voids very small quantities of urine involuntarily while sneezing, coughing or laughing. The condition also develops during pregnancy and immediately after delivery during the early weeks of the puerperium, although the majority of symptoms tend to disappear with time. An important condition that is readily confused with stress incontinence is urge incontinence. In this condition, the patient must pass urine at a moment's notice and, unless she is quick about it, she is unable to control her bladder, which empties some of its contents before she can reach the washroom. As a point of differential diagnosis from stress incontinence, the amount of urine lost in urge incontinence is always considerable and sometimes the bladder is completely emptied involuntarily. This catastrophe is preceded by an extreme desire to pass urine. In stress incontinence, the amount of urine lost is minimal and measurable (a few millilitres), and there is no previous desire to pass urine. Urge incontinence is more common than true stress incontinence. The condition is essentially due to detrusor instability, which overcomes the normal urethral sphincter. Cystoscopy is normal apart from a decreased bladder capacity. The condition is largely functional, but there may be an organic base. For example, urge incontinence is often associated with true cystitis or urinary infection.

CYSTITIS

The female urethra always contains microorganisms such as coliform bacilli, streptococci, staphylococci and Döderlein's bacilli, which should be regarded as its normal inhabitants. These microorganisms neither cause urethritis unless the urethral tissues are damaged nor do they spread upwards to the bladder unless they are transported by catheterization. The catheter is undoubtedly the most common cause of lower urinary tract infection (UTI). However gentle and meticulous aseptic the technique is, no matter of what material the catheter is made of, once it has been passed, there remains a danger of infection.

As the catheterization is almost an integral part of all deliveries and of all gynaecological operations, the incidence of cystitis must be accepted at a figure in the region of 80%, understandably highest in those patients requiring frequent catheterization or an indwelling catheter. The logical answer is to abolish the use of catheters as a routine preoperative measure in minor pelvic surgery and only to use them when strictly indicated, in which case a urinary antiseptic is a prudent prophylactic precaution.

Another cause of infection of the bladder is by a descending infection from the kidney, such as that may occur with renal tuberculosis and chronic pyelonephritis. Organisms may also reach the bladder from adjacent structures such as an inflamed cervix and parametritis infections. The bladder may perhaps be infected by way of the bloodstream and in other cases by lymphatic spread from the genitalia or the bowel. The organisms found in urine in cystitis are *E. coli*, *Klebsiella*, streptococci, staphylococci, *Bacillus proteus*, the tubercle bacilli and occasionally other organisms such as *Pseudomonas pyocyanea*. Gonococcal cystitis is relatively rare. The organism which is found most frequently is *E. coli*. This organism is now supposed to attack the bladder secondarily to an original infection by other organisms and subsequently to overgrow and replace the primary infection. On the contrary, it is well established that cystitis due to a primary *E. coli* infection is occasionally encountered. As the result of antibiotic treatment, *P. pyocyanea* sometimes becomes the dominant infecting organism because of its resistance to antibiotics relative to the other infecting organisms.

SYMPTOMS

The symptoms and signs of cystitis are painful and frequent micturition, pain in the region of bladder, strangury and passage of pus in the urine. As the bladder fills up with urine, its sensitive inflamed mucous membrane causes pain and a desire to micturate. Pain is also experienced at the end of the act of micturition when the adjacent inflamed surfaces of the bladder come into contact. In urethritis, pain is felt as the urine is being voided. Frequency of micturition may be extreme, as the patient has to pass urine every 15 minutes. The symptoms of acute cystitis are severe, and patients are deprived of sleep and soon become exhausted. The temperature is often raised, but it soon falls if proper treatment is given. A persistent high temperature usually due to infection ascending to the kidney, causing pyelonephritis when constitutional symptoms are more marked and rigors may occur. With pyelonephritis, the kidney is always tender to palpation in the costovertebral angle, and the patient will complain of pain localized to the loin which radiates down the ureter into the lower quadrant of the abdomen. In chronic cystitis, pain and strangury are less prominent symptoms, but frequency of micturition and pyuria are always present. Chronic cystitis may persist for months or even years without causing symptoms and signs other than frequency of micturition and pyuria.

DIAGNOSIS

The diagnosis of acute cystitis is based on the characteristic symptoms and by an examination of the urine. Difficulty may be experienced in distinguishing between acute urethritis and acute cystitis. In acute urethritis, pain is experienced during the act of micturition. There is no abdominal pain or tenderness, and frequency is not extreme. In both conditions, the urine contains pus and microorganisms. In acute urethritis, harm may be done by catheterization or cystoscopy, because the instrumentation may carry infection to the bladder. Similarly, the inflamed mucous membrane is readily damaged and bleeds easily. Urethritis can be diagnosed by massaging the urethra against the back of the symphysis pubis when pus will be expressed from the external meatus. Another simple method of distinguishing between acute urethritis and cystitis is the three-glass test; in urethritis, the third specimen will be clear of pus, but more contaminated with pus in cystitis.

TREATMENT

Cystitis must be treated by giving urinary antiseptics along with the administration of large quantities of fluids by mouth, at least 2.5 L every 24 hours. Plain water, alkaline drinks, milk and weak tea should be given. Alcohol in any form is contraindicated, as it aggravates the symptoms. In the acute phase, the patient must stay in the bed and some relief may be obtained by the application of a hot water bottle over the bladder region. The pain is best treated with spasmolytics such as codeine and belladonna. Large quantities of citrates should be given by mouth, as much as 3 g of potassium citrate given three to four times a day.

The organisms which have been cultured are as a routine tested for sensitivity against the various antibiotics, and the bacteriological report will indicate which drug should be used for a given patient. Most of the lower UTIs are due to *E. coli*, which is nearly always sensitive to nitrofurantoin, so this drug is particularly useful as a prophylactic and as specific therapy for the established infection. Drugs such as norfloxacin, ciprofloxacin, pefloxacin and sparfloxacin in appropriate doses have been found to be very effective and are amongst the first-line drugs selected by clinicians in present-day practice.

CHRONIC CYSTITIS

Chronic cystitis caused by descending infection from the kidney is a urological problem, and patients with chronic cystitis should be seen by a urologist.

PYELONEPHRITIS (PYELITIS)

Pyelonephritis is an infection of the upper urinary tract involving kidneys, mostly a complication of the lower urinary tract infections. The urinary infections of postoperative and puerperal cystitis often spread to the kidneys to cause pyelonephritis. Pyelonephritis in pregnancy is not uncommon, and the infective organism is usually *E. coli.* Ascending pyelonephritis is a common complication of advanced carcinoma of the cervix and vagina, either as a result of the growth ulcerating into the bladder or through involvement of the ureter by the growth, and a large number of patients with carcinoma of the cervix, at least 60%, die of uraemia induced by ureteric obstruction. Recurrent attacks of pyelonephritis also occur in patients who have had ureterocolic transplantation, either for the relief of incurable fistula or because the bladder has been removed in exenteration operation for advanced pelvic cancer. The signs and symptoms of pyelonephritis are pain and tenderness in the loins, with high temperature and frequent rigors, headache, vomiting and furring of the tongue. Frequency of micturition is present due to the associated cystitis. In acute pyelonephritis, the affected kidney region is exquisitely tender, whereas in chronic pyelonephritis, tenderness and rigidity along the course of the ureter can often be detected on abdominal examination. The urine is turbid and contains pus cells and bacteria. In acute pyelonephritis, toxaemia is well marked, the blood urea level is raised and casts are found in the urine.

TREATMENT

Treatment consists in keeping the patient in the bed lying on the unaffected side to prevent pressure upon the tender renal angle. Copious fluids must be administered. Systemic antibiotics, followed by oral fluid, should be given for 10–14 days. It often needs a referral to a urologist.

Pyelonephritis which does not respond to the usual methods of treatment or which recurs after initial successful treatment becomes a urological problem, and the patient should be transferred to the care of a urologist.

DISEASES OF THE FEMALE URETHRA

URETHRITIS

AETIOLOGY

Inflammatory disorders of the urethra are fairly common. Sexually transmitted diseases caused by the gonococcus, *Chlamydia trachomatis, Trichomonas, Candida* and certain viruses may lead to this disorder.

The lower urethra is usually affected, as vulvovaginitis is a common accompaniment. Frequent sexual intercourse often aggravates the problem. Honeymoon cystitis is a distinct clinical entity following coital injury to the urethra and the bladder base.

Menopausal women suffer from thinning of the vaginal epithelium and urethral lining due to oestrogen deficiency; these women are more susceptible to trauma and infection, which may lead to urethritis.

Use of chemicals, deodorants, douches, vaginal contraceptives and tampons may lead to allergic or chemical reactions causing vulvovaginitis and urethritis.

SYMPTOMS

The common symptoms of urethritis are frequency of micturition and dysuria. The patient complains of pain during micturition and not at the end of micturition as seen in cystitis. Examination may reveal an inflamed urethral orifice, and milking of the urethra may yield a purulent discharge. Culture and microscopy of the urethral discharge help establish the diagnosis.

TREATMENT

Treatment consists of administration of appropriate antimicrobials. Antibiotics such as ampicillin, nitrofurantoin or cephalosporins may be used as indicated by the culture. The patient should be encouraged to maintain an adequate fluid intake, and menopausal women should be given supplementary vaginal oestrogen cream to improve the atrophic state of the vagina and the urethra. The patient should be advised to avoid all irritants such as deodorants, vaginal contraceptives and douches.

URETHRAL CARUNCLE

Urethral caruncle is not an uncommon condition. It is frequently encountered in postmenopausal women. The atrophic vulva and vagina and introitus leave the urethral meatus exposed to infection. The posterior urethral mucosa becomes swollen, congested and pouts like a cherry from the posterior wall of the external meatus (Figs 30.2 and 30.3).

The patient may present with postcoital bleeding, dyspareunia, pain and dysuria. Before making a diagnosis of urethral caruncle as a cause of these symptoms, it is important to exclude genital tract malignancy by cytology, endometrial histology and sonographic evaluation of the pelvis.

The caruncle is treated by diathermy excision. Simultaneous administration of oestrogen helps in recovery, and this is prescribed on a long-term basis; intermittent progestogens must also be used to avoid uterine and breast cancer development as a result of long-term use of unopposed oestrogen. Local oestrogen cream may be preferred to oral hormone.

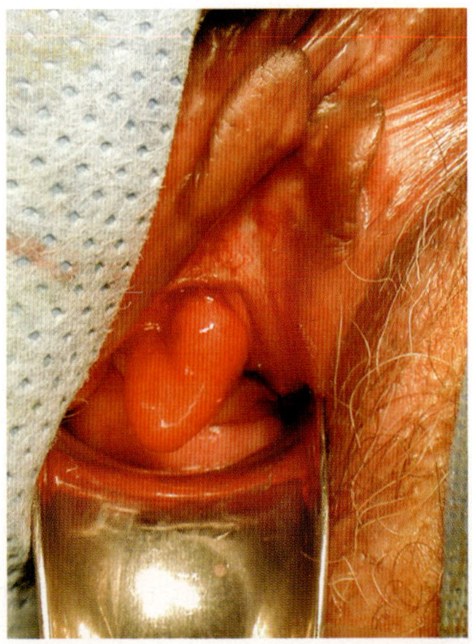

Figure 30.2 A urethral caruncle. (*Source*: V Nitti, N Rosenblum, B. Brucker, Vaginal Surgery for the Urologist. Benign Vaginal Wall Masses and Paraurethral Lesions. Saunders, 2012.)

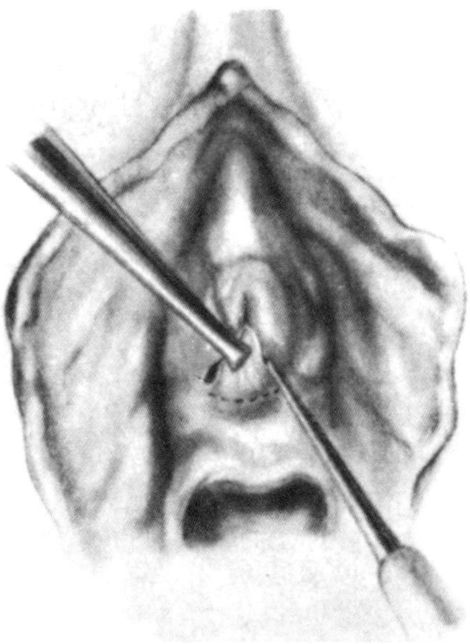

Figure 30.3 Operation for removal of urethral caruncle by diathermy excision.

URETHRAL PROLAPSE

This uncommon condition is seen in the very young and the old. Chronic straining and oestrogen deficiency contribute to its occurrence. Surgical excision of the excess of mucosa, followed by suturing of the urethral mucosa to the circumference of the urethral meatus by interrupted sutures, corrects the condition. Spontaneous prolapse of urethral mucosa is rarely seen in children.

URETHRAL DIVERTICULUM

The woman complains of nonspecific symptoms such as urinary frequency, dysuria, dyspareunia and dribbling, urgency or incontinence of urine. A swelling may be noted in the urethral region. The differential diagnosis includes urethrocele, Gartner's duct cyst or a Skene's gland abscess. Treatment comprises antibiotic therapy, followed by surgical excision or marsupialization. Urethral stricture and fistula are the likely postoperative complications.

URETHRAL STENOSIS

The common sites of narrowing are the region of the bladder neck and the meatus. It may be congenital in origin or as a result of infection, injury, neoplasm or a diverticulum. The patient complains of a poor stream, straining at micturition and repeated UTIs. Urethroscopy may reveal a narrowing of the passage and trabeculation of the walls of the bladder. Treatment consists of control of infection and surgical removal of any existing cyst or tumour. Intermittent urethral dilatation, urethrotomy and reconstructive urethroplasty may be needed in select cases.

URINARY FISTULAE

In women, most urinary fistulae result either from injury to the urinary tract during gynaecological operations or from obstetric damage. In India, obstetric fistulae are more common than the gynaecological or radiological fistulae because of difficult home deliveries conducted by dais when obstructed labour is not recognized. The most common form of fistula is vesicovaginal, in which there is a communication between the bladder and the upper third of the anterior vaginal wall. Next in order of frequency is ureterovaginal fistula, which is usually caused by injury to the ureter during gynaecological operations. Urinary fistulae can be classified as follows:

Vesical fistulae: Vesicovaginal, vesicocervical, vesicouterine, vesicoabdominal and vesicointestinal
Ureteric fistulae: Ureterovaginal and ureteroabdominal

Urinary fistulas have been described in detail in the chapter on Urinary Fistulas.

URETERIC OBSTRUCTION

Ureteric compression and obstruction occur from extraneous sources. Many conditions in the female pelvis are associated with ureteric obstruction. These are discussed as follows:

UTERINE PROLAPSE

In complete procidentia of the uterus, the main supporting structures, namely the Mackenrodt ligaments, are greatly elongated, and in their descent with the uterus, a loop of the ureter is drawn down on either side to lie outside the vaginal orifice. This process causes an acute angulation of the ureters. Hence, it is not surprising that it gives rise to hydroureter and hydronephrosis. The uterine arteries may also compress the ureters as they become elongated by the descent of the uterus. Many of these patients have a chronic urinary infection and this, associated with ureteric obstruction, may seriously impair the renal functions and render them in poor surgical risks for any repair operation. Vaginal tampons soaked in glycerin—acriflavine for several days preceding surgical repair of prolapse helps in decreasing changes in ureters.

PELVIC TUMOURS

Pelvic tumours may cause compression and obstruction to the ureter, and this is especially true of the myoma which lies firmly embedded in the pelvis. Ovarian cysts, benign and malignant, pelvic endometriosis and inflammatory disease, and broad ligament tumours produce the same picture. Such patients should have thorough urological investigations before operation because roughly half of them would show some ureteric obstruction and this may well account for postoperative urinary infection. Removal of these tumours will restore the urinary tract to normal in 70% of cases. The worst offenders are those in whom the obstruction is due to pelvic inflammatory disease or advanced cancer of the cervix where permanent stricture formation may have occurred in a segment of the ureter.

CARCINOMA OF THE CERVIX

Although the ureter is guarded by a tough sheath in the ureteric canal against actual malignant infiltration, its situation in this tunnel is a grave danger because it is particularly subject to compression. It is an absolute dictum that no case of cancer of the cervix should ever be treated by surgery or radiation therapy until a preliminary urographic study has been conducted. Those patients who show ureteric obstruction have a definitely poorer prognosis, and it must be remembered that in 70% of cases, patients with carcinoma of the cervix die not of their primary disease but of bilateral ureteric obstruction. In these patients, the surgeon's knife has been regarded in the past as a great menace to the ureter, but effective irradiation of an infiltrated parametrium is an equal if not greater menace, because the resulting fibrosis eventually strangles the ureter. This postradiation process is not immediate but may develop over months or even years, and the patient may well be cured of the local disease to succumb at a later date to the ureteric obstruction (see the chapter on Cervical Intraepithelial Neoplasia, Carcinoma of Cervix).

OBSTRUCTION AT THE SITE OF FISTULA

Many ureteric fistulae heal spontaneously and, although this is a gratifying process to the surgeon and the patient, the net result of such a cicatrix may be disastrous to the affected kidney. By the same token, ureteroureteric anastomosis of a ureter injured too high to be implanted into the bladder is unfortunately often followed by stricture formation at the site of the junction. Such a patient should be carefully followed up by a competent urologist. A periodic dilatation may well save the kidney, but many of these patients end up with a nephrectomy.

PREGNANCY AND URINARY PROBLEMS

All gynaecologists are conversant with the fact that pregnancy has a profound effect on the ureter and kidney. This is due to the specific action of progesterone on all smooth muscles throughout the body. The gastrointestinal tract and the gall bladder, the musculature of the veins, and the ligaments of the spine and the pelvis are all affected. The changes are most remarkable, however, in the urinary tract and appear by the fourth month to reach a maximum at term. After pregnancy, this process of hydroureter slowly resolves and returns to normal by the end of the puerperium, certainly by the third month. If, however, a severe infection occurs, such as in pyelonephritis of pregnancy, the process of involution may never be completed and permanent damage may result in chronic pyelonephritis. The cause of this ureteric dilatation is not the compression from the growing uterus because it occurs before such an obstruction can operate. It is more frequently noticed on the right than on the left side and is probably due to some distortion of the ureteric canal by dextrorotation and dextroposition of the pregnant uterus, which is so frequent a finding at caesarean section.

KEY POINTS

- Urinary symptoms are commonly encountered in gynaecological practice. The gynaecological diseases, pelvic operations and difficult vaginal deliveries contribute towards most of the urinary complaints.
- Neurological disorder may also be the underlying cause, so the gynaecologist must exclude the neurological cause before undertaking surgery for urinary complaints.
- Apart from postoperative and puerperal retention of urine, other obstructive conditions are haematocolpos, retroverted gravid uterus, fibroids, and an ovarian tumour and bladder neck obstruction in old women.
- Urethral syndrome is noticed in postmenopausal women due to oestrogen deficiency and is effectively treated with short-term oestrogen vaginal cream.
- Urinary fistula in developing countries is mostly obstetric in origin. In developed countries, urinary fistula follows trauma to the bladder during difficult surgery.

SELF-ASSESSMENT

1. How would you investigate and treat acute urinary retention in a woman?
2. Describe the urethral syndrome. How would you treat it?
3. Describe the management of dysuria.
4. Discuss the management of urinary incontinence in middle-aged women.
5. What are the clinical manifestations of infection of the female urinary system? Discuss its management.

SUGGESTED READING

Allen RE, Hosker GL, Smith ARB, et al. Pelvic floor damage and childbirth: A neurophysiological study. Br J Obstet Gynaecol 1990; 97: 770–9.

American College of Obstetricians and Gynecologists. Genitourinary Fistulas. ACOG Technical Bulletin 83. Washington, DC, ACOG, 1985.

Bhatia NN, Bergman A. Cystometry: Unstable bladder and urinary tract infection. Br J Urol 1986; 58: 134–7.

Burgio KL, Matthews KA, Engel BT. Prevalence, incidence and correlates of urinary incontinence in healthy middle-aged women. J Urol 1991; 146:1255–9.

Elia G, Bergman A. Estrogen effects on the urethra: Beneficial effects in women with genuine stress urinary incontinence. Obstet Gynecol Surv 1993; 48: 509–17.

Preminger GM. Acute urinary retention in female patients: Diagnosis and treatment. J Urol 1983;130: 112–3.

Urinary Incontinence Guideline Panel. Urinary Incontinence in Adults: Clinical Practice Guideline. Rockville, MD, Agency for Health Care Policy and Research. Public Health Service, U.S. Department of Health and Human Services, 1992, AHCPR publication no. 92-0038.

Wall LL. Diagnosis and management of urinary incontinence due to detrusor instability. Obstet Gynec Surv 1990; 45(Suppl): 1S–47S.

Urinary Fistula and Stress Urinary Incontinence

31

CHAPTER OUTLINE

The urinary system and the female genital system are closely related embryologically, anatomically and functionally. It is therefore not surprising that urinary fistulae result from obstetric and gynaecological operations and gynaecological diseases. A urinary fistula is one of the most distressing conditions for a woman, for her family members and equally for a gynaecologist who looks after such a patient.

URINARY FISTULAE

Urinary fistulae are abnormal epithelialized communication tracts between the genital tract and the urinary tract (Fig. 31.1).

Injuries to the urethra, bladder and ureter can occur during childbirth or during pelvic surgery. Genital tract malignancy in its advanced form is known to involve these pelvic organs and cause fistulae. Finally, radiation therapy can cause tissue necrosis and may result in fistula formation.

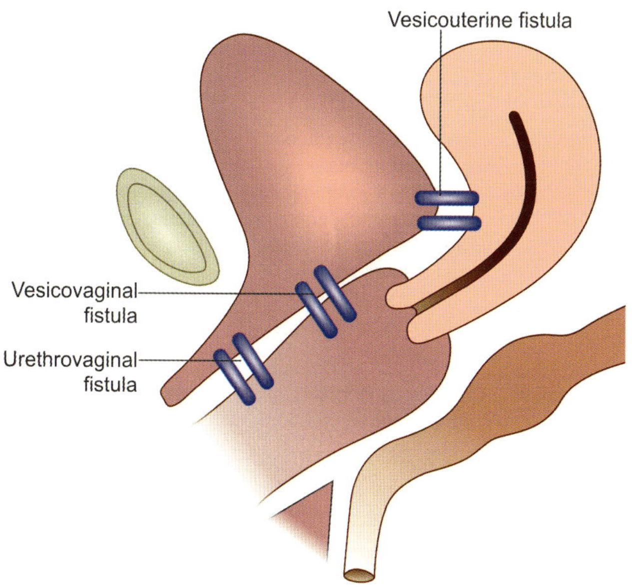

Figure 31.1 Diagrammatic representations of urethrovaginal, vesicovaginal and vesicouterine fistulae.

In developing countries, the vast majority of genital fistulae continue to be obstetric in origin. Even in the present times in rural India, it is not uncommon to encounter obstetric emergency cases of prolonged, neglected and obstructed labour. These potentially infected and dehydrated patients may often narrate the history of attempted manipulation or vaginal instrumentation which has failed to accomplish childbirth or resulted in a difficult traumatic delivery with poor perinatal outcome. In such women, the bladder and vaginal walls which have undergone prolonged ischaemic changes ultimately end up with tissue necrosis and fistula formation.

In developed countries, on the contrary, operative trauma during pelvic surgery constitutes the most common cause of genital fistulae.

AETIOLOGY

The common causes of genital fistulae are as follows:

OBSTETRIC CAUSES

Prolonged obstructed labour, difficult instrumental or manipulative deliveries such as forceps delivery or forceps rotation can cause injury to the bladder neck and the urethra. The surgeon must take care to avoid injury to the urinary bladder during caesarean section. The bladder is most vulnerable (particularly if it is not empty) during its mobilization from the front of the lower segment before making a transverse incision on the stretched lower segment to deliver the fetal head. Bladder injury may follow as a result of extension of the lower segment incision anteriorly to the bladder during delivery of a deeply impacted fetal head in the pelvis. The bladder or ureter may be inadvertently included in the suture line while suturing the lower uterine segment. Women undergoing repeat caesarean sections are at a higher risk for bladder injury. The use of cranial perforators and spicules of bone during craniotomy and symphysiotomy also cause injury. Rupture of uterus is another cause of urinary fistulae if the bladder is involved.

OPERATIVE INJURIES

The bladder and the pelvic ureter are vulnerable to injury during gynaecological surgery. These may result from poor exposure of the organs, faulty technique or due to distorted anatomy caused by tumour or fibrosis, or previous surgery. In Western countries, operative injuries during a gynaecological operation account for most of the urinary fistulae.

Bladder injury may ensue during its dissection from the cervix in abdominal or vaginal hysterectomy and during caesarean section when the bladder needs to be dissected from the lower uterine segment. The injury is most likely to occur in a woman with previous caesarean section. Other causes are pelvic adhesions, cervical fibroid and sling operations for stress urinary incontinence (SUI).

Ureteric injuries. Most of the ureteric injuries occur during gynaecological surgery, especially cancer surgery. Ureteric injuries can be serious if not recognized at operation. Only a third of the ureteric injuries are detected during surgery and repaired. Others are discovered only in the postoperative period.

The causes of ureteric fistula are as follows:

- **Congenital fistula** is rare and occurs in double ureters.
- **Direct injury** such as cutting (partial or complete), clamping, ligaturing or including it in a suture to obtain haemostasis.
- **Devascularization of ureter.** The ureter receives rich vascular supply on the lateral aspect of the ureter below the pelvic brim, and the dissection on the lateral aspect can cause avascularity. Devascularization follows denuding of the ureter and stripping it off its blood supply during cancer surgery.
- **Thermal injury** (cautery or laser cautery during laparoscopic surgery).

Sites of Ureteric Injury are as Follows

- **At the infundibulopelvic ligament.**
- **In ureteric tunnel.** Wertheim hysterectomy while dissecting the ureter in the parametrium.
- **Near the cervix and vaginal vault,** as the ureter is close to it and the uterine vessel also is proximal to it during hysterectomy. Clamping the uterine vessel may include the ureter anteriorly.
- **Near entry of the ureter in the bladder** during bladder dissection.
- **Near the pelvic brim,** during ligation of the internal iliac artery.
- **Near the uterosacral ligament.** During laparoscopic uterosacral nerve ablation, vault closure during hysterectomy and in endometriosis.

The risk of injury is high when the surgery is undertaken for pelvic endometriosis, pelvic inflammatory disease, cervical and broad ligament fibroid, as well as during Wertheim hysterectomy when the anatomy of ureter is distorted. The left ureter is closer to the cervix and is liable to injury, but, overall, it depends upon the position of the ureter.

Other nonsurgical injuries to the bladder occur due to criminal abortion, bladder stone, tuberculosis of the bladder, cancer of the bladder and cervix, radiotherapy for cancer of cervix and, rarely, in infections such as tuberculosis, lymphogranuloma venereum, schistosomiasis and actinomycosis.

RADIOTHERAPY

The bladder cannot tolerate the same dose of irradiation as the cervix. Hence, genital fistulae may follow in the course of time if due precautions are not taken to protect the bladder during radiotherapy.

LAPAROSCOPIC INJURIES

Direct trocar injuries to the urinary bladder have been reported, along with the injury to the ureter, bowel, sigmoid colon and rectum. Their timely identification and prompt repair prevent long-term sequelae.

ANATOMICAL CLASSIFICATION OF URINARY FISTULAE

It is important to group bladder fistulae according to their anatomical location. This has an important bearing on the selection of approach for surgical repair, the technique of repair, complications to be anticipated and prognosis (Fig. 31.1 and Table 31.1).

CLINICAL FEATURES (Table 31.2)

Women with urinary fistula complain of continuous leakage of urine in clothes. In case of vesicovaginal fistula (VVF), the woman is not able to pass urine whereas, in case of ureteric fistula, the woman complains of urinary incontinence in addition to, be able to pass urine. In urethrovaginal fistula, the woman notices incontinence only when she tries to pass urine.

Table 31.1 Classification of Urinary Fistulae

- Bladder: Vesicovaginal fistula
  Vesicocervical
  Vesicouterine
- Ureter: Ureterovaginal fistula
  Ureteroabdominal fistula
- Urethra: Urethrovaginal fistula

Table 31.2 Clinical Features of Fistulae

	Bladder Fistula	Ureteric Fistula
Aetiology	Mostly obstetric causes Prolonged labour – operative – vaginal caesarean section. Sometimes gynaecological causes such as sling operations for stress incontinence, hysterectomy	Mostly following gynaecological surgical procedures, sometimes following caesarean section
Clinical	Continuous dribbling of urine – no micturition	Continuous dribbling of urine but can also micturate
Methylene swab test	Swab stains with methylene blue	Swab stains with urine but not with methylene blue
IVP	Normal	Hydronephrosis on the affected side

The fistulous tract is lined by epithelium, fibrous and granulation tissues, or malignant tissue depending upon the cause.

VESICOVAGINAL FISTULA

In India, 80%–90% of the bladder fistulae are a result of the obstetrical causes. The patient presents with complaints of constant dribbling of urine (true incontinence). The constant wetness in the genital areas leads to excoriation of the vagina, vulva, perineum and thighs. These women are depressed and often treated as social outcasts. Some develop amenorrhoea and may develop bladder stones as well. The most common type of fistula in our country is VVF (Figs 31.2 and 31.3) at the bladder neck region following difficult childbirth. The woman with an obstetric fistula is invariably short statured with a contracted pelvis and suffers from secondary amenorrhoea. Whenever a fistula is suspected, it is a good practice to examine the patient in the knee–chest position under a good light. A speculum introduced to retract the posterior vaginal wall exposes the fistula, and urine is seen collecting in the vagina. It also enables clinical assessment of its size, location and number; a bimanual examination provides information about the size of fistula, its fixity and extent of scarring in the surrounding tissue. A positive methylene blue test confirms the diagnosis in case the fistula is not visible due to scarring in the vagina and helps the surgeon to plan a repair operation (Fig. 31.4).

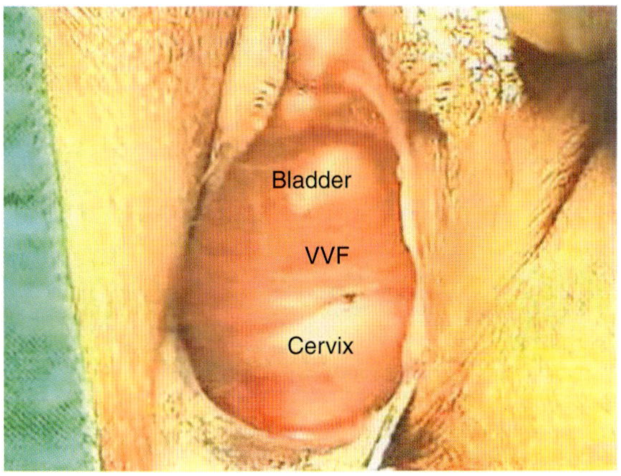

Figure 31.2 Vesicovaginal fistula.

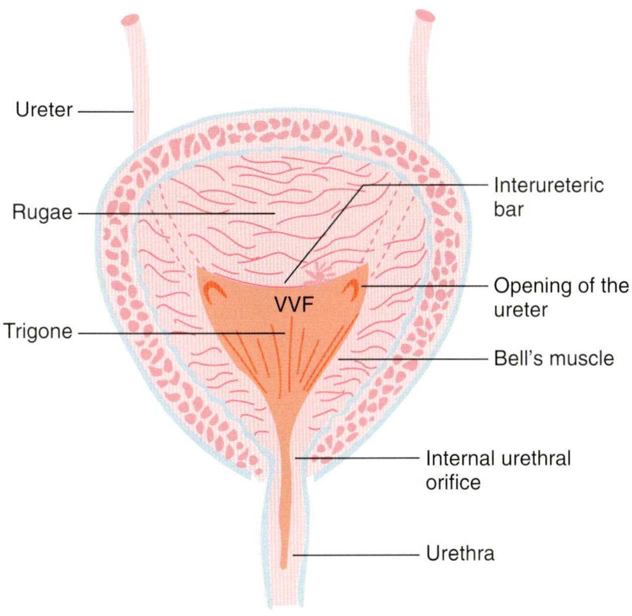

Figure 31.3 Transvesical view of vesicovaginal fistula.

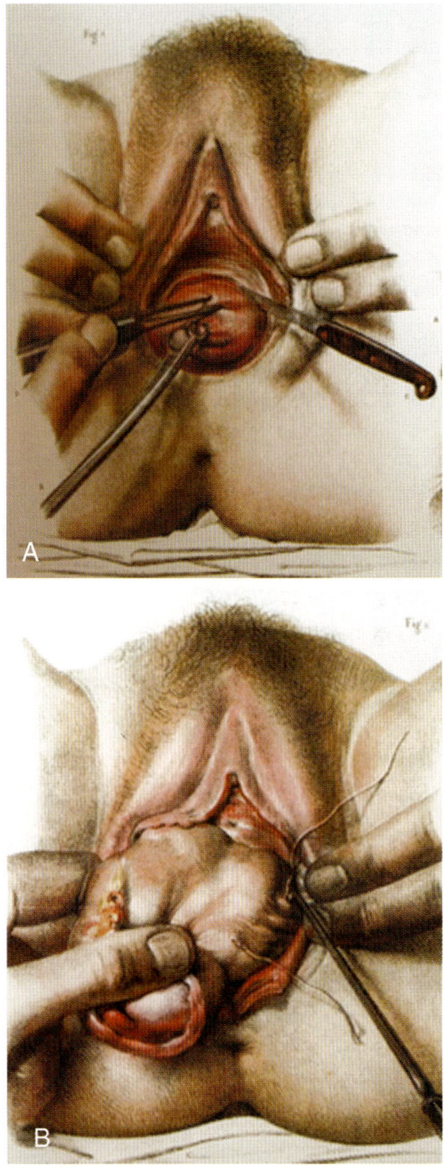

Figure 31.4 **(A)** Repair of a fistula. A circular incision is made through the vagina around the fistula. **(B)** Repair of a vesicovaginal fistula. The vaginal wall is now dissected away from the bladder with utmost care to obtain a maximum degree of mobilization of the bladder. (*Source*: M Walters and M Barber. Hysterectomy for Benign Disease: Female Pelvic Surgery Video Atlas Series, Saunders: 2010.)

URETERIC FISTULA (Figs 31.5–31.8)

Ureteric fistulae result from direct injury or devascularization of the pelvic ureters during gynaecological surgery, especially during Wertheim operation for carcinoma of the cervix.

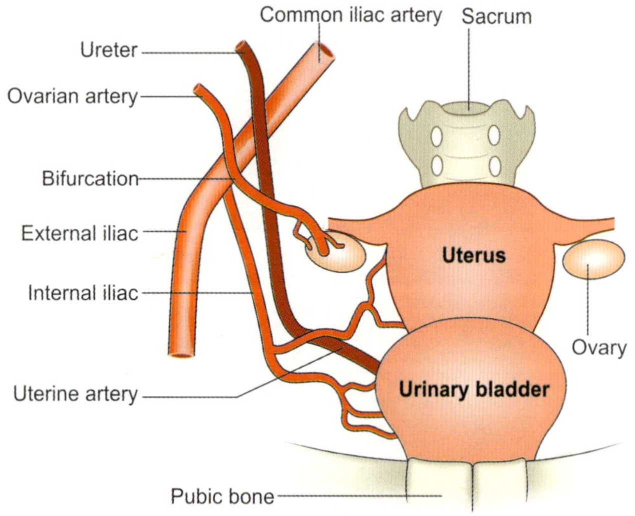

Figure 31.5 Relations of the pelvic ureter. It crosses the bifurcation of common iliac vessels, lies close to ovarian vessels and then crosses the uterine artery to enter the ureteric tunnel.

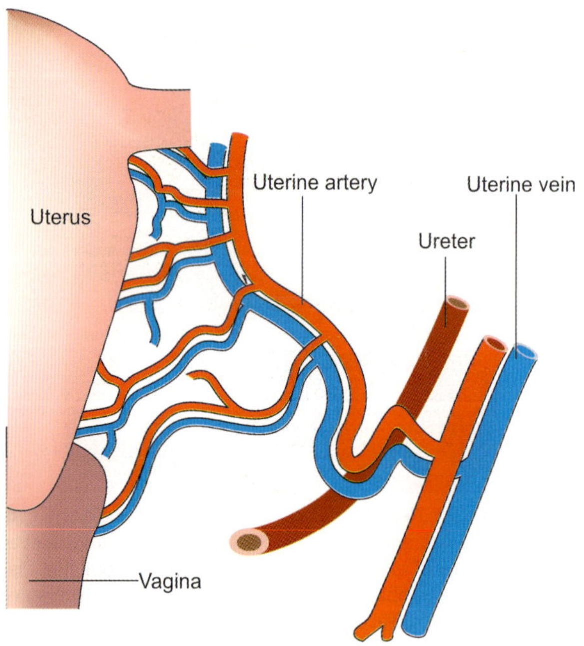

Figure 31.6 Uterine artery and ureter. The ureter crosses under the uterine artery.

In case of transection of the ureter, the woman develops urinary leak into the peritoneal cavity immediately. Because of failure to recognize and repair the trauma at the time of operation, these women have a stormy postoperative course and present with nausea and vomiting, abdominal distension and ileus, associated with the rise of temperature and leucocytosis, and loin pain.

In case of obstruction as a result of ligating one or both ureters, the clinical features differ. If both ureters have been tied (5%–10%), there is no passage of urine and the patient complains of pain in the flanks; palpation in the renal angles reveals tender enlarged kidneys.

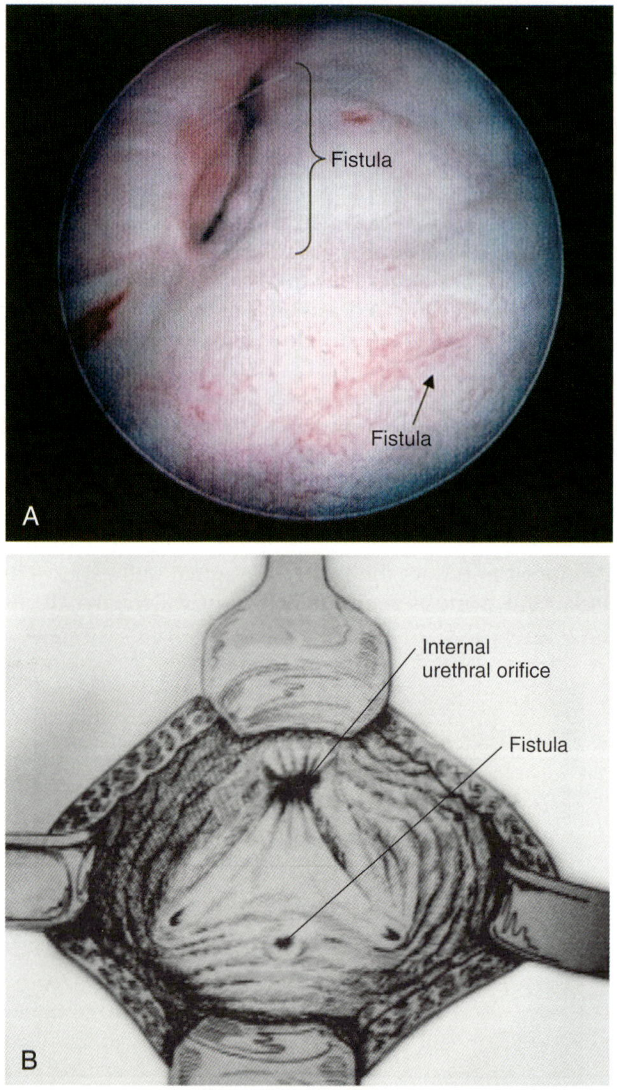

Figure 31.7 **(A)** Cystoscopic view showing relation of vesicovaginal fistula to the trigone. **(B)** Small midline vesicovaginal fistula. (*Source* for (A): AJ Wein, LR Kavoussi, MF Campbell, PC Walsh. Campbell-Walsh Urology: Urinary Tract Fistulae. Saunders: 2012)

The woman develops fever, haematuria, loin tenderness and oliguria.

In case of necrosis of the ureter following denudation, the urinary leak is delayed. It generally starts 2 weeks or later after surgery when the woman starts dribbling urine from the vagina apart from passing urine from the urethra. Unilateral injury causes oliguria, fever and pain in the renal angle on that side, apart from dribbling.

Late complications of ureteric injury includes stricture with hydronephrosis and infection.

INVESTIGATIONS FOR A CASE OF URINARY FISTULA

Investigations for urinary fistulae include the following:

Besides the usual tests of urine examination, complete blood cell count, renal function tests and serum electrolytes, the following special tests are useful in planning surgical procedures: Urine culture is mandatory before surgery, and infection should be treated. The urine is collected by catheterization in case of VVF or by using urine which collects in the well of a sterile Sim's speculum.

Cystoscopy: Cystoscopy with indigo carmine excretion test (5 mL intravenously) enables visualization of the dye from each ureteric orifice individually (Fig. 31.7A and B) and identifies which ureter is damaged. It helps in knowing the site and number of fistulae. During sonography of the kidneys, ureter and bladder, a cystic mass (urinoma) due to collection of urine can be identified.

- *Descending intravenous pyelography* (IVP): IVP may reveal hydronephrosis and hydroureter and indicates the exact site of ureteric obstruction.
- *Ureteric catheterization* will detect the side and site of ureter damage.
- In case the fistula is small and not clearly visible, methylene blue test is applied.
- *Methylene blue – Three-swab test.* A catheter is introduced into the bladder through the urethra. The vaginal cavity is packed with three sterile swabs; 50–100 mL of dilute methylene blue dye is injected into the bladder through the catheter. If there is a VVF present, the methylene blue dye stains the middle swab. If the lowermost swabs get stained, the leak is from the urethra. If the swabs do not take up the stain but get wet with urine, the leak is from the ureter. Oral Pyridium (phenazopyridine) (100 mg) stains urine orange and is easily recognized in the vagina; however, it does not identify the site of fistula.
- Metal catheter not only identifies a fistula but also confirms the patency of the urethra.

MANAGEMENT

VESICOVAGINAL FISTULA

In case bladder damage is suspected following a difficult childbirth, an indwelling catheter for 3–4 weeks is recommended for prolonged draining of the bladder, and antibiotics and supportive therapy are recommended. Spontaneous healing of small fistulae is known to occur. However, in case of an established fistula, it is better to wait for about 3 months for all tissue inflammation to subside, tissue vascularization to improve and local infection to be cleared before surgery is undertaken.

In case of a fistula following cancer, a biopsy should be taken from the edge of the fistula and the presence of cancer ruled out prior to surgery.

- Most VVF can be repaired vaginally. The Latzko procedure involving denuding of the vaginal epithelium all around the fistulous edge, freshening the edge and approximating the wide raw surfaces with rows of absorbable sutures is often successful. This technique is suitable for post - hysterectomy fistulae. It, however, leads to narrowing of the upper vagina or atresia.
- The Chassar Moir technique of widely separating the vaginal and bladder mucosa all around by the flap-splitting method and suturing the bladder and vagina separately in two layers is the most commonly used method. Absence of tension on the suture line promotes healing. It is preferable to see that the suture lines on the bladder and vagina do not overlap. Haemostasis should be meticulous to ensure success. In cases of extensive fibrosis, omental grafts, interpositioning of Martius graft or gracilis muscle graft between the bladder and vaginal walls improves the blood supply at the site of repair and promotes healing. Flap-splitting surgery has the advantage of tension-free sutures. If one attempt fails to heal the fistula, a second vaginal repair can be undertaken after a period of 3 months. In case of a large fistula close to or involving the ureteric orifice, vaginal repair may be difficult; also in cases of failure of previous surgical attempts to repair the fistula by the vaginal route, transabdominal approach is recommended to achieve successful closure.
- In case of extensive loss of bladder tissue, previous repetitive failures to close the fistula or radiation fistula which fails to heal, the surgeon must consider procedures for urinary diversion such as implantation of the ureters into the sigmoid colon, creating an ileal loop bladder into which the ureters are implanted, or a rectal bladder – an operation in which the terminal sigmoid colon is brought out as a colostomy. The distal end of the rectosigmoid is sutured and closed and the ureters implanted into the terminal rectal pouch, which acts as a urinary receptacle. The dangers of ureteric implantation into the large bowel include a high incidence of ascending infection to the kidneys and the risk of electrolyte imbalance leading to **hyperchloraemic acidosis** as well as stricture at the site of implantation.
- If the fistula repair fails, one should wait for at least 3 months before attempting a second repair. A fistula located at the vaginal vault following hysterectomy is the most difficult to repair.
- Fistula caused by cancer cervix may require anterior exenteration.

Postoperative management after VVF repair:

- Continuous bladder drainage for 14–21 days. Some prefer suprapubic drainage.
- Antibiotics – Urine infection should be treated adequately. After removal of the catheter, the woman is advised to pass urine frequently as the bladder capacity may have been reduced.

No vaginal or speculum examination or intercourse is allowed for 2 months after the surgery. In the next pregnancy, a caesarean section is indicated following successful fistula repair. Stress incontinence following VVF repair may be noted, and it results from rigid urethra, loss of vesicourethral angle, small bladder and short urethra.

URETERIC FISTULA (Fig. 31.3)

Most ureteric fistulae are traumatic; rarely, ectopic ureter causes dribbling of urine apart from passing urine from the other kidney.

Only one-third cases of ureteric trauma are recognized intraoperatively. In case of total obstruction following bilateral ureteric ligation, anuria will ensue; sonography will reveal bilateral hydronephrosis and dilated ureters up to the site of the block. The renal function tests reveal a rise in creatinine levels. If the obstruction is detected early, the offending ligatures removed and the ureters stented, recovery is possible. However, if the ureters are damaged, these should be implanted into the bladder. In case the diagnosis is delayed, as happens in cases of unilateral ureteric block, the symptoms of loin pain and fever gradually subside and the kidney on the affected site undergoes atrophy. A procedure of percutaneous nephrostomy (PCN) can save the kidney functions before reimplantation of ureters is undertaken at a later date.

In case of ureteric transection, partial or complete, a pyelography fails to show part or whole of the ureter on the transected site and there may be pooling of the urine in the peritoneal cavity. The immediate treatment is percutaneous nephrostomy and retrograde dye injection under fluoroscopy to help identify the site of transection. If the injury is partial transection, cystoscopic catheterization and stenting of the ureter at the site of injury may be attempted. In case of complete transection, urinary diversion by nephrostomy is advisable to tide over the crisis, followed later with repair surgery. In case the transection is recognized during surgery itself, the surgeon must either undertake anastomosis at the site of injury or implant the cut end of the ureter into the bladder or perform a **Boari flap ureteroneocystostomy**. Ureteroureteric anastomosis is also sometimes possible, but the risk of stricture should be remembered. Fixing the dome of the bladder to the psoas muscle relieves tension on the implanted ureter. Ureteric stricture and infection are the sequelae of ureteric implantation and need to be observed.

When ureteric damage goes unnoticed, following the hectic postoperative period, fever settles down, but patient starts dribbling urine from the vagina around the 10th–14th day. Urine collects in the vagina, but the woman also micturates and oliguria is noticed. It is difficult to visualize the fistulous opening. Methylene blue test recognizes the ureteric fistula. Cystoscopy with retrograde catheterization shows the absence of urine coming from the affected side and the site of blockage, respectively. IVP will be required to detect hydroureter/hydronephrosis. Urine culture and kidney function tests are also required.

One should not wait for the kidney damage to occur and perform laparotomy; it should be performed at the earliest, once the inflammation and infection subside.

The surgery for ureteric injuries comprises the following:

- Ureteroureteral anastomosis with the ureteric stent inserted
- Implantation of the ureter into the bladder
- Psoas muscle stitched to the dome of the bladder to avoid stretching and tension on the ureter
- Boari operation
- Ileal bladder

Prophylaxis

In a difficult gynaecological surgery where injury to ureters is likely, it is prudent to trace the ureter from the pelvic brim downwards before clamping any vessel or cutting the tissues. The ureter is identified by its position (may be distorted or abnormally placed in pelvic diseases), pale glistening appearance and peristaltic movement when stroked.

In a difficult case, some gynaecologists prefer to insert the ureteric stent before starting the surgery, but this does not always prevent ureteric damage if devascularization occurs during its dissection.

Blood supply to the pelvic ureter comes from the lateral side, so dissection of the ureter should be done on its medial side and devascularization and ischaemia should be avoided.

VESICOUTERINE FISTULA

Vesicouterine fistula is a rare variety of fistulae where there is a communication between uterus and bladder, usually caused during caesarean section or uterine rupture or placenta accreta. The patient's symptoms are unlike those of lower urinary tract fistula. The patient remains continent, as urine does not dribble into the uterine cavity. The patient, however, complains of cyclical haematuria – menstrual blood trickling through the fistula into the bladder (Youssef syndrome). The other cause of cyclical haematuria are bladder endometriosis and rarely an intrauterine contraceptive device (IUCD) perforation into the bladder. Cystoscopy will reveal the true pathology. Methylene blue injected into the uterine cavity will show a leak into the bladder. Occasional prolonged bladder catheterization may close the fistula; otherwise, the treatment is by abdominal repair. Omental or gracilis graft is sometimes required.

URETHROVAGINAL FISTULA

The patient is continent and dry but dribbles urine only during the act of micturition. A speculum examination will show the fistulous opening clearly. Vaginal repair is often successful, but urethral stricture may follow. A big fistula may need a graft technique. The urethral fistula is encountered following surgery for paravaginal cyst and urethral diverticulum. Penetrating injury following a fall or during criminal abortion can cause urethral fistula. Urethral reconstructive surgery is required.

STRESS URINARY INCONTINENCE

SUI is a fairly common condition affecting 25%–40% of women. It is more commonly seen among women older than 40 years. The condition may be seen in association with genital organ prolapse or may occur as an isolated condition. It is a very distressing problem, especially among working women, limiting their social activities. The treatment, often a surgical repair, may fail to provide relief from symptoms. The exact aetiology of SUI remains unknown; however, a number of hypotheses have been put forward.

Urinary incontinence may be stress incontinence, urge incontinence or true incontinence. The common type of stress incontinence is associated with cystocele and genital prolapse when the woman voids a small quantity of urine involuntarily while sneezing, coughing or laughing. The condition also develops during pregnancy and soon after delivery.

Stress incontinence is confused with urge incontinence. In urge incontinence, the woman wants to pass urine at a moment's notice, and unless she is quick about it, she passes urine in large quantity before reaching the washroom. The amount of urine passed is considerable. In stress incontinence, there is no desire to pass urine, but escape of a small quantity of urine occurs during coughing, sneezing, lifting heavy weight or change of posture. Both are bothersome symptoms and affect the quality of life.

Urinary incontinence may indicate a symptom, a sign or a condition. The patient complains of involuntary leakage of urine, which is socially and hygienically unacceptable. The sign is the objective demonstration of urine loss, and the condition is the underlying pathophysiologic mechanism responsible for the urine leak.

The symptom of involuntary urine loss may be associated with stressful activity such as coughing, sneezing, straining or other physical activity (stress incontinence). The involuntary urine loss may follow a strong desire and need to void (urge incontinence), or there may be continuous urinary leak (true incontinence) as in a fistula.

MECHANISM OF FEMALE URINARY CONTINENCE

Most women remain continent. It is as a result of normal mechanism of micturition and supports to the urethra provided by surrounding tissues. Ultrasonography and MRI have recently improved our knowledge about the anatomy of the lower urinary tract and validated some of the urodynamic investigations of stress incontinence.

In normal conditions, internal urinary meatus lies above the level of levator ani muscles. Upper half of the urethra lies above and the lower half below the levator ani muscles (Fig. 31.8).

Normal mechanism of continence mainly relies on the internal sphincter at the neck of the bladder and is maintained by the urethral closure pressure. The urethral closure pressure is the intraurethral pressure minus the intravesical pressure (closure pressure is the difference between the vesical pressure and the urethral pressure). Normal urethral closure pressure is more than 20 cm of water (cm H_2O) when the upper urethra and the bladder neck remain above the levator muscles and the urethrovesical angle is more than 100°. Under this condition, the abdominal pressure is transmitted equally to the bladder and the urethra, maintaining the closure pressure.

Because of atony of pelvic floor muscles or damage to the pudendal nerve during vaginal delivery, the bladder neck descends below the level of levator ani muscles and the urethrovesical angle is lost, thus the abdominal pressure is transmitted only to the bladder, resulting in urinary incontinence. The vascular plexus and the longitudinal fibres of the urethra maintain the tone during the filling phase (Figs 31.9–31.11). Extrinsic control of the bladder neck is provided by striated smooth muscles. Internal sphincter consists of two loops of smooth muscle fibres: one loop pulls the sphincter anteriorly and the other loop posteriorly and maintains the urethrovesical angle. The tone of the levator ani muscles, pudendal nerve and pubovesical fascia also contribute to urinary continence. Lateral attachment of the urethra to the arcus tendineus and pubococcygeus muscles limits urethral mobility and maintains continence.

GENUINE STRESS INCONTINENCE OF URINE (SUI/GSI)

Genuine stress incontinence (GSI) of urine occurs when the bladder pressure exceeds urethral pressure during physical stress in the absence of detrusor contraction. It is defined as a small involuntary leakage of urine with increased abdominal pressure in the absence of detrusor contraction.

Aetiology

It is generally due to anatomical changes in the urinary tract such as hypermobility of urethra (80%), loss of posterior urethral angle or sphincteric dysfunction.

- **Age:** Older menopausal women with loss of pelvic muscle tone are liable to develop GSI (oestrogen deficiency).
- **Multiparous women** after repeated childbirths are prone to loss of tone of the pelvic floor muscles.
- **Obesity, smoking, prolapse and constipation.**
- **Pregnancy and puerperium** – during pregnancy, stress incontinence is due to the progesterone hormonal effect and the pressure of the gravid uterus on the bladder neck. During puerperium, the stress incontinence is caused by the descent of the bladder neck, the loss of

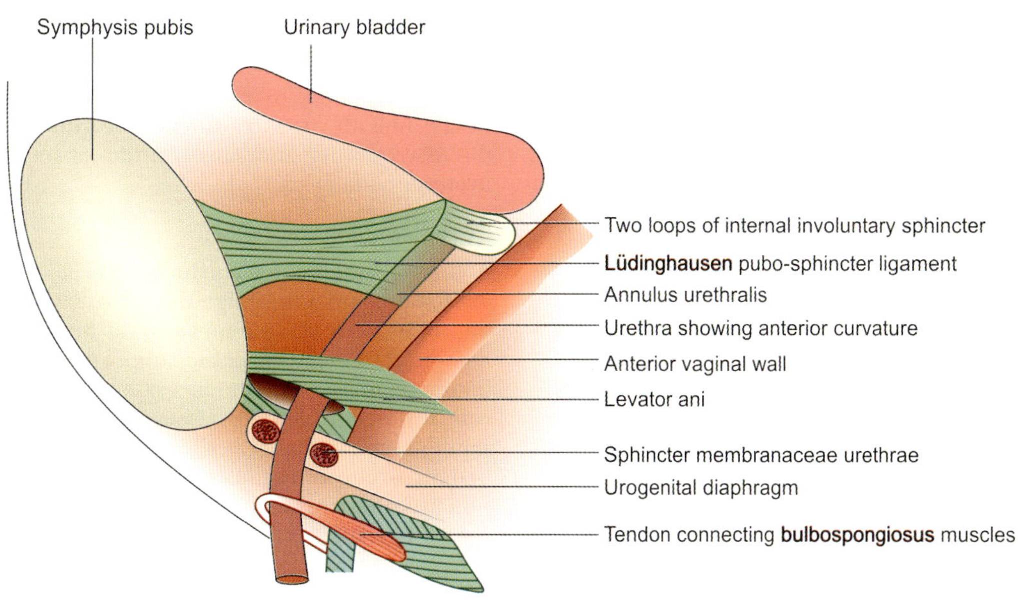

Figure 31.8 Normal support of internal sphincter.

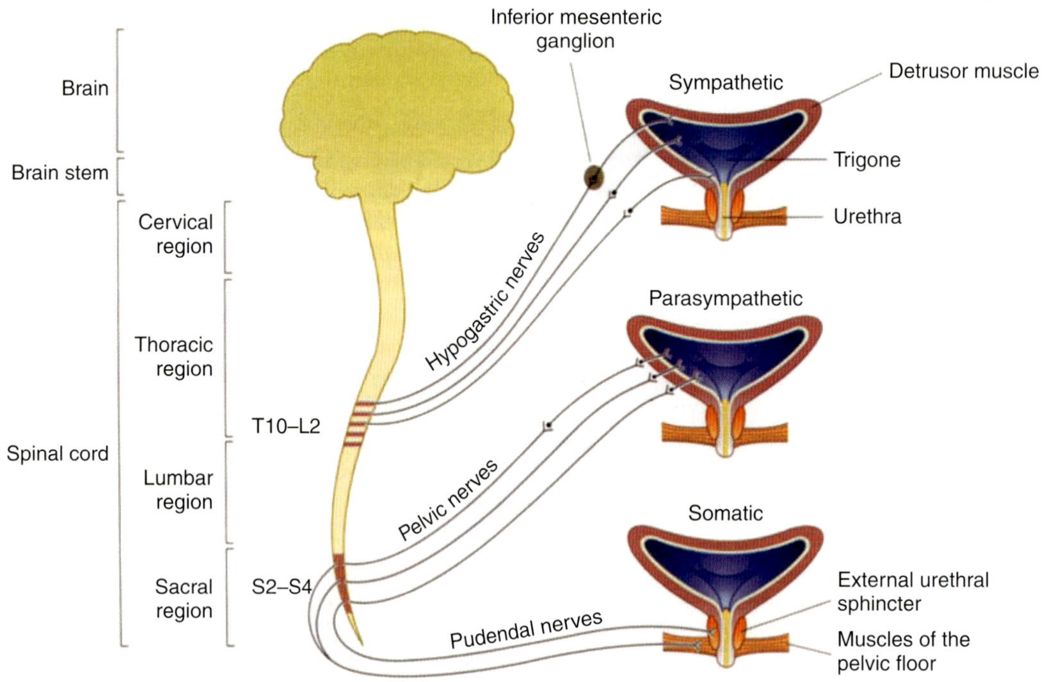

Figure 31.9 Normal control of micturition.

urethrovesical angle due to pudendal nerve denervation, and diminished tone and stretching of levator ani muscles during vaginal delivery.

- **Hereditary** – loss of collagen tissue
- **Repair of VVF** and urethral fibrosis may also cause GSI

GSI is the only type which can be cured by surgical procedures, hence the importance of making a correct diagnosis before planning any surgical repair.

URGE INCONTINENCE

Urge incontinence of urine is involuntary escape of a large amount of urine following a desire to pass urine unless the woman immediately goes to the washroom. Urge incontinence (motor) is commonly the result of detrusor muscle overactivity (detrusor instability, DI). Sensory urgency is an intense desire to void that is not associated with detrusor pressure. Unconscious incontinence is often the result of a neuropathic bladder; the underlying cause of the involuntary urine loss may be retention of urine with overflow.

PRIMARY CLINICAL EVALUATION IN A CASE OF URINARY INCONTINENCE

HISTORY

A carefully taken history can help diagnose urge incontinence and avoid making a wrong diagnosis of SUI. Menopausal obese women with previous vaginal deliveries are at risk of urinary stress incontinence. Patients with GSI usually complain of the passage of a single spurt of urine at the height of physical exertion such as sneezing or coughing without the urge to urinate. Patients with motor urge incontinence admit to a strong desire to void, which if not complied with immediately, leads to a considerable involuntary passage of urine. A history of diabetes and pulmonary disease is relevant.

Local pathology in the bladder and urethra may lead to frequency of micturition, i.e. infection, lowered capacity of the bladder, lowered compliance of the bladder because of chronic fibrosis of the bladder interfering with its contraction pattern following radiotherapy, tuberculosis or diabetes. Organic neurological diseases may adversely affect bladder function. These include multiple sclerosis, tabes dorsalis and subacute combined degeneration of the cord. Major pelvic dissection during radical operations on the uterus and rectum causes widespread damage to the splanchnic nerves in the deeper parts of the cardinal ligaments. The nervi erigentes carry the parasympathetic motor supply to the detrusor muscle of the bladder, and interference with this pathway can cause disturbances of bladder function. Extraurethral causes of urinary incontinence include true continence of genitourinary fistulae discussed earlier and rare conditions such as an ectopic ureter.

PHYSICAL EXAMINATION

A clinical examination, including pelvic and speculum examination, and a thorough neurological assessment should be undertaken. An attempt should be made to assess the anatomical defects of pelvic supports and the tone of the levator muscles. Note the increase in urethral and urethrovesical junction mobility. Assess vaginal wall prolapse and senile vaginal changes. Elderly postmenopausal women benefit from oestrogen therapy when follow-up examination reveals a healthy pliable vaginal wall.

GSI is graded as follows:

- Grade I. Incontinence with only severe stress, such as coughing, sneezing and jogging

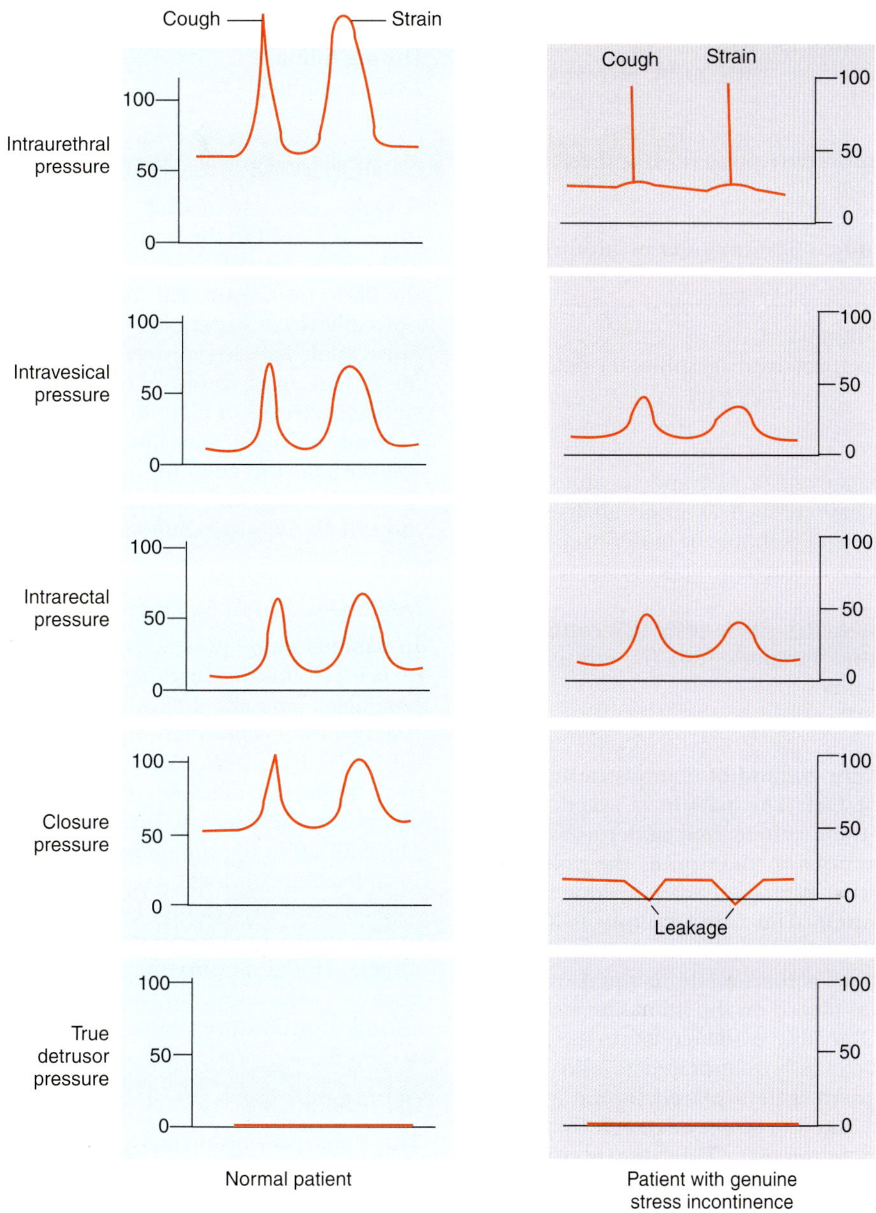

Figure 31.10 Comparison of urethral and vesical pressure in a normal subject and in one suffering from genuine stress urinary incontinence.

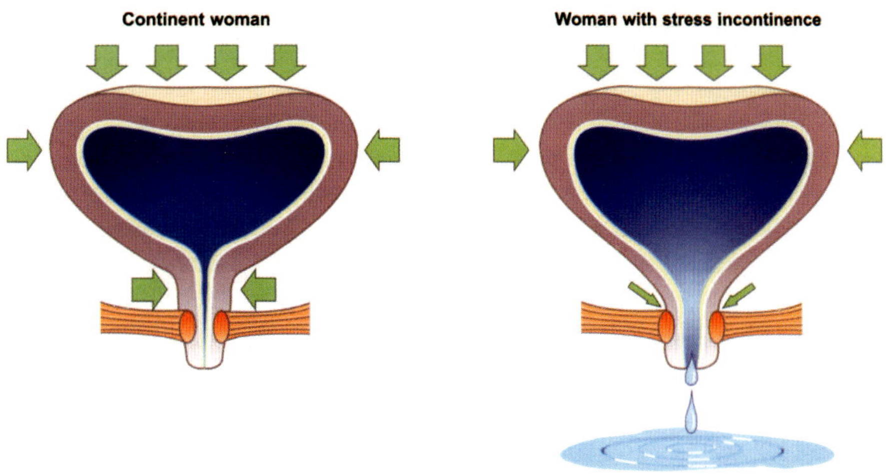

Figure 31.11 SUI mechanism.

- Grade II. Incontinence with moderate stress, such as fast walk, going up and down the stairs
- Grade III. Incontinence with mild stress such as standing

From the surgical procedure point of view, three types of GSI have been described:

- Type I. GSI occurs due to loss of posterior urethrovesical angle alone.
- Type II. Loss of posterior urethrovesical angle as well as urethral hypermobility.
- Type III. This results from intrinsic sphincter deficiency.

INVESTIGATIONS

Prior to surgical management of GSI and in urge incontinence, detailed investigations such as urine analysis, urine culture and urodynamic studies should be undertaken to avoid making a wrong diagnosis and achieve appropriate results.

Urine culture.

Investigations such as (i) stress test, (ii) cotton swab test, (iii) Marshall's and Bonney's test, (iv) urethroscopy and (v) urodynamic studies.

STRESS TEST

Stress test is an excellent method of demonstrating objectively the presence of GSI. The patient is asked to void urine. The patient is then catheterized under aseptic conditions, taking precautions to determine the volume of residual urine present. Ultrasound scan is done and residual urine is measured. The urine sample is sent for culture. Thereafter, 250 mL of sterile saline is instilled into the bladder. The patient is then made to squat on a preweighed absorbent pad placed on the floor. She is asked to cough and strain. Objective evidence of urine leak is noted. The leak can be grossly quantitated as mild, moderate or severe. The patient is then placed supine in the lithotomy position and asked to strain or cough for further evidence of stress incontinence. The absorbent pad is weighed at the end of the test. A net weight gain of 2 g or more is indicative of GSI.

Urine culture before invasive investigations is mandatory. It is necessary to rule out urinary infection by culture before undertaking invasive investigations because of the following reasons:

- The symptoms may be due to urinary infection.
- Invasive procedures should not be undertaken in the presence of infection.
- Urinary infection may interfere with interpretations of invasive procedures.

These tests are also required if the GSI recurs following surgery:

Normal cystometric findings

Parameter	Normal findings
Residual urine	<50 mL
First desire to void urine	150–250 mL
Bladder capacity	500–600 mL

Detrusor pressure

During filling	<15 cm H_2O
During voiding	<70 cm H_2O
Urine flow	>15 mL

COTTON SWAB STICK TEST

A Q-tip cotton swab stick dipped in Xylocaine Jelly (lidocaine) is placed in the urethra. The patient is asked to strain and cough. Initially, the cotton swab stick will be parallel to the floor. In patients with no GSI, the cotton swab stick will normally reach an angle not exceeding 10–15° above the horizontal. This angle increases by 20° or more, commonly 50–70° in most positive cases. A positive test indicates sufficient degree of bladder neck descent. Unfortunately, all patients with GSI may not have a positive test. A positive test obviates the need for a metal bead chain cystourethrogram. However, this test is not very specific and does not indicate the severity and type of surgery the woman requires (Fig. 31.12).

MARSHALL'S AND BONNEY'S TEST

In patients with a positive stress test, the absence of leakage of urine following bladder neck elevation is indicative of beneficial outcome following surgical repair. In Bonney's test, two fingers are placed in the vagina at the urethrovesical junction on either side of the urethra and the bladder neck region is elevated. On straining or coughing, the absence of leakage of urine indicates a positive test. In Marshall's test, the vagina in the region of the bladder neck is infiltrated with local anaesthetic and the area is elevated with an open Allis clamp. Failure to demonstrate leakage of urine on coughing is indicative of a positive test. Instead of fingers, Hodge pessary may be used to elevate the bladder neck. A positive test indicates that woman will benefit from a surgical procedure where elevation of the bladder neck is achieved.

URETHROSCOPY

The Robertson urethroscope using a gas medium permits satisfactory visual evaluation of the urethra, trigone and bladder neck regions. Urethroscopy provides information about the opening pressure, presence or absence of urethritis, presence of diverticulum or a rigid urethra. The urethrovesical junction can be observed during bladder filling with a hold command, during coughing or during Valsalva manoeuvre.

URODYNAMIC EVALUATION

These are a group of tests to study the pattern of storage and evacuation of urine. *These tests are required when clinical diagnosis is not clear prior to surgery.*

Cystometry

Measurement of pressures within the bladder and urethra during artificial filling of the bladder with saline CO_2 or fluid helps differentiate true stress incontinence, DI, urgency instability and other types of incontinence. The relationship between the bladder and urethral pressures can be most helpful in planning the correct treatment.

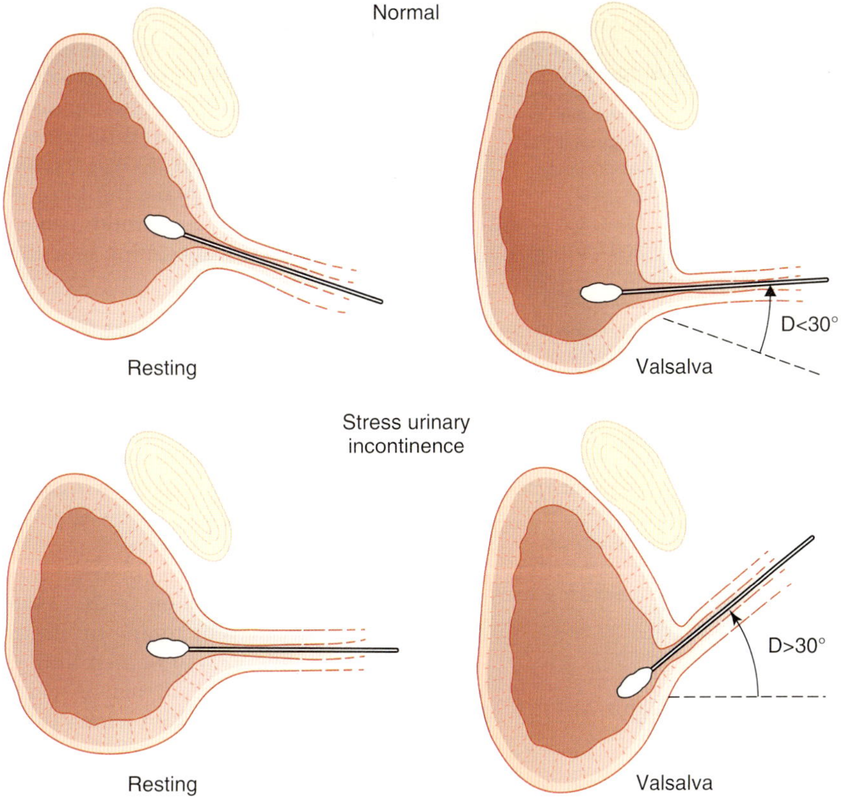

Figure 31.12 Diagrammatic representation of Q-tip cotton swab test. (*Source:* Hacker NF, Gambone JC, Hobel CJ, Hacker and Moore's Essentials of Obstetrics and Gynecology, 5th ed. Philadelphia: Elsevier, 2010.)

Urethrocystometry

Normal findings are as follows: At rest, 150 mL of urine causes 2–8 cm H_2O pressure, which rises to 15 cm H_2O at filling. Urethral pressure averages 40 cm H_2O, and less than 20 cm H_2O pressure leads to incontinence.

Uroflowmetry

Measurement of urine flow rate and volume provides an objective, noninvasive measure of voiding function.

Micturition Cystourethrography

Normally, a continent woman demonstrates a well-marked posterior urethrovesical angle of about 100°. Loss of posterior urethrovesical angle causes stress incontinence in many women. Colposuspension and sling operations are based on restoring this angle surgically.

Uroprofilometry

Uroprofilometry measures the dynamic urethral pressures and diagnoses urethral instability and urethral diverticulum. It is a gold standard in the diagnosis of GSI.

The normal flow is 15–25 mL/s. Flow below 10 mL/s occurs in atonic bladder and during obstruction, which is confirmed by cystometry. Increased bladder pressure of more than 50 cm H_2O and low flow suggest obstruction.

Urodynamic study may not be needed in all cases of urinary incontinence; however, it is desirable when diagnosis is in doubt or the patient continues to have symptoms despite surgical intervention.

Ultrasonography

Ultrasonography is useful in measuring the bladder volume and residual urine. A bladder wall thickness of more than 6 mm suggests DI. Bladder stone can be seen.

Videocystourethrography

Videocystourethrography is the new gold standard urodynamic investigation to study the lower urinary tract dysfunction. It combines the pressure studies with the video position of the bladder neck and urethrovesical angle.

MRI Studies

MRI studies the defects in the pelvic floor muscles and the supporting fasciae. Appropriate surgery to buttress the bladder neck will cure incontinence.

Sophisticated *neurophysiological testing* is required when the neurological component for stress incontinence is suspected.

Residual urine on ultrasound scan shows incomplete voiding.

TREATMENT

It is important to rule out DI before any surgery for SUI is undertaken; otherwise, the symptoms will worsen.

Table 31.3 Management of Stress Incontinence

Conservative	Drugs	Surgery
First line of treatment • Young women • Frail, old women • Postpartum, previous failed surgery 1. Kegel pelvic floor exercises × 4–6 months 2. Electric/magnetic stimulation for nerve damage, magnetic stimulation 3. Artificial urinary sphincter in neurological condition 4. Vaginal cones	• Oestrogen cream in menopausal women • Venlafaxine 75 mg daily • Imipramine 10–20 mg b.d.	If others fail • Vaginal (Kelly) • Abdominal Marshall–Marchetti–Krantz and Pereyra Burch • Combined vaginal and abdominal suspension • Slings • Tension-free sling • Transobturator tape Laparoscopic suspension of the bladder neck

Treatment comprises the following (Table 31.3):

- Conservative therapy
- Surgical repair

The main aim of treatment is to improve the quality of life.

CONSERVATIVE TREATMENT

Conservative treatment should be the first line of treatment, especially in younger women. It is cheap, has fewer complications and does not compromise future surgery if so required.

Conservative therapy is also applied to the elderly and frail women unfit for surgery and during the 6 months after the delivery. It is also applicable in those with previous failed surgery and in women desirous of childbearing.

The treatment comprises the following:

- Physiotherapy
- Drugs
- Intraurethral and vaginal devices
- Electric stimulation
- Artificial urinary sphincter
- Weight loss exercises
- Reduced caffeine intake and smoking cessation
- Bladder training and timed voiding

Physiotherapy

Suited for Grade I GSI. Pelvic floor exercises for 4–6 months with or without electrical stimulation make patient's life tolerable in 60% of cases. Both weight loss and exercise are beneficial. It takes 8–12 weeks before any improvement is seen.

Kegel pelvic floor exercises work best in younger women and in those with mild stress incontinence associated with urethral hypermobility with no damage to internal sphincter. It is also effective in those with urge incontinence, as these exercises tone up the levator ani muscles and internal sphincter.

Drugs

α-Adrenergic drugs may help to constrict the bladder neck and reduce the frequency of stress incontinence. Oestrogen cream is useful in menopausal women. Phenylpropanolamine enhances urethral pressure. Venlafaxine 75 mg daily is a serotonin (5-hydroxytryptamine [5-HT]) and noradrenaline reuptake inhibitor and is the latest drug of choice. It can cause mild transient nausea and mild cardiac effect. Imipramine at a dose of 10–20 mg b.d. is also effective.

Intraurethral and Vaginal Devices

These have been tried with some success. A ring pessary in genital prolapse may reduce stress incontinence in some women. Contiform is a silastic vaginal cone available in India. It is placed during the day and removed and cleaned at night. The cone needs changing every 6 weeks. It is successful in 85% of the cases. Vaginal cones weighing 20–100 g are available. A small cone is used initially, with larger ones used later. The cone is inserted in the vagina and held in position by contraction of the levator ani muscles as long as possible, thereby toning up these muscles. They are not useful in menopausal women with weak levator ani muscles or in the presence of vaginal scar. Toxic shock syndrome can occur if retained for a long period.

Electric Stimulation

Electric stimulation of the pelvic floor muscles has also been tried during physiotherapy if the stress incontinence is caused by denervation of the pudendal nerve during delivery. Magnetic stimulation is lately employed. It is especially useful in old women with weak pelvic floor muscles.

Artificial Urinary Sphincter

Artificial urinary sphincter (AUS) (Fig. 31.13) model-800 is used in those with neurological conditions and in those with previous surgical failure and sphincteric dysfunction. Although an 80% success rate is reported, equipment is

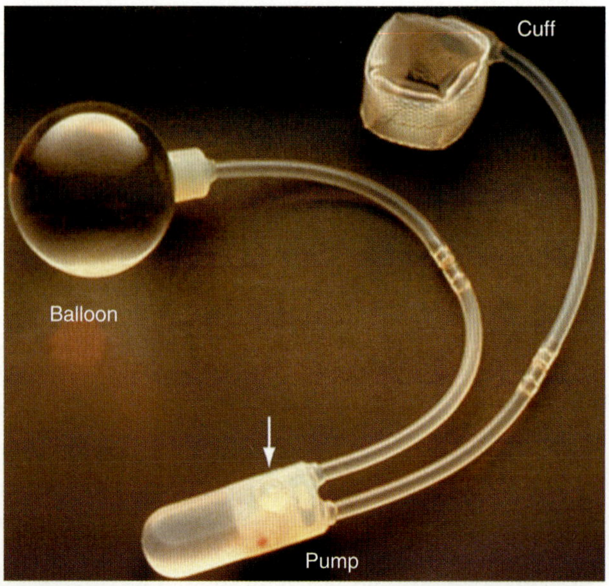

Figure 31.13 Artificial urinary sphincter. (*Source:* R González, L Piaggio. Pediatric Urology: Artificial urinary sphincter. Saunders: 2010.)

expensive, can cause infection and mechanical failure can occur.

Genuine Stress Incontinence

Postmenopausal women with senile changes in the vagina, hypotonic urethra and mild stress incontinence may benefit immensely with oestrogen replacement therapy, preferably cream applied locally. Women with chronic cough, constipation and allergic rhinitis or excessive physical activity may benefit with medical measures. Avoiding aggravating factors such as smoking, straining or undue physical exertion also plays a complementary role. Successful surgery for GSI restores the relationship between the bladder, urethra and the urogenital diaphragm.

The *goals* of surgical repair of GSI include the following:

- Repositioning the proximal urethra to a high retropubic position to maximize proper urethral compression.
- Preserving vesicourethral angle to facilitate urethral compression.
- Preserving compressibility and pliability of the urethra.
- Preserving integrity of the sphincteric mechanism.

SURGICAL REPAIR OF STRESS URINARY INCONTINENCE

Various surgical procedures (>100) have been designed over the years; some of these existing procedures are discussed here. It is, however, recommended that *any surgery should be deferred in a young woman and conservative method employed initially.* Future pregnancy may mar the good result of surgery.

Primary surgery offers the best results; therefore, selection of cases and the procedure should be most appropriate.

Vaginal Operations

These include anterior colporrhaphy with plication of the bladder neck (Kelly's repair) or apposing the medial fibres of the puborectalis muscles in the midline under the bladder neck region to elevate the same (Pacey's repair).

Abdominal Operations

These operations are of retropubic colposuspension such as the Marshall–Marchetti–Krantz operation, in which the bladder neck and vaginal vault are sutured to the periosteum of the back of the pubic symphysis, or the Burch colposuspension, which aims at vaginal suspension using the iliopectineal ligaments rather than the periosteum of the back of the symphysis pubis. Osteitis may follow the Marshall–Marchetti–Krantz operation. Because of this and a low cure rate, this operation has been more or less replaced by the sling operation.

Combined Abdominal and Vaginal Operations

The Pereyra operation is performed by the vaginal route. A Foley catheter is inserted and its bulb distended with 5 mL of saline. Traction on the bulb helps identify the bladder neck and urethra. Two parallel incisions are made on either side of the urethra in the region of the bladder neck. Paraurethral spaces are created by blunt dissection. A helical suture is passed through the paraurethral tissues and its ends threaded into a needle, which is advanced through the endopelvic fascia into the retropubic space. The needle is now advanced close to the back of the pubic bones to penetrate the rectus abdominis muscle where it can be palpated and guided into a small midline transverse suprapubic incision in the abdominal wall. A similar paraurethral tissue sling can be pulled up on the other side with a helical suture. After appropriate traction which elevates the bladder neck adequately, the helical sutures are fixed to the aponeurosis of the anterior abdominal wall. As an extension of this principle, fascial slings or nylon mesh slings placed under the bladder neck region vaginally can be made to sling up the bladder neck like a 'hammock' (Razz and Stamey modifications are becoming increasingly more popular) with a 50% success rate.

Immediate complications of sling operations are as follows:

- Bleeding
- Trauma
- Urinary infection

Late complications are as follows:

- Bladder dysfunction
- Erosion of the sling
- Prolapse of the posterior vaginal wall and enterocele as the intraabdominal pressure is exerted on the posterior vaginal wall

Burch Colposuspension (Figs 31.14 and 31.16)

After the retropubic space is reached, nonabsorbable sutures of (3–4) polyglycolic acid are placed in the lateral fornices (paravaginal tissue) lateral to the bladder base and the bladder neck is fixed to the ipsilateral iliopectineal ligament. An 85% success rate has been reported with this procedure. It is to be balanced against the risk of development of enterocele and rectocele postoperatively due to transmission of intraabdominal pressure. Burch operation, though popular until recently, has now been superseded by tension-free vaginal T-tape. Burch operation causes bleeding in 3% of cases, bladder trauma in 6%, venous thrombosis in 1% and voiding difficulties in as much as 25% of cases.

Laparoscopic Colposuspension

Burch colposuspension has been successfully accomplished laparoscopically through the extraperitoneal or transperitoneal route. Expertise and facilities for laparoscopic Burch operation may not be available at all the centres.

Intravesical Bladder Neck Plication

This operation is used only exceptionally.

Tension-Free Vaginal Tape (TVT)

The tape does not elevate the urethra but provides a resistant platform in the mid-urethra that maintains continence against intraabdominal pressure. It was designed by Petros (1993) and Ulmstem (1996). This technique is good for obese women, as it does not causes detrusor dysfunction.

TVT (Figs 31.15 and 31.16) has been designed from nontissue reactive synthetic material (Prolene). After exposing the region of the bladder neck on vaginal dissection, the hammock of the tape is placed underneath it to provide support at the mid-urethral level, the lateral extensions are brought out paraurethrally onto the skin at the

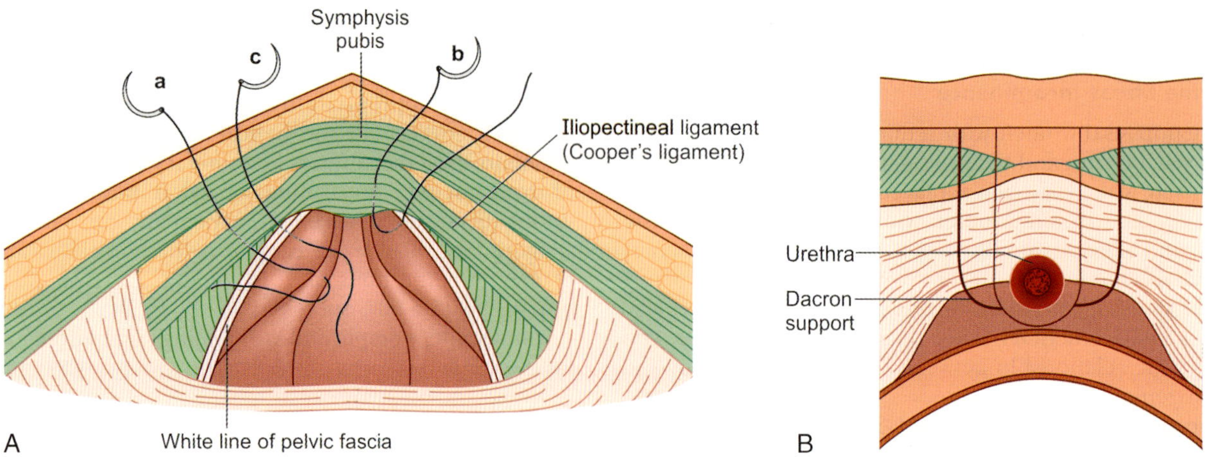

Figure 31.14 **(A)** Colposuspension (Burch operation). (a) Burch colposuspension; (b) colposuspension using the white line of pelvic fascia; (c) MMK procedure. **(B)** Modified Stamey method of endoscopic colposuspension.

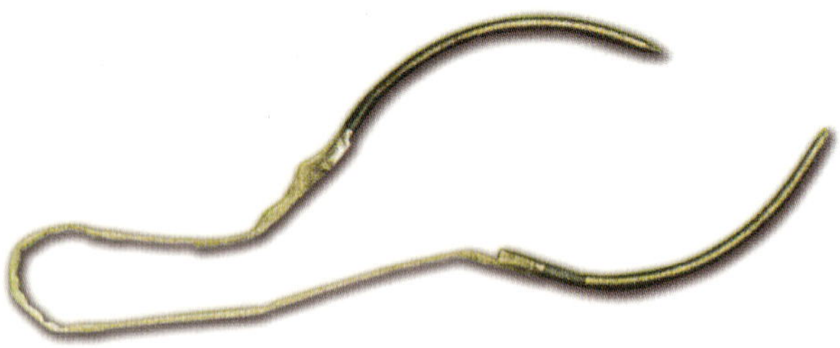

Figure 31.15 Transobturator tape.

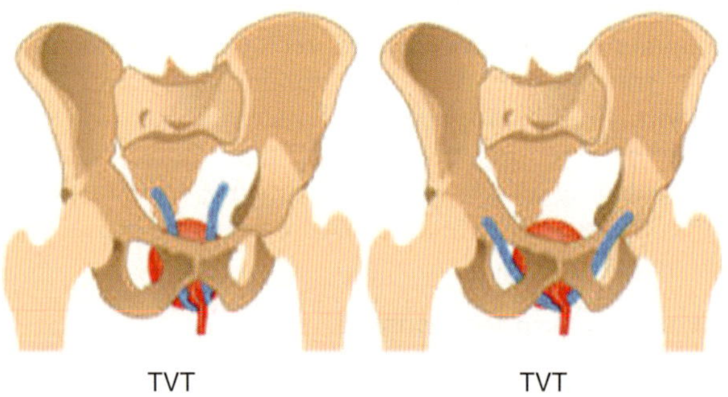

Figure 31.16 Tension-free vaginal tape device.

level of the pubic symphysis and the vaginal incision is closed. After adjusting the proper elevation of the bladder neck region, the extra length of the lateral arms of the tape is cut. The operation can be performed under local anaesthesia. Under local anaesthesia, tension can be checked by asking the woman to cough. Cystoscopy avoids inadvertent bladder entry. Success rate of 88%–90% has been claimed at the end of 3 years. This procedure also does not require catheterization postoperatively. Two per cent of procedures require removal, and 5% have voiding problem.

This surgery is employed in the following cases:

- Previously failed surgery
- Internal sphincter dysfunction
- Mobile urethra

Transobturator Tape (TOT) (Fig. 31.17)

Designed by Delorme (2001), this mid-urethral tape avoids passing through the retropubic space. Instead, a hammock is inserted mid-urethra by passing the trocar from the thigh through the obturator canal. This reduces the risk of bladder perforation and cystoscopy is not required. This technique is good for obese women.

Mid-urethral sling is good for urethral hypermobility, whereas other slings are for internal sphincter dysfunction. Lately, TOT has become more popular than TVT.

Periurethral Collagen Injection

Glutaraldehyde cross-linked bovine collagen (Contigen, Bard) is commercially available for periurethral injection. A dose of 2.5 mL is injected at 3 and 9 o'clock positions into the submucosa of the proximal urethra near the bladder base under cystoscopic vision. It can be undertaken as an office procedure for mild cases but is often reserved for cases of surgical failures. Objective relief is achieved in about 50% of cases. However, allergic reactions to the collagen injection have been reported. The procedure raises the urethral pressure by external compression and is useful in sphincteric dysfunction. It is used in internal sphincter

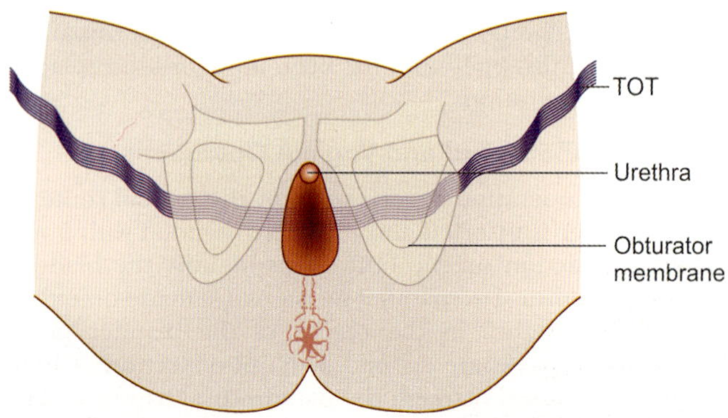

Figure 31.17 Transobturator tape (TOT) procedure. The tape is placed under the mid-urethra, taken through the obturator membrane to be fixed to the thigh.

dysfunction. It can cause retention of urine and may require reinjection.

Recently, micronized silicon rubber particles suspended in nonsilicon gel known as uroplasty has been used with success. Local reaction with fibrosis is less seen with uroplasty than with collagen. Durasphere is nondegradable, nonallergic and longer acting. Bulkamid is a type of hydrogel.

Complications. The following complications can occur with these operations:

- Injury to the bladder, urethra
- Haematoma in the retropubic space
- Infection
- Breakdown of sutures
- Voiding difficulties, retention of urine
- Incomplete bladder emptying and repeated urinary infections
- Late problems include erosion of nonabsorbable sutures into the bladder, urethra or vagina, resulting in infection, fistula or stone formation
- DI follows surgery for GSI in 1%–10% of cases
- Failure

Outcome following surgical repair of GSI. Initial success rates noted with various operations for SUI are followed by failures over a period of time.

Potential reasons for failure include the following:

- Surgical failure – sutures cut out because of poor placement of sutures, inadequate mobilization of the bladder neck and proximal urethra, postoperative haematoma formation/infection.
- Incorrect choice of operation – mainly the result of incomplete or incorrect preoperative assessment of the cause of urinary incontinence.
- Development of incontinence due to other causes such as fistula formation, DI or pipe-stem urethra previously not present.

With the passage of time, the results of all kinds of incontinence surgery tend to deteriorate. Long-term follow-up data suggest (Table 31.4) cure rates of different surgical procedures.

Table 31.4 Cure Rate of Different Surgical Procedures

Operation for Repair of GSI	Long-Term Cure (%)
1. Bladder buttress operation	67.8
2. Marshall–Marchetti–Krantz operation	89.5
3. Colposuspension	89.8
4. Endoscopic suspension	86.7
5. Vaginal sling operations	93.9

Source: Modified from Jarvis (1994) and Leach (1997).

DETRUSOR INSTABILITY

Incontinence occurs when the detrusor muscle contracts spontaneously or on provocation during the filling phase while attempting inhibition of micturition. It is more common in older women with decreased bladder capacity, decreased sensation and central nervous system (CNS) diseases. It is often caused by overactivity of parasympathetic nerves.

AETIOLOGY OF DETRUSOR INSTABILITY

DI may be:

- Functional and psychosomatic.
- Detrusor hyperreflexia (neuropathy) in certain medical conditions such as diabetic neuropathy, a cerebrovascular accident, multiple sclerosis, spinal injury and Parkinsonism.
- It occurs following surgery for GSI if the bladder neck is placed too high and tightly sutured. It is seen in 1% of the cases following anterior vaginal wall repair, 5.8% after endoscopic bladder neck suspension and 10% following colposuspension and sling operation.
- Idiopathic. Ten per cent of men and 30% women older than 40 years have DI.
- Urinary infection.

PATHOPHYSIOLOGY

Increased α-adrenergic and cholinergic activity is responsible for this condition.

SYMPTOMS

A woman develops involuntary escape of urine with urge to urinate. This urge is accompanied by frequency more than seven times during the day and at least once during the night. There could also be bedwetting during sleep. DI also occurs during sexual intercourse and with the sound of flowing water and handwashing.

INVESTIGATIONS

- Neurological examination, especially in older women.
- Blood sugar estimation.
- Urine culture will indicate whether the urinary infection is the cause of frequency and urge.
- Cystometry. The normal pressure of 15 cm H_2O at 200 mL exceeds in DI. Cystoscopy is normal. Bladder capacity may be reduced.
- Other investigations may be required to rule out other causes of associated bladder neck instability.
- Ultrasound scan shows a thick bladder wall more than 6 mm in DI and residual urine, apart from urethrovesical angle posteriorly.

Differential diagnosis – interstitial cystitis, it has urge but no dribbling.

TREATMENT

- Low caffeine intake and avoid smoking
- Bladder training
- Restricted fluid intake and weight reduction

Treatment of DI is medical. Anticholinergic drugs are most useful. Some of them are mentioned in (Table 31.5).

Table 31.5 Dosage and Side Effects of Anticholinergic Drugs

Drugs	Dosage	Side Effects
• Urispas (flavoxate)	200 mg t.i.d. Antispasmodic action on the detrusor muscle, an analgesic	Headache, nausea, dry mouth, blurred vision
• Dicyclomine HCl	100 mg q.i.d.	Headache, nausea, dry mouth, blurred vision
• Pro-Banthine	15–90 mg q.i.d.	Headache, nausea, dry mouth, blurred vision
• Oxybutynin HCl	5–10 mg t.i.d.	Cognitive impairment, not to be given to elderly women. Outflow obstruction, glaucoma, myasthenia gravis
• Imipramine	50–100 mg at night × 3 months	Sedation, constipation, blurred vision
• Tolterodine (Roliten, Terol)	2 mg b.d.	Fewer side effects
• Duloxetine	40–80 mg b.d. × 3 months	Headache, nausea, dry mouth, blurred vision
• Solifenacin (Soliten)	5 mg daily × 12 months	Decreased libido
• Darifenacin (antidepressant [Depsol])	7.5–15 mg daily	Under trial

- Flavoxate (Urispas) is musculotropic and has a direct action on the smooth muscle when given at a dose of 200 mg t.i.d. It has antispasmodic and analgesic action.

Side effects include headache, nausea, constipation, dry mouth and blurred vision. It is contraindicated in the presence of glaucoma and cognitive impairment.

- Dicyclomine HCl: 10 mg four times daily
- Pro-Banthine (propantheline): 15–90 mg four times daily
- Oxybutynin HCl: 5–10 mg t.i.d. or extended release o.d. tablets
- Imipramine (tricyclic antidepressant): 50–100 mg at night for 3 months has a 70% success rate. It causes sedation, constipation and blurred vision in 10% of cases. It is not suitable for elderly women.

The drugs may cure incontinence in 60% of cases. New drugs are tolterodine tartrate 2 mg b.i.d. (extended release o.d. 4 mg) and propiverine. These drugs cause less dry mouth than flavoxate. Darifenacin and trospium chloride are currently under trial.

Duloxetine is a serotonin-norepinephrine reuptake inhibitor (SNRI). Dose of 40–80 mg b.d. orally for 3 months improves the bladder capacity. Nausea and dry mouth are its side effects. It increases the bladder capacity but decreases libido.

If the drugs fail, posterior tibial nerve stimulation (PTNS) should be tried. PTNS – neuromodulation is indirectly applied on the third sacral nerve via a needle electrode and connected to a stimulator. Thirty minutes of stimulation 3 monthly is practised.

If the drugs fail, transvesical injection of phenol is tried. A 10-mL volume of 6% phenol is injected into the trigone; 60% get benefit for a short period, but at the end of 1 year, only 2% get relief. Sloughing and fistula can occur. Acupuncture may be useful in some cases; urethral dilatation is successful in a few cases when the drugs fail. Augmentation 'Clam' cystoplasty involving augmentation of bladder capacity with a (25-cm length) segment of ileum gives a 95% cure rate. It is a major surgical procedure that requires repeated catheterization to empty the bladder; excessive mucus secretion from ileal mucosa can be troublesome. Twenty-five per cent complain of other urinary problems, and 5% develop adenocarcinoma of the ileal segment. Augmentation cystoplasty requires self-catheterization and causes stone formation, urinary infection, as well as electrolyte imbalance and malignancy.

Botox (Botulinum toxin A). Injection of Botulinum toxin A (neurotoxin) produced by anaerobic bacteria *Clostridium botulinum* into the detrusor muscle inhibits acetylcholine release at the neuromuscular junction and increases bladder compliance and capacity; the effect lasts for 9–12 months.

Side effects: Retention of urine and requires self-catheterization, normally in the first 6 weeks. It is recommended in resistant cases of DI and may supersede surgery in future, but more trials are required. Done via cystoscopy, 15–30 different detrusor muscle sites are injected under direct visualization. Though side effects of anticholinergic therapy are avoided, this technique has a higher rate of urinary retention and urinary infection.

- Detrusor myectomy creates a diverticulum and improves bladder capacity.
- Oestrogen cream alleviates symptoms of incontinence in postmenopausal women.
- Restricting fluid intake, especially at night, psychotherapy and treating the cause are also of help.
- Bladder drills or training disciplines the bladder to hold the urine for a longer period.

1-Deamino-8-D-arginine vasopressin (DDAVP) is a synthetic antidiuretic hormone (ADH) analogue. Peptide or intranasal 20–40 mcg at night cures nocturnal enuresis. Nausea, hyponatraemia and fluid retention may occur with this drug. It is contraindicated in coronary heart disease, hypertension and epilepsy in elderly women. Oral tablets are now available.

Medical therapy should be the mainstay of treatment; nerve stimulation and surgery should be employed only if medical therapy fails.

Biofeedback uses visual and auditory signals to demonstrate the strength of detrusor activity. Hypnotherapy helps in women with psychological disorders.

Neuromodulatory – Sacral nerve stimulation is reserved for refractory urge incontinence. It comprises surgical implantation of a generator to provide stimulation to the sacral nerve. It is very expensive, and 60% subjective relief is reported. Pain at the insertion is complained by 40% of women.

PTNS is also attempted.

KEY POINTS

- Incidence of genital fistulae of obstetric origin is decreasing as a result of improved obstetric care. However, they still contribute to a major share of all genital fistulae seen in clinical practice in India.
- Genital fistulae occur following prolonged unsupervised obstructed labour, following difficult vaginal instrumental deliveries and occasionally as a complication of caesarean section.
- Genital tract fistulae have been reported following gynaecological operations. The bladder or ureter may be involved.
- Investigations including methylene blue dye test, descending pyelography, cystoscopy and ureteric catheterization may be required to make a correct diagnosis. Surgical correction is possible in most cases.
- Besides obstetric and surgical trauma, advanced genital cancers and radiation injuries can cause fistulae. To alleviate symptoms, the surgeon may have to resort to palliative procedures such as surgical diversion of the urinary tract in these cases.
- GSI requires to be differentiated from urge incontinence, DI and a neurological bladder. Surgical repair in selected cases gives gratifying results, but the long-term results are not satisfactory. Primary treatment should be conservative.
- Burch operation is recommended for hypermobility of the urethra but is now superseded by TVT and TOT in some countries.
- TOT is considered superior to TVT, as it avoids retropubic space, osteitis and bladder injury.

DI caused by an overactive detrusor muscle is treated with various drugs. Surgery is rarely resorted.

- Botox injection may replace surgery but requires a longer trial in DI.
- Various drugs available (extended release) should be tried first, along with physiotherapy, before surgery is undertaken for DI.

SELF-ASSESSMENT

1. Discuss the causes of vesicovaginal fistula.
2. How will you investigate, diagnose and manage a case of vesicovaginal fistula?
3. What are the causes of ureteric fistula?
4. Discuss the management of ureteric fistulae.
5. What are the causes of genuine stress incontinence?
6. How will you manage a case of genuine stress incontinence in a woman 40 years of age?
7. Discuss the causes and management of detrusor instability.

SUGGESTED READING

Abstracts of the American College of Obstetricians and Gynecologists 53rd Annual Clinical Meeting. May 7-11, 2005, San Francisco, California, USA. Obstet Gynecol 2005; 105:1S.

American College of Obstetricians and Gynecologists. Urinary incontinence in women. Obstet Gynecol 2005; 105:1533.

American Urogynecologic Society and American College of Obstetricians and Gynecologists. Committee opinion: evaluation of uncomplicated stress urinary incontinence in women before surgical treatment. Female Pelvic Med Reconstr Surg 2014; 20:248.

Bonnar J. Recent Advances in Obstetrics and Gynaecology. Vol. 15, Elsevier, 1987.

Bonnar J. Recent Advances in Obstetrics and Gynaecology. Vol. 19, Elsevier, 1996.

FOGSI. Urodynamic assessment of women with urinary incontinence, 2009.

Sengupta et al. Textbook of Gynaecology for Post Graduates and Practitioners. Elsevier, 2007.

Shulman Lee P. Year Book of Obstetrics, Gynecology and Women's Health. Mosby: Elsevier, 2010.

Studd et al. Progress in Obstetrics and Gynecology, Vol. 18, Elsevier, 2008.

Studd J. Mechanical devices in stress incontinence. In Progress in Obstetrics and Gynaecology, Vol. 13: 325, Churchill Livingstone: Elsevier, 1998.

Studd J. Surgery for genuine stress incontinence. In Progress in Obstetrics and Gynaecology. Vol. 14, Churchill Livingstone: Elsevier, 2000.

Studd J. Treatment of detrusor instability and urge incontinence. Progress in Obstetrics and Gynaecology. Vol. 14, Churchill Livingstone: Elsevier, 2000.

Studd J. Ureteric injuries. Progress in Obstetrics and Gynaecology. Vol. 16, Churchill Livingstone: Elsevier, 2005.

32 Injuries of the Genital Tract and Intestinal Tract

CHAPTER OUTLINE

Most of the injuries of female genital tract are obstetrical, gynaecological and traumatic injuries are rare. They need to be recognized and repaired immediately to avoid bleeding, infection, painful scar and symptoms related to the associated injury to the neighbouring structure.

OBSTETRIC INJURIES

Most injuries of the female genital tract occur during childbirth. In a normal delivery, the circular fibres which surround the external cervical os are torn laterally on each side so that an anterior and a posterior lip of the cervix become differentiated. As a result of stretching, the vagina becomes more patulous, and as a result of laceration the hymen is subsequently represented by irregular tags of skin termed as the carunculae myrtiformes. A superficial first-degree laceration of the perineal skin is common even in uncomplicated deliveries.

In abnormal labour and when obstetrical manipulations have been carried out, or as a result of inaccurate technique, injuries of the birth canal are frequent. Severe lacerations of the perineum are perhaps the most common form of birth injury. Tears of the vagina may be caused by rotation of the head with forceps or may take the form of extension of tears either from the perineum or the cervix. Severe lacerations of the cervix are usually caused by strong uterine contractions at the end of the first stage of labour; others result from the delivery of a baby in an occiput posterior position and some from cervical dystocia. A vesicovaginal fistula may result from ischaemic necrosis or a difficult forceps delivery in cases of cephalopelvic disproportion, whereas a rectovaginal fistula is a result of a complete tear of the perineum or a suture which perforates the rectal wall. Extensive vaginal laceration causes fibrosis and narrowing of vagina, which may lead to dyspareunia and even apareunia.

Majority of obstetric injuries are theoretically preventable. A case of cephalopelvic disproportion should be recognized antenatally and treated in time by a caesarean section. Lacerations of the cervix and extensive tears of the perineum, though avoidable, should be treated by immediate suturing. One of the worst injuries in obstetric practice in India is **rupture of the uterus**. It occurs mostly in delivery cases conducted at home when obstructed labour is not diagnosed by the midwife. Uterine rupture carries a very high maternal mortality and subsequent morbidity among the survivors.

Obstetric trauma during childbirth can involve more than one organ. The perineum and the vaginal walls are most vulnerable; however, on occasions, childbirth trauma is known to badly injure the cervix, vaginal fornix, causes colporrhexis and even extends into the uterus resulting in uterine rupture.

PERINEAL TEARS

These are not uncommon; a thorough inspection of the perineum and lower genital tract under a good light is mandatory after any instrumental or assisted vaginal delivery and after spontaneous labour whenever traumatic postpartum haemorrhage is diagnosed. Small lacerations that are not bleeding may be left alone. All other injuries must be surgically repaired, preferably in an operation theatre. The presence of a competent assistant and availability of an anaesthesiologist during the procedure are of immense help. All bleeders should be meticulously tied. The tear should be repaired in layers. Sometimes, a small bleeder may be overlooked; this may lead to a vulval haematoma. In such an event, it is important to evacuate the haematoma at the earliest, ensure haemostasis and repair the wound promptly. At times blood transfusion may be needed to correct shock.

The **common risk factors** predisposing to perineal floor injuries are listed below:

1. **Overstretching of the perineum:**
   - Big-sized baby
   - Prolonged labour (dystocia)
   - Occipitoposterior malposition
   - Vaginal instrumental delivery
   - After-coming head in breech presentations
   - Midline episiotomy
2. **Rapid stretching of the perineum:**
   - Breech presentation
   - Precipitate labour
3. **Rigid perineum:**
   - Elderly primigravida
   - Vulval oedema
   - Scarred perineum following previous surgery
   - Repair of previous complete perineal tear

PREVENTION OF PERINEAL TEARS

Perineal tears can be avoided by timely adoption of the following measures:

1. Supporting the perineum and permitting gradual egress of the presenting part during delivery.
2. Timely episiotomy if the stretched perineum seems likely to tear.
3. It is advisable to perform an episiotomy while undertaking any instrumental-assisted vaginal delivery.
4. It is advisable to perform an episiotomy while conducting assisted vaginal breech delivery.
5. In patients having history of successful repair of complete perineal tear, difficult genital tract prolapse. It will be advisable to go for a caesarean section as the route for delivery in women with previous repair of urinary fistulas.

VAGINAL TEARS

Isolated vaginal tears or lacerations without involvement of the perineum are usually found following instrumental or manipulative vaginal deliveries. These should be promptly repaired after delivery to prevent undue blood loss. Sometimes, it is advisable to pack the vagina with sterile roller gauze soaked in glycerine acriflavine/Betadine to provide local compression; the pack should be removed in 24 hours.

CERVICAL TEARS

These may follow instrumental vaginal delivery, in shoulder dystocia or manipulations during vaginal breech delivery. The fact that there is excessive vaginal bleeding in the presence of a well-contracted uterus, should raise suspicion of genital tract trauma. Speculum examination and packing of the cervix against the vaginal vault permits satisfactory visualization of the vaginal walls. Thereafter, the entire rim of the cervix should be inspected between ring forceps to identify any cervical tear and repair the same.

COLPORRHEXIS

Rupture of the vaginal vault is called colporrhexis. There may be concomitant tear of the cervix. If this injury is extensive, it may lead to formation of broad ligament haematoma requiring laparotomy. Suturing of the rent should suffice. There is danger to the uterine vessels and ureter during repair. Great care should be exercised to avoid complications.

INJURIES DUE TO COITUS

A slight amount of bleeding from the torn edges of the ruptured hymen is normal after defloration, but the haemorrhage can sometimes be severe, particularly when the tear has spread forward to the region of the vestibule. The haemorrhage can usually be controlled by the application of gauze pressure, but occasionally suturing under anaesthesia is required and blood transfusion may be necessary.

Bruising of the vaginal wall is not uncommon in the early days of married life, and a urethritis may result from bruising of the urethra. Such cases (honeymoon cystitis) are seen frequently and it is not uncommon for ascending pyelonephritis to result.

Lacerations of the vagina caused by coitus are occasionally seen. Violent coitus or rape in young girls, forceful penetration in postmenopausal women with atrophy of the vagina or in the presence of malformations such as transverse vaginal septum, extensive and serious injuries are known to occur. These lacerations may be of various types. It often takes the form of a longitudinal tear of the anterior vaginal wall. Cases are on record where the posterior vaginal wall has been torn through and the peritoneal cavity opened up. Both bladder and rectum may be involved in serious coital injuries. Similar injuries may occur in patients who have undergone vaginal operations in the past, especially if coitus takes place soon after the operation. All patients who have had a vaginal operation should be advised to avoid coitus for initial 2 months. A similar injury can occur after the operation of total hysterectomy when the recently stitched vaginal vault may be disrupted by coitus. Large or small bowel and omentum can prolapse into the vagina with resulting shock and peritonitis. Severe haemorrhage follows injuries of this kind. When the injuries are small, treatment consists in plugging the vagina, provided thorough inspection has excluded the possibility of extensive or internal injury. In more severe cases, it is necessary to suture the laceration under anaesthesia. If the bowel has prolapsed, it is imperative to open the abdomen so that a complete inspection of the gut from the jejunum to the rectum can be undertaken. Damage to bowel or mesentery can then be assessed and the correct treatment performed under direct vision. It is interesting to note that quite apart from the coitus or direct injury, a spontaneous rupture of the vagina can occur in the upper posterior one-third. The patients are usually elderly and the vagina is atrophic. The cause is usually a violent bout of coughing or some severe strain associated with a sudden rise in intraabdominal pressure. The treatment is the same as for coital injuries.

DIRECT TRAUMA AND VULVAL HAEMATOMA

Injuries to the vulva as the result of direct trauma are not uncommon. Accidents such as falling astride gates and chairs are frequent and usually produce bruising of the labia majora. In more severe cases, large haematoma develops in the labia majora and the effused blood spreads widely in the lax connective tissues. This is specially seen when the laceration involves the region of the clitoris and the erectile tissue around the vaginal orifice. Compressible haematomas of the vulva are sometimes caused by the rupture of varicose veins of the labia majora during pregnancy, and the large swelling may obstruct the delivery of the head (Fig. 32.1).

The most common cause of the vulvovaginal haematoma is the inadequate haemostasis during suturing of an episiotomy or a perineal tear. The important complications of haematoma of the vulva are haemorrhage with subsequent anaemia and local infection. A vulval haematoma presents as a painful tender swelling, bluish black in appearance. The patient may look pale and she may be in a condition of shock. A small haematoma responds well to bed rest, sitz bath and magnesium sulphate fomentation. Antibiotics are given to prevent infection. With large haematoma, it is necessary to incise the swelling under anaesthesia and to remove the clot. If the haemostasis is difficult to secure, packing and drainage is employed. The deep penetrating injuries require immediate operation, suture and repair of the injured structure. If there is a suspicion of visceral injury or if the pouch of Douglas has been opened, laparotomy must be performed and perforation of the bowel and bladder sutured. A temporary colostomy may be necessary, if the rectum has been injured. Road traffic injuries may involve injury to pelvic bones, vagina and perineum.

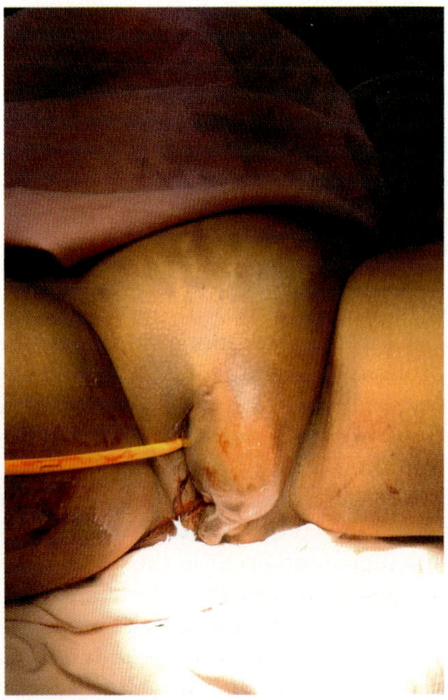

Figure 32.1 Vulval haematoma.

PELVIC HAEMATOMA

Pelvic haematomas are of two types. Infralevator haematoma following a perineal tear or episiotomy, these have been described above.

Supralevator haematoma results in the formation of broad ligament haematoma. It follows cervical tear involving the uterine vessels, uterine rupture (spontaneous or caesarean scar rupture) and uterine artery tear during uterine surgery. The diagnosis may be delayed, if it is small. A large haematoma causes hypotension, tachycardia and pallor. A tender swelling is felt on one side of the uterus in the broad ligament.

Management depends upon the size of the haematoma.

- Conservative treatment with observation: A small haematoma gets gradually absorbed. Antibiotics should be given.
- Laparotomy: If the bleeder cannot be identified as is the usual case, the broad ligament should be packed for 24 hours and one end of the pack brought out of the abdominal wound to be removed later. Blood transfusion may be required.
- Hysterectomy for uterine rupture.
- Internal iliac ligation to control bleeding.
- Embolization of internal iliac artery.

It is important to identify the ureter and avoid trauma to ureters during hysterectomy.

GENITAL MUTILATION

This practice of genital mutilation is still prevalent in African countries, parts of Asia and amongst Arabs. It involves partial or total removal of external genital organs in girls, for nonmedical reasons. It involves partial or total removal of the clitoris and prepuce (type I), clitoris with labia minora (type II), cutting and apposing labia minora (type III) or pricking, piercing, incision and cauterization (type IV).

Immediate complications are as follows:

- Bleeding – haematoma
- Pain
- Infection

Long-term adverse effects are as follows:

- Severe persistent pain due to unprotected nerve endings.
- Dyspareunia, apareunia.
- Haematoma during forceful intercourse.
- Infection with scaring.
- Transmission of HIV, tetanus.
- Retention of urine, haematocolpos.
- Difficult childbirth and need for caesarean delivery.
- Psychological trauma of mutilation and distorted anatomy of the external genitalia.

INJURIES DUE TO FOREIGN BODIES AND INSTRUMENTS

VAGINA

An extraordinary variety of bizarre foreign bodies have been recovered from the vagina including safety pins, hair grips, pencils and small jam jars. The patient is often mentally retarded or a young child, and in both these cases a persistent and a malodorous discharge should always suggest the presence of a foreign body.

Neglected or forgotten objects employed therapeutically. The most frequently found is the ring pessary used in prolapse. Some of these have remained in the vagina for many years and have become encrusted with phosphatic deposits. These neglected pessaries can cause severe ulceration of the posterior fornix and later even vaginal carcinoma. Less traumatic are forgotten swabs and tampons which cause a foul purulent discharge.

Contraceptive devices such as cervical caps and diaphragms, even a mislaid condom when retained, can cause discharge and ulceration.

Instrumental damage is caused during attempted criminal abortion. Sound, gums, elastic bougies, knitting needles and the like have caused perforation of the vagina into the bladder, rectum, the pouch of Douglas and the parametrium.

CERVIX

Obstetric cervical tears occur during precipitate labour or instrumental delivery.

The commonest cause of cervical tear is cervical dilatation with the metal dilators and this causes bleeding and later an incompetent os. Cervical stenosis follows conization and amputation as in Fothergill's operation for prolapse and cauterization of cervix for cervical erosion. This can lead to haematometra and infertility.

UTERUS

Foreign bodies in the uterus are almost always intrauterine contraceptive devices such as copper-T. These may be neglected or forgotten by the patient. They can cause ulceration of the endometrium and give rise to a serious ascending infection with inflammatory tubo-ovarian masses. These foreign bodies may also be a cause of menorrhagia.

The other foreign body met within the uterus has usually been introduced to procure abortion. Serious intrauterine infections often result in pelvic abscess from acute salpingo-oophoritis.

Perforation of the uterus may occur during dilatation and curettage (D&C) and medical termination of pregnancy (MTP). Perforation during hysteroscopic operative procedures, such as transcervical resection of endometrium (TCRE) or division of the uterine septum, is known. These should not be treated lightly; the possibility of injury to hollow viscera, or vessels, must always be borne in mind and necessary surgical measures immediately taken to ensure patient safety.

Sometimes Asherman syndrome with uterine synechiae follows vigorous curettage or uterine packing to control haemorrhage, manual removal of the placenta and uterine infection.

TREATMENT

Treatment for vaginal foreign bodies is to remove them, if necessary, under anaesthesia. Simple local antiseptic douches are sufficient thereafter. If, however, the vagina has been perforated, antibiotics are indicated, and if there are signs of peritonitis or bowel damage, laparotomy should be undertaken.

Uterine foreign bodies should be removed under anaesthesia and, if infection is present, a swab taken and the appropriate antibiotics given. Adnexal involvement if resistant to chemotherapy, e.g. large persistent masses with recurrent fever and constitutional upset, calls for laparotomy and their surgical removal. In young women, it is sometimes possible to conserve the uterus and part of one ovary. When the pelvic organs are grossly damaged by the pelvic inflammatory disease (PID), total hysterectomy and bilateral salpingo-oophorectomy is the only logical answer. Fortunately, these severe infections due to uterine foreign bodies are rare now.

CHEMICAL AND OTHER BURNS OF THE VAGINA

The most common cause of these is the use of strong chemicals such as Lysol, permanganate or corrosive sublimate to induce abortions by untrained persons. The dangerous complication of this type of burn is that during healing, extensive vaginal adhesions and fibrosis will obliterate the canal and prevent coitus, and even cause retention of menstrual discharge with haematometra and pyometra. Plastic reconstruction is the only answer to this problem.

Douches administered at a very high temperature can also cause burn. This is a culpable error on part of the operator.

During the operation of cauterization of the cervix by cautery or diathermy, it is quite easy to burn the vagina directly or by conduction. Fortunately, cryosurgery has nowadays replaced cauterization of the cervix, and burn injuries of this nature are rare. Laser therapy for cervical lesions and vaginal cancer in situ can also result in burns of vagina.

It must be remembered that the radium inserted into the vagina for carcinoma of the cervix always causes radiation burn. During the process of healing, the vaginal vault frequently becomes obliterated by adhesive vaginitis and fibrosis.

TREATMENT

Most vaginal burns, unless severe, heal with expectant treatment. Those resulting in extensive scarring and atresia will require plastic surgery.

PERINEAL INJURIES

A minor degree of laceration of the perineal body often occurs during childbirth. Some degree of perineal laceration occurs in nearly all normal deliveries, whereas the incidence is greater if instrumental deliveries have been performed. Lacerations are five to six times more frequent in primiparae than with multiparae.

It is customary to grade lacerations of the perineum into four degrees. In the **first degree**, the laceration is restricted to the skin of the fourchette. In the **second degree**, the muscles of the perineal body are torn through, whereas in the **third degree** the tear extends partially backwards through the external sphincter of the anus. In the **fourth degree**, the sphincter is torn and anal mucosa is also involved. A rare type of tear is the central tear of the perineum when the head penetrates first through the posterior vaginal wall, then through the perineal body and appears through the skin of the perineum. It usually occurs in patients with a contracted outlet of pelvis.

PERINEAL LACERATIONS

An occult injury to the perineum without noticeable sign occurs in 0.5%–2% of women following vaginal delivery.

Studies have shown that as much as 35% of primiparae sustain occult sphincter injury as shown by ano-endosonogram.

The first-degree lacerations, restricted to the skin of the fourchette, have no influence on the integrity of the pelvic floor, but if the lacerations are not sutured after delivery, the vaginal orifice becomes patulous. In practice, small lacerations of the fourchette are not sutured unless they extend to the skin of the perineum, where they are more likely to become infected and to cause pain.

The second-degree lacerations should always be sutured carefully immediately after delivery. The pelvic floor is weakened unless the injury to the muscles of the perineal body is efficiently repaired. If the decussating fibres of the levator ani muscles are torn through, the hiatus urogenitalis becomes patulous predisposing to prolapse of the vagina and the uterus subsequently.

With the extensive second-degree tears, the patient should be given a local, regional pudendal block or general anaesthesia, placed in the lithotomy position and the torn muscles of the perineum identified and sutured together with catgut. The torn edges of the vagina and the skin of the perineum should then be sutured together with an absorbable suture material. The essential part of the after treatment of perineal lacerations consists in keeping the perineum clean. Frequent swabbing is therefore imperative during the puerperium. The wound should be cleaned with an antiseptic solution such as Betadine after micturition and defecation. Antibiotics are required.

The third- and fourth-degree tears are much more important, because unless they are efficiently repaired immediately after delivery, the patient develops incontinence of faeces and flatus. Amongst the predisposing causes of complete tear of the perineum are forceps delivery in the persistent occipitoposterior positions, and extraction of the aftercoming head in a breech presentation. Large head and precipitate labour are also contributory factors, but the most common cause is vigorous pulling in the wrong direction during forceps delivery, especially with Kielland's forceps. A properly performed episiotomy will very largely eliminate the risk of the third- and fourth-degree tear. This type of tear is more common with median episiotomy than mediolateral episiotomy.

Complete tear of the perineum should be repaired as soon as possible after the delivery. A practitioner should not undertake the repair of a complete tear of the perineum single-handedly. The operation should be undertaken under anaesthesia with the patient lying in the lithotomy position in good light and with good assistance. The operation should be regarded as a surgical emergency and there is no excuse for delay. As facilities may not be available in the patient's home, she should be transferred to a hospital.

The immediate repair of a complete tear of the perineum is a relatively simple procedure, because the muscles of the perineal body, though torn, can be distinguished without much difficulty. The surrounding skin is first cleaned and the operation area isolated with sterile towels. A sterile pack is placed in the vagina and the limits of the laceration defined with tissue forceps. The rectum and the anal canal are first repaired with Vicryl '30' sutures inserted with an atraumatic needle. A few Lembert sutures are then introduced to invaginate the torn edges of the rectal wall. The muscles of the perineal body are now sutured together, and every effort should be made to obtain exact anatomical reposition. Particular attention must be paid to the sphincter ani muscle, and at least two Vicryl sutures should be used to draw the cut edges together. The tears in the vaginal wall and in the skin of the perineum are now repaired with interrupted sutures. Care should be taken to avoid tying the sutures too tightly; otherwise, oedema of the perineum will lead to severe pain and cause the stitches to cut through. If a complete tear of the perineum is treated by immediate suture, the end result is satisfactory if correct anatomical reposition has been attained. If primary union of the vagina and the perineal skin is not obtained, the wound should be kept clean and encouraged to granulate by frequent sitz baths. The end results are often functionally good in spite of the initial breakdown of the suture line. The bowels should be confined for at least 5 days, solid foods withheld and intestinal antiseptics given, along with stool softeners. Systemic antibiotics are necessary.

Lately, instead of end-to-end suturing of the torn sphincter muscles, an overlap technique is recommended to yield a stronger sphincteric control.

OLD, LONGSTANDING COMPLETE PERINEAL TEARS

Various degrees of complete perineal tears, usually resulting from careless attempts at immediate suturing, are not unusual. The rectal wall may be torn through as high as 5 cm or more along the posterior vaginal wall, but in most cases only the anal canal is involved. The appearance of the perineum in cases of old complete tear is characteristic. The red glistening mucous membrane of the anal canal and rectum protrudes and fuse directly with the vaginal wall without any of the perineal tissues intervening. Laterally, on each side, on a level with the anus, is the depression in the skin which corresponds to the position of the severed edge of the torn external sphincter (Fig. 32.2). Behind the anus are the radial folds in the skin which are corrugated by the underlying contracted subcutaneous sphincter. The external sphincter is only present posteriorly and the absence of the sphincteric grip is appreciated by inserting a finger into the anus.

One of the most interesting features of the complete tear of the perineum is that it is very rarely, if ever, associated with

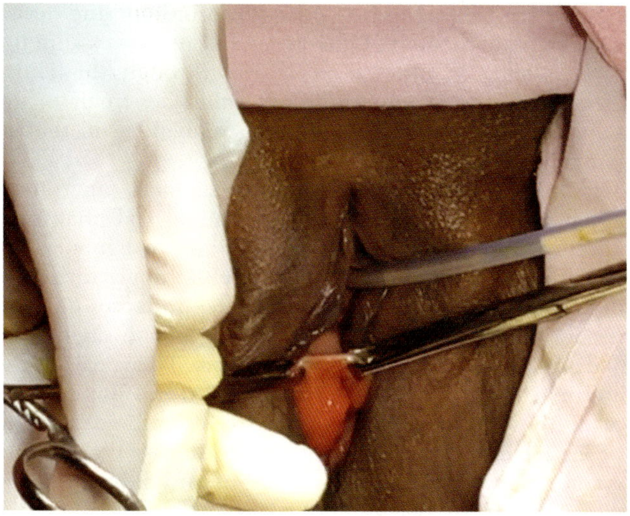

Figure 32.2 Complete tear of the perineum.

uterine prolapse, although the decussating fibres of the levator ani muscles have been torn through. The reason is that the patient continuously draws together the two levator ani muscles in an effort to close the anus so that by constant use the tone of the muscles becomes exceptionally good. This firmness and good development of the levator muscles is found on clinical examination when the levator muscles are palpated.

SYMPTOMS

The patient complains of incontinence of faeces and flatus. A few patients develop the tone of the levator muscles so well that they only suffer incontinence of flatus. These women will complain of incontinence of faeces only if they develop diarrhoea.

Apart from clinical examination, a gap in the sphincter can be identified by perineal ultrasound or magnetic resonance imaging (MRI).

TREATMENT

The treatment of old complete tear of the perineum is operative. The technical difficulties are much greater in old cases than in those operated upon immediately after delivery. The optimum time for operation in the case of old tears is 3–6 months after delivery. If the operation is attempted earlier than this, healing by first intention is exception, whereas if the operation is further delayed, a dense scar tissue forms which adds to the operative difficulties. Preoperative preparation is of importance, and the patient should be kept in the hospital for a couple of days before the operation during which time the bowels should be emptied by aperients and enemas, and the vagina disinfected by douching and by insertion of gauze packs soaked in flavine (1 in 1000) or Betadine lotion. The bacterial flora of the bowel should be controlled by ampicillin or neomycin, given in large doses for 3 days before the operation. The patient should be put on a nonresidual diet such as milk and fluid for 2 days before surgery. Various techniques have been described in the operative treatment of complete tears of the perineum, but the underlying principles are the same in all. The rectum must be dissected from the vagina by incising the intervening scar tissue and by dissecting upwards in the rectovaginal septum.

Perhaps the most important step in the operation is to dissect the rectum clear of scar tissue and to mobilize it so that it can be brought down, without tension to the anal region. The tear in the rectum and anal canal is now repaired by excising scar tissue, freshening the cut edges and suturing them together with fine Vicryl sutures mounted on an atraumatic needle and tied within the lumen of bowel. The needles, forceps and scissors used during this step are discarded. The wound in the bowel is now invaginated with a layer of interrupted Lembert sutures. Next, the deep muscles of the perineal body and the levator ani are identified and sutured together with no. 0 or 1 Vicryl. It is important to ensure that the muscles are dissected clear of scar tissue and are mobilized. The next important step in the operation is to suture together the torn edges of the external sphincter. These must be carefully defined, dissected clear of scar tissue and sutured together with three or four separate Vicryl sutures. The remains of the superficial muscles of the perineum are now sutured together with catgut/Vicryl and then the cut edges of the vagina and the perineum are repaired, interrupted catgut/Vicryl sutures being used. These principles are uniformly followed in the various methods described for the treatment of a complete tear of the perineum. The modifications depend solely on the position of the incisions made in the vaginal walls and in the skin of the perineum, and these, in their turn, depend not on any particular technique, but on the type of complete tear which is to be repaired (Fig. 32.3).

Lately, many gynaecologists believe in the overlap of sphincteric sutures to strengthen the tone and function of the sphincter, though others feel this overlap technique has no advantage on the surgical outcome. This remains a controversial point as of today.

AFTER TREATMENT

The most important part of the after treatment is to keep the wound dry. The perineum should be swabbed after micturition and defecation with an antiseptic solution and subsequently powdered. Betadine is the antiseptic solution of choice, and it is effective. The bowels should be confined until at least the fifth day of the operation. To achieve this, the patient is given only intravenous fluids for the first 2 days and oral fluids the next 2 days. From third day she gets a small dose of laxative so that when she passes stool on fifth day they are not hard. As in all operations on the perineum, retention of urine is a common complication; it may be advisable to leave a Foley's catheter for a few days in the immediate postoperative period. Antibiotics administered preoperatively should be continued for at least a week postoperatively. Systemic chemotherapy is necessary to prevent infection and it should be given for a week. The end result is usually good. Another complication that may develop is a rectovaginal fistula which is usually the result of faulty technique but also may be due to infection and breakdown of sutures.

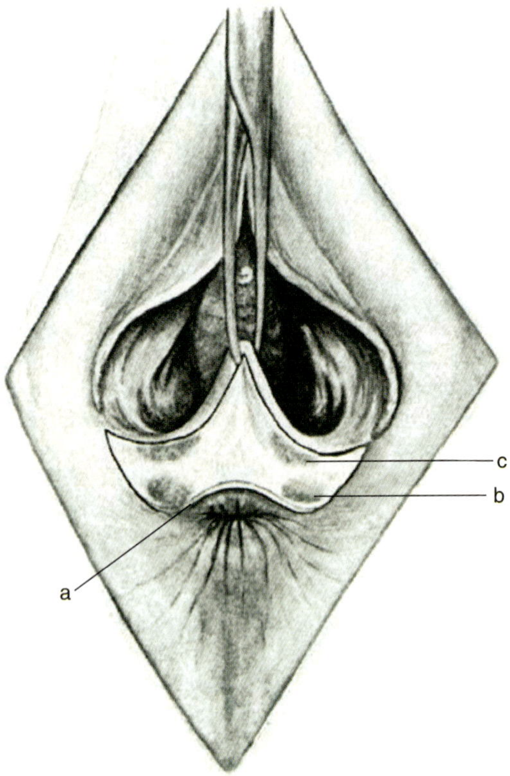

Figure 32.3 Operation for repair of a complete perineal tear. An area of scarred skin is excised and the mucous membrane of the anal canal freshened at the edge. The rectum is then mobilized and pulled down. Three structures must be defined, freed of scar tissue and mobilized, namely (a) the mucous membrane of the anal canal, (b) the external sphincter and (c) the levator ani muscles. First the edges of the anal canal mucosa must be sutured together, then the cut edge of the sphincter and lastly the levator muscles. Afterwards the cut edges of the posterior vaginal wall and the skin of the perineum are sutured.

RUPTURE OF THE UTERUS

Rupture of the uterus is the most dreaded complication in obstetrics, almost entirely a complication of difficult labour. It is common in multiparae, usually following a neglected, obstructed delivery. Misuse of oxytocics, or dehiscence of a previous uterine scar (caesarean section), rarely a haematometra or pyometra, may lead to rupture spontaneously as a result of distension and thinning of the atrophic myometrium. Depending on the cause and extension of tear, repair or hysterectomy is performed at laparotomy.

PERFORATION OF THE UTERUS

In the nonpregnant state, perforation of the uterus may occur during the operation of D&C. The perforation is more common if the uterus is soft as in pregnancy and in malignancy. The atrophic uterus of a menopausal woman can easily be perforated during curettage for postmenopausal bleeding. Spontaneous perforation may also occur with intrauterine contraceptive devices. The intrauterine device may perforate the wall of the uterus, but remains within the myometrium. At times it perforates through the entire thickness of the myometrium and either lies freely in the peritoneal cavity or more often gets embedded in the abdominal viscera.

If the uterus is empty and not malignant, laparotomy may not be necessary. Simple observation is all that is required. In the presence of pyometra and malignancy, immediate laparotomy and hysterectomy is strongly advised. If the abdominal viscera, i.e. the intestine, prolapses through the perforation and is seen protruding in the vagina, immediate laparotomy becomes mandatory. The repair of the intestinal injury by resection and end-to-end anastomosis will be required depending on the extent of the damage to the intestine. If the uterus contains products of conception, repair of the rent after evacuation of uterus under guidance will suffice. If the perforation is large or if the patient has completed her family, hysterectomy is the operation of choice. Uterine injury has been recently reported during hysteroscopic excision of the uterine septum. Excision under laparoscopic supervision can avoid this injury. The uterine perforation can also occur during ablation of endometrium through a hysteroscope in cases of dysfunctional uterine bleeding (DUB).

INJURIES OF THE INTESTINAL TRACT

A close anatomical relation of the lower female genital tract to the rectum and anal canal sometimes results in injury to these structures. This is reported during vaginal delivery and vaginal surgery. Similarly, abdominal gynaecological surgery may inadvertently injure the bowel. The use of cautery in gynaecology may inflict a burn injury to the gastrointestinal tract (GIT), and this becomes noticeable a few days after the procedure.

It is important therefore to realize the risk of injuries to the small and large bowels in obstetrics and gynaecology.

Injuries to the bowel in obstetrics are as follows:

1. Vaginal delivery
   - The third- and fourth-degree perineal tear
   - Rectovaginal fistula
   - Faecal incontinence
   - Stricture of the anal canal and rectum
2. Caesarean delivery
   - Intestinal injury
3. During MTP
4. Other causes of bowel injuries in obstetrics and gynaecology
   - Congenital rectovaginal fistula
   - Penetrating injury – accidents
   - Infective – sexually transmitted infections, septic abortions
   - Rectal abscess, pelvic abscess
5. During surgery
   - Abdominal hysterectomy
   - Vaginal surgery – postvaginal repair and vaginoplasty
   - Endoscopic – laparoscopy and hysteroscopy
6. Genital cancers
7. Radiotherapy for cancer of the female genital organs

VAGINAL DELIVERY

The injury to the anal sphincter, anal canal and sometimes the rectum during vaginal delivery is more common in a primipara. A big baby, prolonged labour, occipitoposterior presentation, breech and forceps delivery are factors leading to higher incidence of bowel injury.

The injury may be a direct muscle trauma, injury to the pelvic floor muscles or to the nerve supply of the anal canal (pudendal nerve).

The symptoms appear soon after the delivery if a tear occurs, or may appear years later due to stretching when a woman develops anal wall prolapse or faecal incontinence.

The injury to the pelvic floor muscles will cause both stress incontinence of urine and faecal incontinence besides genital prolapse.

FAECAL INCONTINENCE

Normal anatomy of the anal canal and maintenance of continence of faeces:

The anal canal is 3–4 cm in length and is surrounded by the internal sphincter above and external sphincter below. The internal sphincter represents the expanded distal portion of the circular smooth muscle of the rectum and is innervated by autonomic nerves. The external sphincter is a striated muscle and is innervated by the pudendal nerve (sacral 2–4). The anal pressure remains above the rectal pressure and internal sphincter remains contracted in a continent woman, and opens only when the rectum distends aided by intraabdominal pressure. The external sphincter muscle is supplemented by the puborectalis muscle of the levator ani and this prevents or defers defecation when the suitable situation does not prevail. In addition, the rectum forms an angle of 60–130° with the anal canal, and this also helps to keep the internal sphincter closed, and prevents stool from entering the anal canal. During defecation, the angle straightens out and allows the faecal matter to enter the anal canal. The levator ani muscles relax, so also the external sphincter. The pelvic floor descends by 2 cm. The anal canal widens and shortens during defecation.

Faecal incontinence is defined as a loss of normal control leading to involuntary leakage of faecal contents. Depending on the degree of incontinence, flatus, loose motion (diarrhoea) or solid stool leaks out.

Faecal incontinence is reported in 0.5%–2% of women following vaginal delivery. Women are more prone to faecal incontinence than men, and elderly women suffer more than younger women. Faecal incontinence may follow some years after the delivery, but many develop it within 6 months of delivery. Primiparae are more inclined than the multiparae. The occult damage to the internal sphincter occurs in 35% of women following first vaginal delivery, though the perineum appears intact. This is revealed by anal endosonography.

AETIOLOGY

Several causes are known to cause faecal incontinence, but the most important factor in women is obstetric trauma during vaginal delivery.

Obstetric trauma during vaginal delivery:

- Prolonged labour which can overstretch the levator ani muscle or damage the pudendal nerve.
- Difficult forceps delivery.
- Occipitoposterior presentation of the fetus, big baby.
- Rigid perineum.
- Episiotomy does not always safeguard against sphincter damage. Midline episiotomy increases risk of injury to the sphincter, compared to mediolateral episiotomy.
- The third- and fourth-degree perineal tears, by tearing the external sphincter, lead to faecal incontinence.

Nonobstetric causes are as follows:

- Neurogenic, dementia, cerebrovascular accident, spinal cord lesion.
- Bowel diseases such as inflammatory disease, cancer and rectal prolapse.
- Radiotherapy for cancer of the genital tract.

Urge incontinence of faeces results from injury to the external sphincter when the woman is unable to hold on until she can reach the toilet.

HISTORY

The woman may develop faecal incontinence soon after the delivery (usually first vaginal delivery) or some years later if the damage is mild. Further weakening of the pelvic floor muscle support and sphincteric control with an advancing age is the cause of delay for the onset of symptoms. Many a times, the woman is reluctant to reveal this history due to shyness, unless directly questioned.

On examination, perineal tears are obvious, but damage to the internal sphincter shows no external injury and certain investigations are required.

Occasionally, faecal incontinence may follow pelvic surgery.

INVESTIGATIONS

- Proctoscopy and sigmoidoscopy for a rectal disease.
- Manometry to measure the anal canal pressure. Normal pressure is 45–100 mm H_2O.
- Electromyelography to detect a nerve injury to the muscle (pudendal neuropathy).
- Ten hertz (10 Hz) ultrasound scanning of the anal canal has now replaced electromyelography. Ultrasound scanning detects a defect in the sphincter (Fig. 32.4).
- MRI.

TREATMENT

Management of faecal incontinence comprises the following:

- Medical – Loperamide and codeine phosphate increase the resting tone of the anal sphincters and also cure urge incontinence.
- Fibre-rich diet makes the stool firm.
- Antidiarrhoeal treatment in inflammatory diseases of the bowel.
- Physiotherapy and biofeedback training are useful though time consuming, but nerve injury recovers in 2 weeks in 60% of early cases.
- Sacral nerve stimulation with a probe improves pudendal nerve stimulation and tones up the levator ani muscles.

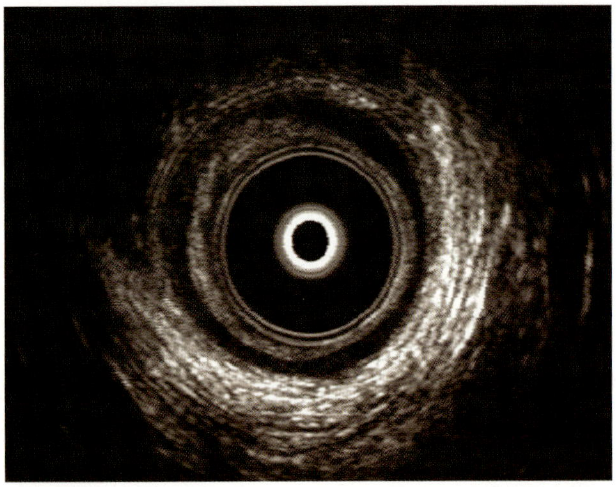

Figure 32.4 Transrectal ultrasonography (TRUS) showing a defect in external anal sphincter.

- Surgery – surgery is required for extensive perineal tears, fistula and anal prolapse. Rectopexy for rectal prolapse cures incontinence. The woman should be delivered by caesarean section following a successful repair in subsequent pregnancy.

RECTOVAGINAL FISTULA

The majority of rectovaginal fistulas result from obstetric injuries, usually a complete tear of the perineum which has been imperfectly sutured immediately after delivery (Fig. 32.5). It has already been pointed out that the repair of a complete tear of the perineum should be undertaken carefully, with the patient in the lithotomy position and under anaesthesia. If, for instance, a few sutures are placed through the lower part of the anal canal and the upper part of the tear in the rectum is not accurately sutured, a fistulous opening may form between the rectum and vagina. Rectovaginal fistula may occur after operation for old complete tears of the perineum if the wound breaks down, or if the rectum is not properly mobilized before the repair of the wound in the rectal wall. These fistulas also occur after the operation of perineorrhaphy in thin, elderly patients when the anterior wall of the rectum is accidentally opened.

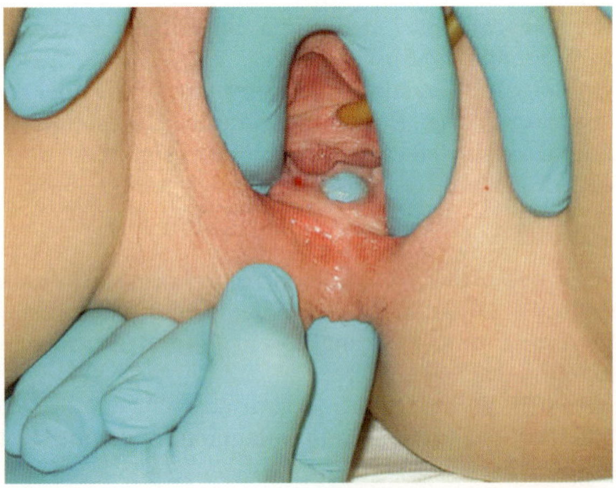

Figure 32.5 Examining finger passed through rectum seen to emerge into the vagina through a rectovaginal fistula. (*Source:* Benjamin Person and Juan J. Nogueras. The Management of Rectovaginal Fistulas in Patients with Inflammatory Bowel Disease. Seminars in Colon and Rectal Surgery,17(2):2006.)

Other causes are tuberculosis, which is not uncommon in India, and lymphogranuloma inguinale. In advanced carcinoma of the cervix, when the growth has spread down the posterior vaginal wall, a rectovaginal fistula eventually results. Such fistulas also occur following radiation treatment of carcinoma of the cervix or vagina, or following Wertheim's operation for the same condition. A fistula following radiotherapy may occur 3 months to several years after radiotherapy and such a fistula is surrounded by extensive fibrosis. It is difficult to cure a malignant fistula and it can only be treated by some form of posterior pelvic exenteration or a palliative colostomy. Primary carcinoma of the rectum can also extend forward and involve the vagina to cause a rectovaginal fistula. A congenital rectovaginal fistula is rarely seen and is the result of maldevelopment of the lower part of the rectum and anal canal. In such cases, it is customary to perform preliminary colostomy before plastic operation. Diverticulitis, rectal abscess and direct trauma are other rare causes of a fistula.

In case of a pelvic abscess when there is collection of pus in the pouch of Douglas, the abscess sometimes bursts into the rectum and a rectovaginal fistula develops, particularly if the abscess is surgically opened up through the posterior fornix. There is a form of a rectovaginal fistula which follows infection in an anal crypt with a resultant abscess formation, which bursts into the vagina. These cases are difficult to treat surgically, and good results cannot be expected until the entire fistulous tract into the anal canal has been excised. This necessitates division of the external sphincter and follows the principles laid down in the treatment of fistula-in-ano. The patient complains incontinence of faeces and flatus. A large fistula can easily be identified, but a small one is very difficult to detect, especially if it is surrounded by dense fibrosis. Proctoscopy, sigmoidoscopy and injection of radiopaque dye will be needed to trace the fistulous tract.

TREATMENT

The traumatic form of a rectovaginal fistula is treated by operation. Preoperative treatment is important and the bowel should be emptied with enema, and the vagina disinfected by douches and gauze packs soaked in antiseptic solutions such as flavine or Betadine. Phthalylsulphathiazole or neomycin should be given for a few days before operation to sterilize the bowel contents. Other drugs such as Ampicillin, Tinidazole can be used for bowel preparation.

With a small rectovaginal fistula above an intact perineal body, an unusual event, it is sometimes feasible to excise the fistulous track and close the defect successfully by a local operation. It will, however, be more commonly found that the perineal body below the fistula is inadequate and that the levators are not approximated. In fact, in many rectovaginal fistulas, there is merely a thin skin bridge below the fistula and often the anal sphincter itself is incompetent. When, in addition to these perineal defects, the fistula is very large, the best treatment is to cut the skin bridge in the midline and convert the fistula into a complete perineal tear. This is then repaired like a complete perineal tear. A **high rectovaginal fistula** may require a preliminary colostomy. The fistula due to cancer of the cervix or rectum requires an exenteration operation. A fistula following radiotherapy for cancer may be successfully closed by colpocleisis. This operation consists of obliteration of the vaginal cavity after denuding the entire vaginal mucosa. However, results are not good.

The surgeon may be involved in complicated rectal surgery.

Optimal mode of future delivery is not defined; and the decision is individualized. However, most gynaecologists believe in performing elective caesarean section to avoid further damage to the sphincter.

BOWEL INJURY

AETIOLOGY

- *While entering* the *peritoneal cavity*, the risk factors are obesity, previous surgery, gynaecological pathology such as pelvic endometriosis, PID, cancer surgery and previous irradiation.
- *Laparoscopy*. It is not uncommon to perforate the bowel with the Veress needle or the trocar. The use of cautery or laser during laparoscopic surgery can cause burns to the intestine. This will be detected about 5–7 days later, when the woman returns with peritonitis and ileus.
- *Hysteroscopic resection of a uterine septum*, or TCRE in DUB, can cause uterine perforation and thermal heat can cause intestinal burn.
- *D&C*. It is rare to damage the intestine during gynaecological D&C, though some cases have been reported.

Types of injury – perforation, laceration and crush injuries are likely to occur in gynaecological surgery.

DIAGNOSIS

Most of the above injuries can be recognized at surgery. Burn injuries, however, may take about a week to present as peritonitis and a fistula.

SURGICAL TREATMENT

Thorough exploration of bowel with the help of a surgical colleague is needed for appropriate treatment. Caesarean section performed following a prolonged second stage can also cause injury to the anal sphincter and anal wall. More commonly, however, it is the small bowel that gets injured during caesarean section, more so if the intestine is adherent to the parietal peritoneum through previous surgery.

MEDICAL TERMINATION OF PREGNANCY

Apart from criminal abortion, the bowel can be injured during MTP if the uterine perforation goes unnoticed and a loop of intestine is pulled through the perforation. Immediate laparotomy is required and bowel injury dealt with. Criminal abortions are responsible for most of the injuries.

Sexually transmitted infections can cause extensive stricture around the anus (i.e. condyloma venereum).

SURGERY

It is rare to injure the bowel during gynaecological surgery and the incidence quoted varies between 0.3% and 0.8%.

1. A small injury less than 5 mm in the small bowel can be effectively closed by a purse-string or transverse sutures in two layers.
2. A larger laceration may need resection and end-to-end anastomosis.
3. Colonic injury needs proximal colostomy.

Rectal injury occurs mainly during vaginal surgery such as posterior vaginal repair for prolapse, repair of perineal tear, exenteration operation and vaginoplasty.

A small tear can be sutured immediately, but a large hole needs proximal colostomy.

Radiation causes a fistula or stricture. Colpocleisis can cure the fistula.

The gynaecologist should not hesitate to ask for a general surgeon's assistance. In case of doubt or a major injury, surgical assistance is necessary.

PREVENTION

Obstetric injuries to intestine can be avoided by proper obstetric management.

During gynaecological surgery, the high-risk factors should be remembered. A sharp dissection in endometriosis and PID can avoid laceration. The surgeon should be careful while using cautery or laser during laparoscopic surgery.

KEY POINTS

- Most genital tract injuries originate from an obstetric cause. Difficult vaginal instrumental-assisted childbirth can cause traumatic injuries.
- Coital injuries may cause alarming haemorrhage. Severe lacerations and penetrating injury entering the pouch of Douglas require emergency surgical attention.
- In young girls with perineal vaginal injury, always keep a possibility of sexual offence (rape) in mind. Follow the steps outlined for examination of a rape victim.
- Vulval haematomas: Small haematomas may be observed. Large haematomas need surgical evacuation.
- Foreign bodies in the vagina cause inflammation and ulceration and rarely lead to a fistula formation.
- Chemical burns generally occur due to use of corrosive substances. Strictures may follow as a sequelae. Laser burn is now the common cause of a vaginal burn.
- Old, healed perineal tears cause faecal incontinence. Timely detection and surgical correction prevent morbidity.
- Cervical tear may cause incompetent os and repeated pregnancy losses. Cervical stenosis can cause haematometra or infertility.
- Uterine rupture occurs during labour and carries a high morbidity and risk of maternal mortality.

- Bowel injuries are observed in 0.3%–0.8% of gynaecological cases.
- Anal canal and rectal injuries are mostly obstetrical, inflicted during a difficult or operative vaginal delivery. It is rarely encountered during an operation on the posterior vaginal wall.
- Intestinal and rectal injuries can occur during gynaecological operations on PID and endometriosis cases, when extensive pelvic adhesions have to be dissected.
- Intestinal injuries are increasingly reported following laparoscopic surgery when cautery or laser are used.
- Hysteroscopic uterine perforation leading to intestinal burn and peritonitis is reported with transcervical endometrial resection and excision of the uterine septum.
- The endoscopic burn injuries are, however, not immediately recognized and symptoms may develop 5–7 days later.
- Treatment of intestinal injury is surgical suturing or resection and end-to-end anastomosis. Bowel injury may require proximal colostomy.
- The help of the general or gastrointestinal surgeon should be sought in major bowel injury.
- Obstetric trauma during vaginal delivery with immediate diagnosis and surgical repair can prevent or minimize the distressful symptom of faecal incontinence.

SELF-ASSESSMENT

1. Describe the common types of pelvic floor injuries encountered in practice.
2. How would you manage a case of vulval haematoma?
3. How would you manage a case of complete perineal tear?
4. Describe the causes and management of chemical burns of the vagina.
5. Describe the practice of genital mutilation. What complications may follow this procedure?
6. Describe the outcome of long-retained foreign bodies in the vagina of children.
7. Describe the genital injuries following coitus.
8. How would you manage a patient of faecal incontinence?
9. How would you manage a patient with a rectovaginal fistula?
10. What are the common causes of bowel injury during obstetric/gynaecologic surgery? How would you recognize the same? What precautions help to avoid intestinal injuries?
11. What are the causes of intestinal injury during laparoscopy? How would you safeguard against the same?
12. Enumerate the situations leading to bowel injury in obstetric practice.

SUGGESTED READING

Boyd ME, Ulster RH, McLean FH, et al. Failed forceps. Obstet Gynecol 1986; 68: 779–86.

Handa VL, Harris TA, Ostergard TR. Protecting the pelvic floor: Obstetric management to prevent incontinence and pelvic organ prolapse. Obstet Gynecol 1996; 88: 470–78.

Leung AS, Farmer RM, Leung EK, et al. Risk factors associated with uterine rupture during trial of labour after cesarean delivery: A case control study. Am J Obstet Gynecol 1993; 168: 1358–63.

Pokorny SF. Long-term intravaginal presence of foreign bodies in children. A preliminary study. J Reprod Med 1994; 39: 931–35.

Robertson PA, Laros RK Jr., Zhao RL. Neonatal and maternal outcome in low-pelvic and midpelvic operative deliveries. Am J Obstet Gynecol 1880; 162: 1436–42.

Smith NC, Van Coeverden de Groot HA, Gunston KD. Coital injuries of the vagina in nonvirginal patients. S Afr Med J 1983; 64(19): 746–47.

Birns MT. Inadvertent instrumental perforation of the colon during laparoscopy: Non-surgical repair. Gastrointest Endosc 1989; 35: 54–56.

Krebs HB. Intestinal injury in gynecologic surgery. A ten year experience. Am J Obstet Gynecol 1985; 155: 509.

Nicholls DH (ed). Clinical Problems, Injuries and Complications of Gynecologic Surgery Baltimore, Williams & Wilkins, 1983.

Pasulka PS, Bistrian BR, Benotti PN, et al. The risks of surgery in obese patients. Ann Int Med 1986; 104: 540.

Reich H. Laparoscopic bowel injury. Surg Laparosc Endosc 1992; 2: 74–78.

Russell TR, Gallaghar DM. Low rectovaginal fistula. Am J Surg 1977; 134: 13.

Schaefer G, Graber EA (eds). Complications in obstetric and gynecologic surgery. Hagerstown, MD, Harper & Row, Publishers, 1981.

Shell JH Jr, Myers RC Jr. Small bowel injury after laparoscopic sterilization. Am J Obstet Gynecol 1973; 115: 285.

Thompson BH, Wheeless CR Jr. Gastrointestinal complications of laparoscopy sterilization. Obstet Gynecol 1973; 41: 669–76.

Wheeless CR. Thermal gastrointestinal injuries. In Phillips JM (ed). Laparoscopy, Baltomore, Williams & Wilkins. 1977, 231–35.

SECTION 7

GYNAECOLOGICAL MALIGNANCIES

SECTION OUTLINE

33 Preinvasive and Invasive Carcinoma of Cervix

CHAPTER OUTLINE

Carcinoma of the cervix is the third most common cancer among women worldwide and is now attributable to infection with human papillomavirus (HPV). However, it is the most common genital cancer among women in India. In certain parts of the country, it remains even more common than carcinoma breast; however, in most of the large metropolitan cities in India, it now ranks second to carcinoma of the breast amongst cancers in women. The median age at diagnosis is 48 years, and the majority of cases are diagnosed between 35 and 55 years. The universal application of Pap smears in Western communities has led to a drastic decline in the number of invasive cancers of the cervix and a higher detection of preinvasive lesions. However, this has not happened in India because of lack of universal screening; a drive against this preventable cancer must continue to keep the disease under control.

Every year 530,000 new cases and 275,000 deaths are reported annually worldwide. In India alone, 130,000 new cases occur with a death toll of 70,000 cases every year. Cancer of the cervix accounts for 15% of all cancers in women.

Prevalence rate is 2.3 million annually globally. In India, it is 13–24 lakh per year and at diagnosis more than 75% are in the advanced stages.

Table 33.1 Predisposing Factors for Cancer of the Cervix

- Coitus before the age of 18 years
- Multiple sexual partners
- Delivery of the first baby before the age of 20 years
- Multiparity with poor spacing between pregnancies
- Poor personal hygiene
- Sexually transmitted diseases
- Poor socioeconomic status
- Circumcision: Exposure to smegma from uncircumcised partners was considered an important factor, accounting for lower incidence of cancer of the cervix; now it is realized that the incidence of human papillomavirus (HPV) is low in circumcised men, and that is the reason for low incidence of cancer in their wives
- Smoking and drug abuse, including alcohol
- Women with STD, HIV infection, herpes simplex virus 2 infection
- Immunosuppressed individuals (following transplant surgery), viral infections and HIV
- Women with preinvasive lesions of cervix
- Women who never had screening for cancer cervix
- Use of oral contraceptive pills

EPIDEMIOLOGY (Table 33.1)

There are many conditions which predispose a woman to development cervical cancer. Most important among these is early age at start of sexual activity. Multiple sex partners, low socio-economic status, multi parity, sexually transmitted diseases and poor personal hygiene are some of these factors.

Average age of development of cancer cervix is 35–45 years in India. However, disease can be seen any time between 21–65 years of age. The precancerous lesion of cervix usually occurs 10–15 years earlier. There is a period of 10 years or larger when a precancerous lesion can progress to invasive cancer.

Now a definitive relationship has been established between HPV infection and development of cancer cervix. (Fig. 33.1).

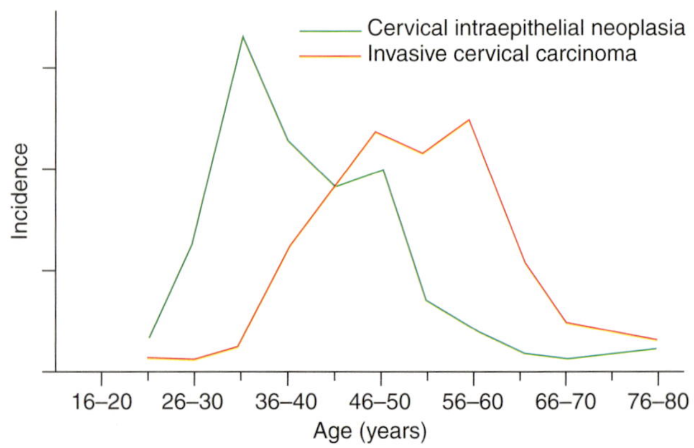

Figure 33.1 Age incidence of cervical carcinoma in situ and invasive cervical carcinoma.

To view the lecture notes scan the symbol or log in to your account on www.MedEnact.com

SQUAMOCOLUMNAR JUNCTION

Most cancers of cervix begin in the region of squamocolumnar junction. This junction has a variable position on cervix during long life phase of a woman.

ORIGINAL SQUAMOCOLUMNAR JUNCTION

- It is a junction in between the columnar epithelium of the endocervical canal and the stratified squamous epithelium of ectocervix.
- The position of the original squamocolomnar junction determines the extent of cervical squamous metaplasia

NEW SQUAMOCOLUMNAR JUNCTION

- With increased oestrogen secretion following puberty, eversion of endocervical columnar epithelium occurs onto ectocervix; this everted columnar epithelium becomes metaplastic because of increasing vaginal acidity.
- This new junction between the squamous metaplastic epithelium and the endocervical columnar epithelium is called new squamocolumnar junction.

THE TRANSFORMATION ZONE

It is the area between the original and the new squamocolumnar junction. Cervical neoplasia almost invariably originates within the transformation zone.

CERVICAL INTRAEPITHELIAL NEOPLASIA (CIN)

Before actual development of cancer cervix, there are changes in the epithelium in the region of transformation zone; these changes can be picked up on cytology. These changes have been named cervical dysplasia, cervical intraepithelial neoplasia (CIN) and lately as squamous intraepithelial lesions. Cervical dysplasia is a cytological term used to describe cells resembling cancer cells. CIN refers to the histopathological description in which a part or the full thickness of the stratified squamous epithelium is replaced by cells showing varying degrees of dysplasia; however, the basement membrane is intact. Dysplasia represents a change in which there is an alteration of cell morphology and disorderly arrangement of the cells of the stratified squamous epithelium. The cells vary in size, shape and polarity. There is an alteration in the nuclear cytoplasmic ratio, and the cells reveal large, irregular, hyperchromatic nuclei with marginal condensation of chromatin material and mitotic figures. Some of these lesions progress with time and ultimately end up as frank invasive cancers. *While 4% reach the invasive stage by the end of 1 year and 11% by the end of 3 years; as much as 22% become invasive by 5 years and 30% by 10 years* (Table 33.2).

Table 33.2 Course of CIN Disease

	Regression (%)	Persistence (%)	Progression (%)	Years
CIN-I	80–90	10–20	1–4	2–10
CIN-II	30–40	40	20	1–5
CIN-III	20–30	50–60	Almost all	6m–2yrs

DYSPLASIA (Figs 33.2–33.9)

Dysplasias are graded as follows:

1. ***Mild dysplasia (CIN-I):*** The undifferentiated cells are confined to the lower one-third of the epithelium. The cells are more differentiated towards the surface. Mild dysplasia is often due to infections such as HPV infection, *Trichomonas vaginitis.* CIN-I is lately described as low-grade squamous intraepithelial lesions (LSIL) according to the Bethesda classification. 'ASCUS' is a term described in the Bethesda system as atypical squamous cells of undetermined significance. The intermediate cells mostly display mild dysplasia with enlarged nuclei and irregular outline. One per cent progress to cancer over the years.
2. ***Moderate dysplasia (CIN-II):*** Undifferentiated cells occupy the lower 50%–75% of the epithelial thickness.

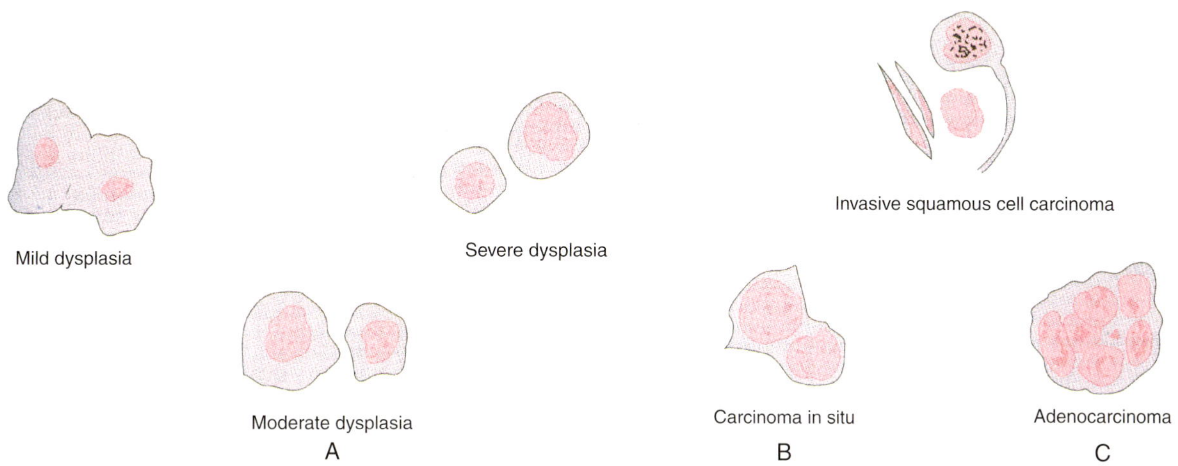

Figure 33.2 Dysplasias. **(A)** Mild and moderate dysplasias. **(B)** Severe dysplasia and carcinoma in situ. **(C)** Invasive cell – carcinoma and adenocarcinoma.

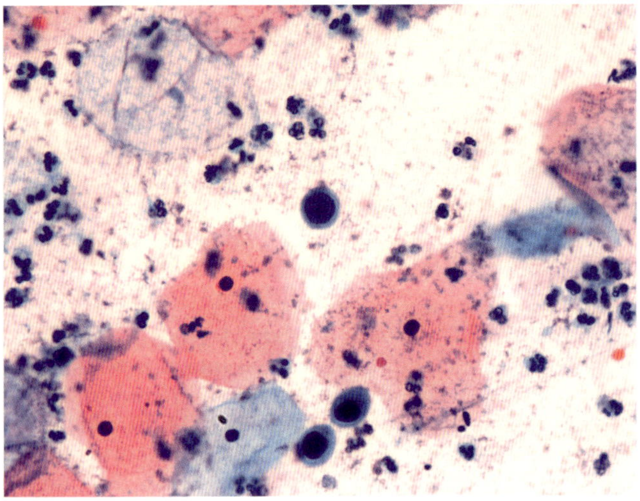

Figure 33.3 CIN-III: cervical smear showing cells with coarse chromatin and increased nuclear to cytoplasmic ratio. (*Courtesy:* Dr Sandeep Mathur, AIIMS.)

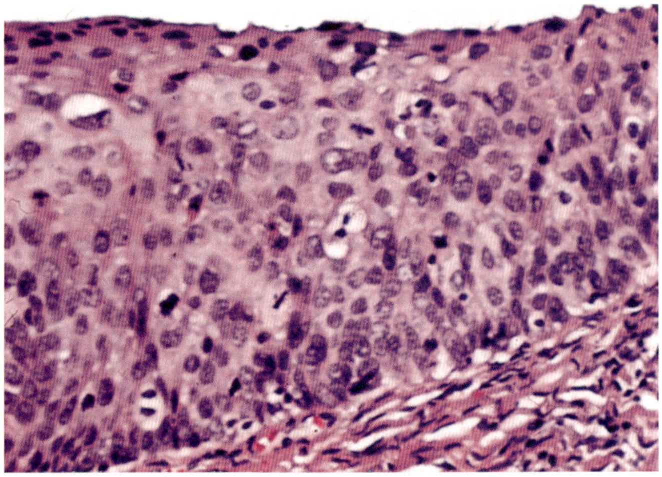

Figure 33.5 Cervical intraepithelial neoplasia 3 (severe dysplasia, carcinoma in situ). There is a lack of squamous maturation throughout the thickness of the epithelium. Almost all the cells have enlarged nuclei with granular chromatin. Note that the basement membrane is intact, showing that this process is confined to the epithelial layer only. (*Source:* Vijaya Reddy, Paolo Gattuso, Odile David Daniel Spitz, Meryl Haber. Differential Diagnosis in Surgical Pathology, Female Reproductive System. Saunders, 2010.)

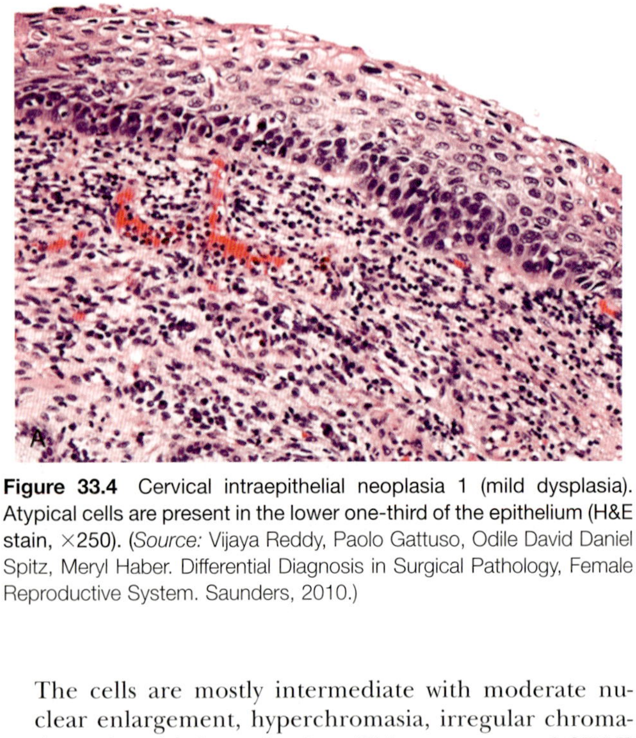

Figure 33.4 Cervical intraepithelial neoplasia 1 (mild dysplasia). Atypical cells are present in the lower one-third of the epithelium (H&E stain, ×250). (*Source:* Vijaya Reddy, Paolo Gattuso, Odile David Daniel Spitz, Meryl Haber. Differential Diagnosis in Surgical Pathology, Female Reproductive System. Saunders, 2010.)

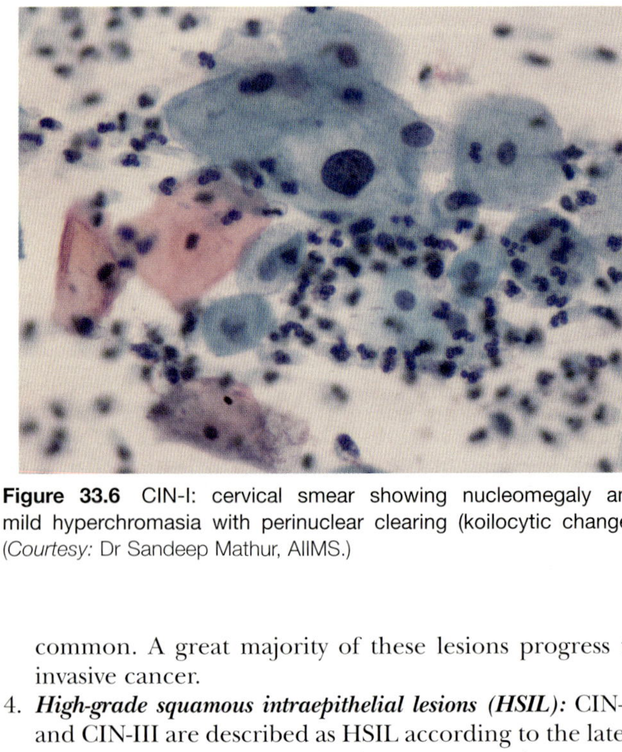

Figure 33.6 CIN-I: cervical smear showing nucleomegaly and mild hyperchromasia with perinuclear clearing (koilocytic change). (*Courtesy:* Dr Sandeep Mathur, AIIMS.)

The cells are mostly intermediate with moderate nuclear enlargement, hyperchromasia, irregular chromatin and multiple nucleation. Thirty per cent of CIN-II regress, 40% persist and the rest progress to invasive cancer.

3. ***Severe dysplasia and carcinoma in situ (CIN-III):*** In this grade of dysplasia, the entire thickness of the epithelium is replaced by abnormal cells. There is no cornification and stratification is lost. The basement membrane, however, is intact and there is no stromal infiltration. Often, an abrupt change in histological appearance from normal to abnormal is apparent (Figs 33.2–33.7). On cytology, cells are mostly parabasal with increased nuclear–cytoplasmic ratio. The nuclei are irregular, with coarse chromatin material; mitosis and multinucleation are common. A great majority of these lesions progress to invasive cancer.
4. ***High-grade squamous intraepithelial lesions (HSIL):*** CIN-II and CIN-III are described as HSIL according to the latest Bethesda classification. HSIL have a propensity to progress and become invasive, and therefore need investigations and treatment.

The term 'CIN' denotes a continuum of disorders from mild through moderate to severe dysplasia and carcinoma in situ. Mild dysplasia is often seen with inflammatory conditions such as trichomoniasis and HPV, and is reversible following treatment, whereas the severe varieties progress to invasive cancer in about 10%–30% of cases in 5–10 years' time. This progression time may be shorter in immunocompromised persons.

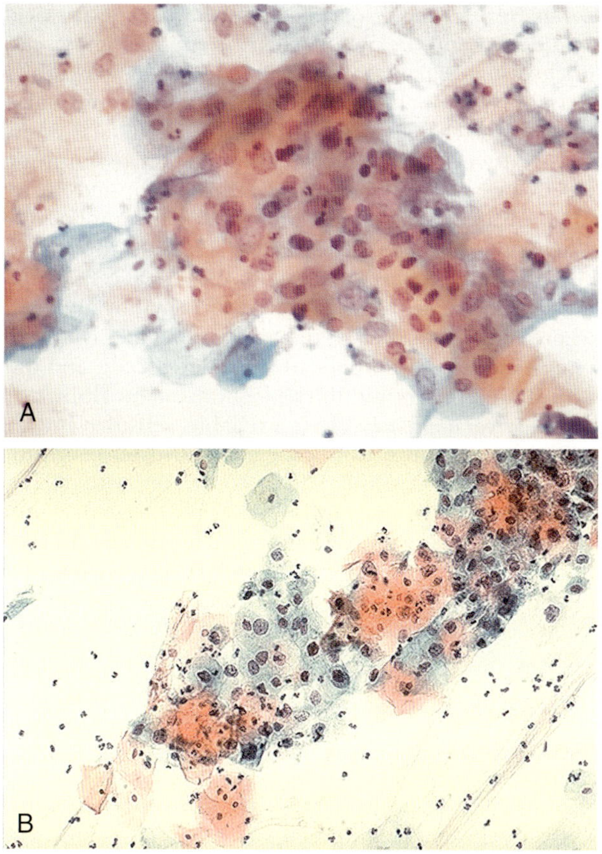

Figure 33.7 **(A)** Cervical cytology smear in CIN. This cytology preparation shows a clump of cervical epithelial cells demonstrating moderate and severe dyskaryosis. **(B)** Cervical squamous dysplasia, Pap smear (*Source* **(A)**: From Figure 19.10. Alan Stevens, James Lowe and Ian Scott: Core Pathology, 3rd Ed. Elsevier, 2009. *Source* **(B)**: From Figure 13-25. Edward C. Klatt: Robbins and Cotran Atlas of Pathology, 2nd Ed. Saunders: Elsevier, 2010.)

A number of studies in India including Indian Council of Medical Research (ICMR) have reported the incidence of cervical dysplasia to be 15:1000 women among cytologically screened women. The incidence of severe dysplasia is reported to be about 5:1000.

Koilocytes. These cells are often seen in young women suffering from HPV infection, and are cells with perinuclear halo in the cytoplasm. Koilocytes disappear as dysplasia advances.

DIAGNOSIS

Diagnosis of cervical dysplasia is mainly based on cytological screening of the population. The peak incidence of occurrence of dysplasias appears to be 10 years earlier than that of frank invasive cancer. Many of these women are asymptomatic. Some women complain of postcoital bleeding or discharge. On inspection, the cervix often appears normal, or there may be cervicitis or an erosion which bleeds on touch. Some women present with postmenopausal bleeding.

The guidelines for screening women for cancer cervix vary from country to country. The currently followed guidelines in the USA are given in the subsequent text (Table 33.3).

Table 33.3 Pap Smear Screening (www.health.ny.gov.)

Age Group	Screening Recommendations
<21 years	Do not screen
21–29 years	Perform cytologic testing alone every 3 years
30–65 years	Perform cytologic and HPV co-testing every 5 years (preferred), or perform cytologic testing alone every 3 years (acceptable)
>65 years	Discontinue screening if there has been an adequate number of negative screening results previously (three consecutive negative cytologic tests or two consecutive negative co-tests in the past 10 years, with the most recent test in the past 5 years) and if there is no history of HSIL, adenocarcinoma. in situ, or cancer
Women who have undergone hysterectomy	Discontinue screening if the patient has undergone a total hysterectomy with removal of cervix and if there is history of HSIL, adenocarcinoma in situ, or cancer

Cytological Screening for Cancer Cervix

DNA study. Diploid or polyploid nucleus is normal. Aneuploidy is a hallmark of malignant potential and mandates treatment.

Cytology alone does not indicate which abnormal cells will progress to cancer. Further tests are required. Usefulness of Pap smear in the screening programme for cancer cervix is shown by the following:

- Long latent period of 10–15 years between the diagnosis of CIN and invasive cancer allows adequate treatment of CIN and prevention of invasive cancer.
- Screening programmes based on cytology have proved successful in reducing the incidence of invasive cancer by 80% and its mortality by 60% in developed countries. Because of 15%–30% false-negative reporting, it is prudent to repeat Pap smear annually for 3 consecutive years. If it continues to remain negative, the Pap smear is repeated 3- to 5-yearly up to the age of 50 years. After 50 years, the incidence of CIN drops to 1%. The presence of endocervical cells in the smear indicates a satisfactory smear. A false-negative report is because of improper technique in smear taking (not through 360°), dry vagina and poor shedding of cervical cells or recession of squamocolumnar junction in endocervical canal in menopausal women.

High-grade squamous intraepithelial lesion. The presence of high-grade squamous intraepithelial neoplastic cells is significant as these have the potential to progress to invasive cancer and need to be treated.

Sensitivity of Pap smear for HSIL is 70%–80% and specificity 95%–98%. While false-positive smear may lead to unnecessary investigations and treatment, false-negative reporting is more ominous as cancer lesion may be missed. Pap smear in postmenopausal women is inaccurate and often negative on account of indrawing of squamocolumnar junction, dry vagina and poor exfoliation of cells. This can be improved by administration of oestrogen cream/oral oestrogen daily for 7–10 days. To reduce the incidence of false-negative reporting, the following procedures are added to Pap screening:

- ***Endocervical scrape cytology by endocervical brush or curettage:*** Endocervical scrape should be obtained first with Pipelle/cotton swab followed by ectocervical smear to avoid the latter from air drying.
- ***Incorporating HPV testing by hybridization or polymerase chain reaction in young women:*** This improves the predictive value of Pap smear to 95% and reduces the number of referrals for colposcopic evaluation. A young woman with HPV infection should be followed up with Pap smear. Incidentally, it is observed that the prevalence of HPV-positive cases drops with advancing age (regression) or is transient, but in persistent HPV infection, the incidence of HSIL rises after the age of 30 years. The specificity of Pap smear in HPV-infected cases is therefore low in young women.
  Cytology with added HPV testing helps to triage ASCUS and CIN cells.
- ***Liquid-based cytology:*** Here the smeared *plastic* (not wooden) *spatula is placed in a liquid fixative* (buffered methanol solution) instead of smearing on a slide. This removes the blood, mucus and inflammatory cells. The suspended cells are then gently sucked onto a filter membrane and the filter is pressed onto a glass slide to form a thin monolayer, and then it is stained. The liquid can also be employed to test HPV infection, making it a cost-effective technique. The cells wash off the plastic device more than the wooden one, and the fixation solution contains haemolytic and mucolytic agents. This improves specificity and sensitivity of the test. Besides HPV testing, the liquid can also be used for genetic study and repeat cytology if required. Disadvantages are increased cost, need of trained personnel and transportation and storage of so many vials.
- ***Automated computerized image processor:*** It eliminates 25% of most likely negative smears and 75% are selected for cytotechnician screening.
  Cytology alone does not give a clue as to which abnormal cell will progress to invasive cancer, and aneuploidy which suggests the risk of progression is not routinely performed, so it is necessary to submit all women with HSIL cytology for colposcopic study and biopsy of suspicious lesions.
- ***Visual inspection of acetowhite areas (VIA):*** Because of lack of cytology-based screening universally and lack of trained manpower capable of reading cytology smears, a newer technique of screening called VIA has been advocated in India and other low-resource countries. In this technique, after exposure of cervix during speculum examination, cervix is painted with 3/5% acetic acid. Areas which turn white after application of acetic acid for 1 minute are suspicious areas and need evaluation by biopsy/colposcopy. VIA has been widely investigated and accepted as a potential alternative to cytology in low-resource settings. Where the facilities for Pap screening do not exist, VIA is able to select abnormal areas on the cervix by applying 5% acetic acid (downstaging) – acetic acid dehydrates the abnormal areas containing increased nuclear material and protein which turn acetowhite. The normal cells which contain glycogen remain normal. Although this has low specificity and high false-positive rates, false-negative, which really matters, is seen in only 0.9% of cases. The abnormal areas are biopsied. Instead of acetic acid, Schiller's iodine can also be employed.
- ***Visual inspection with Lugol's iodine (VILI):*** In this method, cervix is painted with Lugol's iodine. Normal cells containing glycogen take up iodine and turn mahogany brown, whereas abnormal area remains unstained. Dull white plaques with faint borders are considered LSIL and those with sharp borders and thick plaques contain HSIL.
- ***See and treat approach:*** VIA is a reliable, sensitive and cost-effective alternative to cytology in low-resource settings. 'See and biopsy' in one sitting is possible with VIA and VILI. Abnormal areas may be cauterized (or cryotherapy) in the same sitting. Although it may prove 'overtreatment', as a considerable number of women may have benign lesions, this is feasible and convenient in rural and peripheral set-ups where follow-up visits by patients are low.

OTHER SCREENING TECHNIQUES

Speculoscopy. It uses a special disposable, low-intensity, blue-white magnifying device or loupe. This has not proved effective and more false-positive cases are unnecessarily referred for colposcopic study.

Spectroscopy. Cervical impedance or fluorescence spectroscopy is specific and sensitive, and provides instant results unlike Pap smears. It is a noninvasive technique which probes the tissue morphology and biochemical composition.

Magnoscope has a magnifying lens as a built-in source. It magnifies cells five times and enables visualization of punctuation and mosaics. It is portable and useful in rural areas. It has been introduced by ICMR as Magnivisualizer.

Microspectrophotometry is also able to distinguish between benign and malignant cells.

Colposcopy

This technique was introduced in 1936 by Heinselman as a technique to visualize the surface of cervix. Currently this has come to occupy an important step in the diagnosis of preinvasive lesions of cervix.

The aims of colposcopy are as follows (Figs 33.8–33.11):

- To study the cervix when Pap smear detects abnormal cells
- To locate abnormal areas and take a biopsy
- To study the extent of abnormal lesion
- Conservative surgery under colposcopic guidance
- Follow-up of conservative therapy cases

Colposcopy reduces the false-positive findings. In ASCUS cases, it is used as a triage to rule out high-grade lesion. Abnormal areas appear under colposcopy as acetowhite areas, mosaics, punctuation and abnormal vessels (Fig. 33.12).

While Pap smear detects abnormal cells, colposcopy locates the abnormal lesion.

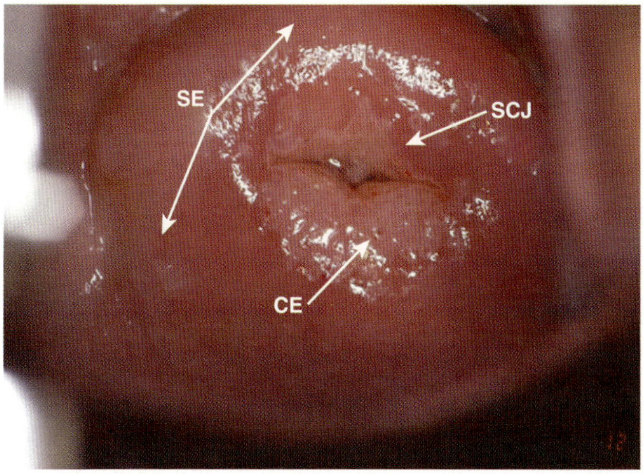

Figure 33.8 Normal colposcopic picture of the transformation zone: squamous epithelium (SE), columnar epithelium (CE) and squamocolumnar junction (SCJ). (*Source:* From Figure 137-2B. John L Pfenninger and Grant C Fowler: Pfenninger and Fowler's Procedures for Primary Care, 3rd Ed. Mosby: Elsevier, 2011.)

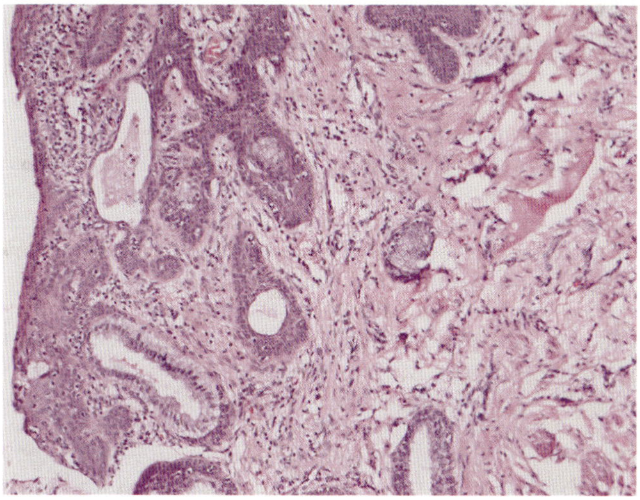

Figure 33.11 Squamous metaplasia of cervical transformation zone: endocervical glands lined by a combination of columnar cells and abrupt stratified squamous epithelium. (*Courtesy*: Dr Sandeep Mathur, AIIMS.)

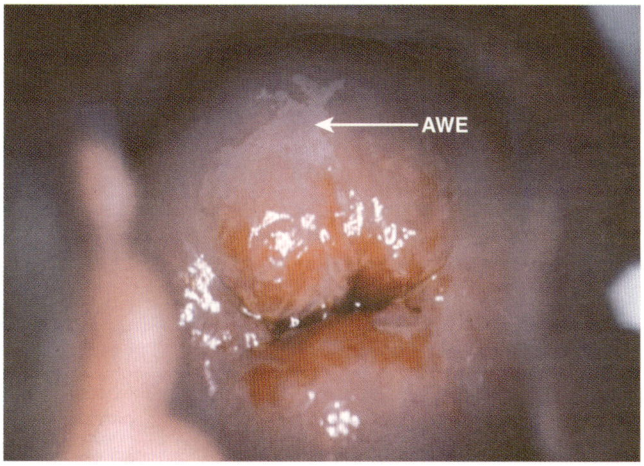

Figure 33.9 Colposcopy showing acetowhite areas. (*Source:* From Figure 137-4E. John L Pfenninger and Grant C Fowler: Pfenninger and Fowler's Procedures for Primary Care, 3rd Ed. Mosby: Elsevier, 2011.)

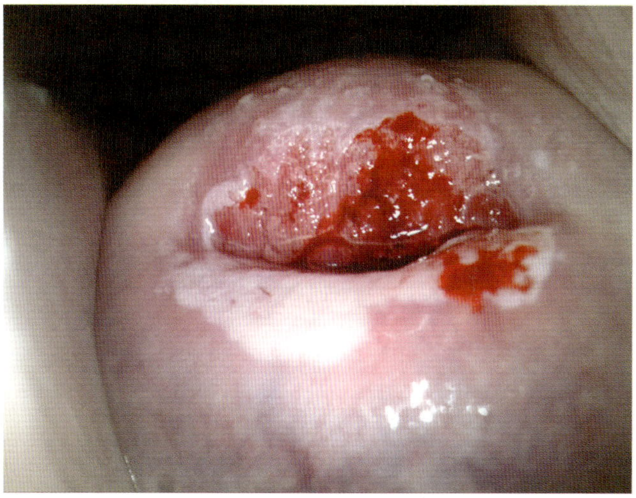

Figure 33.12 Colposcopy showing CIN III Lesion
▶ Scan to play Colposcopy

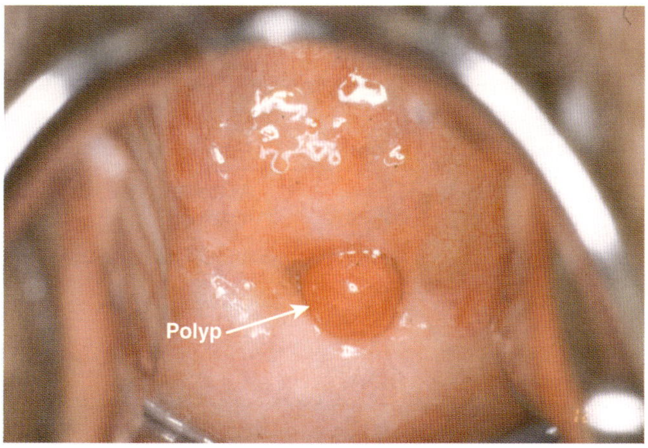

Figure 33.10 Cervical polyp seen. (*Source:* From Figure 137–40. John L Pfenninger and Grant C Fowler: Pfenninger and Fowler's Procedures for Primary Care, 3rd Ed. Mosby: Elsevier, 2011.)

Colposcopic study is challenging in postmenopausal women because of the following reasons: narrow vagina, senile vaginitis, squamocolumnar junction indrawn and not visible, and atropic cervix flush with vagina. Oestrogen cream for 7–10 days and 400 mcg misoprostol 3–4 hours before colposcopy expose the ectocervix better. Colposcopy decides whether a small biopsy or a cone biopsy is required.

Cervicography

This technique was described in 1990s where a photograph of cervix is taken and sent for evaluation. It is useful when a colposcopist is not available for spot evaluation. A photograph of the entire external os is taken with a 35-mm camera after application of 5% acetic acid and sent to the colposcopist for selecting areas for biopsy. Because of 50% specificity and sensitivity, this technique is not cost-effective.

Cone Biopsy

It is both diagnostic and therapeutic. Whenever the area of abnormality is large, or its inner margin has receded into the cervical canal, the squamocolumnar junction is not completely visible on colposcopy, or there is discrepancy between cytology and colposcopy, a wide cone excision biopsy including the entire outer margin of the lesion and the entire endocervical lining is obtained using cold-knife technique under general anaesthesia. A large loop excision of the transformation zone (LLETZ) has become more popular than cone biopsy for obtaining biopsies from transformation zone because of its ease of doing; it is associated with less bleeding, low chances of infection and faster healing, without scar formation.

Cone biopsy (Table 33.3) can cause bleeding, infection, cervical stenosis and incompetent os. However, it is also required if endocervical or microinvasive lesion is suspected.

AgNOR is a new molecular tumour marker which stands for silver-stained nucleolar organizer regions; DNA is present in dysplastic cells. They appear as black dots which increase in number but decrease in size with advancing dysplasia. The lesions with low counts often regress, whereas those with high counts progress and need treatment. This test has been tried only in research settings.

HPV Testing

With the knowledge that most cancer cervix occur as a result of HPV infection, there has been a trend towards screening for HPV infection. Currently most screening programmes for cancer cervix in rich countries use HPV testing as a primary screening method or in combination with cytological screening. Most sexually active women acquire HPV infection following first sexual encounter. However, in most women this infection clears, whereas 80%–90% of HPV infections are transitory and self-limited, and disappear over a period of 18 months or so; only 10%–20% persist and form a high-risk group beyond 30 years of age. Incorporating HPV testing in cytology screening improves the predictive value, and reduces unnecessary colposcopy referral and overtreatment, but justifies follow-up in persistent cases.

The HPV testing is done by either study of cells in liquid-based cytology or endocervical secretion and self-obtained vaginal swab. A combined HPV testing and Pap smear yields 96% sensitivity as compared to only 60%–70% with Pap smear alone. Polymerase chain reaction, Southern blot and hybrid capture technique detect HPV DNA. Out of these, hybrid capture technique is the most commonly used and is commercially available. The test may cost Rs 800–1500 or more.

TREATMENT OF CERVICAL DYSPLASIAS AND CIN (Table 33.4; Figs 33.13–33.19)

Treatment of dysplasia based on cytology or colposcopy alone is not appropriate because of their false findings.

Table 33.4 Comparison of Different Methods of Treatment of Dysplasia and CIN

Characteristics	Cryotherapy	Coagulation	Laser Ablation	Conization Knife	Laser Conization	LLETZ	LEEP
Place	OPD	OT	OPD	OT	OPD or OT	OPD	OPD
Anaesthesia	Nil	GA	Nil analgesia	GA	Local	Local	Local
Instrument's cost and portability	Cheap, portable	Cheap, portable	Expensive	Cheap, not portable	Expensive, not portable	Cheap, portable	Cheap, portable
Risk of equipment	Nil	Nil	Yes	Nil	Yes	Nil	Nil
Complications during surgery	Nil	Bleeding risk	Personnel	Bleeding risk	Personnel	Nil	Nil
Depth of destruction	4–5 mm	8–10 mm	7 mm	–	–	–	–
Pain	Nil	Painful	Slight	–	Slight	Nil	Slight
Bleeding	Nil	+	Nil		Slight	Slight	
Sepsis	Discharge	+	Nil	+	Nil	Slight	Slight
Healing	6–8 weeks	6–8 weeks	4 weeks	6–8 weeks	4 weeks	4–6 weeks	4–6 weeks
Tissue for histology	NA	NA	NA	Available with excision methods	Tissue available	Available histology	Available
Cure rate	90%	90%–95%	90%–97%	90%–95%	90%–95%	90%–95%	90%–95%
Pregnancy complications	Nil	Nil	Nil	Stenosis cervix, abortion, premature labour, cervical dystocia with excisional methods		Cervical stenosis	
Postoperative transformation zone	Indrawn	Indrawn	Seen	Visible with zone excisional method			

GA, general anaesthesia; NA, not available.

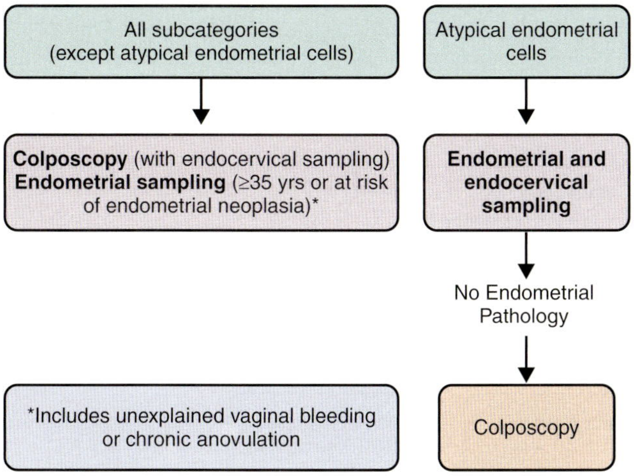

Figure 33.13A Women with Atypical Glandular Cells.

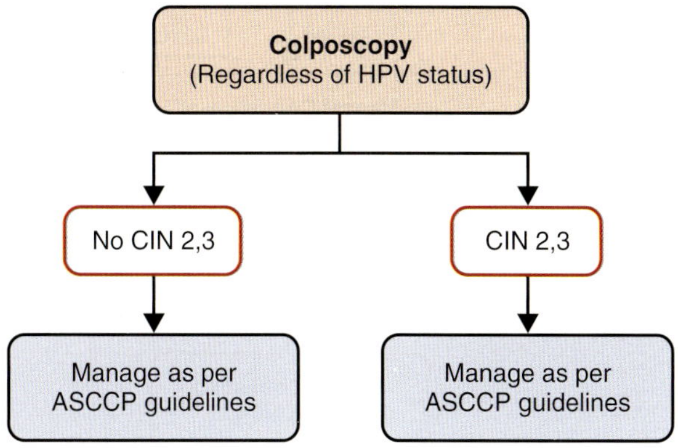

Figure 33.13B Atypical squamous cells-H.

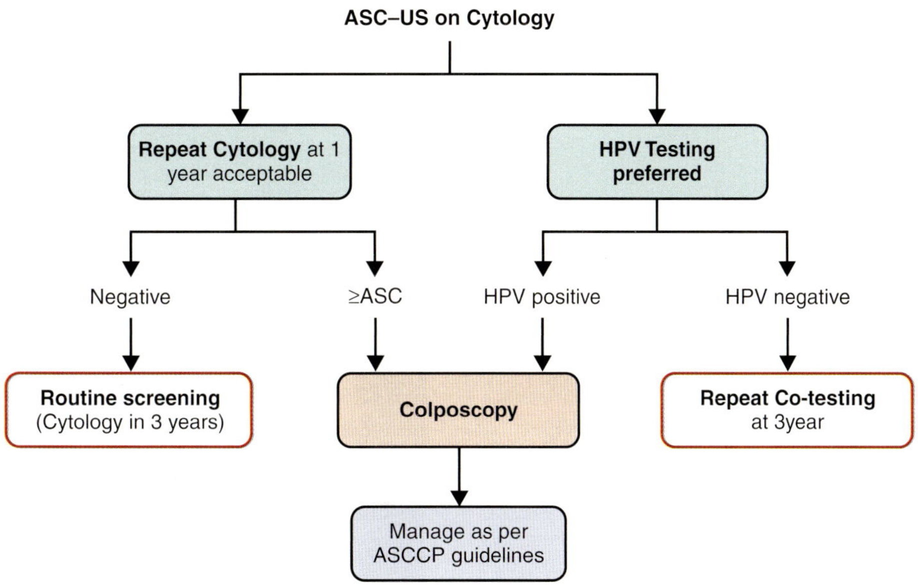

Figure 33.13C Atypical squamous cells-US.

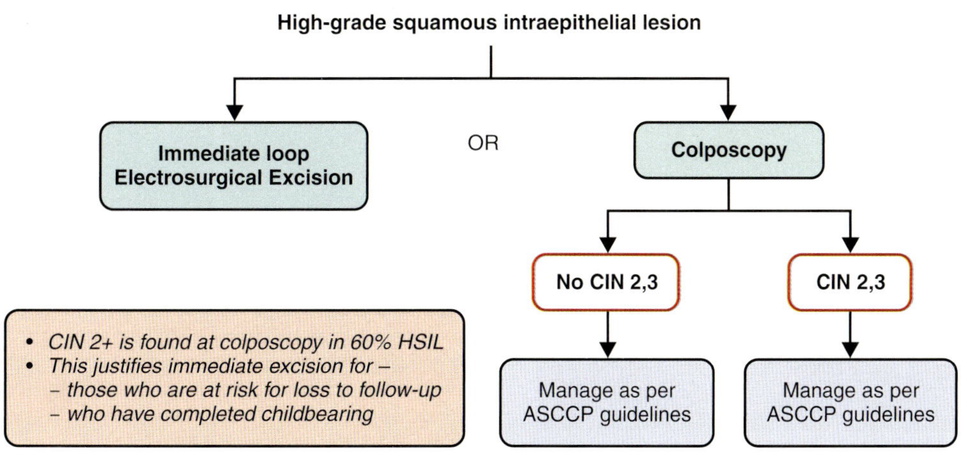

Figure 33.13D High-grade squamous intraepithelial lesion.
Scan to play HPV Testing

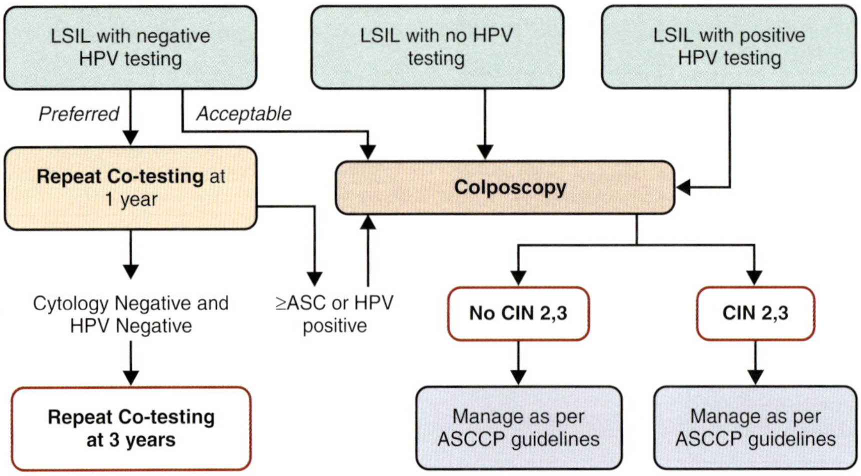

Figure 33.13E Low-grade squamous intraepithelial lesion.

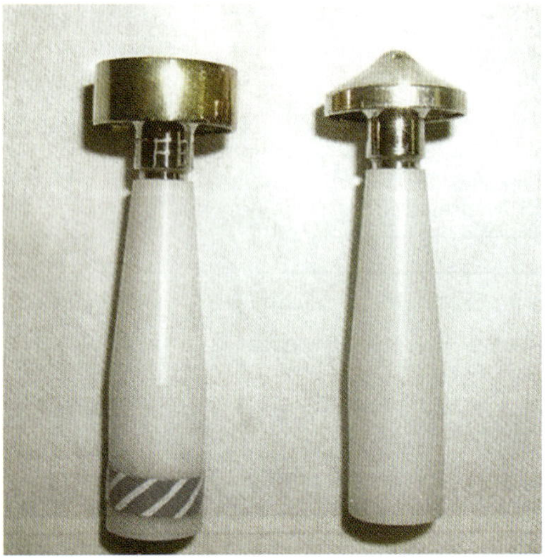

Figure 33.14 Cryotherapy probes with various size tips. (*Source:* From Figure 2. Stephanie Long and Lawrence Leeman: Treatment Options for High-Grade Squamous Intraepithelial Lesions. Obstetrics and Gynecology Clinics, Vol 40(2): 291–316, Elsevier, 2013.)

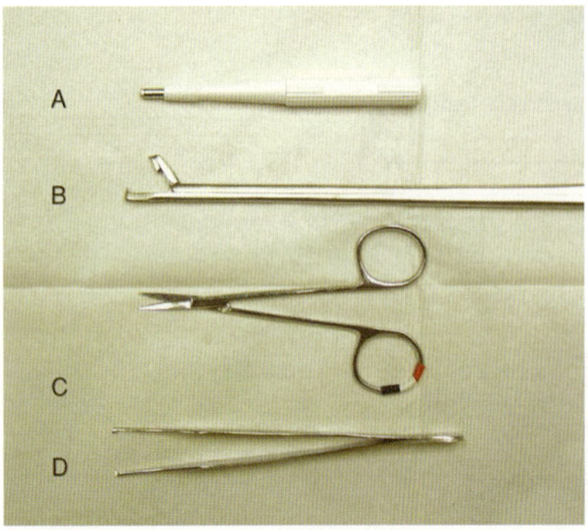

Figure 33.15 **(A)** Keyes punch biopsy. **(B)** Cervical punch biopsy forceps. **(C)** Iris scissors. **(D)** Tissue forceps. (*Source:* From Figure 1A. Pre-procedure. Procedure Consult. Vulvar Biopsy. Editors: Michael L Tuggy, Jorge Garcia.)

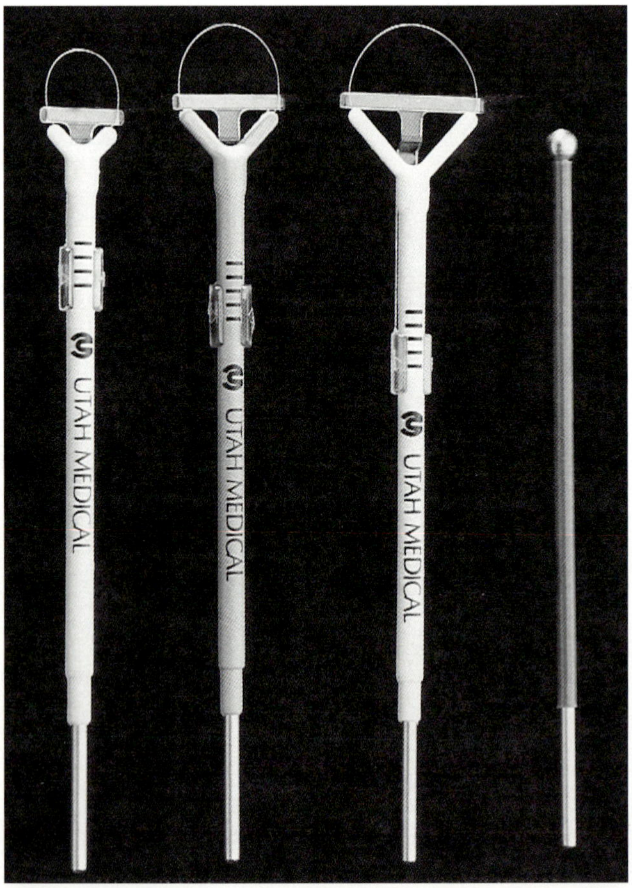

Figure 33.16 Electrodes (Utah Medical, Midvale, UT) used for a loop electroexcision procedure. The width of the excised tissue specimens can range from 1.0 to 2.0 cm, and the specimen depth can be adjusted by sliding the guard attached to the electrode shaft. Following excision, the base of the cervix is often gently cauterized with a ball electrode. (*Source:* From Figure 28.15. Gretchen M Lentz, Roger A Lobo, David M Gershenson, et al. Comprehensive Gynecology, 6th Ed. Mosby: Elsevier, 2012.)

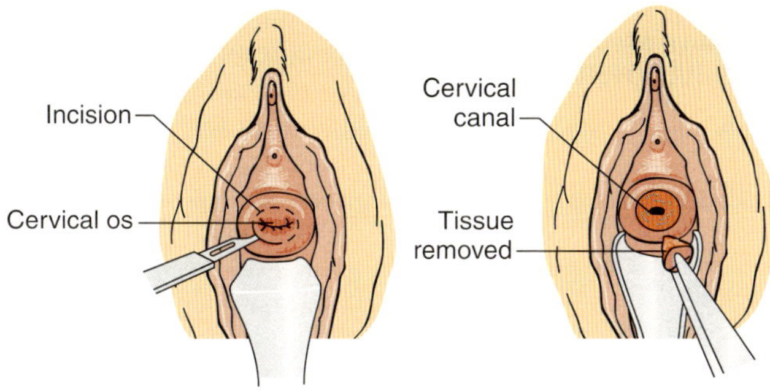

Figure 33.17 Conization technique. **(A)** Incision. **(B)** Removal of tissue. (*Source:* From Figure 134-3. John L Pfenninger and Grant C Fowler: Pfenninger and Fowler's Procedures for Primary Care, 3rd Ed. Mosby: Elsevier, 2011.)

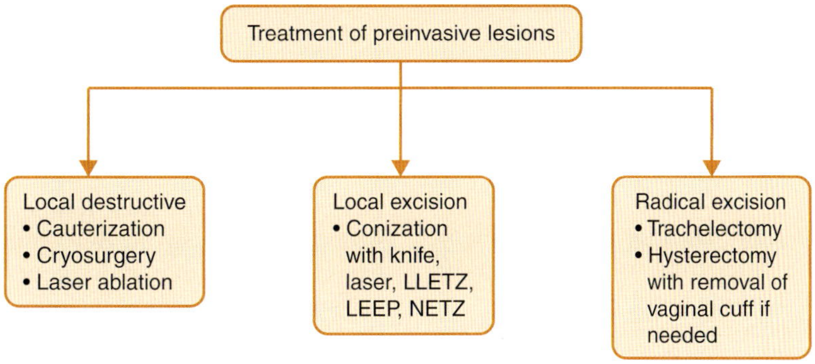

Figure 33.18 Treatment of preinvasive lesions.

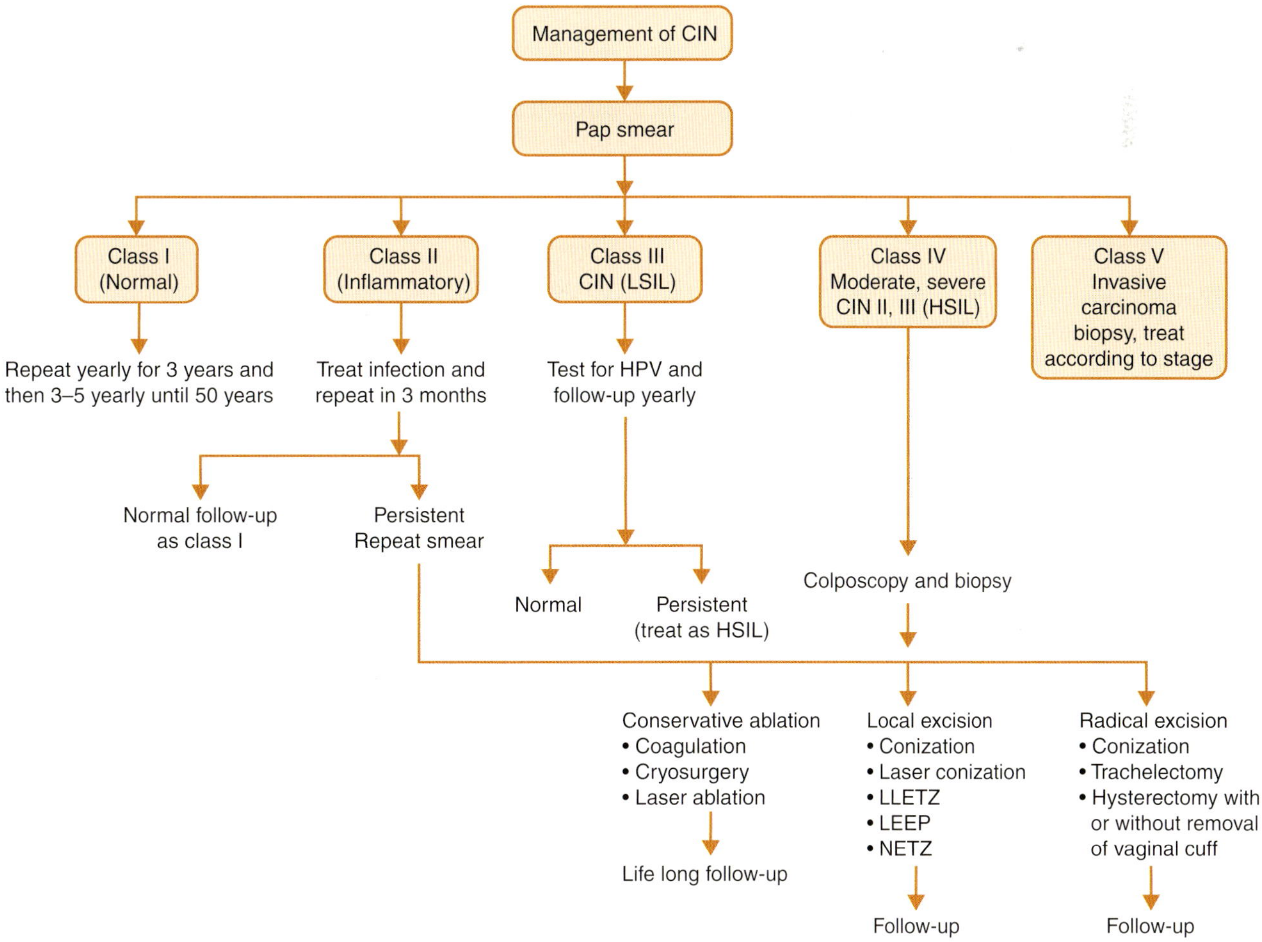

Figure 33.19 Management of CIN.

Table 33.5 Criteria for Conservative Methods of Treatment for CIN-II/III (HSIL)

- The entire lesion should be visible within the squamocolumnar junction.
- There should be no microinvasion or macroinvasion as proved by histological study through biopsy.
- There should be No evidence of endocervical involvement.
- Cytology and histology must correspond.
- In case of a young woman desirous of future child-bearing, conservative methods of treatment for CIN-II/III are followed.

A false-positive finding means unnecessary treatment or overtreatment. As mentioned before, more serious is false-negative finding which undermines the treatment and allows invasive growth to occur. As much as 50% of persistent LSIL (CIN-I) show HSIL (CIN-II, CIN-III). Before resorting to any treatment for cervical dysplasia/CIN, it is mandatory to perform colposcopy and directed biopsy. This approach also helps to rule out invasive cancer.

Mild dysplasia (LSIL) is usually because of infection *by-Trichomonas* or some other infections, which should be treated and cytology follow-up done every 3–6 months.

Indications for colposcopy and treatment of LSIL are as follows:

- Persistent LSIL (CIN-I) over 1 year
- Patient showing poor compliance
- LSIL showing HSIL on colposcopy or LSIL progressing to HSIL during the follow-up.

Moderately severe to severe dysplasias (CIN-II and CIN-III)
The treatment options are the following:

- ***Local destructive methods:***
  - (i) Cryosurgery
  - (ii) Fulguration/electrocoagulation
  - (iii) Laser ablation
- ***Excision of abnormal tissue:***
  - (i) Cold-knife conization,
  - (ii) Laser conization,
  - (iii) Loop electrosurgical excision procedure (LEEP)
  - (iv) Needle excision of transformation zone (NETZ)
- ***Surgery:***
  - (i) Therapeutic conization,
  - (ii) Hysterectomy
  - (iii) Hysterectomy with removal of vaginal cuff if carcinoma in situ extends to the vaginal vault

Criteria for conservative methods are provided in Table 33.5.

CRYOSURGERY

Cryosurgery was introduced by Townsend; it is suited for small lesions. It is done as an OPD procedure without analgesia. Cryosurgery is the best-tolerated technique, least painful and cheap.

MECHANISM OF ACTION

Cryosurgery refers to destruction of cells by crystallization of intracellular water. Freeze–thaw–freeze technique over 9 minutes destroys the tissue up to 4–5 mm depth. It is done as an OPD procedure without analgesia. CO_2 (−60°C), Freon (−60°C) and nitrous oxide (−80°C) are the freezing agents. CO_2 is cheaper, but nitrous oxide has a more cooling effect; hence, depth of penetration and destruction are more. A small lesion can be dealt with in one stroke applied for 3 minutes. A large lesion may require segments to be treated piecemeal. Application of acetic acid, Lugol's iodine or preferably colposcopic view helps to eradicate the entire lesion in one sitting. The woman should abstain from intercourse for 4 weeks. Repeat cryosurgery can be done 3 months later if the entire region is not previously treated as seen by cytology or other alternative method chosen.

Disadvantages are as follows:

- Profuse discharge initially for a period of 7–10 days
- Indrawing of squamocolumnar junction making subsequent screening by colposcopy difficult

ELECTROCOAGULATION

Electrocoagulation uses temperature over 70°C and destroys the tissue up to 8–10 mm deep. The procedure is painful, so it is done under general anaesthesia.

Complications: These include recurrence, bleeding, sepsis, cervical stenosis and indrawing of SCJ.

LASER ABLATION

Laser ablation boils, steams and explodes the cells. The laser is very expensive and can be harmful to the personnel (burn injury to the skin and eyes). *It is an OPD procedure done under local anaesthesia and under colposcopic guidance.* It destroys the tissue up to 5 mm deep. Currently, laser ablation is not advocated as a method of treatment for HSIL. Laser ablation is useful when the CIN extends up to the vaginal vault. Laser causes minimal bleeding, no infection, no post-laser scar formation and no deeper excision. More importantly, laser does not cause indrawal of squamocolumnar junction and, therefore, repeat laser is possible for residual lesion unlike cautery or cryosurgery. Recurrence of 2%–8% is reported.

Excisional and Cone Biopsy

It provides tissue for histopathological study and can be therapeutic but needs to be carried out in an operation theatre under anaesthesia and may have risk of complications such as secondary haemorrhage, cervical stenosis and infections.

Punch Biopsy

If done under colposcopic view, it can remove the entire lesion, if small, and can be performed under sedation or local anaesthesia.

Large Loop Excision of the Transformation Zone (LLETZ/LEEP)

It uses low-voltage diathermy under local anaesthesia. The loop is advanced into the cervix lateral to the lesion until the required depth is reached. It is then taken across to the opposite side and a cone of tissue removed. A loop size of less than 2 cm gives a better cone than a larger one. The low cost of the equipment and harmless effects on personnel make LLETZ more popular than laser. Besides, it takes a shorter time to perform with similar success and recurrence as that of laser.

With the availability of LEEP, a simple and effective method, laser seems to have taken a backseat.

NETZ removes cervical tissue in one piece.

All the excisional procedures should be done in the immediate postmenstrual phase, most of them under colposcopic view and under local anaesthesia; this reduces incomplete excision to only 2%–3%.

Only 0.1%–0.5% of cases of invasive cancer are detected during the follow-up of these cases.

Excisional treatment may cause stenosis of the cervix, so subsequent abortions and preterm labour, ablation therapy may be better suited for young women desiring future childbirth. Recurrence or persistent lesions in 2%–8% can be avoided by application of Schiller's iodine during therapy. Repeat cytology and follow-up is indicated after 3 months, after healing of the cervix.

Conization

It includes the entire outer margin (Fig. 33.20) and endocervical lining short of internal os. A smaller cone is desirable in young women to avoid risk of abortion or preterm labour subsequently. Complications are bleeding, sepsis, cervical stenosis, abortion and preterm labour.

Indications for conization

- (i) In endocervical dysplasia
- (ii) When transformation zone is not completely visualized
- (iii) When there is discrepancy in findings between cytology, colposcopy and biopsy
- (iv) When microinvasion is suspected

Hysterectomy

Hysterectomy as a treatment for HSIL is considered overtreatment; however, it still has a place in the following situations:

- Older and parous women
- When a woman cannot comply with the follow-up
- If uterus is associated with fibroids, DUB or prolapse
- If microinvasion exists
- If recurrence follows conservative therapy or persistent lesion
- In situ adenocarcinoma of the cervix

Follow-Up After Treatment of HSIL

Following conservative therapy, cytology is deferred for 3 months for inflammatory and regenerative changes to settle. In some cases, the squamocolumnar junction may retract within the os – 5% of women progress to invasive cancer during follow-up. Lifelong follow-up is therefore necessary.

Complications of these procedures are charted in Table 33.7

Choosing between various modalities within the group of conservative treatment is a matter of gynaecologist's preference, the availability of the equipment and its cost.

GLANDULAR LESIONS OF CERVIX

Preinvasive glandular endocervical lesion, also known as carcinoma – in situ endocervix, or cervical intraepithelial glandular neoplasm (CIGN) – is now proved to exist, though very rare. Many endocervical cancers arise de novo without passing through the in situ stage. It exists as a low- or high-grade lesion. It may appear anywhere along the endocervix, but is mostly seen near the squamocolumnar junction.

If the woman is young, nulliparous or of low parity, HPV infection and oral combined pills are probable causes of this lesion.

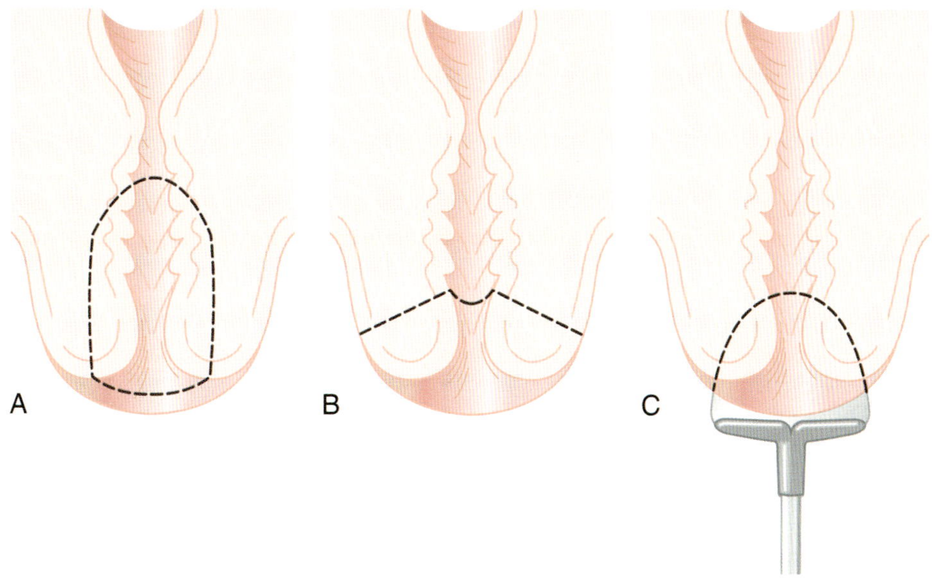

Figure 33.20 Cone biopsy of the cervix. **(A)** Diagnostic conization performed when the squamocolumnar junction is not fully visualized colposcopically. **(B)** Therapeutic conization performed for disease involving the ectocervix and distal endocervical canal. **(C)** Loop electrosurgical excision procedure. The goal of the procedure is to remove the cervical tissue above the squamocolumnar junction, including any visible lesions. (*Source:* Hacker NF, Gambone JC, Hobel CJ: Hacker and Moore's Essentials of Obstetrics and Gynecology, 5th ed. Philadelphia: Elsevier, 2010.)

It is difficult to pick up the cells in routine cytology and difficult to interpret. Similarly, colposcopy may miss the lesion if it is located within the cervical canal. Endocervical brush or endocervical curette is required to detect this lesion. In a suspected case, when cervical cytology shows abnormal glandular cells, cone biopsy is required.

The lesion is best treated with either cold-knife conization or hysterectomy. LLETZ can leave a residual tumour if the lesion is located high up in the cervical canal. Follow-up is necessary, as residual tumour can grow into endocervical cancer. Conization is applicable only in young women after counselling regarding recurrence. Hysterectomy is ideal otherwise.

PREVENTION OF CANCER OF THE CERVIX

The success of screening programme world over shows that it is a preventable cancer. Effective screening by Pap smear, VIA/VILI and HPV testing can detect most of the lesions in preinvasive stage and by appropriate action invasive cancer can be avoided. Majority of cancer cervix are HPV related. Fortunately, HPV vaccine is now available, although it is expensive as of today. Given to adolescents before exposure to the virus (before sexual activity begins), a high protection rate is expected. Such a vaccine also protects against genital warts. Initially, three doses of HPV vaccine were advocated at 0, 0.5 and 6 months but data available show that even two doses of HPV vaccine offer protection rate. What is not known is the duration of immunity and whether booster doses will be needed during the reproductive period.

PROPHYLACTIC HPV VACCINES

Gardasil is a quadrivalent vaccine against HPV 6, 11, 16 and 18 to be given to adolescents at 0, 2 and 6 months intramuscularly in the deltoid muscle.

16, 18 to be given (0.5 mL) at 0, 1 and 6 months.

Immunity is expected to last 10 years, and reimmunization may be required. Nowadays, a nonavalent vaccine (Gardasil 9) has become available which covers HPV 6, 11, 16, 18, 31, 33, 45, 52, 58; these types are responsible for 90% of cervical cancers, 82% of high-grade anogenital precancerous lesions and 90% of genital warts.

There is no need to test the young woman for HPV infections if vaccine is given before the start of sexual activity.

Reported Side Effects of Vaccine

- Local pain and swelling
- Dizziness, headache and myalgia
- Anaphylactic reaction
- Lymphadenopathy

If a patient is in the middle of a vaccination course, when she gets pregnant, all further vaccinations should be stopped until after the delivery. Medical termination of pregnancy is however not required. The woman can continue with remaining vaccination after delivery and to continue breast feeding following vaccination.

HPV Vaccine for Males

The vaccine is also an applicable prophylaxis for male adolescents.

Another prophylaxis is the use of barrier contraceptives to prevent transmission of viral infections and other sexually transmitted infections from man to woman.

INVASIVE CANCER OF THE CERVIX

About 132,000 women develop invasive cancer every year in India. In India, the incidence is 20–35/100,000 women between 35 and 65 years, whereas in developed countries, where screening programmes are on, the incidence of invasive cancer of cervix has fallen to 8/100,000 women. Approximately 74,000 women die of cancer cervix in India every year. Cumulative lifetime risk of development of cancer cervix is 2.5% among Indian women and cumulative lifetime risk of dying from cancer cervix is 1.4% among Indian women. In most cases, invasive disease is preceded by a preinvasive lesion of several years' duration. Certain women are at a higher risk of development of cancer cervix. These include immunocompromised persons, start of sexual activity at an early age, multiple sex partners, poor genital hygiene, poverty and low socioeconomic status, use of hormonal contraception and lack of access to health facilities.

PATHOLOGY

Majority of the invasive cancers of cervix are squamous cell carcinomas; however, in 10%–20% of cases, these carcinomas are adenocarcinoma in histology. Majority of the cancers start from ectocervix but in 10%–20% of cases they may be located in the endocervix. For a growth or lesion visible on ectocervix, cervical biopsy remains the method of establishing diagnosis. Occasionally, a diagnosis may be made by a Pap smear in case there is no visible lesion on cervix but the patient presents with symptoms of irregular vaginal bleeding. In a Pap smear, invasive cancer shows tadpole cells, fibres and malignant cells and haemorrhage, and necrosis in the background.

Commonly two types of carcinoma of the cervix are seen; first and more common variety is the **epidermoid carcinoma**. It arises from the stratified squamous epithelium of the cervix, and accounts for almost 80% of all cancers in the cervix. The second variety, endocervical carcinoma, arises from the mucous membrane of the endocervical canal, and accounts for 20% of all cervical cancers. Histologically, 95% of cervical cancers are squamous carcinomas and only 5% are adenocarcinomas. This is because the columnar epithelium of the endocervix often undergoes squamous metaplasia (Figs 33.21–33.24), before undergoing malignant change.

Incidence of endocervical cancers of the cervix has recently increased because of prolonged use of oral combined contraceptive pills and progestogen pills which have a profound effect on glandular epithelium (Fig. 33.22).

HISTOLOGICAL CLASSIFICATION

- Squamous cell carcinoma
- Adenocarcinoma
- Adenosquamous carcinoma
- Clear cell carcinoma
- Rare types such as neuroendocrine carcinoma

Squamous cell cancers of the ectocervix appear as proliferative growths, ulcers or flat indurated areas. The common proliferative or cauliflower-like growth is vascular, friable and bleeds on touch. It undergoes ulceration and necrosis, which is associated with an offensive foul-smelling vaginal discharge. The mucoid discharge is often blood-stained.

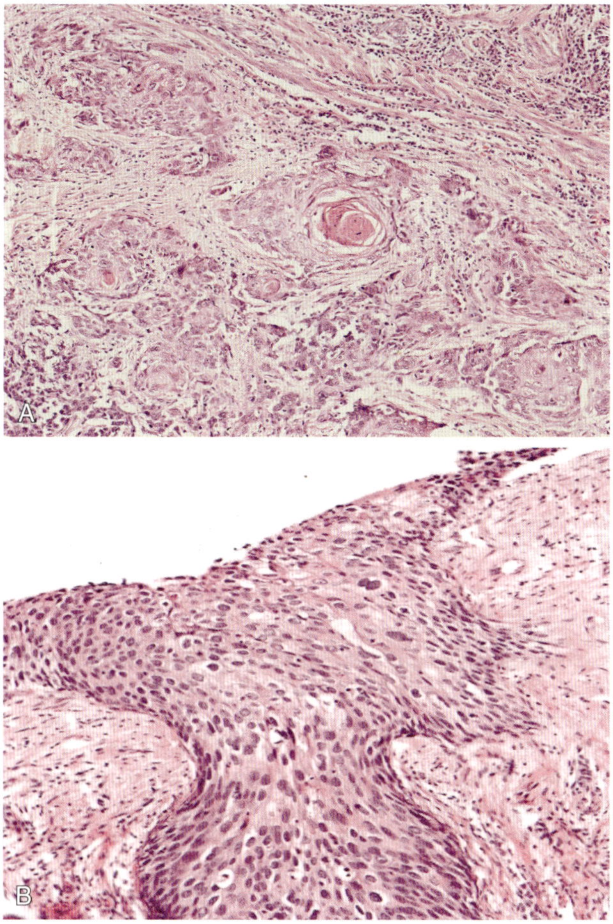

Figure 33.21 **(A)** Keratinizing squamous cell carcinoma of cervix: nests of atypical squamous cells infiltrating into the stroma. Keratin pearls are seen. **(B)** Carcinoma in- situ (CIN III) (*Source:* for **(B)** Dr Sandeep Mathur, AIIMS)

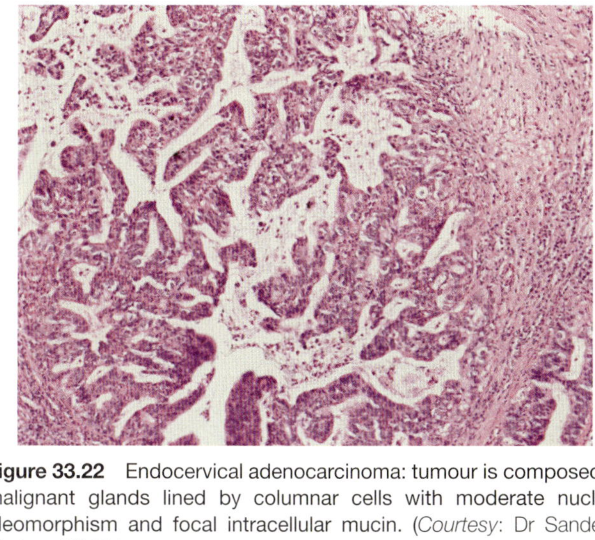

Figure 33.22 Endocervical adenocarcinoma: tumour is composed of malignant glands lined by columnar cells with moderate nuclear pleomorphism and focal intracellular mucin. (*Courtesy*: Dr Sandeep Mathur, AIIMS.)

Histologically, the tumour is graded as well-differentiated (showing epithelial pearl formation – see Fig. 33.21), moderately differentiated or poorly differentiated. A squamous cell carcinoma of cervix usually is nonkeratinizing but at times can have keratin pearl formation.

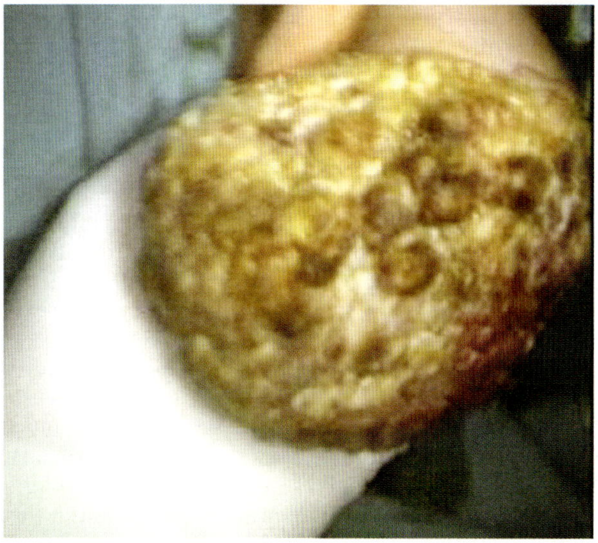

Figure 33.23 Large fungating carcinoma of the cervix in a case of procidentia.

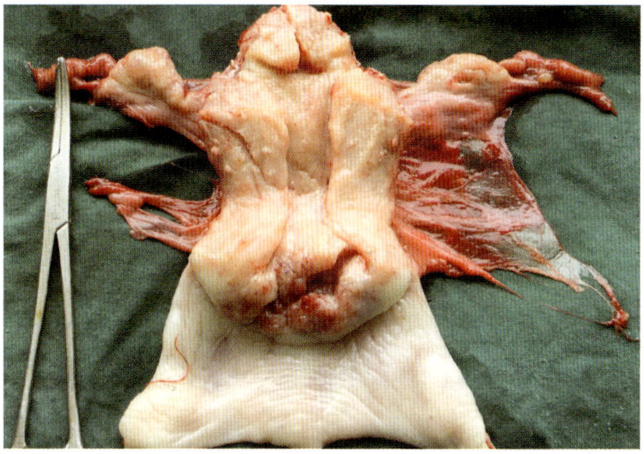

Figure 33.24 Ulcerative carcinoma of cervix, the specimen was removed by radical hysterectomy. Note also the parametrium and 2 cm of vagina removed.

The endocervical growth remains confined to the cervical canal for a long time causing a **barrel-shaped enlargement** of the cervix, and only at a late stage growth protrudes beyond the external cervical os and become visible.

MODE OF SPREAD

In initial stages, the cancer of cervix spreads by its continuity to adjoining structures (involving the vagina, parametrium and body of uterus); in advanced stages, it spreads to urinary bladder and rectum. Lymphatic spread occurs to draining lymph nodes (parametrial nodes, obturator, hypogastric and rarely distant nodes). Vascular spread occurs in late stages to distant sites such as lungs, liver, bones, kidneys and brain. *Ovarian metastasis occurs in only 1% in cases of squamous cell cancer but occurs in 10% in cases of adenocarcinoma of cervix.*

CLINICAL FEATURES

Most patients with invasive cancer of cervix present with the complaints of irregular menses, menometrorrhagia, continuous bleeding, postcoital bleeding, leucorrhoea and blood-stained or offensive discharge. It is not uncommon to encounter disease in postmenopausal women where the presenting symptom is postmenopausal bleeding.

On per speculum examination, cervix reveals a growth which bleeds on touch or an ulcer with edges that bleed on touch. On per vaginal examination, the uterus may appear bulky because of pyometra in the advanced stage when the cervix gets blocked by growth. In lateral fornices induration is felt, and on per rectal examination thickening of uterosacral ligaments may be noted.

In all suspected cases, a biopsy is needed to confirm the diagnosis.

Tissue biopsy in a case of frank invasive cancer reveals loss of stratification and cellular polarity; the cells show alteration of morphology, the nuclear:cytoplasmic ratio is increased and the tumour cells show hyperchromatism. Thickening of the nuclear membrane, clumping of the chromatin material, penetration of the underlying basement membrane and presence of the cancer cells into the underlying stroma are noted (Figs 33.25 and 33.26).

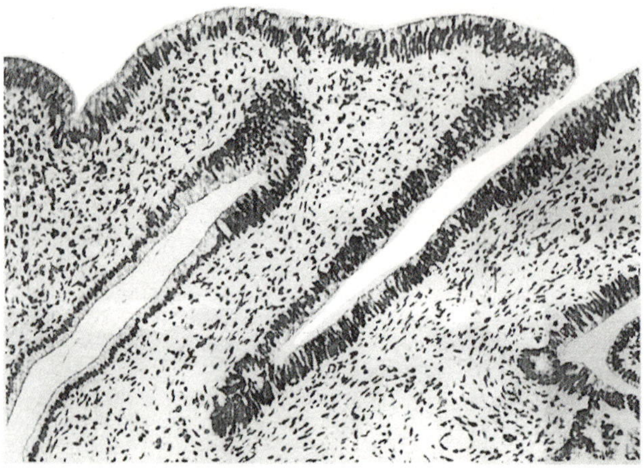

Figure 33.26 Adenocarcinoma in situ. The superficial parts of the crypts are lined by epithelium which shows loss of polarity and nuclear atypia (×155). (*Source:* From: Haines & Taylor's Obstetrical and Gynaecological Pathology, 3rd ed. Churchill, 1987.)

DIFFERENTIAL DIAGNOSIS

The cervical growth and ulcer may at times be mistaken for tubercular and syphilitic ulcer, mucus and fibroid polyp and rarely sarcoma of the cervix. Biopsy helps in ruling out other conditions.

STAGING OF CANCER OF THE CERVIX (Figs 33.27–33.39; Table 33.6)

Staging of cancer of cervix is based on revised FIGO staging given in year 2009. This staging is a clinical staging. For the purpose of staging, a careful clinical examination of the patient including per vaginal examination, per rectal examination and a combined per rectal–per vaginal examination is performed. Commonly done investigations include chest X-ray, an ultrasound of the abdomen and pelvis and liver and kidney function test. Presence of hydronephrosis makes a clinical stage as stage IIIb. Use of newer imaging techniques such as CT scan, MRI and positron emission tomography (PET) scan is not routinely recommended nor is the clinical stage changed based on results of these investigations.

Early invasive cancer of cervix (stage Ia) is diagnosed by histological examination of biopsy. Depending on the depth of stromal invasion and horizontal extent of the spread, the disease is further classified as stage Ia1 or stage Ia2. If the invasion is less than 3 mm in depth and less than 5 mm in horizontal spread, it is labelled as stage Ia1. When the depth of invasion is 3–5 mm and horizontal spread more than 5 mm, it is labelled as stage Ia2.

The surgical treatment and other modes of treatment depend on the exact clinical staging.

The staging of invasive carcinoma of the cervix is essentially based on clinical findings (chest radiograph, IVP, cystoscopy and proctoscopy are permitted). Because of wider availability of CT and MRI, these are now included in pretreatment strategy. **MRI is more sensitive than clinical examination in detecting parametrial involvement and regional lymph nodes** but FDG-PET is considered the gold standard in the investigation (see Chapter 40).

INCIDENCE OF LYMPH NODE METASTASIS IN CANCER CERVIX

Both pelvic and para-aortic lymph nodes can be involved in cancer cervix. Incidence varies with the stage of the disease.

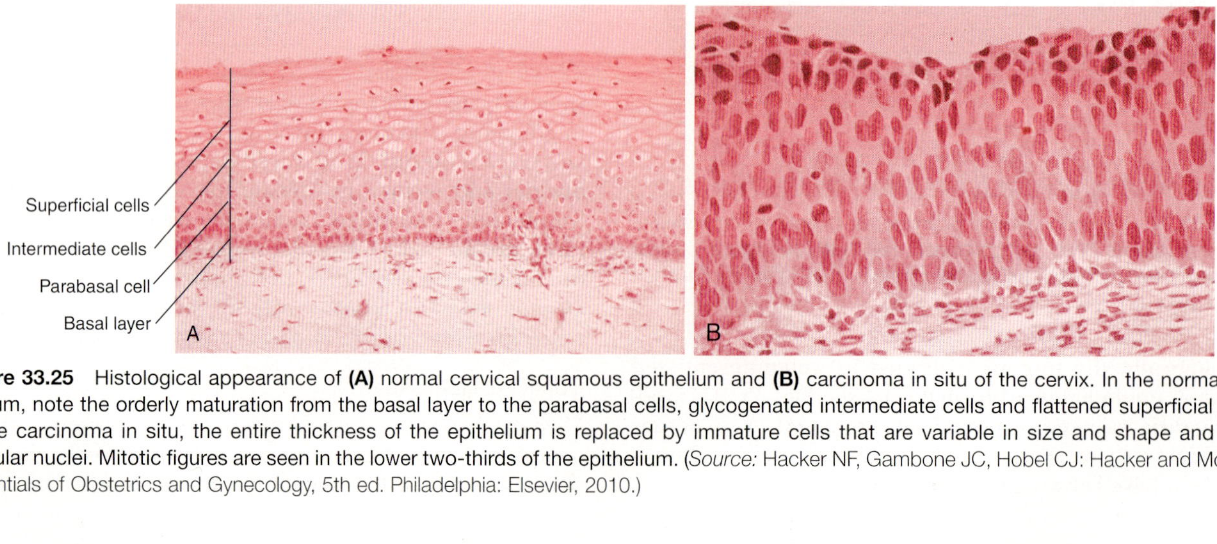

Figure 33.25 Histological appearance of **(A)** normal cervical squamous epithelium and **(B)** carcinoma in situ of the cervix. In the normal epithelium, note the orderly maturation from the basal layer to the parabasal cells, glycogenated intermediate cells and flattened superficial cells. In the carcinoma in situ, the entire thickness of the epithelium is replaced by immature cells that are variable in size and shape and have irregular nuclei. Mitotic figures are seen in the lower two-thirds of the epithelium. (*Source:* Hacker NF, Gambone JC, Hobel CJ: Hacker and Moore's Essentials of Obstetrics and Gynecology, 5th ed. Philadelphia: Elsevier, 2010.)

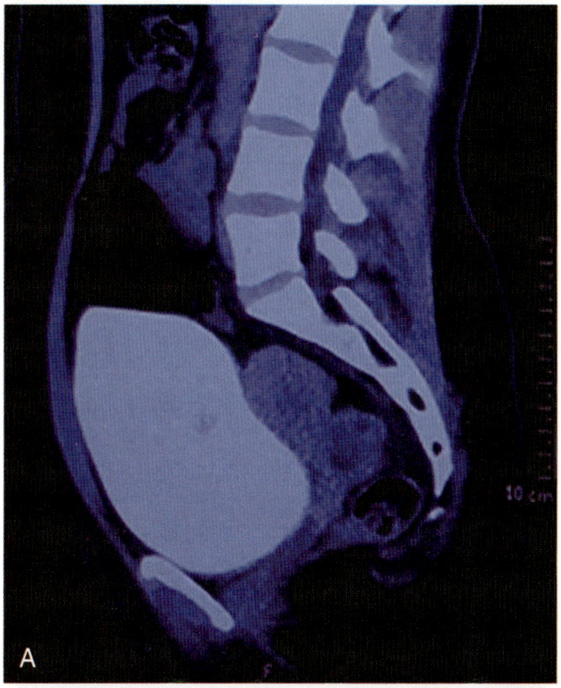

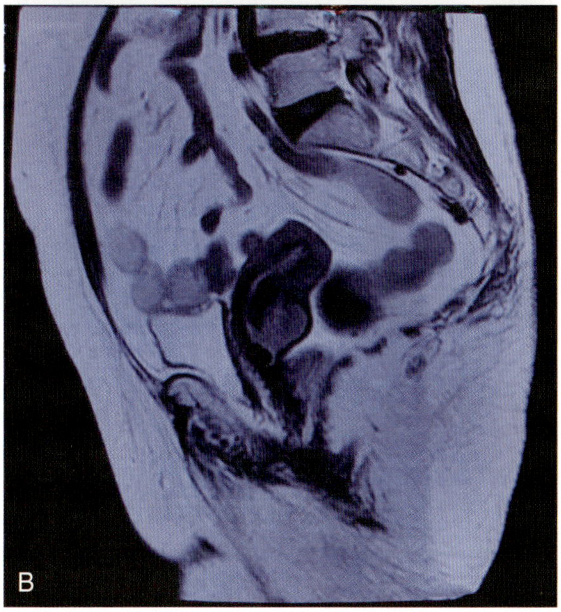

Figure 33.27 **(A)** MRI showing noninvasive cervical carcinoma with no parametrial invasion. **(B)** MRI showing carcinoma of the cervix with parametrial invasion.

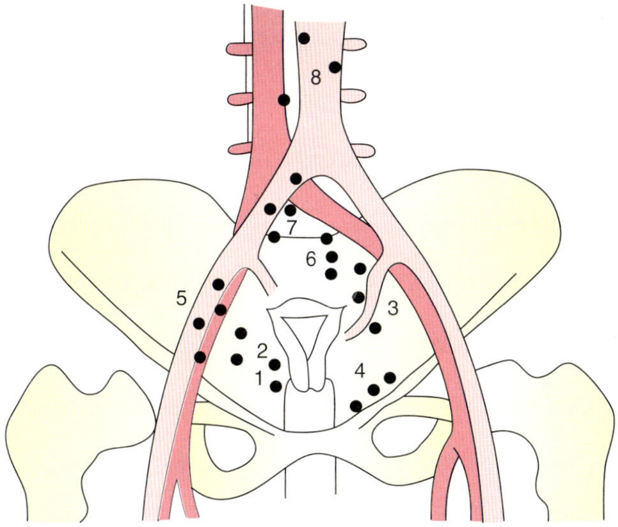

Figure 33.28 The distribution of pelvic nodes draining lymphatics from the cervix. Lymph node of drainage of the cervix: (1) paracervical, (2) parametrial, (3) internal iliac, (4) obturator, (5) external iliac, (6) presacral, (7) common iliac and (8) para-aortic.

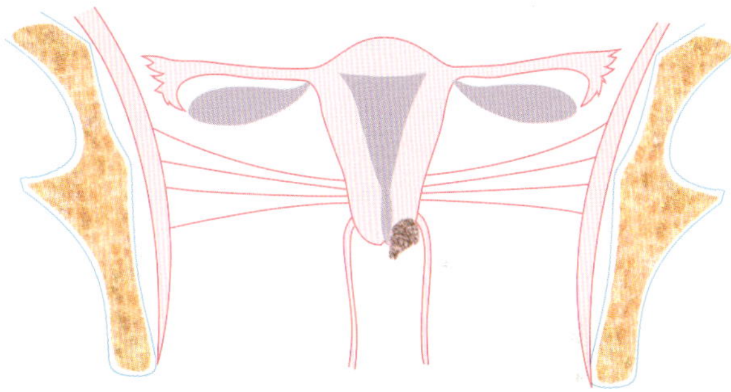

Figure 33.29 Carcinoma of the cervix. Stage I: ulcerative type.

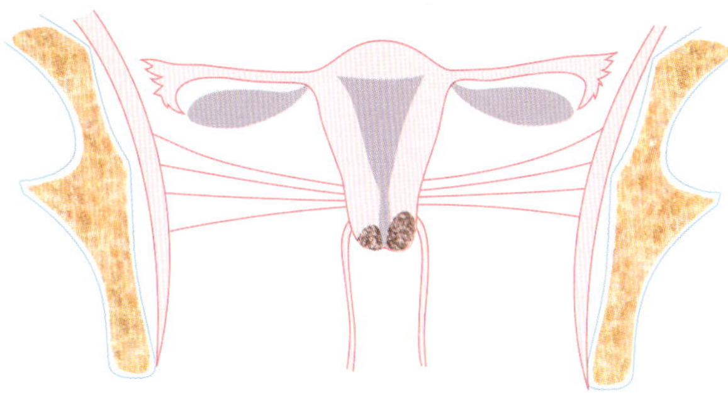

Figure 33.30 Carcinoma of the cervix. Stage I: infiltrating type.

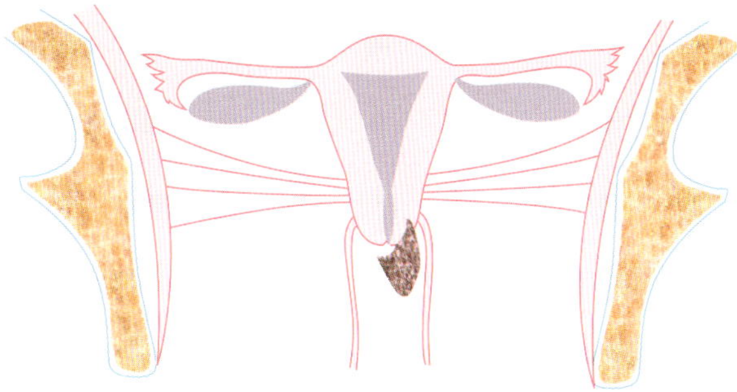

Figure 33.31 Stage I: cauliflower type.

In the presence of lymphovascular invasion, the incidence of lymph node metastasis further increases.

Incidence of lymph node metastasis in carcinoma of the cervix

Stage Ia1	Less than 1%
Stage Ia2	2%–7%
Stage Ib1	10%–15%
Stage Ib2	15%–35%
Stage II	15%–25%
Stage III	25%–40%
Stage IV	40%–65%

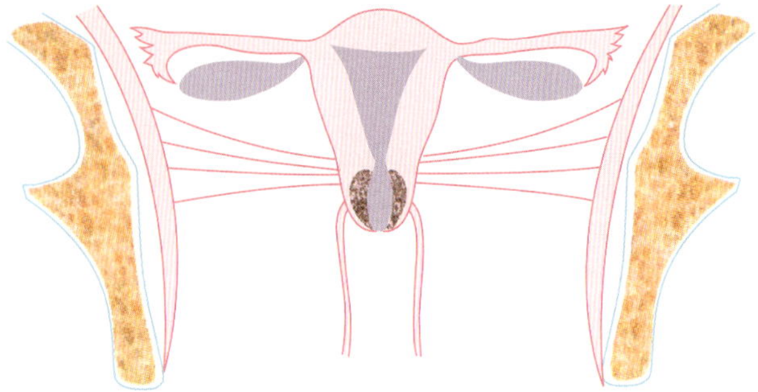

Figure 33.32 Stage I: endocervical type.

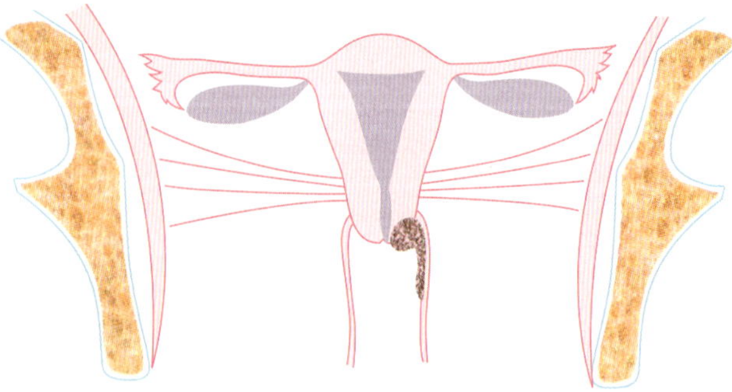

Figure 33.33 Stage IIa: infiltration of the vagina.

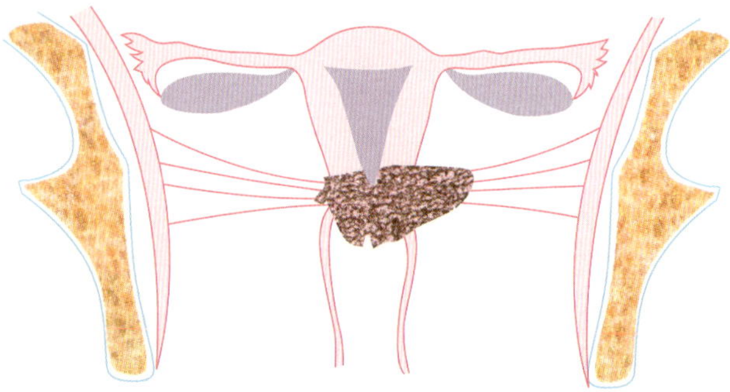

Figure 33.34 Stage IIb: infiltration of the parametrium.

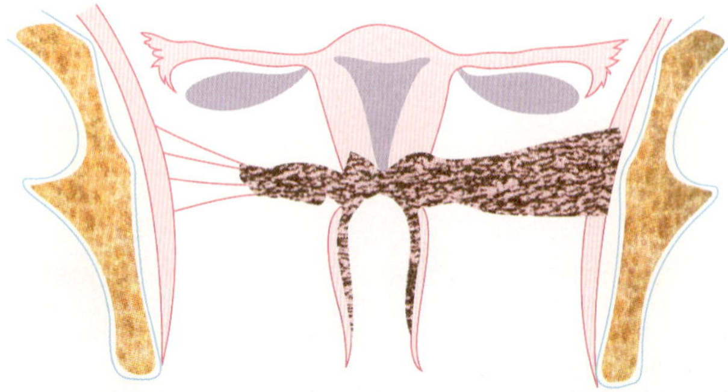

Figure 33.35 Stage IIIb: infiltration of the parametrium together with the whole of the vagina. Fixity of the parametrium by malignant invasion into the pelvic wall.

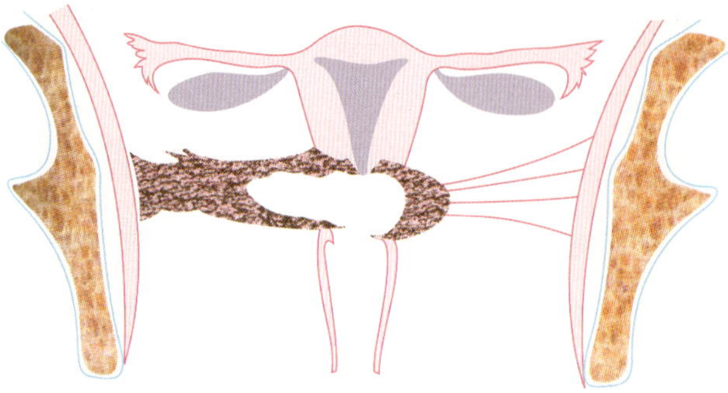

Figure 33.36 Stage IIIb: infiltration of the parametrium. The vagina is not involved.

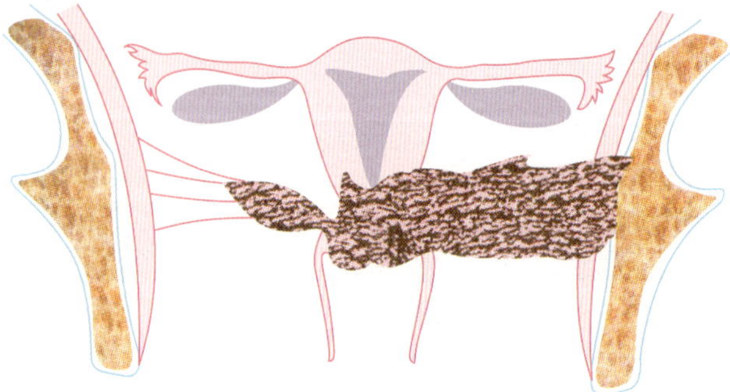

Figure 33.37 Carcinoma of the cervix. Stage IIIb: infiltration of the parametrium as far as the periosteum, but not through it.

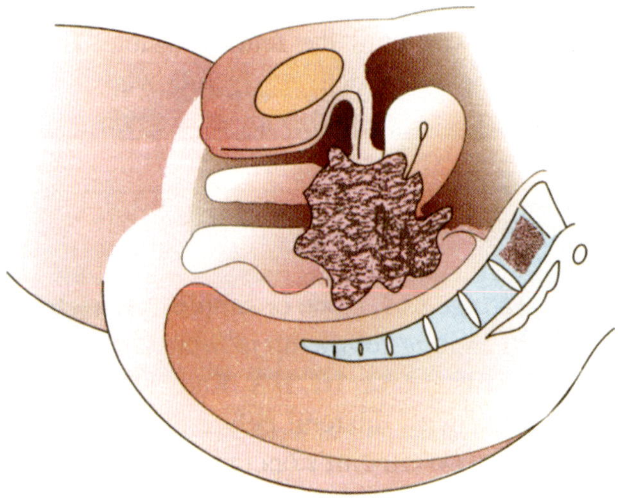

Figure 33.38 Carcinoma of the cervix. Stage IVa: infiltration into the rectum and bladder, together with bone metastases.

PARA-AORTIC LYMPH NODE METASTASIS

Para-aortic nodes are infiltrated in advanced cases (20% in Stage II, 30% in Stage III). Ureteric obstruction occurs in 30% in Stage III and 50% in Stage IV. Hypercalcaemia indicates bone metastasis.

DIAGNOSIS

Biopsy and histopathological evidence of invasive malignancy should precede any treatment modality. This may be

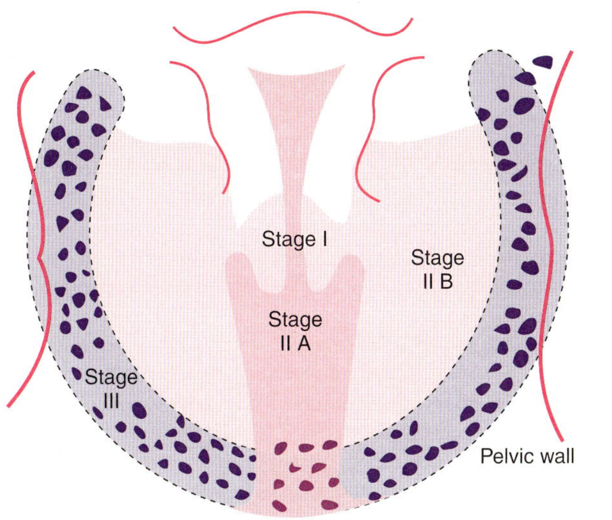

Figure 33.39 Staging of cancer cervix. (*Source:* From: Wilson et al. Textbook of Gynaecology and Obstetrics. BICL.)

from a suspicious growth, edge of an ulcer or colposcopy-directed biopsy from suspicious areas.

INVESTIGATIONS

Basic investigations include a haemogram, urinalysis, blood sugar levels – both fasting and postprandial – liver function tests, renal function tests and serum electrolytes. In advanced disease, ultrasonography, intravenous pyelography and cystoscopy should also be undertaken. A radiography of chest helps to exclude lung metastasis. A cystoscopy and proctoscopy may be required to assess the involvement of the bladder and rectum prior to finally assigning the stage of the disease.

- *CT and MRI* are now employed in routine investigations of invasive cancer of the cervix. While they detect lymph node enlargement more than 1 cm, multiplanar MRI offers improved imaging in staging and in pretreatment assessment of the growth and its spread as compared to CT. MRI can identify parametrial infiltration, but cannot always differentiate between inflammatory fibrotic and

Table 33.6 Carcinoma of the Cervix Uteri – Staging (FIGO, 2009)

Stage I	The carcinoma is strictly confined to the cervix (extension to the corpus would be disregarded)
IA	Invasive carcinoma which can be diagnosed only by microscopy, with deepest invasion ≤5 mm and largest extension ≥7 mm
IA1	Measured stromal invasion of ≤3.0 mm in depth and extension of ≤7.0 mm
IA2	Measured stromal invasion of >3.0 mm and not >5.0 mm with an extension of not >7.0 mm
IB	Clinically visible lesions limited to the cervix uteri or preclinical cancer greater than Stage IA[a]
IB1	Clinically visible lesion ≤4.0 cm in the greatest dimension
IB2	Clinically visible lesion >4.0 cm in the greatest dimension
Stage II	Cervical carcinoma invades beyond the uterus, but not to the pelvic wall or to the lower third of the vagina
IIA	Without parametrial invasion
IIA1	Clinically visible lesion ≤4.0 cm in the greatest dimension
IIA2	Clinically visible lesion >4 cm in the greatest dimension
IIB	With obvious parametrial invasion
Stage III	The tumour extends to the pelvic wall and/or involves lower third of vagina and/or causes hydronephrosis or nonfunctioning kidney[b]
IIIA	Tumour involves lower third of the vagina, with no extension to the pelvic wall
IIIB	Extension to the pelvic wall and/or hydronephrosis or nonfunctioning kidney
Stage IV	The carcinoma has extended beyond the true pelvis or has involved (biopsy proven) the mucosa of the bladder or rectum. A bullous oedema, as such, does not permit a case to be allotted to Stage IV
IVA	Spread of the growth to adjacent organs
IVB	Spread to distant organs

[a]All macroscopically visible lesions – even with superficial invasion – are allotted to Stage IB carcinomas. Invasion is limited to a measured stromal invasion with a maximal depth of 5.00 mm and a horizontal extension of not >7.00 mm. Depth of invasion should not be >5.00 mm taken from the base of the epithelium of the original tissue – superficial or glandular. The depth of invasion should always be reported in millimetres, even in those cases with 'early (minimal) stromal invasion' (−1 mm).
[b]On rectal examination, there is no cancer-red space between the tumour and the pelvic wall. All cases with hydronephrosis or nonfunctioning kidney are included, unless they are known to be because of another cause.
Source: FIGO guidelines.

malignant infiltration. Because of intestinal peristalsis, para-aortic lymph nodes are not clearly visible on MRI. MRI is safe during pregnancy, but CT is not so because of radiation. A small lymph node less than 1 cm cannot be picked up by CT or MRI. It is important to emphasize that CT and MRI findings should not alter the clinical staging.

- *PET*, a noninvasive scan, detects tissue biochemical changes and para-aortic node involvement, and maps the area of concern. In PET scan, the whole body is scanned for an area of increased uptake of radioactive tracer.

FDG-PET using F-18 fluoro-2-deoxy-D-glucose is useful in the determination of primary disease, lymph node detection and local recurrence detection. The test is based on the fact that malignant tissue exhibits greater glycolysis than normal tissue, and FDG accumulates in the malignant tissue resulting in increased tumour contrast. While CT and MRI show anatomical changes, PET shows biochemical changes in the tissues. A combination of PET and CT would predict the presence of malignant tumour and its anatomy better than either singly. FDG-PET is now considered a gold standard in the investigation of cancer cervix.

TREATMENT OF INVASIVE CANCER

Treatment depends on the stage of the disease. However, in case there is a need to preserve fertility, a conservative surgical procedure is possible in early stage disease.

Better understanding of early lesions has permitted a more conservative surgical treatment without compromising the success, at the same time reducing the morbidity and retaining the fertility potential in younger women.

SURGICAL TREATMENT

Stagewise Treatment of Cancer of the Cervix

- **Stage Ia1:** The diagnosis is by cone biopsy. The lymph node involvement in this stage is only 0.5%. Therefore, conization with a clear margin is considered adequate and is diagnostic as well as therapeutic. Hysterectomy in a young woman is considered rather a radical surgical approach with increased morbidity but without improved survival. Hysterectomy (extrafacial hysterectomy – Type I hysterectomy) is appropriate in elderly and parous women, or those having an associated disease in the uterus. Lymphadenectomy is not required, but long term follow-up is necessary. Lymphatic or vascular channel infiltration however mandates treatment as in Stage Ib.
- **Stage Ia2:** Lymph node involvement and recurrence rate is 2%–7%, provided vascular and lymphatic channels are not involved. Extended hysterectomy and lymph node sampling are recommended (Type II hysterectomy). Nodal involvement requires postoperative radiotherapy. In a young woman desirous of child-bearing, conservative treatment comprising laparoscopic lymphadenectomy followed by vaginal trachelectomy introduced by Daniel Dargent(1987) is appropriate and does not compromise on its success. **Fertility-conserving trachelectomy** consists of whole or at least 80% removal of the cervix and upper vagina and cutting Mackenrodt's ligament on either side. Involvement of lymphatic or vascular channel needs similar treatment as in Stage Ib. Before conservative surgery, MRI mapping for local extension and lymph node involvement is needed. Obturator gland is the sentinel node – if negative, no further lymphadenectomy is required. Injection of blue dye into the cervical tissue before surgery identifies lymph nodes. Conception rate of 30%–40% at the end of 1 year, with miscarriage (20%–30%), preterm labour (18%) and chorioamnionitis, is reported. Recurrence rate of 5% is also reported. Contraindication to fertility-preserving operation is a lesion more than 2 cm. Cervical cerclage at the time of primary surgery may reduce the pregnancy complications of abortion and preterm labour (Fig. 33.40).

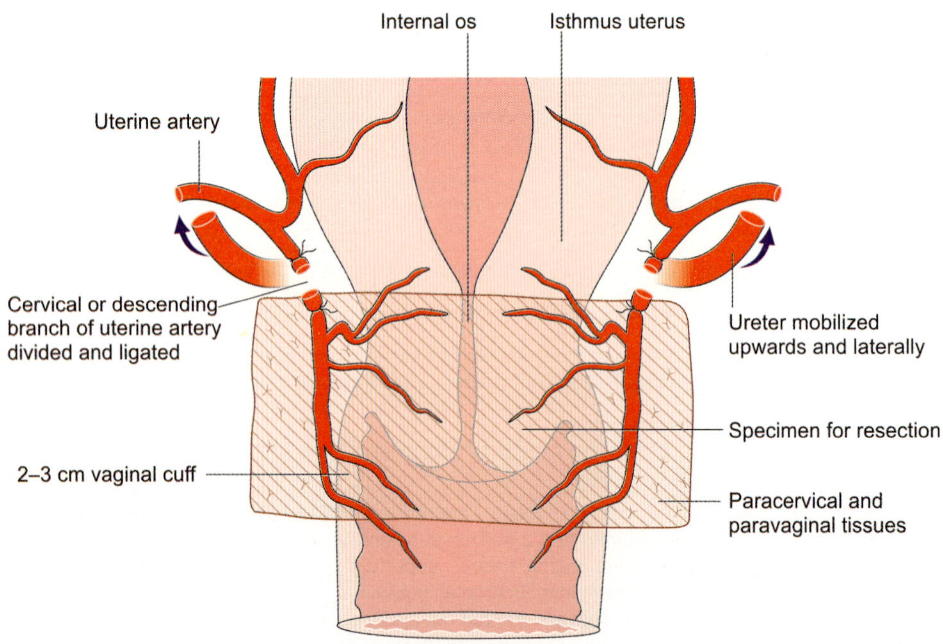

Figure 33.40 The technique used for radical trachelectomy. Area of tissue for resection (shaded) including cervix and upper vagina with paracervical and paravaginal tissues up to the level of the uterine isthmus.

- **Stages Ib and IIa:** The treatment options are as follows:
  - Radical Abdominal hysterectomy (Type III radical hysterectomy)
  - Schauta's vaginal hysterectomy (known as Mitra operation in India) and Taussig's or laparoscopic lymphadenectomy
  - Primary radiotherapy with concurrent chemotherapy
  - Combined surgery and radiotherapy

Injection of blue dye into the cervical tissue before surgery identifies lymph nodes during surgery (sentinel lymph node). Negative sentinel lymph node (obturator lymph node) helps avoid extensive pelvic lymphadenectomy.

Wertheim's hysterectomy, also known as Meigs–Obayashi hysterectomy, is the surgical treatment in Stage Ia2, with lymphovascular invasion and tumour size of 2 cm. Whereas for Stages Ib and IIa is slightly more radical procedure (Type III-radical hysterectomy). It comprises exploratory laparotomy, removal of the entire uterus, both adnexa, pelvic lymph nodes, medial one-third of the parametrium on either side and upper one-third of the vagina, sparing sacral glands. The ovaries are involved in only 1%, so they may be retained if appear healthy in a young patient. In such a case, the ovaries maybe transposed outside the pelvis to avoid damage in case radiotherapy is required later. Lately, radical hysterectomy is performed laparoscopically by experts, a robotic radical hysterectomy is done in specialised centres.

Schauta's operation is an extended vaginal hysterectomy consisting of removal of the entire uterus, adnexa, most of the vagina and medial portion of the parametrium. This is combined with pelvic lymphadenectomy which can be done by extraperitoneal approach. The original vaginal radical hysterectomy has been reintroduced with modification by a number of surgeons in France where a laparoscopic approach or laparoscopic-assisted operation is done. Alternatively, postoperative pelvic radiotherapy may be employed. With the possibility of laparoscopic lymphadenectomy and lesser morbidity of vaginal approach, this modified laparoscopic-assisted radical vaginal hysterectomy is gaining popularity among many oncologists.

Complications of Radical Hysterectomy

- Haemorrhage during surgery
- Trauma to the bladder and ureter (1%–2%) causing fistula
- Dysfunction of bladder because of nerve damage
- Damage to the obturator and genitofemoral nerve
- Sepsis
- Thromboembolism, pulmonary and urinary tract infection
- Paralytic ileus, peritonitis, wound sepsis, burst abdomen and scar hernia
- Lymphocyst formation in the broad ligament
- Lymphoedema (10%–20%)

A radical abdominal hysterectomy is a major surgical procedure associated with major and minor complications as mentioned above; this procedure also has a risk of primary mortality in the region of 1%. Not all centres and not all surgeons are capable of doing this major surgical procedure.

Radiotherapy

Advances in radiotherapy techniques have made it possible to treat cases of cancer cervix with equally good results as seen with surgery. In addition, radiotherapy is applicable in stages such as Stages IIb, IIIa and IIIb where surgery is not feasible. Primary radiotherapy consists of intracavity brachytherapy and external radiation to the pelvis. It yields the same 5-year cure rate as that of surgery, i.e. 80%–90%. It is, however, observed that many surgical cases show positive lymph node metastasis which requires additional postoperative radiotherapy anyway, and this combined therapy increases the morbidity in the woman. Therefore, some oncologists prefer to avoid surgical approach and employ primary radiotherapy (see chapter 39 on Radiation Therapy and Chemotherapy).

Addition of chemotherapy with cisplatin 40 mg^2 weekly to radiotherapy improves the radiation effect, as cisplatin acts as a radiosensitizer agent. Current standard of radiation therapy is to combine it with weekly cisplatin when the patient is undergoing external beam radiation. Young women in this group warrant special consideration because of risk of destruction of ovaries, stenosis of vagina and occurrence of pyometra following radiotherapy. Primary surgery therefore is the treatment of choice in young women. In case of a large lesion, external radiotherapy is used first, followed by two applications of brachytherapy 2 weeks apart. This shrinks the tumour, and allows insertion of internal applicator.

The advantages and disadvantages of surgery and radiotherapy are mentioned in Table 33.7.

Indications for Postoperative Radiotherapy

In case surgery was the first line of treatment of early stage cancer cervix, postoperative radiotherapy will be needed for the following indications:

- Positive lymph nodes for metastasis
- Positive resected margin of vagina or parametrium
- Evidence of lymphovascular invasion or deep stromal invasion
- Poorly differentiated tumour

Preoperative Chemotherapy

Currently giving preoperative chemotherapy to a case of carcinoma of the cervix is not a standard method of treatment; however, people are exploring this as a mode of treatment in women with bulky disease.

- Neoadjuvant paclitaxel 90 mg and injection ifosfamide 2000 mg plus mesna 400 mg weekly for three cycles
- Cisplatin 50 mg weekly followed by surgery yields 94% success in early stages

Recurrence of Cancer

Advanced stage diseases such as Stages IIB, III and IV are at a risk of recurrences. Recurrence can also occur in early stage disease managed by surgery or chemoradiation. Most patients tend to develop recurrences in the first 5 years after treatment. Chemoradiotherapy can improve the survival and allow the woman to spend a comfortable life or increase the duration of remission. A centrally placed growth, a bladder and rectal fistula may be subjected to exenteration operation.

Recent trend is to treat stage IIb with chemoradiation or chemotherapy for the first 3 months followed by surgery.

Table 33.7 Advantages and Disadvantages of Surgery Compared with Radiotherapy

Surgery	Radiotherapy
Advantages	
• Accurate surgical staging possible • Pelvic lymphatic glands can be removed • Conservation of ovaries – transposition of ovaries in case post-operative chemotherapy is required • A more pliable, but short vagina retained • Applicable if fibroids, adnexal masses present • Failed surgery can be treated with radiotherapy	• Survival rates for surgery and radiotherapy are similar • Applicable to all stages between Stages IB and IV • OPD procedure • No immediate mortality
Disadvantages	
• Surgical mortality – 1% • Anaesthesia complications • Haemorrhage, trauma during surgery • Sepsis – wound, pelvic, chest, urinary tract, burst abdomen • Bladder atonicity, fistula, ureteric injury, bladder dysfunction because of denervation • Paralytic ileus, thrombophlebitis, embolism • Lymphocyst formation • Many require radiotherapy postoperatively • Scar hernia, pelvic adhesions • Obturator nerve damage	• Anaemia • Ovarian destruction • Pyometra • Decreased libido because of ovarian failure • Vaginal stenosis • Bladder – cystitis, fistula, ureteric stenosis • Bowel – chronic diarrhoea, proctitis, rectal stricture, fistula – skin burn • Avascular necrosis of femoral head • Not applicable in the presence of ovarian tumour, adnexal mass, fibroids, prolapse • Risk of sarcoma a few years later

Recurrent Lesion

Twenty to twenty-five per cent of early lesions recur within 2 years of primary treatment. This may be centrally located or on the lateral pelvic wall with lymph node involvement or distal in the para-aortic nodes, lungs, liver or bones. Most recurrences are related to the size of the primary growth of more than 2 cm, stage of cancer, lymph node involvement and tissue differentiation.

The symptoms appear late, but are similar to those of early cancer. The development of sciatic pain, lymphoedema of the leg and fistula are sure signs of recurrence. It is important to differentiate inflammatory from malignant, parametrial thickening. On pelvic examination, inflammatory infiltration is smooth, whereas malignant infiltration is nodular.

Follow-Up of a Treated Case of Cancer of the Cervix

Pap smear is difficult to interpret. The cells appear large with cytoplasmic vacuolation, multinucleation and nuclear shrinking with inflammatory cells in the first few months of radiotherapy. Clinical examination and combination with investigations if indicated can detect recurrences. Fine-needle aspiration cytology (FNAC) and tricot needle biopsy confirm the recurrence. Cystoscopy, sigmoidoscopy, CT, MRI and PET are required to study the extent of the growth.

MRI is superior to CT in identifying malignant infiltration in the parametrium, but in case of difficulty, MRI is repeated 3 months later; PET also helps. CT is specific in 60%–70% of cases, but MRI is specific in 70%–90% of cases. PET–CT is more specific than the two.

Management of Recurrences

Recurrent growth following radiotherapy can be treated by hysterectomy in a small central growth or exenteration operation. Most recurrences are centrally placed and 30% are fit to be managed by pelvic exenteration operation. Anterior exenteration comprises hysterectomy and removal of the bladder with ureteric implantation in the ileal conduit. Posterior exenteration removes the uterus and the rectum with low rectal anastomosis, avoiding permanent colostomy. In total exenteration, both bladder and rectum are removed in addition to the uterus. Vaginoplasty may be required in young women. Exenteration operation is indicated in recurrent and residual tumours centrally located.

Exenteration surgery makes the life of the woman comfortable, with 5%–15% surgical mortality but 60% 5-year cure rate. The following are the contraindications to this operation:

- Age over 80 years
- Woman not accepting colostomy
- Presence of lymph node or distal metastasis
- Fixed tumours

Lateral recurrence is managed by radiotherapy in a previous surgical case, but repeat radiotherapy can cause fistula unless radiotherapy was applied more than 1 year ago.

Distal metastasis has a 5-year survival rate of only 5%, but chemotherapy has recently shown considerable improvement in short-term remission in 20%–40% of cases. Of all drugs, cisplatin proves most promising, singly or in combination.

The details of radiotherapy and chemotherapy are given in chapter on Radiotherapy and Chemotherapy.

Stagewise Treatment of Cancer of the Cervix

Stage Ia1	Conization or extrafacial hysterectomy (Type I)
Stage Ia2	Modified radical hysterectomy (Type II) Or Radical trachelectomy in young women
Stage Ib1	Radical hysterectomy (Type III) Or Radical trachelectomy in young women
Stage Ib2	Radical hysterectomy (Type III) Or Chemoradiation
Stage IIa	Radical hysterectomy (Type III) Or Chemoradiation
Stages IIb, IIIa, IIIb	Chemoradiation
Stage IV	Palliative radiotherapy
Recurrent carcinoma of the cervix	Exenteration operation/ chemotherapy

Conservative Surgery in a Young Woman

In a young woman diagnosed to have early stage cancer cervix (Stages Ia, Ib1), it is possible to preserve her uterus for future childbearing. In a young woman wishing to conserve fertility potential, the following measures are recently being tried:

1. Trachelectomy with lymphadenectomy and cervical cerclage
2. Transposition of the ovaries outside the pelvis in case radiotherapy is required
3. Oocyte and embryo cryopreservation prior to chemoradiation

CARCINOMA IN PREGNANCY

PREINVASIVE CANCER IN PREGNANCY

When a young woman presents with bleeding during pregnancy or postcoital bleeding, it may be a sign of early stage disease of cervix.

The cervix may appear normal or show chronic cervicitis or erosion. Pap smear and colposcopy-directed biopsy confirm the diagnosis. Cone biopsy should be avoided in pregnancy whenever possible, because of risk of postbiopsy bleeding and abortion. Besides, transformation zone is usually clearly visible during pregnancy for biopsy. In case of preinvasive lesion and Stage Ia1 lesion, the woman is allowed a vaginal delivery, provided invasive lesion is excluded. Six weeks postpartum, another Pap smear followed by colposcopy will help to evaluate the case for any further treatment (Fig. 33.41).

INVASIVE CANCER OF THE CERVIX IN PREGNANCY

The incidence of cancer of the cervix is reported in 1:2500 pregnancies.

The woman presents with antepartum haemorrhage. The cervix presents a similar picture as in the nonpregnant condition. Confirmation of diagnosis is based on a cervical

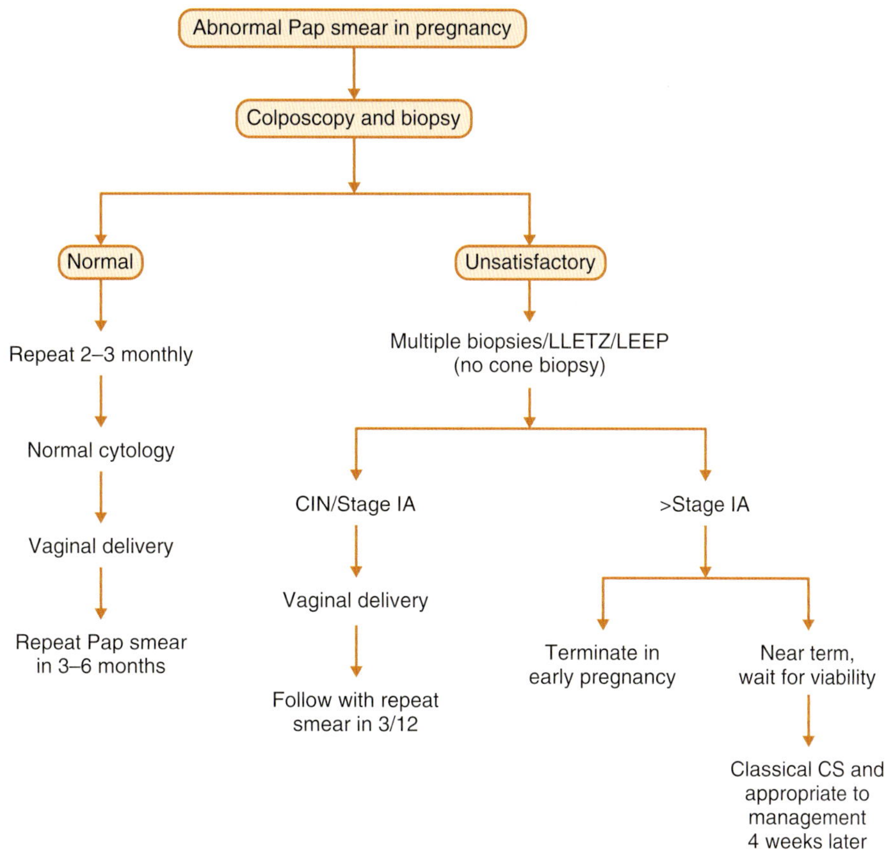

Figure 33.41 Abnormal Pap smear in pregnancy.

biopsy. Cone biopsy can cause profuse bleeding; therefore, the diagnosis is confirmed on multiple biopsies or colposcopy-directed biopsies. MRI is permissible as it does not cause radiation. CT is contraindicated. Staging of invasive cancer of cervix in pregnancy is done on the same lines as in nonpregnant state.

MANAGEMENT IN PREGNANCY

The pregnancy does not appear to alter the biological behaviour of the tumour, and treatment, therefore, depends on stage of the disease and duration of pregnancy.

For Stage Ib or IIa cancer of the cervix detected before 20–24 weeks of pregnancy, a surgical treatment by Wertheim's hysterectomy (Type III radical hysterectomy) is desirable. Alternately, primary radiotherapy is also feasible after termination of pregnancy by upper segment hysterotomy.

If pregnancy is more than 24 weeks or approaching term, it may be prudent to wait until the fetus is viable. Elective classical caesarean delivery is followed by radical hysterectomy in the same sitting or radiotherapy as in a nonpregnant state. Breast-feeding is usually avoided during radiotherapy or chemotherapy.

For advanced disease, it is better to terminate pregnancy by upper segment hysterotomy or a classical caesarean section followed by radical chemoradiation.

ENDOCERVICAL ADENOCARCINOMA OF CERVIX

Endocervical cancer occurring in younger woman around 35 years, nulliparous or of low parity. Viral infections and combined oral pills probably cause this cancer. The symptoms, similar to those of squamous cancer, appear late. The cervix appears barrel-shaped with the growth pouting through the external os in the advanced stage. The parametrial infiltrations occur early, so also the spread to the uterus.

Pap smear has low sensitivity, but endocervical cytology, curettage or cone biopsy improves the detection rate.

In invasive cancer, chemoradiation for 6 weeks should be followed by Wertheim's hysterectomy. The ovaries should be removed because of the advanced growth at diagnosis and distal spread. They are involved in 10% of cases.

HRT can be prescribed following oophorectomy in cancer cervix.

RESULTS

Refer to Table 33.8.

Table 33.8 Comparison of FIGO Staging and 5-year Survival Rate

FIGO Staging	5-Year Survival Rates (%)
Stage I	>90
Stage IIA	>80
Stage IIB	>65
Stage IIIA	About 45
Stage IIIB	About 35
Stage IV	<15

PROGNOSIS

Prognosis is related to tumour volume, staging, lymph node involvement and grading of the tissue. It is worse than that of squamous cell carcinoma. Raised carcinoembryonic antigen (CEA) level indicates bad prognosis.

Stump Cancer

Stump cancer cervix occurs in 1%–2% of cases following subtotal hysterectomy performed for benign lesions. If it occurs within 2 years of surgery, it is likely that it was present at the time of hysterectomy. Pap smear prior to hysterectomy reduces its risk. Management is difficult, involving both surgery and radiotherapy. Conization with external radiotherapy is recommended.

PALLIATIVE TREATMENT IN TERMINAL STAGES OF CANCER OF THE CERVIX

- Pain relief with morphine and tramadol; oral morphine 5–60 mg
- Vomiting: Dehydration and electrolyte imbalance corrected; neutropenia, uraemia and chemoradiation are the causes of vomiting
- Haloperidol 1.5–3 mg (dopaminergic antagonist)
- Appetite improved by metoclopramide, domperidone and corticosteroids for bowel oedema (60–100 mg daily prednisone); dexamethasone 4–8 mg daily for 3–5 days
- Lymphatic leg oedema stockings, garments and massage
- Diuretics and spironolactone for ascites
- Vaginal discharge – Betadine douche or metronidazole irrigation
- Ondansetron 4 mg t.i.d. for radiation vomiting
- Ascites tapping

For profuse vaginal bleeding, packing and administration of tranexamic acid 500 mg i.v. 6–8 hourly are helpful. Rarely, embolization/ligation of internal iliac artery is needed.

FUTURE DEVELOPMENT

A new line of approach in the form of VEGF factor such as bevacizumab is being tried along with standard treatment protocol to achieve better survival rates. Other forms of chemotherapy such as paclitaxel + carboplatin are also being evaluated for treatment of advanced disease. Gene therapy may have a role in locally advanced disease. It is possible for the direct injection of DNA–liposomal complexes and human leucocyte antigen, which may promote a favourable cytotoxic immune response. This may have a role in reducing local recurrence.

KEY POINTS

- Carcinoma of the cervix is the most common genital tract cancer in women and ranks next to breast cancer. It is a disease of young women between the age of 35 and 50 years.

- Human papillomavirus (HPV) infection is now proved to be the most important cause of preinvasive and invasive cervical cancer. It is sexually transmitted. Other contributory factors are early age of sexual activity, multiple partners, poor hygiene, multiparity and immunosuppressive conditions such as HIV.
- Use of barrier contraceptives prevents transmission of viral infection to a woman and prevents preinvasive and invasive cervical cancer. Prolonged use of oral combined pills increases the risk of cancer cervix, especially endocervical cancers.
- Ninety per cent of young women with HPV infection show spontaneous resolution within 2 years and do not develop cancer. Only those with persistent infection after the age of 30 years are at a high risk for preinvasive and invasive cancer.
- Stepwise development of cancer cervix from HPV infection and its persistence leading to preinvasive and invasive cancer takes 10–15 years. This long period allows routine screening and treatment of preinvasive cancer, so that invasive cancer does not develop.
- Routine Pap smear and colposcopic study and biopsy pick up preinvasive lesions (CIN) effectively in 90% of cases. Adding HPV testing further improves the pick-up rate.
- Ablative therapy for early stage disease is a successful fertility-conserving therapy in young women, but lifelong follow-up is necessary to detect recurrence. Hysterectomy is reserved for elderly and multiparous women. Follow-up is necessary irrespective of treatment for preinvasive cancer.
- Endocervical cancer is difficult to diagnose in its early stage, as the tissue is not available for cytology and colposcopy. Endocervical scrape and cone biopsy are required for diagnosis. Treatment is chemoradiation followed by Wertheim's hysterectomy.
- Radiotherapy is applicable in all stages of invasive cancers. However, because of ovarian atrophy, vaginal stenosis and pyometra, primary surgery is preferred in young women.
- Prognosis in invasive cancer depends on the size of the lesion, stage of the disease, involvement of lymph nodes and cell differentiation.
- Prophylactic vaccine against HPV is now available. Given before the start of sexual activity, the vaccine is expected to reduce the incidence of cervical cancer in future.

SELF-ASSESSMENT

1. Discuss the causes of carcinoma of the cervix.
2. Discuss the clinical features and management of preinvasive cancer of the cervix.
3. Describe the clinical features of invasive cervical cancer and the differential diagnosis.
4. How will you investigate a case of cancer of the cervix?
5. Discuss the management of stage Ib cancer of the cervix.
6. Describe the FIGO staging of cancer cervix.
7. Discuss the diagnosis and management of endocervical cancer.
8. Discuss management of a case of cancer cervix with pregnancy.

SUGGESTED READING

Duncan J, Shulman P. Yearbook of Obstetrics, Gynaecology and Women's Health; 40: 423, 2010.

Studd J. HPV role in cancer cervix: In: Progress in Obstetrics and Gynaecology Vol: 14, 2000.

Studd J. Prognosis in cancer cervix. Progress in Obstetrics and Gynaecology 15, 2003.

Studd J. Progress in Obstetrics and Gynaecology 7: 1989.

Studd J. Screening cancer cervix. Progress in Obstetrics and Gynaecology 16: 323, 2005.

34 Cancer of the Body of the Uterus

CHAPTER OUTLINE

The body of the uterus is the site of endometrial cancer, the most frequent genital tract cancer in rich countries; however, it ranks third in India after cancer of cervix and cancer of ovary.

ENDOMETRIAL CANCER

Endometrial cancer has recently emerged as the more frequently encountered gynaecological cancer accounting for 20%–25% of all genital cancers in the developed countries, not only because of the longer survival of women, but mainly because of the marked decline in cervical cancer by screening programme (Figs 34.1–34.5). In developing countries including India, the incidence has remained low at 5%–7% of all genital cancers; cervical cancer continues to predominate and is seen in 1.8 per 100,000 population.

The majority of the endometrial cancer is seen in the 55–70 years age group, 20%–25% of cases occur in perimenopausal women and only 5% of cases develop in women younger than 40 years when they these cancers are well-differentiated with good survival. Women are either nulliparous or of low parity. An early menarche and late menopause is a characteristic of women suffering from this cancer, indicating the prolonged exposure to oestrogen hormone. Seventy-five per cent of the tumours are localized in the uterus when diagnosed, and surgery is the cornerstone in its management. Surprisingly, oestrogen-dependent endometrial cancer can develop in atrophic endometrium in a postmenopausal woman when the level of the hormone is lowest. However, the behavioural pattern differs; endometrial cancer is poorly differentiated in postmenopausal women, whereas in young women it is well-differentiated and curable. After the age of 80 years, the incidence drops. Two types of endometrial cancers have been identified: The Type I cancer occurs mostly in obese persons with excess of endogenous or exogenous oestrogens and is histologically endometrioid adenocarcinoma. The Type II endometrial cancer is histologically a clear cell variety or papillary serous variety seen in elderly women without any evidence of a hyperoestrogenic state and is associated with poorer prognosis.

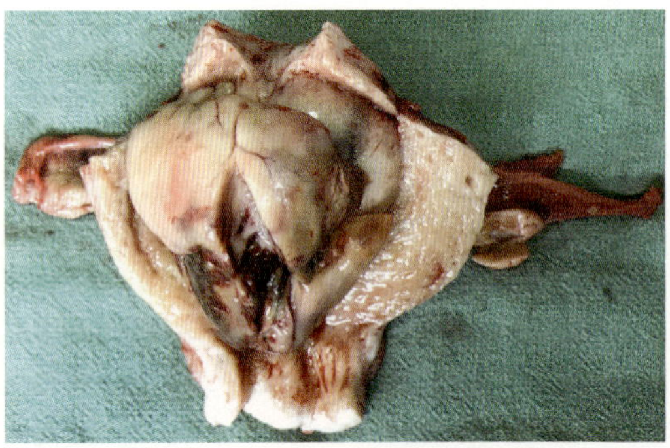

Figure 34.1 An adenocarcinoma of the endometrium. The growth forms a large tumour projecting into the cavity of the uterus.

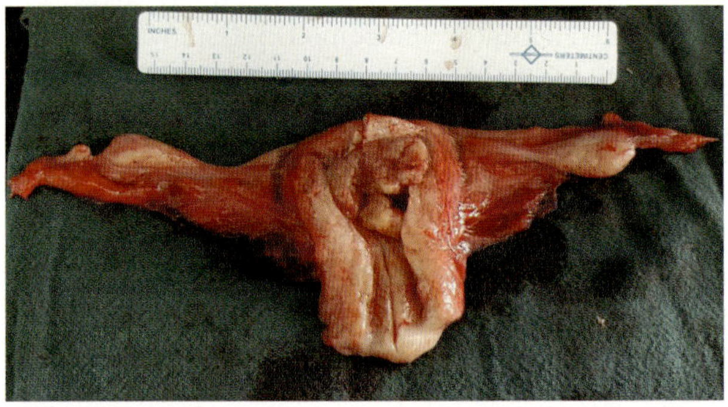

Figure 34.2 Stage II carcinoma of the endometrium. The muscle is deeply and extensively infiltrated, but has not yet reached the serosa.

PREDISPOSING FACTORS (Table 34.1)

Any factor that increases the exposure of endometrium to unopposed or high oestrogen level, either endogenous or exogenous, increases the risk of endometrial cancer. This is

---

To view the lecture notes scan the symbol or log in to your account on www.MedEnact.com

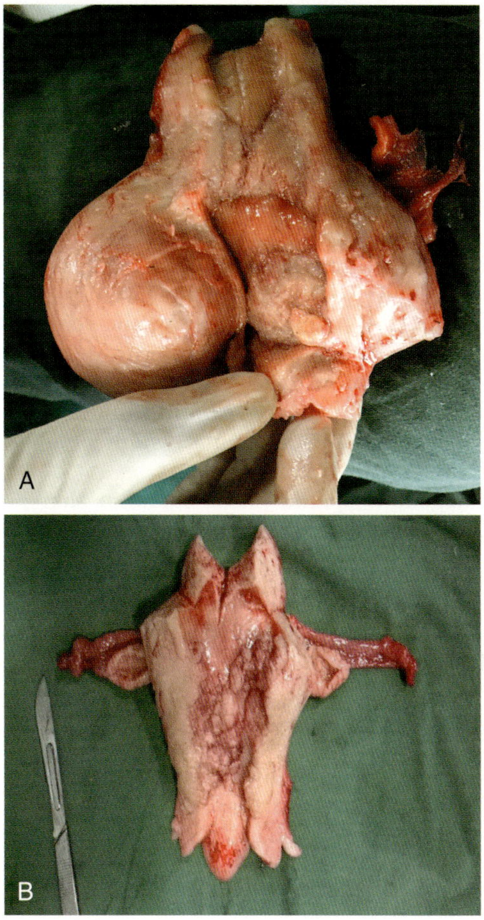

Figure 34.3 **(A)** and **(B)** Invasive cancer of endometrium – localized and diffuse varieties.

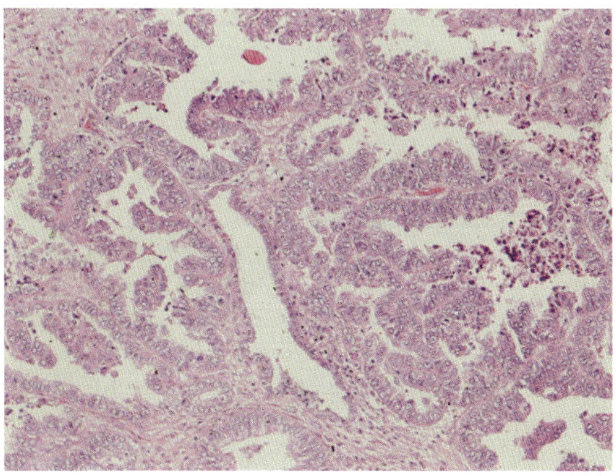

Figure 34.4 Well-differentiated endometrial adenocarcinoma (back-to-back glands with minimal intervening stroma and the gland-within-gland pattern). (*Courtesy*: Dr Sandeep Mathur, AIIMS)

also linked to dose and duration of exposure; the risk persists for 10 years after the hormone exposure. The endometrial cancer therefore is encountered in the following conditions:

- Unopposed and unsupervised administration of hormone replacement therapy after menopause predisposes the woman to endometrial hyperplasia and cancer.

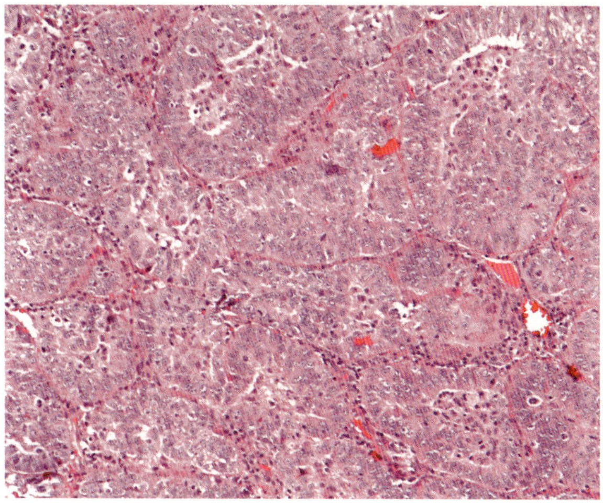

Figure 34.5 Endometroid adenocarcinoma Grade 3, Endometrium: Tumour cells arranged in glands as well as solid seeds, showing a marked nuclear pleomorphism and prominent nucleoli. (*Courtesy*: Dr Sandeep Mathur, AIIMS.)

  Fortunately, the malignancy is well-differentiated with good prognosis.
- Chronic anovulatory cycles as seen in PCOS.
- In some families, a strong familial predisposition is noticed. This may be due to genetic or dietetic habits such as animal protein and fat. The oestrone is derived by peripheral aromatization in the fat tissue from androstenedione and contributes to a high level of oestrogen. Women with the familial Lynch II syndrome suffering from anorectal and breast cancer are also likely to suffer from endometrial cancer.
- Tamoxifen given to women suffering from breast cancer increases the risk of endometrial hyperplasia and cancer to two- to threefold. Raloxifene has no adverse effect on the endometrium.

Table 34.1 Risk Factors for Endometrial Cancer

Risk Factor	Relative Risk
Long-term unopposed oestrogen	10–20
Lynch syndrome	6–20
Oestrogen-producing tumour	>5
Older age	2–3
Higher income and education	1.5–2
White race	2
Nulliparity	3
Menstrual irregularity	1.5
History of infertility	2–3
Late age at menopause	2–3
Early age at menarche	1.5–2
Tamoxifen	2–3
Obesity	2–5
History of type 2 diabetes mellitus (T2DM), hypertension (HTN) or thyroid disorder	1.3–3

- Obesity, hypertension and diabetes are seen in 30% of cases of endometrial cancer. Obesity reduces the level of serum sex hormone–binding protein and allows free oestrogen to circulate in the body. Moreover, a peripheral conversion of epi-androstenedione is aromatized to oestrone in the peripheral fat.
- Infertile women and women with polycystic ovarian syndrome on account of nonovulation have high oestrogen. These women have more chance of developing endometrial hyperplasia and endometrial cancer than normal women. The uterine fibroid is associated with endometrial cancer in 3% of cases after the age of 40 years.
- Feminizing ovarian tumour such as granulosa cell tumour or theca cell can have associated endometrial cancer in 15% of cases.
- Combined oral contraceptive pills have a protective effect and reduce its risk by 40%–50%; adding progestogens for 12 days each cycle to oestrogen in hormone replacement therapy (HRT) reduces its risks to 2%.

PATHOLOGY (FIG. 34.6)

Endometrial cancer may be localized or diffuse. It may appear as a nodule, polyp or diffuse lesion involving the entire uterine cavity. Histologically most endometrial cancers are adenocarcinomas and are called endometroid adenocarcinoma. About 10%–15% endometrial cancers can have other histological variants such as papillary serous, clear cell, adenosquamous or pure squamous variety.

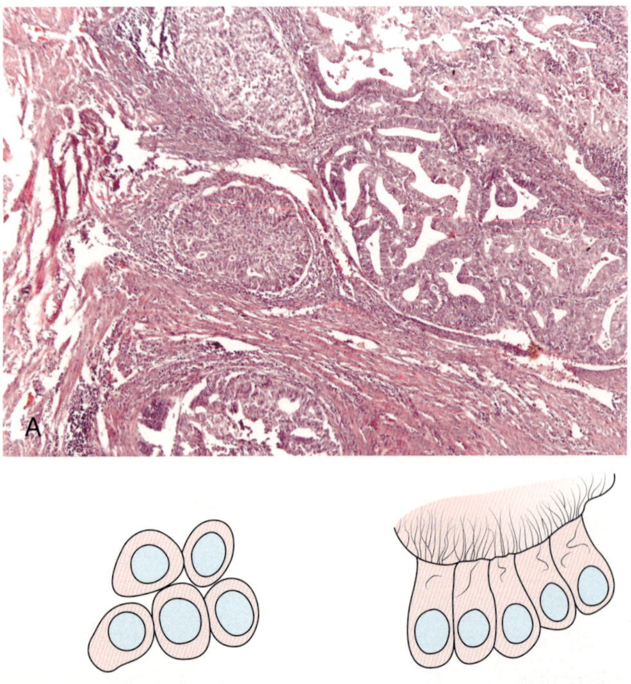

Figure 34.6 **(A)** Endometroid carcinoma: Malignant endometrial glands showing moderate nuclear atypia infiltrating the myometrium. **(B)** Normal endometrial and endocervical cells. (*Courtesy*: for (A) Dr Sandeep Mathur, AIIMS.)

MODES OF SPREAD

Endometrial carcinoma spreads by following routes:

1. **Direct extension to adjacent structures**: Most common mode of spread is by penetration of the myometrium and eventually the serosa of the uterus. The cervix, fallopian tubes and ultimately the vagina and parametrium may be invaded.
2. **A transtubal passage of exfoliated malignant cells** into adjoining ovary, pelvis and peritoneal cavity.
3. **Lymphatic dissemination**: Lymphatic channels pass directly from the fundus of the uterus to the para-aortic nodes. It can spread to the obturator nodes and other pelvic lymph nodes, if the growth is in the lower half of the uterus. Spread to inguinal lymph nodes can take place through the round ligament.
4. **Hematogenous spread**: Most common sites are lung, liver, brain and bone. Rarely, other sites can be involved.

Histologically, endometrial cancers are endometrioid adenocarcinoma in 75% of cases. The rest are clear cells, squamous and serous variety, which are more malignant than adenocarcinoma.

TUMOUR DIFFERENTIATION

The grading of these tumours is based on differentiation, glandular architecture and anaplasia of the cells. Adenoacanthoma is the least malignant (Figs 34.4–34.6). Necrosis in the tumour has an adverse effect on women's survival. This grading is part of International Federation of Gynaecology and Federation (FIGO) staging for endometrial cancer.

Grade 1: The glandular pattern is maintained, but cells show atypia.
Grade 2: Some glands show a papillary pattern and are solid.
Grade 3: The glands are solid with cellular proliferation, and glandular architecture is lost. The endometrium is packed with glands and little stroma.

TYPES OF ENDOMETRIAL CANCERS

There are two varieties of endometrial cancer.

Type I is oestrogen dependent and accounts for 90% of the cases. The source of oestrogen may be endogenous or exogenous. This type is mostly well-differentiated with good prognosis.

Type II is oestrogen independent and develops in atropic endometrium. This type is mostly undifferentiated with poor prognosis. P_{53} mutations are recognized in Type II tumours. Histologically, these tumours may be papillary serous or clear cell variety, metastasis occurs relatively early and tumour may metastatize to omentum, lymph node and other structures.

As mentioned earlier, oestrogen-stimulated endometrial cancers are well-differentiated, whereas cancers developing in atrophic endometrium in menopausal women are poorly differentiated.

CLINICAL FEATURES

Endometrial cancer may be asymptomatic in 7%–10% to begin with. The most common presentation of endometrial cancer is in the form of postmenopausal bleeding or discharge. It may manifest as menorrhagia or irregular periods in perimenopausal women. Past history of PCOS or HRT may be elicited. The woman may be obese, hypertensive or diabetic. Pain and lumps appear late in the advanced stages.

On per vaginal examination, the uterus may appear bulky or may be normal in size. The clinical features of a bulky uterus may not always be present. A bulky uterus is due to growth itself or due to associated fibroid or pyometra. An adnexal mass, if present, is often a feminizing tumour of ovary or a metastasis to the ovaries. In the advanced stage, the cervix is bulky and the os is patulous with the growth protruding through the os. Rarely a metastatic vaginal nodule is visible in the suburethal area. Discovering a lower genital tract lesion in a postmenopausal woman does not rule out endometrial cancer. Both may exist and investigations are required to rule out endometrial cancer.

INVESTIGATIONS

Various investigations confirm the diagnosis and assess its stage and extent of the disease, so that an appropriate and optimal treatment may be planned. Obtaining a sample of endometrial tissue for histopathology helps to confirm the diagnosis.

Unlike cancer of cervix, a cost-effective screening programme is not available for endometrial cancer. In high-risk cases a periodic transvaginal ultrasound combined with an endometrial tissue sampling may be used to pick up disease in an early stage.

- **Pap smear** is not a good method to pick up endometrial cancers as it is only 50% sensitive and not reliable. The presence of normal or abnormal endometrial cells in Pap smear increases the prevalence of premalignant uterine disease or endometrial carcinoma.
- **Endometrial aspiration** from the uterine cavity is effective in screening high-risk cases, and those on tamoxifen and HRT if presented with bleeding per vaginum. The aspiration is done with a Pipelle curette, Isaac aspirator, Vibra aspirator, Gravely jet wash and Novak curette as an OPD procedure (Fig. 34.7). A simple cost-effective method is to aspirate endometrial cavity with a fine 4-mm Karman's cannula attached to a disposable 20 mm syringe.
- **Fractional curettage** comprises obtaining endocervical scraping before dilating the cervix, followed by cervical dilatation and curettage from the whole endometrial cavity. Two specimens are examined separately for the presence of cancer. ***Hysteroscopy and biopsy.*** **On hysteroscopy,** one visualizes the entire uterine lining and obtains biopsy from suspicious areas; it reduces the chances of missing a lesion. Even then, this is not 100% predictive, as an early lesion ***can be missed.*** Some people have raised the concern regarding spilling of cancer cells into the peritoneal cavity during hysteroscopy.
- **Transvaginal sonography** is useful in studying the endometrial thickness before resorting to endometrial tissue sampling. Increased endometrial thickness, an irregular line and the presence of polyps are helpful in indicating the need for endometrial tissue sampling. Occasionally associated ovarian tumour or ovarian metastasis can be picked up. The extension to the endocervix can also be recognized. In a postmenopausal woman, the normal endometrium should not exceed 4 mm in thickness and this cut-off value is 10 mm in a perimenopausal woman. In a menopausal woman with vaginal bleeding, even an endometrial thickness of less than 4 mm has the risk of cancer and the entire endometrium should be subjected to a histopathology study (Fig. 34.8).
- **Doppler ultrasound** revealing a low resistance index of 0.37–0.7 or below is seen in endometrial malignant lesions.
- **Sonosalpingography.** In the absence of facility for hysteroscopy, sonosalpingography is useful in detecting endometrial polyp which could be malignant.
- **CA-125.** This tumour marker if raised above 35 IU/mL in a case of endometrial cancer suggests extrauterine spread of the disease.
- **Contrast-enhanced computed tomography (CECT)** has a predictable rate of 85% in studying the extent of the lesion spread. Hypodensity in the myometrium suggests myometrial infiltration. The pelvic and aortic nodes are defined if enlarged to more than 1 cm. CT is superior to MRI in detecting ascites, bowel and omental metastasis, but radiation exposure is the disadvantage.
- **MRI** is superior to CT in detecting myometrial involvement and nodal enlargement with a 90% detection rate and without a radiation hazard. Normally, between the endometrial and myometrial junction, a low-intensity zone exists and if this zone is intact, myometrial invasion can be ruled out, and the tumour is staged as Stage I. MRI is more expensive and time-consuming, but accurate

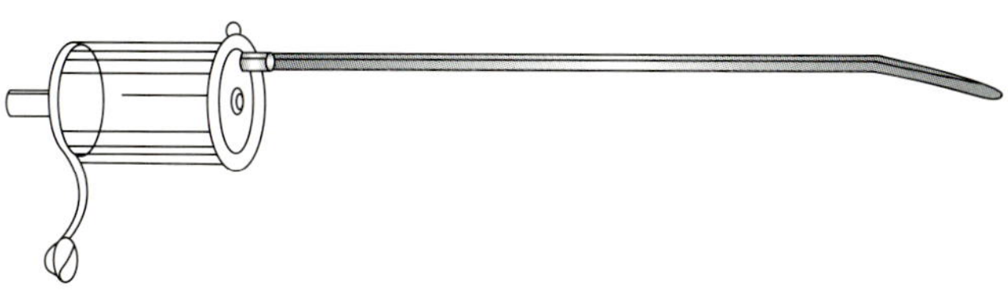

Figure 34.7 Vibra aspirator for suction curettage.

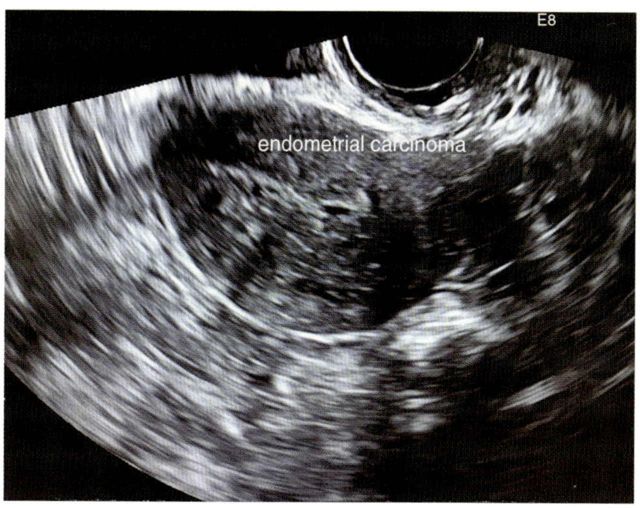

Figure 34.8 Transvaginal ultrasound showing heterogenous growth in the cavity with infiltration into the myometrium suggestive of carcinoma endometrium.

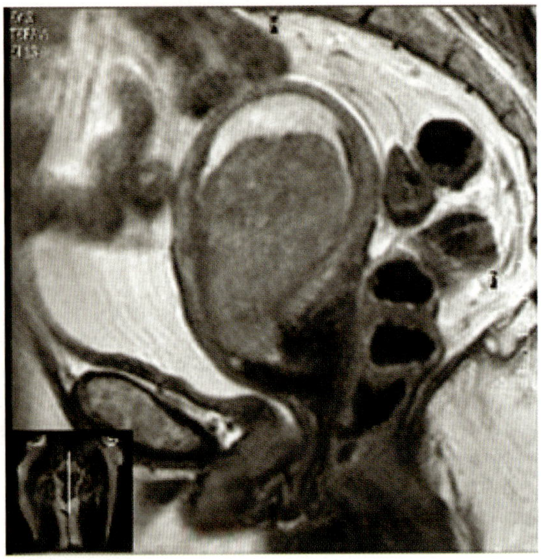

Figure 34.9 MRI showing extension of endometrial cancer into the cervix. (*Courtesy*: Dr Parveen Gulati, New Delhi.)

staging is possible in 80%–90% (sensitivity 72% and specificity 96%) (Fig. 34.9). MRI is also useful to know endocervical stromal invasion by the disease.

- **X-ray** of the chest is done as a routine to rule out lung metastasis. For bone and liver metastasis, radioisotope scanning is useful.
- **PET–CT can** reveal a metabolic activity in the tissue and lymph nodes. Although it is a gold standard for staging, but is not indicated as a routine preoperative investigation due to radiation hazards and limited availability of this facility.

DIFFERENTIAL DIAGNOSIS

Endometrial cancer can be mistaken for the following entities:

1. Senile endometritis
2. Tubercular endometritis
3. Atypical hyperplasia
4. Endometrial polyp

ENDOMETRIAL HYPERPLASIA

Endometrial hyperplasia appears to be a precursor to the development of endometrial carcinoma in Type I endometrial cancers. Presence of increased exogenous or endogenous oestrogen levels results in hyperplasia of endometrium. Longstanding hyperplasia can result in the development of endometrial cancer.

2014 REVISED WHO CLASSIFICATION OF ENDOMETRIAL HYPERPLASIA

New classification simply classified endometrial hyperplasia into the following two groups based on the presence or absence of cytological atypia:

(i) Hyperplasia without atypia
(ii) Atypical hyperplasia

The complexity of architecture is no longer part of the classification. The diagnosis of endometrial intraepithelial neoplasia (EIN) in the new WHO classification is considered interchangeable with atypical hyperplasia.

TREATMENT

Endometrial hyperplasia without atypia: Progesterone given both orally or as intrauterine (Levonorgestrel-releasing intrauterine system [LNG-IUS]-Mirena) is effective in achieving regression of endometrial hyperplasia without atypia. The **LNG-IUS should be the first-line medical treatment,** because compared with oral progestogens it has a higher disease regression rate with a more favourable bleeding profile and is associated with fewer adverse effects. Continuous progestogens should be used (medroxyprogesterone 10–20 mg/day or norethisterone 10–15 mg/day) for women who decline use of LNG-IUS. **Treatment** with oral progestogens or the LNG-IUS should be for a minimum of 6 months to induce histological regression of endometrial hyperplasia without atypia.

Atypical hyperplasia: Women with atypical hyperplasia have a substantial risk of developing endometrial carcinoma. It can be as high as 8%–29%; therefore, they should undergo a total hysterectomy to reduce the risk of developing malignancy. Rarely, in a young woman desirous of fertility atypical hyperplasia may be treated with high doses of progesterone with frequent evaluation of endometrial biopsy to rule out progression to cancer.

TREATMENT OF CARCINOMA OF THE ENDOMETRIUM

Almost all patients diagnosed to have endometrial carcinoma are initially treated by surgery except those with advanced disease or found unfit for surgery on account of associated medical conditions such as cerebrovascular accident (CVA), coronary artery disease or morbid obesity.

STAGING (FIGO STAGING 2009) (Table 34.2)

Surgical staging is now recommended, but clinical staging is applicable in inoperable cases. A staging laparotomy is recommended through a midline lower abdominal incision and any peritoneal ascitic fluid or washing is collected for cytology. The complete abdominal exploration followed by total abdominal hysterectomy (TAH) along with bilateral salpingo-oophorectomy (BSO), pelvic and para-aortic lymph node sampling remains the cornerstone in the management of early endometrial cancer.

TREATMENT

SURGERY

The main modality of treatment in carcinoma endometrium is surgery, if the patient is medically fit for surgery.

Surgical staging, abdominal hysterectomy, bilateral salpingo-oophorectomy, omentectomy and pelvic as well as para-aortic lymph node sampling remain the cornerstone in the management of early endometrial cancers.

1. Steps of surgery: The abdomen is opened by a vertical incision which allows a thorough intraabdominal exploration.

Table 34.2 Carcinoma of the Endometrium Staging (FIGO 2009)

Stage I[a]	Tumour confined to the corpus uteri
IA[a]	No or less than half myometrial invasion
IB[a]	Invasion equal to or more than half of the myometrium
Stage II[a]	Tumour invades cervical stoma, but does not extend beyond the uterus[b]
Stage III[a]	Local and/or regional spread of the tumour
IIIA[a]	Tumour invades the serosa of the corpus uteri and/or adnexae[c]
IIIB[a]	Vaginal and/or parametrial involvement[c]
IIIC[a]	Metastases to pelvic and/or para-aortic lymph nodes[c]
IIIC1[a]	Positive pelvic nodes
IIIC2[a]	Positive para-aortic lymph nodes with or without positive pelvic lymph nodes
Stage IV[a]	Tumour invades bladder and/or bowel mucosa, and/or distant metastases
IVA[a]	Tumour invasion of bladder and/or bowel mucosa
IVB[a]	Distant metastases, including intraabdominal metastases and/or inguinal lymph nodes

[a]Either G1, G2 or G3.
[b]Endocervical glandular involvement only should be considered as Stage I and no longer as Stage II.
[c]Positive cytology has to be reported separately without changing the stage.
Source: FIGO guidelines.

2. Peritoneal washings are obtained from subdiaphragmatic areas, paracolic gutters and the pelvis, and sent for cytology.
3. Hysterectomy and BSO,
4. Omentectomy only if the histopathology report suggestive of nonendometrioid variety.

After removal, the uterus is cut opened to look for tumour size, myometrial invasion and cervical extension are assessed. The frozen section is preferred. Lymph node sampling or lymphadenectomy is indicated, if tumour is more than 2 cm in size, it invades more than half the thickness of endometrium or the extension of the disease is up to endocervix and if the preoperative grading of the tumour was grade 2 or 3. All grades 2 and 3 in Stage I, clear cell, serous and adenosquamous cancers and myometrial invasion require pelvic lymphadenectomy and para-aortic lymph node sampling. There is no need to remove the vaginal cuff. However, omentectomy is advisable in the advanced stages.

Although for surgery an abdominal route is conventionally used, a vaginal route can be preferred in obe se diabetic women and women with prolapse because it results in lesser morbidity. This is combined with laparoscopic lymphadenectomy or postoperative radiotherapy. With increased experience in laparoscopic surgery, most cases of endometrial cancer can be managed by this technique. A robotic endoscopic surgery is gaining popularity as a method of surgical treatment.

POSTOPERATIVE RADIOTHERAPY

Application of postoperative radiotherapy depends on the surgicopathological findings and staging.

The commonest local metastasis occurs in the vaginal vault in 15% of cases. The incidence now has been reduced to 1%–2% by delivering radiation to the vaginal vault with the help of the colpostat 4 weeks after the surgery (brachytherapy). A dose of 6000–7000 cGy is delivered over a period of 6 weeks. Vaginal stenosis and dyspareunia are the complications.

Pelvic postoperative radiotherapy (external) in a dose of 6000 cGy over a 6-week period is also recommended in high-risk cases such as undifferentiated tumour, myometrial infiltration, pelvic node involvement and in serous, clear cell and adenosquamous carcinoma. The postoperative radiotherapy is required in Stages IA (Grade 3), IA2, IB and II. For stage III and IV, chemoradiation therapy yields a better effect.

Whole-abdomen radiation is required when para-aortic lymph nodes are involved, while protecting the liver and kidneys.

It is observed that women who receive pelvic radiotherapy often develop distal metastasis. Therefore, some advocate pelvic as well as abdominal radiotherapy to improve their survival.

The most important factors in considering the **need for postsurgical radiotherapy** are as follows:

(1) Histology
(2) Grading as studied by biopsy
(3) Depth of myometrial invasion as seen by ultrasound, MRI and at the time of surgery

PRIMARY RADIOTHERAPY

Stages III and IV are not operable. They are treated with brachytherapy followed by external radiation. The uterine cavity can be packed with Heyman capsules. Adjuvant chemotherapy and progestogen therapy prolong remission and improve quality of life. Hormonal therapy is nontoxic and does not need hospitalization.

PROGESTOGENS

- Medroxyprogesterone acetate (MDPA) 1 g weekly or 200 mg orally daily.
- 17-α progesterone or norethisterone 1 g i.m. weekly. Norethisterone is stronger than MDPA and suppresses oestrogen receptors. Thirty per cent response with hormone is reported, especially with lung metastasis. Tamoxifen 10 mg twice daily is also useful in reducing oestrogen receptors (for chemotherapy, refer to chapter 39).

Doxorubicin, platinum and taxane/carboplastin are under trial.

Stage-wise treatment of carcinoma of the endometrium	
Stage IA G1	Surgery only
G2, G3	Surgery + vaginal brachytherapy
Stage IB G1, G2	Surgery + vaginal brachytherapy
IB G3	Surgery + vaginal brachytherapy + external beam radiotherapy (RT) to pelvis
Stage II	Surgery + external RT + vaginal brachytherapy
Stage III	Surgery + external RT + brachytherapy+ chemotherapy
Stage IV	Palliative RT + chemotherapy + high-dose progesterone

RECURRENCE OF CARCINOMA OF THE ENDOMETRIUM

Recurrences are not common with the early stage disease (Stage IA, IB); however, recurrences may be seen with more advanced stage of the disease.

Most recurrences are observed in first 2 years; may occur as late as 5 years or longer.

SITES OF RECURRENCE

The most common site of recurrence is upper vagina. The metastasis occurs in the vaginal vault, lateral pelvic wall, lymph nodes, lungs, liver, brain and bones. Distal metastasis occurs mostly in women who have undergone surgery and postoperative pelvic radiotherapy.

Postoperative vaginal vault radiotherapy reduces the recurrence in the vaginal vault.

Recurrences are managed by palliative chemotherapy. There is a place for radiotherapy in case patient did not receive radiotherapy initially.

Prognosis: It depends on the histology of the tumour, grading, myometrial infiltration, pelvic node involvement and staging. Although a 5-year survival rate in Stage I is 75%, it reduces to 10%–20% in Stage IV. A survival rate of 55% in Stage II and 30% in Stage III has been reported.

Stage-wise 5-year survival rates in carcinoma endometrium	
Stage I	75%
Stage II	60%–70%
Stage III	25%
Stage IV	10%–20%

It is important that a woman who has been treated for uterine malignancy should not be offered HRT for menopausal symptoms.

PREVENTION OF ENDOMETRIAL CARCINOMA

- Adding progestogen for 12 days in HRT reduces the risk of endometrial hyperplasia and cancer to 2%.
- A woman on tamoxifen needs a periodical ultrasound scanning to study the endometrial thickness. Raloxifene has no adverse effect on the endometrium.
- Mirena IUCD is effective against simple endometrial hyperplasia.
- Oral combined pills reduce cancer risk by 40%–50%.
- Tibolone also reduces the risk.
- The complete treatment of PCOS avoids the risk.

SARCOMA OF THE UTERUS

Sarcomas arising from the body of the uterus are far less common than endometrial carcinoma. A sarcoma can arise either from myometrium or from stroma of endometrium. The uterus can be a site of rare types of sarcoma such as rhabdomyosarcoma, osteosarcoma, chondrosarcoma; the tissues which are normally not found in the uterus.

Uterine sarcomas are rare mesodermal tumours comprising 3%–7% of all malignant growths of the uterus and 1%–3% of all genital tract cancers. About 0.5% of all myomas undergo a sarcomatous change (Fig. 34.10). The tumours arise most frequently in women between the ages of 40 and 50 years, and are rare before 30 years. The incidence of premenopausal and postmenopausal sarcoma is almost equally divided. Twenty-five per cent of patients are nulliparous, but parity is unrelated in the aetiology. About 8% of sarcomas occur in women who received radiation for carcinoma cervix 8–10 years earlier.

Historically, uterine sarcomas have been classified into carcinosarcomas, accounting for 40% of cases, leiomyosarcomas (40%), endometrial stromal sarcomas (10%–15%) and undifferentiated sarcomas (5%–10%)

Leiomyosarcoma is the most common type, it is a spindle-celled tumour arising from a smooth muscle of myometrium. To the naked eye, the cut surface of the tumour is haemorrhagic and irregular, without the whorled appearance of a myoma. The consistency is friable and soft. The outline is irregular with invasion into the surrounding structures without a demonstrable capsule. The mucosal form sometimes tends to project in the form of a polyp into the cavity of the uterus, whereas in other cases it spreads around the cavity of the uterus to produce a uniform enlargement. Two-thirds of cases are intramural, one-fifth of cases are submucous and one-tenth of cases are subserously located.

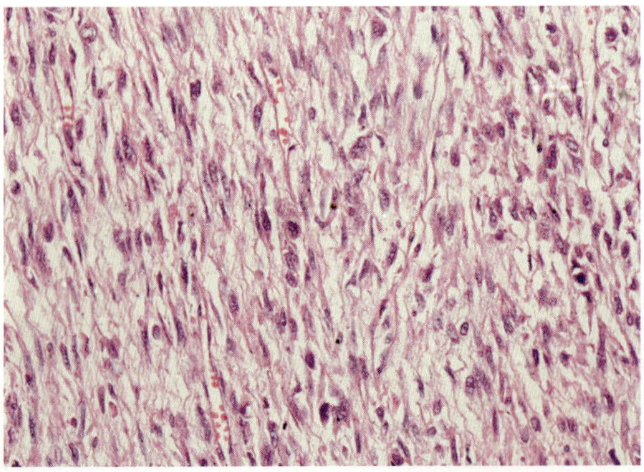

Figure 34.10 Histological picture of leiomyosarcoma (showing mitotic figures >10/HPF). (*Courtesy*: Dr Sandeep Mathur, AIIMS)

Metastasis occurs relatively early; the spread occurs by the bloodstream, by lymphatics, by direct spread and by an implantation. As a result of bloodstream dissemination, it can metastasize to lungs and kidneys and other organs. Lymphatic spread involves pelvic lymph nodes in 35% of cases in Stages I and II, and para-aortic glands in 15% of cases. Direct spread into the peritoneal cavity leads to multiple metastases over the peritoneum with accompanying ascites and large deposits in the omentum. Most patients have poor survival after the diagnosis of leiomyosarcoma is made, with an average duration of life of about 2 years from the commencement of symptoms.

In most cases, a diagnosis of a sarcoma comes to light on the basis of histopathology of a specimen of the uterus or myoma removed at myomectomy or hysterectomy. Failure to respond and shrink in size following GnRH administration in a case of fibroid should strongly suggest the possibility of malignancy. Positron emission tomography (PET), Doppler ultrasound and MRI may help in the diagnosis. With submucosal tumours which produce continuous bleeding, a histological examination of curettings may enable a diagnosis to be made. Again, a rapid enlargement of a quiescent myoma in a woman of postmenopausal age is almost pathognomonic of a sarcomatous change. A sarcoma of the uterus usually causes a rapid enlargement of the uterus with profuse and irregular vaginal bleeding. Pain is present in 60% of cases and fever due to degeneration or infection may also occur in about one-third of the patients. If the tumour has encroached upon the cavity of the uterus and caused postmenopausal bleeding, diagnosis may be made by curettage. The interpretation of the histology is very difficult because of the presence of degenerative and infective changes. However, a mitotic count more than 10 per 10 high-powered fields and an atypical cell would suggest a diagnosis of leiomyosarcoma.

Staging of leiomyosarcoma

Stage	Description
Stage I	Tumour limited to the uterus
IA	<5 cm
IB	>5 cm
Stage II	Tumour extends to the pelvis
IIA	Adnexal involvement
IIB	Tumour extends to extrauterine pelvic tissue
Stage III	Tumour invades abdominal tissues (not just protruding into the abdomen)
IIIA	One site
IIIB	More than one site
IIIC	Metastasis to pelvic and/or para-aortic lymph nodes
Stage IV	
IVA	Tumour invades bladder and/or rectum
IVB	Distant metastasis

TREATMENT

The treatment of a sarcoma of the uterus consists of **total hysterectomy with bilateral salpingo-oophorectomy**, followed by a full course of radiation therapy. If the growth is in the region of the isthmus or cervix, a radical hysterectomy of the Wertheim type with a bilateral lymph node excision probably offers the best chance of cure, because in many cases the glands may be involved. This is followed by radiation therapy. The 5-year cure rate is under 30% and largely depends on the type of growth, being the worst in the round cell variety where the growth originates in the endometrium. Metastasis such as lung, liver or brain metastasis is a contraindication to surgery.

Radiotherapy is ineffective in distal metastasis. Chemotherapy is the only hope and comprises a combination of cyclophosphamide, vincristine, doxorubicin and dacarbazine or vincristine, actinomycin and cyclophosphamide (VAC). It reduces the recurrence rate. The conservation of ovaries does not adversely influence the prognosis, and it is a wise decision to leave them behind during hysterectomy in a young woman. Breast cancer is seen associated with leiomyosarcoma, so it is prudent to screen the woman's breasts.

Rhabdomyosarcoma is a rare, highly malignant tumour in children. It is now managed by chemoradiotherapy. The prognosis is poor with a 5-year survival rate of 40%. A 50% response is reported with docetaxel and gemcitabine. Progestogen and aromatase inhibitor hold future promise.

MALIGNANT MIXED MULLERIAN TUMOURS

These uncommon tumours of the uterus comprise elements of mesodermal and ectodermal origin. In the past, these tumours were commonly named as carcinosarcomas; however, now a preferred term is malignant mixed Mullerian tumours (MMMT). Although the uterus is a common site for these tumours; however, these can be seen in vagina, cervix or ovaries.

MESODERMAL MIXED TUMOUR (INCLUDING BOTRYOID AND GRAPE-LIKE SARCOMA)

Uterine sarcoma arises typically in the body of the uterus, whereas a sarcoma of the cervix is very rare. Eight per cent of cases follow pelvic radiotherapy. Pathologically, the tumours should be regarded as mesodermal mixed tumours as they often contain cartilage, striated muscle fibres, glands and fat. The stroma is embryonic in type, similar to the embryonal mesenchyme. A grape-like sarcoma of the cervix arises typically in adult women, metastases develop rapidly and local recurrence follows their removal.

Somewhat similar tumours are known to develop in the vagina in children at a very early age, and such tumours contain striated muscle fibres and an embryonic stroma. Rather similar tumours sometimes develop in the body of the uterus in old women, and in this way three types of mixed tumours, namely the vaginal tumours of children, the grape-like sarcoma of the cervix and the mixed tumours of the body of the uterus of old women can be distinguished. In all cases, the prognosis is bad and a rapid recurrence follows their removal.

ENDOMETRIAL STROMAL TUMOURS

Sarcomas can arise rarely from the stroma of endometrium. These stromal tumours have a variable course and have been classified as follows:

1. Stromal nodules/stromal hyperplasia
2. Low-grade stromal sarcomas
3. High-grade stromal sarcomas

In most cases, diagnosis is made on the basis of histology of hysterectomy specimen conducted for irregular, abnormal uterine bleeding. Sometimes diagnosis can be suspected on the basis of D&C material submitted for histopathology in a case of abnormal uterine bleeding (AUB). Although a low-grade stromal sarcoma does not require any adjuvant treatment, patients with a high-grade stromal sarcoma require radiotherapy and chemotherapy as an adjuvant treatment. A high-grade stromal sarcoma is associated with poor prognosis.

Staging of endometrial stromal tumours (FIGO 2009)

Stage I	Tumour limited to the uterus
IA	Tumour limited to endometrium/endocervix with no myometrial invasion
IB	Less than or equal to half myometrial invasion
IC	More than half myometrial invasion
Stage II	Tumour extends to the pelvis
IIA	Adnexal involvement
IIB	Tumour extends to extrauterine pelvic tissue
Stage III	Tumour invades abdominal tissues (not just protruding into the abdomen)
IIIA	One site
IIIB	More than one site
IIIC	Metastasis to pelvic and/or para-aortic lymph nodes
Stage IV	
IVA	Tumour invades bladder and/or rectum
IVB	Distant metastasis

KEY POINTS

- Endometrial cancers account for 20%–25% of all genital tract cancers. In rich countries, this is the most common genital tract cancer, whereas in India it ranks third after cancer of cervix and cancer of ovary.
- The risk factors are elderly age, unopposed oestrogen therapy, tamoxifen, obesity and hypertension, diabetes as well as chronic anovulation seen in PCOS.
- Although simple endometrial hyperplasia leads to endometrial cancer in 2% of cases, atypical hyperplasia leads to endometrial cancer in 8%–29% of cases.
- Early stage of endometrial cancer is treated by hysterectomy, bilateral salpingo-oophorectomy. Lymphadenectomy is required in case of deep myometrial infiltration, endocervical involvement, poorly differentiated tumours.
- CT, MRI are helpful in mapping the myometrial invasion and lymph node involvement.
- Surgery is the primary mode of treatment. Postoperative radiotherapy is required in the advanced stages, and for reducing the recurrence in the vaginal vault.
- Progestogen and Mirena can prevent endometrial hyperplasia. Progestogens are effective in 30% of cases with lung metastasis.
- Sarcomas are rare tumours arising from the body of the uterus. They can be leiomyosarcoma, endodermal stromal sarcomas, malignant mixed Mullerian tumours or rarely rhabdomyosarcoma, osteosarcoma, chondrosarcomas. In most cases, diagnosis comes to light on the basis of histopathology on a hysterectomy specimen.

SELF-ASSESSMENT

1. Describe the clinical features of endometrial cancer. How will you investigate the case?
2. What are the high-risk cases for endometrial cancer?
3. Discuss the management of endometrial cancer.
4. Write short notes on:
   - Endometrial hyperplasia
   - Mixed mesodermal tumours
   - Sarcoma of the uterus

SUGGESTED READING

Berek and Novak's Textbook of Gynaecology, Adashi EY, Hillard PA (eds). Novak's Gynecology. 15th ed. Philadelphia, PA: Williams & Wilkins, 2014.

Duncan J, Shulman P. Yearbook of Obstetrics, Gynaecology and Women's Health 41: 437, 2010.

Studd J. Progress in Obstetrics and Gynaecology 14: 2000.

Studd J. Progress in Obstetrics and Gynaecology 7: 1989.

Studd J. Progress in Obstetrics and Gynaecology 16: 343, 2005.

Pathology of Ovarian Tumours and Benign Ovarian Tumours

35

CHAPTER OUTLINE

PATHOLOGY OF OVARIAN TUMOURS

Ovaries can be the site of a variety of benign and malignant tumours. These tumours can be cystic or solid, often a combination of the two. They can vary in size from as small as 3–5 cm to as big as equal to a full-term pregnant uterus. They can be seen in any age group starting from prepubertal to adolescent during reproductive life and postmenopausal age group. Malignant tumours can develop in any age group. Ovaries are the site of three common types of tumours: (i) epithelial tumours: those which arise from surface lining of ovaries; (ii) germ cell tumours: those which arise from germ cells within ovaries; and (iii) sex cord stromal tumours: those which arise from sex cords present in ovaries.

Ovarian tumour is not a single entity, but a complex wide spectrum of neoplasms involving a variety of histological tissues ranging from epithelial tissues, connective tissues and specialized hormone-secreting cells to germinal and embryonal cells. The most common are epithelial tumours forming 80% of all tumours. Eighty per cent are benign tumours and 20% are malignant. Of all the malignant tumours, 90% are epithelial in origin, 80% are primary in the ovary and 20% secondary from breasts, gastrointestinal tract and colon. Benign tumours can become secondarily malignant. Mucinous cyst becomes malignant in 5%–9% but papillary cyst adenoma becomes malignant in 30%–50% if left untreated.

Unfortunately, patients with ovarian tumours are often symptom-free for a long time, and the signs are often nonspecific. By the time diagnosis of ovarian malignancy is established, about two-thirds of these are already far advanced and the prognosis in such cases is unfavourable.

An ovarian tumour in adolescent and postmenopausal women is more often malignant. Most germ cell tumours occur in young girls younger than 25 years of age.

PATHOLOGY

In an attempt to standardize the nomenclature used in describing the diverse varieties of ovarian tumours, the World Health Organization (WHO) devised a classification listing nine major groups for benign and malignant tumours (Table 35.1).

Epithelial ovarian neoplasms arise from the mesoepithelial cells on the ovarian surface. Epithelial cancers constitute about 80% of all ovarian cancers. The most common histological type is the papillary serous cystadenomas and carcinomas accounting for almost 50% of all epithelial tumours. Mucinous tumours account for 12%–15% of the cases, clear cell and endometrioid combined about 10% of the cases, and the unspecified types 25%–27% of the cases. If the lining of tumours resembles the lining of epithelial tumours of fallopian tubes, they are labelled as serous tumours; if the lining of epithelium resembles endocervical epithelium, they are labelled as mucinous tumours; if the lining of epithelium resembles endometrium, they are labelled as endometrioid tumours; and if the lining of epithelium resembles bladder epithelium, they are called clear cell variety.

The degree of cellular differentiation of the epithelial ovarian neoplasm expressed as histological grade has an important significance in prognosis as well as in identifying malignancy.

The criteria of grading used include mitotic count, stratification, cellular pleomorphism, nuclear atypism and proportion of solid areas within the tumour.

Grade '0' tumours, also known as borderline malignancies or tumours of low malignant potential (LMP), may demonstrate papillary tufting, stratification, epithelial atypia, exfoliation of cellular clusters and minimal mitotic activity, but no stromal invasion. The 5-year survival of patients with Stage I Grade '0' tumours is more than 90%

Table 35.1 WHO Classification of Ovarian Tumours (Major Groups)

I. Common epithelial tumours: • Serous tumours • Mucinous tumours • Endometrioid tumours • Clear cell (mesonephroid tumours) • Brenner tumours • Mixed epithelial tumours • Undifferentiated carcinoma • Unclassified epithelial tumours
II. Sex cord (gonadal stromal) tumours: • Granulosa stromal cell tumours, theca cell tumours • Androblastomas: Sertoli–Leydig cell tumours • Gynandroblastomas • Unclassified
III. Lipid (lipoid) cell tumours
IV. Germ cell tumours: • Dysgerminoma • Endodermal sinus tumour • Embryonal carcinoma • Polyembryoma • Choriocarcinoma • Teratoma • Mixed forms
V. Gonadoblastoma: • Pure • Mixed with dysgerminoma or other germ cell tumours
VI. Soft-tissue tumours not specific to ovary
VII. Unclassified tumours
VIII. Secondary (metastatic) tumours
IX. Tumour-like conditions

compared to 54% survival for patients with Stage I Grade 3 serous cystadenocarcinomas.

Besides histological tumour grading, flow cytometry analysis of tumour DNA content provides another method of assessing tumour differentiation and prognosis.

TUMOURS OF THE SURFACE EPITHELIUM

SEROUS CYSTADENOMA AND CYSTADENOCARCINOMA

Serous cystadenoma and cystadenocarcinoma are amongst the most common of cystic ovarian neoplasms, accounting for about 50% of all ovarian tumours; of these, 60%–70% are benign, 15% borderline and 20%–25% are malignant.

Serous cystadenomas occur in the third, fourth and fifth decades of life; malignant cystadenocarcinomas tend to occur more frequently with advancing age; however, no age is barred. In about half of the cases, they are bilateral.

Delicate papillary excrescences may be seen on the surface and within the loculi in a benign cyst. In case of serous cystadenocarcinoma, coarse papillary growths spread to the peritoneal surfaces. The papillae are friable unlike their benign counterparts. Histologically, the benign variety shows cystic spaces, and the lining of the tumour consists of tall columnar ciliated epithelium resembling the endosalpinx. The loculi contain a serous straw-coloured fluid, which may be blood stained when malignant transformation occurs. Unless cellular atypia exceeds four-cell-layer thickness or stromal invasion occurs, the tumour is classified as borderline or benign (Fig. 35.1).

MUCINOUS TUMOURS

Mucinous tumours are multiloculated cysts lined by epithelium resembling the endocervix (Figs 35.2 and 35.3). Formerly, they were referred to as pseudomucinous cysts, as their contents are not chemically true mucin. The cut surface shows multiloculi and honeycomb appearance. The tumours are not infrequent, can grow to a large size and often weigh as much as 5–10 kg; they are often pedunculated. These may be combined with a dermoid cyst or a Brenner tumour (Fig. 35.4). They are usually unilateral; only 5%–10% are bilateral. The tumours are mostly benign; only 5%–10% become malignant and 10%–15% are of LMP. Bilateral tumours are often metastatic from the gastrointestinal tract, mainly mucocele of appendix or primary adenocarcinoma of appendix or stomach.

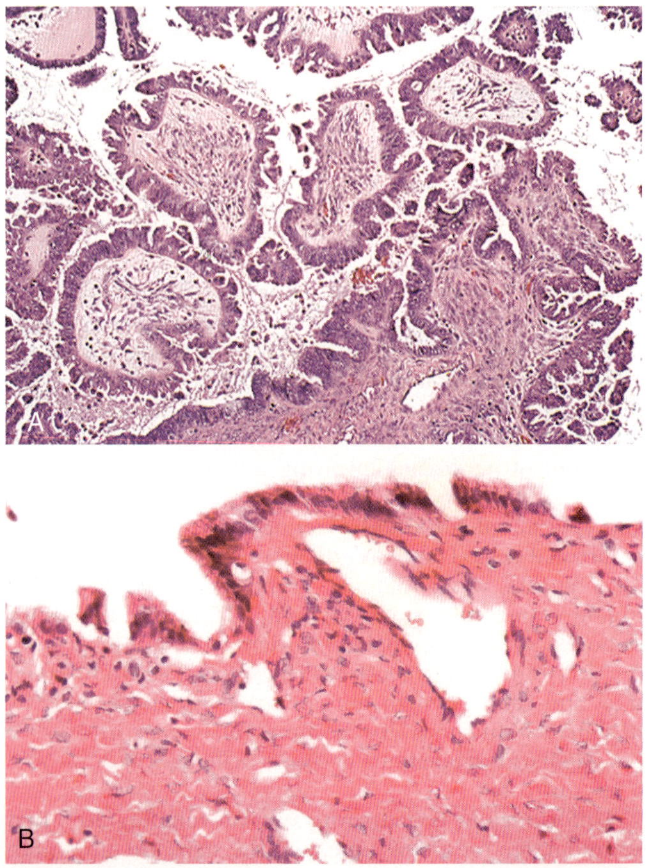

Figure 35.1 (A) A papillary form of serous cystadenoma of the ovary. The epithelium, though hyperplastic, is undoubtedly benign (×60). **(B)** High-power serous cystadenoma. (*Source:* for (A) Rao KA: Textbook of Gynaecology. India: Elsevier, 2008. *Courtesy* (B): Dr Sandeep Mathur.)

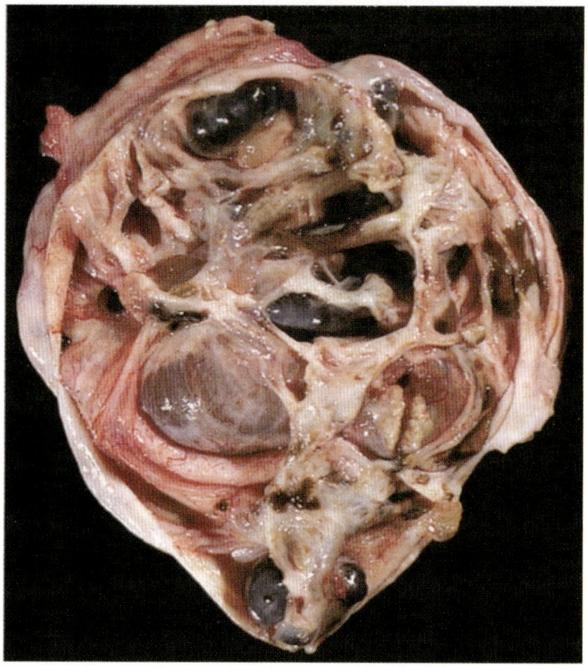

Figure 35.2 Mucinous tumour.

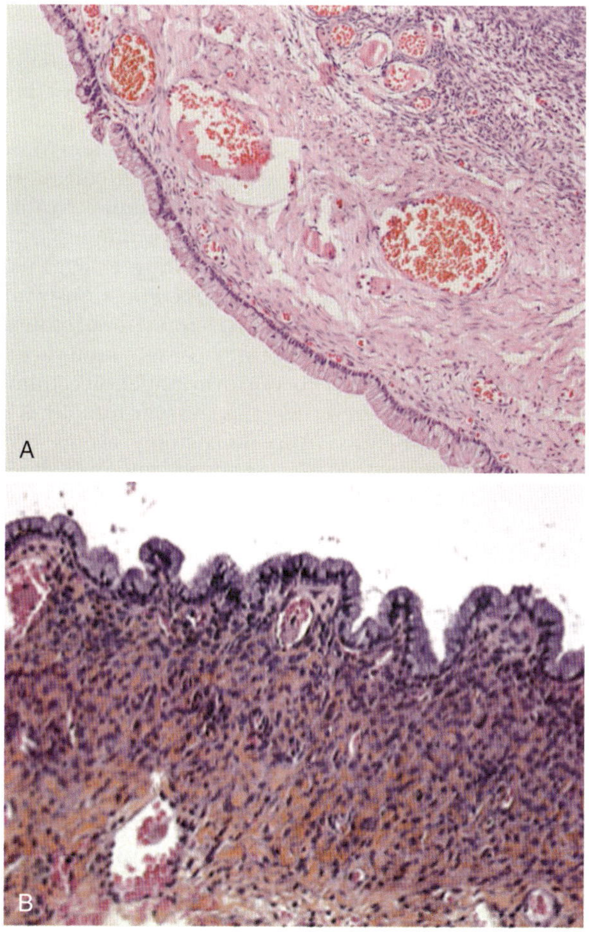

Figure 35.3 **(A)** Mucinous cystadenoma. **(B)** Mucinous cystadenoma. High power shows cells resembling endocervix. (*Courtsey:* Dr Sandeep Mathur)

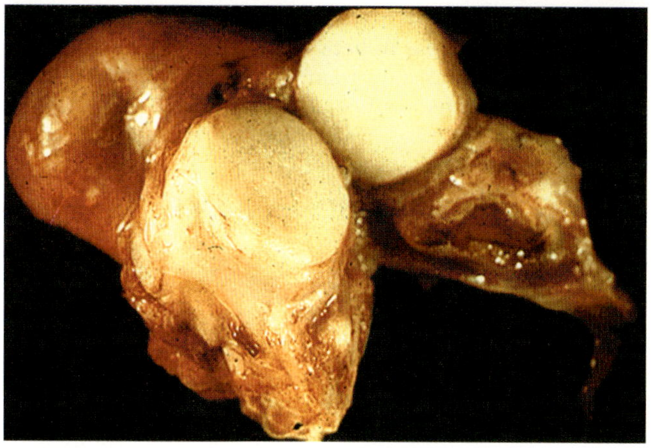

Figure 35.4 A combined Brenner tumour (solid area) and multilocular mucinous cystadenoma.

Mucinous tumours occur in women between 30 and 60 years. They have a glistening surface, and the cut section reveals loculi filled with mucinous contents (Fig. 35.5). If the tumour ruptures, it may lead to formation of pseudomyxoma peritonei and the viscera show extensive adhesions. Appendicectomy at the time of primary surgery prevents pseudomyxoma peritonei, as often mucocele of appendix is known to cause this complication.

ENDOMETRIOID TUMOUR

Endometrioid tumours are mostly malignant and account for about 20% of all ovarian cancers. They are lined by a glandular epithelium resembling the endometrium.

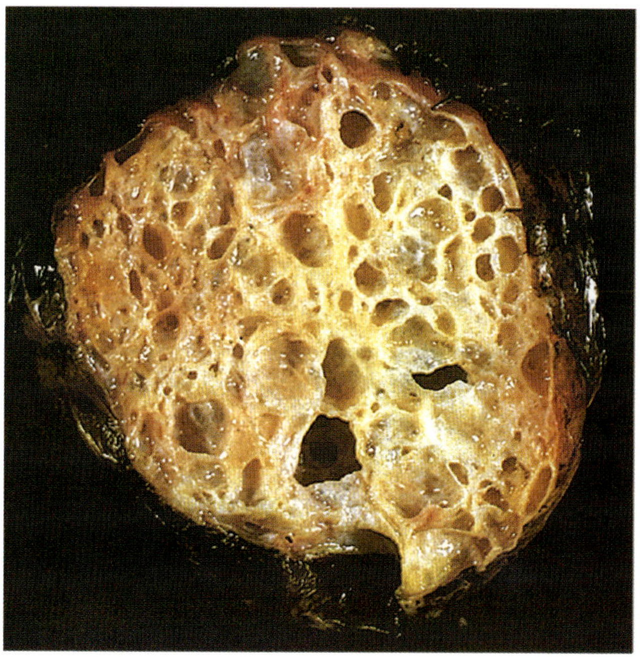

Figure 35.5 A mucinous cystadenoma with its multicystic appearance and delicate septa. (*Source*: The Female Genital System and Breast. Robbins Basic Pathology, Elsevier, 2007)

The tumours are of moderate size, and are essentially solid, with cystic areas in between filled with haemorrhagic fluid. In 15% of cases, ovarian endometriosis may coexist. They are associated with endometrial cancer in 20% of cases.

CLEAR CELL (MESONEPHROID) TUMOUR

Mesonephroid tumour, also called clear cell carcinoma, is an uncommon tumour of the ovary. It is composed of large cuboidal epithelial cells with abundant clear cytoplasm characteristically forming tubules, glands and small cystic spaces lined by clear cells showing large, dark nuclei protruding into the lumen (hobnail cells). The tumour is highly malignant.

BRENNER TUMOUR

Brenner tumour is an uncommon solid fibroepithelial tumour accounting for about 1%–2% of all ovarian neoplasms. On gross appearance, it resembles a fibroma of the ovary (Fig. 35.4); its cut surface appears gritty and yellowish grey. It is generally unilateral, small to moderate in size, mostly benign and has no endocrine function. Brenner tumour can occasionally be malignant.

The tumour is generally seen in women around menopause, and causes postmenopausal bleeding. Occasionally, it may be associated with ascites and hydrothorax (pseudo-Meigs syndrome). In rare cases, it becomes malignant.

Histologically, the tumour shows a background of fibrous tissue – interspersed within it are nests of transitional epithelium (Walthard cell rests). These cells demonstrate a longitudinal groove resembling puffed wheat. As mentioned earlier, this tumour may be combined with a mucinous adenoma of the ovary.

SPREAD OF EPITHELIAL TUMOURS OF THE OVARY

When these tumours become malignant and extend through the capsule, they may be seeded on to the peritoneal surface, omentum and intestinal viscera and by transcoelomic spread reach the subdiaphragmatic space. The ascitic fluid is often blood-stained and shows the presence of clusters of tumour cells. The tumour cells may spread to the para-aortic lymph nodes, and metastasize to the liver, lungs, gastrointestinal tract and other areas. In over half of the cases, the opposite ovary is also involved.

BORDERLINE OVARIAN TUMOURS

Borderline ovarian tumours or ovarian epithelial tumours of LMP were first described by Taylor in 1929. There is a broad agreement that a category of borderline tumour exists. Histologically, these tumours are intermediate between truly benign neoplasms and those with invasive characteristics. Clinically these tumours tend to have LMP.

They are prevalent in 2.5/10,000 women and account for 10%–20% of all epithelial tumours. No matter how malignant the epithelial cells appear, unless they invade the stroma or are at least four cells high in the mucinous tumour, they must be classified as of LMP. Mitotic figures should be less than 4 per 10 high-power fields.

CHARACTERISTICS OF BORDERLINE OVARIAN TUMOURS

- Patients have a high survival rate of 90%.
- Tumours run a typical indolent course. It may however progress to malignancy in 10-15% cases.
- Spontaneous regression of peritoneal implants is known to occur.
- Diagnosis must be based exclusively on the histological examination of the ovarian tumour.
- Multiple sections must be examined to exclude invasion.

Nonepithelial tumours (germ cell and gonadal stroma) do not lend themselves to a diagnosis of LMP tumour. Borderline malignant tumours occur in younger women (35–55 years), 10 years younger than their malignant counterparts.

RISK FACTORS

Low parity, infertility and failure to lactate increase the risk of developing these tumours. Unopposed oestrogen and obesity are also likely risks. Smokers are prone to LMP tumours. Induction of ovulation may also be a risk factor. Oral combined pills do not provide any protection against development of a borderline ovarian tumour.

PATHOLOGY

Borderline ovarian tumours are mainly serous (endosalpinx and endocervical type) and mucinous, the former being more common than the latter.

The clinical features are similar to those of benign ovarian tumours, so also are the investigations. The diagnosis is entirely dependent on several sections studied histologically; frozen section is necessary in young women.

Management is individualized according to age, parity and desire to conserve the fertility function. Conservative surgery in the form of ovarian cystectomy, ovariotomy or salpingo-oophorectomy is performed. In mucinous borderline tumour, it is prudent to perform appendicectomy as well, because many believe that this ovarian tumour is secondary to the appendix. Appendicectomy avoids occurrence of pseudomyxoma peritonei. No adjuvant chemotherapy or radiotherapy is necessary, but follow-up is mandatory, as recurrence of 10%–30% is reported. Routine lymphadenectomy is also not required.

GERM CELL TUMOURS

Germ cell tumours are usually seen in young adolescent girls before the age of 25 years. They account for 15%–20% of all ovarian tumours. The majority of tumours (about 95%) are benign cystic teratomas, also called dermoids. Below the age of 20 years, 60% of the tumours are of the germ cell origin, and in girls younger than 10 years, almost 85% belong to this group and are invariably malignant.

DYSGERMINOMA

Dysgerminoma corresponds to the seminoma of the testis and accounts for 3%–5% of all ovarian tumours. It usually

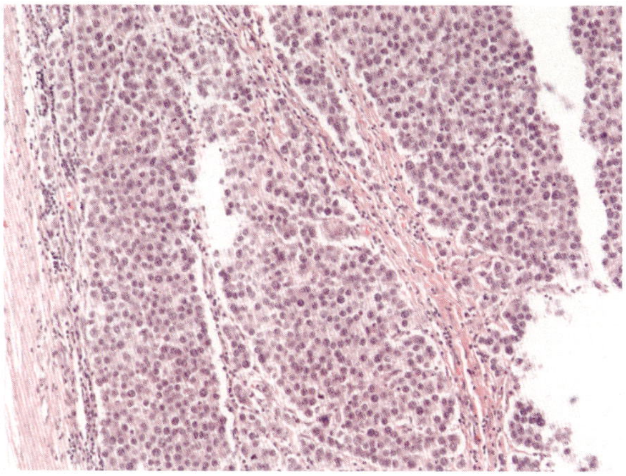

Figure 35.6 Ovarian dysgerminoma. (*Courtesy:* Dr Sandeep Mathur, AIIMS.)

arises in young girls or in children, with an average age of 20 years. The tumour tends to be solid with a peculiar elastic rubbery consistency and a smooth, firm capsule. The cut surface is yellow or grey with areas of degeneration and haemorrhage. The size is variable, usually moderate usually moderate (10-15cm), although large tumours have been described. It is usually unilateral, bilateral in 10% of cases, occasionally undergoes torsion and may, like all solid tumours, be associated with ascites. The tumour consists of large cells arranged in bunches or alveoli. Lymphocytes and giant cells are always found amongst the tumour cells. This appearance of large dark-staining nuclei with clear, almost translucent, cytoplasm and lymphocytic infiltration of the fibrous septa is diagnostic (Fig. 35.6). The tumour is neutral and does not secrete either male or female sex hormones but secretes placental alkaline phosphatase (PLAP), lactate dehydrogenase (LDH) and β-human chorionic gonadotropin (hCG). A number of patients with a dysgerminoma of the ovary have been reported to show genital abnormality, with hypoplasia or absence of some part of the genital tract. It has been reported in pseudohermaphrodites. Such congenital abnormalities are not caused by the dysgerminoma and its removal has no beneficial effect on them. The malignancy rate is 30%–50% and depends largely on the findings at laparotomy:

- A unilateral tumour confined to one ovary may behave in relatively benign manner.
- Extra capsular spread of disease indicates poor prognosis.
- The presence of extrapelvic metastases in the general peritoneal cavity, lymph glands or omentum indicates advanced disease. Conservative surgery is recommended as most patients are young girls. Though highly radiosensitive, ovarian destruction contraindicates the use of radiotherapy in young girls. Postoperative chemotherapy yields 90% success. Chemotherapy comprises:
- Injection bleomycin 15 mg i.v. or i.m. weekly for 12 weeks
- Injection etoposide 100 mg/m^2 1–5 days every 3 weeks
- Injection cisplatin 20 mg/m^2 1–5 days every 3 weeks

Alternate chemotherapy regimen are as follows:

- Vincristine, adriamycin and cyclophosphamides (VAC) for 12 cycles cure 86% in Stage I disease.
- Vincristine, bleomycin and cisplatin (VBP) are also effective.
- Carboplatin and ifosfamide combination is better and less toxic than cisplatin.
- Radiotherapy is employed only for residual and recurrent tumours.

TERATOMA

Germ cell tumours that show differentiation along embryonic rather than extraembryonic pathways are grouped together as teratomas, and divided into three categories: (i) mature (benign), e.g. dermoid cyst; (ii) immature (essentially malignant), e.g. solid teratoma; and (iii) monodermal or highly specialized, e.g. struma ovarii.

DERMOID CYSTS (BENIGN CYSTIC TERATOMA)

Of all cystic tumours of the ovary, 5%–10% are dermoids. A dermoid cyst is usually unilocular with smooth surface, seldom attaining more than 15 cm in diameter. It contains sebaceous material and hair, and the wall is lined in part by squamous epithelium which contains hair follicles and sebaceous glands. Teeth, bone, cartilage, thyroid tissue and bronchial mucous membrane are often found in the wall (Fig. 35.7). Sometimes, the sebaceous material collects together in the form of small balls, and as many as 1000 sebaceous balls have been recovered in a dermoid cyst. The inner surface is called a 'focus' or 'embryonic node' from which the hair project and in which the teeth and bone are usually found. The nomenclature 'dermoid cyst' is inaccurate, for in addition to ectodermal tissues, tissues from both the mesoderm and the endoderm are also seen in some part of the tumour. Moreover, although squamous epithelium usually lines the cyst, columnar and transitional types are also found. It is extremely rare for pancreas, liver tissue and intestinal mucous membrane to be present in the wall of a dermoid cyst (Figs 35.8 and 35.9).

Dermoid cysts frequently arise in association with mucinous cystadenomas to form a combined tumour, part of which consists of a dermoid cyst whereas the rest has

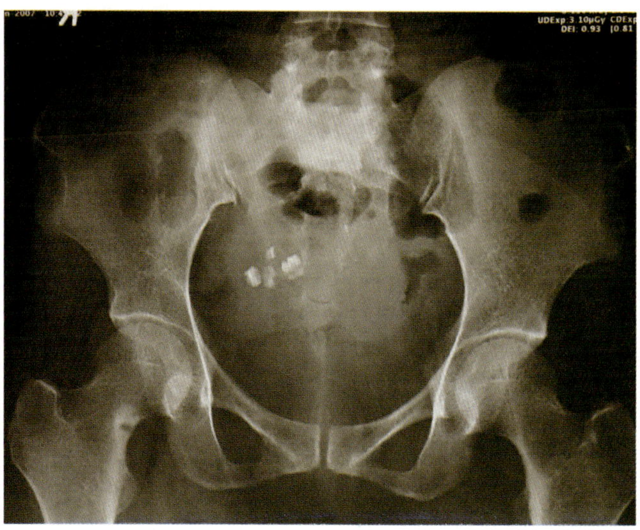

Figure 35.7 Dermoid cyst showing a tooth. (*Courtesy*: Dr KK Saxena, New Delhi.)

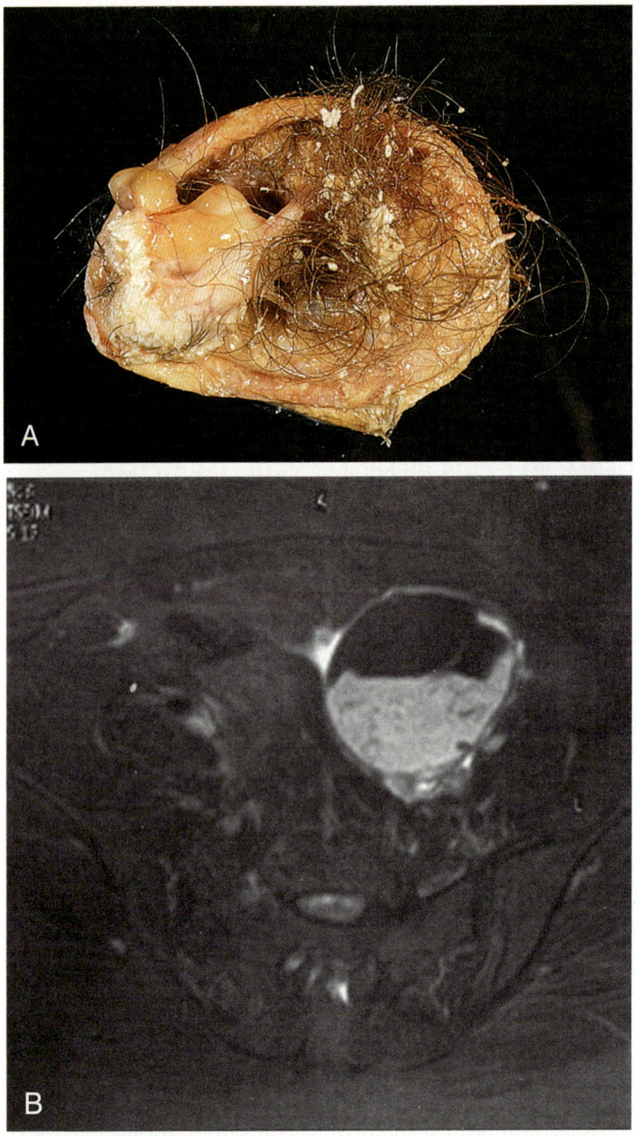

Figure 35.8 **(A)** Gross appearance of a cut-open dermoid cyst. Note the presence of hair-bearing skin. **(B)** MRI showing a dermoid cyst. **(C)** Tooth-like calcifications seen in the right hemipelvis suggestive of dermoids. (*Source* **(A)**: Hacker NF, Gambone JC, Hobel CJ: Hacker and Moore's Essentials of Obstetrics and Gynecology, 5th ed. Philadelphia: Elsevier, 2010; Courtesy **(B)**: Dr Parveen Gulati, New Delhi.)

the characteristic structure of a mucinous cystadenoma. Perhaps as many as 40% of dermoid cysts are combined tumours of this kind. This association suggests the common origin of the two forms.

Multiple dermoid cysts in the same ovary are well recognized and it is not uncommon to find two to three separate dermoids. Extraovarian dermoid cysts arise occasionally in the lumbar region, uterovesical area, parasacral region and rectovaginal septum. Combined tumours tend to arise in patients between the ages of 20 and 30 years, whereas simple dermoid cysts have the highest age incidence between 40 and 50 years. Tumours may, however, arise at any age. Dermoids are bilateral in 12%–15% of cases.

Dermoid cysts are innocent ovarian tumours but epidermoid carcinoma occurs in 1.7% of cases and sarcomatous

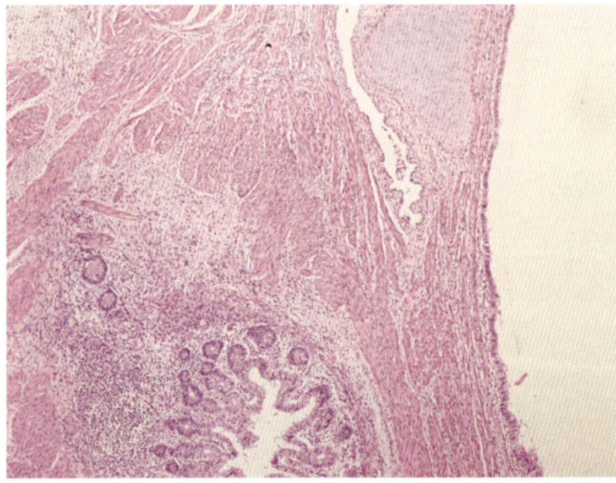

Figure 35.9 Histological appearance of the Dermoid cyst of the ovary (Mature cystic teratoma). The cyst is lined by squamous epithelium, Sebaceous glands open into the cavity of the cyst, hair follicles are also present. (*Courtesy:* Dr. Sandeep Mathur, AIIMS.)

changes have been described. Usually, a squamous cell carcinoma develops from the ectodermal tissues but mammary carcinomas and malignant thyroid tumours have also been described.

SOLID TERATOMA OF THE OVARY

These tumours are rare. They are mostly solid and the cut surface has a peculiar trabeculated appearance. Invariably large loculi are found beneath the capsule. The solid part of the tumour contains cartilage and bone, whereas hair and sebaceous material are found in the cystic spaces. The solid area also contains plain muscle, brain tissue, glia, pia mater and intestinal mucous membrane. The attempted formation of a rudimentary eye has been described and even the recognizable pattern of a fetus has been simulated, the so-called embryoma. As a rule, however, the formation is a conglomerate, without order or arrangement. Most solid teratomas of the ovary are malignant tumours because of sarcomatous change, but about 20% are innocent (Fig. 35.10).

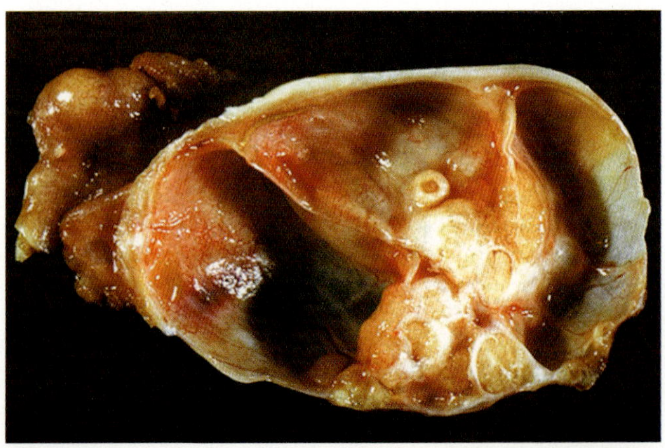

Figure 35.10 Benign cystic teratoma. (*Source*: Diagnostic Gynecologic and Obstetric Pathology. Germ Cell Tumors of the Ovary. Saunders, 2011.)

ENDODERMAL SINUS TUMOUR (YOLK SAC TUMOUR)

This is the second most common type of ovarian germ cell tumour. It is mostly unilateral and is characterized by the secretion of a large amount of alpha-fetoprotein (AFP) in circulation. It is one of the fastest growing tumours in the human body. Most patients tend to be young girls between 15 and 25 years of age. Grossly these tumours tend to be 10–20 cm in size with solid–cystic feel. Cut section shows a variegated appearance of solid and cystic areas. Microscopically diagnosis is made based on the presence of tissue similar to yolk sac contents. The presence of Schiller–Duval bodies under microscope is a diagnostic feature. They tend to spread rapidly by local spread, vascular and lymphatic routes. Before the use of chemotherapeutic agents, these tumours were considered highly malignant. However, with effective therapeutic regimen such as 'BEP regimen'. Now a days cure can be expected with preservation of menstrual and reproductive functions.

STRUMA OVARII

Struma ovarii (Fig. 35.11) consists of thyroid tissue similar to that of a thyroid adenoma. The tumour is solid, consisting almost entirely of thyroid tissue, and should be clearly distinguished from a dermoid cyst with thyroid tissue in its wall. To the naked eye, the tumour resembles a small mucinous cystadenoma, but the material contained in the vesicles is colloid and gives reaction to iodine. Some cases develop thyrotoxicosis. Most of the tumours are innocent, but malignant thyroid tumours have been recorded. The histogenesis is supposedly a dermoid in which the thyroid tissue dominates at the expense of the other elements.

CARCINOID TUMOURS

An interesting tumour of the ovary, sometimes primary and sometimes metastatic, is the argentaffinoma. It occurs as a malignant change in a benign dermoid cyst and presents as a solid yellow tumour with the histological property of reducing silver salts derived from the specialized Kulchitsky cells of the intestine. It produces 5-hydroxytryptamine which causes attacks of flushing and cyanosis.

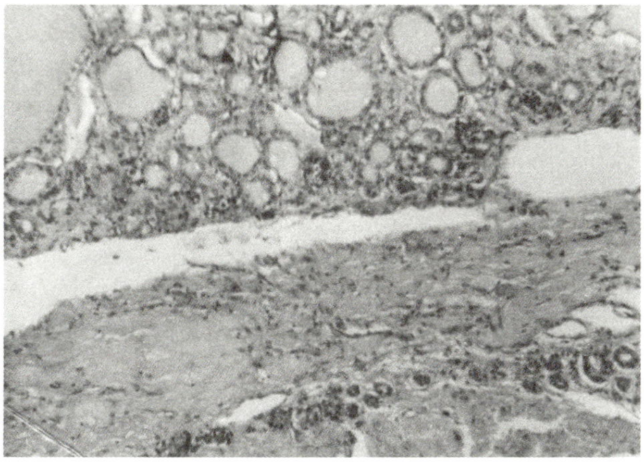

Figure 35.11 Struma ovarii showing space filled with colloid.

MIXED GERM CELL TUMOUR

Mixed germ cell tumours contain two or more recognizable germ cell entities, e.g. combination of dysgerminoma, gonadoblastoma, teratoma, endodermal sinus tumours and choriocarcinoma. Gonadoblastoma contains calcified elements, and Y chromosome is detected in 90% of tumours. Fifty per cent turn malignant.

Tumour markers secreted by germ cell tumour

	AFP	*hCG*	*LDH*
Dysgerminoma	–	+	++
Yolk sac tumour	++	–	–
Embryonal cell carcinoma	+/–	+/–	–
Choriocarcinoma	–	+	–

SEX CORD STROMAL TUMOURS

Sex cord stromal tumours originate either from the sex cords of the embryonic gonad (before the differentiation of the gonadal mesenchyme into male or female) or from the stroma of the ovary. Theca cells are the source of ovarian steroids, so many of these are functional and exert feminizing effects. The embryonic sex cords may differentiate along the male line, giving rise to Sertoli or Leydig cell tumours called androblastomas. The sex cord tumours are also referred to as *mesenchymomas*.

FEMINIZING TUMOURS

GRANULOSA CELL TUMOUR

Granulosa cell tumours are interesting growths of the ovary composed of cells closely resembling the granulosa cells of the Graafian follicle.

CLINICAL FEATURES

Granulosa cell tumours are fairly common and represent 10% of all solid ovarian tumours. They can occur at any age. Of all the tumours, 80% occur in women older than 40 years and 5% in prepubertal girls. The main clinical feature depends on the oestrogenic activity of the tumour and only the larger ones cause pain and abdominal swelling. Feminizing tumours secrete oestrogen.

- When this tumour occurs before puberty, a precocious puberty (see Fig. 6.5) results with the development of secondary sexual characteristics, hypertrophy of breasts and external genitalia, pubic hair and myohyperplasia of the uterus. The endometrium shows an oestrogenic, anovulatory pattern. Removal of the tumour causes regression of all these manifestations.
- When occurring in adult life, the oestrogenic effect is less marked than in the prepubertal stage. There is no change in the secondary sexual characteristics because these are already established. The effect on the endometrium is that of hyperoestrogenism in general, i.e. an exaggerated proliferative pattern, endometrial hyperplasia or endometrial carcinoma (Fig. 35.12). Superthreshold level of serum oestrogen may lead to amenorrhoea,

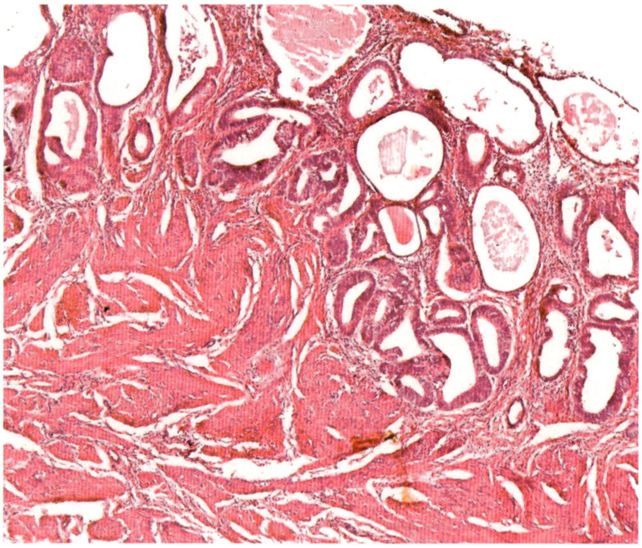

Figure 35.12 Cystic glandular hyperplasia. (*Courtesy:* Dr Sandeep Mathur, AIIMS.)

followed by prolonged bleeding. In fact, the behaviour of the endometrium closely resembles that of metropathia haemorrhagica.

- In the postmenopausal patient, the most remarkable feature is postmenopausal bleeding (Fig. 35.12). The secondary sexual characteristics are less affected, although hypertrophy of the breast is sometimes seen. The uterus shows myohyperplasia and cystic glandular hyperplasia similar to metropathia. Removal of the tumour causes regression of all these symptoms.

MACROSCOPIC FEATURES

The tumour varies in size from tiny to gross, the average being 10 cm in diameter. The shape is oval and the consistency soft. The cut surface is reticular or trabeculated with areas of interstitial haemorrhage, and shows yellow areas. The outer surface is smooth and lobulated.

The cells are arranged either in cords or in trabeculae, and are often surrounded by structureless hyaline tissue, which resembles the glass membrane of an atretic follicle. Moreover, small **Call–Exner bodies** can usually be found in some part of the tumour. These small cyst-like spaces are characteristic features of the granulosa cells of the Graafian follicle. **Three histological types of granulosa cell tumours have been identified:** (i) an early undifferentiated form which consists of a solid mass of granulosa cell, (ii) a trabecular form and (iii) a folliculoid type in which the granulosa cells are grouped around spaces filled with secretion. Most granulosa cell tumours are encapsulated and appear to be clinically benign. Both this appearance of the gross specimen and the histological picture may be misleading as judged by the subsequent recurrence of the tumour. Recurrence may be delayed for many years. Kottmeier reported that malignant recurrence occurs in 50% of granulosa cell tumours and the term granulosa cell carcinoma is justified.

There is a certain correlation between the histological appearance and malignancy. A well-differentiated folliculoid appearance has 10% malignant potential, whereas an anaplastic, almost sarcomatous appearance has 65% malignant potential.

The metastases are interesting, because the opposite ovary first becomes involved, and then metastases develop in the lumbar region; secondary deposits become scattered in the mesentery, liver and mediastinum.

ASSOCIATION OF CARCINOMA OF THE ENDOMETRIUM WITH GRANULOSA CELL TUMOURS

Excess production of oestrogen can lead to endometrial hyperplasia and development of endometrial carcinoma. There is a strong evidence that carcinoma of the endometrium may be associated with feminizing tumours of the ovary in postmenopausal women. It has been estimated that in one-fifth of oestrogenic ovarian tumours, an endometrial cancer will develop. A theca cell tumour is four times more commonly associated with endometrial cancer than the granulosa cell tumour, because of its high oestrogen secretion.

THECA CELL TUMOUR

This tumour is usually seen after menopause. It is nearly always unilateral and forms a solid mass. The cut surface is yellow in colour and, if stained selectively, lipoid material is characteristically present. The tumour consists of spindle-shaped cells reminiscent of an ovarian fibroma together with fat-laden polyhedral cells which resemble the theca lutein cells of the Graafian follicle. The tumour is intensely oestrogenic and causes postmenopausal bleeding. It usually runs a benign course but malignant forms have been described. It has been shown that both granulosa cell tumours and theca cell tumours may show luteinization of their cells, with the result that progesterone is secreted and secretory hypertrophy can be demonstrated in the endometrium.

VIRILIZING TUMOURS

The ovarian tumours which produce male sex hormones are called virilizing tumours. Virilizing mesenchymoma and other virilizing tumours of the ovary are grouped together here for convenience.

ARRHENOBLASTOMA (SERTOLI-LEYDIG TUMOUR)

Arrhenoblastoma are rare tumours that secrete androgens which cause defeminization followed by masculinization. Women in the childbearing age may complain of altered body contours, flattening of the breasts, and scanty and irregular menstruation ending ultimately in amenorrhoea. Later signs of masculinization such as increased hair growth on the face (hirsutism) appear. Coarsening of the features, enlargement of the clitoris (Fig. 35.13) and even breaking of the voice may occur. Removal of the tumour reverses most of the above-mentioned features of endometrial carcinoma except the voice change.

The gross appearance of the tumour is like that of other mesenchymomas. Generally, only one ovary is affected. Its

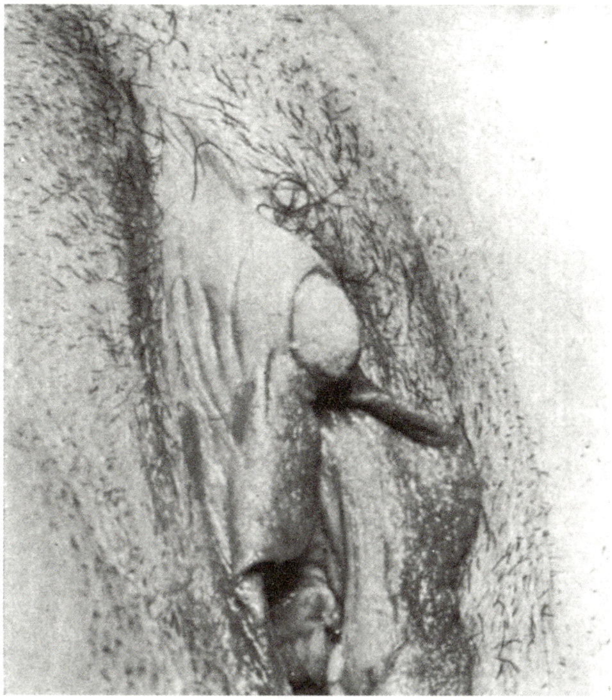

Figure 35.13 Hypertrophy of the clitoris in a patient with arrhenoblastoma.

association with pregnancy has been reported. The incidence of malignant transformation is rated to be higher than with feminizing tumours.

Histologically, the tumour reveals all grades of differentiation from the testicular adenoma showing perfectly formed seminiferous tubules to a sarcomatous anaplastic variety, wherein lipoid-containing cells are seen. The diagnosis is usually made on the basis of the endocrine behaviour of the tumour.

ADRENAL CORTICAL TUMOURS OF THE OVARY

Adrenal cortical tumours of the ovary have a resemblance to the adrenal cortex when examined microscopically and have been called hypernephroma, masculinovoblastoma, virilizing luteoma or clear-celled tumours. These various appellations show that the constituent cells resemble the large clear cells of the adrenal cortex or lutein cells of the corpus luteum. Whatever may be their true origin, they are very rare tumours. They are sometimes masculinizing.

HILUS CELL TUMOUR

A rare virilizing tumour arising from cells in the ovarian hilum has been described in women after menopause. One interesting feature of the hilus cell tumour is the presence of Reinke crystals in the cells, a distinguishing feature of the Leydig or interstitial cells of the testis.

GYNANDROBLASTOMA

A gynandroblastoma combines the characteristics of the granulosa cell tumour and an arrhenoblastoma. This rare tumour sometimes arises in dysgenetic gonads.

TUMOURS ARISING FROM CONNECTIVE TISSUES OF THE OVARY

Of the innocent connective tissue tumours of the ovary, fibromas are the most common.

OVARIAN FIBROMA

Ovarian fibroma comprises about 3% of ovarian neoplasms and has no particular age incidence. The tumour is oval in shape with a smooth surface and large veins always noticeable in the capsule. The consistency is firm and harder than that of a uterine myoma. The tumour frequently undergoes degeneration so that cystic spaces are found towards the centre. Calcareous degeneration is not uncommon. The tumours are usually about 15 cm in diameter but sometimes become much larger than this and may weigh as much as 25 kg. Torsion may occur with the larger tumours.

Microscopic examination shows the tumour to be composed of a network of spindle-shaped cells which closely resemble the spindle cells of the ovarian cortex. The cellular pattern is strikingly uniform and there is no attempt at nuclear activity. The association of Brenner tumours with ovarian fibroma is known. In large tumours, the connective tissue cells are elongated and an intercellular matrix becomes prominent. The tumours are often accompanied by ascites. Sometimes, the patient has hydrothorax. **The combination of an ovarian fibroma with ascites and hydrothorax, usually right-sided, is known as Meigs syndrome.** It is now accepted that the diaphragm is porous either by reason of minute foramina or via the lymphatics. Meigs syndrome can occur with other solid ovarian tumours such as granulosa cell tumour and Brenner tumour.

Three types of fibromas are recognized. In the first type, the tumour takes the form of a surface papilloma on the ovary. In the second type, there is a small encapsulated fibroma arising in an ovary so that normal ovarian tissue can be recognized at one pole of the tumour. In the third type, the fibroma replaces the ovary completely.

HISTOGENESIS OF OVARIAN TUMOURS

FIBROMAS

Small ovarian fibromas form white, rounded excrescences in the cortex of the ovary. The tumour arises from the stroma cells of the ovarian cortex. Histologically, a fibroma and a Brenner tumour have a close resemblance, apart from the inclusion of the epithelioid Walthard rests in the latter. With subsequent growth, a capsule becomes differentiated and the tumour grows at the expense of the normal ovarian tissue, so that finally the ovary is completely replaced by the fibroma. The structure of a large ovarian fibroma is not unlike that of the stroma of the ovarian cortex, except that the constituent cells are more primitive in type.

PAPILLARY SEROUS CYSTADENOMA

Papillary serous cystadenomas almost certainly originate from downgrowths of the surface epithelium of the ovary into the cortex. Small downgrowths of this sort are extremely common, even in normal ovaries, and small cysts, only recognized by microscopic examination, are fairly frequent. Papillary forms result from intracystic growths into these tumours. Papillary serous carcinomas of the ovary arise when the intracystic growths become malignant.

The origin of the tumours from downgrowths of the surface epithelium of the ovary is generally accepted and the tumours are regarded as examples of ovarian Müllerianosis, with epithelial cells resembling endosalpinx.

GRANULOSA CELL TUMOURS

Granulosa cell tumours consist of cells identical to the granulosa cells of Graafian follicles and theca cell tumours similar to the theca interna cell (Fig. 35.14). As both types of tumours may arise after menopause, when there are no Graafian follicles in the ovaries, the tumours cannot be regarded as being derived from mature cells of this type. They are therefore regarded as originating in mesenchymal cells which are differentiated sexually. The arrhenoblastoma is regarded as being derived from mesenchymal cells of the male type. The theca cell is regarded as the master hormone producer in the ovary.

TERATOMAS

Teratomas probably arise from totipotent cells, i.e. cells which are capable of producing ectodermal, mesodermal and endodermal structure.

MUCINOUS CYSTADENOMAS

The cells of the tumour resemble those of the cervix and the large intestine. The two present-day theories are (i) the tumour represents an example of ovarian Müllerianosis, with metaplasia of the ovarian surface epithelium into cervical epithelium and (ii) the tumour arises from large intestine elements of a dermoid cyst.

BRENNER TUMOUR

Brenner tumours are often associated with a mucinous cystadenoma, where there is probably some relation between their origins. The similarity to Walthard inclusions has already been noted and this suggests that Brenner tumours, like Walthard inclusions, are derived from the germinal epithelial layer of the ovary.

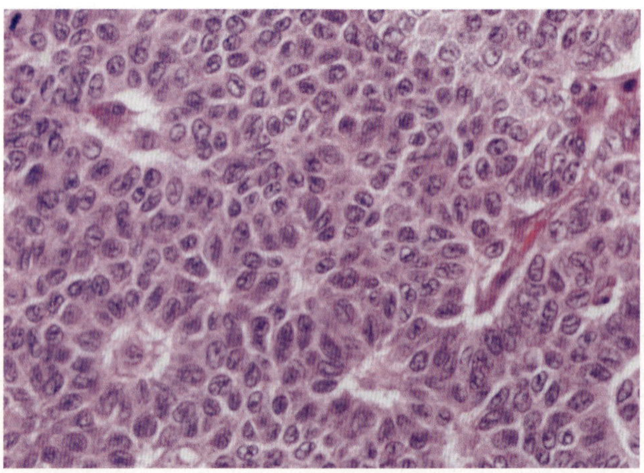

Figure 35.14 Granulosa cell tumour, folliculoid pattern. (*Courtesy:* Dr Sandeep Mathur, AIIMS.)

COMPLICATIONS OF OVARIAN TUMOURS (Table 35.2)

AXIAL ROTATION: TORSION

Torsion of an ovarian cyst is a common complication, and occurs in about 12% of cases. Dermoid cyst is the most common ovarian cyst to undergo torsion. Chocolate cysts and malignant ovarian tumours are usually fixed by adhesions, so it is very rare for these ovarian tumours to undergo torsion. On the contrary, paraovarian cysts and broad ligament cysts are the most likely pelvic tumours to undergo torsion, probably because they develop in the outer part of the broad ligament and come to lie above the infundibulopelvic fold and above the pelvic brim so that they have a greater degree of mobility than other ovarian tumours. In most cases, the cyst is about 10 cm or more in size when it undergoes torsion. Because of the high incidence of mucinous cystadenomas, dermoid cyst torsion is most frequently seen with these tumours. There is no particular age incidence. The right and left sides are involved with equal frequency. Usually, the tumour rotates so that its anterior surface turns towards the patient's right side. It is not uncommon for the tumour to be rotated through three or more complete circles. As a result of rotation, the veins in the pedicle become occluded, the tumour becomes congested, and there is interstitial haemorrhage in the wall of the tumour and into the loculi. The increased tension causes severe abdominal pain and the signs of peritoneal irritation. Subsequently, adhesions form with surrounding structures, so that the omentum and intestines become attached to the tumour. On occasions, the cyst may become infected.

The most probable explanation of rotation of an ovarian cyst is haemodynamic. It is suggested that some violent movement, a history of which is almost invariably obtained, initiates the twist and as a result the ovarian artery itself becomes twisted. The pulsation in the vessel will then cause a series of tiny impulses to be transmitted to the pedicle, each of which will aggravate the twist. After a time, the degree of torsion will be such that the veins in the pedicle become occluded and the patient complains of severe abdominal pain (Fig. 35.15).

CLINICAL FEATURES OF TORSION OF OVARY

The woman often presents with acute abdominal pain, fever and vomiting. Sometimes, she complains of intermittent abdominal pain referred along the obturator nerve to along

Table 35.2 Complications of an Ovarian Tumour

- Torsion
- Rupture
- Haemorrhage
- Infection
- Pseudomyxoma peritoneum
- Malignancy

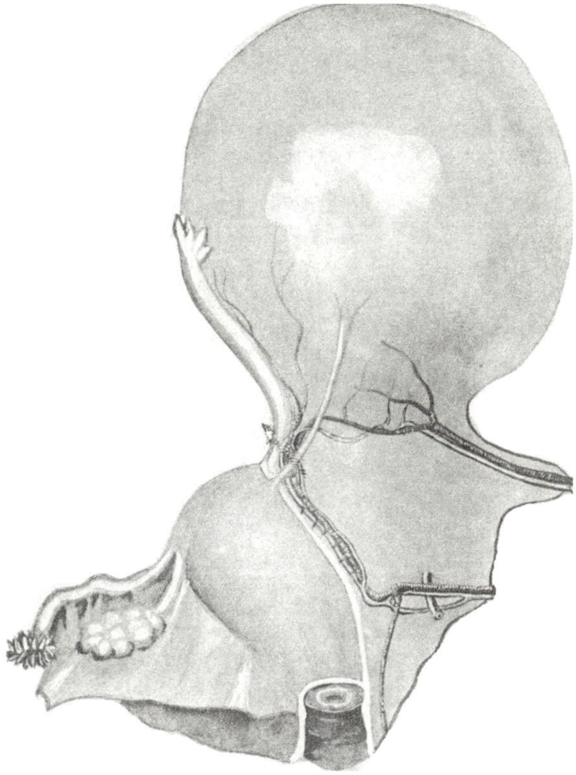

Figure 35.15 The pedicle of an ovarian cyst showing the relations of the ovarian vessels, the ovarian ligament and the fallopian tube, together with the anastomosing branch of the uterine artery.

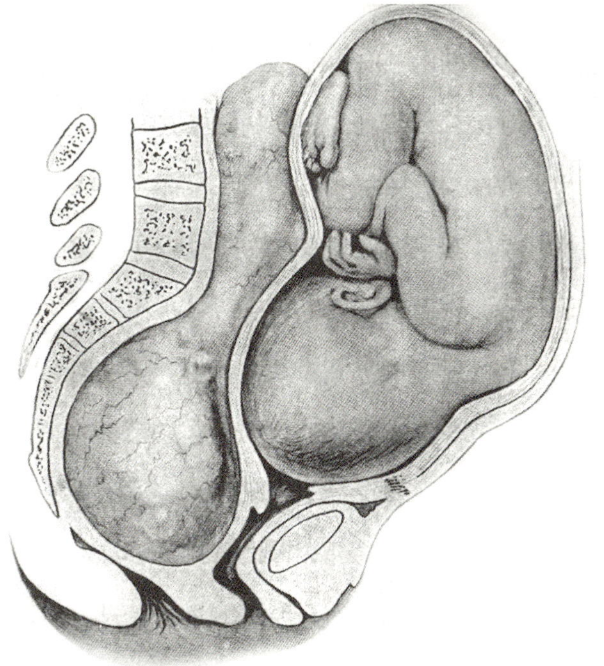

Figure 35.16 Ovarian cyst obstructing labour. (*Source:* From Eden and Holland's Manual of Obstetrics.)

the medial aspect of the thigh. Symptoms may start after emptying of bowel in the morning.

Ultrasound shows a swollen oedematous ovary, globular in shape, and free fluid in the peritoneal cavity. The pelvic findings reveal a tender mass separate from the uterus.

This is an emergency requiring urgent laparotomy. The appearance of torsion of the ovarian tumour does not correlate with the ovarian viability, even when the tumour appears blackish. Therefore, one is advised to try and conserve the ovary if possible, unless gangrene has set in. Detorsion of the ovary and ovariopexy, after removal of the tumour, should be attempted. The ovary should be observed for colour change from bluish black appearance to its normal appearance. The theoretical risk of embolism with detorsion does not normally occur. The ovary recovers and becomes functional. This approach is especially important in a young woman.

RUPTURE

Rupture of an ovarian cyst may be traumatic or spontaneous. Traumatic rupture results from direct violence to the abdomen. It may happen during labour when a cyst is impacted in the pouch of Douglas in advance of the presenting part (Fig. 35.16). It is not uncommon for a small thin-walled retention cyst to rupture during bimanual examination.

Spontaneous rupture of an ovarian cyst is not uncommon. With malignant ovarian tumours, particularly those of the papillomatous type, the carcinoma cells infiltrate through the connective tissue capsule to ulcerate into the peritoneal cavity. With innocent papillary serous cystadenomas, a similar process may take place. The most interesting cases of spontaneous rupture are those arising with actively growing mucinous cystadenomas. The epithelial elements of the growth grow so rapidly that the connective tissues of the capsule are unable to keep up with them, and spontaneous rupture of the tumour is the result. The mucinous material is discharged into the peritoneal cavity. In most cases, with a small leak there is no serious after-effect, but in rare cases, the condition called pseudomyxoma of the peritoneum develops (pseudomyxoma peritonei).

HAEMORRHAGE

Haemorrhage may occur in an ovarian cyst. It mostly occurs spontaneously, giving rise to acute pain similar to pain because of torsion. Occasionally, haemorrhage in cyst can occur following aspirations of cyst.

PSEUDOMYXOMA OF THE PERITONEUM

In this condition, the peritoneal cavity is filled with coagulated mucinous material adherent to the omentum and intestines. The findings at laparotomy almost exactly resemble a boiled sago pudding. The material cannot be removed completely at operation because of its attachment to the bowel, and the condition tends to recur after operation. Pseudomyxoma of the peritoneum usually occurs with a mucinous cystadenoma of the ovary, but it has also been reported with a mucocele of the appendix and carcinoma of the large intestine in men. In pseudomyxoma of the peritoneum, the mesothelium of the peritoneum is converted, in part, into high columnar cells which are histologically similar to those lining a mucinous cystadenoma of the ovary, and these cells secrete mucinous material into the peritoneal cavity. The prognosis in pseudomyxoma of the peritoneum is bad, even after the ovaries and the appendix are removed, as it is to recur again and again. It is now believed that mucocele of the appendix may induce secondary ovarian tumour. *Therefore, there is a tendency amongst gynaecologists to remove the appendix as well, when encountered with mucinous ovarian tumour, and avoid pseudomyxoma of the peritoneum.* Pseudomyxoma may be treated with palliative chemotherapy.

INFECTION

Infection of an ovarian tumour is infrequent. Most cases follow acute salpingitis or when the cyst becomes infected during the puerperium as part of an ascending genital tract infection. Infection may also follow torsion when, as a result of adhesions to the intestine, the tumour becomes directly infected. Infection by the bloodstream is very uncommon. Infected ovarian tumours are always adherent to adjacent viscera and occasionally discharge their contents into the rectum. Sebaceous material in a dermoid cyst also causes infection in the tumour; it may also cause peritonitis.

EXTRAPERITONEAL SPREAD

Some ovarian tumours burrow extraperitoneally during their development and may spread upwards into the perinephric region. The removal of these tumours is extremely difficult and there is danger of injuring the ureter. During dissection and removal of such a cyst, large vessels may be torn in the retroperitoneal space and subsequent leakage of blood will form a retroperitoneal haematoma giving rise to shock and requires drainage.

Malignant change: Secondary malignant changes occur in 50% of serous cystadenomas and 5% of mucinous cystadenomas, but only in 1.7% of dermoid cysts. A longstanding ovarian cyst may become the site of malignant change.

BENIGN OVARIAN TUMOURS

Three commonly seen benign ovarian tumours are Serous Cystadenoma, Mucinous Cystadenoma and Benign Cystic Teratoma. These can be seen in any age group, however, more commonly seen between 20-25 yr of age. These three common benign tumours can present with a variety of symptoms such as lump abdomen, pain abdomen or detected incidentally at the time of ultrasound being done for some other indications.

SYMPTOMS

Although benign ovarian cysts occasionally attain enormous tumours, they cause relatively few symptoms. Indeed, in innocent ovarian tumours, the patient's attention is first directed to the abdominal swelling. The average pseudomucinous cystadenoma removed at operation is about the size of a football, and it is not until the tumour has reached this size that it causes sufficient abdominal enlargement to make the patient realize that something is wrong (Figs 35.17 and 35.18; Table 35.3).

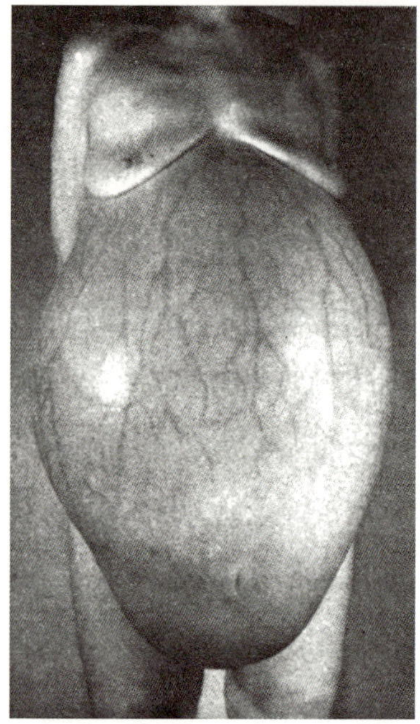

Figure 35.17 A very large benign mucinous ovarian cyst which weighed about 50 kg. Note the prominent veins, displacement of the umbilicus and oedema of the lower abdomen.

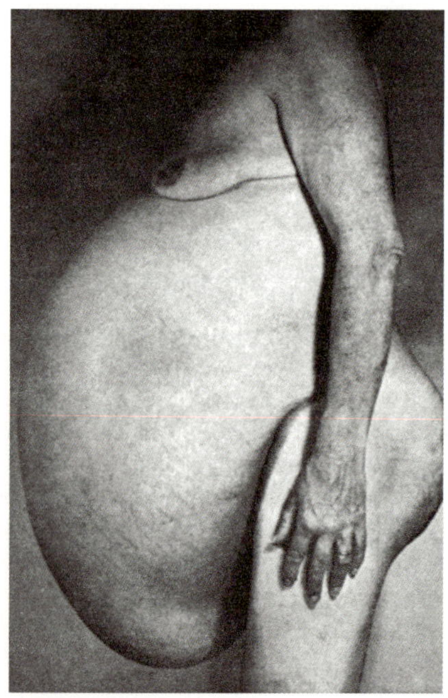

Figure 35.18 A lateral view of the same patient as in Fig. 35.18. Note the lumbar lordosis.

MENSTRUAL IRREGULARITIES

Ovarian tumours, even bilateral, do not generally affect the menstrual cycles. The only tumours causing menorrhagia are granulosa and theca cell tumours by virtue of their oestrogen hormone secretion. Similarly, masculinizing tumours cause amenorrhoea and virilization. Postmenopausal bleeding may occur in benign Brenner and feminizing tumours.

Table 35.3 Features of Benign and Malignant Ovarian Tumours

Benign Ovarian Tumours	Malignant Ovarian Tumour
History	
• Not related to age or parity, though most common during childbearing period • Slow-growing tumour, no pain. No menstrual disorder unless it is a feminizing tumour or masculinizing tumour	• Seen most commonly in adolescents and elderly women – mostly after 50 years of age; low parity or infertile woman • Rapidly growing tumour, pain in advanced stage; postmenopausal bleeding • Family history of breast, ovarian or colonic cancer
Examination	
• Usually unilateral, cystic, well-defined and mobile; no ascites (except in Meigs syndrome); no nodules in the abdomen or pouch of Douglas	• May be bilateral and solid, fixed; ascites may be present; metastatic nodules may be felt per abdomen; nodules in the pouch of Douglas
Ultrasound	
• Cystic well defined with or without echoes; no ascites (except in Meigs syndrome)	• Often solid and bilateral fixed with internal echoes, ascites may be present; metastatic nodules may be seen
Doppler Ultrasound	
• No increased vascularity	• Increased vascularity • Pulsatile index <1 • Resistance index <0.4
MRI and CT	
• Similar to ultrasound findings • CA-125 normal	• Metastatic and enlarged lymph nodes may be detected • CA-125 raised more than 35 IU/mL
Operative Findings	
• Well-defined ovarian cystic or solid tumour; no ascites or metastatic nodule; often mobile	• Fixed solid tumour, often bilateral – with blood-stained ascites; metastatic growth over the omentum and peritoneal cavity; lymph nodes may be enlarged

PRESSURE SYMPTOMS

The ovarian tumour placed in the uterovesical pouch anterior to the uterus and those impacted in the pouch of Douglas may cause increase in frequency of micturition and even urinary retention. Pressure on the rectum is hardly ever noticed. Mammoth tumours such as mucinous tumours may cause dyspnoea and palpitation, and bilateral pitting oedema of the feet.

PAIN

Normally, benign ovarian tumours cause no abdominal pain and are comfortably placed in the abdominal cavity which is distensible. The mammoth tumour may however cause abdominal discomfort and difficulty in walking. Acute abdominal pain develops if the ovarian tumour undergoes torsion, rupture or haemorrhage. An infected dermoid cyst is likely to lead to pain and fever.

With torsion, the woman develops acute abdominal pain, vomiting and at times low-grade fever. The patient may be in shock, with thready pulse. The abdomen is distended, and moves poorly with respiration. The cyst is tense and tender. Immediate laparotomy is required to remove the tumour.

Occasionally, the germ cell tumours occurring in adolescent and young women grow rapidly and cause abdominal pain, which may be the first symptom noticed by these young girls.

PHYSICAL SIGNS

The ovarian cyst may present as an abdominal swelling detected by inspection. The abdominal wall can be seen to move over the swelling when the patient takes a deep inspiration. The tumour is symmetrically situated in the abdomen. On palpation, the upper and lateral limits of the tumour can be defined, but it is impossible to identify the lower pole of the tumour except in case of a relatively small cyst with a long pedicle. The surface of the tumour is smooth, or it may be slightly bossed with multilocular cysts. Small cysts are usually movable from side to side, but large tumours filling the abdomen and tumours which have burrowed extraperitoneally are fixed. The consistency of the cystic tumour is tense and cystic and a fluid thrill can be elicited. Sometimes, a cyst is flaccid, when a well-marked fluid thrill is obtained. It is not uncommon for hard areas to be palpated, even in large ovarian cysts. These areas in mucinous cystadenomas are composed of small loculi which give the tumour an almost solid feeling on palpation. All patients with an ovarian cyst should be examined carefully for ascites, because the presence of ascites is a strong evidence that the tumour is malignant. Exception is the Meigs syndrome associated with fibroma, Brenner tumour and occasionally granulosa cell tumour. An ovarian tumour on percussion is dull over the centre of the tumour but resonant in the flanks which are occupied by the displaced large and small bowel. This sign is reversed in ascites. The legs should be examined for oedema (Fig. 35.19).

The physical signs on bimanual examination vary according to the size of the tumour. With small tumours, the uterus can be identified without difficulty, and the ovarian cyst outlined bimanually. The cyst usually displaces the

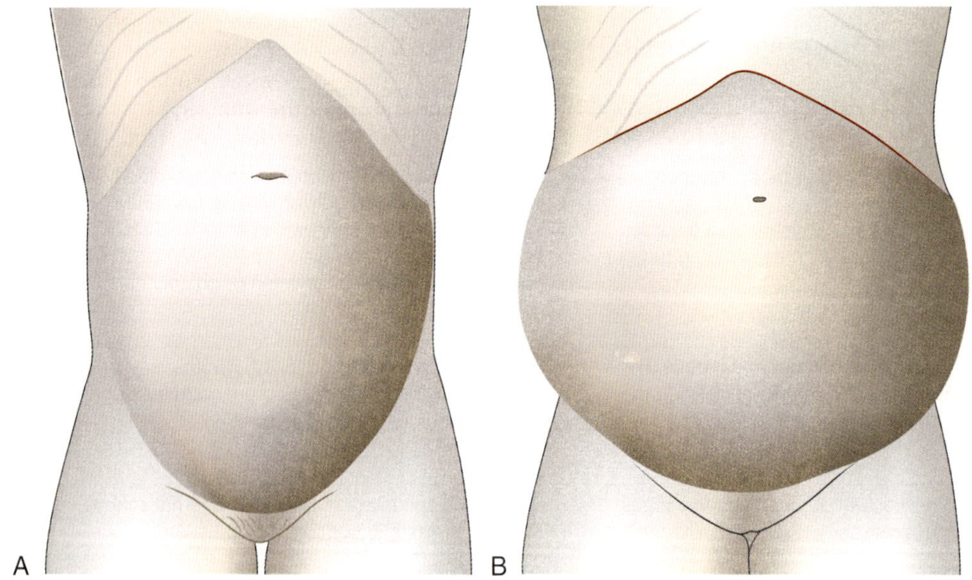

Figure 35.19 On the left is a case of ovarian cyst **(A)**, whereas on the right is the abdomen **(B)** of a case of ascites. In ascites, the abdomen spreads much more laterally than in the case of an ovarian cyst.

uterus to the opposite side. With large cysts, it may be difficult to outline the uterus. Even with a large cyst, the lower pole of the tumour may be palpable through one of the fornices. The firm, rounded lower pole of the tumour has a characteristic feel, and fluctuation can usually be detected between the fingers placed in the vagina and the external hand. It is important to identify the position of the uterus if possible, as mistakes in diagnosis with innocent ovarian cysts are almost always because of failure to identify the body of the uterus separate from the tumour. An ovarian cyst may simulate very closely a cystic degenerated myoma and the diagnosis cannot be made with accuracy unless the position of the body of the uterus is established. The cardinal sign that distinguishes a mobile ovarian tumour from a uterine tumour is when the ovarian tumour is raised up by the abdomen and the cervix remains stationary to the vaginal fingers. In all cases, the pouch of Douglas should be examined carefully as the presence of hard nodules is a strong evidence that the tumour is malignant. Per-rectal examination can help to differentiate an ovarian mass groove between uterus and adnexal mass.

DIFFERENTIAL DIAGNOSIS

The abdominal physical signs of an ovarian cyst may be simulated by a full bladder, a pregnant uterus, a myoma, ascites and other abdominal tumours such as hydronephrosis, mesenteric cyst, retroperitoneal tumour and tuberculous peritonitis, especially if encysted by coils of adherent intestines.

FULL BLADDER

Full bladder is tense and tender, fixed in position, anterior to the uterus and projecting anteriorly more than an ovarian cyst, and a catheter should be passed to establish the diagnosis.

PREGNANT UTERUS

A pregnant uterus should be thought of whenever a tumour is found arising from the pelvis. The exclusion of pregnancy offers no difficulty if a careful bimanual examination is made and signs of pregnancy looked for. Appropriate investigations such as ultrasonic examination and a pregnancy test will help to rule out pregnancy. Mistakes are made because this possibility is not considered, especially in an unmarried girl who denies history of amenorrhoea.

MYOMA

A myoma is usually hard or firm, without the tense cystic consistency of a typical ovarian cyst. Pedunculated and degenerated fibroid may however be mistaken for an ovarian tumour. Imaging studies such as ultrasound or MRI will help to rule out such a possibility.

ASCITES

Sometimes great difficulty is felt in distinguishing between a large ovarian cyst and ascites. With a large ovarian cyst, the percussion note over the tumour is dull, whereas both flanks are resonant. In ascites, the note is dull over the flanks, while the abdomen is tympanitic in the midline. Moreover, the physical signs of shifting dullness may be obtained. Even with large ovarian cysts, the lateral borders of the tumour may be palpable and the tumour may have some degree of mobility (Figs 35.19 and 35.20). Ultrasound distinguishes these two conditions.

The most difficult cases are those of encysted tuberculous peritonitis with ascites. Often, a history of oligomenorrhoea or amenorrhoea can be elicited. The tympanic note over the tumour suggests intestinal adhesions over the cyst. The cyst is also fixed. In most cases of tuberculous peritonitis, the patient has lost weight and is pyrexial, and there may be other signs of tuberculosis in the body. A diagnostic curettage may reveal tuberculous involvement of the endometrium.

In rare cases, obesity can be mistaken for an ovarian cyst. The surest method of excluding an ovarian cyst is to percuss the abdomen below the level of the umbilicus. If the note is

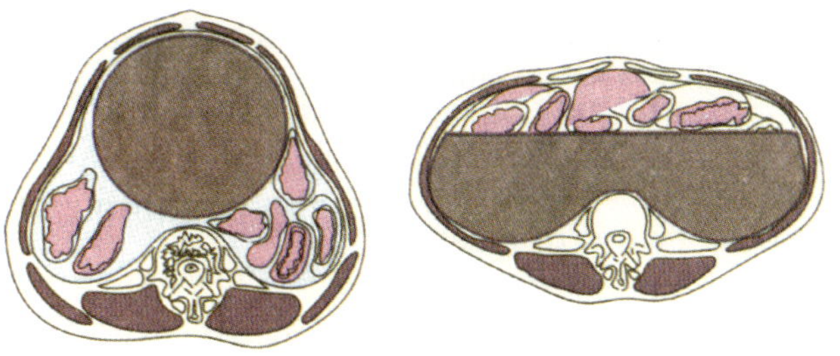

Figure 35.20 On the left, a cross-section of the abdomen is shown from a case of an ovarian cyst, whereas on the right is a cross-section from a case of ascites. With an ovarian cyst, the intestines are displaced dorsally, whereas with ascites, the intestines lie immediately beneath the abdominal wall.

tympanitic, an ovarian cyst can be excluded. An ultrasound scan may be necessary in a few cases.

OTHER TUMOURS

Other tumours may cause difficulty in diagnosis. For example, a large hydronephrosis may project forwards into the abdomen. Such a tumour always penetrates back into the loin and is situated high up in the abdomen, well above the pelvis. Investigations by intravenous or retrograde pyelography will establish the diagnosis. Other tumours such as enlarged spleen, mesenteric cyst, mucocele of the appendix or gallbladder, hydatid cysts and pancreatic cysts should be considered if the physical signs of an ovarian cyst are atypical, and if the tumour lies in mid or upper abdomen.

Small ovarian cysts which lie in the pelvis are palpated without much difficulty. They are movable, with a tense consistency and a smooth rounded surface. It may be difficult to establish the diagnosis with accuracy if the tumour is fixed.

INVESTIGATIONS

- **Ultrasound**: A transabdominal or transvaginal ultrasound (TVS) is the most important investigation. Transabdominal transducer is employed if the tumour is abdominal. Otherwise TVS gives more detailed features of the tumour.
- A benign cyst is characteristically unilateral, unilocular or multilocular with a thin wall and thin septa of less than 5 mm in a multilocular cyst. The contents are nonechogenic. These findings along with normal CA-125 level (below 35 U/mL) indicate the benign nature of the epithelial tumour in 95% of cases.
- A raised CA-125 level is also reported in abdominal tuberculosis and pelvic endometriosis. On the other hand, only 50% of Stage I epithelial ovarian malignant tumours have raised levels.
- A solid tumour suggests malignancy except in a fibroma and Brenner tumour. Dermoid can be identified by solid areas in a cystic tumour and occasional presence of a tooth on ultrasound scanning.
- A menopausal ovary measures not more than 2 × 1.5 × 1 cm in size (volume 8 mL). A size more than this is suspicious of an ovarian growth.

A malignant ovarian tumour is suspected if ultrasound reveals bilateral or a solid tumour with ascites. The tumour wall is usually thick with echogenic areas within the tumour. The septum is more than 5 mm thick with papillary projections from its wall. Except in Meigs syndrome, the presence of ascites as shown on ultrasound strongly points to the malignant nature of the tumour.

Colour flow Doppler, which adds further information of neovascularization, indicates increased blood flow to the tumour and probability of the tumour being malignant. Low pulsatile index also suggests increased blood flow in a malignant tumour.

Additional information may be provided by the following:

- Radiograph of abdomen/pelvis may demonstrate a soft-tissue shadow, or teeth in a dermoid (molar tooth).
- Diagnostic laparoscopic examination may be needed in a few cases.
- In all suspected metastatic ovarian cancers, an upper gastrointestinal endoscopy and colonoscopy meal should be performed to exclude gastrointestinal primary carcinoma.
- Radiograph of chest will rule out pulmonary metastasis and also hydrothorax in case of Meigs syndrome.
- Breast examination will rule out a primary disease in breast.

CT and MRI are useful in identifying a dermoid cyst, haemorrhagic cyst, fibroma, endometriosis and hydrosalpinx (Fig. 35.10).

In a malignant tumour, CT and MRI identify the spread of the tumour and enlargement of pelvic and para-aortic lymph nodes. This helps in planning surgery and postoperative chemotherapy.

Tumour markers such as CA-125 and carcinoembryonic antigen (CEA) are useful mainly in the follow-up of certain tumours. CA-125 is a glycoprotein and surface cell antigen which is secreted by the malignant epithelial tumours. A level more than 35 U/mL suggests malignancy. CA-125 is also raised in abdominal tuberculosis and endometriosis. CEA more than 5 ng/ml is seen in a mucinous ovarian tumour. It should be emphasized that CA-125 is raised in only 50% of cases in Stage I ovarian cancer and in 90% of cases in Stage II ovarian cancer.

Germ cell tumours produce hCG, AFPs, PLAP and LDH, and, when combined with ultrasound, improve predictability of the type of tumour.

Cytology of ascitic fluid or aspirated cyst fluid either laparoscopically or under ultrasound guidance may reveal malignancy, but false-negative rates are high. Fine-needle aspiration cytology (FNAC) of a solid tumour may give a clue to the nature of the tumour.

TREATMENT

A simple unilocular cyst less than 7 cm is often a functional cyst and should be observed. Most functional cysts resolve spontaneously over 4–6 months. A repeat ultrasound will pick up a persistent cyst which requires laparoscopic evaluation. To expedite its resolution, oral combined pills may be prescribed for 3–4 months in women of reproductive age as this may help in its resolution.

Simple aspiration of a cyst is not advisable, because of the high risk of recurrence. Besides, if the cyst proves malignant, the outcome will be compromised.

Laparotomy or laparoscopy is required in other cases to obtain the specimen for histology and for definitive treatment. Even a benign ovarian tumour more than 7 cm requires removal; otherwise, it may grow in size, undergo complications or turn malignant.

Open laparotomy is preferred to laparoscopic excision, although lately some expert laparoscopists are carrying out surgery for an ovarian tumour laparoscopically.

PROPHYLACTIC OOPHORECTOMY

Bilateral removal of ovaries at hysterectomy is also desirable in a high-risk woman with a family history of ovarian cancer, colonic and breast cancer, and previous hyperstimulation of ovaries in infertility, and in a woman carrying *BRCA-1* and *BRCA-2* gene mutation.

The exact age when prophylactic oophorectomy is beneficial is difficult to decide and depends on the following considerations:

- At what age does the ovary cease to function? This is difficult to determine.
- Does the preserved ovary continue to function after hysterectomy? It is observed that following hysterectomy, ovarian blood supply is compromised and at best it may retain its function for about 4 years.
- Following oophorectomy, is HRT effective? Though effective, it is advisable not to continue HRT for more than 5 years because of the risk of breast cancer.
- It can cause ovarian remnant syndrome.

SURGICAL TREATMENT OF BENIGN OVARIAN TUMOURS

The treatment comprises:

- Abdominal hysterectomy and bilateral salpingo-oophorectomy
- Unilateral ovariotomy
- Ovarian cystectomy
- Laparoscopic cystectomy–ovariotomy
- Laparoscopy/ultrasound-guided aspiration and removal of the cyst

Abdominal hysterectomy and bilateral salpingo-oophorectomy is recommended in a perimenopausal woman, even if the tumour is benign and unilateral. The probability of discovering microscopic evidence of malignancy in histological specimens and thereby the need for second surgery can be avoided.

Ovariotomy/cystectomy. In a young woman, irrespective of parity, conservation of a healthy ovary is highly desirable. Therefore, the ovarian cyst should be enucleated (cystectomy), and if this is not possible, ovariotomy should be done by clamping the infundibulopelvic ligament laterally, mesovarium in the middle, and fallopian tube and ovarian ligament medially. It is important to be certain that the tumour is benign and the other ovary healthy by frozen section biopsy.

Laparoscopic cystectomy–ovariotomy is a minimal invasive surgery in vogue for small cysts.

Because of the risk of spillage of cyst content in a dermoid cyst resulting in peritonitis and mucinous material spillage causing pseudomyxoma peritonei in a case of mucinous cyst, some prefer open surgery. In a laparoscopic surgery, retrieval of the tumour in a plastic bag reduces the risk of spillage of cyst contents.

Laparoscopy carries a low morbidity and allows a quick recovery without a conventional abdominal scar.

Laparoscopic ovarian cystectomy is performed by first aspirating the cyst fluid followed by dissection of the cyst wall or by ablation. Mere aspiration of fluid is not recommended on account of recurrence of the tumour. Aspirated material/cyst wall should be subjected to histopathology to rule out cancer. Ablation of the cyst wall carried out with cautery or laser carries the risk of recurrence of the cyst. While dissection or peeling off of the cyst wall avoids recurrence, bleeding during dissection, adhesion formation and reduction in the ovarian reserve (because of destruction of a portion of the ovary) are the disadvantages.

OVARIAN TUMOURS ASSOCIATED WITH PREGNANCY

A variety of cysts or tumours may be discovered in association with pregnancy. These include corpus luteum cyst, dermoid cyst, germ cell tumours or rarely epithelial ovarian carcinoma. An asymptomatic tumour is discovered during routine ultrasound scanning in early pregnancy. Symptomatic tumour however presents with abdominal pain in pregnancy.

Corpus luteal cyst regresses after the 12th week and can therefore be observed. The benign tumour should be removed in the second trimester between the 14th and 16th weeks. Earlier surgery may increase the risk of abortion, whereas laparotomy in the third trimester increases the surgical difficulty because of the growing uterus; preterm labour is also a possibility. The tumour discovered late in pregnancy should be removed in early puerperium to avoid torsion and infection. The malignant ovarian tumour requires laparotomy at the earliest, irrespective of the duration of pregnancy.

OVARIAN CYST IN A MENOPAUSAL WOMAN

A simple unilocular cyst measuring less than 5 cm can be observed with repeat ultrasound and CA-125 every 3 months. Many a time the cyst resolves in 6 months. A persistent cyst calls for its removal laparoscopically or by laparotomy. Aspiration of the cyst is contraindicated because of low yield of malignant cells (false-negative) and possibility of spread of malignancy if the cyst proves malignant. Many perform bilateral oophorectomy and hysterectomy in perimenopausal women with persistent ovarian cyst.

OVARIAN REMNANT SYNDROME

Ovarian remnant syndrome follows hysterectomy in 1.4% of cases. It is caused by ovarian adhesions to the vaginal vault, and causes cyclical abdominal pain and deep dyspareunia. It requires oophorectomy. The retained ovary may also develop malignancy in 1% of cases. Apart from these, it is also

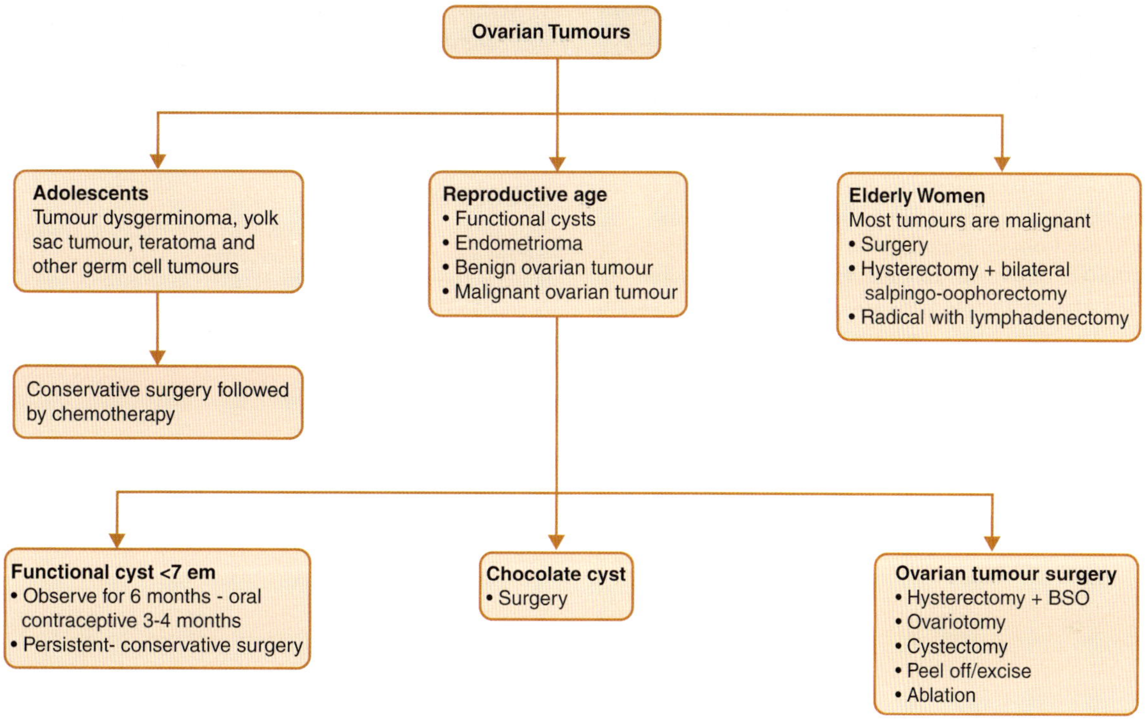

Figure 35.21 Flowchart of ovarian tumours in adolescents.

observed that many ovaries atrophy prematurely (within 4 years) following hysterectomy, if the ovarian vessels get kinked and obliterated during hysterectomy.

OVARIAN TUMOURS IN ADOLESCENTS (Fig. 35.21)

Before the age of 20 years, of all ovarian tumours, 60 - 80% are germ cell tumours and most of them are malignant.

Epithelial tumours are uncommon in adolescent period. Dysgerminoma is the commonest tumour in this age group. Conservative surgery followed by chemotherapy is the best approach in management. It helps in preserving menstrual and reproductive functions.

Differential diagnosis of adnexal masses

Premenarchial	*Reproductive Age*	*Postmenopausal*
Germ cell tumours	Functional ovarian cyst	Ovarian malignancies
Tubercular masses	Pelvic inflammatory disease	Subserous fibroid
Pelvic kidney	Endometrioma	Pyometra
	Ectopic pregnancy	Colonic carcinoma
	Broad ligament tumour	
	Tubercular masses	
	Ovarian tumours	

Often to make a correct diagnosis ultrasound, CT, MRI and tumour marker are needed. Treatment depends upon age of patient, underline pathology and her desire to preserve reproductive organs.

KEY POINTS

- A variety of ovarian tumours are known to arise from the ovary. Many of these are malignant potential. The tumours are often asymptomatic to begin with, and are often far advanced by the time they are diagnosed. These tumours can be cystic or solid.
- In young girls below the age of 25, most tumours are germ cell tumours. Conservative surgery followed by chemotherapy (BEP) helps to cure these tumours.
- Sex cord tumours have a potential to secrete hormones which may present with clinical symptoms such as precocious puberty, menstrual disturbances and postmenopausal bleeding. Virilizing effects may be observed in masculinizing tumours.
- Bilateral tumours, rapidly growing tumours and presence of ascites are suggestive of malignancy and require investigations.
- Tumour markers such as CA-125 and CEA are particularly useful in postmenopausal women suspected of having a malignant epithelial cell tumour. Markers such as alpha-fetoproteins, LDH and hCG are helpful in making a diagnosis of germ cell tumours.
- Imaging modalities such as ultrasonography, CT scan and MRI help to detect ovarian neoplasms, and assist in staging of ovarian cancers.
- It is important to differentiate between benign and malignant enlargements of the ovary to institute timely and effective treatment without delay.
- Benign ovarian tumours are surgically dealt with by ovarian cystectomy, ovariotomy, laparoscopic dissection of the cyst in a young woman and hysterectomy with bilateral removal of adnexa in an older woman.

SELF-ASSESSMENT

1. An 18-year-old girl presents with an abdominal tumour and slight abdominal pain. Discuss the differential diagnosis and management.
2. A 36-year-old parous woman presents with ascites and abdominal lump. Discuss the differential diagnosis.
3. A 30-year-old woman, para 2, presents with menorrhagia of 6 months' duration. An abdominal tumour is palpable abdominally. Discuss the differential diagnosis and management.
4. Write short notes on:
   - Brenner tumour
   - Mucinous epithelial tumour
   - Arrhenoblastoma
   - Theca cell tumour

SUGGESTED READING

Sengupta S, Chattopadhyay, Varma. Gynaecology for Postgraduate and Practitioners, 2nd Ed. Elsevier, 2007.

Studd J. The adnexal mass. In: Progress in Obstetrics and Gynaecology 17: 306, 2006.

Ovarian Malignancies 36

CHAPTER OUTLINE

Ovarian cancer is the fourth most common cancer among women after breast cancer, cervical cancer and gall bladder cancer. In India 45,231 ovarian cases occurred in 2015 and estimated 59,276 cases will occur in 2020. Ovarian cancer is the second most common of all genital cancers with high case-fatality rate and accounts for 10%–15% of all gynaecological cancers in developing countries including India. Over the past two decades, there has been an increase in the incidence as well as survival rate amongst women with ovarian cancer. The risk of a woman developing cancer of the ovary in her lifetime is around 1:70 to 1:100. Women of low parity, decreased fertility and delayed childbearing appear to be more predisposed. There appears to be a familial predisposition to the disease. Association between ovarian cancer, colon, breast cancer and endometrial adenocarcinoma has also been recognized. In such families, cancers tend to occur at a younger age (less than 40 years). Five to ten per cent malignant ovarian tumours are genetic, and BRCA-1 and BRCA-2 gene mutations are implicated. BRCA-1 gene mutation on chromosome-17 and BRCA-2 gene mutation on chromosome 13 are noted. BRCA-1 is more carcinogenic than BRCA-2, it occurs earlier in life. With one family member affected, the lifelong risk is 2.7%, but it goes up to 13% with two or more relations. The risk increases with age up to 70 years. The pattern of inheritance is autosomal dominant, and ovarian tumour occurs at a younger age below 50 years, associated with a risk of breast and colonic cancer. Occurrence of mumps before menarche and multiple ovulations in IVF (in vitro fertilization) programme appear to increase the risk of ovarian malignancy in later life. Geographical variations are suggestive of the fact that high dietary fat intake, the use of talc on the perineum and industrial pollution are environmental factors implicated in the high incidence in the West. Protective factors include multiparity, breastfeeding, anovulation and use of oral contraceptive pills. These contraceptive pills reduce the incidence of ovarian cancer by 40%–50% and the beneficial effect extends for about 10 years after stoppage of pills. The effect is also dose dependent. Repeated ovulation as seen in induction of ovulation, IVF, low parity suggests ovulation trauma to the epithelial lining to be carcinogenic. Late diagnosis and early metastasis are responsible for the poor survival rates. No satisfactory method of mass screening has as yet been developed, so only 20% of cases are confined to the ovaries at the time of diagnosis. Eighty per cent of ovarian malignancies are of epithelial origin and almost 80% are in Stage III or IV at the time of diagnosis. In younger patients, germ cell tumours are more frequently encountered when tumour markers such as alpha-fetoproteins (AFPs), carcinoembryonic antigen (CEA) and human chorionic gonadotropin (hCG) are useful. In ovary eighty per cent are primary and 20% are secondary from the breast, colon, stomach and uterus. Risk of malignancy increases with age. Bilateral tubectomy or hysterectomy reduces the risk of ovarian cancer, if the theory of mutagen ascending the genital tract is correct (Table 36.1).

New Histologically ovarian tumours have wide variations. They are grouped as follows:

1. Epethilial Ovarian Tumours: 80-90%
2. Germ Cell Tumours: 10-15%
3. Sex Cord Tumours: 5%
4. Metastatic Tumours: 5-8%
5. Unclassified Tumours

Table 36.1 Risk Factors for Ovarian Cancer

- Age – between 45 and 60 years
- Nulliparous or of low parity
- Woman with previous PCOS, or on tamoxifen
- High-calorie, high-fat diet
- Genetic predisposition BRCA-1 and BRCA-2 gene mutation
- Late menopause
- Family history of breast and gastrointestinal cancers
- Multiple cycles of ovulation induction

Non epithelial ovarian tumours: These include malignancies of (i) germ cell origin, (ii) sex cord stromal cell origin, (iii) metastatic cancers and (iv) rare malignancies such as lipoid cell tumours, sarcomas.

EPITHELIAL CANCERS OF THE OVARY

Seventy-five per cent of epithelial cancers are of the serous histologic type, about 10% are mucinous and 12%–15% are endometrioid. Brenner tumour, clear cell carcinomas and undifferentiated cancers account for 1% or less each. Each tumour type has a histologic pattern similar to a part of the upper genital tract, e.g. serous or papillary (Figs 36.1–36.3) pattern resembles the lining of the fallopian tube, mucinous tumours have lining resembling the endocervical glands and the endometrioid tumours have a pattern resembling the endometrium.

As much as 50% of benign serous epithelial tumours undergo secondary malignant change, but only 5% mucinous cysts undergo malignant transformation.

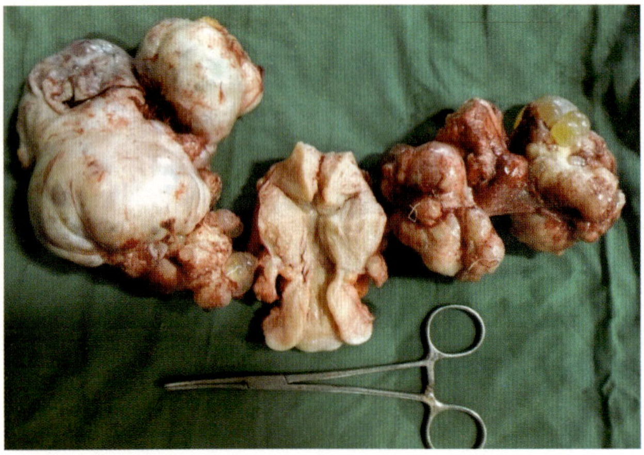

Figure 36.1 Bilateral papillary ovarian carcinoma.

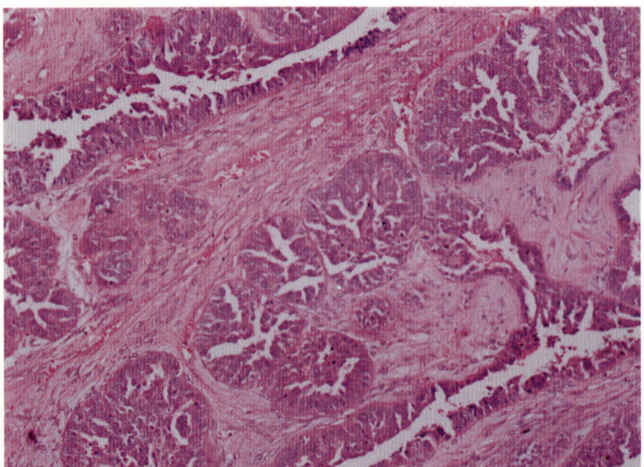

Figure 36.2 Serous carcinoma of the ovary: Tumour cells arranged in papillae and nests with marked nuclear atypia and the presence of stromal invasion. (*Courtesy*: Dr Sandeep Mathur, AIIMS.)

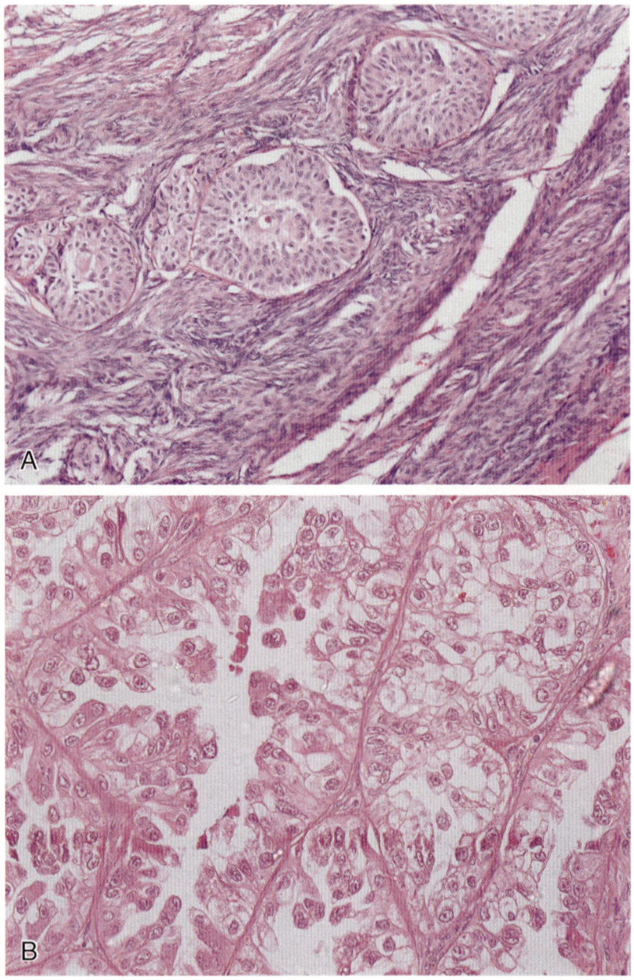

Figure 36.3 **(A)** Brenner tumour nests of transitional type cells within a fibromatous stroma. **(B)** Clear cell: Tumour cells arranged in a papillary and glandular pattern with moderate to abundant clear to eosinophilic cytoplasm, vesicular nucleus with prominent nucleoli and hob nailing. (*Courtesy*: Dr Sandeep Mathur, AIIMS.)

Ten to twenty per cent of these tumours are of low malignant potential (LMP) and are labelled as borderline tumours (Grade 0). They tend to remain confined to the ovaries for long and predominantly occur in the premenopausal age groups (30–50 years). They are associated with a good prognosis. Five-year survival is 90%. In contrast, invasive cancers are often seen in women aged 50–70 years, and they spread rapidly.

CRITERIA FOR DIAGNOSIS OF BORDERLINE TUMOURS (SEE ALSO CHAPTER 34 ON OVARIAN TUMOURS)

- Epithelial proliferation with papillary formations and pseudostratification.
- Nuclear atypia and increased mitotic activity.
- The absence of true stromal invasion.
- Borderline tumours can be either epithelial or mucinous variety (Fig. 36.4).

These tumours are described in the chapter on Ovarian Tumours. Only serous and mucinous epithelial tumours fall into this group of borderline ovarian tumours.

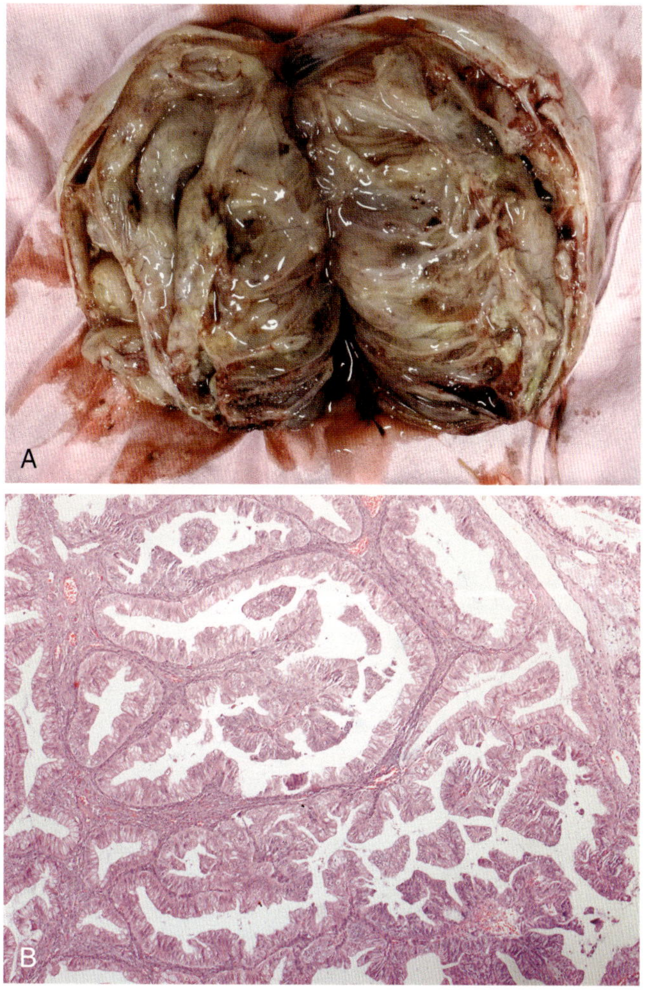

Figure 36.4 **(A)** Mucinous tumour of ovary. **(B)** Mucinous cystadenocarcinoma of ovary: Ovarian cyst lined by a single layer of mucinous cells. (*Courtesy*: Dr Sandeep Mathur, AIIMS.)

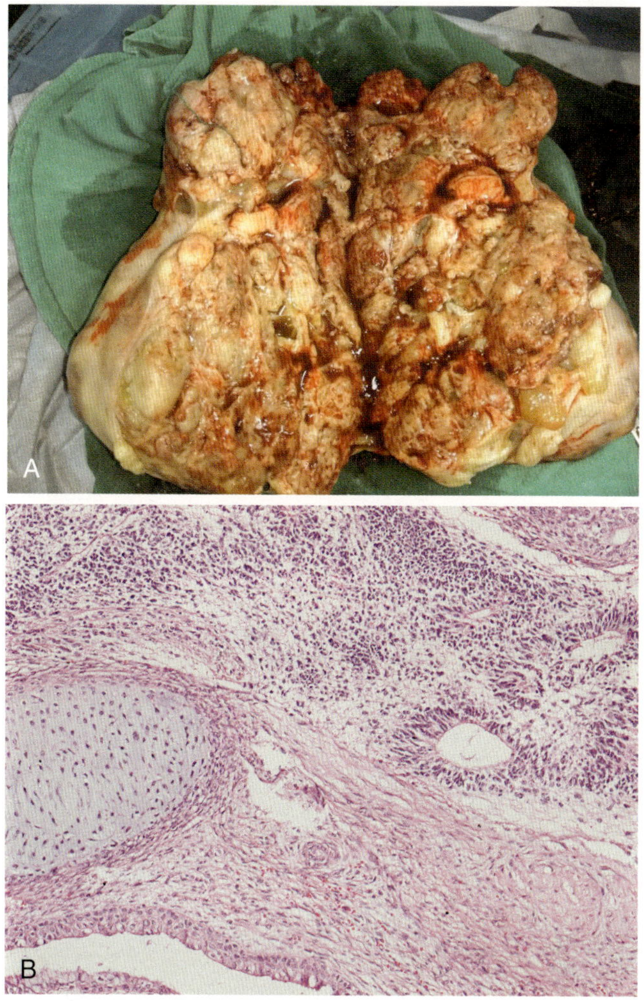

Figure 36.5 **(A)** Immature teratoma. **(B)** Immature teratoma: Tumour composed of mature elements (hyaline cartilage, glandular lining) as well as immature neuroectoderm.

NONEPITHELIAL MALIGNANCIES OF THE OVARY

Nonepithelial malignancies of the ovary account for 10%–20% of all malignancies of the ovary. The details of these types are as follows:

Germ cell malignancies are derived from the primordial germ cells of the ovary. These include:

- Dysgerminoma (refer to Chapter 35; Fig. 36.6)
- Teratoma; (a) mature, dermoid cyst, (b) immature – solid/cystic and (c) monodermal teratomas such as struma ovarii, carcinoid, mixed and others (Figs 36.5 and 36.8)
- Endodermal sinus tumour (Fig. 36.7)
- Embryonal carcinoma
- Polyembryoma
- Choriocarcinomas
- Mixed forms

GERM CELL TUMOURS

DYSGERMINOMA

Dysgerminoma are the commonest germ cell tumours of ovary. They account for 45-50% of all germ cell tumours. They are mostly seen in young adolescent girls, occasionally they may be seen in association with pregnancy. These tumour are female counterpart of seminomas same in boys. Most of these tumours do not produce any tumour marker, however, elevated levels of LDH and alkaline phosphate may be seen in most of these tumours. In 10-15% cases of dysgerminoma low level of HCG may be noted. Most of the tumours are unilateral but in 15-20% cases may be bilateral. In most cases tumour size is between 10-25 cm, rarely tumour can attain large size. This tumour has propensity to disseminate by lymphatic spread. In 5% of girls with dysgerminoma external genitalia may be ambiguous. Dysgerminoma can also occur in dysgenetic gonads, especially if chromosomal pattern is 46XY. At laparotomy tumour is found to be well and capsulated in most cases. At cut section tumour is predominantly solid with few cystic areas. The under microscope tumour consists of large cells arranged in groups of alveolar fashion. Lymphocytes and giant cells are diffusely present among tumour cells. Presence of large dark staining nucleus with clear cystoplasm and lymphocytic infiltration of fibrous septa is diagnostic of dysgerminoma.

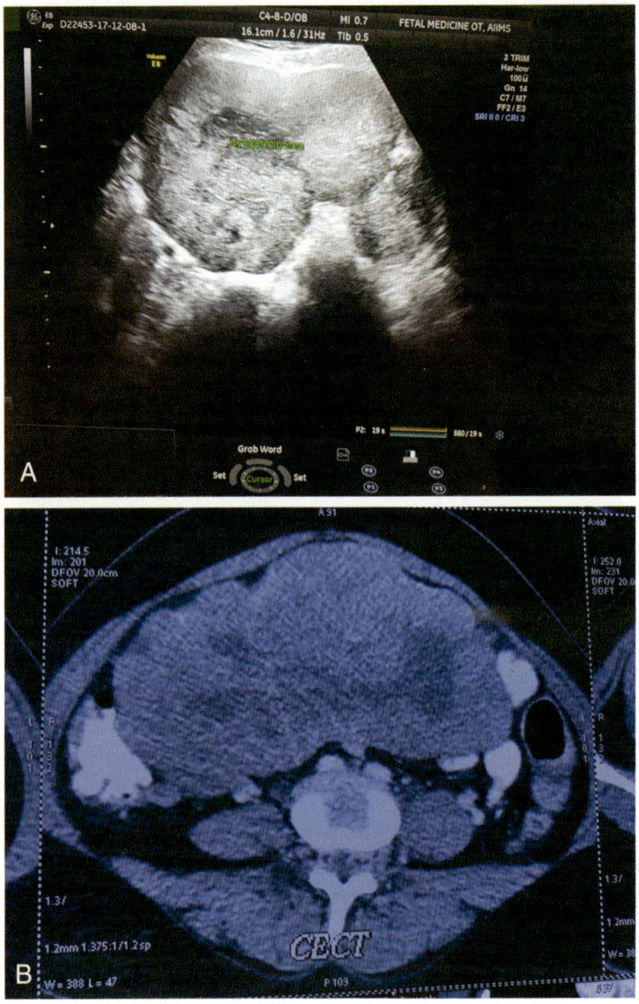

Figure 36.6 **(A)** Ultrasound appearance of dysgerminoma of the ovary showing solid tumour with mixed echogenicity. **(B)** CECT image of germ cell tumour of ovary showing a solid tumour with intact thick capsule.

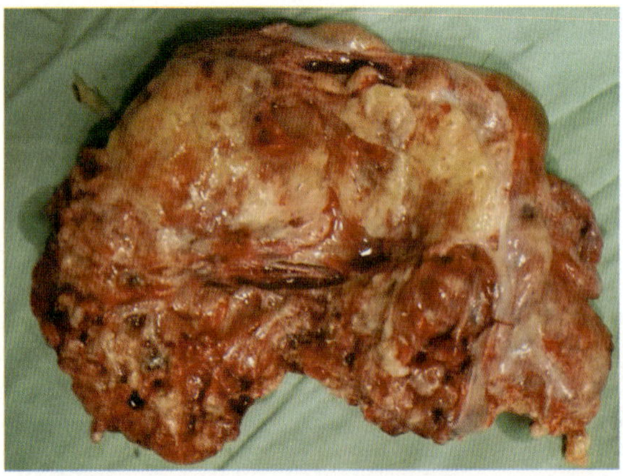

Figure 36.7 Endodermal sinus tumour of ovary.

Dysgerminomas are highly radiosensitive (though radiotherapy leads to future infertility). They also respond well to chemotherapy without interfering with future fertility and therefore chemotherapy is preferred.

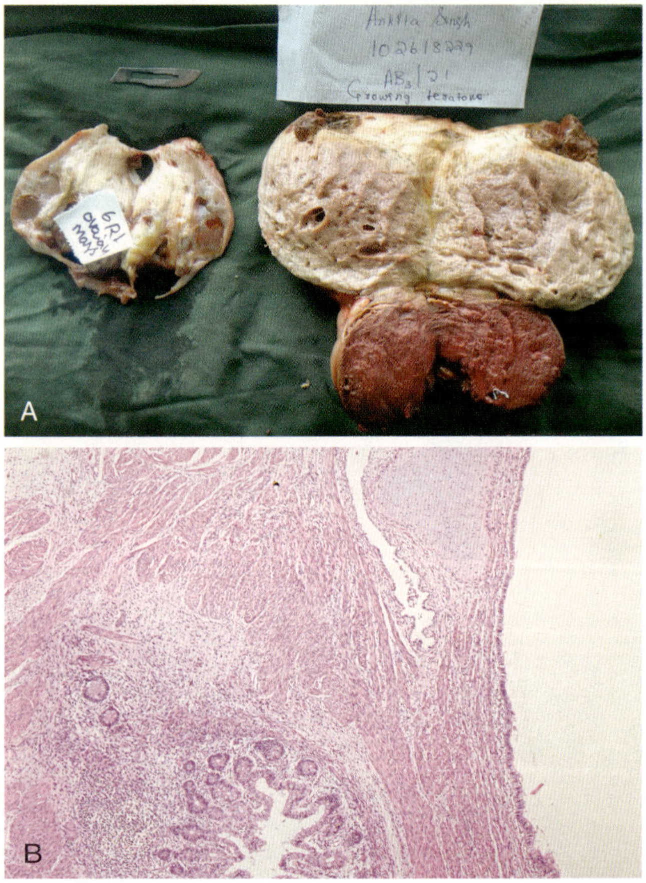

Figure 36.8 **(A)** Solid teratoma of the ovary. **(B)** Teratoma of ovary showing mesodermal (hyaline cartilage and smooth muscle) and endodermal (intestinal epithelium) elements. No immature component is seen. (*Courtesy*: Dr Sandeep Mathur, AIIMS.)

ENDODERMAL SINUS (YOLK SAC) TUMOUR

Endodermal tumour although a rare tumour is the second most common germ cell tumour. It is thought to **originate from a multipotent embryonal tissue** as a result of selective differentiation of yolk sac structures (Fig. 36.9). This explains why the tumour is rich in AFPs and alpha-l-antitrypsin. In most cases this tumour tend to be unilateral. Histologically, the tumour characteristically presents with papillary projections composed of a central core of blood vessels enveloped by immature epithelium. Intracellular and extracellular hyaline droplets are present in all tumours, **Schiller–Duval bodies**. The AFP content can be stained by immunoperoxidase techniques. Most of these patients are children or young women, presenting with abdominal pain and a pelvic mass. The tumours are known to grow rapidly. Although considered to be highly malignant, they respond to chemotherapy with good survival rate.

CHORIOCARCINOMA

Rarely seen in a pure form, generally choriocarcinoma is a part of a mixed germ cell tumour. Its origin as a teratoma can be confirmed in prepubertal girls, when the possibility of its gestational origin can be definitely excluded. The tumours are very vascular.

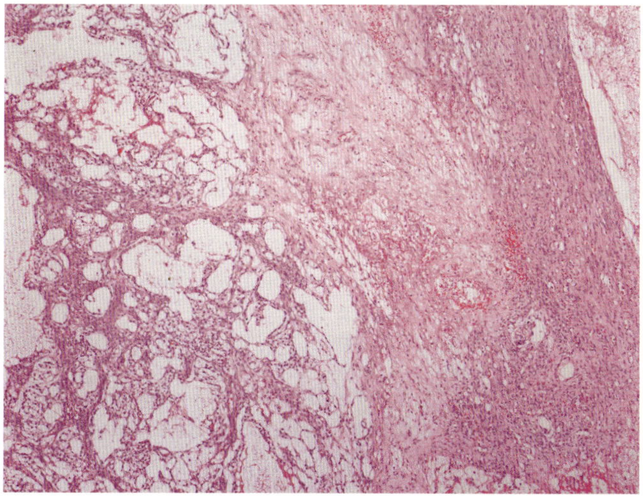

Figure 36.9 Yolk sac tumour: Tumour cells arranged in a reticular pattern in a loose, hypocellular stroma. (*Courtesy*: Dr Sandeep Mathur, AIIMS.)

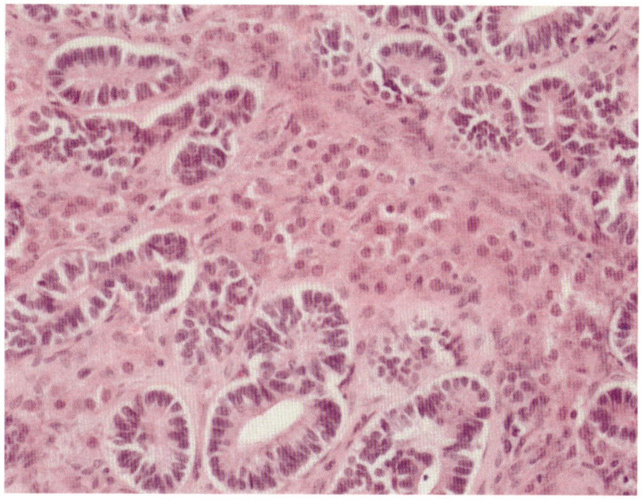

Figure 36.10 Arrhenoblastoma. (*Courtesy:* Dr Sandeep Mathur, AIIMS)

Histologically, the tumour shows a dimorphic population of syncytiotrophoblasts and cytotrophoblasts. It secretes large quantities of hCG hormone, which forms an ideal tumour marker in the diagnosis and management of the tumour. The tumour is highly malignant, and metastasizes by bloodstream to the lungs, brain, bones and other viscera.

EMBRYONAL CELL CARCINOMA

Embryonal cell carcinoma is a rare tumour accounting for about 5% of all germ cell tumours, and occurs in prepubertal girls. It elaborates both AFPs and chorionic gonadotropins. It is associated with the symptoms of precocious puberty and menstrual irregularities. It is highly malignant. The condition may be associated with fever due to torsion, rupture and haemorrhage.

CLINICAL FEATURES OF GERM CELL TUMOURS

Of all ovarian tumours 10-15% are germ cell tumours. Most of these tumours are malignant except mature cystic teratoma. The incidence of malignant germ cell tumours is lower in Caucasian whites, but threefold higher in Asians and Afro-Americans. Many of these secrete biochemical substances which are used as tumour markers; for example, embryonal carcinomas (AFP, hCG), endodermal sinus tumour (AFP) and choriocarcinoma (hCG). Dysgerminoma and pure germinomas do not secrete these markers, but secrete lactose dehydrogenase.

Although dysgerminomas are highly radiosensitive (though radiotherapy leads to future infertility). They also respond equally well to chemotherapy. In young patients use of chemotherapy is desirable for preserving future fertility and ovarian function.

SEX CORD STROMAL TUMOURS

Sex cord stromal tumours are either benign or malignant. The benign tumours are described in Chapter 35. These account for about 5%–8% of all ovarian malignancies. This group of ovarian neoplasms is derived from the sex cords and the ovarian stroma or mesenchyme. These tumours are composed of various combinations of cells consisting of 'female cells' (granulosa, theca cells) and 'male cells' (Sertoli, Leydig cells) as well as morphologically indifferent cells (Fig. 36.10). They are also called mesenchymomas. The tumours of clinical interest are the following.

GRANULOSA CELL TUMOURS

Granulosa cell tumours secrete oestrogens. Depending on the age of their appearance, they may cause precocious puberty. Menometrorrhagia and episodes of abnormal uterine bleeding (AUB) are not uncommon in women of childbearing age and postmenopausal bleeding in elderly women. Endometrial hyperplasia occurs in 25%–50% of patients, and endometrial carcinoma occurs in about 5% of cases. Theca cell tumour is more oestrogenic and more likely to cause endometrial cancer. A granulosa cell tumour secretes inhibin, a marker for this tumour. Often tumour has component of granulosa cell tumour and theca cell tumour. Hence, these tumours are also called as Theca Granulosa Cell Tumour.

ANDROBLASTOMAS OR ARRHENOBLASTOMAS (SERTOLI–LEYDIG CELL TUMOURS, Fig. 36.10)

Androblastomas or arrhenoblastomas occur commonly in the third and fourth decades of life. These tumours are very rare and account for 0.2% of all ovarian neoplasms. They secrete androgens and cause defeminization followed by masculinization. The women experience oligomenorrhoea followed by amenorrhoea, flattening of the breasts, acne, hirsutism, enlargement of the clitoris and finally a change in voice. On removal of the tumour, all the above changes reverse except voice change.

UNCOMMON OVARIAN CANCERS

Uncommon ovarian cancers comprise only 0.1% of all ovarian malignancies. The chief representative types in this subgroup are **lipid or lipoid cell tumour, sarcoma of the**

ovary and chorioepithelioma. The lipid cell variety arises from the adrenal cortical cell rests that reside in the vicinity of the ovary. These tumours are often benign or of low-grade malignancy. They may be associated with virilization, obesity, hypertension and glucose intolerance.

Malignant mixed mesodermal sarcomas are rare tumours of the ovary. They occur in postmenopausal women. The tumours are very aggressive and metastasize early. Chemotherapy offers the best hope.

SARCOMA

Ovarian sarcomas are rare. Many tumours labelled as sarcomas have been misdiagnosed histologically and are in reality granulosa cell tumours or anaplastic carcinomas. Sarcomas arise most frequently after menopause, particularly in multiparae. They give rise to multiple metastases. Rhabdomyosarcoma of the ovary has also been described.

METASTATIC CARCINOMAS

Ovarian metastases are commonly from the primary growth in the gastrointestinal tract, notably the pylorus, colon and, rarely, the small bowel; they occasionally occur from the gall bladder and pancreas. They may also occur in late carcinoma of the breast, as seen in 30% of all autopsy material from breast cancer. Carcinomas of the corpus (10%) and cervix (1%) also metastasize to the ovary owing to the close relationship of their lymphatic drainage. Carcinoma of the corpus is 10 times more likely to metastasize to the ovary than the cervix. The reason for this is that the ovarian lymphatics drain the corpus directly, whereas the cervical metastases tend to bypass the ovarian lymphatics and travel by way of the hypogastric and aortic glands. About 20% of clinically malignant ovarian tumours are secondary deposits from primary growths elsewhere. Two forms of secondary carcinoma of the ovary are recognized. In the first, the growth corresponds in its histology with the primary growth. Dissemination to the ovaries takes place either by implantation from metastases within the peritoneal cavity or by retrograde lymphatic spread. Both ovaries are replaced by solid carcinomas and multiple secondary deposits are usually disseminated over the peritoneum. A curious feature is that the ovarian tumours are much larger than the other secondary deposits, which is explained by assuming that the ovaries offer a much better environment for the growth of malignant cells than the other intraperitoneal viscera.

These secondary ovarian cancers have the following features. They are solid with irregular surface, and nearly always bilateral. Ascites is common and other obvious peritoneal metastases are present, notably in the omentum which is often replaced by an enormous solid malignant plaque. The method of ovarian infiltration is either by surface implantation or by retrograde lymphatic permeation. Both methods are probably operative, and histological examination is rarely able to reveal the route through which the metastases occurred.

The second type of secondary ovarian carcinoma is the Krukenberg tumour.

KRUKENBERG TUMOUR

This type of tumour should be diagnosed only if it conforms to the following pattern. Krukenberg tumours are almost bilateral. They have smooth surfaces which may be slightly bossed; they are freely movable in the pelvis (Fig. 36.12). There is no tendency to form adhesions with neighbouring viscera and there is no infiltration through the capsule. The tumour retains the shape of the normal ovary and has a peculiar solid waxy consistency although cystic spaces due to degeneration of the growth are common. **Histologically, the tumour has a cellular or myxomatous stroma amongst which are scattered large signet-ring cells.** These cells are ovoid in shape with a granular cytoplasm and the nucleus is compressed against one pole of the cell so that the outline of the cell resembles a signet ring (Fig. 36.11). The tumours are secondary growth in the ovary and most often arise from a primary carcinoma of the stomach (70%), large bowel (15%) and breast (6%). The Krukenberg tumour outstrips the primary growth in size, and unless the histology of the tumour is known, the case may be regarded as one of primary malignant ovarian carcinoma, particularly as the tumours are usually freely movable without obvious intraperitoneal metastases. The tumours almost certainly arise by retrograde lymphatic spread; the carcinoma cells pass from the stomach to the superior gastric lymphatic glands which also receive the lymphatics from the ovary. Retrograde lymphatic spread can be demonstrated in early cases when carcinoma cells are found infiltrating the ovary by way of the lymphatics in the medulla.

COINCIDENT CARCINOMA OF THE OVARIES AND THE BODY OF THE UTERUS (SYNCHRONOUS CARCINOMA)

Cases of coincident carcinoma of the ovaries and the body of the uterus are known. In some cases, the growth is primary in the body of the uterus and forms secondary deposits in the ovaries. In other cases, the primary growth is in the ovaries and secondary deposits reach the cavity of the uterus either by lymphatic permeation or by retrograde spread through the fallopian tube. Another group of cases is well-recognized in which the ovarian carcinomas are histologically different from the carcinoma of the body of the uterus. Any postmenopausal bleeding associated with an ovarian tumour should suggest the possibility of a coincident endometrial carcinoma, and this possibility always demands the removal of the uterus as well as the ovarian

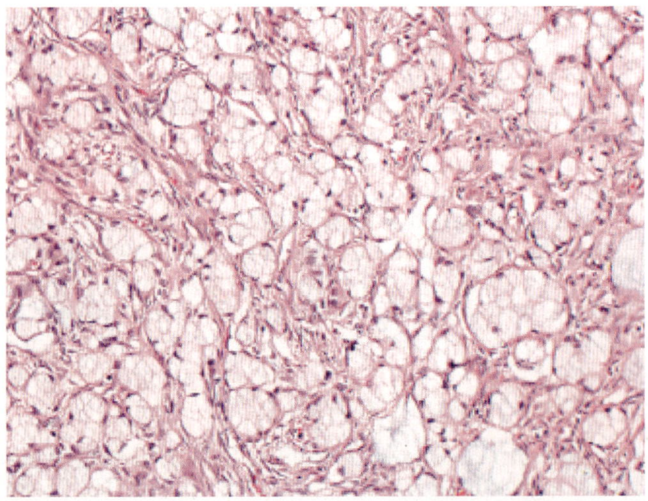

Figure 36.11 Microscopic appearance of Krukenberg tumour showing signet ring appearance of cells.

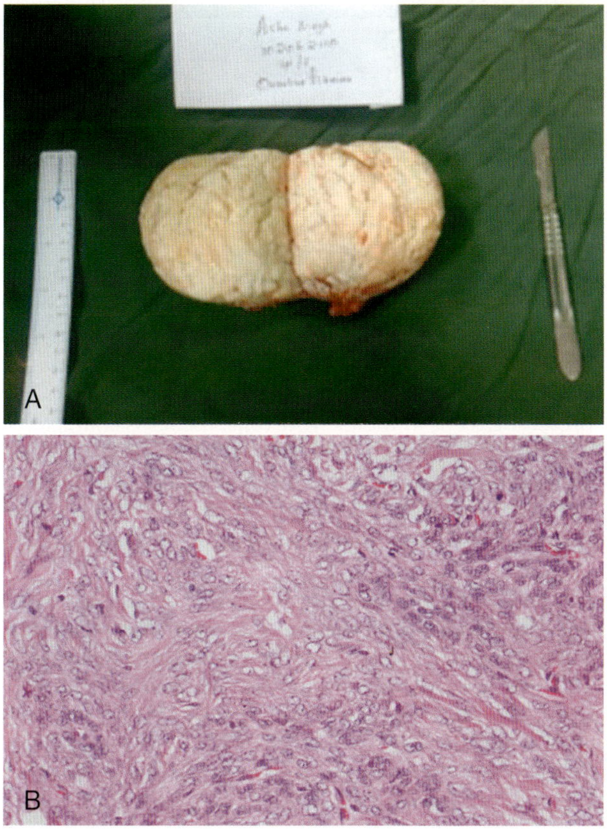

Figure 36.12 (A) Ovarian fibroma showing a solid tumour. **(B)** Histological appearance of Fibroma:Tumour comprises fascicles of spindled cells with mild nuclear atypia. Few collagen bundles are seen between the cells. (*Courtesy* for (B): Dr Sandeep Mathur, AIIMS.)

tumours. In case it becomes difficult to make out cyto primary tumours these cases are labelled as Synchronous carcinoma.

METASTASES IN THE UTERUS

Advanced carcinoma of the ovaries becomes adherent to the surrounding structures so that the uterus is directly infiltrated by the growth. The peritoneal surface of the uterus is also infiltrated in some cases by carcinoma cells disseminated over the peritoneum. In rare cases, metastases form in the endometrium as a result of carcinoma cells passing along the fallopian tube into the cavity of the uterus. In some cases of carcinoma of the ovaries, secondary deposits are formed in the vaginal walls, and such metastases correspond to those found in cases of chorioepithelioma and of carcinoma of the body of the uterus, when metastases form by retrograde lymphatic spread.

Direct spread of the tumours occurs in the pouch of Douglas, paracolic gutter, subdiaphragmatic on the right side, liver and peritoneal lining.

SPREAD BY WAY OF BLOODSTREAM

It is rare for carcinoma of the ovaries to spread by way of the bloodstream, but with very malignant tumours, metastases may be disseminated in this way. It is therefore important to obtain a chest radiograph in all cases with malignant ovarian tumours.

LYMPHATIC SPREAD

The regional lymphatic glands of the ovaries are the para-aortic and the superior gastric which are impalpable clinically. Sometimes, the malignant cells reach the mediastinal glands when they may ulcerate into the pleural cavity and cause pleural effusion. Sometimes, secondary deposits may be found above the left clavicular region, where they have arrived via the main lymphatic ducts in the mediastinum. Once the peritoneum is involved, pelvic lymph nodes will be infiltrated with metastases.

METASTASES IN OPERATION SCARS

It is not uncommon after the removal of malignant ovarian tumours for metastases to form in the operation scar and to spread to the adjacent skin. This may be more common with laparoscopic surgery.

BILATERAL CHARACTER OF OVARIAN TUMOURS

Seventy per cent of primary ovarian cancers are bilateral, whereas nearly all secondary growths are bilateral. Both ovaries may be involved in 16% benign tumours. Even with malignant ovarian tumours, the two ovaries are involved simultaneously by the disease and the involvement of one by secondary deposits from the other is exceptional. With secondary ovarian carcinomas, if the involvement is by retrograde lymphatic spread, one would expect both ovaries to be involved simultaneously. Similar may be the pathogenesis when implantation of carcinoma cells is the cause of development of secondary deposits in the ovaries.

The most important metastases of malignant ovarian tumours are those which form on the peritoneum and lead to the development of large tumours in the omentum. The secondary deposits of carcinoma of the ovaries rarely involve the liver, because the ovarian vessels belong to the systemic system and not to the portal system like those of the intestine and stomach.

CLINICAL FEATURES

The clinical features are usually nonspecific in early stages, resulting in late diagnosis in 70% cases. A woman with malignant ovarian tumour is usually a post menopausal woman of low parity. A family history of breast or ovarian tumour may be relevant.

Initially, the woman is asymptomatic. Initial symptoms are in the form of fullness of abdomen after meals, alteration in bowel habits or vague pain abdomen. These symptoms often make woman to visit general physician or gastroenterologist or a surgeon. This results in delay in diagnosis of carcinoma ovary in early stages.

The malignant ovarian tumours are often bilateral, solid and present with ascites. The benign tumour that cause ascites (Meigs syndrome) are ovarian fibroma (Fig. 36.13), Brenner tumour and rarely granulosa cell tumour. The tumours are often fixed in the late stage and intraperitoneal metastasis may be palpable abdominally.

The vaginal examination may reveal fixed nodules in the pouch of Douglas, apart from adnexal masses felt separate from the uterus.

Unilateral nonpitting oedema of the leg, pleural effusion and enlarged liver are suggestive of the advanced stage of the disease. *Peritoneal tuberculosis mimics ovarian cancer with raised CA-125.*

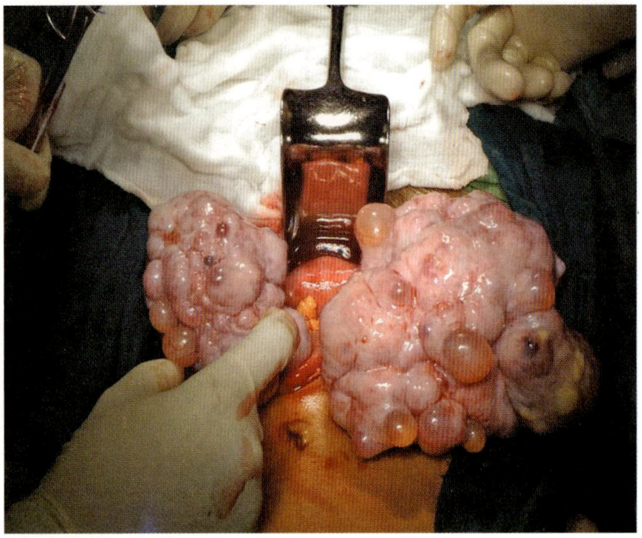

Figure 36.13 Krukenberg tumour of both ovaries. The tumour has an intact capsule and surface free of all adhesion.

SCREENING FOR OVARIAN CANCER

There is no satisfactory screening for ovarian malignant tumour. CA-125 and ultrasound have low detection rates in picking up the tumour (Table 36.2). However, a high-risk woman should be under observation. A palpable ovary in a menopausal woman is likely to be malignant and should be investigated.

In a woman with family history of ovarian or breast cancer, screening of ovarian cancer should be carried out by periodic ultrasound for ovaries and CA-125.

INVESTIGATIONS

The investigations to confirm the diagnosis and nature of the tumour are described in the chapter 35. Following investigations are commonly done to diagnose ovarian cancer:

- Ultrasound shows a solid tumour with echogenic or cystic areas, a thick capsule with papillary projectors and a thick septum measuring more than 5 mm in a malignant tumour. The other ovary may be enlarged or bilateral tumours seen. An endometrial lining more than 4 mm in thickness with papillary projections in a perimenopausal woman is seen in a feminizing tumour and if endometrial secondaries are present. Except in Meigs syndrome, ascites is characteristic of a malignant tumour. 3D ultrasound is useful.
- Tissue markers mentioned earlier suggest the histological nature of the tumour, as well as decide the duration of postoperative chemotherapy or need for radiotherapy. CA-125 is raised in epithelial tumours.
- CT and MRI indicate the extent of the tumour spread.
- Barium meal, barium enema and breast examination are required when metastatic tumour is suspected. X-ray of chest and liver scan are required to detect metastatic growth.
- Doppler ultrasound showing a low pulsatile index less than 1 and a resistance index less than 0.4 suggest malignancy. In a benign tumour, blood flow and vascularity is from the periphery to the centre. In a malignant tumour, neovascularity is initiated in the centre of the tumour.
- D&C is required if the woman develops postmenopausal bleeding.
- Tissue markers.
  - CEA more than 5 ng/mL (normal 2.5–5 ng/mL) is reported in endometrioid, Brenner tumour, mucinous tumour, colonic, liver, breast and lung metastasis.

Table 36.2 FIGO Staging for Carcinoma of the Ovary: 2014

State I: Tumour Confined to Ovaries
IA: Tumour limited to one ovary, capsule intact, no tumour or surface, negative peritoneal washing IB: Tumour involves both ovaries, otherwise like IA IC: Tumour limited to one/both ovaries IC1: Surgical spill IC2: Capsule rupture before surgery or tumour on ovarian surface IC3: Malignant cells in ascetic or peritoneal washing
Stage II: Tumour Involves One or Both Ovaries with Pelvic Extension (Below Pelvic Brim) or Primary Peritoneal Cancer
IIA: Extension and/or implants on the uterus and fallopian tube IIB: Extension to other pelvic intraperitoneal tissue
Stage III: Tumour Involves One or Both Ovaries with Cytologically or Histologically Confirmed Spread to the Peritoneum Outside the Pelvis and/or Metastasis to Retroperitoneal Lymph Node
IIIA: Positive retroperitoneal lymph node only IIIA1: (i) Metastasis < 10 mm (ii) Metastasis > 10 mm IIIA2: Microscopic extrapelvic peritoneal involvement + positive retroperitoneal lymph node IIIB: Macroscopic extrapelvic, peritoneal metastasis > 2 cm + positive retroperitoneal lymph node, extension to capsule of liver/spleen
Stage IV: Distant Metastasis
IVA: Pleural effusion with positive cytology IVB: **Hepatic and/or splenic parenchymal metastasis, metastasis to extra-**abdominal organs (inguinal lymph node, lymph node outside abdomen)

Source: FIGO guidelines.

- CA-125 is a glycoprotein surface antigen raised in 80% epithelial tumours, but is not very specific, as it is also raised in abdominal tuberculosis and endometriosis as well. It is normal in 50% Stage I epithelial carcinoma. Some have observed raised CA-125 levels, 18 months to 3 years before clinical detection of malignant ovarian tumours.
- AFP, hCG, NB/70K, placental alkaline phosphatase and lactase dehydrogenase (1000 U/L) are the tissue markers for germ cell tumours. Inhibin is raised in granulosa cell tumour. NB/70K is a glycoprotein raised in 60% epithelial tumours (above 11 kU/mL), but also seen in liver and renal failure. The tissue markers are useful during chemotherapy to decide the response and the duration of therapy in postoperative follow-up. Recently CA - 19.9 and HE-4 are being utilised as tumour markers for making diagnosis of ovarian cancer.
- Fine-needle aspiration cytology (FNAC) and ascitic fluid cytology yield a high false-negative report.
- CT and MRI diagnose dermoid, endometriosis and extent of spread of ovarian malignancy as well as assess lymph node involvement. Because these only pick up lymph nodes enlarged more than 1 cm, some employ lymphography if CT and MRI give negative lymph node involvement, because lymphography can pick up nodes as small as 5 mm.
- Debulking surgery is undertaken even in the advanced stages, so diagnostic laparoscopy has lost its importance.

SURGICAL TREATMENT OF CARCINOMA OVARY

MANAGEMENT OF EPITHELIAL OVARIAN CANCER

Most patients need a combined modality of treatment, maximum possible debulking surgery followed by chemotherapy. In most cases, surgery is the initial step in the management, it provides opportunity to know stage of the disease, exact spread of the disease and also helps in removing maximum possible amount of the disease from abdomen and pelvis. Such a surgical procedure is called **debulking surgery (cytoreductive surgery).** Prognosis depends on amount of residual disease left at the end of cytoreductive surgery. Following are the standard steps followed while operating a case of carcinoma ovary.

STEPS OF SURGERY FOR OVARIAN CANCER

1. Open abdomen by vertical midline incision.
2. Obtain ascetic fluid for cytology. If ascites is absent peritoneal washings are obtained by instilling 200 mL of saline in pelvis and aspirating this fluid with a disposable syringe.
3. Evaluate extent of disease: By careful inspection of all pelvic and abdominal organs try to make out extent of the disease. Make special efforts to feel liver surface, subdiaphragmatic area, stomach, spleen, small intestine, large bowel, surface of bladder and the pouch of Douglas.
4. Obtain small peritoneal biopsy from subdiaphragmatic area, right and left paracolic gutters, surface of bladder and the pouch of Douglas.
5. Perform total abdominal hysterectomy with bilateral salpingo-oophorectomy.
6. Perform intracolic omentectomy.
7. Obtain lymph nodes from pelvic and paracolic area for sampling.
8. Remove any other structure which may be involved by the disease.
9. At the end of surgery make a careful note of tumour which is left in spite of maximum possible surgical effort (Residual tumour).

CONSERVATIVE SURGERY FOR EPITHELIAL OVARIAN CANCER

On rare occasion if one finds cancer limited to one or both ovaries in a young patient who is desirous of pregnancy in future, a conservative surgical approach in the form of **unilateral salpingo-oophorectomy** or bilateral salpingo-oophorectomy with preservation of the uterus can be carried out. Such patients if remain disease free for 2 years or more during follow-up can be allowed to attempt pregnancy spontaneously or by IVF approach.

INTERVAL DEBULKING SURGERY

On occasions where a newly diagnosed case of carcinoma ovary is found to have advance disease and is considered unfit for anaesthesia on account of a coexisting cardiac, respiratory or other disease, these patients are managed by initially giving three cycles of chemotherapy (Paclitaxel + Carboplatin) at the three weekly intervals followed by debulking surgery. Such a surgical procedure is called 'interval debulking surgery'. By such an approach, often general condition of patients improves, ascites reduces and she becomes fit for anaesthesia and surgery. A patient managed by this approach gets remaining chemotherapy (three cycles) after surgery.

SECONDARY DEBULKING SURGERY

If a treated case of carcinoma ovary develops recurrence, she can be managed by a second operation with the aim of removing recurrences. However, with wide spread recurrences treatment with the second-line chemotherapy is usually the preferred approach.

PROGNOSIS

Ovarian cancers are one of the most lethal tumours. In spite of maximum possible surgery and chemotherapy, a great majority of women experience recurrences and may die subsequently of disease recurrences. Although recurrence rates depend on stage of disease at diagnosis, surgical procedure and chemotherapy, but up to 80% patients experience recurrences within 3 years. Following Table 36.3 shows stagewise 5-year survival rates.

CHEMOTHERAPY FOR OVARIAN CARCINOMA

After initial surgical management almost all cases need 'adjuvant chemotherapy'. Only patients who can be kept on follow-up by avoiding postoperative chemotherapy are the ones who had Stage Ia disease. Patients who were reported to have 'borderline ovarian malignancy' on histopathology are also kept on follow-up only without giving any chemotherapy.

Table 36.3 FIGO Staging and 5-Year Survival Rate in Carcinoma Ovary

Staging	5 year Survival Rate
Stage I:	90%
Ia:	94%
Ib:	92%
Ic:	85%
Stage II:	70%
IIa:	78%
IIb:	73%
Stage III:	39%
IIIa:	59%
IIIb:	52%
IIIc:	39%
Stage IV:	17%

DRUGS USED FOR CHEMOTHERAPY

In the past, several chemotherapy drugs either given singly or in combination have been tried with variable success rates. Currently most commonly used combination of drugs in the treatment of epithelial ovarian cancers is Paclitaxel + Carboplatin. These drugs are given intravenously every 3 weeks for six cycles. Doses and side effects of these two drugs are given below:

Paclitaxel: Dose 175 mg/m^2, intravenously over 3 hours.
Main side effect: Neurotoxicity.

Carboplatin: Dose is calculated by area under curve (AUC) which is generally taken as 5–6. However, in subjects with compromised renal function a smaller dose is given.
Side effects: Nephrotoxicity, bone marrow suppression.

OTHER CHEMOTHERAPY REGIMENS

1. Paclitaxel 80 mg/m^2 every weekly + Carboplatin every three weekly.
2. Paclitaxel 60 mg/m^2 + Carboplatin AUC-2 given weekly.
3. Docetaxel 60–75 mg/m^2 + Carboplatin AUC 5–6 every three weekly.

NEWER DRUGS FOR TREATMENT OF EPITHELIAL OVARIAN CANCER

In case patient is found to be platinum resistant, following newer drugs can be used:

1. Topotecan 1.5 mg/m^2/day × 5 days
2. Pegylated liposomal doxorubicin (PLD) 50 mg/m^2 orally × 28 days.
3. Gemcitabine 1000 mg/m^2 on day 1, 8 and 15.
4. Nanoparticle albumin bound Paclitaxel (Nab-paclitaxel)
5. Etoposide 50 mg/m^2 orally × 21 days
6. Trabectedin 1300 mcg/m^2 over 3 hours every three weekly.
7. Bevacizumab (Avastin): It is an anti-angiogenic 'Human Monoclonal Antibody to VGEF (vascular growth endothelial factor)'. It is not chemotherapy, but addition of this agent to the standard chemotherapy helps in improving result of chemotherapy. This new approach has been tested in ovarian cancers and is being tried in other tumours also (breast cancer). Drug is initially given weekly for 20-21 cycles, but can be extended up to 22 weeks. At present, high cost of treatment with bevacizumab prevents its routine usage.

FOLLOW-UP OF EPITHELIAL OVARIAN CANCERS

Cases of epithelial ovarian cancers treated by surgery and chemotherapy are seen at regular interval of 3 months for initial 2 years and subsequently every 6 month for next 3 years for any recurrences. Clinical examination and serum CA-125 every 3 months help in detection of recurrences. Imaging studies are carried out in case of any suspicion of recurrences.

GERM CELL TUMOURS OF OVARY

Germ cell tumours of the ovary comprise 5%–10% of all ovarian malignancies. They tend to arise from germ cells with the ovary. Although they originate from the ovary, they differ from epithelial ovarian cancers in many respects. Most often these tumours are seen in young adolescent girls, it is rare to find these tumours after the age of 25 years. Most of these tumours are usually fast growing and highly malignant, yet with timely diagnosis and appropriate surgical management good outcome can be expected. Currently postoperative management of these patients with chemotherapy in the form of Bleomycin Etoposide-Cisplatin (BEP) has almost ensured cure for these tumours. With effective and timely chemotherapy, most of these young girls can be expected to resume their normal menstrual function and achieve reproductive outcome in the form of normal live births.

STAGING SYSTEM

For staging of germ cell tumours of the ovary, same staging system as given by International Federation of Gynaecology and Obstetrics(FIGO) of ovarian cancer (2014) is followed.

PREOPERATIVE WORK UP

In addition to commonly done investigation such as haemogram, chest X-ray, imaging of abdomen by ultrasound and CT/MRI; a panel of tests including hCG, AFP and LDH are conducted. These investigations help in knowing type of germ cell tumour. Raised AFP is noted in yolk sac tumours, raised hCG points towards choriocarcinoma. Raised LDH is noted in dysgerminomas. A combination of tumour markers, when raised, points towards the possibility of embryonal carcinoma or mixed germ cell tumour.

SURGICAL MANAGEMENT

Surgery is the first line of treatment in most cases of ovarian germ cell tumours. Majority of cases are young girls, so preservation of the uterus and normal ovary or ovarian tissue is desirable. With a careful approach and surgical efforts it is always possible to preserve normal-looking ovarian tissue in one or both ovaries.

SURGICAL STEPS

Same surgical steps are followed as described for epithelial ovarian cancers.

1. Vertical midline abdominal incision.
2. Peritoneal washings/ascites fluid for cytology.
3. Exploration of abdominal and pelvic organs.
4. Unilateral salpingo-oophorectomy with preservation of the uterus and normal-looking ovary.
5. Pelvic and para-aortic lymph node sampling.
6. Infracolic omentectomy
7. Removal of any other tumour mass in the abdomen

CHEMOTHERAPY

All patients with germ cell tumours of ovary need postoperative chemotherapy with the exception of Stage Ia dysgerminoma. Bleomycin-Etoposide-Platinum (BEP) regimen as given below is the best regiment for germ cell tumours of ovary.

BEP Regimen
Bleomycin 15 mg i.v. on day 1, 2
Etoposide 100 mg/m^2 on day 1–5
Cisplatin 20 mg/m^2 i.v. on day 1–5

Follow-up: All treated case of ovarian germ cell tumours are followed by three monthly by clinical examination, tumour markers for initial 2 years.

SEX CORD STROMAL TUMOURS

Sex cord stromal tumours are uncommon. They comprise 3%–5% of all ovarian tumours. They can occur in any age group. These tumours by virtue of excess production of female sex hormones or male sex hormones are easy to diagnose. They mostly are small sized (5–15 cm) and tend to grow slowly. In most cases, surgery alone is the treatment except those which have metastasize or are recurrent. Their symptoms may vary depending on the age group in which they occur. Granulosa cell tumours which are associated with excess production of oestrogen may cause precocious puberty in young premenarchal girl; it may cause menstrual irregularities such as menorrhagia, in a woman in a reproductive age and cause postmenopausal bleeding in women with excess production of inhibin A. Similarly, male hormone–producing sex cord tumours (Sertoli–Leydig Cell tumours) may cause features of defeminization followed by masculinization in the form of breast atrophy, change in voice, amenorrhoea, hirsutism and clitoromegaly. If suspected diagnosis is easily made based on levels of sex hormones and imaging.

STAGING SYSTEM

A similar staging system as given for epithelial ovarian cancers is used. In most cases, disease is unilateral limited to ovary.

SURGICAL TREATMENT

Surgery remains the cornerstone of treatment. Removal of ovary harbouring tumour will suffice in most cases. However, in case of bilateral tumours or tumours with spread to other structures an operative procedure on the lines of epithelial ovarian cancers is carried out in the form of total abdominal hysterectomy with bilateral salpingo-oophorectomy and infracolic omentectomy.

CHEMOTHERAPY

Early stage cases are usually kept on follow-up and do not require adjuvant chemotherapy. However, for the advanced disease and for recurrences chemotherapy can be considered. Both regimens (Paclitaxel + Carboplatin) and BEP have been used. However, a response to chemotherapy varies and is not as good as for germ cell tumours.

Prognosis: Most patients have early stage disease at diagnosis and have good prognosis. However in the advanced disease and recurrences prognosis is compromised.

FALLOPIAN TUBE CANCER

Cancer of the fallopian tubes is rarest of all genital tract malignancies. More often the fallopian tubes are involved by extension of disease from ovaries or uterus. Primary carcinoma of the fallopian tube is uncommon and accounts for only 0.3% of all cancers of the female genital tract, though metastatic growths from the uterus, ovaries and gastrointestinal tract are common.

The tumour is bilateral in one-third of cases when it resembles a pyosalpinx or tubercular lesion. The tumour is often an adenocarcinoma though choriocarcinoma may develop in a tubal ectopic pregnancy or in a tubal mole. The tumour is highly malignant and spreads rapidly to the surrounding areas, and via lymphatics to the pelvic organs. Very often, the tumour is in the advanced stage when diagnosed and mostly it is diagnosed only on a histological study after the surgery.

The distal portion of the tube is the common site of cancer.

Staging of fallopian tube carcinoma (FIGO)

Stage	*Description*
0	Carcinoma *in situ* (limited to tubal mucosa)
I	Growth limited to fallopian tubes
IA	Growth limited to one tube with extension into the submucosa and/or muscularis but not penetrating the serosal surface; no ascites
IB	Growth limited to both tubes with extension into the submucosa and/or muscularis but not penetrating the serosal surface; no ascites
IC	Tumour either stage IA or IB with tumour extension through or onto the tubal serosa; or with ascites present containing malignant cells or positive peritoneal washings
II	Growth involving one or both fallopian tubes with pelvic extension
IIA	Extension and/or metastasis to the uterus and/or ovaries

Continued

IIB	Extension to other pelvic tissues
IIC	Tumour either stage IIA or IIB with ascites present containing malignant cells or with positive peritoneal washings
III	Tumour involves one or both fallopian tubes with peritoneal implants outside the pelvis and/or positive retroperitoneal or inguinal nodes; superficial liver metastasis equals stage III; tumour appears limited to true pelvis but with histologically proven malignant extension to the small bowel or omentum
IIIA	Tumour grossly limited to the true pelvis with negative nodes but with histologically confirmed microscopic seeding of abdominal peritoneal surfaces
IIIB	Tumour involving one or both tubes with histologically confirmed implants of abdominal peritoneal surfaces, none >2 cm in diameter; lymph nodes are negative
IIIC	Abdominal implants >2 cm in diameter and/or retroperitoneal or inguinal nodes
IV	Growth involving one or both fallopian tubes with distant metastases; if pleural effusion is present, there must be positive cytology to be stage IV; parenchymal liver metastases equals stage IV

STAGING

Erez classification of the fallopian tube cancer is as follows:

- Stage I: The tumour is limited to the mucosa and muscle.
- Stage IIA: The serosa is breached, but the tumour has not spread to other organs.
- Stage IIB: The tumour invades the pelvic organs.
- Stage III: Metastasis outside the pelvis, but within the abdominal cavity.
- Stage IV: Extraabdominal metastasis is present. Para-aortic lymph nodes are involved in the advanced stages.

CLINICAL FEATURES

The tumour occurs in menopausal women, 50% of these women are nulliparous. The early symptom is a watery discharge per vaginum, which may at times be amber coloured. Sooner or later, postmenopausal bleeding develops. A lump may be too small to be felt on clinical examination. Pain is a late symptom. A fallopian tube carcinoma may be suspected in a woman with a persistent excessive vaginal discharge where pap smear shows abnormal cells, but evaluation of cervix and endometrium does not reveal any abnormal area. In such a situation, the presence of a small adnexal mass should strongly raise possibility; a rare situation of the fallopian tube carcinoma. In most cases, diagnosis of the fallopian tube carcinoma comes as a surprise at laparotomy being conducted for a diagnosis of ovarian pathology.

DIFFERENTIAL DIAGNOSIS

The condition is often mistaken for uterine or ovarian malignancy, and tubercular adnexal mass.

INVESTIGATIONS

The clinical diagnosis is difficult and often missed.

- Pap smear: The adenomatous cancer cells are very rarely seen and Pap smear screening is unreliable.
- Uterine curettings are negative in postmenopausal bleeding so also hysteroscopic examination. Negative curettings in postmenopausal bleeding should arouse the suspicion of the fallopian tube malignancy.
- Laparoscopy shows adnexal mass.
- Ultrasound showing an adnexal mass in a postmenopausal woman with postmenopausal bleeding suggesting tubal cancer.
- Doppler flow velocity shows low-resistance blood flow.
- Sometimes serum level of CA-125 is raised in adenocarcinoma.

MANAGEMENT

Surgical staging is important. In operable cases, surgery is similar to that of ovarian malignancy and consists of hysterectomy, bilateral salpingo-oophorectomy, pelvic lymph node sampling and omentectomy.

Postoperative radiotherapy, chemotherapy and progestogen hormonal therapy are often required.

PROGNOSIS

Prognosis is poor and overall 5-year cure rate is 25%.

- Stage I survival is 60%.
- Stage II survival is 40%.
- In the advanced stage, survival is 10%.

KEY POINTS

- Epithelial ovarian tumours are the commonest tumours, and account for 80% of all ovarian malignant tumours.
- Borderline epithelial tumours with low malignant potential occur in younger women, and respond well to the conservative surgery.
- Germ cell tumours of ovary produce tumour markers such as hCG, AFP and LDH making diagnosis easy.
- The common malignant tumours in adolescents are dysgerminoma, teratoma, embryonal tumours and granulosa cell tumour. The conservative surgery followed by chemotherapy yields good results and retains fertility potential in young women.
- Primary surgery followed by postoperative chemotherapy is the cornerstone in the management of epithelial ovarian malignant tumours. Hysterectomy, bilateral salpingo-oophorectomy and omentectomy are the standard surgical procedure. Some include lymphadenectomy as well.
- Chemotherapy (Paclitaxel + Carboplatin) is most preferred regimen given three weekly for six cycles.
- In an advanced stage, a 3-weekly course of chemotherapy followed by debulking surgery has improved the outcome and survival rate.

- A woman with genital cancer also needs guidance in nutrition, pain relief and psychological support.
- In case of bilateral ovarian malignant tumours in young women, conservation of the uterus will enable pregnancy by oocyte donor and IVF.
- PET and CT improve the early diagnosis in detecting location and recurrence of the tumour, and assessing the response to chemotherapy.
- The gold standard is abdominal hysterectomy and bilateral salpingo-oophorectomy with omentectomy in the early and operable cases of ovarian cancer. Debulking and chemotherapy prolong life and duration of remission.
- Primary fallopian tube cancer is very rare and is difficult to differentiate from ovarian and endometrial cancers clinically. Prognosis is poor.

SELF-ASSESSMENT

1. Describe the clinical features of malignant ovarian tumours.
2. Discuss the management of malignant ovarian tumour.
3. A 50-year-old woman presents with postmenopausal bleeding, abdominal pain and a lump in the lower abdomen. Discuss the differential diagnosis and management.
4. A 10-year-old girl is brought with abdominal pain and a lump felt during the last 1 month. Discuss the differential diagnosis and management.
5. Short notes on:
   - Teratomas Krukenberg tumour
   - Borderline ovarian tumour

SUGGESTED READING

Bonnar J (ed). Recent Advances in Obstetrics and Gynaecology, Paul Donnellan and David Fennelly. In: Recent advances in ovarian cancer. 20: 179, 1999.

Bonnar J (ed). Recent Advances in Obstetrics and Gynaecology 16: 357, 2005.

Duncan J, Shulman P. Yearbook of Obstetrics, Gynaecology and Women's Health 2010.

Jonathan S (ed). Gynecologic Oncology, Berek and Hackers.12: 530, 2015.

Studd J. Progress in Obstetrics and Gynaecology. In: P Norman, P Schwartz. Prophylactic oophorectomy in BRCA carrier Vol 17: 369, 2007.

37 Vulval and Vaginal Cancer

CHAPTER OUTLINE

CANCERS OF THE GENITAL TRACT

Genital tract cancers are important in gynaecology because of the high mortality, morbidity and shortening of lifespan in women. The detection of the preinvasive and microinvasive stages and the near-100% survival by the conservative surgery now adds to the success story of genital tract cancers. Although breast cancer predominates in the developed countries, genital tract cancers remain the main killers in developing countries, including India.

Table 37.1 shows that cancer of the cervix holds the prime position in developing countries, followed by that of the uterus, ovary, vulva, fallopian tube and vagina in that order of frequency and forms a major health problem despite it being potentially preventable.

Burden of gynaecologic and breast cancers in Southeast Asia: Nandakumar A et al. (2000) reviewed the cancer burden amongst women living in the Indian subcontinent. Their findings have been briefly shown in Table 37.2 for a quick comparison.

Table 37.2 shows that cancer of the cervix continues to be the leading cause of cancer in our subcontinent. Breast cancer comes up as the second most common cancer, except in Pakistan, where breast cancer leads the list of cancers in women. Fortunately, both these cancers are amenable to early diagnosis and cure.

Table 37.1 Incidence of Genital Tract Cancers in Developed and Developing Countries

Organ	Developed Countries	Developing Countries
Cervix	60%	80%
Uterus	25%–30%	5%
Ovary	10%	10%–15%
Vulva	4%–5%	1%–5%
Fallopian tube	0.3%–0.5%	0.3%
Vagina	0.2%	0.2%

Table 37.2 Common Gynaecologic Cancers and Breast Cancer in Southeast Asian Countries

Cancer Site	India (ASR)	Pakistan (ASR)	Bangladesh (ASR)	Sri Lanka (ASR)
Cervix	30.7	6.5	27.6	28.8
Corpus uteri	<1.5	5.8	<1.5	<1.5
Ovary	4.9	9.8	3.3	5.1
Breast	19.1	50.1	16.6	19.3
Others	<1.0	<1.0	<1.0	<1.0

ASR, age-standardized rates per 100,000 female population.

CANCER OF VULVA

Cancer of the vulva is a rare entity and accounts for 1%–5% of all genital tract cancers. In developing countries incidence is lower as compared to rich countries.

Malignant tumours of the vulva are grouped as follows:

1. **Preinvasive lesions**—intraepithelial cancer usual type VIN and Differentiated VIN
   Bowen disease
   Paget disease
   Microinvasive
   Melanoma in situ
   } Intraepithelial carcinomas

2. **Invasive lesions**
   - Squamous cell carcinoma – most common 90%
   - Melanoma 1%–5%
   - Adenocarcinoma 1%
   - Sarcoma 2%
   - Rodent ulcer or basal cell carcinoma 1%.

The vulva can also occasionally be the site of metastatic cancer. Cancer of the vulva and the cervix may coexist in case it is caused by papilloma virus. Most of these malignant lesions are located on the labia majora. In 5% of cases, the lesions are multifocal, and are seen in younger women below 40 years.

A single lesion is seen in older women.

PREINVASIVE LESIONS

INTRAEPITHELIAL VULVAL NEOPLASIA (VIN)

Definition

Intraepithelial vulval cancer is defined as a cellular abnormality limited to the epithelium of the vulval skin, excluding the keratinized layer. The cancer cells are restricted by the basement membrane and do not spread to the dermis.

Histopathological characteristics

- The presence of **acanthosis**
- Intraepithelial **pearl formation** at the rete pegs
- Inflammatory reaction in the dermis

Classification

The classification is comparable to that of preinvasive carcinoma of the cervix.

In 2004, the International Society for the Study of Vulvovaginal Disease officially divided VIN into two types:

(i) **Usual type VIN**, which is related to human papilloma virus (HPV) infection.
(ii) **Differentiated VIN**, which is unrelated to HPV infection.

The term VIN 1 is no longer used, because of lack of reproducibility of histopathology and difficulty in differentiating from the normal cases, and VIN 2 and VIN 3 are simply called VIN. In young patients, it is related to HPV and there are 90% chances of regression and 10% progress, whereas in elderly it is associated with lichen sclerosis and higher chances of progression to invasive cancer.

It is, however, important to remember that invasive cancer need not always be preceded by preinvasive lesion and it can develop de novo.

Incidence

A rise in the incidence of VIN in the recent times is attributed to greater awareness of its existence, better diagnosis and the longer survival of woman beyond the age of 70 years, when the carcinoma of the vulva prevails. The intraepithelial cancer also increasingly affects women younger than 40 years, who are often affected by sexually transmitted diseases and viral infections such as HPV (70%–80%) and herpes simplex virus II (HSV). HPV (type 16, 18, 31, 33) as well as smoking predisposes one to cancer. Type 16 is the most common and is present in 60%–90% of cases.

Aetiology

The aetiological factors are similar to those of vulval dystrophy (see Chapter 25 on Benign Diseases of the Vulva), and therefore it is not surprising to see the lesions of VIN amongst the dystrophic areas.

Chronic vulval irritation, immunosuppressive conditions such as pregnancy, **HIV** infection and **smoking** suppress the immune system and predispose the patient to VIN lesions. **Condyloma**, **sexually transmitted diseases** and **dystrophies** are the other risk factors. Poor nutrition and hygiene, and local moisture are the contributing factors. The association with carcinoma of the cervix and breast cancer in the same woman indicates the common aetiological factors.

Fifty per cent of VIN cases have sequential or concomitant neoplasia in the lower genital tract, especially cancer of the cervix.

The VIN lesions are observed in relatively young women below 40 years. Obesity, diabetes, chronic pruritus and dermatitis are often linked to this disease.

Histology

A loss of polarity, and stratification and dystrophic changes are confined to the epidermis, and the basement membrane remains intact.

Clinical Features

Many early lesions may remain asymptomatic for a long period, and VIN I is not visible macroscopically. **Pruritus** may be the only symptom in the early stage. It may be mistaken and treated for fungal infection. Later, soreness, dysuria and dyspareunia develop. The preexisting leucoplakia, condyloma and dystrophic areas may now show white, or red, flat warty or papular lesions, single or multiple with well-defined edges. Multiple widespread lesions are more common in younger women, and occur in 5%–25% of cases. Some develop pigmentation. The lesions mainly affect the labia majora, but may also be seen over the perineum and perianal regions. The clitoris and labia minora are not spared. The inguinal glands are not palpable (Figs 37.1 and 37.2).

Investigations

It is impossible to diagnose VIN and differentiate it from dystrophies without a biopsy. Exfoliative cytology does not yield satisfactory results because of keratinization and poor exfoliation of cells. Colposcopic study too does not always show punctuation, mosaic and abnormal vascular pattern, if the vulval skin is hypertrophied and thick. Application of K-Y jelly improves visualization of the vasculature of vulval skin. Five per cent acetic acid causes white areas and staining the

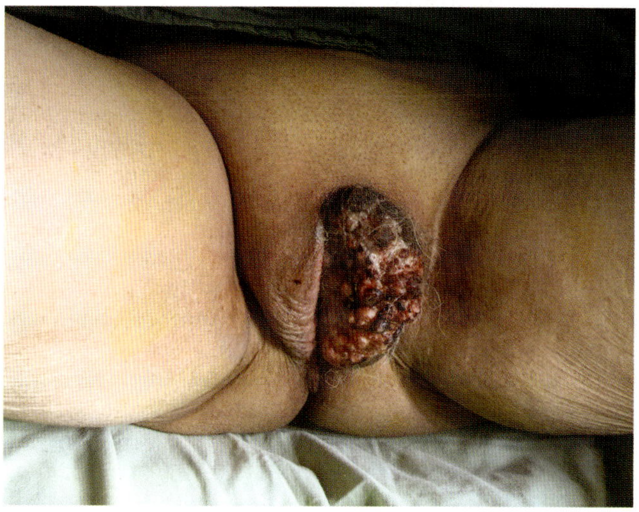

Figure 37.1 Basal cell carcinoma. (*Source:* From Figure 8-30. Clinical Gynecologic Oncology. In: Invasive Cancer of the Vulva, 2007.)

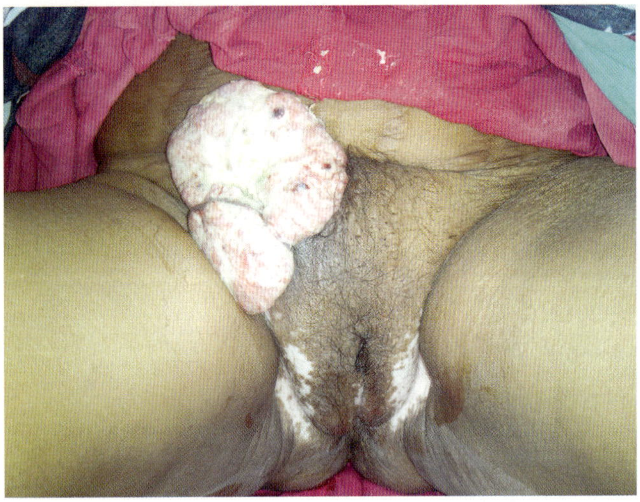

Figure 37.2 Squamous cell carcinoma of vulva with groin metastasis.

area with 1% toluidine blue marks abnormal areas royal blue, thus enabling selective biopsies from the dark-stained areas. Excisional biopsy of a localized lesion picks up VIN. Colposcopy and Pap smear of the cervix are also required to rule out concomitant preinvasive cancer of the cervix.

Proctoscopy and anoscopy may be required, if the perianal region is involved in the lesion. This will show the extension into the anal wall. **Vaginal and Pap smear become mandatory in the diagnosis as well as in the treatment of these multifocal lesions.**

DNA study is useful so far as aneuploidy is concerned. Aneuploidy strongly suggests the possibility of VIN progressing to invasion and should be treated, whereas euploidy in young women can be observed over a period of 6 months, with a hope of regression.

Human papilloma virus DNA detection combined with cytology improves the detection test to 95%.

Vulvoscopy defines a vascular pattern, but is not so clear because of keratinization. Condyloma which does not respond to treatment should be investigated for VIN.

Management (Table 37.3)

The purpose of treating VIN lesions is threefold:

- To relieve the symptoms of pruritus and soreness.
- To prevent cancer developing in the area. *Five to ten per cent VIN III progresses to invasive cancer within 8 years.*
- To avoid mutilating surgery and sexual dysfunction in young women; radical vulvectomy is mutilating and causes genital disfigurement and dyspareunia.

The treatment is therefore based on the age of the woman, sexual activity, site and extent of VIN and grading.

With more young women developing VIN, there is a tendency to shift from the earlier radical approach to a very conservative management with success of 90%–94%. However, a long follow-up is required to watch for recurrence and progression to invasion.

The management is as follows:

1. **Young women with multiple focal lesions and showing euploidy** on DNA study may be observed for up to 6 months, because such lesions often disappear by then. This occurs more commonly in young women who develop VIN during pregnancy, during an immunosuppressive period and following viral infection, especially HPV 16, 18.
2. With **unifocal lesion**, wide excision of the lesion going 2 cm beyond the margin is found adequate and vulvectomy is not warranted. The skin edges can be approximated with or without undermining the excised margins. Local recurrence is the risk to be watched for. Excision is performed with a knife, cautery or laser.
3. **Persistent VIN and VIN III** require **excision**, **skinning vulvectomy** (Rutledge and Sinclair) with a split-skin graft to avoid disfigurement of the introitus and dyspareunia. Skinning vulvectomy is desirable, if the involved area is widespread. CO_2 laser vaporization (Townsend) or laser excision, cryosurgery, application of dinitrochlorobenzene, 5% testosterone cream and corticosteroids are also conservative treatment, but they do not guarantee recurrence or invasion and need a lifelong follow-up. Laser therapy avoids pain and scar formation without disfigurement; the cut heals in a few weeks. Periurethral and perianal lesions are, however, not amenable to laser, and require excision.

   Cryosurgery up to a depth of 2 mm can cause extensive sloughing. *Prophylactic HPV vaccine* is now available.

   Photodynamic therapy (PDT) uses a tumour photosensitizer 5-amino-levulinic acid (ALA) combined with nonthermal light of an appropriate wavelength to generate oxygen-induced cell death. Quick healing and minimal tissue destruction are its advantages.

   Conservative therapy requires that invasive lesion should be excluded by multiple or adequate biopsy.
4. Elderly women should be dealt with by simple vulvectomy.

A lifelong follow-up is required in all cases.

Table 37.3 Management of VIN

- Observe young women with multiple lesions and HPV positive for 6 months. Persistent lesion requires treatment.

Excision
- Wide excision
- Skinning vulvectomy

Ablative
- CO_2 laser
- Photodynamic therapy

Surgery
- Simple vulvectomy in older women and in Bowen disease

Medical
- Local application of dinitrochlorobenzene, 5% testosterone cream, Fluorouracil (5-FU) mainly for local recurrence
- Lifelong follow-up

Follow-Up

Recurrence around the excised lesion or fresh recurrence occurs in 20%–30% of cases. Five to ten per cent of cases progress to invasive cancer in 8 years, after which invasion is less likely, unlike that in carcinoma in situ of the cervix which may take 10–15 years to develop to invasive cancer. Pap smear, colposcopy three to six monthly and later yearly will be required. Recurrent tumour is treated with 5-Fluorouracil.

Bowen Disease

Bowen disease is an intraepithelial carcinoma of the vulva. It presents as a slow-growing hard reddish indurated patch. Initially, it is well-circumscribed, with a dry or eczematous surface. This verrucous lesion rarely metastasizes. Pruritus is the main complaint. The biopsy reveals typical prickle cells invading the epidermis. The presence of **giant cells** and **corps ronds** is a characteristic of the lesion. The vagina and the cervix may also show similar lesions in the colposcopically directed biopsy. The treatment consists of simple vulvectomy.

Paget Disease

A rare extramammary disease, Paget disease, is comparable to intraductal carcinoma of the breasts, because the apocrine sweat glands are involved. It occurs in a postmenopausal woman as a sharply demarcated and slightly elevated white indurated or eczematous lesion and causes pruritus. The biopsy reveals the characteristic large, pale, vacuolated cells in the epidermis (Fig. 37.3). Perianal and perineal areas are rarely involved. Paget's cells are adenocarcinomatous mucus-secreting cells, round cells with pale cytoplasm and vesicular nuclei. Mitosis is rare. Unlike Paget disease of the breast, the underlying carcinoma is reported in only 20% due to adenocarcinoma of Bartholin's gland. In the perianal region, it is associated with adenocarcinoma of the anus. It is important to search for the underlying malignancy which may be involved in 30% of cases. The treatment is local excision or vulvectomy, if no underlying lesion is detected. With underlying lesion, treatment is as of invasive cancer. Radiotherapy is employed for women unfit for surgery, but a prolonged follow-up for recurrence is obligatory. Local and systemic 5-FU and bleomycin are also tried. The tumour recurs in 20% of cases.

Microinvasive Cancer

Microinvasive melanoma is rare and detected only histologically.

Superficially invasive vulval cancer (microinvasive – SIVC) is defined as a single lesion measuring 2 cm or less in the maximum diameter with a depth of invasion not greater than 1 mm.

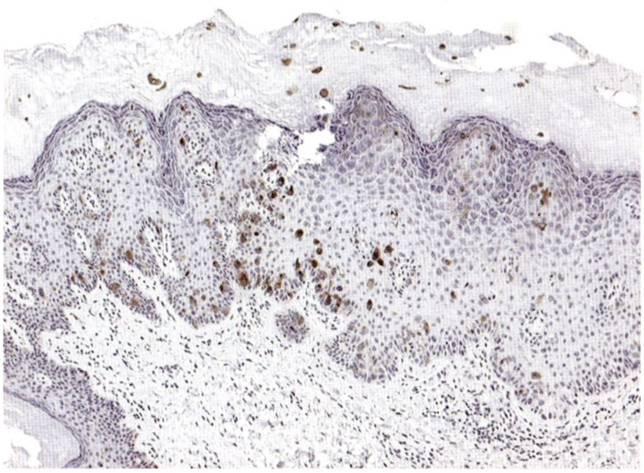

Figure 37.3 Paget disease of the vulva. (*Source:* David Dabbs, University of Pittsburgh School of Medicine, Department of Pathology.)

It represents Stage IA of the FIGO classification. Multiple foci even of depth less than 1 mm do not fall under this classification. Avoiding radical surgery while maintaining the same survival rate has reduced the surgical morbidity of extensive lymphadenectomy and improved sexual and general quality of life. A sentinel lymph node mapping and accurate staging is therefore very necessary. Wide excision or vulvectomy is done.

When the lymph nodes are involved, surgery is better than radiation for groin lymph nodes. However, radiotherapy yields better survival rates for pelvic lymph nodes.

INVASIVE CARCINOMA OF THE VULVA

EPIDEMIOLOGY

Vulval cancer accounts for 2%–4% of all malignancies of the female genital tract. The women are generally elderly, in the sixth or seventh decade of life. Thirty per cent of cases are older than 70 years, and 40% of cases are between the age of 60 and 70 years. Increasing number of lesions are now seen in younger women, and most of them suffer from sexually transmitted diseases such as HPV and HIV infection. Smoking is also a risk factor in these young women. However, only 2% of cases are younger than 30 years. Nulliparous and women of low parity are disposed to vulval cancer. Vulval cancer is associated with cervical and ovarian cancer in 20% of cases. This may be related to viral infection in the genital tract in the former and low parity and older age group in the ovarian cancer.

AETIOLOGY

The causes are the same as those of in situ carcinoma. The lesion associated with VIN and atypical dystrophy often progresses to invasive cancer. VIN however does not always precede invasive cancer as is seen in cervical cancer. Squamous cell carcinomas account for 90% of all vulval cancers.

CLINICAL FEATURES

Eighty per cent women complain of pruritus, vulval swelling, lump or an ulcer. The lump may be papular, raised pigmented area. The ulcer has often an everted margin. The surrounding skin may be fissured, cracked and indurated. Leukoplakic or dystrophied area may be present, and these may be single or multifocal. The lesion is more commonly encountered over the labia majora (70%), but the clitoris and perineal area may be involved. The anterior two-thirds of the vulva is usually involved. The lesion is single in 98% of cases, and multiple lesions are seen in only 2% of cases, in elderly women.

The ulcerative lesions bleed, and cause offensive vulval discharge. Pain is a late feature of the disease. When the urethra is involved, the woman complains of dysuria and micturition difficulty. When the anal area is affected, rectal symptoms in the form of rectal bleeding and painful defecation develop. The inguinal lymph nodes may or may not be palpable. A woman may be diabetic, hypertensive or obese.

DIFFERENTIAL DIAGNOSIS

(i) Tubercular or syphilitic ulcer
(ii) Elephantiasis vulva
(iii) Soft sore
(iv) Lymphogranuloma

STAGING

Refer to Table 37.4.

Table 37.4 Staging of Vulval Cancer (FIGO 2009)

Stage I	Tumour confined to the vulva
IA	Lesions ≤2 cm in size, confined to the vulva or perineum and with stromal invasion ≤1.0 mm[a], no nodal metastasis
IB	Lesions > 2 cm in size or with stromal invasion > 1.0 mm[a], confined to the vulva or perineum, with negative nodes
Stage II	Tumour of any size with extension to adjacent perineal structures (one-third lower urethra, one-third lower vagina, anus) with negative nodes
Stage III	Tumour of any size with or without extension to adjacent perineal structures (one-third lower urethra, one-third lower vagina, anus) with positive inguino-femoral lymph nodes
IIIA	(I) With 1 lymph node metastasis (≥5 mm), or (II) 1–2 lymph node metastatis(es) (<5 mm)
IIIB	(I) With 2 or more lymph node metastases (≥5 mm), or (II) 3 or more lymph node metastases (<5 mm)
IIIC	With positive nodes with extracapsular spread
Stage IV	Tumour invades other regional (two-thirds upper urethra, two-thirds upper vagina), or distant structures.
IVA	Tumour invades any of the following:
IVB	Any distant metastasis including pelvic lymph nodes

[a]The depth of invasion is defined as the measurement of the tumour from the epithelial–stromal junction of the adjacent most superficial dermal papilla to the deepest point of invasion.

SPREAD OF THE TUMOUR

The tumour proliferates mainly by following:

(i) Direct spread to the adjacent organs
(ii) Lymphatic spread
(iii) Haematogenous spread rare

Parry Jones was the first to describe the lymphatic spread that occurs in a systematic manner. At first, the superficial inguinal nodes are involved through lymphatic emboli, but later lymphatic channel permeation occurs causing lymphatic blockage and leg oedema. The malignancy spreads to deep nodes and via the gland of Cloquet (uppermost of the femoral or the lowermost of the external iliac gland) to the external iliac glands, obturator and common iliac nodes in the advanced stages.

Laterally placed tumours rarely spread to the contralateral inguinal glands, but centrally located lesion involves the lymph nodes of the opposite side in 25% of cases and this is because of crossing of lymphatics in the midline.

Lymph nodes not clinically suspicious may show metastasis in about 25% of cases.

Inguinal lymph nodes are involved in 10% in Stage I, 30% in Stage II, 70% in Stage III and 100% cases in Stage IV.

See Fig. 37.4 for lymphatic drainage of the vulva.

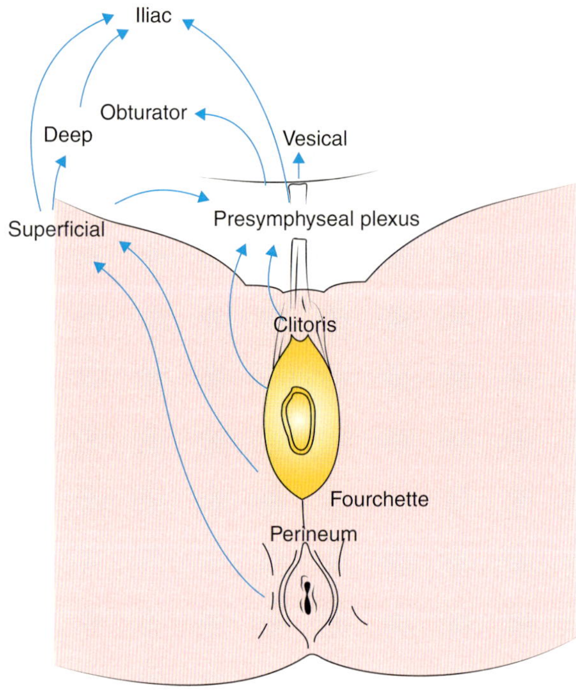

Figure 37.4 Lymphatic drainage of the vulva.

Lymphatics of the clitoris drain directly into the pelvic lymph nodes. The regional lymph nodes are assessed by MRI and PET. The involvement of the lymph nodes depends on the site of the lesion, its size and depth of invasion.

INVESTIGATIONS

Diagnostic investigations include following:

- Punch or excision biopsy depending on the size of the lesion.
- Cystoscopy if urethra is involved.
- Anoscopy and proctoscopy if the perianal area is involved.
- X-ray of chest and bones.
- CT and MRI scans for lymph node metastasis.
- Lymphography is superior to CT scan and can detect metastasis in the lymph nodes 2–5 mm in size, whereas CT can pick up metastasis only if it is more than 1 cm.

Restricting unnecessary lymph node dissection reduces the surgical morbidity in early cancer. However, to do this, determination of the extent of primary lymph node (sentinel) involvement is necessary. Lymphatic mapping and sentinel node biopsy (frozen section) before or during surgery help in carrying out an adequate surgical procedure with good prognosis.

Mapping is done by:

- An intraoperative intradermal injection of blue dye around the tumour (Fig. 37.5); a detection rate of 100% is reported.
- Labelling tissues with radioactive tracer and localization with a handheld detector.
- Lymphoscintigraphy has also a 100% detection rate.

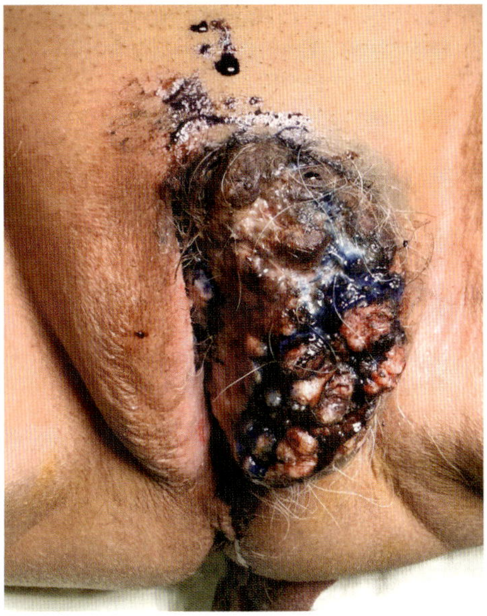

Figure 37.5 A picture showing infiltration of methylene blue dye into the subdermal tissue of the tumour to facilitate sentinel lymph node identification.

Microinvasive vulval cancer Stage IA is applicable only to a single lesion of squamous cell carcinoma up to 2 cm in size and less than 1 mm invasion below the epithelium with no evidence of vascular space invasion and lymph nodal involvement. Adenocarcinoma and melanoma are not included in this group of tumours, because of their high propensity for nodal involvement. Microinvasive tumours can be treated by local excision with a margin of 2 cm beyond the lesion, provided the surrounding skin is not dystrophic. If it is dystrophic, vulvectomy is recommended because of the possible recurrence of cancer in the dystrophic tissue. Multiple foci do not come under this classification and require more radical surgery.

Treatment

The traditional treatment by radical vulvectomy with bilateral lymphadenectomy of inguinal, femoral and pelvic nodes, as described by Way and Taussig in 1935, has undergone a radical modification in the recent years. This is based on the observation of high primary mortality of radical surgery, a high percentage of negative lymph node involvement and satisfactory 5-year cure rate with the conservative approach (Table 37.5). Besides, invasive cancer encountered in young women has also

Table 37.5 Results of Treatment and 5-year Survival Rates for Cancer of the Vulva

FIGO Staging	5-Year Survival Rates
Stage I	90%
Stage II	80%
Stage III	About 50%
Stage IV	About 15%
Total	About 60%

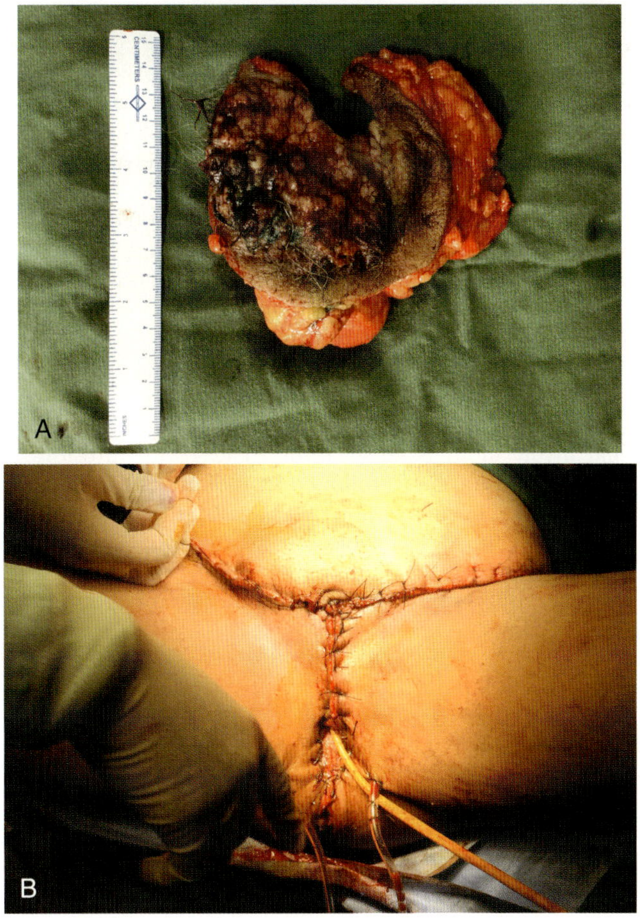

Figure 37.6 **(A)** Radical vulvectomy specimen of carcinoma of the vulva. **(B)** Post vulvectomy reconstruction.

welcomed this conservative surgery, there is a multidisciplinary approach for the treatment and it should be individualized (Fig. 37.6).

The factors to be considered before individualizing the surgical treatment are the general condition of the woman, stage and site of the tumour, tumour histology and differentiation. The surgery is now performed with a separate groin incision rather than extensive skin incision over a wide area which is mutilating and difficult to heal. Primary mortality of surgery is 1%–5%.

Stage I. Stage 1A – Lateral lesions can be dealt with by **simple partial vulvectomy** with a margin of at least 2 cm beyond the growth, or **unilateral vulvectomy, accompanied by ipsilateral inguinal node dissection**. If the frozen section reveals the absence of involvement of glands, nothing more is required. This is because, in this case, the contralateral lymph nodes are involved in only 0.4% and extensive surgery will not improve survival, but add to morbidity. Ipsilateral lymph node involvement demands contralateral removal of inguinal glands. The pelvic lymph nodes are removed only if the gland of Cloquet (femoral) shows malignant cells. Alternatively, a woman is subjected to postoperative radiation, in place of extensive pelvic node dissection. A central tumour requires bilateral inguinal node dissection.

Stage II. Radical/modified radical vulvectomy and bilateral inguinofemoral lymph node dissection. If these are positive, pelvic node dissection or postoperative radiotherapy is required to the pelvic nodes.

If the tumour is more than 4 cm in size, poorly differentiated or it is a melanoma or adenocarcinoma, nothing less than radical vulvectomy and bilateral lymphadenectomy with pelvic node dissection are required. A separate vulval incision and two groin incisions are employed.

Stage III. Megavoltage radiotherapy 4000–5000 rad over a period of 5 weeks causes shrinkage and at times the total disappearance of the tumour. Local excision of the shrunken tumour is then adequate and eliminates the need for exenteration operation. Local recurrence can be dealt with by chemotherapy. Forty per cent survival and 30% recurrence have been reported.

Stage IV. It is treated by chemotherapy or radiotherapy. Anal involvement is satisfactorily treated with infusion of 5-FU and mitomycin-C, followed by radiotherapy 3000 rad, over 3 weeks. Local excision of residual tumour may be required. Chemotherapy avoids exenteration operation with its associated high mortality and morbidity. Fifteen per cent 5-year survival is reported. Other chemotherapy agents used area as follows:

- Bleomycin 5 mg days 1–5
- Methotrexate 15 mg days 1–4
- Trastuzumab 440 mg days 5-7

This regime is administered weekly for 6 weeks.

BARTHOLIN's GLAND TUMOUR

Bartholin's gland tumour is a rare unilateral tumour, commonly an adenocarcinoma, and carries a poor prognosis. Radical vulvectomy is the treatment of choice.

VULVAL SARCOMA

Vulval sarcoma is a rare tumour which occurs in younger women (Fig. 37.7). Treatment is local excision. Metastasis is common. The prognosis is poor.

VULVAL MELANOMA

Malignant melanoma accounts for 3%–5% of all vulval tumours. It occurs at all ages, and may develop in a mole or occur de novo. The lesion is pigmented and presents as either nodular or superficial spreading tumour. The edges of the lesion are often irregular, and frequently ulcerate and bleed. The treatment is managed by vulvectomy and bilateral node dissection. Postoperative radiotherapy may be required. Prognosis is poor.

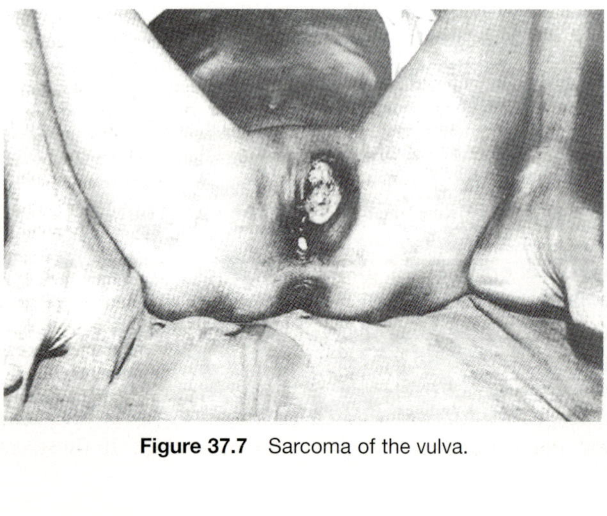

Figure 37.7 Sarcoma of the vulva.

RODENT ULCER

This uncommon lesion presents as an ulcer which keeps invading the deeper tissues of the vulva. Biopsy shows basal cell carcinoma. It is locally malignant and responds well to wide local excision.

PERSISTENT CANCER (RESIDUAL)

Persistent cancer is one which develops within 6 months of primary treatment. Local excision with wide margin is required.

SECONDARY GROWTH OF THE VULVA

Secondary growths of the vulva are metastases from choriocarcinoma, endometrial and ovarian cancer. They are treated by radiotherapy or chemotherapy.

Distal metastatic growths are rare. They are treated with radiotherapy and chemotherapy.

Fifty per cent recurrent growths are seen at the local site within 2 years of primary treatment, and occur with large growths and lymph node involvement. They are treated by exenteration operation, radiotherapy and chemotherapy.

Recurrent growths. Recurrent growths occur in 30% of cases within 2 years. Local recurrence is seen in 75% cases. Lymph node and distal metastasis are rare. If the growth is small, local excision with a wide margin over 2 cm is adequate; otherwise, radiotherapy or chemotherapy is employed as palliative treatment.

Exenteration operation with removal of bladder/rectum with vulvectomy is very rarely performed these days.

PROGNOSTIC FACTORS

Prognostic factors are the size of the tumour, grading, histology, lymph node involvement and immune status of the woman. Groin node status is the best prognostic predictor.

When the lymph nodes are not involved, 5-year survival is 90%. Lymph node involvement diminishes the survival rate proportionate to the number of lymph nodes involved.

VULVAL CANCER IN YOUNG WOMEN

Vulval intraepithelial neoplasia is mostly encountered in young women. Using barrier contraceptives and maintaining hygiene can reduce the transmission of HPV infection which normally causes VIN. Early diagnosis and conservative therapy can cure the disease, avoid mutilating surgery and improve the survival rate. HPV vaccine can prevent malignancy in these cases in future.

VAGINAL CANCER

Primary vaginal cancer is a rare cancer accounting for less than 0.2% of all cancers in women. It occurs in elderly women often older than 70 years when sexual activity has generally ceased. Unfortunately, only about one-third of the patients have regional disease at the time of diagnosis; therefore, late diagnosis is not uncommon (Fig. 37.8). An unusual tumour clear cell adenocarcinoma was seen in young women who were themselves exposed to diethylstilboestrol (DES) in utero.

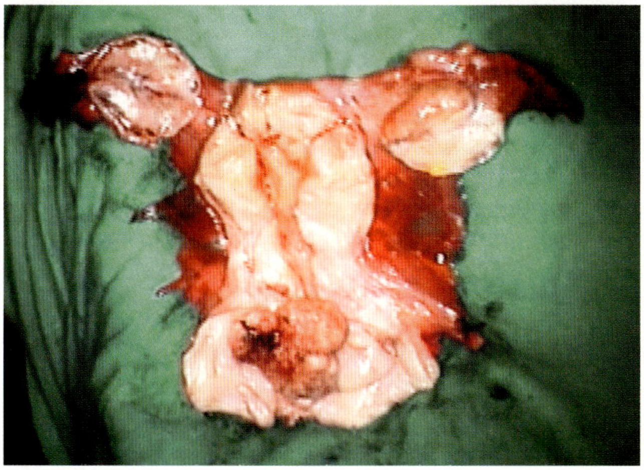

Figure 37.8 Carcinoma of the upper-third of the vagina removed by extended hysterocolpectomy.

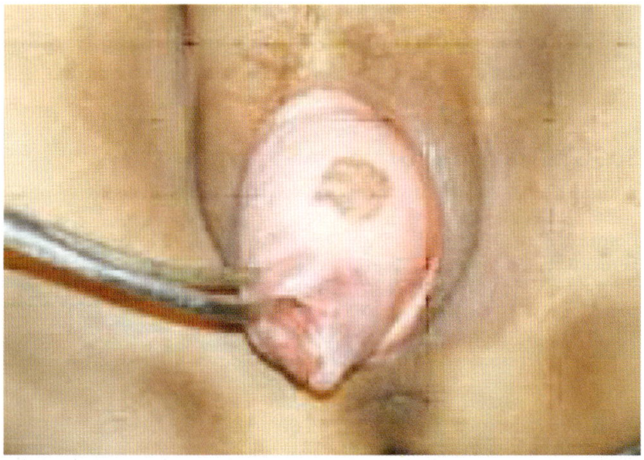

Figure 37.9 Carcinoma in a case of prolapse. (*Source:* From: Sengupta et al. *Gynaecology for Postgraduates and Practitioners, 2nd ed.* Elsevier, 2007.)

However, such cases are fast disappearing with withdrawal of the drug. Cancer of the cervix, bladder and urethra, vulva and lower bowel may spread to involve the vagina. Metastases from cancer of the uterus, ovary and trophoblastic tumours have been known to occur in the vagina. Cancer over a decubitus ulcer in prolapse is also known to occur (Fig. 37.9).

CLINICAL FEATURES

Vaginal cancer is generally asymptomatic in its earlier stages. The usual complaints are the presence of watery discharge, or postcoital bleeding; the lesions may be diffuse, raised velvety patches bleeding on touch, a whitish patch or ulcer. Cytology/Schiller's iodine test/colposcopy and biopsy help settle the diagnosis. The lesions are often multifocal and in the upper-third of the posterior wall. The extent of spread may be determined by combined vaginal and rectal examination. Diffuse spread may involve the urethra and bladder anteriorly and the large bowel posteriorly when urinary and bowel symptoms may occur. Cancers may arise de novo in younger women

Table 37.6 Vaginal Cancer Staging

Stage 0	Vaginal intraepithelial neoplasia (VAIN)
Stage I	Carcinoma limited to the vaginal wall
Stage II	Carcinoma extending beyond the vagina, but not extending to the pelvic side walls
Stage III	Carcinoma extends up to the pelvic walls
Stage IVA	Carcinoma extending beyond the true pelvis/or involving the bladder and/or rectum, or evidence of distal metastasis
Stage IVB	Spread to the distal metastasis

exposed to DES in utero, when the upper one-third vagina is involved, following trophic ulcers in women with procidentia, following prolonged and neglected use of ring pessary for prolapse or as spread from other pelvic organs. Virus infection may be a causative factor.

It may also develop years later following radiation for cancer of the cervix.

The lesion is squamous cell carcinoma in 90% cases, rarely adenocarcinoma arising from vaginal adenosis in young girls. The tumour in the upper vagina drains into pelvic lymph nodes and that in the lower part drains into inguinal lymph nodes (Fig. 37.5).

Vaginal intraepithelial neoplasia (VAIN) is rare, and always progresses to invasive cancer.

STAGING

Refer to Table 37.6.

DIAGNOSIS

Suspicious areas of plaque/white patch should be subjected to Schiller's test and colposcopic biopsy. All gross lesions such as nodule, papule, ulcer or mole should be biopsied. Local application of oestrogen in old women enhances a colposcopic view. Colposcopy is difficult on account of a large vaginal area, multiple lesions and vaginal folds.

MANAGEMENT

PRETREATMENT WORK-UP

Complete history and examination, WBC, urinalysis, blood sugar estimation, liver function test (LFT), renal function test (RFT), chest radiography, ECG, cystoscopy, proctoscopy and barium enema may be required. CT and MRI are done for a nodal study.

TREATMENT

VAIN. It is treated with **local excision biopsy**, **CO_2 laser** and local application of **5-fluorouracil cream**. Electrocautery and cryotherapy are best avoided. Invasive cancer is treated with local radiotherapy, Wertheim hysterectomy with total colpectomy, or exenteration operation for the advanced cases involving bladder/bowel. Overall survival is 30%–40%. Creation of neovagina is required in young women.

Prophylaxis. Treating a decubitus ulcer and proper care of a ring pessary in a prolapse can avoid cancer of vagina.

Sarcoma. Sarcoma botryoides is a rare tumour seen in children.

This tumour arises in the mesenchymal tissues of the vagina and in rare cases, in the cervix before the age of 2 years. It presents as a haemorrhagic grape-like polyp or as a fleshy mass and consists of rhabdomyoblasts with vacuolated cytoplasm, myxoedema and stroma with fusiform cells. The tumour spreads by local infiltration, lymphatics and bloodstream.

Examination is done under anaesthesia; biopsy confirms the diagnosis. CT and MRI indicate its spread.

Treatment. Chemotherapy with VAC (vincristine, adriamycin and cyclophosphamides) is the gold standard in treating this tumour. Other drugs used are cisplatin, actinomycin, cyclophosphamide and ifosfamide.

Surgery is limited to the local residual tumour. Interstitial radiation is used in the advanced stage.

KEY POINTS

- Preinvasive cancer of vulva (VIN) is caused by human papilloma virus in young women.
- VIN is usually a multifocal lesion in young women, but a single lesion in older women.
- In young women, 90% regress, 10% progress to invasive cancer within 8 years. Careful follow-up is recommended.
- VIN in older women invariably progresses to invasive cancer and should be treated by vulvectomy.
- The conservative surgery ablative as well as local wide excision is adequate in young women. Simple vulvectomy should be performed in elderly women. Follow-up is necessary.
- Radical vulvectomy is required if the regional lymph nodes are involved.
- Prognosis depends on the lymph node involvement which in turn depends upon the site, size and depth of the lesion.
- Vaginal cancer is rare and difficult to diagnose in its early stage.
- Radical surgery is usually required. Radiotherapy is palliative in the advanced stages.

SELF-ASSESSMENT

1. A 55-year old woman presents with a vulval ulcer. Discuss the differential diagnosis and management.
2. Discuss the management of vulval cancer Stage I.
3. Discuss the management of vulval cancer Stage II.

SUGGESTED READING

Bonnar J (ed). Recent Advances in Obstetrics and Gynaecology Vol 17: 223, 1992.

Bonnar J (ed). VIN. Recent Adv Obstet Gynaecol 1998; 20: 167.

Duncan J, Shulman P: Yearbook of Obstetrics, Gynaecology and Women's Health 1989; 417: 7, 2010.

Jonathan S (ed). Gynecologic Oncology, Berek and Hackers.13:560, 2015.

Studd J. Role of viruses in gynaecological oncology: In: AB Macleao, et al. Progress in Obstetrics and Gynaecology Vol 12: 403, 1996.

Gestational Trophoblastic Diseases

38

CHAPTER OUTLINE

Gestational trophoblastic diseases (GTDs) comprise a variety of biologically interrelated conditions which form a clinical spectrum from a benign partial hydatidiform mole at the one end to the highly malignant choriocarcinoma at the other without any precise line of demarcation. This spectrum extends from a very early pregnancy (hydatidiform mole) to years after the pregnancy is over (choriocarcinoma).

Trophoblastic tumours may be categorized into three broad groups (Table 38.1):

1. **Hydatidiform Mole:** It may be a complete or a partial mole. The tumour sometimes invades the wall of the uterus and the surrounding structures, when it is called an **invasive mole (chorioadenoma destruens)**.
2. **Persistent trophoblastic disease (PTD)**, also known as residual trophoblastic disease (RTD), includes the invasive mole.
3. **Choriocarcinoma:** This is truly a malignant tumour. It could be a nonmetastatic trophoblastic disease (NMTD) or a metastatic trophoblastic disease (MTD).
   Metastatic tumour may be of low or high risk.

Table 38.1 Classification of Trophoblastic Diseases

1. Molar pregnancy
   - Partial
   - Complete
2. Persistent or residual mole
   - Invasive
   - Placental site
3. Choriocarcinoma
   - Nonmetastatic
   - Metastatic: Low and high risk metastatic

HYDATIDIFORM MOLE

INCIDENCE AND AETIOLOGY

The incidence of the disease is higher in the Eastern countries than in the West. Its geographical distribution is as follows: in the UK and the USA 1:2000 to 1:3000, India and the Middle-East 1:160 to 1:500, China 1:150, Philippines 1:173, and Indonesia and Taiwan 1:82 pregnancies. Likewise, the malignant potential of this disease is higher in Southeast Asia, where it is as high as 10%–15% compared to 2%–4% in the Western countries. Some immigrants from Southeast Asia to a developed country lose the potential to develop hydatidiform mole once they settle down in the new environment. This proves that the condition is not racial, but may be related to geographical and environmental influences.

Vitamin A, β-carotene and folic acid deficiency in the diet are also implicated in the occurrence of trophoblastic disease.

Women belonging to blood group A are susceptible to this disease, but the reason is not known. Very young and women older than 40 years are prone to it. Repeat molar pregnancy occurs in 2%–10% of cases. In contrast to a complete mole, maternal age and nutrition do not appear to influence the incidence of a partial mole.

A mole is considered partial if there is coexisting pregnancy and it is labelled as complete mole when there is no evidence of normal pregnancy. Complete mole is far more common than partial mole.

The diagnosis of complete and partial moles is based on morphological, histological and karyotype findings (Table 38.2).

PATHOLOGY

A complete hydatidiform mole resembles bunches of grape-like vesicles, pearly white in colour and translucent, containing watery fluid (Fig. 38.1A and B). The vesicles vary in size

Table 38.2 Features of Complete and Partial Moles

S. No.	Features	Complete Mole	Partial Mole
1.	Fetus	Absent	Present, malformed or IUGR
2.	Fetal vessels	Absent	Present
3.	Hydropic changes	Diffuse and placenta not present	Focal
4.	Trophoblastic hyperplasia	Marked	Mild to moderate
5.	β-hCG level	Very high	Comparatively low
6.	Karyotype	46XX mostly and paternally derived	69XXY
7.	Malignant potential	15%–20%	Rare

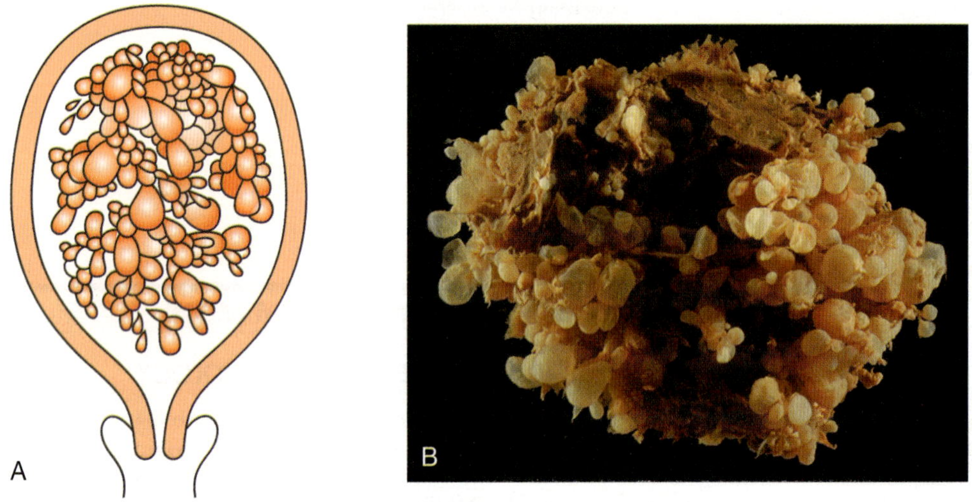

Figure 38.1 **(A)** Hydatidiform mole. **(B)** Specimen of hydatidiform mole from a 43 yr old woman. (*Source:* From Figure 31-2. Physiology in Childbearing. Elsevier, 2005; Figure 16-22. Nicholas Vardaxis: A Textbook of Pathology. Elsevier, 2010.)

from a few millimetres to 2–3 cm in diameter and are attached to the main stalk by thin pedicles. A few haemorrhagic areas are seen in between the bunches. The fetus, amniotic sac and the placenta are conspicuously absent. The size of the mole depends on the duration of pregnancy and degeneration.

Histologically, the disease is characterized by (i) hydropic degeneration and swelling of the villous stroma, (ii) absence of villous blood vessels and (iii) proliferation of both syncito and cyto trophoblastic epithelial. The vesicle demonstrates irregular proliferation and pleomorphism of epithelial cells whose nuclei are hyperchromatic and actively mitotic. The villous structure is, however, well preserved and identifiable. Irrespective of trophoblastic cell proliferation, it is the preservation of a villous structure that determines the benign nature of the trophoblastic disease (Fig. 38.3).

In a very early pregnancy, it is difficult to differentiate between a molar pregnancy and a missed abortion. Histology of products of conception alone can identify molar pregnancy. In complete mole mostly karyotype is 46XX and both sex chromosomes are paternal in origin.

A partial mole resembles the placenta, but contains a few vesicles on its maternal surface. A fetus is identifiable in this case. One of the twins may be a mole and another a normal fetus. Even an ectopic pregnancy has been reported to contain a molar pregnancy. In a partial mole, some or most of the villi appear normal. The fetus most often shows gross malformation, intrauterine growth retardation (IUGR) and in utero death. Very few live babies have been born in a case of partial mole. The fetal blood vessels are seen on ultrasound scan. Karyotype is usually 69XXY.

The average gestational age when a partial mole is diagnosed is at a later date than that for a complete mole; it could be in the second trimester or as late as around 24–26 weeks of pregnancy. The enlargement seen in a complete mole is rarely observed in a partial mole, and it may be of a normal size or smaller for the gestational period on account of intrauterine fetal growth retardation. It rarely metastasizes and does not require prophylactic chemotherapy, as the level of human chorionic gonadotropin (hCG) is comparatively low (<10,000 IU). Despite this, follow-up is necessary, as choriocarcinoma may, in rare cases, follow a partial mole.

The uterine wall is hypertrophied in a hydatidiform mole as in a pregnancy and is lined by a thick decidua. The ovaries contain theca lutein cysts in 60% of cases, and the cysts are usually 6-8 cm in size and tend to be bilateral. Rare complications of a torsion of this ovarian cyst and haemorrhage into the cyst necessitating laparotomy have been reported.

Features of complete and partial moles have been described in Table 38.2.

INVASIVE MOLE

Some hydatidiform moles (about 5%–10%) are invasive moles that invade the wall of the uterus, burrow into the myometrium and, in some cases, even perforate through the uterus into either the peritoneal cavity or the broad ligament when dangerous internal haemorrhage may ensue. It should be emphasized that, though behaving as locally malignant, the invasive mole does not kill by distal metastasis and, therefore, cannot be considered a cancer. The relative proportion of invasive moles to the benign noninvasive type is in the region of 1:12. The invasive mole occupies an intermediate position between a benign hydatidiform mole and a malignant choriocarcinoma (Table 38.3).

An invasive mole is likely to be mistaken for a choriocarcinoma, but histologically there is one distinguishing feature – an invasive mole will show evidence of chorionic villi, whereas in a choriocarcinoma, all evidence of villous formation is lost. Trophoblastic tumour diagnosed up to 6 months following an abortion or a mole is often an invasive mole, but tumour diagnosed later than 6 months is usually a choriocarcinoma. Eighty per cent of hydatidiform moles resolve following treatment in the form of evacuation of uterus, 15% persist as persistent or residual mole and 5% develop into choriocarcinoma.

Invasive or persistent mole is diagnosed clinically by persistent vaginal bleeding and pain following evacuation of a hydatidiform mole, but more often by follow-up with ultrasound scan and serial β-hCG levels (persistently raised level). Chemotherapy is usually effective, but hysterectomy may be required to control bleeding if perforation occurs (Fig. 38.2).

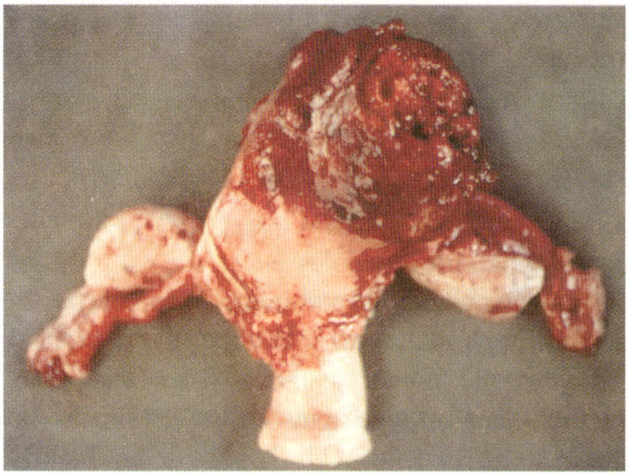

Figure 38.2 Perforation of uterus by hydatidiform mole.

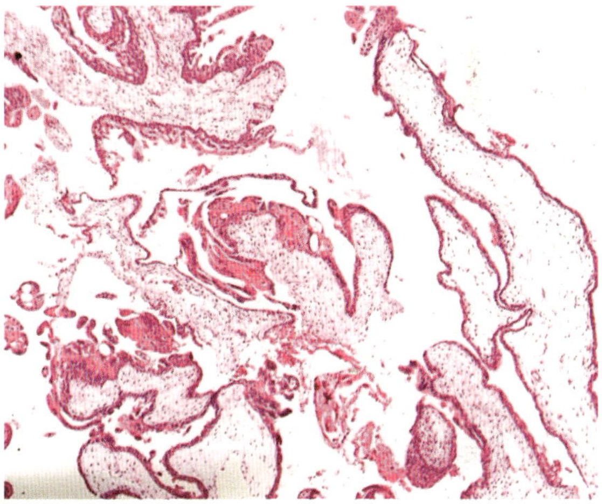

Figure 38.3 Histology of Molar pregnancy.

PLACENTAL SITE TROPHOBLASTIC TUMOUR

It constitutes 1% of all trophoblastic diseases. Placental site trophoblastic tumour arises from the placental bed trophoblast and invades the myometrium. It follows a full-term normal delivery in 95% of cases, although in rare cases, it may follows a mole (5%). hCG levels are lower than those observed in choriocarcinoma, and rarely exceed 2000–3000 IU/L. Most of these tumours run a benign course, malignancy being rare. This tumour contains mainly cytotrophoblasts with few or no syncytiotrophoblasts. For this reason, β-hCG level is low and serum human placental lactogen (HPL) levels are high.

Table 38.3 Spread of Choriocarcinoma

Lungs	80%	X-ray chest, CT
Vaginal metastasis	30%	Speculum examination, β-hCG
Pelvis	20%	Pelvic examination, ultrasound, CT
Liver	10%	Ultrasound, CT
Brain	10%	CT, β-hCG
Gastrointestinal kidney, spleen	Rare	Ultrasound, β-hCG

AETIOLOGY OF GESTATIONAL TROPHOBLASTIC DISEASES

The disease can be seen in women between 18-50 years of age, however, may be more common at extreme of reproductive life. The incidence is higher amongst women belonging to the low socioeconomic group subsisting on a poor rice diet and vitamin deficiency. Diet deficient in protein, folic acid and iron, and environmental factors are incriminated in the aetiology. Folic acid is essential for the cellular metabolism of rapidly growing cells, and it is hypothesized that its deficiency in the diet predisposes to abnormal trophoblastic proliferation.

The cytogenic study of a hydatidiform mole displays typical chromosome patterns. A complete mole is composed of 46XX, and all the chromosomes are of paternal origin. The phenomenon is known as androgenesis, in which the empty ovum is fertilized by a haploid sperm which then duplicates after meiosis to produce 46XX. The chromosomes in the ovum are either absent or inactivated. Infrequently, when 46XY chromosome pattern

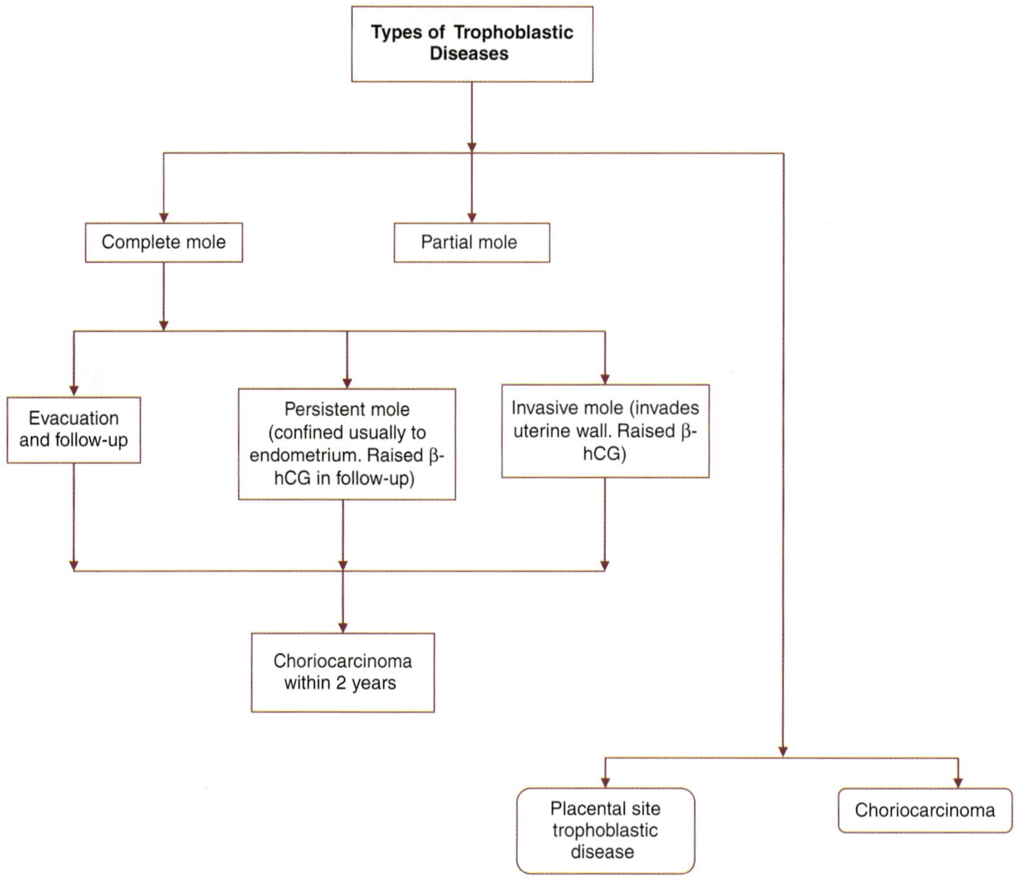

Figure 38.4 Types of trophoblastic diseases.

is detected, it is hypothesized that two sperms have fertilized an empty ovum which itself is lacking chromosomes. The partial mole demonstrates triploid karyotype (69 chromosomes XXY).

CLASSIFICATION (Fig. 38.4)

Histological features are not reliable guides to future clinical behaviour of the tumour as well as therapeutic decisions. In persistent invasive tumour, the tissue may not be available for histology, as previous surgical management by hysterectomy is now replaced by chemotherapy.

WHO has therefore recommended the clinical classification of gestational trophoblastic neoplasia (GTN) as follows (Table 38.4):

I. **Benign GTN**
  A. *Hydatidiform mole*
    - Complete
    - Partial
  B. *Other types*
    - Placental site trophoblastic disease
    - Invasive and persistent trophoblastic disease

II. **Nonmetastatic malignant GTD**: Choriocarcinoma

III. **Metastatic malignant GTD**
  A. *Low risk*
    - Duration of disease from termination of pregnancy to initiation of chemotherapy less than 4 months
    - Pretreatment urine hCG level less than 1000 IU/24 hours or serum β-hCG 40,000–50,000 mIU/mL
    - Metastatic disease limited to the pelvis or lungs
    - No significant prior chemotherapy
  B. *High risk*
    - Duration of the disease from termination of pregnancy to initiation of chemotherapy more than 6 months
    - High serum hCG level – 50,000 mIU/mL or more
    - Brain and liver metastasis
    - Metastatic choriocarcinoma following a term pregnancy

Table 38.4 Symptoms of GTN

- Amenorrhoea
- Irregular bleeding per vaginum
- Expulsion of grape-like structures
- Features of hyperemesis
- Features of thyrotoxicosis
- Asymptomatic but diagnosed on ultrasound

SYMPTOMS AND SIGNS OF GESTATIONAL TROPHOBLASTIC DISEASE

A woman with a complete mole presents with amenorrhoea of less than 24 weeks' gestation, usually 3–4 months. Nowadays a number of cases are diagnosed on the basis of ultrasound done in early pregnancy. A history of vaginal bleeding and abdominal pain is present in 70% of cases. The vaginal bleeding may be slight and intermittent or prolonged. Profuse haemorrhage occurs usually with the onset of spontaneous expulsion, but brisk haemorrhage without abortion is not unknown. The passage of vesicles is rarely observed except when the woman is aborting. Prolonged or heavy bleeding leads to anaemia. The abdominal pain is because of abortion, concealed haemorrhage, sudden distension of the uterus or, in rare cases, perforation. Hyperemesis is reported in about 30% of cases. Pregnancy-induced hypertension (PIH) before 24 weeks is noted in one-third of the cases. Thyrotoxicosis resulting in supraventricular tachycardia, dyspnoea and raised T_3 and T_4 levels is seen in 3% of cases and is because of the fact that subunits of both thyroid-stimulating hormone (TSH) and hCG share a similar structure. One per cent of women are asymptomatic and the condition is suspected by palpating an unduly enlarged uterus. Lately, with routine ultrasound screening performed in early pregnancy, more asymptomatic cases are being diagnosed and treated before bleeding occurs (Table 38.4).

The symptomatic patient may look pale and ill, and she may be febrile. The uterus is larger than would be expected from the calculated date of gestation in 70% of cases. In 15% of the cases, the uterine size corresponds to the period of gestation, and in the remaining 15%, it is smaller than expected because of missed abortion or a partial mole. The uterus feels doughy in consistency because of the absence of amniotic fluid. External and internal ballottement cannot be elicited and the fetal heart cannot be heard on the Doppler. Ovarian theca lutein cysts more than 6 cm and bilateral are often present, but may be difficult to feel because the enlarged uterus occupies most of the pelvis. The cervix feels soft as in a normal pregnancy. Serum hCG levels are raised. Hydatidiform mole usually leads to abortion between the third and sixth months of pregnancy. A partial mole often presents with oligohydramnios, intrauterine growth retarded fetus or malformed fetus as detected on ultrasound scanning, during the second trimester. Few vesicles may be seen in the placenta on ultrasound scanning.

DIFFERENTIAL DIAGNOSIS

MISTAKEN DATE

Undue enlargement of the uterus may be because of the patient stating the wrong date of her last menstrual period (LMP). The fetal parts are palpable. Ultrasound scan reveals a fetus and ultrasonic fetal maturity corresponds to uterine size.

MULTIPLE PREGNANCY

Ultrasound scanning will reveal multiple pregnancies as a cause of uterine size bigger than period of gestation.

ACUTE HYDRAMNIOS

Acute pain, sudden enlargement of the uterus and slight bleeding may simulate a hydatidiform mole with concealed haemorrhage. Ultrasound scan will reveal hydramnios, a fetus and perhaps multiple pregnancy with which acute hydramnios is commonly associated.

FIBROID WITH PREGNANCY

A uterine fibroid may contribute to undue enlargement of the uterus in pregnancy. The presence of fetal parts and fetal heart establishes the diagnosis of a normal pregnancy. Ultrasound scan will show a fibroid in addition to a fetus.

THREATENED ABORTION

Ultrasonic study distinguishes a normal pregnancy from a molar one.

COMPLICATIONS OF GTN

- Hyperemesis gravidarum and PIH
- Haemorrhage and anaemia
- Infection
- Thyroid storm – 3%
- Embolization with acute pulmonary insufficiency and coagulation failure – 2%
- Uterine perforation – spontaneous but more commonly during suction evacuation
- Delayed – recurrent mole and choriocarcinoma

INVESTIGATIONS

SERUM β-hCG

This condition is characterized by marked elevation of serum hCG values. These values may often exceed 40,000–100,000 mIU/mL.

Serum β-hCG level is very high in a complete mole, but is not very much raised in a partial mole. A serum level of more than 40,000 mIU/mL as determined by radioimmunoassay is reported. For diagnostic purpose, ultrasound scan alone is confirmative, quick and a safe procedure. Hormonal assays are now mainly confined to postmolar and postchemotherapy follow-up. HPL is low in a complete mole, but raised in a partial mole, pulmonary metastasis and placental site tumour.

Urinary hCG, though commonly used in the past, is not as reliable as serum hCG.

FETAL HEART DETECTION BY DOPPLER

Ultrasound remains the most reliable investigation to diagnose the hydatidiform mole. The auscultation of fetal heart by Doppler can rule out a complete molar pregnancy. The absence of a fetal heart goes in favour of a molar pregnancy.

ULTRASOUND

Ultrasound examination shows the 'snow-storm' appearance in the uterus and the absence of fetal shadow in a complete molar pregnancy (Fig. 38.5). In a partial mole, the fetus (malformed or IUGR) and placenta are visualized. The placenta shows scattered cysts.

Ultrasound scanning is also required during the follow-up to see if the corpus theca cyst regresses in size and to

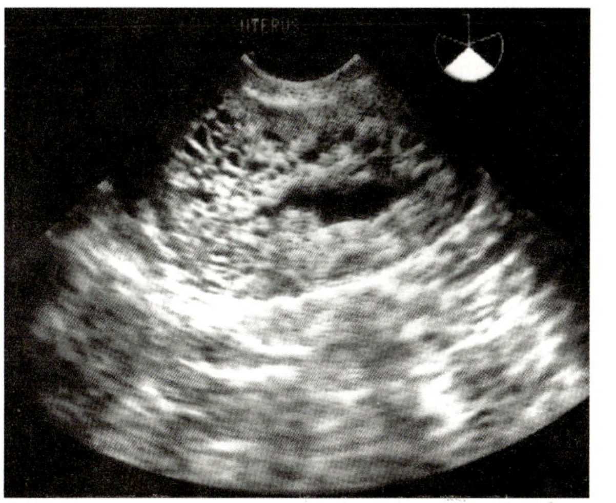

Figure 38.5 Ultrasound scan shows 'snow-storm' appearance of a mole.

detect persistent mole, invasive mole and development of choriocarcinoma. The metastasis in the liver can be picked up on ultrasound scan. Doppler ultrasound shows abnormal vascularization.

Chest X-ray is done to rule out lung metastasis. CT scan is required in liver and brain metastasis and sometimes to detect pulmonary metastasis if chest X-ray is normal.

In the early stage of pregnancy, combined ultrasound scanning and serum β-hCG estimation improves the diagnostic accuracy.

TREATMENT

When a woman comes in the process of abortion, vesicles can be identified amongst the products passed. Blood should be transfused if required and intravenous oxytocin drip of 10–20 units or more in 500 mL of 5% glucose should be set up. Surgical evacuation with a suction evacuation machine (as in medical termination of pregnancy [MTP]), using no. 8-10 Karman cannula, reduces the blood loss in the spontaneous expulsion of a mole. A digital exploration or a gentle curettage will remove any remnants of chorionic tissue. The evacuation can be assisted by administration of intravenous Methergine 0.2 mg. Completeness of evacuation can be confirmed by simultaneous ultrasound. The operation can be associated with considerable blood loss which can be minimized by fast evacuation with an oxytocin drip running and i.v. Methergine, the evacuation can be completed with minimal blood loss.

With the availability of ultrasonic facilities and routine screening in early pregnancy, a molar pregnancy is now diagnosed before a spontaneous abortion begins. In such cases, termination of hydatidiform mole should be done under a planned and controlled situation using a suction evacuation machine. An incomplete evacuation of chorionic tissue will cause the hCG levels to remain elevated and interfere with the proper follow-up of the patient. Besides, it will cause continuous bleeding. *Nowadays, many prefer to evacuate a mole under ultrasonic guidance to ensure complete evacuation and to avoid uterine perforation.* This also avoids a repeat check curettage 7–10 days later, as was practised earlier. One hundred micrograms Rh anti-D globin should be given to an unimmunized Rh-negative woman to prevent isoimmunization in subsequent pregnancies.

Cervical ripening with prostaglandin is effective in dilating the cervix prior to evacuation. Prostaglandin vaginal pessary (400–600 mcg) for ripening the cervix or cervical gel (Cerviprime containing 0.5 mg dinoprostone, PGE_2) may be warranted in a few cases in whom cervical dilation with a metal dilator may be undesirable or difficult because of a tight cervical os. A sudden unexplained collapse during evacuation is attributed to excessive blood loss or because of massive disseminated intravascular coagulation (DIC) or to massive pulmonary embolization by the molar tissue leading to acute pulmonary hypertension and cardiac failure. Hysterectomy is generally not required except for its prophylactic value in preventing choriocarcinoma in patients older than 40 years and who have completed their family. It must be remembered, however, that hysterectomy, while preventing development of local choriocarcinoma, does not obviate the need for careful follow-up because a metastatic tumour can still develop in the distal organ. With the present-day management of hydatidiform mole, the mortality because of a molar pregnancy is very low. Death is invariably associated with profuse haemorrhage. Hyperthyroidism and congestive cardiac failure are seen in 3% of cases. The patient may recover from a molar pregnancy but develop metastasis in the lungs, brain and liver at a later date. Whether it is a benign or a malignant metastatic lesion, haemorrhage in this lesion can cause sudden death. Postabortal anaemia and sepsis are not uncommon.

Choriocarcinoma develops in 2%–10% of cases following evacuation of mole. As the risk of development of choriocarcinoma remains for initial 6month to 2 years a woman who had a molar pregnancy requires careful follow up.

Medical termination with prostaglandin alone is not desirable because of the risk of pulmonary embolization, and surgical evacuation is needed following cervical dilatation. In a partial mole, however, medical termination is the method of choice.

FOLLOW-UP AFTER EVACUATION OF HYDATIDIFORM MOLE (Fig. 38.6)

Following evacuation hydatidiform mole 10-14% people develop persistent gestational Trophoblastic disease. There is no marker to decide which molar pregnancy will proceed to choriocarcinoma. Histological features alone do not provide a reliable clue to the future behaviour of the mole and its progression to carcinoma. Therefore, the therapeutic decision in the follow-up should not be influenced by histology. However, fibrinoid deposition in the tissue does suggest host's favourable immunological response. *Follow-up for 1–2 years remains the only option for detecting early choriocarcinoma.* During this period, an effective method of contraception should be practiced. Serum hCG remains the best test to know status of the disease.

All patients should be kept under careful observation for 1–2 years because choriocarcinoma, if it occurs, develops within this period of evacuation of the mole.

A method of detecting persistent moles and development of choriocarcinoma is by estimating the hCG level in the serum and urine. Normally, the test becomes negative in about 6–8 weeks' time following evacuation of a molar

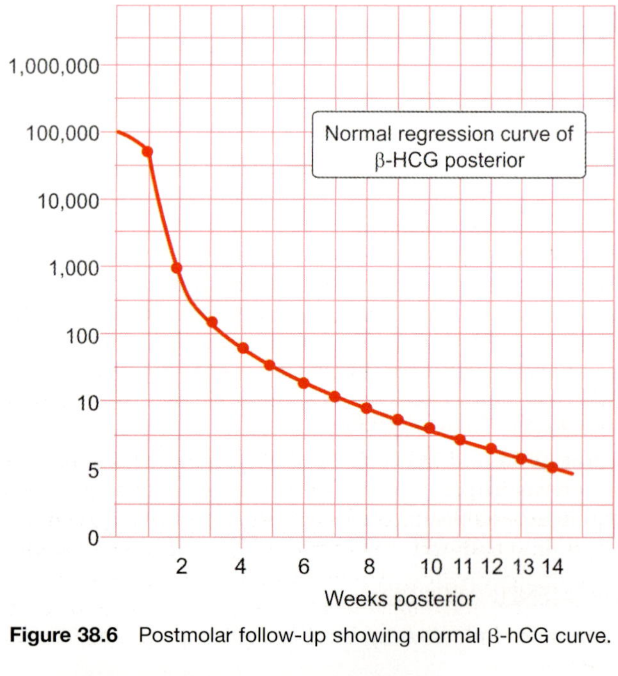

Figure 38.6 Postmolar follow-up showing normal β-hCG curve.

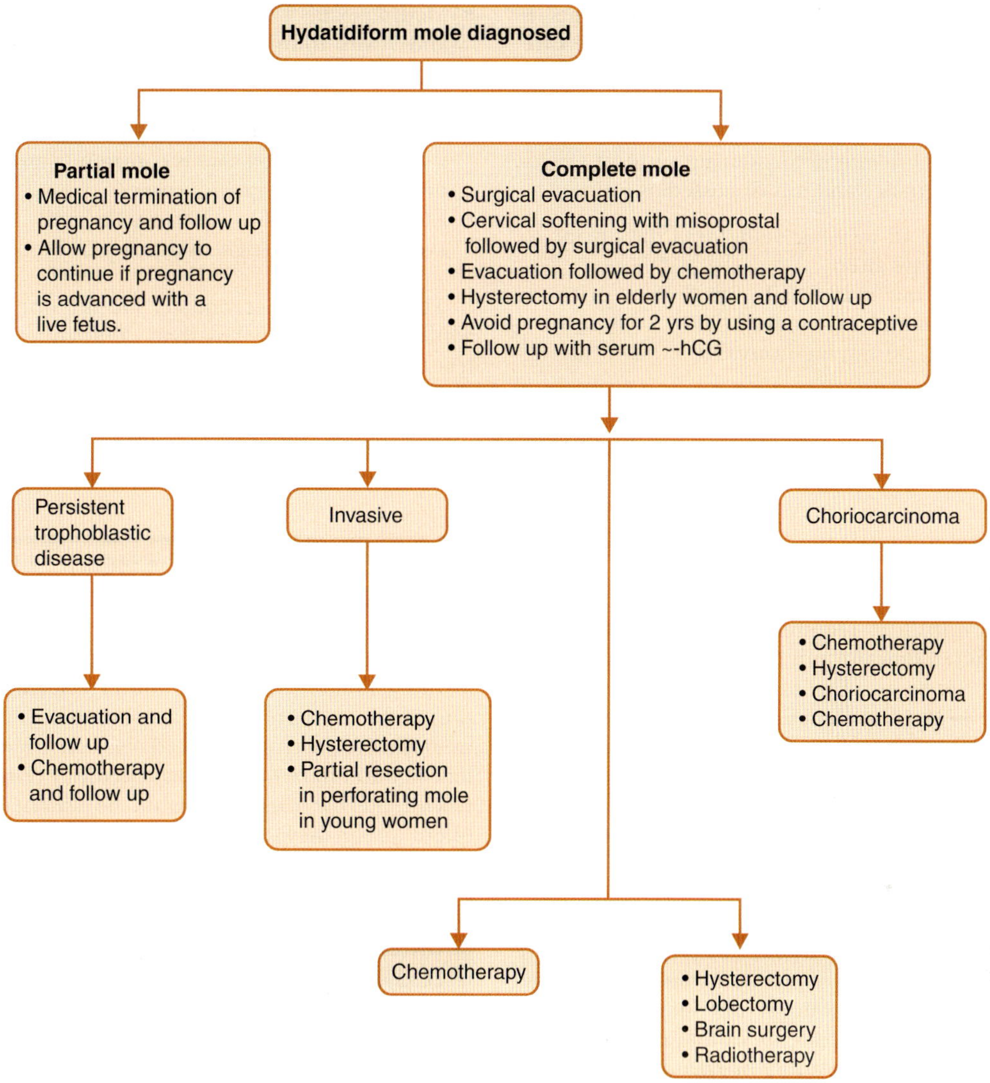

Figure 38.7 Management of hydatidiform mole.

pregnancy. The patient is called at weekly intervals for this test. Once the test becomes negative, the patient is followed up monthly and 3 monthly in the first year and 6 monthly in the second year. Radioimmunoassay techniques have revolutionized the follow-up of patients with molar pregnancy (Fig. 38.7).

Pelvic examination is done to detect any vaginal metastasis, and to assess the uterine size. The size of any ovarian cyst and reduction in its size are noted. A radiograph of the chest is taken to rule out lung metastasis at baseline, after 3 months and subsequently when needed. Persistent uterine bleeding calls for a detailed evaluation and curettage should only be done if retained tissue is suspected and the curettage are sent for histopathological examination to detect choriocarcinoma. Pelvic ultrasound scan can detect residual or locally invasive tumour as well as theca lutein ovarian cyst.

Pregnancy should be avoided preferably by barrier methods for at least 1 year (preferably 2 years) as a fresh pregnancy would interfere with the hCG levels. Intrauterine device and progestogen-only pills cause irregular bleeding and are best avoided. Combined oral pills can be offered once the β-hCG level becomes undetected. Oral combined pills lower the luteinizing hormone (LH) level and, thereby, the hCG level and can cause misinterpretation of results.

Pregnancy should also be avoided for 1 year after stoppage of chemotherapy because of the teratogenic effect of drugs.

Because histopathology of molar tissue does not give a clue as to in which patient molar pregnancy will progress to choriocarcinoma, prophylactic chemotherapy has been used in the following situations:

- High-risk case, i.e. a very young woman and a multiparous woman older than 40 years who refuses hysterectomy.
- A patient with an initial very high level of hCG, where the initial size of uterus was more than 16 weeks' size.
- If a woman cannot come for the follow-up, prophylactic chemotherapy is better than no follow-up.

A partial mole has a very low malignant potential and does not require chemotherapy. All the same, the woman needs a follow-up in the same manner as a complete mole. The hCG level should return to normal within 6–8 weeks.

Prophylactic chemotherapy comprises administration of methotrexate or actinomycin-D.

Routine prophylactic chemotherapy in all patients is not advocated because 80% of molar pregnancies resolve following evacuation. If chemotherapy is prescribed for all molar pregnancies, 80% would be exposed to unnecessary morbidity and toxicity of the drugs.

Some recommend chemotherapy during surgical evacuation of a molar pregnancy and it is discussed as follows:

- Actinomycin-D: i.v. 12 mcg/kg daily for 3 days prior to evacuation and 2 days after
- Methotrexate: 15 mg orally daily for 3 days prior to planned evacuation and 2 days after
- During evacuation, 50 mg methotrexate i.v. drip lasting for 3–4 hours

Use of oral methotrexate may be associated with severe oral/gastrointestinal tract (GIT) ulceration; intramuscular route is the preferred route for administration of methotrexate.

This is expected to reduce the risk of pulmonary emboli and dissemination.

Prophylactic hysterectomy is not recommended today, because (i) it is not often required, (ii) it does not avoid follow-up and (iii) follow-up with β-hCG levels is effective and decides the course of subsequent management.

Because of 2%–10% incidence of recurrent mole, it is necessary to perform an ultrasound scan in subsequent early pregnancies.

PERSISTENT TROPHOBLASTIC DISEASE

PTD is diagnosed when during follow-up at least three weekly values of hCG show persistence of β-hCG level or a rise. About 15%–20% of women with a hydatidiform mole show persistence of the tumour in the uterus following surgical evacuation. Persistence of theca lutein cyst, continued vaginal bleeding and plateauing or raised level of hCG in serum or urine during the follow-up are suggestive of the persistence of chorionic tissue. The International Federation of Gynecology and Obstetrics (FIGO) 2002 criteria of PTD are as follows:

- The plateau of hCG levels of four readings over 3 weeks
- A rise in hCG level of 10% or more over 3 weeks
- Detection of hCG at 6 months
- Persistence of irregular vaginal bleeding

Careful follow-up and hCG monitoring are the keys to identifying PTD:

- Pelvic ultrasound scan will detect PTD in the genital tract.
- Chest X-ray, brain CT scan and liver scan will pick up metastatic growth. Negative chest X-ray does not rule out lung metastasis; CT scan can detect an occult lesion in the lung.

TREATMENT OF PERSISTENT TROPHOBLASTIC DISEASE

Once diagnosed, treatment is chemotherapy:

- Methotrexate 0.5 mg/kg i.v. or i.m. daily for 5 days – repeated every 2 weeks until hCG is undetectable
- Methotrexate 1.0–1.5 mg/kg i.m. or i.v. on days 1, 3, 5 and 7 with folinic acid 0.1–0.15 mg/kg i.m. on alternate days (the course is repeated every 2 weeks as long as required)
- Actinomycin-D 10–12 mcg/kg i.v. daily for 5 days every 2 weeks if methotrexate is contraindicated (liver damage) or fails, and in high-risk cases
- Etoposide (VP-16) – 200 mg/m^2 daily for 5 days orally every 2 weeks in high-risk group or i.v. over 3 hours

Haemoglobin percentage should not fall below 8 g, white cell count not less than 3000/mm^3 and platelet not less than 100,000/mm^3. Blood transfusion will be required if the blood parameters fall below the critical levels. Raised serum glutamic pyruvate transaminase (SGPT), serum glutamic oxaloacetic transaminase (SGOT) and alkaline phosphatase levels indicate liver dysfunction.

PERFORATING MOLE (CHORIOANGIOMA DESTRUENS)

Perforating mole was treated by hysterectomy in the past. In a young woman wishing to conserve fertility, partial resection of the uterus and newer techniques to control bleeding by occlusive instruments and ligation of uterine/internal iliac ligation have now been successfully done. However, the risk of uterine rupture should be watched during subsequent pregnancy, and elective caesarean section is often advocated. Post surgery chemotherapy may also be required for a residual tumour.

RECURRENT MOLAR PREGNANCY

Recurrent molar pregnancy is reported in 2%–10% of cases, with as many as nine consecutive molar pregnancies as reported by WHO in 1973. Following two molar pregnancies, the risk of recurrent mole rises to 28%. A woman with one molar pregnancy faces 20 times the risk of suffering another molar pregnancy and choriocarcinoma. *It is therefore mandatory to perform an ultrasonic screening in this woman in subsequent early pregnancy.*

In a rare case with recurrent molar pregnancies, pregnancy with her husband should be avoided. Instead, in vitro fertilization with a donor sperm is the option to avoid not only subsequent molar pregnancy but also the risk of choriocarcinoma.

COEXISTING MOLAR PREGNANCY

Coexisting molar pregnancy with another uterine pregnancy is reported in 1:10,000 to 100,000 pregnancies. In the vast majority, the fetus shows gross structural and genetic anomalies, and 30% terminate in intrauterine fetal death. Termination of pregnancy is therefore recommended. In rare cases, if the fetus proves normal by ultrasonic scanning and genetic study, pregnancy may be allowed to continue, but hCG monitoring has no value during pregnancy. Vaginal delivery is possible. Placental site tumour does not respond to chemotherapy and requires hysterectomy.

CHORIOCARCINOMA

Choriocarcinoma is rare, but it is one of the most malignant tumour arising in the body of the uterus. The nongestational choriocarcinoma appears as part of a germ cell gonadal neoplasm, both in males and in females. The nature of choriocarcinoma can be identified by DNA study of the tumour. In nongestational choriocarcinoma, DNA is of maternal origin, whereas in molar pregnancy choriocarcinoma, DNA is of paternal origin.

In a woman, this neoplasm follows a pregnancy, 50% of cases follow evacuation of a hydatidiform mole, 25% follow an abortion and 20% follow full-term pregnancy, whereas 5% follow extrauterine pregnancy. The malignancy may appear many years after a full-term pregnancy or an abortion. However, in most cases it develops within next 2 years of a molar pregnancy. The long period that elapses between the pregnancy and the development of choriocarcinoma makes the clinical suspicion of malignancy rather difficult. A primary choriocarcinoma arising in the placenta during pregnancy that led to fetal metastasis in the liver has been reported.

About 4%–10% of molar pregnancies develop choriocarcinoma, within 2 years. Postmolar GTD may be an invasive mole or choriocarcinoma, but nonmolar GTD is always a choriocarcinoma.

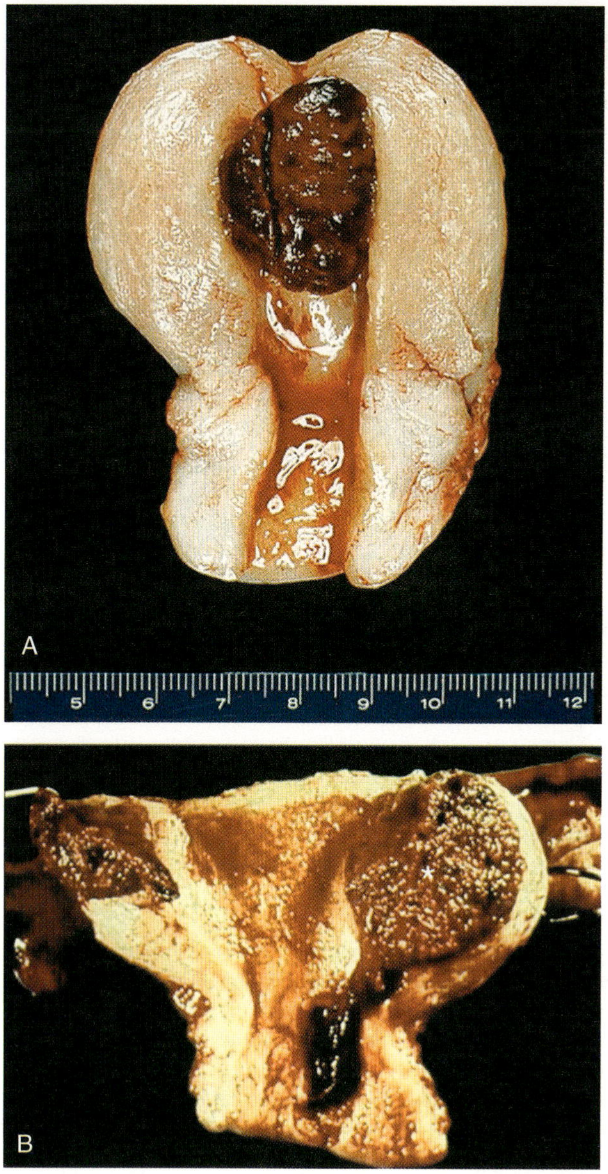

Figure 38.8 Choriocarcinoma of the uterus. **(A)** The tumour has infiltrated the myometrium and presents as a polypoid excrescence into the cavity of the uterus. It is, therefore, readily diagnosed on exploratory curettage. **(B)** Patient came with massive intraperitoneal haemorrhage. (*Courtesy*: Dr Narayan M Patel, Ahmedabad.)

INCIDENCE

Choriocarcinoma exhibits a geographical distribution very similar to that of a hydatidiform mole. The incidence in the UK and the USA is of the order of 1:50,000 to 1:70,000 pregnancies, and it is 10 times more common in Southeast Asia. An older woman with high parity and belonging to a low socioeconomic group runs a high risk of developing this malignancy.

MORBID ANATOMY

To the naked eye, the growth appears as a solid purple friable mass. The majority of primary growth arises in the body of the uterus and develops first within the endometrial cavity (Fig. 38.8). In such cases, the growth projects into the cavity of the uterus, quickly ulcerates and causes a blood-stained discharge, which later becomes offensive and purulent as the growth becomes infected and necrotic. There may be periodic episodes of fresh haemorrhage. Growths of this kind superficially resemble placental polyp, but choriocarcinoma always infiltrates the wall of the uterus, whereas a placental polypus is clearly demarcated from the myometrium and can be easily detached. Choriocarcinoma does not necessarily develop primarily in the endometrium, and it is not uncommon for the growth to start in the myometrium in the deeper tissues of the uterine wall. Primary choriocarcinoma of the uterus may erode through into the broad ligament or peritoneal cavity and cause profuse bleeding, or it may cause enlargement of the uterus to such a degree that the fundus of the uterus reaches upwards to the level of the umbilicus. Metastasis occurs early and dissemination usually occurs by way of the bloodstream. Ones which can be detected easily are those found in the lower third of the vagina and at the vulva. Such metastases form purple haemorrhagic projections either into the vagina or around the vaginal orifice. Their appearance is characteristic and pathognomonic of choriocarcinoma. These metastases are interesting pathologically, for they are comparable to the vaginal metastases sometimes found with carcinoma of the body of the uterus and malignant ovarian tumours. Such metastases are produced by retrograde spread along the venous channels of the vaginal plexuses of veins. The general metastases probably develop early, the growth disseminating by way of the bloodstream. Multiple metastases may form in the lungs and cause haemoptysis (Fig. 38.9). Vaginal metastasis forms in 30% of cases. Deposits are frequently found in the kidneys, brain, spleen and liver, but when the dissemination is widespread, almost any organ

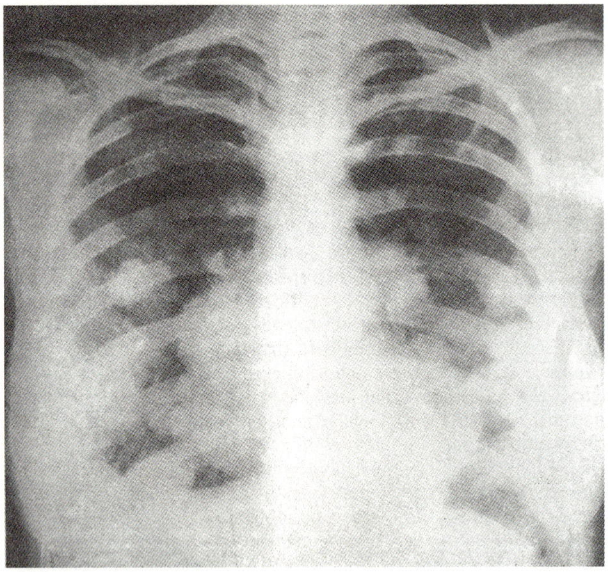

Figure 38.9 Multiple 'cannon ball' metastases in lungs from choriocarcinoma.

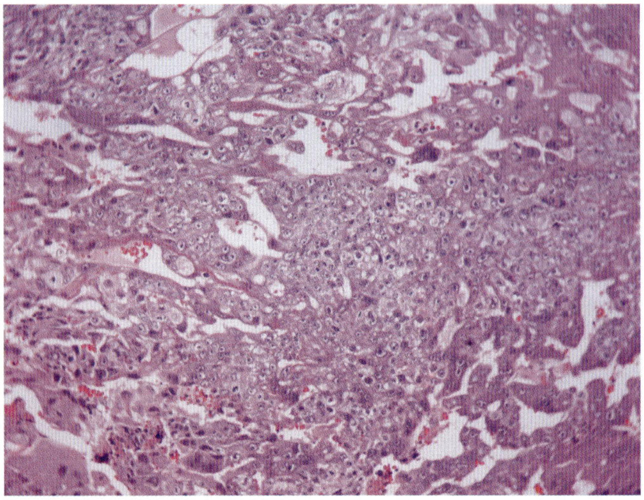

Figure 38.10 Choriocarcinoma: sheets of tumour cells showing marked nuclear pleomorphism. A biphasic pattern with mixture of cytotrophoblastic and syncytiotrophoblastic cells is seen. *(Courtesy:* Dr Sandeep Mathur, AIIMS.)

may be affected and large emboli may get lodge in the large arteries of the systemic circulation. The most common sites of metastasis are lungs (80%), brain and liver (10% each). Less common sites are GIT, kidney, spleen, genital tract and the lymph nodes (10%). In advanced cases, the parametrium may be extensively infiltrated with growth. Invasion of the ovaries is usually by the way of the bloodstream. Ovarian cysts of the theca lutein cyst are found in about 9% of cases (Table 38.4).

The histological appearance is very typical. Syncytium, cytotrophoblast and degenerated red blood cells constitute the growth. The cells are actively growing and show such malignant characteristics as typical mitotic division and anaplastic changes. In some areas, the cells are translucent or vacuolated and may resemble decidual cells. No evidence of chorionic villi can be detected, the growth consisting solely of embryonic syncytium, cytotrophoblast and degenerated blood cells. The absence of villi must be stressed as a diagnostic feature which separates the malignant choriocarcinoma from the benign and invasive mole in which villi are demonstrable. This is because the trophoblast grows in such extensive columns as to completely obliterate the villous pattern. The other distinguishing feature of malignancy is invasion of the uterine wall by trophoblastic cells, with destruction of muscle tissues accompanied by necrosis and haemorrhage (Fig. 38.10). The primitive infiltrating properties of the embryonic cytotrophoblast are retained in choriocarcinoma so that vessels are eroded and local haemorrhages are produced, which cause the typical macroscopical appearances. As a result of erosion of vessels, the growth penetrates into the systemic bloodstream, and generalized metastases are apt to develop early.

There is clinical evidence that metastases may regress after the removal of the primary growth but this is rare. The radiograph of lungs presents the haemorrhagic metastasis as a 'cannon ball' (see Fig. 38.9), whereas, in reality, they may be only zones of haemorrhage. It may also present a woolly appearance because of diffuse haemorrhage. It must be remembered that vaginal nodules resembling the metastases of choriocarcinoma can occur with benign hydatidiform mole and even normal pregnancy, according to Magnus Haines. This concept of benign trophoblastic embolism must considerably influence our thinking on the question of spontaneous regression of the so-called malignant metastases in choriocarcinoma. Choriocarcinoma, as with hydatidiform moles, shows high levels of β-hCG in the urine and serum.

SYMPTOMS AND SIGNS

These are dependent on the site of growth. Persistent or irregular uterine haemorrhage following an abortion, a molar pregnancy or a normal delivery should always raise the suspicion of choriocarcinoma. The bleeding is usually profuse, but sometimes there may be only blood stains. An offensive vaginal discharge develops when secondary infection supervenes; pyrexia and cachexia will be the accompanying symptoms. *When amenorrhoea occurs, it is because of a very high level of hCG secreted by the tumour.* The perforation of the uterus with intraperitoneal haemorrhage simulates an ectopic pregnancy. The other symptoms may vary depending upon cyto metastasis. Dyspnoea and haemoptysis are noticed with lung metastasis. The appearance of neurological symptoms such as hemiplegia, epilepsy, headache and visual disturbances suggests brain metastasis.

On examination, a vaginal metastasis appears as a bluish red vascular tumour which bleeds easily on touch. The uterus may be enlarged. The theca lutein cyst in ovary are palpable in some cases. The liver and brain metastases are often seen in cases with lung metastasis.

DIFFERENTIAL DIAGNOSIS

- Both postdelivery and postabortal retained placental tissue or placental polyp cause secondary postpartum haemorrhage (PPH). Histopathology of curettings will help to diagnose choriocarcinoma. However, the diagnosis can be missed if the growth is in the myometrium. β-hCG level in serum and the urine will establish the correct diagnosis. Ultrasound and CT scans are useful to determine spread of the disease.

- When choriocarcinoma develops many years later following a pregnancy, its clinical diagnosis is difficult to make. Irregular bleeding mandates curettage which will reveal the cause of bleeding. Ultrasound will reveal the uterine growth.
- Intraperitoneal haemorrhage following spontaneous uterine perforation by the tumour growth may simulate ectopic pregnancy. The treatment is laparotomy in both these conditions when the true nature of the lesion becomes obvious.
- **Pulmonary Metastasis.** The pulmonary symptoms may resemble pulmonary tuberculosis. The 'cannon ball' metastasis is typical of a malignant lesion.
- **Brain Metastasis.** The neurological symptoms point towards a brain lesion. The elevated hCG level in the serum or preferably in cerebrospinal fluid (CSF) and CT/MRI scan will establish the diagnosis.

When the metastasis develops more than 1 year following abortion, diagnosis of choriocarcinoma becomes difficult. Think of choriocarcinoma if a young woman develops neurological symptoms with a history of past abortion or pregnancy, in such cases estimate β-hCG level in CSF, serum.

STAGING

Disease is staged into four stages (Stages I–IV) by FIGO. Furthermore, to risk score the disease, a WHO risk scoring system is commonly used. Refer to Tables 38.5 and 38.6.

DIAGNOSIS

The diagnosis is based on clinical features and histological evidence when available. Serum β-hCG level, X-ray of lungs as well as CT scan of lungs and brain, and ultrasound scan of liver and pelvis help in establishing the correct diagnosis. PET is employed in difficult cases with unusual symptoms and signs.

Table 38.5 FIGO Classification of Gestational Trophoblastic Diseases

Stage I	Disease confined to the uterus
Stage II	GTD extends outside of the uterus but is limited to the genital structure
Stage III	Lung metastasis with or without genital tract involvement
Stage IV	Other metastasis
IVA	No risk factor
IVB	One risk factor
IVC	Two risk factors
Risk factors:	
1.	Serum β-human chorionic gonadotropin (hCG) level >100,000 mIU/mL
2.	Duration of disease >6 months

Note: Lately, risk factors are not included in staging.

TREATMENT

CHEMOTHERAPY

One of the biggest triumphs of medical science is effective chemotherapy in choriocarcinoma. Histopathological evidence may not be available in every case, especially in invasive and metastatic tumours. β-hCG is a very specific marker, so the chemotherapy can be administered based on this alone.

Unlike other malignant lesions, the treatment of choriocarcinoma is mainly chemotherapy, for both local and distant metastases.

The most effective chemotherapeutic agent is methotrexate, a folic acid antagonist. It is a mixture of 4-amino-10-methyl folic acid and related compounds. This drug interferes with the formation of nucleic acid and mitosis in the malignant cells and thereby arrests the growth. The staging decides whether single or multiple drug therapy is required.

Table 38.6 Modified WHO Prognostic Scoring System

Prognostic Factors	0	1	2	4
Age (years)	<39	>39	–	–
Antecedent pregnancy	Mole	Abortion	Term pregnancy	
Interval (months)	<4	4–6	7–12	>12
Pretreatment hCG (mIU/mL)	$<10^3$	10^3–10^4	10^4–10^5	$>10^5$
Size of tumour (cm)	<3	3–5	>5	
Site of metastasis	Lung	Spleen, kidney	GI liver	Brain
Number of metastasis	–	1–4	5–8	>8
Previous failed chemotherapy			Single drug	2 or more
Low risk– </=6, high risk>6				

Methotrexate is given orally 5 mg five times a day for 5 days earlier but was associated with significant GIT side effects. It is now given by intramuscular/intravenous injections. To reduce side effects with the use of methotrexate, therapy is usually given on days 1, 3, 5 and 7. On alternate days (days 2, 4, 6, 8), injection folinic acid is given. The course of chemotherapy is repeated at intervals of 10–14 days depending on the blood picture and side effects of the drug. The patient should completely recover from any toxic side effect before the second course is started. These courses are continued until complete regression of the primary tumour and all metastases are achieved – indicated when three consecutive weekly radioimmunoassays for hCG in serum are negative. Thereafter, one more course is administered. This is done because even radioimmunoassay cannot detect β-hCG level below 1 mIμ/mL, and the last course hopefully destroys any minute trophoblastic tissue that might have been left untouched.

Methotrexate has the following side effects: (i) ulcerative stomatitis and gastric haemorrhage; (ii) skin reaction; (iii) alopecia; (iv) bone marrow depression, leading to anaemia, leucopenia and agranulocytosis; and (v) liver and kidney damage.

It is advisable check on haemoglobin, white cell count and platelet count and carry out liver function tests, kidney function tests and radiograph of chest before instituting this chemotherapy. Methotrexate is contraindicated in liver disease. To avoid or to reduce toxicity, 'folinic acid rescue regime' is recommended. This regime consists of citrovorum factor (folinic acid) 15 mg intramuscularly and methotrexate administered on alternate days, so that one course of treatment lasts for a total of 10 days.

COMBINATION CHEMOTHERAPY REGIMEN

Combined chemotherapy is recommended in high-risk cases. A variety of combinations of chemotherapeutic agents are being used, such as (i) methotrexate, actinomycin-D and cyclophosphamide (MAC) and (ii) methotrexate, actinomycin-D and adriamycin (MAA). The number of courses depends on the severity of the disease and response of the patient.

Bagshaw treated cases with a combination of etoposide, methotrexate and actinomycin-D and claimed equally good results with less side effects. All authors agree that it is more effective to treat the high-risk cases with combined therapy ab initio than to treat them with combined therapy only after a failed attempt with a single agent. Currently EMA-CO regimen is the most commonly used combination chemotherapy regimen in the management of high risk.

The course is repeated every 2 weeks depending on recovery from toxicity.

MAC treatment comprises the combination of methotrexate 50 mg i.v., actinomycin-D 0.5 mg i.v. and cyclophosphamide 250 mg i.v. daily for 5 days and repeat every 3 weeks (Table 38.7).

The placental site trophoblastic disease is often resistant to chemotherapy, and hysterectomy is recommended.

In brain and lung metastases, previous treatment with radiotherapy is now replaced by chemotherapy, because the results are good and radiotherapy causes extensive fibrosis.

Table 38.7 MAC Regimen and EMA-CO Regimen

(A) MAC Regimen	
Day 1-5	Methotrexate 1mg/kg
Day 1-5	Actinomycin-D 12/ug/day
Day 1-5	Cyclophosphamide 3mg/kg
(B) EMA-CO Regimen	
Day 1	Etopocide 100mg/m² iv infusion over 30 min in 200ml saline Actinomycin - D : 500/μg iv stat Methotrexate 100mg/m² iv over/2hr
Day 2	Etopocide 100mg/m² iv infusion over 30 min Actinomycin - D 500μg/iv stat Folinic Acid 15mg im × 4 does every 12 hr
Day 8	Vincristine (Oncovin) 10mg iv stat Cyclophosphamide 600mg iv infusion in saline

*Next course repeated after 2-3 wks.

Methotrexate 12.5 mg can be injected intrathecally at every 2–4 weeks' interval until hCG level becomes negative.

Newer drugs such as Taxol, typotecan and gemcitabine (antimetabolite) have been used in resistant cases. Gemcitabine 1250 mg/m^2 on days 1–8 with cisplatin is effective.

Rarely, leukaemia has been reported with the use of Etoposide several years later.

SURGERY

Surgery is rarely indicated in the management of choriocarcinoma.

Hysterectomy is indicated in the following conditions:

- High-risk cases older than 40 years, multiparous
- Chemotherapy ineffective/chemotherapy resistance
- Haemorrhage because of uterine perforation
- Large-sized growth in the uterus
- When placental site trophoblastic disease does not respond to chemotherapy and hysterectomy is the only solution

Hysterectomy is usually followed by chemotherapy. There is no need to remove the ovaries as ovarian metastasis is rare and can be effectively treated by chemotherapy. Hysterectomy reduces the number of chemotherapy courses.

Role of radiotherapy is limited to only acute bleeding from vaginal metastasis, brain and liver metastasis. The post-radiotherapy fibrosis is the disadvantage.

A solitary lung metastasis can be dealt with by thoracotomy and lobectomy. Craniotomy is rarely resorted to in a solitary brain tumour.

The role of high dose chemotherapy with autologous bone marrow transplant is being explored.

Table 38.8 Management of Metastasis

Vagina	Vaginal pack for bleeding, avoid excision, chemotherapy
Lungs	Chemotherapy, Lobectomy if the growth is localized or resistant to chemotherapy
Liver	Chemotherapy, Radiation
Brain	• Chemotherapy • Intrathecal chemotherapy • Surgery • Radiation

CEREBRAL METASTASIS (Table 38.8)

A focal lesion detected by CT/MRI can be excised to prevent haemorrhage in the tumour and death. A large lesion is treated with radiation given in a dose of 30 Gy in 10 fractions 5 days a week for 2 weeks along with EMA/CO and this yields 80% response. Liver metastasis should receive whole-organ radiation over 10 days in a dose of 20 Gy.

Lobectomy is required in a chemotherapy-resistant case.

FOLLOW-UP OF A CASE OF CHORIOCARCINOMA

Serum β-hCG is done every week till it becomes negative. Once negative it is repeated every 2 weekly for 3 month, thereafter every month for one year and then 6 monthly for rest of life.

PROGNOSIS

Overall cure rates in recent years have been excellent with chemotherapy alone, and surgery is undertaken only in selective cases described earlier. With chemotherapy, 100% success has been claimed in low-risk group (J Lewis, 1980) and 90% success in high-risk group. A successful pregnancy has followed treatment with chemotherapy. However, it is advisable for the patient not to conceive for 2 years after the drug treatment is over. The lifelong follow-up of the woman, however, should be encouraged.

KEY POINTS

- Trophoblastic diseases comprise a spectrum of clinical conditions varying from hydatidiform mole, invasive mole and choriocarcinoma.
- Hydatidiform mole is more prevalent in Southeast Asia, diagnosed clinically and confirmed by ultrasound scan and raised β-hCG levels.
- Treatment of hydatidiform mole is surgical evacuation. Six month up to two-years monitoring is required to detect persistent moles and development of choriocarcinoma. Pregnancy during this period should be avoided. Prophylactic chemotherapy is beneficial in selective cases.
- Serum hCG level is the key marker in follow-up.
- Histology is not able to indicate the potential of molar pregnancy for development of malignancy. Therefore, follow-up with serum β-hCG is necessary for 2 years. Thereafter, the risk of malignancy is negligible.
- Persistent trophoblastic disease and choriocarcinoma are treated effectively by chemotherapy. Surgery is rarely required.
- Choriocarcinoma and metastatic growths developing several years after pregnancy render the diagnosis difficult.
- Placental site trophoblastic disease with low hCG but raised HPL level fails to respond to chemotherapy and requires hysterectomy.
- Following molar pregnancy, the woman needs counselling regarding recurrent mole and choriocarcinoma, and should be counselled for follow-up.
- Prognosis has greatly improved because of specific hCG marker and effective chemotherapy.
- Choriocarcinoma is uncommon, but highly malignant.
- Choriocarcinoma may follow a molar pregnancy, abortion, term pregnancy and ectopic pregnancy.
- Fifty per cent cases of choriocarcinoma occur following molar pregnancy and occur within 2 years.
- The long interval of years between pregnancy and choriocarcinoma makes the diagnosis difficult.
- Primary treatment of choriocarcinoma is chemotherapy and is effective in 90%–100% of cases. Surgery is reserved for selective cases.
- Pregnancy is possible following treatment with chemotherapy. However, conception should be delayed for 2 years to avoid teratogenic effect on the fetus.

SELF-ASSESSMENT

1. A 25-year-old woman presents with 3 months' amenorrhoea, abdominal pain and vaginal bleeding. The uterus is 20 weeks' size. How will you investigate the case?
2. How will you manage a case of hydatidiform mole at 16 weeks' pregnancy?
3. What are the complications of hydatidiform mole? How will you prevent them?
4. Describe the clinical features of choriocarcinoma.
5. Discuss the management of choriocarcinoma.

SUGGESTED READING

Dalya Alhamdan, Tommaso Bignardi, George Condous. Recognising gestational trophoblastic disease. In: Best Practice and Research: Clinical Obstetrics and Gynaecology, Vol 20(5): 565–573, Elsevier, 2006.

Ma HK, Wong LC, Ngan JYS. In: The modern management of trophoblastic disease. Bonnar J. In: Recent Advances in Obstetrics and Gynaecology. Vol 16: 1–23, Churchill Livingstone, London, 1990.

39 Radiation Therapy, Chemotherapy and Palliative Care for Gynaecological Cancers

CHAPTER OUTLINE

Most gynaecological malignancies need adjuvant treatment in the form of radiotherapy and chemotherapy. Advances in the field of radiation oncology and medical oncology have helped in achieving optimal results while treating cancer of the cervix, cancer of the ovary, endometrial cancers, gestational trophoblastic diseases and other rare types of genital tract cancers.

RADIATION THERAPY

Radiation therapy plays an important role in the management of gynaecological malignancies. Its specific curative role has been established beyond doubt in the management of cervical cancer, the most commonly seen gynaecological cancer in clinical practice. Radiation treatment may also be curative for localized endometrial cancer and when surgery is not possible. It improves prognosis if used as adjuvant postoperative therapy in advanced cervical and endometrial cancer. The scope of radiation therapy has been enhanced in the management of cancers of the vulva and vagina. In selected cases of cancer of the ovary, postoperative adjuvant radiotherapy may be beneficial in controlling the disease. In many cases, a judicious combination of radiotherapy and cancer chemotherapy has contributed significantly in improving the patient's prognosis and survival period.

Cell death in terms of radiation biology is defined as the loss of clonogenic capacity or 'cell reproductive potential'. Ionizing radiation produces free radicals which disrupt the reproductive integrity of DNA-producing cells and thus control cell division and neoplastic growth. Radiation affects both normal cells and tumour cells. However, the dividing mitotic cells are most vulnerable. Hence, by grading the dose of irradiation, a differential effect can be attained by forcing the cancer cells to differentiate and thus lose their malignant potential, stimulating angioblasts and fibroblasts to grow into the tumour cell mass, dividing them into smaller nests of neoplastic cells and, finally as the connective tissue fibroblasts constrict, cutting off the tumour cell blood supply causing tumour necrosis. Anaplastic tumours therefore respond better compared to well-differentiated squamous cell tumours. Adenocarcinoma and sarcoma are poor responders.

PHYSICAL PRINCIPLES OF RADIATION THERAPY

BASIC PHYSICS

Radiation physics deals with the measurement of energy that is transferred from the radiation source to the target tissue being irradiated.

The therapeutic activity of radiation is mainly related to the process of ionization. There are two forms of *photons* (quanta of radiation whose energy is proportional to their frequency and inversely proportional to their wavelength). One form of ionizing radiation is electromagnetic, which refers to X-rays. These sources of energy have no mass and no electrical charge. They are produced in discrete quanta or photons. A second source of photon radiation comes from the production of gamma rays (similar to X-rays) which result from the decay of radioactive isotopes.

Electromagnetic radiation with shorter wavelengths has a higher frequency, hence higher energy. The energy produced is measured in electron volts (eV); 1 eV = 1.6×10^{-12} erg. The X-ray radiotherapy units can range from 50,000 eV (50 kV) to over 30 million eV.

Photon radiation is measured in curies (Ci). One curie is defined as 3.7×10^{10} disintegrations/second, which is equivalent to the disintegration of 1 g of radium.

Irrespective of the source of electromagnetic or photon radiation, the transmitted energy diverges from the source of origin and diminishes inversely as the square of the distance traversed ($1/d^2$).

X-rays and photons can be generated as a result of rapidly accelerated electrons in vacuum striking a target. Modern generators that accelerate these electrons to a high speed may do so in a circular fashion (betatron) or linearly (linear accelerator).

Another type of radiation energy, known as particulate radiation, is produced by subatomic particles having a discrete mass. These particles are derived as a result of disintegration of radionuclides. Four different types, namely alpha particles, neutrons, protons and electrons, are produced.

Neutrons are highly penetrative and have no charge but have a large mass. They cause high-energy collisions with atomic nuclei, principally hydrogen in the tissues. The resultant recoil proton loses energy to the surrounding tissue by ionization, causing cell death.

Photons are positively charged particles and can be produced directly by generators. The high-energy beams produced are used for special applications such as the treatment of pituitary tumours.

Alpha particles (helium nucleus) have very little penetrating power and therefore are not of much practical use.

Electrons, also referred to as beta rays, can be produced at different energies by machines for various therapeutic uses.

RADIATION BIOLOGY

Photons (gamma rays or X-rays) act by dislodging orbital electrons of the tissue through which they pass. This collision produces a fast electron (Compton effect) which then ionizes molecules along its path producing secondary electrons and free hydroxyl (OH) radicals. This process continues until the photon loses all of its energy. About 80% of the cell contains water, so cellular radiation damage is mediated by the ionization of water and production of free radicals, hydrogen (H) and hydroxide (OH).

The free OH radical causes DNA cell damage. The effect may be lethal and kill the cell or it may be sublethal, in which case the cellular DNA may undergo repair and the cell recovers.

The free molecular OH radicals react with molecular oxygen to form peroxides, which in turn further damage the tissues. *Oxygen is therefore important to enhance photon effects.* Large tumours with poor blood supply have poor photon effect in hypoxic areas and are radioresistant. *Radiation in the presence of anaemia, infection and scarred tissue produces poor results.*

The rate of loss of energy of an ionizing particle as it traverses a unit length of medium is known as linear energy transfer (LET). In case of photons, energy transfer from an X-ray or electromagnetic source, the LET is low; hence, multiple tissue bombardments are required to achieve a lethal dose. In case of particulate irradiation with large particles (neutrons), the ionization achieved is high, leading to high LET, more intense ionization and production of more toxic hydroxyl radicals, achieving greater lethal tissue effect independent of tissue oxygenation.

Successful radiotherapy requires a good balance between the dosage to the tumour and to that of the surrounding structure (radiation tolerance) so that least damage is inflicted to the normal tissues, while maximal radioeffect reaches the tumour cells. The aim is to deliver a high dose to the tumour and minimal dose to the normal tissues. Radiosensitizers, cisplatin and 5-fluorouracil, enhance the lethal effect of radiation when given concomitantly. *This combination is called chemoradiation.*

An important principle to remember is that a given dose of radiation kills a constant fraction of tumour cells; hence, each repetitive sitting achieves a similar reduction of tumour cell activity.

There are four phases of a cell cycle: resting phase, RNA and protein synthesis, DNA synthesis and cell division or mitosis. Rapidly dividing cells are the most radiosensitive. This explains the higher response of anaplastic tumours compared to a well-differentiated one.

Fractionation of radiation treatment permits effective treatment of the tumour, and minimizes complications which could result from exposure of normal tissues (bone marrow, normal intestine) to a single large dose. The more effective repair of normal tissue occurring between treatment fractions allows recovery of normal cells which is a therapeutic advantage.

The clinician must be familiar with the unit of measurement of amount of energy absorbed by the tissue, called the rad. Rad is defined as 100 ergs of energy absorbed per gram of tissue.

Lately the term *gray* (1 J/kg) has been introduced. One gray (Gy) is equivalent to 100 rad.

Summary

Radiation biology produces the following effects:

- Radiation (photons or gamma rays) is transferred from the radiation source to the tissues undergoing irradiation. The process of ionization occurs (Compton effect) along the path of radiation. The free radicals liberated produce tissue damage. Mitotic cells are killed (lethal effect) or undergo differentiation (rendered nonlethal). Proliferation of angioblasts and fibroblasts breaks up the mass into smaller islands of tissue tumours. Finally, the fibroblasts constrict and cause necrosis of tissue by way of decreasing vascularity.
- The effect of transmitted energy, irrespective of the source of irradiation as it diverges from the source of origin, rapidly diminishes inversely as the square of the distance travelled.
- Success of radiotherapy requires a good balance of dosage between the tumour tissue and the healthy surrounding tissue.

RADIATION SOURCES: EXTERNAL AND INTERNAL THERAPY

In general, two techniques are utilized in radiation treatment, brachytherapy (internal) and teletherapy (external).

BRACHYTHERAPY

Brachytherapy is a form of radiation therapy in which the source is placed close to the tumour. The application may be in the form of needles implanted into the tumour (interstitial) or placed in the vagina, cervical canal or uterine cavity (intracavitary) in tandem with vaginal ovoids or use of colpostat.

In the case of cervical and uterine cancer, brachytherapy comprises a central uterine tandem and two ovoids in the vaginal vault. This positioning irradiates the primary growth as well as the parametrium and the obturator lymph nodes (Fig. 39.1).

Preradiation preparation includes:

- Checking haemoglobin and WBC
- Rectal enema or suppository
- Antibiotic cover

Method. Under general anaesthesia, a self-retaining catheter is inserted into the bladder. The cervix is dilated to allow the insertion of the uterine tube. After inserting the long empty device, two rubber ovoids or platinum boxes are placed in the vaginal fornices. The vagina is then packed

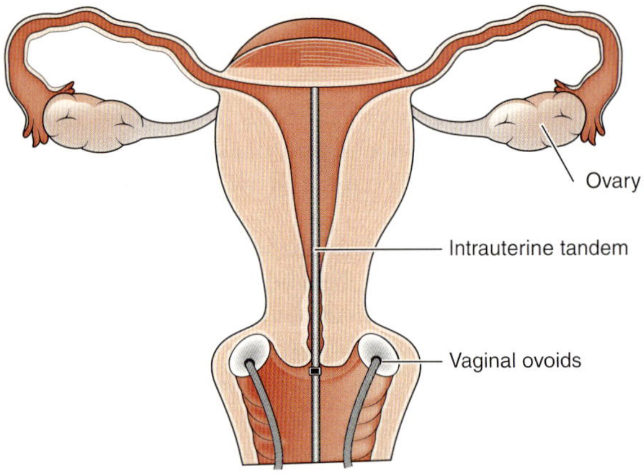

Figure 39.1 Intracavitary source of irradiation in cancer cervix.

with sterile gauze in such a way that the bladder and the rectum are displaced away from the radiation source. Anteroposterior and lateral X-rays of the pelvis are taken to check the correct position of the devices (Fig. 39.2). The radioactive substance is then loaded into the device by remote control of 'afterloading technique'. It is unloaded when nursing medical staff enters the patient's room. This reduces the radiation exposure to nurses and doctors (safety method).

Three methods are in vogue (Table 39.1). In the *Paris method*, the radium (which is removed daily for cleaning) is applied continuously for 5 days. In the *Stockholm method*, the radium is inserted on three occasions, with intervals of 7 days between the first two insertions and 2 weeks after the last insertion, each insertion lasting 48 hours (Fig. 39.3). In the *Manchester technique*, two insertions 72 hours each are applied at a week's interval (Fig. 39.4).

In brachytherapy, various radioisotopes are used depending on their half-life (Table 39.2). In general, those with a short half-life may be placed in the patient and left permanently (e.g. radioactive gold-198), whereas those with a longer half-life are left temporarily in the patient, and removed after a prescribed dose of irradiation has been administered (caesium-137).

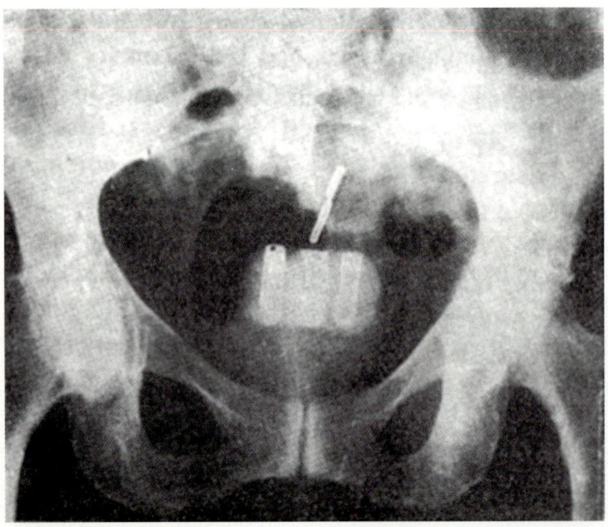

Figure 39.2 X-ray of pelvis, showing positioning of radium in a Manchester insertion. Note that the central opacity between the two ovoids is, in fact, a space and not a third radium-containing ovoid. (*Source:* From: Macleod and Read, Gynaecology. 5th ed. Churchill, 1955.)

Table 39.1 Brachytherapy

Technique	Amount and Type of Radium	Number of Applications	Duration
Paris technique	Intrauterine tube 33.3 mg – two vaginal ovoids 13.3 mg	One	Five days, each day, radium is removed, cleaned and replaced
Stockholm technique	Intrauterine tube 50 mg – two vaginal ovoids 50–60 mg	Three	48 hours each with a gap of 1 week between the first and the second, and 2 weeks between the second and the third
Manchester technique	Intrauterine tube 50 mg and vaginal colpostat 30–50 mg	Two	72 hours each at intervals of 1 week

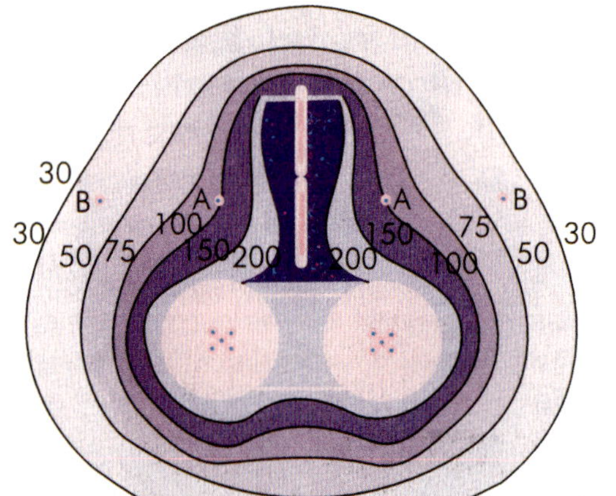

Figure 39.3 Isodose curves of a standard radium insertion using the Manchester technique for carcinoma of the cervix uteri. The dose at point A is taken as 100%. (*Source:* From: Paterson R. The Treatment of Malignant Disease by Radium and X-Rays. Edward Arnold.)

During brachytherapy, it is important to achieve a uniform distribution of radiation in the adjacent tissues to avoid 'hot spots' which can cause excessive damage to the normal tissues, and 'cold spots' which can lead to undertreatment of the tumour. In brachytherapy for cancer of the cervix, the limiting factor to be kept in mind is point A, a point 2 cm above the lateral fornix and 2 cm lateral to the cervical canal. It is the anatomical location of the ureter;

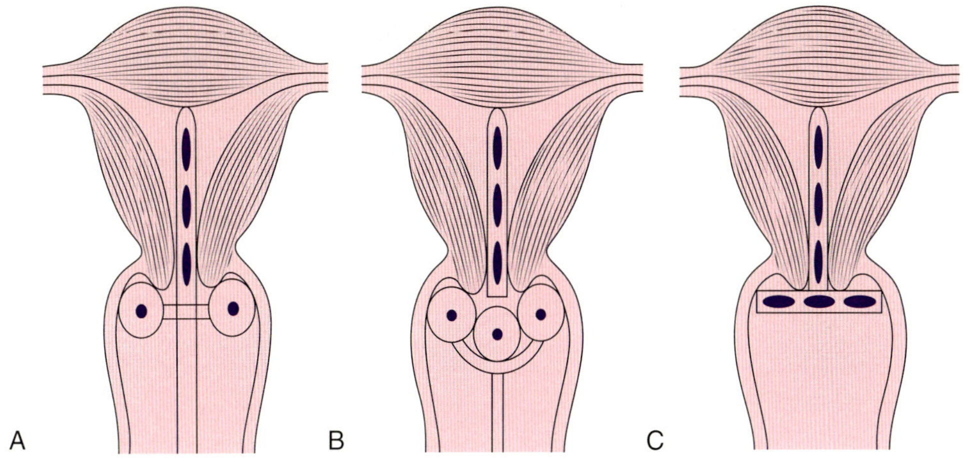

Figure 39.4 Different methods of brachytherapy. **(A)** Manchester technique. **(B)** Paris technique. **(C)** Stockholm technique.

Table 39.2 Half-lives of Commonly Used Isotopes

Radionuclide	Half-Life (Days)
Gold-198	2.7
Phosphorus-32	14.3
Iodine-125	60
Iridium-192	74.4
Cobalt-60	5.3
Caesium-137	30
Radium-226	1620 years

hence, a dose exceeding 8000 rad should not reach this point. The second objective should be to irradiate maximally point B, located 5.0 cm from the uterine axis, laterally and at the same level as point A, and dose is 5000 rad. This point represents the lateral pelvic wall. However, the radiation dose achieved at the lateral pelvic wall would be low because of the inverse square law (1000 rad).

The bladder and rectal mucosa cannot withstand overirradiation (rectum: 5000 rad; bladder: 6000 rad); hence, adequate packing of the vagina and keeping the bladder and rectum empty are mandatory. Optimal safe dose depends on the 'radiation tolerance' of the normal surrounding structures: bladder, rectum, intestines, liver and kidneys.

TELETHERAPY

It is a form of radiation therapy where the radioactive source is placed at a distance from the patient (external therapy). The source of radiation is placed at a distance 5–10 times greater than the depth of the tumour to be irradiated, in order to achieve uniform distribution of radiation to the tumour, and thereby avoid the large dose variations attributable to the inverse square law. This distance is also called source-to-skin distance (SSD). External radiotherapy irradiates mainly the parametrium and the pelvic lymph nodes. Brachytherapy is followed by teletherapy over a period of 4–6 weeks. In a few cases, where the primary tumour is large or the tumour has distorted the cervical canal and prevents the insertion of a uterine device, it is prudent to apply teletherapy first (3000 rad). This shrinks the primary tumour and enables the application of brachytherapy. Cobalt-60 and caesium-137 are the common sources of teletherapy (external radiotherapy).

Selectron reduces the period of application and shrinks the tumour quickly. Megavoltage therapy has the following advantages:

- Greater penetration which allows deeper tissues to be effectively radiated
- Spares the skin effect
- Shorter treatment time
- No bone necrosis
- Can cover a larger field in the abdomen

Supplementary teletherapy through four or more portals is necessary to achieve uniform and adequate cancericidal dose or irradiation to the entire pelvis.

The tumour tissue recovers more slowly or not at all as compared to the normal tissue. Therefore, fractionated course of radiotherapy (four to five times a week) allows normal tissues to recover before the next dose and reduces the toxicity.

In pelvic radiation, each fraction is 180–200 cGy. In abdominal radiation, it is reduced to 100–120 cGy to avoid damage to the liver, kidneys and intestines. A total of 25–30 fractions over 5–6 weeks are administered. This fractionation minimizes the side effects of radiation.

INTERSTITIAL RADIOTHERAPY

In this, the radioactive source is placed directly into the tissue tumour. It may be removable implants or permanent implants which are placed in inaccessible tumours, such as radioactive iodine at the time of surgery. Removable implants can be used in the vagina and cervix. Iridium-192 is the radioactive isotope of choice in these cases. As with intracavity, afterloading devices are now available as safety methods. Other sources are caesium-137 and cobalt-60.

COMPLICATIONS OF RADIOTHERAPY

Complications of radiotherapy are divided into early and late complications.

1. *Early complications*: These include:
   - Transient nausea and vomiting; antiemetic drugs help
   - Bladder irritation causing frequency; dysuria or haematuria is treated with anticholinergic drugs or chlorpromazine
   - Rectal irritation causing tenesmus and diarrhoea (1%); anticholinergic drugs help
   - Irritation of small intestine causing anorexia, nausea, vomiting, diarrhoea and weight loss (5%); octreotide is used to relieve these symptoms
   - Malaise and irritability, nervous depression and headache
   - Flare-up of sepsis, tubo-ovarian mass, pyometra, peritonitis and septicaemia
   - Pyelitis, pyelonephritis and cystitis
   - Pyrexia
   - Pulmonary embolism
   - Skin reaction

   Megavoltage therapy reduces these complications.
2. *Late complications*: These include:
   - Persistent anaemia
   - Chronic pelvic pain because of fibrosis involving nerve trunks
   - Pyometra because of cervical stenosis
   - Proctitis, followed later by radiation ulcers, rectal bleeding, rectal strictures and occasionally rectovaginal fistula
   - Postirradiation ulcers in the bladder, causing dysuria, haematuria and vesicovaginal fistula
   - Small bowel strictures, obstruction, ulceration and gut perforation
   - Colonic ulcer, telangiectasia, perforation, stricture or obstruction
   - Atropic vaginitis, fibrosis and vaginal stenosis causing marital discord
   - Ureteric stricture and obstructive uropathy
   - Osteoporosis and fracture neck of the femur
   - Disturbed psyche
   - Ovarian destruction causing severe menopausal symptoms and osteoporosis; this can be avoided by translocation of ovaries above the pelvic brim during primary surgery, or prescribing HRT
   - Sarcoma reported in 8% of cases some years after radiotherapy, as some are suspected to be carcinogenic

CONTRAINDICATIONS TO RADIOTHERAPY

- Severe anaemia
- Poor general health
- Sepsis
- Pregnancy
- Presence of fibroids in the uterus
- Tubo-ovarian mass
- Uterovaginal prolapse
- Presence of genital fistulae
- Radioresistant tumour

Certain chemotherapeutic agents, such as cisplatin, carboplatin, 5-FU, paclitaxel and interferon (IFN), are radiosensitizers and potentiate the radiation effect on hypoxic cells. They have been used concomitantly to improve the results of radiotherapy. *This is known as chemoradiation.*

Table 39.3 Preoperative and Postoperative Radiation: Advantages and Disadvantages

Advantages	Disadvantages
Preoperative radiation	
1. Surgically undisturbed tumour bed. Intact vascularity (good oxygenation)	1. Precludes accurate pretreatment staging of the disease
2. May facilitate surgical dissection, allowing a lesser procedure by shrinking the tumour	2. May be considered unnecessary in hindsight, in cases with high chances of cure with surgery alone
3. May decrease the likelihood of risk of implantation or dissemination of viable tumour cells during surgical handling of tissues	3. Interferes with tissue healing 4. Combined therapy increases the morbidity
Postoperative radiation	
1. Accurate surgical staging	1. Surgery may alter the kinetics of tumour proliferation
2. Extent of locoregional disease accurately defined	2. Surgery often disturbs tumour vascularity causing hypoxia
3. Choice of omitting or selective use of radiation in some patients	

NEWER TECHNIQUES SPARING ADJACENT TISSUES

Normal tissue sparing with optimal target tissue radiation is known as 3D conformal radiotherapy. RapidArc is better than 3D.

Intensity-modulated radiation therapy is being attempted.

3D conformal radiotherapy uses CT, MRI and PET to place the beam of radiation to conform only to the target area, maximize dose to the tumour and minimize dose to the normal tissues.

Tomotherapy and cone-beam CT also allow precise localization of the beam to the target tissue.

ROLE OF PREOPERATIVE AND POSTOPERATIVE RADIATION

Role of preoperative and postoperative radiation is summarized in Table 39.3.

CLINICAL APPLICATIONS OF RADIOTHERAPY

CANCER OF THE CERVIX

Primary radiation therapy for cancer of the cervix combines teletherapy with brachytherapy. Radiation, like surgery, is a local therapy. It therefore influences only the tumour cells falling within the radiation volume. Intracavitary radiation by itself may therefore not be curative for patients in whom the tumour spread involves tissues beyond the effective radiation range and those with distant metastases. Additional external supplementary radiation to the pelvis is required to treat the pelvic lymph nodes. The tolerance of the normal tissues within the pelvis acts as the limiting factor in planning radiation therapy. Cervical cancer requires a radiation dose of 6000 cGy. The tolerance dose of irradiation for the urinary bladder is about 6000 cGy and for the rectum, it is about 5000 cGy. Doses in excess can damage these hollow viscera and cause radiation fistulae. The intracavitary radiation source is so calculated that it does not deliver a dose in excess of 8000 cGy to the point A located 2.0 cm above and lateral to the external cervical os. This point denotes the point of crossing of the ureter in the pelvis. The second point of consideration is point B located 5.0 cm laterally on the pelvic sidewalls where the obturator gland is located. The radiation dose at point B should not exceed 4500 cGy. This is to safeguard the bladder and rectum from overirradiation. *Preoperative brachytherapy* is used in barrel-shaped endocervical growth of more than 2 cm. This is followed within a week or 4 weeks later by Wertheim's hysterectomy. Cisplatin prior to or during brachytherapy improves the response rate (Fig. 39.4).

Cisplatin acts as a radiosensitizer and is employed as a neoadjuvant or concomitant chemoradiation.

Cisplatin 40 mg/m^2 i.v. given within 1 hour prior to radiotherapy weekly improves the response rate of the latter. Other radiosensitizers are 5-FU, gemcitabine, paclitaxel and carboplatin.

Postoperative external radiotherapy is required when the surgery has been incomplete or lymph nodes prove positive for malignancy.

Primary radiotherapy is mainly applied in advanced cancer of the cervix, but also preferred in Stages I and IIA by some gynaecologists as an alternative to Wertheim's hysterectomy. The cure rates achieved in early stages are comparable by either method. However, realizing that radiotherapy causes vaginal stenosis leading to dyspareunia, ovarian destruction with menopausal symptoms, and osteoporosis and cervical stenosis causing pyometra, the choice of treatment in young women is surgery in the form of Wertheim's hysterectomy. In a few cases, radiotherapy fails to irradiate the pelvic nodes completely, and recurrence occurs. In such cases, surgery is preferable to repeat radiotherapy, provided the woman is surgically fit. In primary radiotherapy normally, brachytherapy is applied first followed by external teletherapy. If the growth is large, first teletherapy is applied to shrink the tumour followed by brachytherapy.

ENDOCERVICAL CANCER

In endocervical cancer, the best survival is seen when concomitant cisplatin weekly combined with pelvic radiotherapy for 6 weeks is followed by surgery. Postoperative radiotherapy is required if pelvic lymph nodes prove positive for cancer.

ENDOMETRIAL CANCER

The importance of radiation therapy in the management of endometrial cancer is listed as follows:

- It is performed as an adjunct to surgery comprising of TAH-BSO and lymph node sampling.
- By administering vaginal radiation via colpostat, vaginal vault recurrence drops to 2% from the previous 13%.
- The survival improves in Stages IC and II when postoperative radiotherapy is administered to sterilize the pelvic lymph nodes. Radiation is indicated in uterine sarcoma, although outcome is poor.
- It is used to treat patients who are unfit for surgery.
- It helps to treat patients with vaginal/pelvic recurrences.
- It is performed for palliation in cases of nonresectable intrapelvic or metastatic disease.

OVARIAN CANCER

The primary treatment for ovarian cancer is cytoreductive surgery(total abdominal hysterectomy, removal of both ovaries and omentectomy). In advanced cases, maximal debulking surgery is followed by chemotherapy in epithelial tumours, and most of the other malignant ovarian tumours. In few selected cases radiation therapy in the form of 'Moving Strip' technique is applied to para-aortic lymph nodes and abdominal metastasis. Dysgerminoma and granulosa cell tumours, although highly radiosensitive are not being routinely used as advances in chemotherapy has resulted in chemotherapy being the first line of treatment for these tumours.

In the 'moving-strip' technique, a strip of 2.5 cm area is irradiated front and back over 2 days, and the strip moved upwards, until the entire abdomen receives radiation. With the liver and kidneys shielded, the total tumour dose of 2600–2800 cGy is administered. CT and MRI are useful in detecting para-aortic lymph node involvement prior to radiotherapy.

The earlier instillation of radioactive gold, thiotepa and other chemotherapy drugs at the end of surgery is not widely used, because the drug needs to be evenly distributed to avoid intestinal adhesions. Besides, cyclophosphamide needs to be activated in the liver before its effect is felt. Therefore, systemic chemotherapy is more effective.

Five years survival rates in ovarian cancer depend on a number of factors including residual tumour, grade of disease and use of effective chemotherapy in the form of paclitaxel-Carboplatin.

VULVAR CANCER

The aim of integrated multimodality therapy including surgery, radiation and possibly chemoradiation therapy is to reduce the risks of locoregional failure in patients with advanced primary or nodal disease, and to obviate the need for exenteration operations in women in whom the anus or lower urethra will be involved. The dose of radiation given is 4500–5000 cGy to women with microscopic disease and 6000–6400 cGy to women with macroscopic disease.

Preoperative radium needles (60 Gy in 6 days) shrink the tumour and facilitate extirpation of the tumour at a later date.

Postoperative pelvic radiotherapy is preferred to pelvic lymphadenectomy as it reduces the surgical morbidity. Pelvic radiotherapy is administered only if the inguinal lymph nodes prove histologically positive.

VAGINA

Radiotherapy is often chosen in place of radical surgery, especially in children. If the tumour is located in the upper one-third of vagina, radiotherapy is similar to that of the cervix. If it is located in the middle one-third, interstitial needles (iridium-192) are placed in the vaginal tissue.

CHORIOCARCINOMA

Choriocarcinoma responds extremely well to chemotherapy which has replaced surgery and radiotherapy in young women. Radiotherapy is applicable in the distal metastasis in a few cases.

CANCER CHEMOTHERAPY FOR GYNAECOLOGICAL CANCERS

The use of drugs to treat disseminated cancer has developed into a specialized discipline. The first successful effort to control cancer with the help of drugs is attributed to Mm Chiu Li et al. (1956), who demonstrated permanent remission in trophoblastic disease. The understanding of the mode of action of the drugs at DNA level has brought out newer effective drugs with less toxicity and has improved and prolonged the survival of women with genital cancers.

TUMOUR CELL KINETICS

A fundamental characteristic of malignant tumours is the rapid proliferation of malignant cells. These rapidly proliferating cells keep repeating a cycle of biochemical events continuously which culminate in cell division (Fig. 39.5).

Each proliferative cell gives rise to two daughter cells that continue the proliferative process, so the cell population increases geometrically.

A tumour is described as consisting of four types of cells (Figs 39.5 and 39.6).

Dividing tumour cells: This is the only compartment that adds to the cell population. Cells in this compartment are most sensitive to cytotoxic agents.

Resting cells: These are nondividing cells resting temporarily (cells in G_0 phase). They are refractory to chemotherapeutic agents.

Differentiated cells: These cells have lost their dividing potential and are awaiting natural death. They do not have malignant potential, so they are of little concern to the chemotherapist.

Dying cells: These are terminal cells.

Small rapidly growing tumours have many more rapidly dividing and growing cells; hence, the doubling time is short. However, these are the same tumours which have a

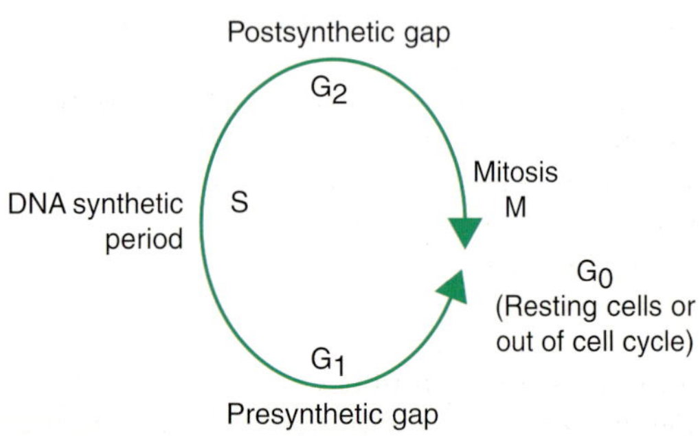

Figure 39.5 Scheme representing cell cycle: G1 → S → G2 → M phase.

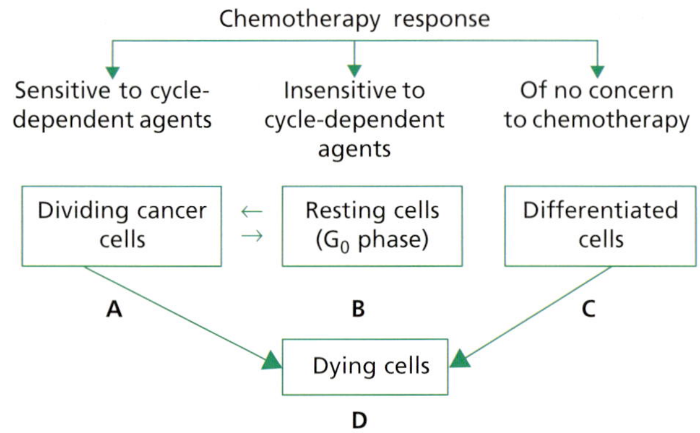

Figure 39.6 Cell types constituting tumour mass.

high number of cells sensitive to cell cycle-specific cytotoxic drugs. As the tumour mass enlarges, the growth rate progressively slows down, doubling time becomes longer and the cell input may equal loss; hence, a stationary size may be reached, and the sensitivity to cell-specific drugs diminishes.

Another factor to be considered during cancer chemotherapy is the tumour load present at the commencement of therapy. Reduction in the burden of tumour cell load will bring an apparent remission, but during the interval between successive courses of cancer chemotherapy, the tumour growth recurs. This results in stepwise decrease in tumour cell mass.

To attain maximum tumour cell kill, the following principles must be considered:

- The chemotherapist must be well aware of the 'total tumour cell kill concept'.
- Tumour cell kill by cytotoxic drugs follows the pattern demonstrated by Skipper HE and Perry S (1970) that the killing of tumour cells by cytotoxic agents occurs in an exponential fashion, so that a given dose kills a constant fraction of the population, irrespective of its initial size.
- There is a clear dose–response relationship.
- Prolonged treatment may be necessary to reduce the malignant cell population to a low number which will then be dealt with by the host immune mechanism.
- Chemotherapy is most effective when it is started early because the number of tumour cell population is low and the rapidly growing and dividing cells are sensitive to cancer chemotherapy.
- Chemotherapy must aim at different cell kill. The dose must be so adjusted that maximum destruction of tumour cell is achieved with minimal damage to normal cells.
- Many cytotoxic drugs in present use show some degree of tissue selectivity.
- Combination drug regimens and/or sequential drug regimens achieve superior tumour cell control with lowered side effects. Drugs with different actions yield better response and reduce drug resistance.
- The problem of drug resistance must be constantly borne in mind. This often happens with a single-drug therapy. Drug resistance may be temporary because of poor vascularity not allowing drugs to reach the tumour cells caused by fibrosis or bulky tumour, or permanent when it is either spontaneous or drug-induced mutation.

Chemotherapy has advanced tremendously in recent years, and is being increasingly used in the management of gynaecological malignancies. The drugs by virtue of prolongation of life and prolonged remission period allow a woman to live a nearly normal life.

CHEMORADIATION

It is now recognized that some chemotherapy drugs act also as radiosensitizers and lead to superadded cell kill prior to or preferably along with radiotherapy and prior to surgery. They are thus used as 'neoadjuvants' in a bulky tumour and locally advanced cancer in the pelvis. The most common drug used for this purpose is cisplatin either singly or as in combination. Cisplatin 40 mg^2 weekly is given 1 hour before radiotherapy. The renal functions should be normal before instituting this regime. Other chemoradiation drugs in use are 5-FU, gemcitabine and cisplatin combined with gemcitabine 40 mg^2 in 200 mL saline 2 hours before radiation – it takes 1 hour to administer. *Postradiation chemotherapy is not effective and poor response occurs on account of poor tissue oxygenation and poor vascularity not allowing the drugs to reach and penetrate the tumour.* In addition, myelosuppression of radiotherapy and high drug toxicity because of decreased renal function and ureteric obstruction (radiation fibrosis) caused by radiotherapy limit the use of chemotherapy drugs as postradiation drugs.

Chemotherapy is also used for recurrent and advanced diseases that are not amenable to surgery or radiotherapy, to reduce the tumour volume and provide short-term palliation.

Combined agents are superior to a single-agent therapy; they enhance tumour cell kill, reduce dose toxicity and resistance, and yield a better therapeutic response with longer remission. They also yield better response than drugs acting similarly. Chemotherapy, however, does not prevent occurrence of distal metastasis. It must also be remembered that chemotherapy yields better response in distal metastasis as compared to in postradiated recurrence, as its vascularity is not compromised.

Role of chemotherapy:

- Total response and cure is seen in 10%–20% of cases.
- Remission with partial response is seen in 40%–50% of cases.

Some drugs are nonspecific agents, i.e. alkylating agents, cisplatin, carboplatin and paclitaxel. These drugs damage the cells at any phase of cycle, although dividing cells are most vulnerable. The specific agents are methotrexate and Adriamycin in gestational trophoblastic disease, 5-FU in vulval cancer, and hydroxyurea, bleomycin and etoposide in cancer cervix.

Route. Drugs can be given orally (alkylating agents), intravenously or intraperitoneally at the end of surgery (but are not very effective).

Investigations required prior to chemotherapy:

- Hb%, WBC and platelet count
- Serum electrolytes
- Kidney function tests
- Cardiac function with doxorubicin
- Pulmonary function test with Bleomycin
- Liver function test with Methotrexate

CONTRAINDICATIONS

- Hb% less than 10 g%, WBC less than 3000/mm^3 and platelet count less than 100,000/mm^3
- Liver and renal dysfunction

COMPLICATIONS OF CHEMOTHERAPY

- Anaemia, thrombocytopenia and leucopenia
- Alopecia (reversible)
- Renal damage
- Liver damage
- Cardiac (doxorubicin)
- Pulmonary (bleomycin)

CLASSIFICATION OF DRUGS

- *Alkylating drugs:* These include cyclophosphamide, ifosfamide, chlorambucil, melphalan, thiotepa (nonspecific drugs prevent DNA synthesis or its division) and 6-mercaptopurine
- *Antimetabolites:* Methotrexate and 5-fluorouracil interfere with enzymes required for DNA synthesis.
- *Antibiotics:* Actinomycin-D, bleomycin, Adriamycin, mitomycin (nonspecific) and doxorubicin. These inhibit RNA and DNA synthesis and hence arrest mitosis.
- *Plant alkaloids:* These include vincristine, vinblastine, Taxol, docetaxel and etoposide (cell specific) – antimitotic.
- *Hormones:* These include high dose preparations in endometrial cancer and Tamoxifene in treated cases of carcinoma breast.
- *Miscellaneous:* These include cisplatin, carboplatin, hydroxyurea and topotecan.
- *Biological:* IFN improves host immune defence and maintains remission.

NEWER ANTICANCER DRUGS

The development of new chemotherapy drugs has improved the disease-free interval and prolongs survival.

They are as follows:

1. Vascular targeting agents (VTA)
   a. Angiogenesis inhibitors
   b. VEGF ligand bevacizumab (Avastin, GeneTech)
   c. Receptor targeting VEGF
      Receptor tyrosine kinase inhibitor, cediranib, nintedanib and anti-VEGF antibody
      The former primarily prevent development of new vessels in the tumour. The latter damage the established vessels in the tumour with cediranib 30 mg daily orally; 30% benefit is reported in recurrent epithelial ovarian tumours and fallopian tube cancer.
      Complication includes hypertension.
      Bowel perforation is seen in intraperitoneal tumours involving the bowel.
      Vascular disrupting agents (VDA) fosbretabulin, olaparib (oral 100–600 mg daily).
2. Farletuzumab – a monoclonal antibody against ovarian cancer.
3. Novel cytotoxic agents
   (a) Trabectedin
   (b) Epothilone analogues
   (c) Topoisomerase 1 inhibitors
   (d) Pemetrexed
   (e) Aurora kinase inhibitors

VULVA

5-FU is effective in cancer involving the anus. It shrinks the tumour which may even disappear.

Local excision of the residual tumour is then successful.

VAGINA

The metastasis of choriocarcinoma responds to methotrexate and actinomycin-D.

CERVIX

The use of cisplatin concomitant with radiotherapy and prior to surgery in endocervical growth is mentioned in Chapter 33. It also reduces the incidence of lymph node metastasis in bulky cervical tumour in Stages IB and IIB and improves the surgical outcome, although the survival rate has not shown improvement.

The drugs most effective are as follows:

- Doxorubicin 120 mg/m^2 + cisplatin 50 mg/m^2 i.v. over 24 hours weekly for six cycles (three cycles as radiosensitizers)
- PVB:
  - Cisplatin 100 mg/m^2 i.v. on day 1
  - Vinblastine 6–12 mg/m^2 bolus on day 1
  - Bleomycin 15–30 mg i.m. on days 1, 8 and 15 given 3-weekly for not more than eight cycles

Cisplatin requires adequate hydration.

Response rate of 50%–70% is seen.

Chemoradiation also improves survival in distal metastasis.

ENDOMETRIAL CANCER

Chemotherapy drugs are less commonly used because of poor response in endometrial cancer and surgery and radiotherapy being the cornerstone in its management. Metastatic tumours respond better to progestogens.

Medroxyprogesterone acetate (MDPA) 1 g i.m. weekly or 400 mg orally daily, 1 g norethisterone i.m. weekly or 17-alpha-hydroxyprogesterone i.m. are effective in well-differentiated tumours containing oestrogen and progesterone receptors. Anaplastic tumour does not contain these receptors and fails to respond. Tamoxifen 10 mg b.d. by its antioestrogen action is also effective in advanced cases. Thirty per cent response is seen in lung metastasis with progestogens.

Sarcoma of the uterus is treated with cisplatin and ifosfamide. Doxorubicin is used as single-agent therapy following surgery. Recently, drugs such as doxorubicin, platinum, taxane, carboplatin and paclitaxel have been tried.

OVARIAN CANCER

Chemotherapy plays a major role after surgery in the management of ovarian cancer. Nowadays, new drugs with less toxicity has improved the survival as well as remission period. Multiple-drug therapy yields better survival.

Indications are as follows:

- Prophylactic postoperative chemotherapy in Stage IC to prevent recurrence. Carboplatin alone is adequate prophylactically.
- In advanced stage, chemotherapy as palliative therapy keeps the woman comfortable.
- In unresectable tumour, chemotherapy for 3–6 months followed by debulking surgery is recommended.

Chemotherapy for 3–6 months followed by debulking surgery and monitoring with tissue markers for regression and deciding on duration of therapy is the routine practice in residual tumour, and in recurrent and advanced cancer.

Cisplatin and Taxol are the main drugs useful in ovarian cancer. Carboplatin is superior to cisplatin with less nephrotoxicity and less emetic potential. Myelosuppression is reduced if used with granulocyte colony-stimulating factor (G-CSF, 175–200 mg/m^2). Corticosteroid and antihistamine prevent hypersensitivity reaction to paclitaxel. Carboplatin requires less hydration than cisplatin. Six cycles are usually given.

Second-line drugs when woman fails to respond to cisplatin are cyclophosphamide, topotecan, ifosfamide and doxorubicin.

The woman should be monitored not only for the regression of the disease but also for myelosuppression, vomiting, diarrhoea, nephrotoxicity, neurotoxicity and fungal infection.

The drugs used are as follows:

- Doxorubicin (Adriamycin 120 mg/m^2 weekly for 6 cycles is cardiotoxic)
- Cisplatin 50 mg/m^2 i.v. over 24 hours with good hydration 3-weekly for six cycles (30% response)
- Ifosfamide 1.2 g i.v. over 30 minutes
- Methotrexate 50 mg/m^2 i.v. bolus weekly for 6 weeks
- Topotecan 1–2 mg/m^2 days 1–5, 3-weekly
- Paclitaxel 135–200 mg/m^2 over 3-hour has infusion, followed by cisplatin 75 mg^2 over 1 hour 3-weekly; cisplatin causes nausea, renal failure, peripheral neuropathy and myelosuppression, but no alopecia
- BEP
  - Bleomycin 15 mg i.v. on day 1, 2
  - Etoposide 100 mg/m^2 on day 1–5
  - Cisplatin 20 mg/m^2 i.v. on day 1–5
- Carboplatin 300–400 mg/m^2 4-weekly; response rate 30%
- VAC
  - Vincristine 1.5 mg/m^2 i.v. day 1
  - Actinomycin-D 0.5 mg i.v. 1–5 days
  - Cyclophosphamide 150 mg/m^2 i.v. on days 1-5 weekly
- PVB
  - Cisplatin 100 mg/m^2 i.v. day 1
  - Vinblastine 6–12 mg/m^2 bolus i.v. day 1
  - Bleomycin 15–30 mg i.v. days 1, 8 and 15, maximum of eight doses 3-weekly
- Cyclophosphamide 500 mg/m^2, doxorubicin 50 mg/m^2 bolus i.v. and cisplatin 50 mg/m^2 infused over 30 minutes 3-weekly for six cycles
- Taxol derived from the bark of Pacific yew tree is expensive and available in semisynthetic form; it promotes assembly and stability of microtubules and inhibits mitosis; a dose of 175–250 mg/m^2 i.v. is infused over 3 hours is useful in cisplatin-resistant cases; side effects are neutropenia, paraesthesia, scotoma, myalgia, bradycardia, alopecia, vomiting and diarrhoea
- Alpha-Interferon three times a week subcutaneously, maintains emission period and improves survival

- Gemcitabine 100 mg/m^2 + carboplatin on first and eighth days 3-weekly for six cycles

Extravasation should be avoided by using angiocatheter when giving doxorubicin, actinomycin-D and vincristine.

Topotecan is another new drug which inhibits nuclear enzyme DNA topoisomerase and is well tolerated.

Germ cell tumour responds well to Bleomycin, etoposide (85%) and Cisplatin (BEP regiment).

CHORIOCARCINOMA

See Chapter 38.

SARCOMA

Cisplatin, ifosfamide and doxorubicin are used as single or combination therapy.

BREAST CANCER

Although tamoxifen improves the survival period, it causes endometrial hyperplasia and cancer, and requires regular monitoring with ultrasound study of endometrium and endometrial biopsy.

The gynaecologist should be aware of the limitations of chemotherapy as well as its effectiveness. Tumour markers should be employed during chemotherapy to watch the effectiveness and decide the duration of chemotherapy in an individual case.

IMMUNOTHERAPY

Realizing that immunosuppressed women are more likely to develop cancer, this therapy is receiving consideration. HPV vaccine is now available for cancer cervix prevention.

The best results are obtained if the tumour size is initially reduced by surgery, chemotherapy or radiation.

Immunotherapy includes:

- Vaccine against human papillomavirus for cancer cervix (prophylactic)
- Chemical immunostimulants – levamisole and cimetidine
- Cytokines, IFN, interleukin (IL)-2 and tumour necrosis factor (TNF)
- Chemotherapeutic drugs – cisplatin and doxorubicin
- Passive immunization – immunological active substances directly transferred to the host:
  - Cytoner, IFN and TNF
  - Monoclonal antibodies
  - Activated macrophages
- Drug immune modifiers:
  - Anti-CA-125 antibody (oregovomab) is given as a drug immune modifier.
  - Bevacizumab-24 MAB antibody is not toxic, but bowel perforation and proteinuria are reported and the drug is very expensive. Also helpful are bevacizumab-15 recombinant humanized monoclonal antibody directed towards VEGF-A and antiangiogenesis 15 mg/kg body weight every weekly for 6-21 cycles.

GENE THERAPY

Familial cancer of ovary and endometrium has been observed in 5%–10% of cases. The genes *BRCA-1* and *BRCA-2* are responsible for ovarian malignancy. Gene study and gene therapy are under research. Stem cell therapy may play a major role in the future.

Taxane. Apart from being antimitotic, it is also a radiosensitizer. It causes neutropenia, paraesthesia, myalgia, cardiac arrhythmia and alopecia.

The dosage is 135 mg/m^2 over 3 hours followed by 75 mg cisplatin.

Cisplatin sensitivity is the key predictor of response and survival. It is now replaced by carboplatin, because of its lesser toxicity. Cisplatin/carboplatin with paclitaxel is the first line of chemotherapy treatment in advanced cancer.

In ovarian cancer, chemotherapy is used as:

- Neoadjuvant therapy
- Concomitant therapy
- Adjuvant therapy

Neoadjuvant therapy is employed before surgery.

The drug shrinks the tumour and reduces micrometastasis.

Disadvantage of neoadjuvant therapy is that it delays the specific therapy.

Drugs used are cisplatin, carboplatin, bleomycin and ifosfamide – with 50%–70% response.

The dose is 100 mg cisplatin + 1.2 g/m^2 ifosfamide.

Concomitant therapy (during treatment) acts as radiosensitizer, and enhances radiotherapy effect, but increases toxicity (Table 39.4).

Adjuvant therapy (drugs mentioned earlier) is employed following surgery or radiotherapy but response to local residual/recurrence is low, because of poor vascularity of the tumour. The distal metastasis however responds better to adjuvant chemotherapy, because of its intact vascularity.

With so many new drugs becoming available, tissue sensitivity test to various drugs may improve our decision regarding the best line of chemotherapy in the future.

PALLIATIVE CARE

It is not enough to treat cancer disease per se. Apart from palliative radiotherapy and chemotherapy in the advanced stage of the disease, other adjuvants are necessary in the management of cancers. These are as follows:

- Nutrition
- Relief of pain
- Relief of symptoms
- Psychological support

Table 39.4 Toxicity of Drugs

Drugs	Toxicity
Cisplatin	Vomiting, myelosuppression, renal toxicity, peripheral neuropathy, ototoxicity; no alopecia, hydration required
Carboplatin	Myelosuppression
Taxane	Hypersensitivity, myelosuppression, cardiac arrhythmia, alopecia

NUTRITION

It is necessary to maintain the woman's nutrition before, during and after surgery, radiotherapy and chemotherapy to obtain a good response and successful cure, longer remission and survival as well as a feeling of well-being. The nutritional problem arises in the advanced stage when cachexia sets in, or following radiotherapy and chemotherapy. The optimal nutritional status is a prerequisite to cancer treatment.

Assessment of Nutritional Status

- Weight of the woman: Weight loss more than 10% of previous weight is considered malnutrition.
- Haemoglobin should be more than 10 g%, ideally 12 g%. Low haemoglobin before surgery can cause sepsis, thromboembolism and poor wound healing. Nonresponse to radiotherapy and chemotherapy is seen in anoxic tissues.
- Protein: Normal serum albumin is 4.0-5.0 mg/L and hypoproteinaemia is a sign of malnutrition.

Management

The woman should receive adequate calories, i.e. 2000–2400 kcal, daily along with adequate protein and micronutrients. Anaemia is treated with blood transfusion prior to any treatment. Daily fluid intake should be at least 1500–2000 mL. If the woman cannot tolerate oral diet, intravenous amino acids, glucose and vitamins should be provided. Tube feeding is not always tolerable and is uncomfortable. Initially 50 mL/hour, it is increased gradually to the required amount. Hydration is especially important in chemotherapy with cisplatin.

Apart from those mentioned earlier, neutropenia resulting from radiotherapy and certain chemotherapy drugs requires blood transfusion.

RELIEF OF PAIN

It is important to detect the cause and pathology of pain to deliver appropriate painkillers. Even when cure is not possible, painless days reduce the suffering of the woman and allow her to reach her end in peace and serenity. This palliative treatment should be instituted along with the definitive or other palliative therapy including nutrition mentioned earlier, and not resorted to only in the terminal stage.

Pain may be because of local infiltration, nerve or bone involvement, or psoas muscle spasm. Muscle spasm is relieved with diazepam. Mild pain can be relieved with paracetamol 1 g q.i.d. It provides mild sedation and may cause constipation in long-term therapy.

Opiates. Morphia one-fourth grain or diamorphine (heroin) 1 mg orally is effective when given 4-hourly. Diamorphine is stronger than morphine; 1 mg of diamorphine is equivalent to 3 mg oral morphine. Subcutaneous injection of heroin (2 mg) can also be given and repeated as required in severe pain. Spinal injection of opiates has also been employed.

Synthetic opiate syrup (methadone) is useful for cough in pulmonary metastasis. The side effects of opiates are vomiting, sedation and constipation which should be managed by haloperidol (3–5 mg) for vomiting at night or metoclopramide. Overdose of opiates leads to visual hallucinations, myoclonic jerks, respiratory distress, pinpoint pupils and addiction which is not a problem in the terminal ill women. Laxatives will relieve constipation.

Bony Pain

Morphine is not effective against bone metastasis. It requires a nonsteroidal anti-inflammatory drug (NSAID) such as naproxen 500 mg b.d. and diclofenac 50 mg t.i.d. orally or rectally if gastritis occurs. Subcutaneous injection can also be given.

Bisphosphonate, 4-hourly infusion every 3–4 weeks, protects against osteoporosis. Hypocalcaemia should be watched for during this therapy.

When NSAIDs fail to relieve pain, steroids are recommended. Steroids promote the feeling of well-being and improve appetite. Prednisone 20 mg daily in divided doses should be administered not too late in the evening, as it can disturb the sleep pattern. High-dose dexamethasone 16–24 mg daily is useful in liver and brain metastasis – it relieves the pressure of the metastasis in these organs. It is also effective in bladder and bowel pain. A single morning dose is adequate because of its long half-life. Diabetes, hypertension, obesity and osteoporosis are its side effects.

Bowel and Bladder Pain

Anticholinergic drugs such as Buscopan 20 mg q.i.d., oxybutynin 5 mg b.i.d. chlorpromazine 25–50 mg are effective against bladder and rectal pain.

Nerve Pain

Sodium valproate 200–300 mg t.i.d. and carbamazepine 100–200 mg t.i.d. cure nerve pain. Antidepressants such as amitriptyline 10 mg at night are effective too, but renal function needs observation. In nonresponders, epidural, sacral or pudendal blocks are required. Sympathectomy may be the last resort. Ketamine is effective as an analgesic.

RELIEF OF SYMPTOMS

Vomiting

Vomiting is because of drugs, chemotherapy or radiotherapy, or may be because of cachexia in the terminal stage. Haloperidol 3–5 mg at night or metoclopramide 10 mg t.i.d. controls vomiting. Cerebral vomiting is treated with cyclizine 50 mg t.i.d. or domperidone 20 mg t.i.d. Octreotide reduces intestinal secretion and promotes absorption with the effect that gastric volume is reduced and vomiting stops. It is also effective in diarrhoea. Subcutaneously 300–1200 mg b.d. is given but the drug is very expensive. Thrush infection is not uncommon and can be treated with fluconazole. Ondansetron 4 mg t.i.d. is effective against radiation vomiting.

PSYCHOLOGICAL SUPPORT

Psychological impact may be considerable. More time involvement, sharing emotions and compassion form the holistic care in the management of a woman suffering from terminal cancer.

Other problems are as follows:

- Decreased sex libido can occur because of vaginal discharge, bleeding and fear of cancer dissemination.
- Dyspareunia follows surgery and radiotherapy (short vagina and vaginal stenosis).
- Ovarian removal with menopausal symptoms requires hormone replacement therapy.

- Mental depression may occur because of oestrogen deficiency or fear of a painful death.
- Ascites requires tapping.

Hormone therapy in tumours possessing oestrogen and progesterone receptors does well with progestogens and tamoxifen. Well-differentiated tumours possess oestrogen and progesterone receptors than poorly differentiated tumours, so response is good.

Role of Special Hospitals. Temporary hospitalization gives respite to relatives and provides change of environment for the patient. There are number of special hospitals and care centres which look after these terminally sick cancer patients.

The ultimate goal of palliative treatment is to allow the woman to meet her end gracefully and with serenity. Special hospitals and nursing care for terminally sick cancer patients are of immense help.

KEY POINTS

- Radiotherapy and chemotherapy play an important role in the management of genital tract malignancies.
- Primary radiotherapy can be applied in cancer of the cervix as an alternative to Wertheim's hysterectomy in early stages, with equally good results, and is the treatment in advanced inoperable cases. Surgery is however preferred in young women, because radiotherapy causes vaginal stenosis, pyometra, destruction of ovaries and menopause.
- Preoperative radiotherapy with cisplatin is recommended in endocervical cancer of more than 2 cm, and this shrinks the tumour.
- Postoperative radiotherapy is useful if surgery has been incomplete or lymph nodes are involved in cancer of the cervix and uterine cancer.
- Ovarian cancer is dealt with by primary surgery. Chemotherapy is the choice in the postoperative treatment. Granulosa cell tumour and dysgerminoma are highly radiosensitive and chemosensitive. However, chemotherapy is the preferred treatment in young women.
- 'Moving-strip' technique of radiotherapy is safe in dealing with abdominal and para-aortic lymph node metastasis.
- Choriocarcinoma responds well to chemotherapy which is considered the primary treatment. About 90%–100% success is reported with chemotherapy.
- Chemotherapy is now employed as neoadjuvant, concomitant and adjuvant therapy.
- The limitations and harmful effects of radiotherapy and chemotherapy should be understood.
- Chemoradiation is also used in residual and recurrent tumours as palliative measures.

SELF-ASSESSMENT

1. Discuss the role of radiotherapy in cancer of the cervix.
2. Discuss the side effects of radiotherapy.
3. Discuss the role of chemotherapy in ovarian cancer.

SUGGESTED READING

Aalders J. Textbook of Oncology. WB Saunders: Elsevier, 1991.
Bonnar J. Recent Advances in Obstetrics and Gynaecology Vol 20, 1998.
Maggino J, et al. Gynecol Oncol Vol 68: 274–279, 1998.
Studd J. Progress in Obstetrics and Gynaecology Vol 16, 2005.

SECTION 8

IMAGING MODALITIES, ENDOSCOPIC PROCEDURES AND MAJOR AND MINOR OPERATIONS IN GYNAECOLOGY

SECTION OUTLINE

Imaging Modalities in Gynaecology

40

CHAPTER OUTLINE

PLAIN RADIOGRAPHY

Advances in imaging modalities have revolutionized the practice of gynaecology in recent times. Plain radiograph was the first modality used in older times but has limited place in current gynaecological practice. Advent of ultrasonography, CT and MRI has made virtual real time imaging possible in gynaecology. Sonography especially, transvaginal sonography provides excellent view of anatomy of pelvic organs. In gynaecological practice 80-90% need for imaging is met by ultrasonography. More advanced techniques such as CT scan, MRI imaging having added newer dimensions in the management of gynaecological conditions specially malignancies. The latest addition to imaging techniques is PET scan which is of immense value in managing cancers.

An abdominal radiograph is not used in the diagnosis of pelvic pathology. However, an incidental radiograph taken for other medical or surgical conditions may reveal unsuspected pelvic pathology such as the presence of a tooth in a dermoid cyst or a calcified fibroid (Fig. 40.1).

A plain radiograph of the pelvis in anteroposterior (AP) and lateral views taken after placing a uterine sound in the uterine cavity help to locate an intrauterine contraceptive device (IUCD; commonly a Copper-T in present times) (Fig. 40.2).

A plain radiograph of the chest is required in suspected tuberculosis, to determine the presence of metastasis in gynaecologic malignancies, and finally, as a part of the work-up before undertaking any major gynaecological surgery.

A plain x-ray of skull (Sella view) may be of help in women with galactorrhoea to rule out a pituitary macroadenoma.

HYSTEROSALPINGOGRAPHY

Hysterosalpingography (HSG) where a radio opaque dye is injected in uterine cavity is employed for the following:

- To study the patency of the fallopian tubes in infertility cases and following tuboplasty (Fig. 40.3A–E).
- To assess the feasibility of tuboplasty by studying the location and extent of tubal block.
- To study uterine anomalies such as septate and bicornuate uterus.
- To detect uterine synechiae.
- To detect uterine polyp.
- To study incompetence of internal os. HSG has also been described in Chapter 16.

TECHNIQUE

- It is done as an outpatient procedure, without any anaesthesia, in the Department of Radiology.
- Premedication with atropine and analgesia may be required in an apprehensive woman to prevent tubal spasm.

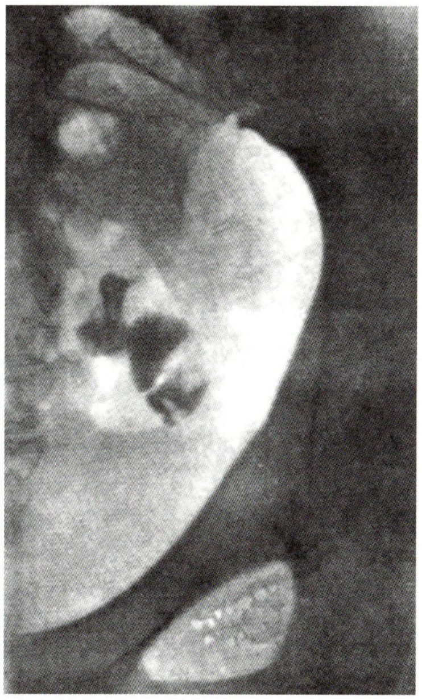

Figure 40.1 X-ray of pelvis showing teeth in an ovarian dermoid cyst.

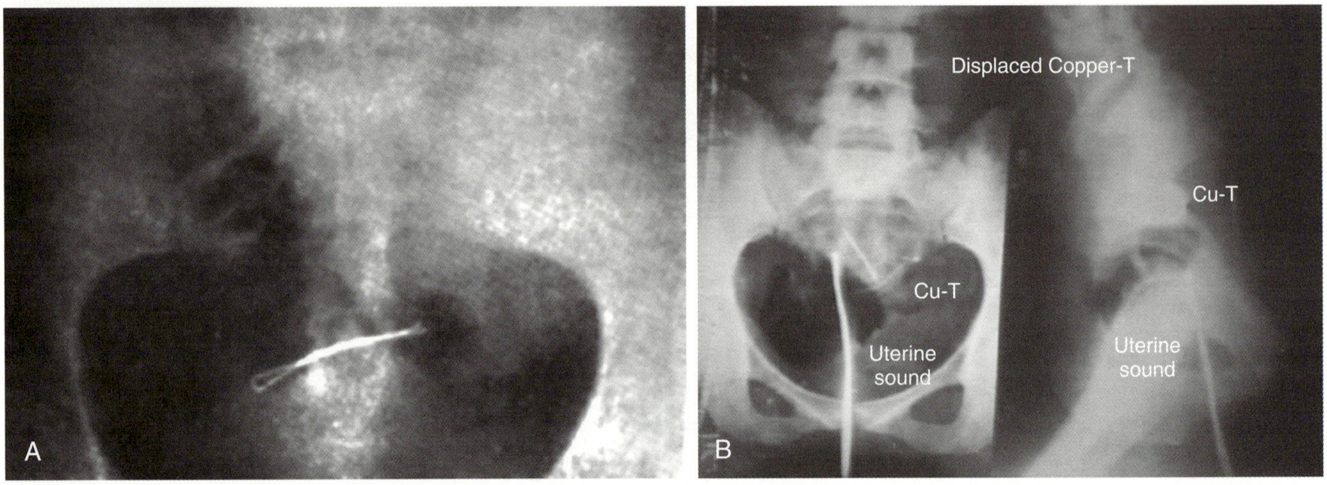

Figure 40.2 **(A)** showing presence of foreign body, and **(B)** shows a migrated Copper-T outside uterus. An **anteroposterior** (AP) and lateral view of the pelvis with a uterine sound in situ confirm the extrauterine location of the IUCD.

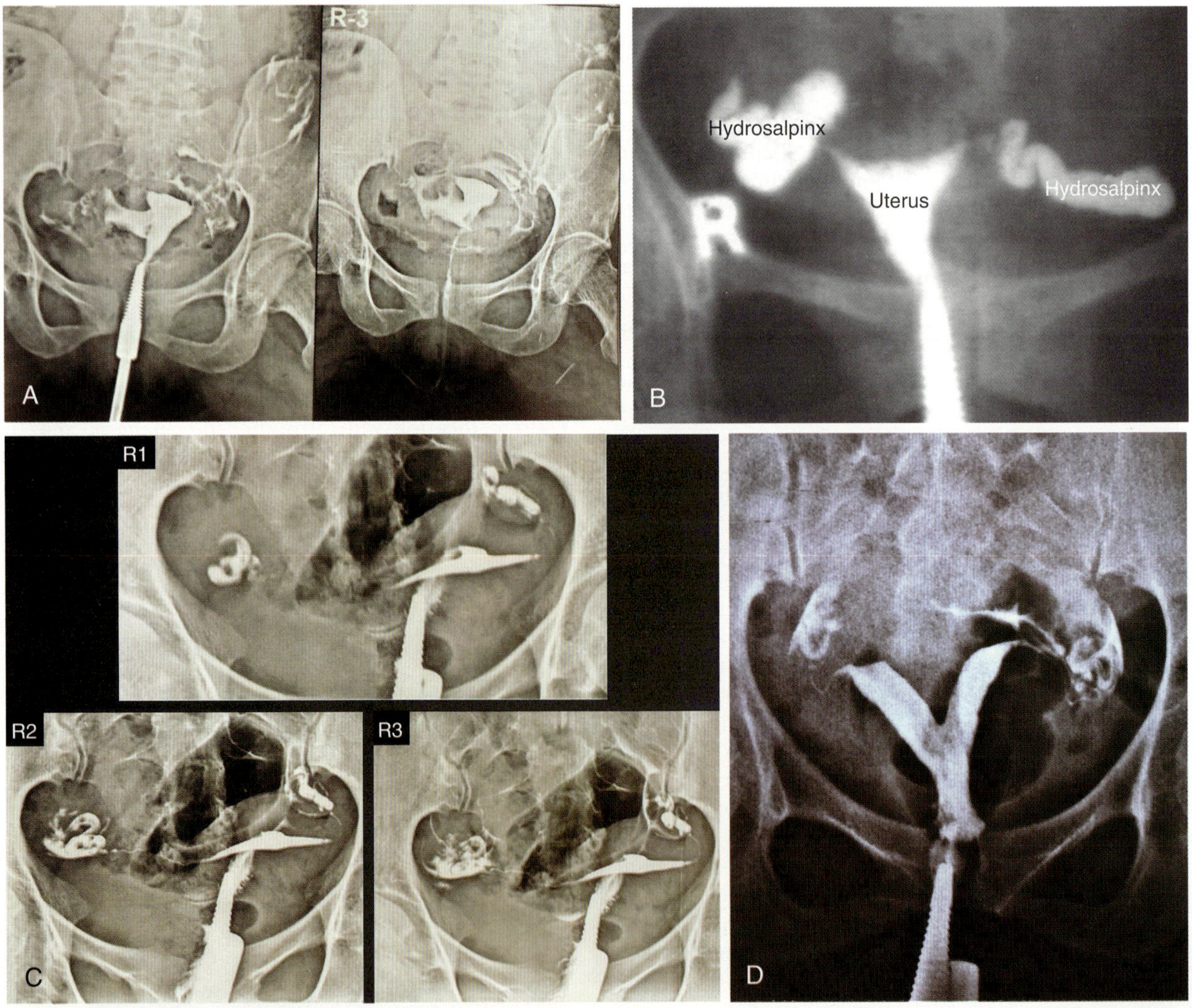

Figure 40.3 **(A)** HSG showing patent fallopian tubes with free peritoneal spill and intravasation of dye. **(B)** HSG showing bilateral hydrosalpinx. **(C)** HSG showing genital tuberculosis– typically beaded blocked tubes seen. **(D)** HSG showing septate uterus with normal corresponding fallopian tubes and free peritoneal spill.

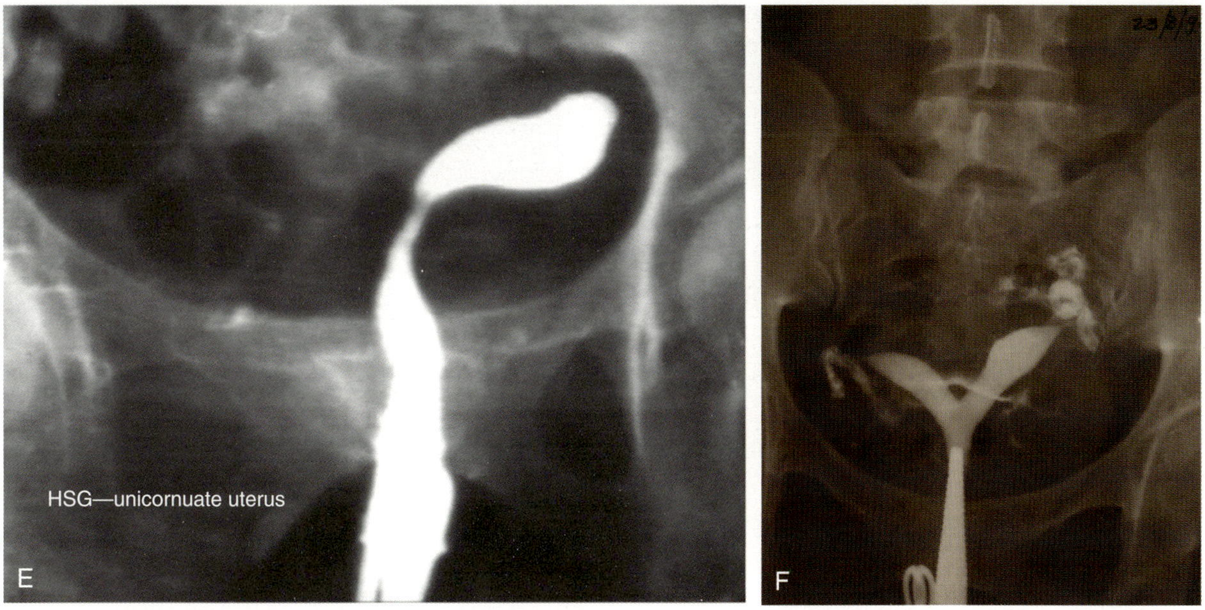

Figure 40.3, cont'd (E) HSG showing unicornuate uterus. **(F)** HSG showing bicornuate uterus. Both fallopian tubes are normal and show free peritoneal spill. (*Courtesy* **(D)** and **(F)**: Dr K.K. Saxena, New Delhi.)

- The woman is asked to empty her bladder.
- She is placed in the lithotomy position, perineal area cleaned with Betadine and draped.
- Bimanual examination is done to note the size and position of the uterus.
- The cervix is exposed and held with an Allis forceps.
- Rubin's cannula, Leech Wilkinson cannula or Foley catheter No. 14 is introduced gently into the uterine cavity beyond the internal os (bulb of the catheter distended to prevent leakage). The cone of Rubin's cannula snugly fits into the external os.
- The radiopaque dye (usually water soluble, rarely oil based), 10–15 mL, is gently injected by attaching the loaded syringe to the cannula or Foley catheter.
- The uterine cavity and fallopian tubes are visualized as the dye passes through them during fluoroscopy.
- At a specific time desired, X-rays are taken for a permanent record.
- The instruments are withdrawn, and the woman is observed for half an hour.

CONTRAINDICATIONS

- The presence of genital tract infection and bleeding.
- Premenstrual phase. Avoid doing test in premenstrual phase as there are chances that pregnancy may have occurred. Thick endometrium may prevent smooth flow of the dye at the cornual end. The risk of endometriosis also precludes doing HSG in the premenstrual phase.
- Suspected genital tuberculosis because of risk of spread of infection following the procedure.
- Allergy to the dye.

COMPLICATIONS

HSG is usually a safe procedure, however, following complications can occur at times.

- Ascending infection, spread of tubercular infection.
- Pelvic irritation and pain due to dye (chemical peritonitis).
- Allergic reaction to the dye.
- Pelvic endometriosis, if done premenstrually or while the woman is menstruating.

ADVANTAGES

- Provides a permanent record.
- Shows the uterine pathology and exact site of tubal blockage.
- Dye may dislodge the mucus plug in tube, thus clearing the tubal block.

SONOSALPINGOGRAPHY

Sonosalpingography is described in chapter 16 on Infertility – Male and Female. It is of particular use in the diagnosis of uterine polyp.

INTRAVENOUS UROGRAPHY

Urography outlines the urinary tract following the administration of an intravenous iodinated contrast medium.

INDICATIONS

Intravenous urography (IVU) is useful in the following indications:

- Gynaecologic malignancy to determine the normality of the urinary tract. In the advanced cancer cervix, the ureters may get involved leading to partial or complete obstruction. The advanced cancer of the cervix involving the parametrium constricts the ureter in its passage through the ureteric tunnel causing obstruction, and back pressure initially leading to hydroureter and hydronephrosis and finally renal atrophy.

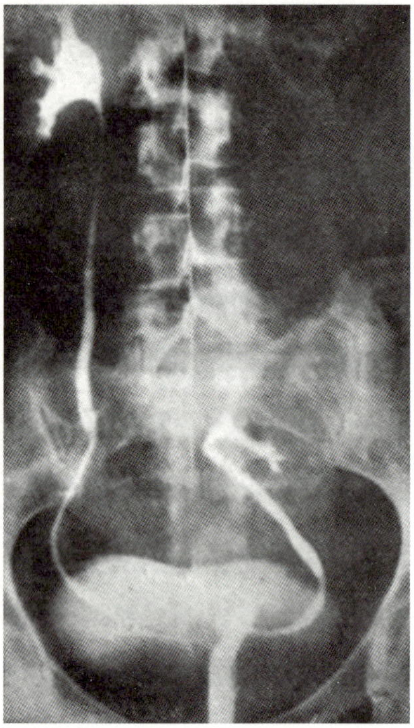

Figure 40.4 Composite X-ray showing ectopic pelvic left kidney demonstrated by retrograde pyelography (clinically diagnosed as left ovarian tumour).

- In ovarian cancers and in the presence of other pelvic masses such as broad ligament fibroids, the ureters may get displaced and are prone to injury during pelvic surgery.
- Rarely, an unidentified pelvic mass turns out to be a solitary pelvic kidney. Instances of removal of such kidneys by the unsuspecting surgeon leading to disastrous consequences have been reported.
- In ureteric injury during difficult pelvic surgery, a descending pyelography may help to confirm and locate the site of injury (Fig. 40.4).
- Renal tract anomalies often coexist with Müllerian duct anomalies; hence, in every case of congenital malformation of the genital tract, it is wise to perform IVU to exclude urinary tract abnormalities.
- Urinary incontinence in young girls may be due to an ectopic ureter: this can be demonstrated on urography.
- In genitourinary fistulae, the relationship of the ureteric orifice to the site of fistula is important in planning any surgical repair.
- To study the anatomy of the ureter in a difficult pelvic surgery.

PRECAUTIONS AND CONTRAINDICATIONS

- IVU is contraindicated in women with iodine sensitivity.
- It should be undertaken with caution in women with impaired renal functions. Renal function should be assessed before undertaking IVU.
- Exercise caution before the test in women with allergic diathesis, asthmatics and diabetics on metformin. It is mandatory to perform a sensitivity test before the investigation.
- Suspicion of pregnancy. Radiation is harmful to the fetus.

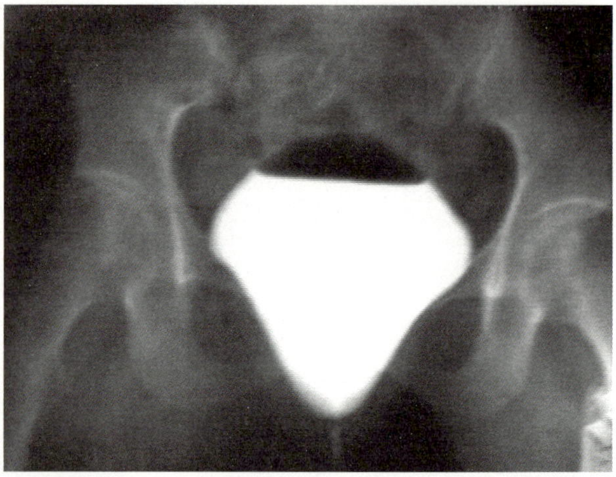

Figure 40.5 Cystography showing altered shape of the full bladder in case of a large cystocele. Note the descent of the bladder neck and proximal urethra which predisposes to stress incontinence.

CYSTOGRAPHY AND URETHROGRAPHY

Cystourethrography is useful in the investigation of urinary incontinence (Fig. 40.5). Most of the information is obtained by combining video studies and pressure studies (simultaneous video cystometrography). This investigation permits the evaluation of the anatomical disorders of bladder neck and proximal urethral displacement and inappropriate detrusor contraction in a patient with incontinence of urine.

GASTROINTESTINAL IMAGING STUDIES

BARIUM MEAL AND FOLLOW THROUGH

This examination and gastroscopy are useful in suspected ovarian metastatic disease. Carcinoma of stomach is often the primary site of malignancy in patients with bilateral ovarian masses. Visualization of the ileocaecal region may help to differentiate a pelvic mass due to ileocaecal tuberculosis from an adnexal mass. Advances in endoscopy have resulted in greater reliance on upper GI and lower GI endoscopy in comparison to barium meal studies.

BARIUM ENEMA

This examination allows the visualization of the colon. Many gynaecological conditions such as ovarian malignancy, pelvic endometriosis, pelvic inflammatory disease (PID), genital and abdominal tuberculosis and previous radiotherapy may all be associated with small and large bowel disturbances. Large bowel inflammation, Crohn disease, chronic amoebiasis, worms and diverticulitis can all confuse the clinical picture and complicate gynaecological procedures.

ARTERIOGRAPHY AND ARTERIAL EMBOLIZATION

The arterial supply of the uterus and appendages can be demonstrated by aortography or internal iliac arteriography. In modern-day practice, the use of ultrasonography, computed tomography (CT) scan, magnetic resonance imaging (MRI) and Doppler blood flow studies have minimized the need for arteriography. However, arteriography can establish the cause of heavy abnormal uterine bleeding not responding to the conventional therapy, such as due to an arteriovenous aneurysm, or varicose veins. Selective embolization of the same can result in cure.

Embolization of the anterior division of internal iliac artery has been successfully used in the treatment of uncontrolled bleeding from the advanced cervical cancer, secondary haemorrhage after a hysterectomy, cervical ectopic pregnancy and for embolization of uterine artery in menorrhagia and in fibroids.

ULTRASONOGRAPHY (Figs 40.6–40.16)

This imaging modality was first pioneered by Ian Donald (1974) in gynaecology and obstetrics. Sonography is generally the first and often the only imaging modality used to demonstrate pelvic anatomy and to document physiological (ovulation monitoring) and pathological changes. Ultrasound examination may be performed by the transabdominal/transvaginal/transrectal or transperineal approach. *The vaginal probe is considered a natural extension of bimanual examination with better and precise pelvic findings.*

Advantages of ultrasound are as follows:

- Noninvasive technique.
- Soft tissue imaging possible unlike X-rays.
- No ionizing radiation, so it can be repeated.

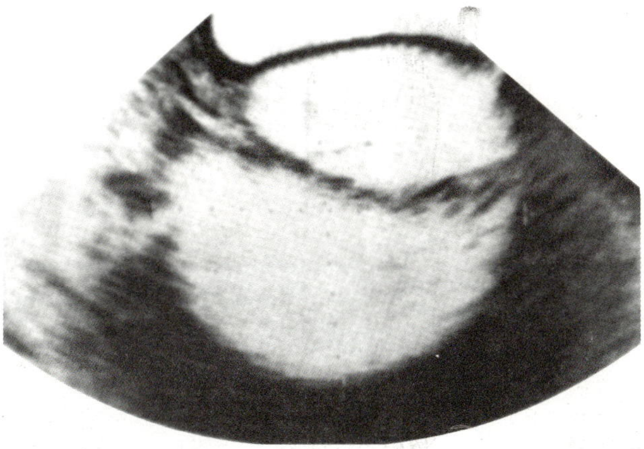

Figure 40.6 USG showing a septate ovarian serous cystadenoma. (*Courtesy*: Diwan Chand Satyapal Aggarwal Imaging Research Center, New Delhi.)

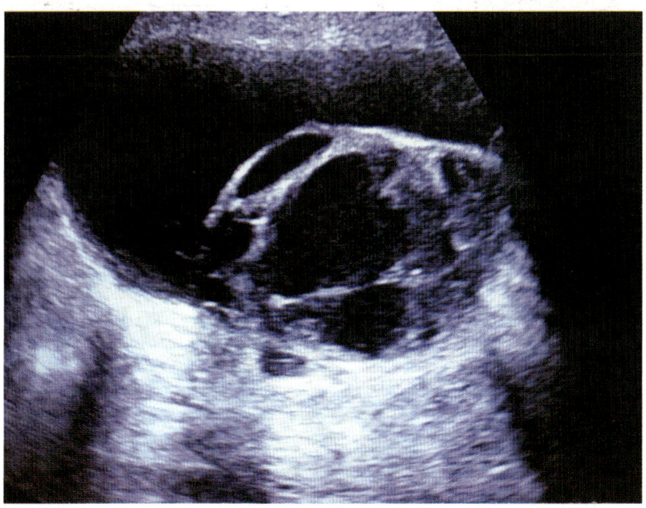

Figure 40.7 USG showing a multiloculated ovarian cyst.

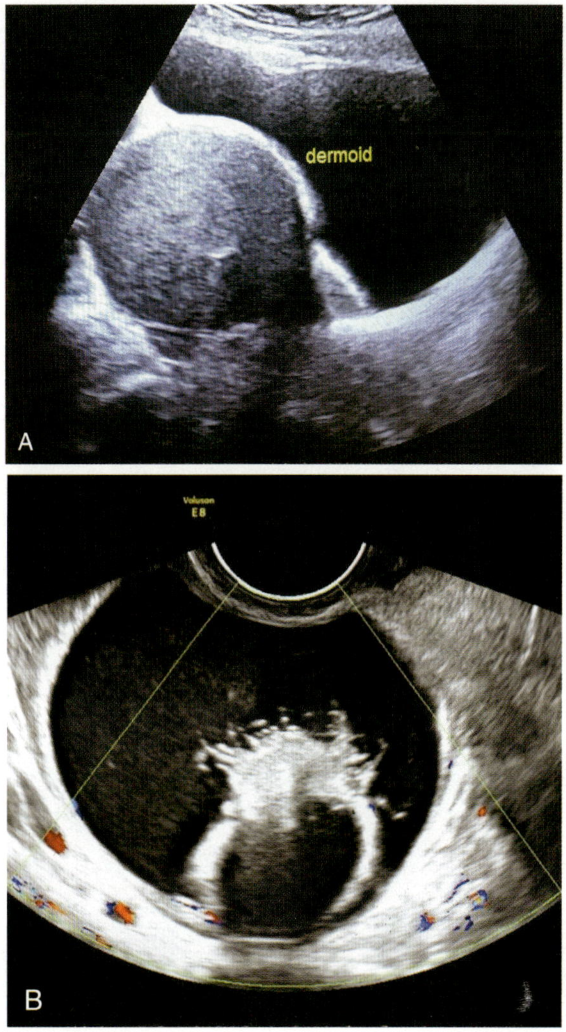

Figure 40.8 **(A)** USG showing dermoid cyst of the ovary with hyperechoic area suggestive of cartilage. **(B)** USG showing a dermoid cyst of the ovary with tuft of hair.

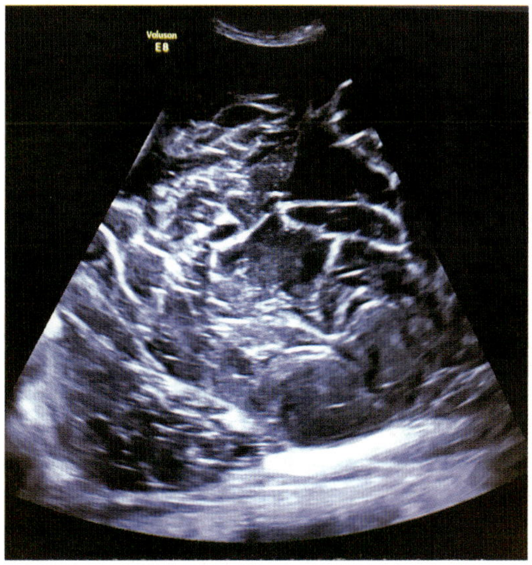

Figure 40.9 USG showing ovarian carcinoma. (*Courtesy*: Dr. Sunesh Kumar, AIIMS.)

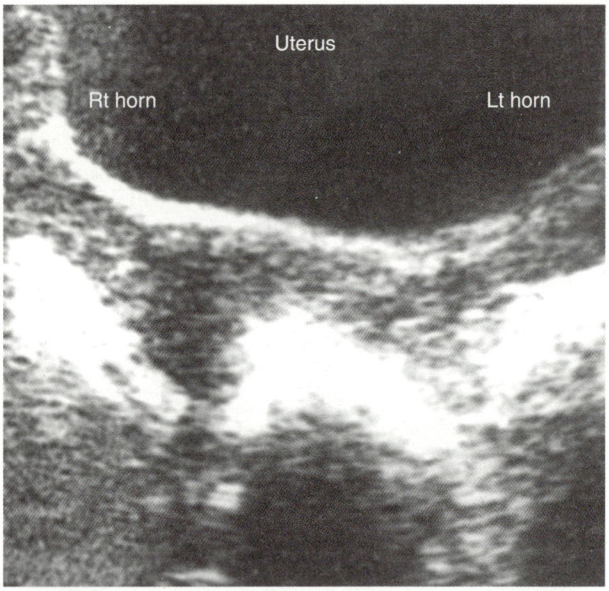

Figure 40.10 USG showing a bicornuate uterus. (*Courtesy*: Dr Ashok Khurana, New Delhi.)

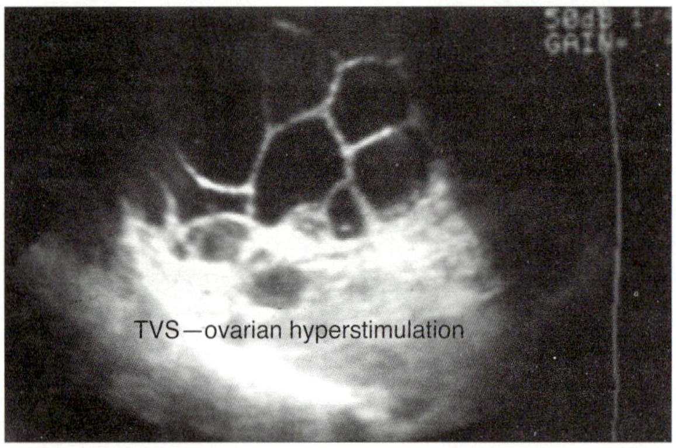

Figure 40.11 Ovarian hyperstimulation.

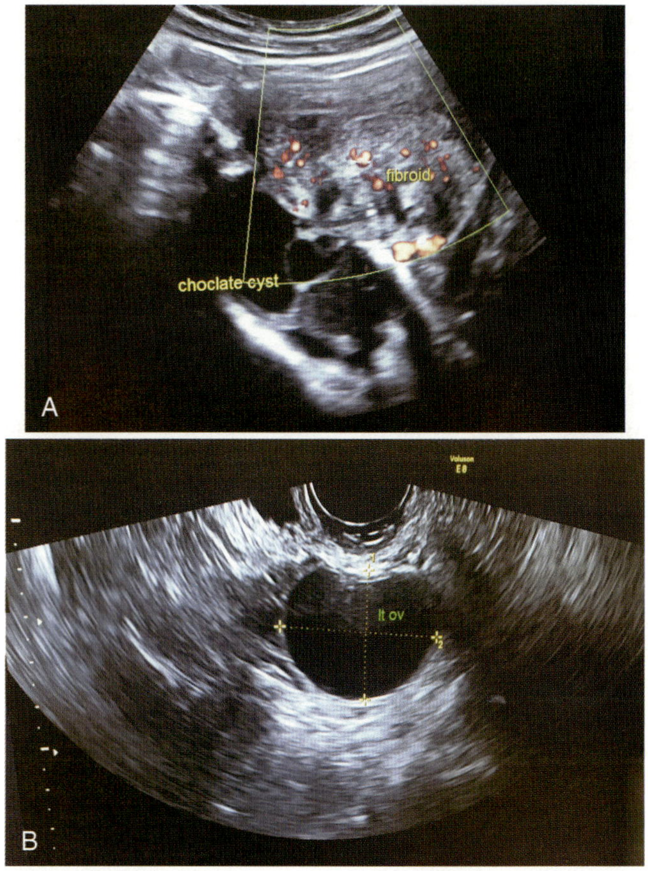

Figure 40.12 **(A)** Fibroid with endometrioma. **(B)** Left ovarian simple cyst.

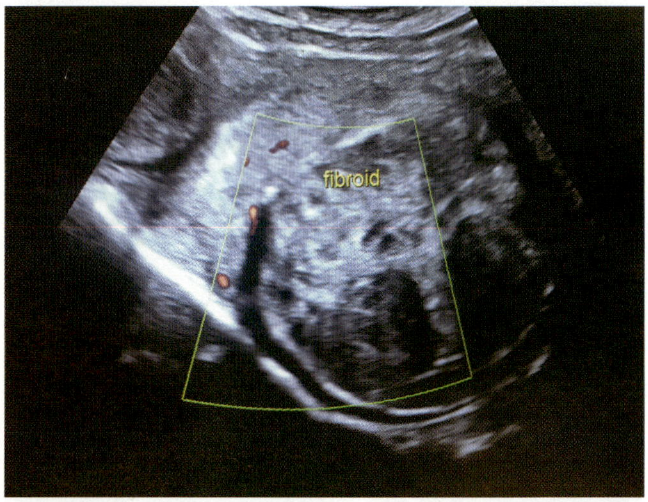

Figure 40.13 Uterine fibromyoma.

Standard examination of the female pelvis is performed by transabdominal approach (TAS) and by the transvaginal route (TVS). TAS is performed with 3.5 MHz convex transducer with a full urinary bladder, which provides an acoustic window as well as displaces the bowel loops away from the path of the ultrasonic beam. The structures deep and away from the vagina are better assessed by TAH approach.

Transvaginal sonogram (TVS) is performed with a high frequency probe of 7.5 MHz which demonstrates better anatomic details of the pelvic organs compared to TAS. The proximity with which the high-frequency TVS probe can be placed on the pelvic contents produces vastly superior resolution. In addition, demonstration of local tenderness and organ mobility yields information equivalent to a gynaecological examination (pain mapping).

The ultrasonic scan should be initiated with TAS and then followed up with TVS after the woman empties her bladder. This also gives the information of residual urine in investigation of urinary dysfunction. TVS should not be performed in virgins, or when TVS is refused by the woman. It is also difficult in a menopausal woman and in stenosed vagina.

Lately, perineal and anal ultrasounds are being employed in faecal incontinence and when TVS is not possible. They are also useful in studying the pelvic floor muscles and plan surgery in genital prolapse. The ultrasound may reveal breaks in the pelvic floor muscles, and helps to determine appropriate surgical approach in women with prolapse.

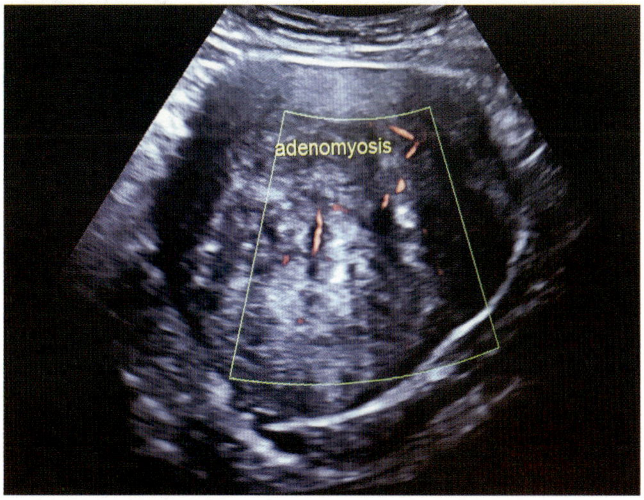

Figure 40.14 Adenomyosis of the uterus

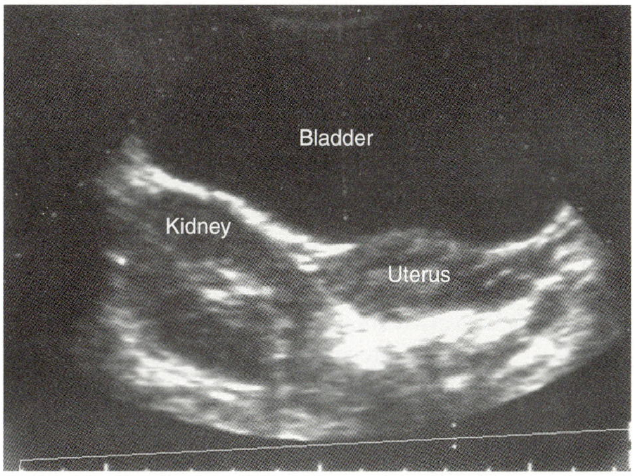

Figure 40.15 Ectopic pelvic kidney.

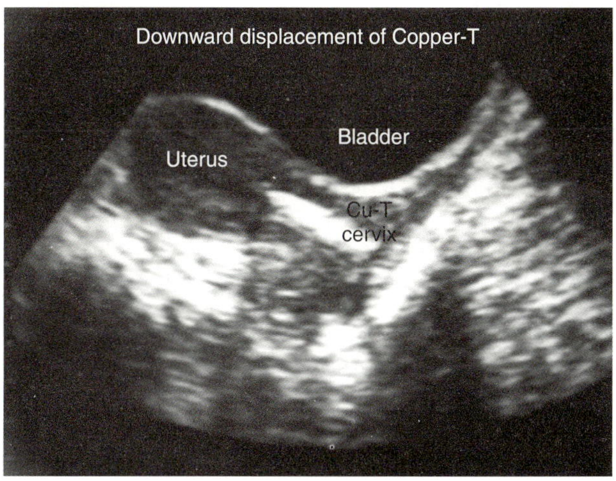

Figure 40.16 Downward displacement of Copper-T.

Advantages of TVS over TAS are as follows:

- Full bladder is not required.
- Better resolution and imaging of pelvic organs.
- In obese women, sound waves are attenuated by subcutaneous fat, and TAS gives a poor image.
- Sonography is the diagnostic modality of choice in pelvic imaging to determine and confirm the presence or absence of pelvic pathology, determine the size, texture and contour of the lesion and to establish the origin and anatomic relationship of the lesion with other pelvic structures. It also helps to determine the presence of absence of abnormalities associated with malignant diseases such as ascites or metastasis. It also provides guidance to the gynaecologist in performing aspiration and biopsy under sonographic control, and selective therapeutic procedures. Transvaginal sonography in infertility practice helps in monitoring follicular maturation, oocyte retrieval and embryo transfer.

Colour flow Doppler studies with spectrum are added to the examination depending on the clinical situation and pathology demonstrated on a grey scale.

- 3D ultrasound accurately measures the uterine and ovarian volume and blood supply.

NORMAL ULTRASONIC FINDINGS

The mean dimensions of the uterus of reproductive age are 7 cm in length and 4 cm in width in a nulliparous woman. It is 8.5 cm in length and 5.5 cm in width in a multiparous woman. After menopause, reduction in the uterus occurs proportionate to the duration of menopause. The location of the uterus is used as a road map in locating adnexal structures.

Ovaries are oval shaped measuring $3.0 \times 2.0 \times 1.0$ cm located laterally in the pelvis. Visualization of the ovary improves the detection of follicles within.

Ovaries have a marked variation in size and shape, so ovarian volume is considered a more reproducible parameter (S Campbell et al. 1982). Mean ovarian volume in reproductive age is 9.5 ± 5.0 mL.

Mean ovarian volume in perimenopausal age is 6.8–9 mL. In postmenopausal woman, it diminishes from 8 mL to 2 mL with advancing age.

A dominant follicle that ovulates is 18-20 mm or more.

Corpus luteum is recognized in the postovulatory phase and a small hemorrhagic cyst may be recognized. Corpus luteum cyst is occasionally seen in women with amenorrhoea but is absent in the postovulatory cycles.

Endometrial changes: These vary according to the different phases of the menstrual cycle.

Proliferative phase: It is thin and starts growing up to 6 mm before ovulation.

Secretory phase: The endometrium thickness further grows and may reach 10 mm in the late secretory endometrium. The glands have a cork-screw appearance and the vascularity increases. In endometrial hyperplasia, the endometrium grows beyond 10 mm, shows irregular margins with folds projecting into the uterine cavity as a sessile single or multiple polypi of same echogenicity.

After menopause, the endometrium atrophies and shrinks to less than 4 mm. The endometrial thickness of more than 4 mm, irrespective of postmenopausal bleeding, is considered abnormal, and requires investigations. However, in a woman taking tamoxifene, this cut off value is taken as 8 mm.

Subendometrial halo is demonstrated in late proliferative phase and its infiltration by endometrial tissue suggests adenomyosis or cancer of the uterus.

DIAGNOSTIC INDICATIONS

- Suspected congenital anomalies of the uterus.
- To diagnose haematocolpos, haematometra.
- To diagnose ectopic pregnancy. Absence of intrauterine sac, presence of adnexal mass with increased vascularity goes in favour of ectopic pregnancy. Occasionally, free fluid may be noted in Pouch of Douglas. On the other hand, in an *intrauterine pregnancy* – the gestation sac is generally eccentric in location. It grows at the rate of 1.0 mm/day. In an ectopic pregnancy, the pseudosac is centrally located.
- To diagnose adnexal mass.
- To diagnose uterine pathology – fibroids, adenomyosis, uterine synechiae.
- To monitor ovulation.
- In abnormal uterine bleeding – to study the endometrial pattern.
- To study endometrial lining in postmenopausal bleeding and its vascular pattern.
- To study ovarian pathology, i.e. polycystic ovarian disease (PCOD), ovarian cyst, ovarian tumour.
- Location of misplaced IUCD.
- Infertility – to detect submucous polyp, fibroid.
- Endometriosis.
- Fine-needle aspiration cytology (FNAC) in suspected gynaecological malignancy.
- Falloposcopy to study the medial end of the fallopian tube.
- In a male with low sperm count to detect varicocele by Doppler.

Details have been described in chapters 11, 13, 14, 16 and 17 respectively.

INTERVENTIONAL ULTRASOUND IN GYNAECOLOGY

- Oocyte retrieval in in vitro fertilization (IVF) programme.
- Drainage of chocolate cyst/simple benign cyst of the ovary. Laparoscopic surgery is superior to ultrasonic guided procedure, though more invasive.
- Drainage of pelvic abscess.
- To break uterine synechiae in Asherman syndrome.
- Evacuation of molar pregnancy, and MTP under ultrasound guidance. This avoids uterine perforation.
- Transcervical cannulation and sperm injection into the fallopian tube in infertility.
- Retrieval of embedded IUCD
- Injection of methotrexate into the ectopic gestational sac in unruptured ectopic pregnancy. Now, i.m. injection is preferred as it is noninvasive and equally effective.

Colour Doppler ultrasound is useful in suspected malignant ovarian tumour and endometrial carcinoma. Neovascularization and decreased resistance index (<0.4) suggest malignancy. Doppler ultrasound is useful to diagnose a rare case of arteriovenous malformation causing menorrhagia. Red colour indicates blood flow towards the transducer, and blue colour away from it.

INDICATION OF 3D/4D ULTRASOUNDS: They provide multiple images used mainly to detect fetal anomalies. In gynaecology, these ultrasounds are used for effective therapeutic procedures.

Some descriptions are mentioned below:

1. **Congenital Müllerian anomalies** (American Fertility Society Classification System)
   - Class I (agenesis, hypoplasia). Uterus is absent in total agenesis. Partial agenesis is identified as unicornuate uterus. In hypoplasia, the endometrial cavity is small with reduced intercornual distance of less than 2 cm.
   - Class II (unicornuate uterus) appears banana-shaped without the rounded fundus and triangular-shaped uterine cavity. If present, rudimentary horn presents as a soft tissue mass with similar myometrial echogenicity. Obstruction in the rudimentary horn is recognized as haematometra on one side.
   - Class III (uterus didelphys). The two horns are widely separated, with no vaginal septum.
   - Class IV (bicornuate uterus) shows two uterine cavities, with concave fundus, with fundal cleft greater than 1 cm, and this differentiates between the bicornuate and the septate uterus. The intercornual distance is more than 4 cm.
   - Class V (septate uterus) shows a convex or flattened fundus. The intercornual distance is normal (<4 cm) and each cavity is small.
   - Class VI (arcuate uterus) with no fundal indentation is of no clinical importance.
2. **Uterine polyp.** Endometrial polyp is sessile, single or multiple, less than 1 cm in size and homogenous with the surrounding endometrium, as it is formed by folding in of endometrial hyperplasia. Submucous fibroid on the other hand is larger than 1 cm, sessile or often pedunculated, mobile. It has a different texture compared to the endometrium. Sonosalpingography reveals a polyp, but cannot differentiate between submucous and endometrial polyp. TVS yields better image than TAS.
3. **Endometrial cancer.** Apart from endometrial thickness, endometrial irregularity, increased blood flow by Doppler and disruption or absence of subendometrial halo suggests myometrial invasion best seen on TVS.
4. **Uterine fibroids.** It is not only important to confirm clinical diagnosis of uterine fibroid but also necessary to assess the number, size and location to plan the management and decide on the type of surgery required. A rapid increase in the size of the fibroid in a perimenopausal woman suggests sarcomatous change in a fibroid.
5. **Ovaries.** In ovaries with heterogenous morphology, several pathological changes can be identified by ultrasound.
   - Functional cyst. It is the most common ovarian finding in the reproductive age group. A follicular cyst may be persistent at times, but never grows more than 5 cm and spontaneously resolves within a month or so. A Graafian follicle starts growing soon after

menstruation, and grows by 1–2 mm near ovulation, reaching about 20 mm in size or little larger. Ovulation is recognized by its disappearance at ovulation and the presence of free fluid in the pouch of Douglas. This is followed by growth of corpus luteum. The corpus luteum cyst has a thick, hypoechoic, sometimes, irregular wall and has echogenic content. Haemorrhage in the cyst reveals as low-level internal echoes.

- **Ovarian hyperstimulation syndrome (OHSS)** has been described in chapter 16.
- PCOD is characterized by more than 12 small follicles, 2–9 mm in size placed peripherally giving a necklace like appearance
- Endometriosis. Ultrasound shows varied appearance ranging from an anechoic cyst, with low echoes with or without solid components to a solid-appearing mass, resembling dermoid cyst, benign neoplasm or a fibroid.

6. **Fallopian tubes (PID).** Ultrasound shows one or more of the following features:
   - Thickening of the tube wall of more than 5 mm.
   - 'Cogwheel' sign, defined as cogwheel-shaped structure visible in cross-section of the tube with thick walls in acute salpingitis.
   - Incomplete septa with a dilated tube, which is sonolucent or contains low-level echoes.
   - Beaded appearances measuring 2–3 mm seen in a fluid distended structure. Cul-de-sac may show the presence of free fluid in the pouch of Douglas in acute infection.
   - Hydrosalpinx appears as a retort-shaped or tubular structure showing incomplete septa and the ovary is seen in the vicinity of the lesion.
7. **Infertility.** Ultrasound has a vast role in the infertility work-up. It is used for:
   - Sonosalpingography which delineates the uterine cavity and studies the patency of the fallopian tube.
   - Detecting unsuspected endometriosis.
   - IVF – To monitor ovulation, to retrieve ova and embryo transfer under ultrasound guidance.
   - In a male, to detect varicocele.

To decrease the cost and invasiveness of gamete intrafallopian transfer technique (GIFT), some employ transvaginal ultrasound to retrieve ova and transfer oocytes and sperms into the fallopian tube by ultrasound-guided catheterization transcervically.

Sometimes, the abnormal findings on ultrasound are incidental and have no bearing on a woman's symptoms and clinical features. It is important therefore, to correlate these findings with clinical features. The role of ultrasound is discussed in Table 40.1.

Table 40.1 Role of Ultrasound in Gynaecology

Diagnostic	Therapeutic
• Endometrial study – endometrial thickness irregularity, polyp, haematocolpos, haematometra	• IVF – ova retrieval
• Uterus – fibroid, adenomyosis, misplaced IUCD, Asherman syndrome, intermenstrual bleeding, postmenopausal bleeding, menorrhagia, uterine abnormality, absent uterus	• Drainage of pelvic abscess
• Falloposcopy	• During falloposcopy
• Tubal ectopic pregnancy	• Retrieval of IUCD
• Tubo-ovarian mass	• Injection of methotrexate, KCl in ectopic pregnancy
• PID, ovary: PCOD, ovarian cyst, differentiate between benign and malignant ovarian tumour	• MTP under ultrasound guidance
• Ovarian follicle monitoring	• Evacuation of a molar pregnancy
• Pelvic endometriosis	• Drainage of a simple ovarian cyst
• Chronic pelvic pain	
• Infertility	
• Varicocele in male	

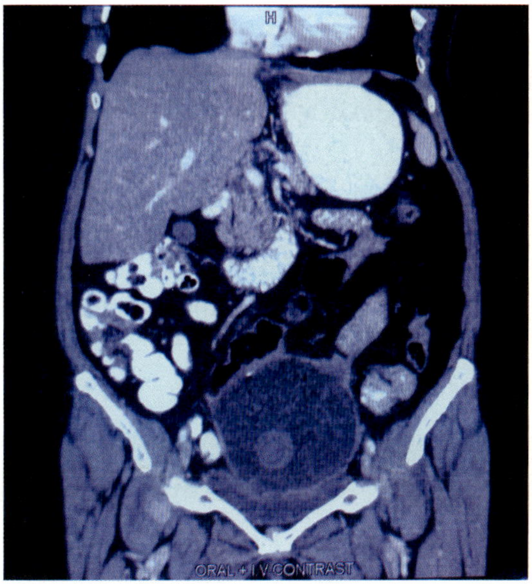

Figure 40.17 CT scan showing dermoid cyst.

COMPUTED TOMOGRAPHY SCAN

In gynaecology, CT scan supplements information obtained on ultrasound examination. The advantage of CT is its easy availability and the ability to survey the whole abdomen and pelvis accurately and rapidly in one sitting. CT is accurate in assessing local tumour invasion and enables accurate localization for biopsy. CT can also demonstrate other masses (Figs 40.17 and 40.18) and abnormalities of extragenital origin. However, both CT and the MRI cannot detect small peritoneal metastatic implants and lymph nodes in malignancies that are less than 1 cm in size.

Recently, *spiral CT* has been introduced into clinical practice. This enables continuous volumetric data acquisition in a single breath-hold. This potentially offers improved lesion detection, optimization of contrast media enhancement and multiplanar or 3D image information.

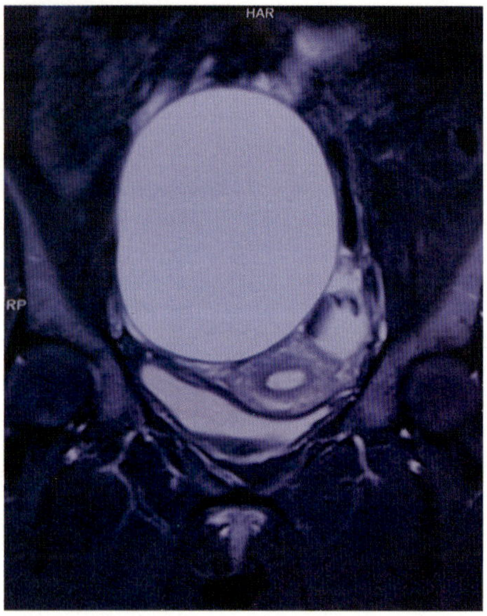

Figure 40.18 CT scan showing right ovarian cyst filling the Pouch of Douglas.

TECHNIQUE

Before undertaking a CT scan, exclude the possibility of pregnancy. The patient is required to have a full bladder. The patient is given 600–800 mL of a dilute oral contrast medium about 1 hour before the commencement of the procedure. Just before starting, a vaginal tampon is inserted to help delineate the position of the vaginal vault and cervix, and a rectal contrast medium given. The oral and rectal contrast media help to differentiate bowel loops from other pelvic organs. The patient is scanned in a supine position. In gynaecologic malignancies, intravenous injection of iodinated contrast medium is recommended to improve tumour delineation, characterization, assess vascularity and lymph node identification.

Advantages of CT are as follows:

- It is useful in the diagnosis of intraabdominal abscess.
- It is useful to diagnose pelvic vein thrombophlebitis.

Disadvantages of CT are as follows:

- It is expensive.
- Radiation up to 2–10 cGy does not permit its use in obstetrics.
- CT scan does not pick up lymph nodes less than 1.0 cm in size.

INDICATIONS

- Cancer of the cervix - to detect local spread, parametrial infilteration and lymph nodes metastasis.
- Endometrial cancer - to detect myometrial invasion and lymph nodes metastasis.
- Ovarian cancer - to detect intrahepatic, omental involvement and para-aortic lymph node metastasis.
- Choriocarcinoma - to detect brain metastasis and metastasis to other organs.
- In infertility - to detect hyperprolactinaemia and amenorrhoea.
- To diagnose intraabdominal abscess, pelvic vein thrombosis

MAGNETIC RESONANCE IMAGING

MRI is the well-established cross-sectional imaging modality. It provides multiplanar imaging capability with high soft tissue contrast resolution without interference from air or bone. There is no need for administration of oral contrast or for injection of intravenous dye for vascular contrast. MRI, unlike CT, has no adverse effects on pregnancy, embryo, fetus or future reproductive potential of the ovary as it has no radiation effect. The major limitations are availability, time taken for procedure and cost. It cannot be done in women with prosthetic valve and other prosthetic transplant.

INDICATIONS

- To assess pelvic anatomy in women with endometriosis and adenomyosis.
- To evaluate Müllerian anomalies.
- Localize the position and size of the fibroids (Fig. 40.19A and B) and sarcomatous change.

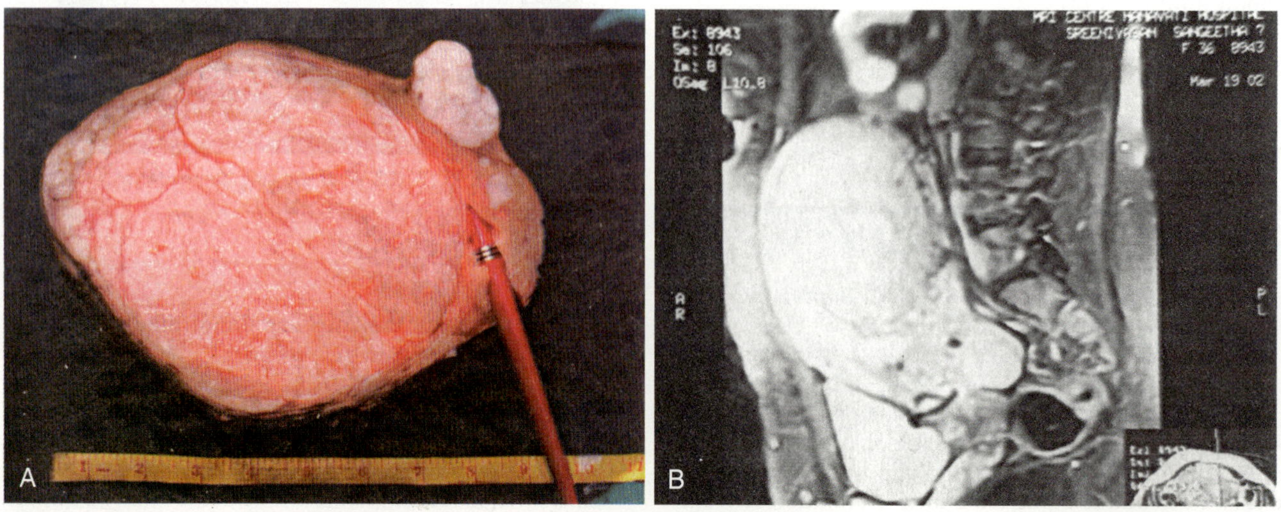

Figure 40.19 **(A)** Mirror image of fibroid seen on MRI. **(B)** MRI showing fibroid uterus.

Table 40.2 Indications of CT and MRI in Gynaecology

CT	MRI

Diagnostic
• Endometrial cancer staging, lymph node assessment, recurrence
• Cancer cervix extension, lymph node involvement recurrence
• Ovarian cancer staging, lymph node involvement, recurrence
• Pituitary tumour
  ◦ Hyperprolactinaemia
  ◦ Amenorrhoea
  ◦ Cerebral metastasis
• Abdominal abscess
• Pelvic vein thrombosis
Contraindicated in pregnancy due to radiation
	• Endometrial cancer – myometrial invasion and endocervical extension
	• Müllerian anomalies
	• Endometriosis
	• Fibroid, sarcoma
	• Cancer of the cervix – involvement of parametria and lymph nodes
	• Ovarian cancer
	• In obstetrics – to detect fetal anomalies
	THERAPEUTIC
	MRI-guided procedures in uterine fibroids and adenomyosis

- Staging and assessment of pelvic neoplastic diseases such as cancer cervix, endometrial carcinoma and other cancers.
- Assess adnexal pathology, endometriosis and chocolate cyst.
- To assess depth of myometrial invasion and endocervical extension in a case of endometrial carcinoma.
- Staging of cervical cancer and detection of recurrence.
- Assess recurrent pelvic disease and metastasis.
- In obstetrics, it can pick up fetal anomalies.
- Detection of lymph nodes metastasis.
- MRI-guided therapeutic procedures used in leiomyomas and adenomyosis.

CONTRAINDICATIONS

- Patients with a pacemaker or cochlear implant.
- Metallic foreign body in the eye.
- Paramagnetic aneurysm clips.
- Overanxious patients need prior sedation.
- Those who suffer from claustrophobia may not tolerate the procedure well. However, newer open machines are now available which overcome this disadvantage.
- Epileptic and women with atrial fibrillation, because electroconvulsions can occur.

Indications of CT and MRI are listed in Table 40.2

RADIONUCLIDE IMAGING

This form of imaging in gynaecology is used for specific clinical situations. Bone scans using *technetium*-99 m diphosphonate are used to detect bone metastasis in patients with malignancies. *Ventilation perfusion scans* are used for detecting pulmonary emboli. *Radio-labelled white cell* scans can be used for locating abscesses.

DUAL-PHOTON DENSITOMETRY

The use of this new imaging technique is becoming increasingly popular in determining the risk of osteoporosis in postmenopausal women. It is recommended in women who suffer from early menopause or who undergo oophorectomy. The lumbar spines and hip are scanned with a dual-photon densitometer, which produces computerized graphs and measurements of bone density and relates them to age-related normal values.

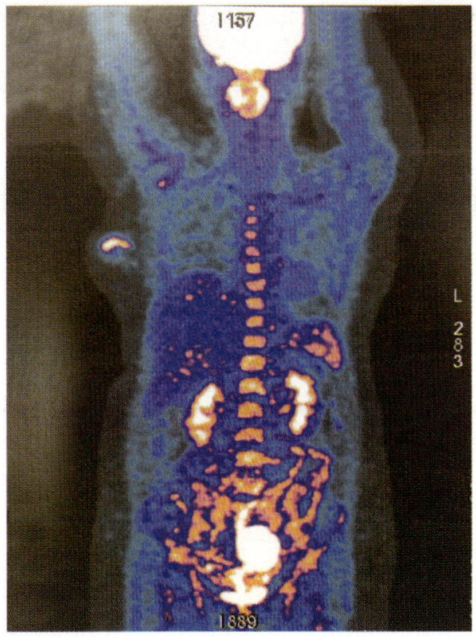

Figure 40.20 PET scan showing increased FDG uptake in uterus, bilateral kidneys and brain.

Positron emission tomography (PET) is a functional diagnostic imaging technique, taking advantage of the fact that malignant cells have a greater glycolysis compared to normal tissue. It helps in initial staging, management and follow-up of cancer growths (Fig. 40.20). PET–CT combines the metabolic status with the anatomical details of the patient, respectively.

[F-18]-fluoro-2 deoxy-D-glucose (FDG) is used as a radiopharmacological agent which is an analogue of glucose. Glucose uptake by malignant cells is higher than that of normal cells. PET maps the tissue spread. It also helps to distinguish cell death following radiotherapy from tumour recurrence, and helps in posttreatment management.

PET scan is a nuclear biological modality and functional diagnostic image technology using radioactive material given orally, injected into the body or inhaled. It is now used in the diagnosis of cancer in its early stage, detect its extent and severity and also assess the patient's response to therapeutic interventions by studying the molecular activity in the tissues. It is noninvasive. PET scan measures the blood flow to the organ, oxygen consumption and glucose metabolism, which is high in the cancer cells.

Combining with CT, which provides anatomical details and PET showing metabolic status, it improves the accuracy of the tests.

'Hot-spots' are detected where large amounts of radiotracer have accumulated, and these spots are mapped in planning therapy.

Preparation:

The woman should not eat food for a few hours as this causes misinterpretation of the test, but take plenty of oral fluids. PET takes 30 minutes to perform, and CT about 2 minutes.

PET is contraindicated in the following:

- Pregnancy and lactation, because of the use of radiotracer.
- Diabetes – one should be careful, as tissue blood sugar is usually high.

- An obese woman as she may not fit into the narrow machine.
- All metals, i.e. hairpins, jewellery and metal implants should be removed.

Sensitivity of PET is 80%–90%. Currently PET scan is used to detect recurrences in women treated for cancer cervix, endometrial cancer and ovarian cancers. Some people are exploring usefulness of PET scan in pre-operative workup of cases of carcinoma cervix, endometrial cancer and other genital tract cancers.

KEY POINTS

- Several newer imaging modalities have come into vogue for accurate assessment of the clinical problems, however, ultrasound remains the most commonly used technique.
- A plain radiograph in gynaecological practice involves a posterior anterior (PA) view of the chest as part of the preoperative work up of patients undergoing surgery. X-ray of the chest is required in suspected lung metastasis in choriocarcinoma and other malignancies.
- A hysterosalpingogram is performed to test tubal patency in infertility, intracavitary uterine lesion and to demonstrate Müllerian anomalies of the uterus.
- Ultrasonography has now become the first line of imaging investigation in the management of gynaecological problems because of its wide availability and low cost. It is an excellent first-line investigation to determine the location and nature of the pelvic pathology. Ultrasound is noninvasive and the report is available on the spot.
- CT scan and MRI are used as additional tools to define the extent of neoplasia and to determine spread to adjacent structures and lymph nodes. These have a great role to play in staging of genital cancers.
- A Doppler examination helps to determine the pattern of blood flow in the organ, identify an ectopic pregnancy and detect suspicious malignant tumours.
- Sonosalpingography is indicated in suspected cases of endometrial polyp and submucous fibroid.
- PET is the latest technology which studies the metabolic status of the tumour, and when combined with CT which gives anatomical details also.

SELF-ASSESSMENT

1. What is the role of hysterosalpingography in the practice of gynaecology?
2. Discuss the importance of ultrasonography as an imaging modality in obstetric practice.
3. What is the role of TAS and TVS in gynaecological practice?
4. Write short notes on (a) colour Doppler and (b) role of CT and MRI scans in gynaecology.
5. What is the role of dual-photon bone densitometry in gynaecological practice?

SUGGESTED READINGS

Guidelines for diagnostic Imaging during pregnancy. American College of Obstetricians and Gynecologists Committee, Opinion No. 299, Sept 2004.

Kamel HS, Darwish AM et al. Comparison of transvaginal ultrasound and sonohysterography in the detection of endometrial polyps. *Acta Obstet Gynecol Scand*, 2000, 79(1): 60.

Rosen CJ. Postmenopausal osteoporosis. *N Eng J Med*, 2005; 353(6): 595–606.

Report on Ultrasound Screening – Supplement to Ultrasound Screening for Fetal Abnormalities London. The Royal College of Obstetricians and Gynaecologists Working Party. RCOG, 2000.

Stanford E. Prevention and Management of Osteoporosis. OB/GYN 6th Edition, 2006: 31.

Endoscopy in Gynaecology

41

CHAPTER OUTLINE

Endoscopes are telescopes designed to view the interior of body spaces or viscera. Although attempts at endoscopy date back to over 100 years, the potential of this method as a diagnostic and therapeutic tool was appreciated and came to the forefront only in the past three decades. When used appropriately, endoscopic surgery offers the advantages of a more accurate diagnosis, less invasiveness, reduced pain, faster recovery and shortened hospital stay or a day care. Advances in instrumentation and techniques now enable the endoscopist to accomplish several operative procedures hitherto performed only by open surgery, including cancer surgery. Some of the advances are harmonic scalpel, suture materials and laser.

Minimal invasive surgery (MIS) implies avoiding an abdominal scar, minimal handling of pelvic and abdominal organs, less pain and thereby fast recovery.

Advantages of laparoscopy: (i) lesser pain, (ii) few analgesics, (iii) short hospital stay, (iv) quick return to daily work, (v) no scar – no scar site hernia, (vi) good cosmetic and (vii) less pelvic adhesions.

Disadvantages of laparoscopy: (i) longer procedure time, (ii) more anaesthesia, (iii) expensive and (iv) expertise required.

LAPAROSCOPY

Laparoscopy was developed in late 1970s, and operative laparoscopy has started gaining ground in the past two decades. Advances in technology led to the development of high-resolution cameras, video laparoscopy, the development of safe instruments permitting the use of electrical and laser energy and harmonic scalpel for cutting and cauterizing tissues or achieving haemostasis.

Its role in the management of infertility stands undisputed, so also the benefits of laparoscopy over laparotomy of being minimally invasive and having a lower incidence of adhesion formation. Low incidence of infection render endoscopy to be an attractive alternative procedure in many gynaecological diseases.

Despite these advantages, there are potential limitations. For example, the exposure to the operative field may be reduced, manipulation of the pelvic viscera often restricted and tissue apposition during suturing is as accurate. Moreover, the feel of tissues experienced by the surgeon during open surgery lacks during endoscopic surgery.

The endoscopic surgeon in the making has to go through supervised training and acquires the skills over a period of time. There is a longer learning curve during which the endoscopist in training understands the limitations of the procedure and knows when to stop. Thereafter, the incidence of complications during endoscopy begins to decline and progressively more complex procedures can be successfully undertaken.

Laparoscope (Fig. 41.1)**.** Laparoscope is a rigid telescope varying in diameter between 4 and 10 mm and it is 30 cm long, incorporating an optical system as a means of illumination. The light is transmitted from an external source to the distal lens by means of fibreglass cables. Light source of 300 W is used for illumination of abdominal cavity. Photography requires light source of 1000 W. Other instruments include Veress needle, trocar- cannula and accessories to perform therapeutic procedures (Fig. 41.1). A long Veress needle is available for obese women and for posterior colpopneumoperitoneum. CO_2 pneumoperitoneum machine to create pneumoperitoneum is specially designed for laparoscopy. About 0.5-1L/minute is instilled into the peritoneal cavity, maintaining intraperitoneal pressure below 15 mm Hg. About 1000 mL is required for adequate pneumoperitoneum (Fig. 41.2).

INDICATIONS FOR LAPAROSCOPY

The laparoscope has emerged as an invaluable tool in the armamentarium of the gynaecologist, both for diagnostic and for therapeutic uses (Table 41.1).

DIAGNOSTIC LAPAROSCOPY

The common indications for diagnostic laparoscopy are described below (Figs 41.3 ▶–41.7).

Infertility and Tubal Disease

Laparoscopy is indicated if hysterosalpingography reveals abnormal or ambiguous findings. It can reveals block tubes or ambiguous findings, salpingography and presence of endometriosis. Chromopertubation using methylene blue dye is a part of diagnostic laparoscopy for infertility evaluation to determine tubal patency.

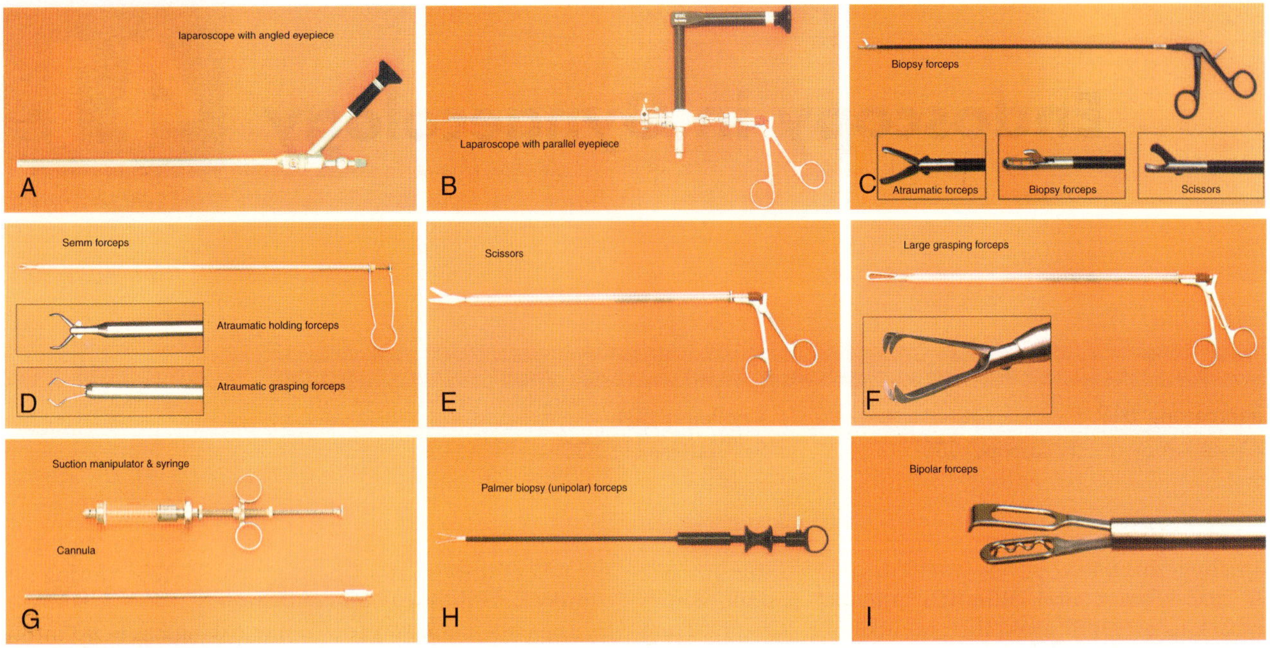

Figure 41.1 Laparoscope and commonly used accompanying instruments. **(A)** Laparoscope with angled eyepiece. **(B)** Laparoscope with parallel eyepiece. **(C)** Biopsy forceps. **(D)** Semm forceps. **(E)** Scissors. **(F)** Large grasping forceps. **(G)** Suction manipulator and syringe. **(H)** Palmer biopsy (unipolar) forceps. **(I)** Bipolar forceps.

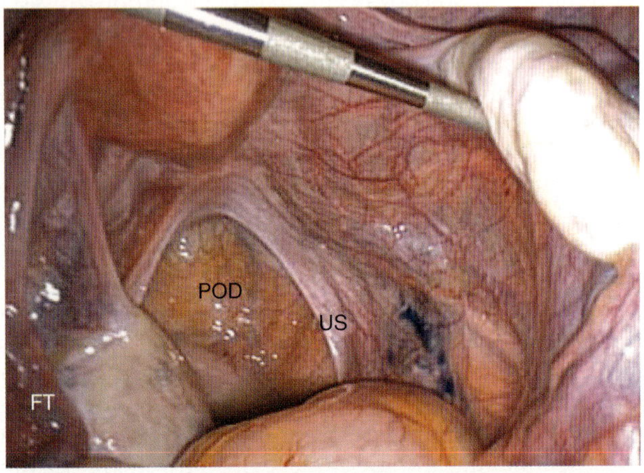

Figure 41.2 View of the pelvis with uterus anteverted from laparoscopy. Right ovary turned over with probe to expose right pelvic sidewall. FT, fallopian tube; POD, pouch of Douglas; US, uterosacral ligament. (*Source:* From Figure 1-1, Robert W Shaw, David Luesley and Ash Monga: Gynaecology, Fourth Edition, Elsevier, 2011.)

Occasionally a fibrous band is recognized extending from the right tube to the undersurface of the liver in pelvic inflammatory disease (PID) caused by gonococcal and *Chlamydia* infection. This goes by the name Fitz-Hugh–Curtis syndrome. The relationship between the ovary and the ovarian fimbria can be studied in infertility. The laparoscopy helps to choose treatment between tuboplasty and in vitro fertilization (IVF). Salpingoscopy through laparoscope studies the ampullary portion of the tube and extent of tubal damage.

Endometriosis

In about 20% of patients with infertility, endometriosis is present without any symptoms. It remains undetected until demonstrated at laparoscopy.

Table 41.1 Indications of Laparoscopy

Diagnostic	Therapeutic
• Infertility – tubal patency adhesions, pathology uterine disease ovulation, PCOD • Ovary – PCOD, size, volume, adhesions • Pelvic endometriosis • Chronic pelvic pain • Ovarian malignancy, nature of the tumour – benign, malignant, extent, staging of carcinoma, second-look surgery • Uterus – malformations, absent uterus, septate, fibroid, adenomyosis, perforation during surgery • Tubal – patency, PID, ectopic pregnancy • Pelvic tuberculosis • Prior to tuboplasty to study the feasibility	• Pelvic adhesiolysis • Ablation of endometriosis • PCOD – drilling • Ovarian cystectomy ovariotomy, surgery • Lymphadenectomy in cancer cervix uterus, ovary • Myomectomy • Myelinolysis • GIFT in infertility • Septate uterus • Ectopic pregnancy • Tuboplasty • LAVH • Hysterectomy • Removal of hydrosalpinx and pyosalpinx • Vault prolapse • Stress urinary incontinence • LUNA (laparoscope uterosacral nerve ablation in dysmenorrhoea)

Chronic Pelvic Pain

In patients complaining of chronic pelvic pain, not responding to usual therapeutic measures, laparoscopy is indicated. Often unsuspected pathology is brought to light such as adhesions, cysts, chronic PID, tubal hydrosalpinx, endometriosis, pelvic congestion, window tears in the broad ligaments and varicosity of the pampiniform plexus of veins. Even a negative finding is valuable to reassure a patient that there is no pelvic pathology.

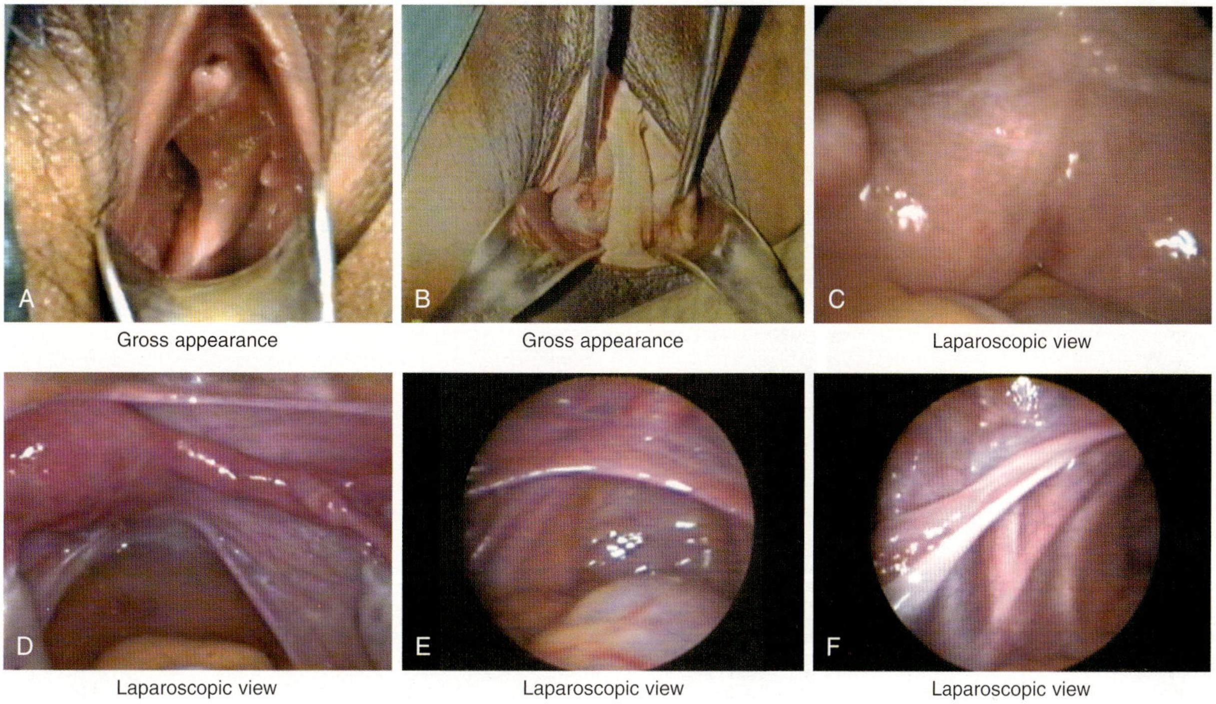

Figure 41.3 Gross and laparoscopic appearance of genital tract abnormalities. **(A)** Septate vagina. **(B)** Two cervices with two vaginas. **(C)** Bicornuate uterus. **(D)** Bicornuate uterus with rudimentary horn. **(E)** Rudimentary uterus (RKH syndrome). **(F)** Streak ovary. ▶ Scan to play Diagnostic Laparoscopy

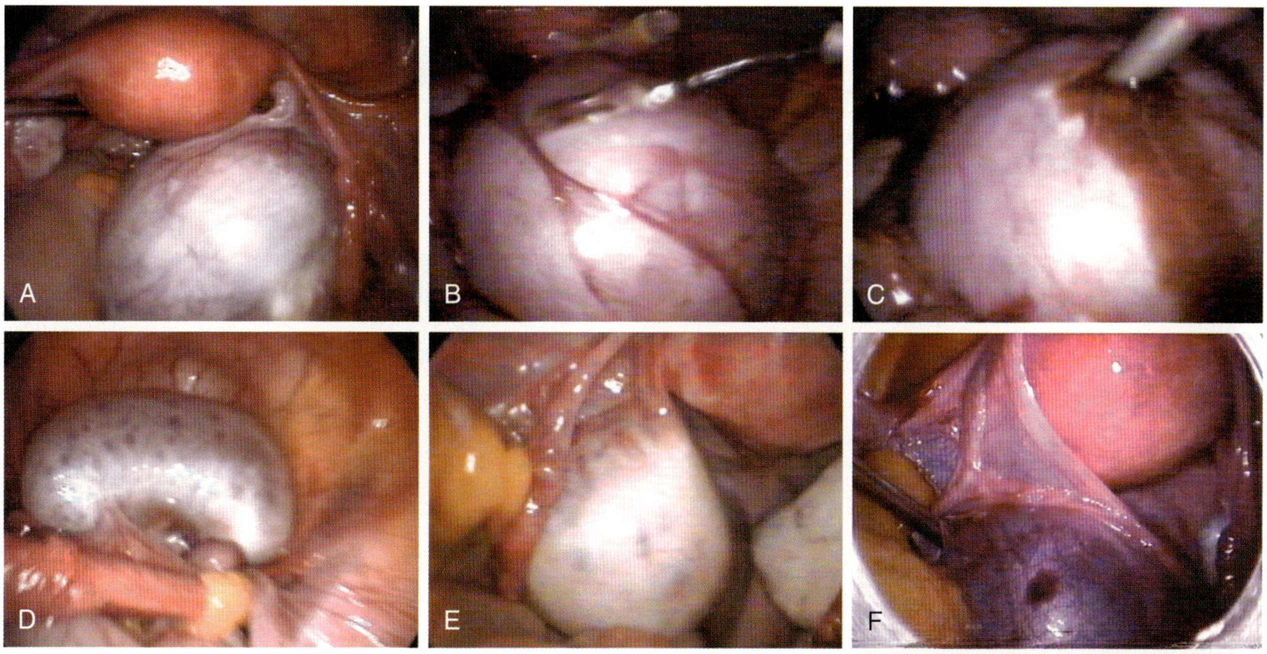

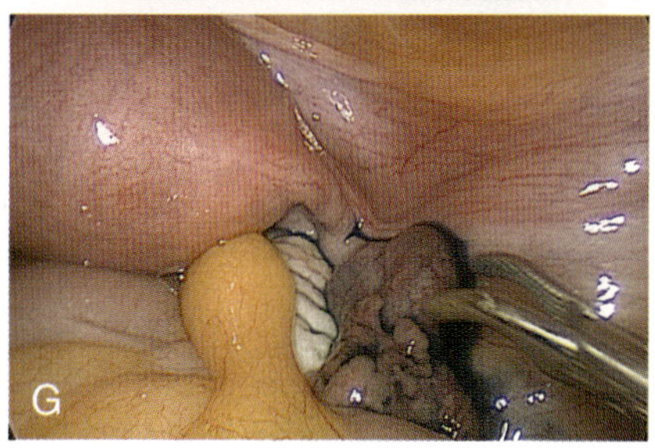

Figure 41.4 **(A–F)** Laparoscopy in ovarian and parovarian pathology. **(A)** Dermoid cyst. **(B)** Intact endometrioma. **(C)** Draining of chocolate cyst. **(D)** PCOD – multiple follicles. **(E)** Polycystic ovaries, bilateral enlargement in size – multiple follicles and thickened tunica albuginea seen. **(F)** Fimbrial cyst with fallopian tube stretched on its surface. **(G)** Laparoscopic view of spillage of dye through fimbrial end. (*Courtesy* (G): Dr Vivek Marwah, New Delhi.)

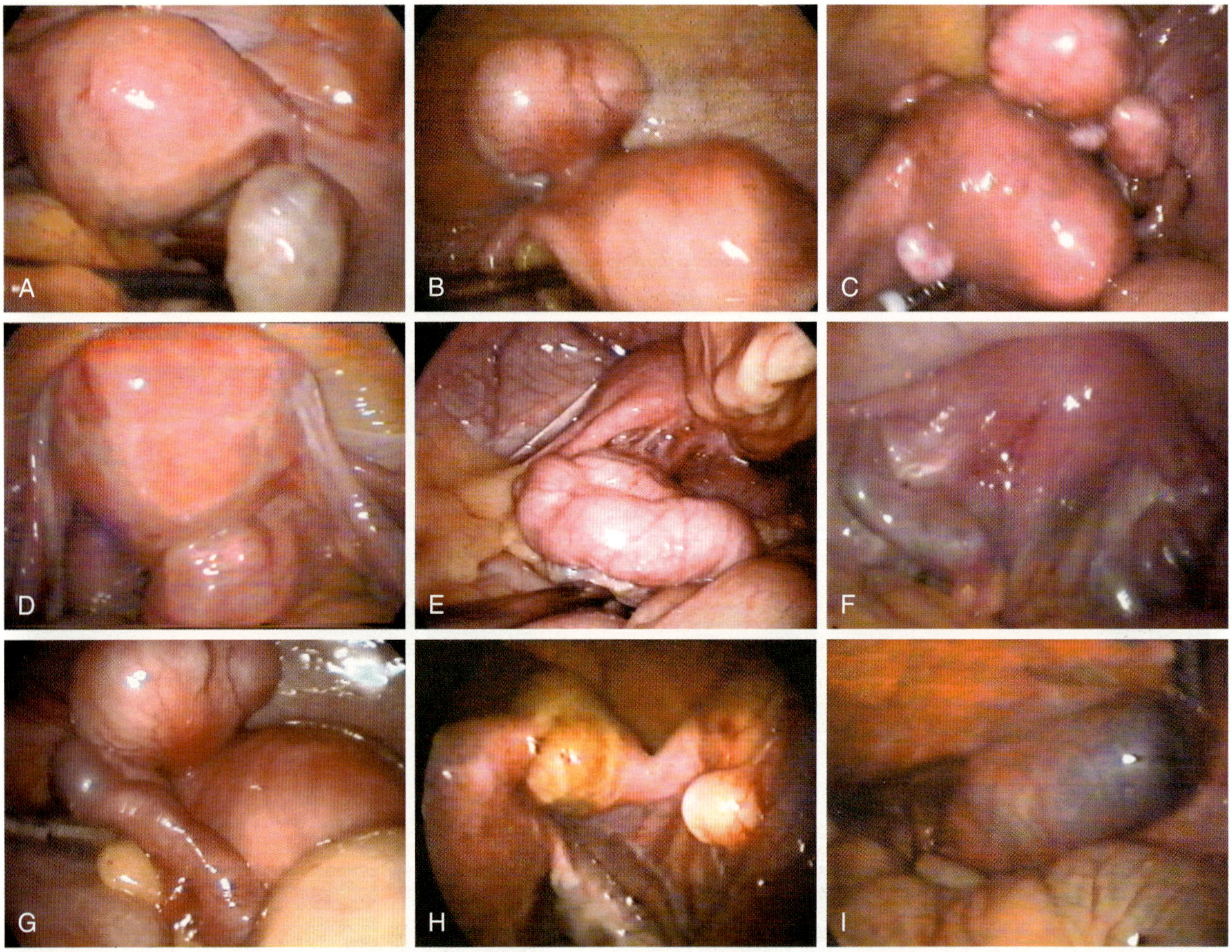

Figure 41.5 Laparoscopy in uterine and tubal pathology. **(A)** Diffusely enlarged uterus because of adenomyosis. **(B)** Anterior wall subserous pedunculated fibromyoma of the uterus. **(C)** Multiple fibroids – uterus subserous and intramural. **(D)** Posterior isthmical fibromyoma. **(E)** Tubal pyosalpinx. **(F)** Bilateral tubal hydrosalpinx. **(G)** Tubo-ovarian mass. **(H)** Genital tuberculosis – tuberculous pyosalpinx. **(I)** Unruptured tubal ectopic pregnancy.

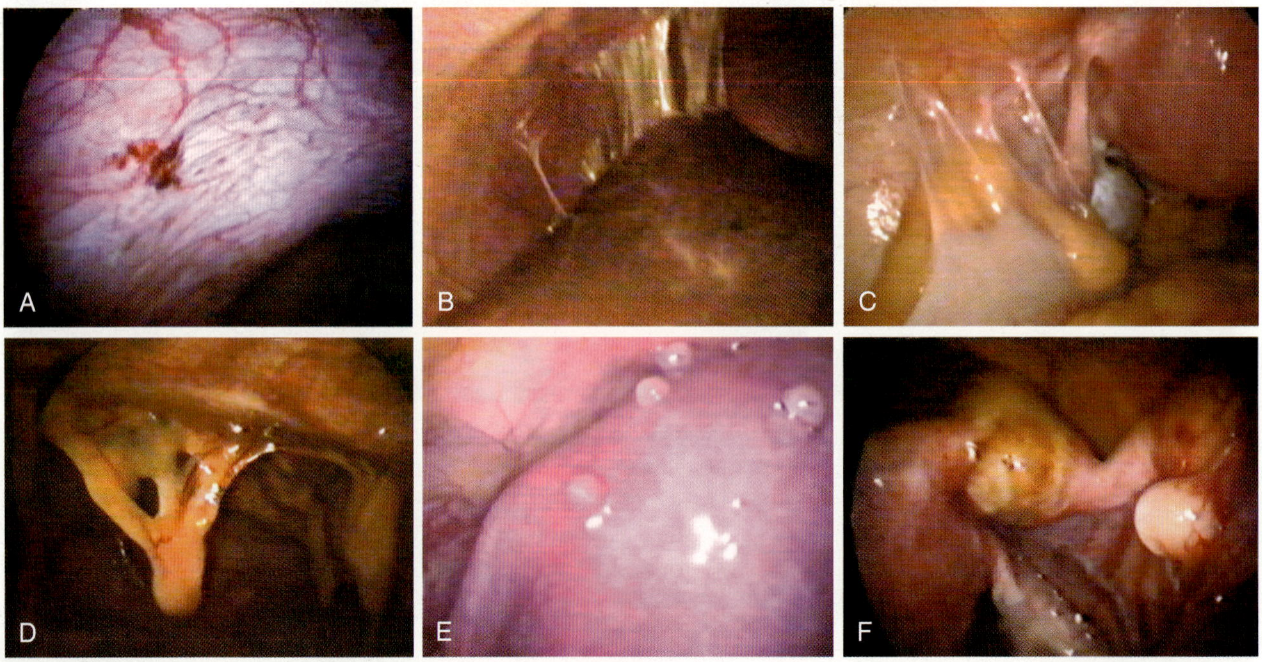

Figure 41.6 Laparoscopy: miscellaneous. **(A)** Endometriosis: peritoneal implant. **(B)** Chronic PID: perihepatic adhesions. **(C)** Chronic PID: pelvic adhesions. **(D)** Abdominal Koch's disease: peritoneal adhesions. **(E)** Genital Koch's disease: tubercles on the uterine serosa. **(F)** Genital Koch's disease: beaded tuberculous fallopian tube.

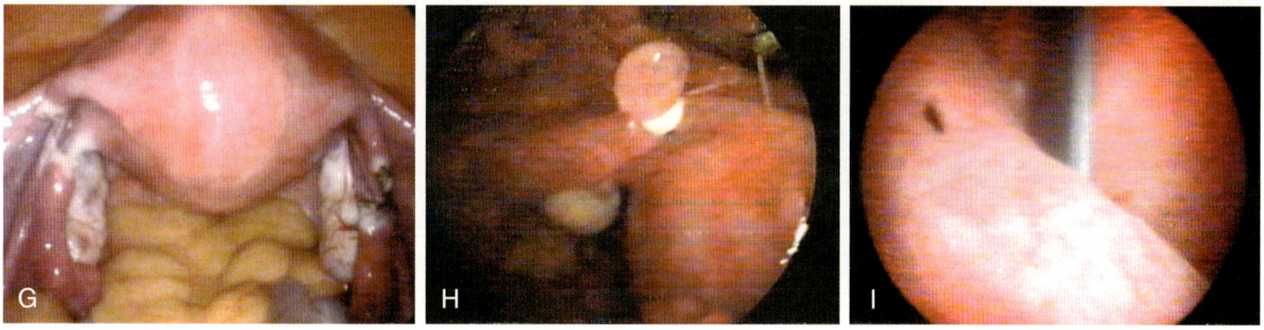

Figure 41.6, cont'd (G) Family planning: tube occlusion with bipolar cautery and cutting. **(H)** Family planning: tube occlusion with silastic band. **(I)** Cystoscopy: ureteric orifice seen – probe in vesicovaginal fistula.

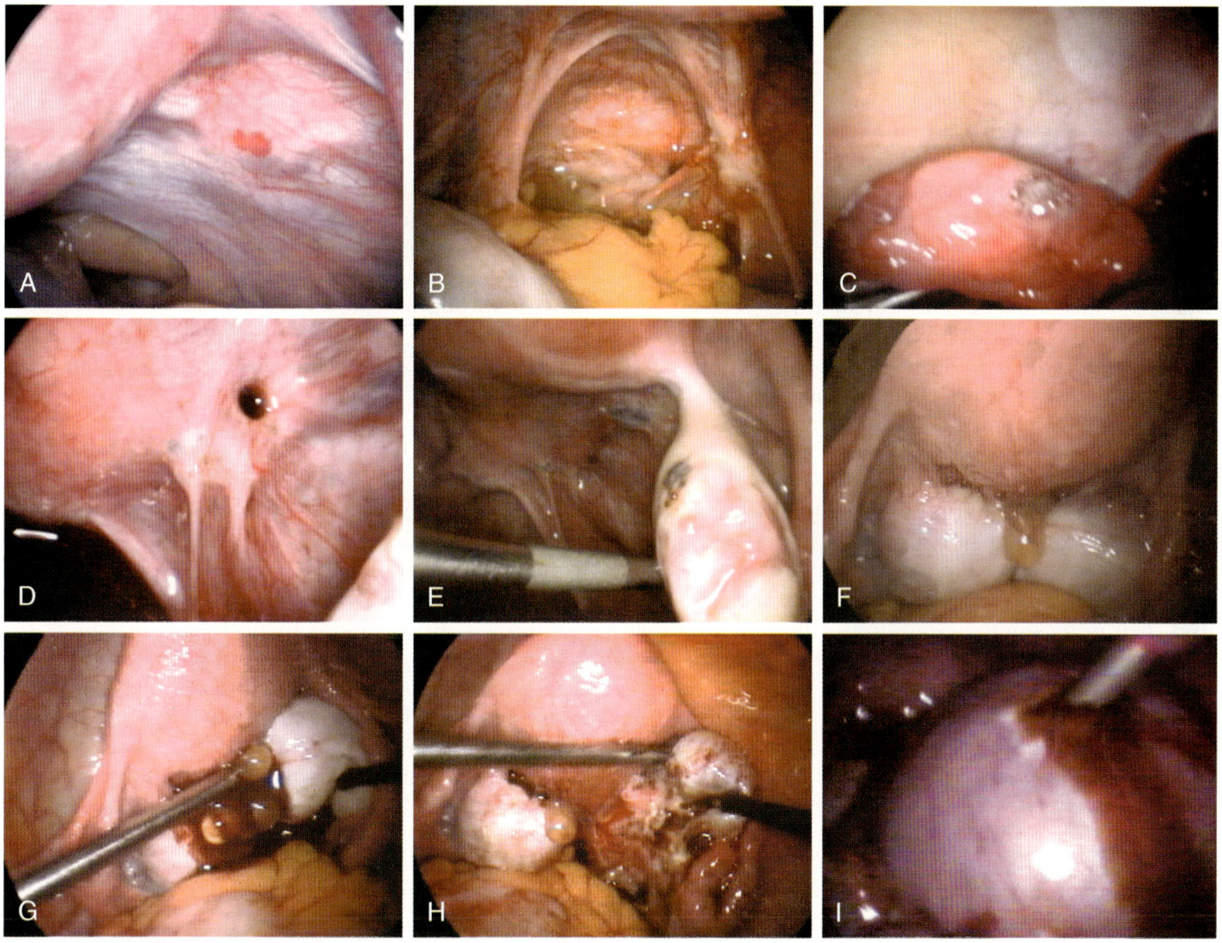

Figure 41.7 Laparoscopic appearance of endometriosis – manifestations. **(A)** Superficial peritoneal flame-like patch. **(B)** Nodular uterosacral endometriosis with adhesions. **(C)** Endometriotic patch on anterior surface of the uterus. **(D)** Endometriotic nodule and powder burn marks in ovarian fossa. **(E)** Superficial endometriosis on ovarian surface and ovarian fossa. **(F)** Endometriotic adhesions binding down the ovaries into the pouch of Douglas, 'kissing ovaries'. **(G)** Chocolate material drained from small chocolate cyst. **(H)** Endometriotic adhesions on posterior uterine surface and the ovaries. **(I)** Large chocolate cyst of the ovary (endometrioma), chocolate material drained.

'Conscious pain mapping' helps to identify the organ which causes pain.

Ovarian Disorders

Most reproductive endocrine disorders of the ovaries do not need a diagnostic laparoscopy, ovarian surgery or biopsy. Ultrasonography and blood hormonal assays usually suffice in arriving at a diagnosis. However, in case of polycystic ovarian disease (PCOD), laparoscopy is useful to confirm the diagnosis, and to further investigate the patient for other causes of infertility. The operation of ovarian drilling is performed to improve the results of ovulation induction therapy. Ovarian cyst, extent and spread of malignant tumour can be assessed by laparoscopy. Second-look surgery is now replaced mostly by ultrasound, MRI and tissue markers.

Suspected Adnexal Masses

Ultrasonography, CT scan or MRI helps in detecting adnexal masses and establishing their site of origin. However, often it is not possible to differentiate a pedunculated fibroid from a solid ovarian tumour, and laparoscopy may be necessary. Laparoscopy helps to distinguish a pelvic mass of uterine in origin, commonly a fibromyoma from an ovarian mass. An asymptomatic fibroid may require observation, whereas an ovarian solid mass needs prompt surgical removal.

Suspected Ectopic Pregnancy

In a patient with abdominal pain, irregular menstruation and a positive pregnancy test, a laparoscope can detect an ectopic pregnancy even before it has ruptured and enable conservative surgery, thereby preserving her future reproductive potential.

Pelvic Inflammatory Disease

In PID, the diagnosis can be confirmed on laparoscopy. Peritoneal fluid or pus can be obtained for culture, and other causes such as acute appendicitis and pelvic tuberculosis considered in the differential diagnosis can be ruled out with certainty.

Ovarian Malignancy

In advanced ovarian malignancy, a laparoscopy may be useful in staging the disease and in obtaining a biopsy from the affected tissue, which confirms the type of tumour and helps the oncologist to select chemotherapy or radiotherapy as the alternative therapy in an inoperable case.

Ascites

In ascites, laparoscopy helps to obtain ascitic fluid for cytology and biochemical analysis. It also helps to determine the cause of ascites as attributable to tumour, tuberculosis or hepatic cirrhosis. A biopsy from the tumour establishes the diagnosis. Ultrasonic-guided aspiration of fluid and biopsy is however a simpler procedure as compared to laparoscopy.

Tuberculosis

Genital tuberculosis accounts for 5-10% of patients with unexplained infertility in our country. The fallopian tube is the most commonly affected site. Presence of tubercles on the serosa, multiple constrictions, thick rigid tubes, presence of violin-string adhesions and tobacco-pouch appearance of the terminal parts of the tubes should arouse suspicion. Presence of tubercles on the bowel serosa or peritoneal surface can be biopsied to arrive at the diagnosis.

Uterine Abnormalities

Laparoscopy reveals uterine abnormalities:

- These include the Müllerian anomalies such as absent uterus as in cases of Rokitansky–Küster–Hauser (RKH) syndrome, bicornuate uterus, septate or presence of a rudimentary horn, testicular feminizing syndrome.
- Laparoscopy can distinguish between a septate uterus and a bicornuate uterus.
- An enlarged uterus because of fibromyomas or adenomyosis can be diagnosed.
- Adhesions to the uterus and its retroverted fixity can also be diagnosed.

Uterine perforation during MTP/D&C can be confirmed or refuted laparoscopically, and decision made regarding the need for laparotomy.

Inspection of the Pouch of Douglas

This can be inspected; often endometriosis is present at this site, so also adhesions to the rectum present. This can be a site of pelvic abscess and ovarian metastasis.

OPERATIVE LAPAROSCOPY

Minimally invasive surgery is replacing conventional surgery as the procedure of choice in selective gynaecological surgeries.

General Indications

Pelvic Adhesions

These adhesions are often postinflammatory, postsurgical or endometriotic in nature. Laparoscopic adhesiolysis restores the anatomy of pelvic organs and their mobility, and relieves pain and discomfort arising out of binding of the organs by adhesions. Pelvic endometriosis may affect many pelvic structures such as the ovaries, tubes, uterosacral ligaments, serosal surface of the uterus, pelvic peritoneum and the pouch of Douglas, as also the rectum, bladder and ureters. Adhesiolysis is done by ablation with cautery, laser or surgical excision of the lesions within the limits of safety and relieves symptoms.

Adhesiolysis is especially required in tubal infertility to restore the patency and mobility of the fallopian tubes and its fimbria.

Ovaries

The various MIS procedures on ovaries are:

- PCOD: The medical hormonal therapy cures PCOD in most women. In those who fail to respond and in infertile women, laparoscopic puncture of cysts by cautery or laser improves the response to hormonal ovulation stimulation, avoids hyperstimulation syndrome and improves the fertility rate to 60%–70%. However, because of possible subsequent adhesion formation and thereby impaired tubal fertility, women are advised to try conception in the first year of ovarian puncture. It is strongly recommended that no more than four cysts should be punctured in each ovary. More punctures may increase the ovarian adhesions and ovarian destruction leading to premature menopause later.
- Ovarian cyst: A simple cyst less than 5 cm is usually a functional cyst, and it disappears in 3 months' time and needs only observation. A large benign cyst can be aspirated laparoscopically and fluid sent for cytology. The cyst wall is then peeled off by aqua suction and tissue sent for histopathology.
- Chocolate cyst: The chocolate cyst is incised, the content aspirated and the cyst wall cauterized or peeled off (Chapter 14). Pelvic endometriosis is also ablated.
- Gamete intrafallopian transfer (GIFT) technique in assisted reproduction is performed laparoscopically by placing 2 ova and 50,000 sperms at each ampullary portion in an infertile woman with patent tubes.
- Second-look surgery laparoscopically is undertaken following primary surgery and a complete course of chemotherapy for ovarian cancer, before deciding whether further chemotherapy or excision of residual tumour is required.

Lately, however, tumour markers are relied upon and this procedure is avoided.
- Pelvic lymphadenectomy is now performed laparoscopically in early cancer cervix and followed by vaginal hysterectomy or trachelectomy. This inflicts less surgical morbidity and allows quicker recovery, especially in an obese woman.

Expert oncologists are now performing Wertheim's hysterectomy laparoscopically safely with equally good results.

Uterus

Operative procedures on the uterus include myomectomy, laparoscopy-assisted vaginal hysterectomy (LAVH), total laparoscopic hysterectomy (TLH), excision of a rudimentary horn and Wertheim's radical abdominal hysterectomy for cancer cervix.

- Myomectomy is indicated planned for young women. Ideally it is rewarding in cases with not more than four fibroids, preferably subserous, and of moderate size not exceeding about 5.0 cm in size. After enucleating the myomas from their beds, the cavity is obliterated with interrupted apposing endosutures to achieve haemostasis and prevent adhesion formation. Large fibroids may be removed by morcellation or through a small suprapubic incision. Small myomas can be removed piecemeal after shredding (myelolysis) or by the vaginal route through the posterior colpotomy incision (Chapter 29).
- LAVH and TLH are performed in women in need of a hysterectomy for benign conditions (myomas, adenomyosis, menorrhagia and abnormal uterine bleeding) in women with in situ cancer of the cervix in whom there is no descent of the uterus to facilitate vaginal surgery, and in women older than 45 years in whom concomitant removal of the ovaries is desirable. The purpose of LAVH is to convert an abdominal hysterectomy to vaginal hysterectomy or a difficult vaginal hysterectomy to an easy surgery. Realizing that LAVH carries a higher morbidity in terms of prolonged anaesthesia and restricted view, many laparoscopists now perform vaginal hysterectomy even on undescended uterus and are able to remove both the ovaries from below as well. In TLH the entire procedure is carried out laparoscopically and at the end of procedure uterus is delivered vaginally. The vaginal vault is closed laparoscopically.

Other uterine surgeries done under laparoscopic guidance are excision of uterine septum and synechiae in Asherman syndrome. A rudimentary noncommunicating horn may be the site of a haematometra, ectopic pregnancy or torsion. Laparoscopic removal is feasible in such cases.

Laparoscopic Radical Hysterectomy

Oncologists now perform Wertheim's hysterectomy laparoscopically (radical abdominal hysterectomy and bilateral extraperitoneal dissection and excision of the iliac and pelvic lymph nodes for cancer of the cervix).

Fallopian Tube

The most common operation performed on the tube is sterilization for family planning. The tubal occlusion is achieved through occlusion with 'Falope rings' or 'Filshie clips'.

Ectopic Pregnancy

An early unruptured ectopic pregnancy can be treated effectively laparoscopically. The surgeon may attempt milking out the gestational sac, particularly so if it is close to the fimbrial end. An ampullary ectopic pregnancy can be treated by linear salpingostomy and enucleating the tubal gestational sac. An early unruptured ectopic pregnancy can be treated by local injection of methotrexate into the gestational sac. All these procedures are conservative measures aimed at preserving the woman's reproductive potential.

Hydrosalpinx of the tube can be treated by lateral salpingostomy and fimbrioplasty with eversion of the inverted fimbriae by fashioning a cuff. In blocked tubes, segmental resection and anastomosis has been successfully performed laparoscopically. Hydrosalpinx is also removed prior to IVF to improve the pregnancy rate (Chapter 16).

OTHER INDICATIONS

Amongst the other operative procedures accomplished laparoscopically, those given in the subsequent text deserve to be noted.

Genital Prolapse

Conservative procedures for second-degree uterine prolapse such as abdominocervicopexy and uterine sling operation have been successfully performed laparoscopically. Vaginal vault prolapse is corrected by sacropexy.

Stress Urinary Incontinence

The operation of colposuspension has been successfully performed laparoscopically. Both the Marshall–Marchetti–Krantz procedure and the Burch operation can be undertaken laparoscopically.

Pelvic Floor Repair

This has been performed laparoscopically to restore the anatomy of the pelvic floor (laparoscopic colposacropexy).

Dysmenorrhoea

Laparoscopic uterosacral nerve ablation (LUNA) aims at cautery and cutting of both the uterosacral ligaments close to their uterine attachment. The uterine pain-carrying nerve fibres travel along the uterosacral ligaments to reach the pelvic autonomic ganglia. Division of these ligaments interrupts the pain pathway and provides relief. However, there is risk of damaging the ureters, and in due course of time, the nerves regenerate, so that dysmenorrhoea often returns. The presacral nerve lies in front of the sacral promontory. Exposing the nerve bundles laparoscopically and dividing the same is possible. However, with the availability of efficient analgesic drugs, there is seldom any need to have recourse to such drastic surgical procedures except in endometriosis.

Others

Procedures such as repair of herniae, appendicectomy and pelvic lymph node biopsies are being performed laparoscopically.

TECHNIQUE OF LAPAROSCOPY

Laparoscopy has become a safe MIS; therefore, it is employed more liberally than before, both for diagnostic and for certain therapeutic procedures. However, bearing in mind that a rare but a serious complication may develop during therapeutic procedures such as myomectomy, hysterectomy and ablation of endometriosis, certain preoperative preparations are required. These are:

- Fibroid: It is desirable to shrink a huge fibroid to reduce bleeding and make it easier to perform myomectomy. This is done by gonadotropin-releasing hormone (GnRH) injection administered monthly for 3 months (Chapter 13).
- Bowel preparation and intestinal antibiotics (metrogyl) are safe precautions in case bowel injury occurs.
- Bladder should remain empty throughout the procedure using a catheter.
- Systemic antibiotics should be started a day before surgery.
- Signature for open surgery should be obtained in the case of complication or inability to complete the procedure laparoscopically.

PROCEDURE

- Whereas diagnostic procedure may be carried out under sedation and local anaesthesia, the therapeutic procedure always requires general anaesthesia because of prolonged time taken and intra-abdominal manipulations required.
- Position: The patient is placed in semilithotomy and slight Trendelenburg position.
- Pneumoperitoneum is created with a Veress needle using carbon dioxide (CO_2) gas through a small infraumbilical incision. Air and nitrous oxide (N_2O) should not be employed, because of the risk of air embolism in the former and combustion with N_2O if electrocautery is used. The proper pneumoperitoneum is confirmed by noting the uniform distension of the abdomen and Palmer test, which consists of injecting 5 mL of saline through Veress needle. Failure to aspirate saline indicates proper placement of the needle.

Continuous flow of CO_2 is maintained at the rate of 100 mL/minute and pressure at 15–25 mm Hg. Trocar and laparoscope insertion follow, through the same skin incision. Under fibre optic illumination, the pelvic organs are inspected, and feasibility of the procedure under consideration confirmed.

- Bipolar cautery is safer than monopolar cautery as it does not spread the burn to the surrounding structures. Laser is even safer and does not form postoperative adhesions, but is expensive. Lately, harmonic scalpel is available and, though very expensive, is very safe and cuts the tissues well.

Additional portals and instruments are used in therapeutic procedures. Suction and irrigation are also provided to clear the blood and fluid from the abdominal cavity.

At the end of the procedure, after making sure haemostasis is secured and no gut injury has occurred, gas is expelled from the peritoneal cavity and the skin cuts sutured.

During the procedure, the uterus is manipulated in different directions by using uterine manipulator inserted transcervically before the start of the surgery.

COMPLICATIONS

Complications (0.5%–1%) are observed in minor procedures, but the incidence as high as 5%–15% is reported with major procedures. Death is reported in 0.08/10,000 of cases.

Major complications are as follows:

- Cardiopulmonary arrest and gas embolism
- Acidosis, arrhythmia and cardiac arrest caused because of CO_2
- Haemorrhage
- Cautery burns to various viscera
- Sepsis
- Injury to the bowel, small intestine, blood vessels, bladder and ureter with the sharp instruments and burn injuries
- Failure to complete the procedure

Cardiopulmonary arrest is an anaesthetic complication. Embolism occurs with the use of air, but excess CO_2 and accidental insertion of Veress needle into a blood vessel can also cause embolism. This mishap is avoidable if pneumoperitoneum is checked by Palmer test.

Haemorrhage

Injury to the epigastric vessel occurs during insertion of the Veress needle and trocar. Injury to the aorta, inferior vena cava, iliac vessels and mesenteric vessels mainly occurs with a sharp instrument such as a trocar. Prolonged surgery during myomectomy can also cause loss of blood.

Careful insertion of the trocar can avoid the injury. Uncontrolled haemorrhage requires laparotomy.

Cautery Burns

Accidental burn to the surrounding structures occurs with unipolar cautery and sometimes with laser. The injury may go unnoticed during surgery and may not manifest clinically as peritonitis for 24 hours or even more. The abdominal distension and vomiting are then the first indications of gut injury and peritonitis. The bowel injury requires laparotomy, resection of the bowel and end-to-end anastomosis.

Sepsis is avoided by preoperative antibiotics and aseptic precaution.

Traumatic injury to the viscera and ureter occurs with sharp instruments (bladder, ureter and intestines) or burn.

OTHER COMPLICATIONS

The other complications include surgical emphysema and haematoma.

- Postoperative peritoneal adhesions occur less commonly with laparoscopy than with laparotomy, because the viscera are not handled and are not exposed to air dryness as in open surgery.
- Hernia at the site of portals with omental protrusion rarely occurs. The uterine perforation with the uterine manipulator does not normally require laparotomy. Metastatic cancer has been reported at the port site.
- Emergency therapeutic procedures which are done laparoscopically for torsion and haemorrhage of ovarian cyst or rupture of endometrioma carry greater risk than planned surgery since preoperative preparation may not be adequate.
- Failed procedure: Because of adhesions, extensive pelvic lesions or uncontrolled haemorrhage, laparoscopic procedure needs to be abandoned and converted to laparotomy. The prior consent to this effect avoids medicolegal problems.

CONTRAINDICATIONS TO LAPAROSCOPY

- Extreme obesity makes laparoscopic procedure and pneumoperitoneum difficult if not impossible. Alternatively, pneumoperitoneum can be created through posterior culdocentesis.
- Cardiac and respiratory diseases contraindicate Trendelenburg position and CO_2 pneumoperitoneum.
- Diaphragmatic hernia precludes Trendelenburg position.
- Umbilical hernia. The trocar can injure the bowel if the latter is adherent to the hernial sac.
- Previous abdominal scar also exposes the bowel to injury during trocar insertion.
- Acute pelvic infection can spread during laparoscopy.
- A large uterus (puerperal) and an abdominal tumour can be injured by the sharp instrument.

ADVANTAGES OF LAPAROSCOPY OVER LAPAROTOMY

- Avoidance of abdominal scar, wound sepsis and scar hernia
- Reduced pain and quick recovery
- Short hospital stay
- Less peritoneal adhesions postoperatively

LATELY, robotic surgery is gaining popularity.

HYSTEROSCOPY (Fig. 41.8)

Hysteroscopy, which started first in 1869 with Pantaleoni as a means of inspecting the uterine cavity, is today functioning as an extended gynaecological armamentarium in various therapeutic procedures. Despite the initial poor light source and nonavailability of distending media, hysteroscopy was not abandoned, and its improvement developed into an important MIS and has led to a resurgence of interest worldwide in recent years.

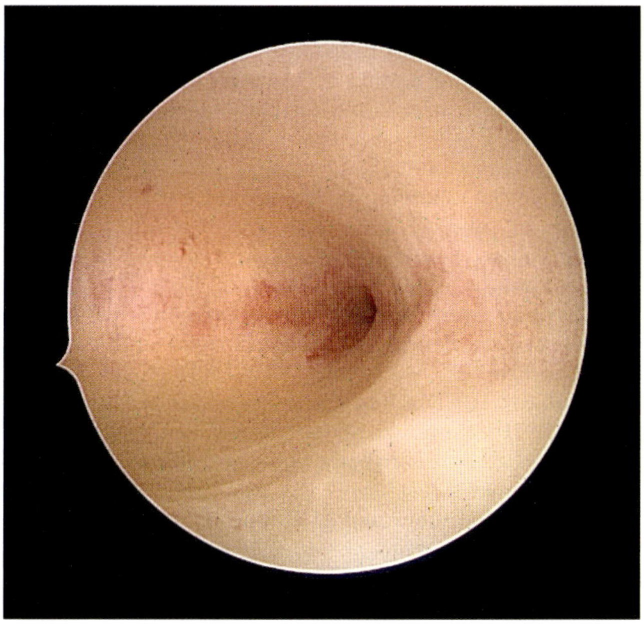

Figure 41.8 Hysteroscopic view of the patent cornual end. (*Courtesy*: Dr Vivek Marwah, New Delhi.)

Hysteroscope

Hysteroscope comprises a rigid 4-mm telescope with Hopkins rod lens optical system having a wide viewing angle and fibre optic illumination cable. Camera and television system enables video study and therapeutic procedures. The sheath is of 5 mm diameter, in the centre of which the telescope is fitted. The uterine cavity is distended with CO_2 at the rate of 70 mL/minute and pressure less than 100 mm Hg, or with saline, dextrose, Hyskon or glycine 1.5%. The scope is covered by inner sheath for inflow of distending medium, and outer sheath for its outflow.

Types of Hysteroscopes

- Microhysteroscope provides magnification of 30–150 times.
- Contact hysteroscope is a diagnostic tool without distending medium.

Flexible hysteroscopy can be directed to all parts of the uterine cavity and extensive inspection is possible.

TECHNIQUE

Hysteroscopy should be performed *in the preovulatory phase when the endometrium is thin and bleeding is less likely to occur*. In transcervical resection of endometrium (TCRE), shrinkage of endometrium is achieved with progestogen, danazol or GnRH given continuously for 6–8 weeks prior to surgery. Diagnostic hysteroscopy can be performed under local (paracervical) anaesthesia and sedation, but the therapeutic procedures mandate general anaesthesia (Fig. 41.9 ●). The cervical dilation is not always required.

In a postmenopausal woman, cervical or misoprostol vaginal tablet (prostaglandin E_1) will soften the cervix and cervical dilatation with the metal dilator made atraumatic as and when required.

The woman is placed in lithotomy position, and bimanual examination confirms the position and size of the uterus and also rules out adnexal mass. The cervix is dilated up to 4–5 mm. The hysteroscope is connected to the source of distending media. As the distension medium distends the cervical canal and uterine cavity, the telescope is progressively advanced into the uterine cavity under direct vision. This precaution avoids perforation. The endocervical and uterine lining are studied, and both uterine ostia identified. Gas inflating machine used in laparoscopy should not be employed in hysteroscopy, since high pressure of the former can cause gas embolism.

The hysteroscope is provided with a cervical adaptor which fits snugly on to the cervix and prevents backflow of the uterine-distended medium.

Distending Media

CO_2 obscures the vision in the presence of blood and cannot be employed in the presence of bleeding. Its use is therefore limited only to diagnostic hysteroscopy.

Five per cent glucose is cheap, and is miscible with blood.

Hyskon and glycine are used mostly nowadays. Hyskon (32% dextrose) coalesces with blood into globules while the medium remains clear.

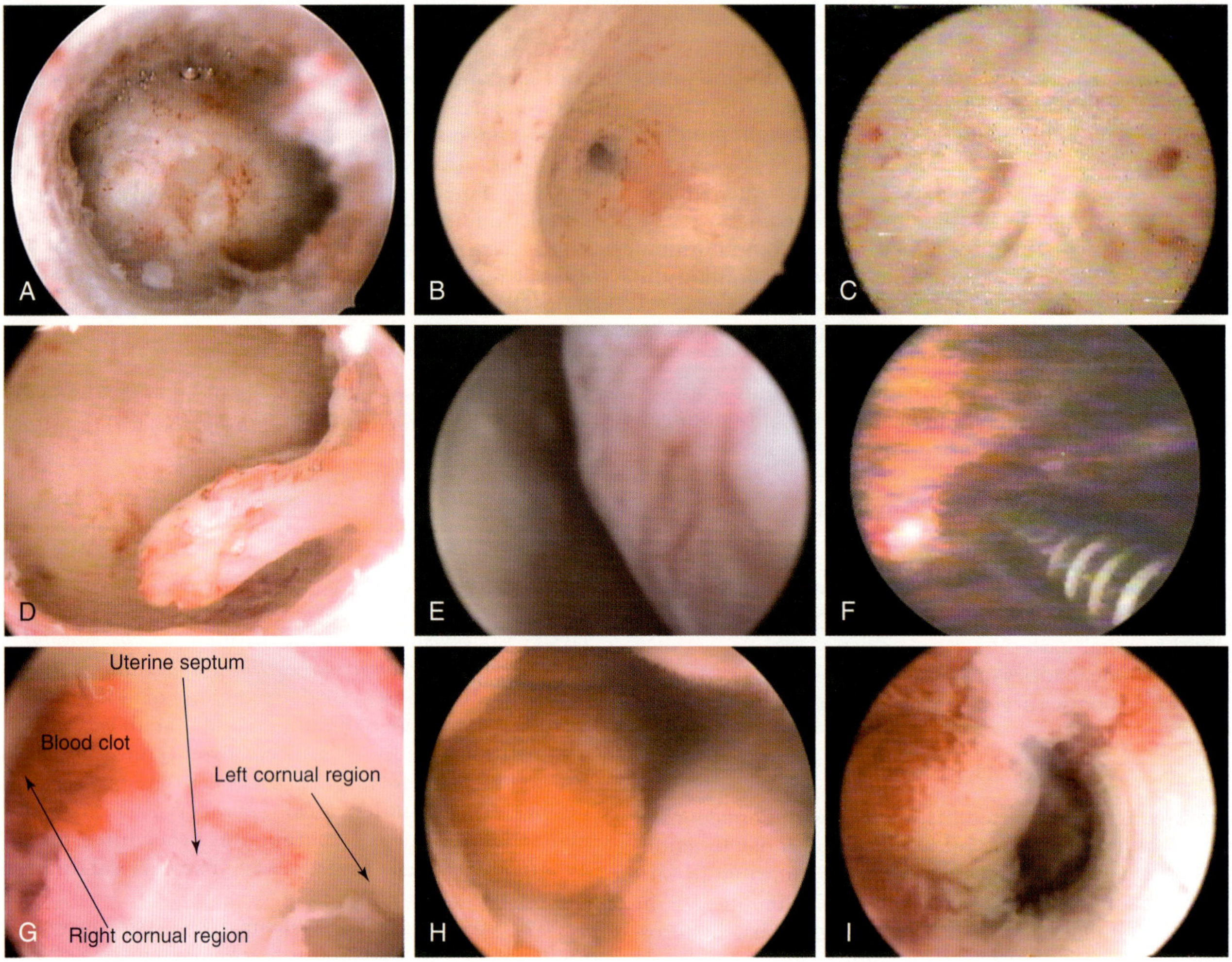

Figure 41.9 Diagnostic hysteroscopy. **(A)** Panoramic view of uterine cavity. **(B)** Normal view of left tubal ostium. **(C)** Appearance of uterine wall in adenomyosis. **(D)** Endometrial polyp. **(E)** Submucous fibromyomatous polyp in uterine cavity. **(F)** IUCD-Cu-T in uterine cavity. **(G)** Müllerian anomaly, intrauterine septum. **(H)** Polyp protruding into the endocervical canal. **(I)** Polyp restricted to endocervix.
▶ Scan to play Diagnostic Hysteroscopy

NORMAL APPEARANCE OF ENDOMETRIUM

The appearance of endometrium changes with the phase of the menstrual cycle. During follicular phase, the endometrium looks thin and pale with a smooth surface and minimal vascularization; the glands are not easily seen. At ovulation, the endometrium appears oedematous, and the glands are seen. In the luteal phase, the increased vascularity causes oedema, and endometrium looks pink with glands seen. Postmenopausal endometrium is thin, pale in colour. The glands are hardly seen even with higher magnification.

DIAGNOSTIC INDICATIONS

1. **The study of endocervical mucosal lining:** Panoramic or contact hysteroscope allows inspection of endocervical epithelium in dysplasia and carcinoma in situ of the cervix, to trace the neoplastic process into endocervix and map the extent of neoplasm. A biopsy can be taken from the suspicious areas. Endocervical polyp can also be identified and removed. Staging of cancer of the cervix and endometrium is done by endocervical biopsy.
2. **Congenital malformation of the uterus:** Hysteroscopy combined with laparoscopy confirms whether the uterus is septate or bicornuate, enables the assessment of the capacity of each horn and also studies the depth and thickness of the septum in planning corrective surgery. The presence of the fundus seen laparoscopically indicates that it is a septate uterus. In a bicornuate uterus, the fundus is absent.
3. **Endometrial tuberculosis:** The presence of caseous areas, ulcers or tubercles on the endometrial lining suggests tuberculosis. Selective biopsies are required to confirm the diagnosis or curettage done.
4. **Asherman syndrome:** Hysteroscopy confirms uterine synechiae, and type (flimsy or fibrous) and extent of adhesions.
5. **Misplaced IUCD:** Although ultrasound can locate a misplaced IUCD, hysteroscope determines whether it is embedded in the endometrium and allows its safe retrieval under direct view.
6. **Endometrial lesions and AUB:** Endometrial and placental polyp, submucous fibroid polyp, endometrial hyperplasia and carcinoma can be identified by hysteroscopy. Selective biopsy and downward extension of endometrial cancer can be assessed and staging done. In a suspected case of cancer, it may be prudent to perform

contact hysteroscopy which avoids the risk of peritoneal spillage of cancer cells when distended medium is used. Negative findings for cancer can be very assuring to the woman.

7. **Polyp:** Endometrial polyp may be single or multiple, less than 1 cm in size, and its appearance is identical to the surrounding endometrium. It is usually sessile and immobile, and is caused by folds of endometrium in hyperplasia. Therefore, the polyp disappears during follicular phase. On the contrary, a mucus polyp is often bigger than 1 cm, sessile or pedunculated, mobile and permanent. A fibroid polyp is a firm, permanent and of various sizes, paler than a mucus polyp.
8. **Cornual tubal blockage:** When hysterosalpingography shows blockage of the corneal end of the tube, hysteroscope enables the falloscope to be inserted into the cornual end and study its patency and mucosa. The decision regarding the feasibility of tubal surgery can then be taken. Cannulation and adhesiolysis are also possible.

THERAPEUTIC INDICATIONS

In therapeutic procedures, cervical dilation up to no. 10 may be required to insert the operating channel, and because of prolonged surgery, general anaesthesia is necessary.

INDICATIONS

- **Uterine septum** (Fig. 41.10) is cut with scissors, cautery, laser or resectoscope. It is not necessary to excise the entire septum, as the fibrous tissue retracts and shrinks after cutting. Bleeding is minimal. Done under laparoscopic guidance, uterine perforation can be avoided. Seventy per cent pregnancy rate is observed following operation.
- **Asherman syndrome:** The adhesiolysis under laparoscopic view prevents uterine perforation. Insertion of IUCD for 3 months and oestrogen therapy prevent reformation of adhesions and helps to build up the endometrium. Lately, many omit the insertion of IUCD. Resectoscope, scissor, laser or cautery is used to break up adhesions.
- **Embedded IUCD** can be retrieved hysteroscopically.
- **Polypectomy**: The polyp can be grasped and twisted off with the grasping forceps. If the pedicle is broad, it can be ablated by cautery and polyp removed.
- **Submucous fibroid**: Type 0 fibroid (pedunculated) and type I fibroid with 50% intramural location can be morcellated or destroyed by coagulation. The leftover myometrial portion of the fibroid can be removed in the second stage when it protrudes further into the uterine cavity. Infection and bleeding are the risks of this operation.

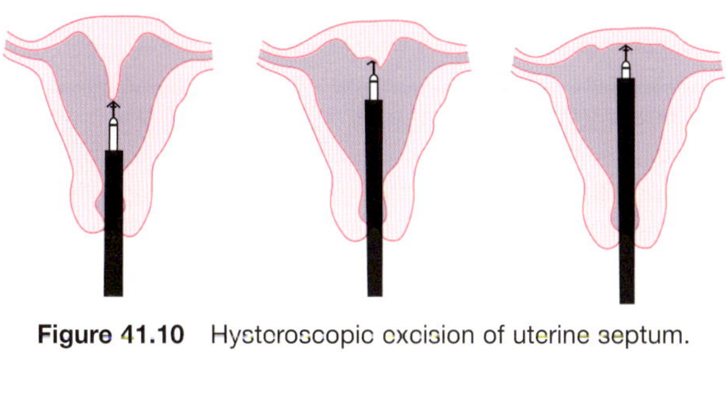

Figure 41.10 Hysteroscopic excision of uterine septum.

- **AUB** is now treated by TCRE in premenopausal women and hysterectomy is avoided. Prior to TCRE, malignancy and hyperplasia should be excluded. The endometrium is resected or ablated with cautery, laser or roller-ball coagulation. Sixty per cent of women become amenorrhoeic and 20% develop oligomenorrhoea at the end of 1 year. Recurrence of menorrhagia by the end of 3 years in 25% of women requires either repeat TCRE or hysterectomy. The details of TCRE and other ablative procedures are given in the chapter on AUB. Partial TCRE is done to procure oligomenorrhoea. Lately, because of availability of MIRENA, TCRE has become less popular.
- **New technique of tubal sterilization** using sclerosing agents, cautery or intratubal plugs is not universally accepted and not legalized in India, because of high failure rate, irreversibility of the procedures and complications.
- **Tubal blockage**: Tubal cannulation and breaking up of flimsy adhesions of the cornual end, removal of polyp and balloonoplasty are possible through hysteroscope.
- In IVF programme, it is now routine to perform diagnostic hysteroscope to study the endometrium prior to IVF.
- Intrafallopian insemination in infertility is practiced by a few.
- Indications of hysteroscopy are explained in Table 41.2.

CONTRAINDICATIONS

Contraindications to therapeutic hysteroscopy are as follows:

- Genital tract infection present.
- Pregnancy
- During menstruation, as view is obscured and infection rate increases.
- Scarred uterus and enlarged uterus more than 12 weeks' size form relative contraindications.
- Cervical stenosis can cause cervical tear and uterine perforation.
- Cardiopulmonary disorders: These include anaesthesia risks, fluid over blood and pulmonary oedema.

DISTENSION MEDIA IN HYSTEROSCOPY

Several distension media are in current usage for hysteroscopy. The choice of medium depends on its availability, safety, effectiveness and cost as well as whether cautery and laser are to be used. The media in common usage include

Table 41.2 Indications of Hysteroscopy

Diagnostic	Therapeutic
• Endocervical study in suspected endocervical malignancy, preinvasive cancer and biopsy • Uterus – malformations, endometrial TB, Asherman syndrome, misplaced IUCD, menorrhagia, intermenstrual bleeding, submucous fibroid, polyp • Falloposcopy	• Endometrial polypectomy • Submucous fibroid • Septate uterus • Asherman syndrome • Removal of IUCD • Tubal sterilization • Balloonoplasty • IVF intrafallopian insemination

carbon dioxide gas delivered through the Hysteroflator at a maximum rate of 70 mL/minute and pressure less than 100 mm Hg. This gives a clear panoramic view of the interior of the uterine cavity, but flattens soft pedunculated polyp against the uterine lining as against those seen as floating objects when liquid media are used.

The popular liquid media used in practice include normal saline, 5% dextrose and Ringer's lactate solutions. To provide adequate uterine distension, the intrauterine pressure needs to be 40–50 mm Hg. More sophisticated pressure systems are available for use during prolonged hysteroscopic operative procedures such as myomectomy, septum cutting or endometrial ablation where continuous flow of fluid is essential. In the above-mentioned procedures, the use of electrocautery is necessary. In such cases, the distension medium must be nonionic (not normal saline) to prevent the of electrical energy; also, the medium should not get admixed with blood as this would interfere with proper visualization of the ongoing operative procedure. The distending media in common use are Hyskon and glycine. Hyskon 1.5% is very thick and sticky; hence, immediately after the operation, the hysteroscope and its sheath must be thoroughly cleaned and the sheath scrupulously brushed of all traces of the medium. Delay may lead to jamming of the instrument. Hyskon is a concentrated dextran solution (32% dextrose), not miscible with blood and with good optical qualities. It can cause anaphylactic reaction and infection. Glycine is absorbed from the uterine cavity and peritoneum. Excess glycine can lead to problems of fluid overload and electrolyte disturbances. Hence, it cannot be overemphasized that strict monitoring of the amount of glycine used, its input and output must be accurately documented. Also, a record of the electrolyte readings before commencement of surgery and at the end of the same must be documented as safety precautions.

CONTACT HYSTEROSCOPY

This 4-mm contact hysteroscope (Hamou type) can be inserted into the uterine cavity without prior dilatation. On light contact with the endometrial surface, and systematic examination of all the uterine walls and the fundus, it enables assessment of the normality of the endometrial tissue lining, and helps to diagnose any early neoplastic change.

COMPLICATIONS OF HYSTEROSCOPY

The following complications are reported during hysteroscopic surgery:

- Anaesthesia complication, more with CO_2 used as a distending medium. Gas embolism can occur.
- Uterine perforation occurs in 1%–10% of cases, mostly during insertion of the hysteroscope through the cervix and during operative procedures. This can be avoided by introducing the telescope under direct vision and performing surgery under laparoscopic guidance. Perforation is suspected when the distending medium escapes into the peritoneal cavity and uterine walls collapse with poor vision and fall in the intrauterine pressure. The perforation is managed by observation, laparoscopic coagulation of the bleeder or laparotomy.
- Organ injury to the bowel and intestine is rare.
- Thermal injury to the bowel occurs with cautery and laser. The injury is not diagnosed at the time of surgery unless perforation also occurs. Delayed diagnosis increases the morbidity. Bipolar cautery is safe from this point of view.
- Bleeding occurs in 1%–2% of cases. Bleeding can be minimized by performing the surgery in the preovulatory phase and thinning the endometrium by hormones prior to TCRE. The bleeding normally occurs as the medium is released and intrauterine pressure drops. It can be controlled by inserting the Foley catheter, distending its balloon with 30 mL saline and leaving it in the uterine cavity for 24 hours for haemostasis.
- Sepsis occurs usually following myomectomy.
- Embolism with CO_2 can be avoided by using the proper instrument, not increasing the flow to more than 70 mL/minute and pressure less than 100 mm Hg. Avoiding head-low position also reduces the morbidity when embolism occurs.
- Distending media cause complications in 4% of cases. While allowing proper view and surgical procedures, the various distending media can increase the procedure morbidity.
- Allergic reaction is noted with dextran and glycine.
- Fluid overload occurs in 4% of cases, and leads to pulmonary oedema if deficit of fluid is more than 1000 mL and electrolyte imbalance occurs. Diuretics are required. Saline and dextrose cause hyponatraemia, hypokalaemia, haemolysis and encephalopathy. Hyskon causes anaphylactic reaction, pulmonary oedema and encephalopathy, brain herniation and temporary blindness. Fluid overload occurs when the intrauterine pressure exceeds 100 mm Hg. Cerebral oedema and cardiac failure may occur.
- There may be failure to perform therapeutic procedure.

LATE COMPLICATIONS

- Haematometra following cervical stenosis may occur.
- Unwanted pregnancy may be present following TCRE.
- Cancer endometrium may go unnoticed for a long time. Delayed diagnosis worsens the prognosis.
- Infection may lead to PID.
- Dysmenorrhoea following TCRE requires hysterectomy.
- Amenorrhoea following TCRE may not be desirable in some women.
- Treatment failure may occur.
- Repeat surgery for treatment failure is seen in 12% of cases at the end of 1 year and in 25% of cases following TCRE at the end of 3 years. Either repeat TCRE or hysterectomy is indicated.
- Uterine rupture during pregnancy and late diagnosis of endometrial pathology are other complications.

SALPINGOSCOPY AND FALLOSCOPY

In salpingoscopy, a fine salpingoscope 1 mm in diameter is introduced through the fimbrial end of the fallopian tube via the laparoscope, and ampullary portion studied after distending its lumen with saline. Flattening of mucosa, adhesions and mucus polyp can be recognized, and feasibility of tuboplasty considered. Hysteroscopic falloposcopy reveals the tubal pathology of the cornual and interstitial end of the fallopian tube. The risks of these endoscopes are perforation, damage to the tubal mucosa, infection and difficulty in inserting the catheters.

KEY POINTS

- Various endoscopic telescopes have been designed to enable the visualization of body cavities. Of particular use in the practice of gynaecology are the laparoscope and hysteroscope.
- The laparoscope has been very useful in the diagnosis of uterine, tubal, ovarian and generalized diseases affecting the pelvic organs such as endometriosis, chronic PID and genital tuberculosis, and in staging of genital cancers and chronic pelvic pain.
- The role of the laparoscope in the evaluation of infertility is undisputed. It is now a common practice to combine laparoscopy with hysteroscopy in its evaluation.
- Operative laparoscopy has made great inroads into clinical practice, making minimally invasive surgery a valid and safe therapeutic option in many situations.
- Diagnostic hysteroscopy helps in the evaluation of a patient presenting with the menstrual disturbances, endometrial polyps, submucous fibromyomatous polyps, a misplaced IUCD and endometrial malignant growth. The indications have expanded in therapeutic procedures.
- Operative hysteroscopy is also performed effectively to correct several menstrual problems, mainly abnormal uterine bleeding.

SELF-ASSESSMENT

1. Discuss the diagnostic indications of laparoscopy in gynaecology.
2. Discuss the therapeutic procedures done laparoscopically.
3. Discuss the contraindications and complications of laparoscopy surgery.
4. What are the diagnostic indications of hysteroscopy?
5. Discuss the therapeutic role of hysteroscopy.
6. Mention the complications and contraindications of hysteroscopy.

SUGGESTED READING

Tulandi T (ed). Advances in laparoscopy and minimal invasive surgery. Obstet Gynaecol Clin N Am Vol 31, 2011; 38.

Studd J (ed). Progress in Obstetric Gynaecology Vol 7, Edinburgh: Elsevier, 1988.

Studd J (ed). Progress in Obstetric Gynaecology Vol. 16, London: Elsevier, 2005.

42 Major and Minor Operations in Gynaecology

CHAPTER OUTLINE

Surgical procedures have become very safe nowadays, because of improved anaesthesia, availability of blood transfusion, antibiotics as well as good preoperative and postoperative care of the woman. The advanced surgical technologies have also contributed to reduced surgical morbidities and operation-related complications.

A number of major and minor procedures are commonly done in the specialty of gynaecology. Although most of the minor procedures are done to establish a diagnosis, majority of major operations such as abdominal and vaginal hysterectomy or laparoscopic hysterectomy are done to treat underlying disorders such as fibroid uterus, endometriosis, adenomyosis, gynaecological cancers or prolapse of the uterus.

Following section describes commonly done minor and major operations in gynaecology.

MINOR PROCEDURES

Pap Smear: It remains most commonly done procedure, and it is done to screen a sexually active woman to detect preinvasive lesions of cancer cervix. It is part of gynaecological examination in most of the countries; however, lack of facility and trained manpower limit its availability for opportunistic screening in developing countries. A detail description of procedure has been described in chapter 1 on Gynaecological Diagnosis.

Cervical biopsy: Obtaining a small tissue from cervix in a suspected case of cancer of the cervix and submitting for histopathology is a commonly done procedure. Indications include, a visible growth on cervix, abnormal Pap smear report suggesting an underlying carcinoma or an abnormal colposcopy suggestive of CIN II/III (HSIL) or frank carcinoma.

Steps: This procedure is usually done on an out-patient department OPD basis, with vaginal speculum in place showing cervix biopsy is taken with the help of a cervical punch biopsy forceps. Any undue bleeding can be controlled by pressure at a biopsy site with a gauge piece.

Loop electrosurgical excision procedures (LEEP): It is a procedure done to obtain cervical tissues for biopsy. A wire loop attached to a diathermy is used to excise entire transformation zone (squama columnar function) on the surface of cervix for biopsy purpose. It avoids crushing of tissues which may happen with the use of cervical punch biopsy. Indications include Pap smear showing HSIL, carcinoma in situ or when there is a disparity between clinical findings, Pap smear report and colposcopic findings. This procedure can be done on an OPD basis in a minor operation theatre (OT), but requires an electrosurgical diathermy and fine-wire loops.

Complications: Mostly a simple and short procedure of few minutes, any bleeding from the surface of cervix after LEEP can be controlled by pressure, application of Monsel's paste or cautery of bleeding points. Patients are advised to avoid sexual relations for next 2–3 weeks to avoid any risk of bleeding.

Conization of cervix: Conization of cervix is required when Pap smear and colposcopy reveal CIN II or CIN III. It is done under general anaesthesia, using cold knife or laser to cut into the tissue. The vaginal wall is incised all round 1 cm above the external os or above the visible lesion and dissected off the cervix. The cone is dissected extending up to or short of the internal os. Haemostasis is secured and the area is left to granulate and not covered with the vaginal flap, as this gives a wrong reading on the follow-up Pap smear (Figs 42.1 and 42.2).

Conization causes bleeding, so it is now mostly replaced by colposcopic directed biopsy or large loop excision of the transformation zone (LLETZ) and LEEP (see Chapter 38 on Cancer of the Cervix). Conization is used as a therapeutic procedure in CIN III in young women desirous of future pregnancy.

COMPLICATIONS

Apart from bleeding and infection, conization can cause cervical stenosis and incompetent os. This can lead to haematometra, habitual abortions and cervical dystocia during labour.

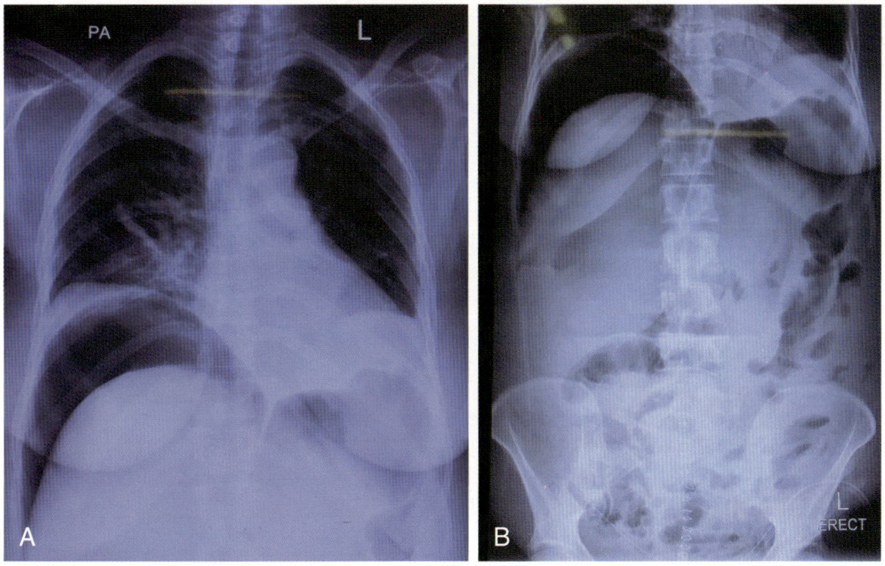

Figure 42.1 (A) Immediate postoperative chest and upper abdominal X-ray showing gas under the diaphragm. (B) X-ray erect abdomen showing dilated bowel loops on postoperative day 2.

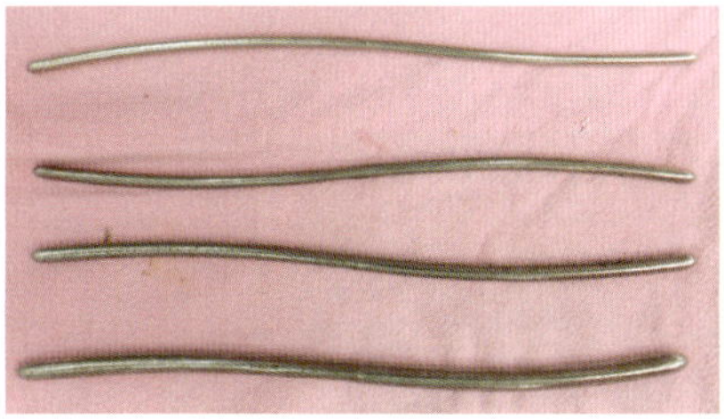

Figure 42.2 Hegar's double-ended dilator used to dilate the cervix.

With the advent of LEEP, conization of cervix has become less popular as LEEP is associated with fewer complications, is an outdoor procedure and provides equally good specimen for histopathology.

Endometrial Tissue Sampling: Obtaining endometrial tissue for biopsy is indicated for cases of abnormal uterine bleeding (AUB), cases of infertility, cases of postmenopausal bleeding and before a woman is subjected to a major procedure such as abdominal or vaginal hysterectomy. There are number of procedures by which endometrial tissue can be obtained for histology. Following is the description of such procedures:

Endometrial Biopsy (Endometrial Aspirate): After initial steps (making woman void urine, placing her in lithotomy position on an operation table, cleaning the vulva and vagina with antiseptic solution and pelvic examination) a Sims speculum is introduced to retract posterior vaginal wall, anterior lip of cervix is held with a vulsellum or tenaculum or a long Allis forceps. Uterine sound is introduced to accurately measure uterine length as well as confirmation of position of the uterus. A 4 mm plastic cannula (Karman's type, Fig. 42.3) is introduced in the uterine cavity and attached to a 20 cm^3 disposable plastic syringe. By sucking with syringe, endometrial tissue so obtained is sent for histopathology and if indicated for bacteriological examination. Previously, a rigid metal cannula was used for the same purpose. Procedure is a short OPD-based test and can be done without any anaesthesia. However, for an apprehensive patient, local anaesthesia with mild sedation given by intramuscular or intravenous route suffices. *Complications*:

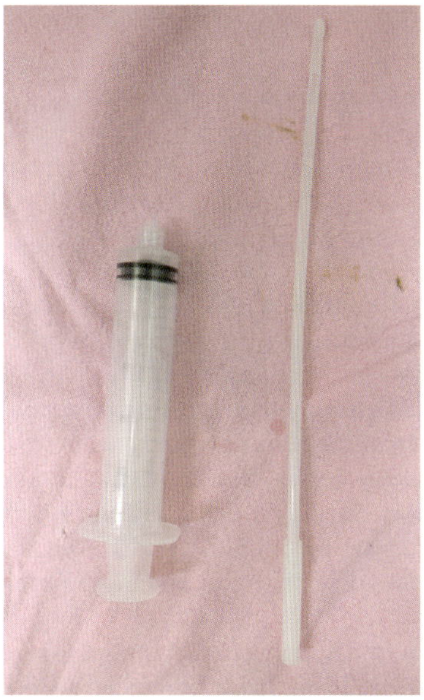

Figure 42.3 Karman's cannula.

Rarely, there may be difficulty in negotiating interval cervical os, while introducing uterine sound or Karman's cannula. Suspected perforation of the uterus should be managed by immediately stopping the procedure, careful observation of patients for possible intraabdominal bleeding and by giving antibiotics to prevent infections.

DILATATION OF THE CERVIX AND ENDOMETRIAL CURETTAGE (DILATATION AND CURETTAGE)

Dilatation and Curettage (D&C) remains one of the most often carried out procedure in gynaecology.

D&C is a minor gynaecological procedure of dilating the cervix and curetting (scraping) the endometrial tissue from the uterine cavity.

It is mainly a diagnostic procedure; however, can be therapeutic in certain obstetric conditions. Dilatation of the cervix alone is required in the following conditions:

- Before curettage (commonest).
- For cervical stenosis.
- To prevent cervical stenosis following Manchester operation for prolapse of the uterus.
- To prevent postoperative cervical stenosis in cauterization of cervical erosion and conization.
- To drain haematometra.
- To drain pyometra.
- Before insertion of radium into the uterine cavity in cancer of the cervix and endometrial cancer.
- Before removal of embedded intrauterine contraceptive device (IUCD).
- Before breaking uterine adhesions in Asherman syndrome.
- Before endocervical curettage (ECC) for endocervical cancer.
- Before hysteroscopy.
- To diagnose incompetent os. If No. 8 dilator goes in easily, the internal os of the cervix is considered as an incompetent os with the risk of habitual abortion and preterm labour.

Obstetric indications are as follows:

- Before evacuation in missed abortion, incomplete abortion, evacuation of a hydatidiform mole. It is also necessary for medical termination of pregnancy.

Curettage of endometrium is mainly diagnostic. This is indicated for following:

- *AUB* to obtain endometrium to study the hormonal pattern causing abnormal bleeding.
- *Secondary amenorrhoea* to detect tubercular endometritis.
- *Postmenopausal bleeding* to rule out endometrial cancer.
- *Endometrial cancer* to study the endocervical tissue and the extent of spread. This helps in staging and deciding on treatment.
- *Infertility.* Now a days, ultrasound is used for monitoring ovulation. However, if genital tuberculosis suspected then this procedure is indicated. The endometrial tissue is preserved in saline for culture. The tissue is also subjected to polymerase chain reaction. Corpus luteal phase defect is diagnosed when the endometrial histology lags behind the menstrual date by 2 days.
- *Hormone Replacement Therapy (HRT).* If a woman on HRT complains of bleeding per vaginal, she should be subjected to D&C to rule out endometrial hyperplasia or carcinoma.
- A woman on Tamoxifen for breast cancer, D & C is indicated if endometroid thickness is more than 8 mm or if she has irregular bleeding.

Therapeutic D&C is indicated for following:

- Missed abortion, incomplete abortion and retains of products of conception.
- To remove endometrial polyp (polypectomy).
- Obstetric indications mentioned for dilatation of cervix.

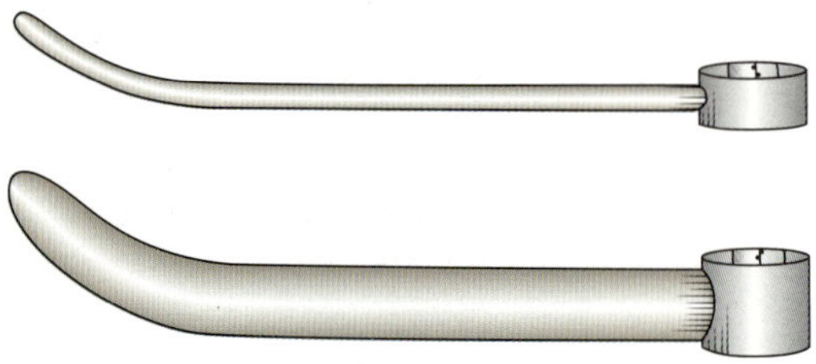

Figure 42.4 Hawkin's single-ended dilator.

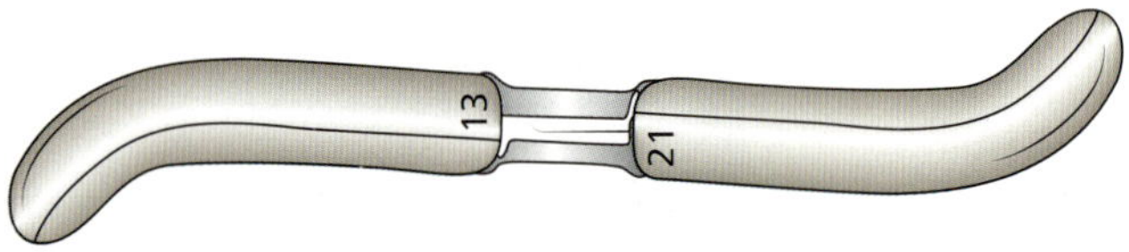

Figure 42.5 Fenton's dilator.

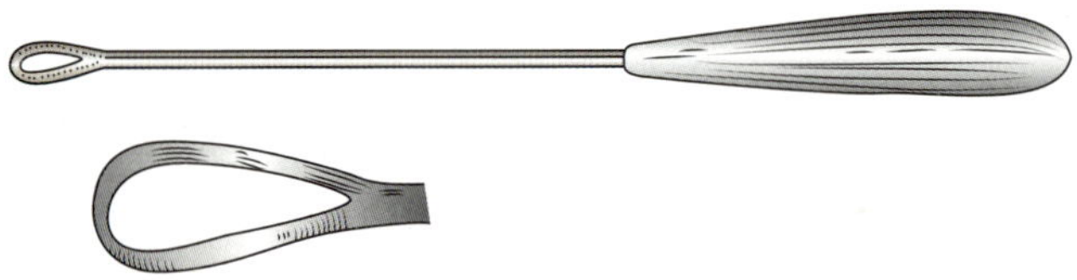

Figure 42.6 Metal Curette.

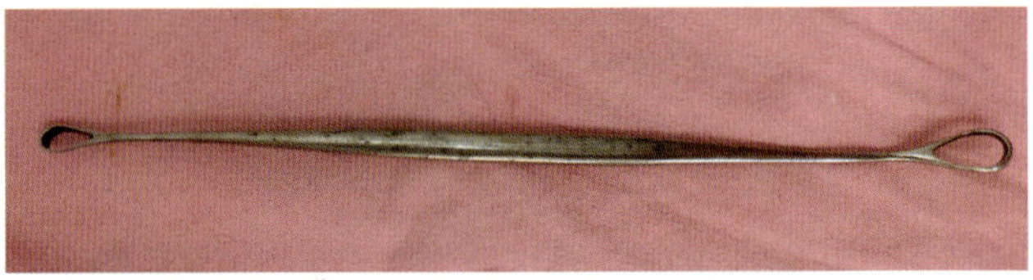

Figure 42.7 Blunt and sharp curettage.

The dilators used are as follows:

- Hegar's double-ended dilator (Fig. 42.2).
- Hawkins' single-ended dilator (Fig. 42.4).
- Fenton's dilator (Fig. 42.5). They come in different sizes (No. 3–10 dilators).

Slow cervical dilatation can be performed with prostaglandin E_1 (misoprostol) vaginal pessary (200–400 mcg). The pessary is inserted in the vagina 3 hours before D&C, and this slow dilatation avoids cervical trauma.

Curettage is performed usually with a sharp curette. The blunt curette is used in obstetric conditions to avoid uterine perforation (Figs 42.6 and 42.7).

Karman's plastic curette is mainly used for suction evacuation in medical termination of first-trimester pregnancy. These come in sizes No. 3–10.

PROCEDURE OF D&C

The equipment required are as follows:

- Sims speculum (Fig. 42.8)
- Anterior vaginal wall retractor
- Vulsellum or Allis forceps to hold the anterior lip of the cervix
- Uterine sound

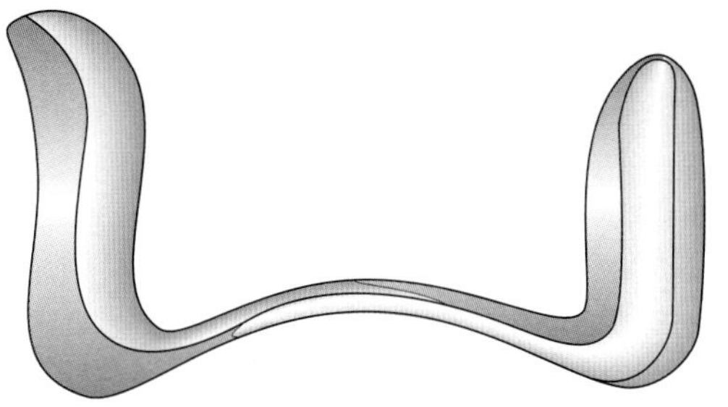

Figure 42.8 Sims speculum.

- Cervical dilators
- Curette
- Sponge-holding forceps and sponges to clean the area and vagina
- Savlon, Betadine
- 10% formalin to preserve the endometrial tissue
- Saline to preserve endometrial tissue for culture

D&C is performed under sedation, paracervical block or general anaesthesia. Local anaesthesia is adequate in a multiparous woman, but a nulliparous or an apprehensive woman may require general anaesthesia.

- The woman is put in the lithotomy position. The perineal and inner thigh area and vagina are cleaned with Savlon or Betadine. The area is draped with sterile sheets.
- Bimanual examination is done to ascertain the size of the uterus and its direction and to rule out adnexal mass.
- With the help of Sims speculum and anterior vaginal wall retractor, the cervix is exposed and the anterior lip held with Vulsellum or Allis forceps.
- The uterine sound confirms the size of the uterine cavity and its direction (normal length is 7-8 cm).
- The cervix is dilated starting from No. 3 up to 8 mm.
- The curette is introduced into the uterine cavity and the uterine lining scraped from above downwards.
- A gritty sensation indicates the end of curettage.
- The tissue is preserved in 10% formalin. For culture and polymerase chain reaction (PCR), the tissue is sent in saline. Other methods of obtaining endometrial tissue for the histological study are as follows:
  - *Fractional curettage*
  - *Endometrial biopsy*

Fractional curettage is indicated in suspected endometrial carcinoma. In this procedure, ECC is done before cervical dilatation. Following dilatation, the isthmic portion is curetted and the tissue kept in a separate bottle. Thereafter, the uterine cavity is curetted and sent separately.

Normal endometrium appears pink and healthy. Profuse, pale looking and friable tissue suggests malignancy. Fractional curettage determines the extent of spread of malignancy down the uterine wall, so that staging can be done and appropriate treatment planned. Involvement of endocervical lining places the malignancy in Stage II of the disease.

Endometrial biopsy is performed as an outpatient procedure without anaesthesia or under sedation. The cervix is not dilated and a biopsy curette is inserted and a strip or two of endometrial tissue is obtained for histological study.

CONTRAINDICATIONS

Contraindications to D&C are as follows:

- Suspected pregnancy
- Lower genital tract infection

This surgical procedure is performed only after the infection clears up with antibiotics.

COMPLICATIONS ASSOCIATED WITH D & C

Dilatation of cervix can cause following:

- Ascending infection.
- Cervical tear and bleeding.
- Incompetent os.
- Uterine perforation occurs mainly in a soft uterus, i.e. pregnant, puerperal uterus, and in atrophic postmenopausal or scarred uterus. It can also occur in a malignant uterus.

Perforation is suspected when the dilator or curette goes further in without resistance beyond the measured length of the uterine cavity. The first thing to do is to remove the instrument and postpone surgery. If the bleeding is slight, the woman is observed for internal bleeding. Heavy bleeding requires immediate laparoscopy and sometimes laparotomy. Laparotomy is required when intestinal injury occurs.

Curretage Can Cause Following Complications

- Infection of upper genital tract.
- Asherman syndrome – In Asherman syndrome band of adhesions develop between anterior and posterior uterine wall. This condition is caused by vigorous curettage, in tubercular endometritis and following packing of the uterine cavity to control postpartum haemorrhage. It also follows uterine sepsis.

Asherman syndrome is classified as mild, moderate or severe depending on the degree and extent of adhesion. The woman presents with hypomenorrhoea, secondary amenorrhoea, infertility or habitual abortions.

- Infertility due to ascending infection causing tubal block.
- Ectopic pregnancy due to PID.
- Rupture uterus during subsequent pregnancy or labour.
- Adherent placenta in subsequent pregnancy.

INSTRUMENTS USED

Sims speculum is a double-ended speculum which retracts the posterior vaginal wall, in dorsal and left lateral positions (Fig. 42.8). It comes in different sizes.

Sims anterior vaginal wall retractor is a double-ended instrument with a loop at either end (Fig. 42.9).

Vulsellum forceps is a long forceps with teeth at one end which ensures a firm grip on the cervix when the Vulsellum is locked. It is applied to the anterior lip of the cervix during D&C, Fothergill's operation and vaginal hysterectomy. It can also be applied to the posterior lip during culdocentesis

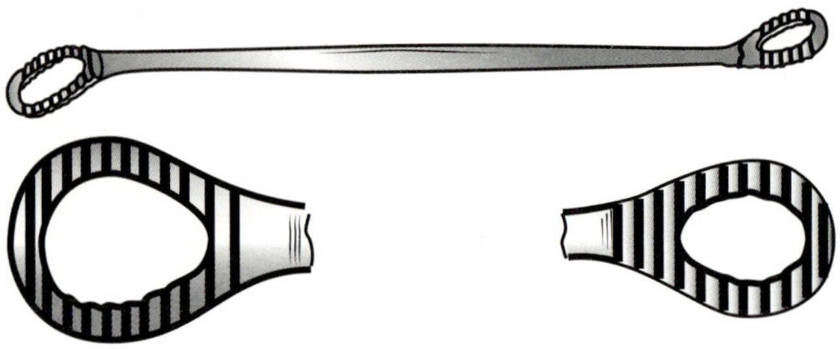

Figure 42.9 Anterior vaginal wall retractor.

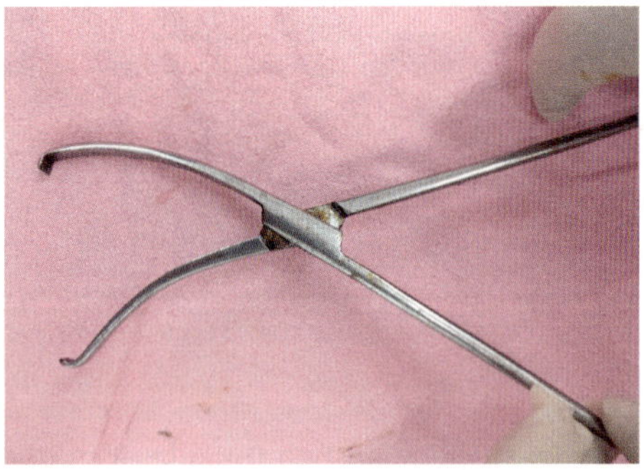

Figure 42.10 Vulsellum forceps. It is used to grasp the cervical lip and steady the cervix during vaginal surgery.

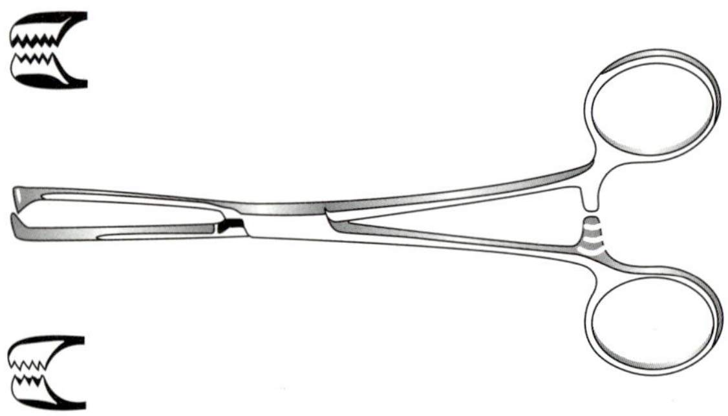

Figure 42.11 Allis forceps. It can also hold the cervix, edges of the vagina during colpography and edges of the rectus sheath during abdominal surgery.

for aspirating pus in pelvic abscess and blood in ectopic pregnancy. In a pregnant uterus and menopausal uterus, it is safer to use Allis forceps – this will avoid cervical trauma and bleeding (Figs 42.10 and 42.11).

Sponge-holding forceps is used to hold the soft cervix during obstetric D&C. Apart from its use to clean the area with sponge, the sponge forceps is also used to hold the cut edges of the lower uterine segment in caesarean section and the cut edges of the cervical tear following vaginal delivery and as a haemostatic as well.

Uterine sound is a 30 cm long angulated instrument with a handle at one end and a rounded blunt tip at the other. It is marked in inches or centimetres. The angulation accommodates for flexion of the uterus (Fig. 42.12).

USES OF UTERINE SOUND

- It measures the uterine cavity and the cervical length.
- It is used to diagnose cervical stenosis.
- It is used to sound a polyp, IUCD or uterine septum.

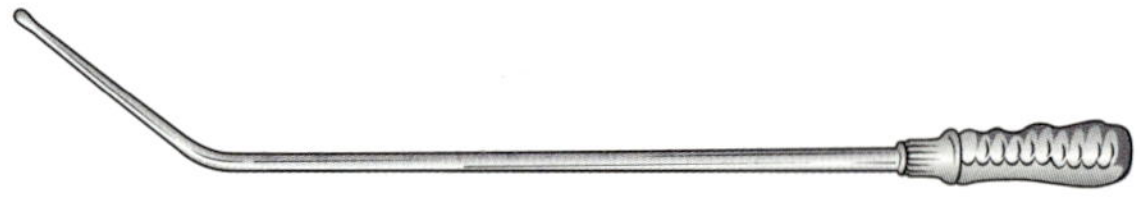

Figure 42.12 Uterine sound. It measures the uterine cavity, sounds a polyp and IUCD.

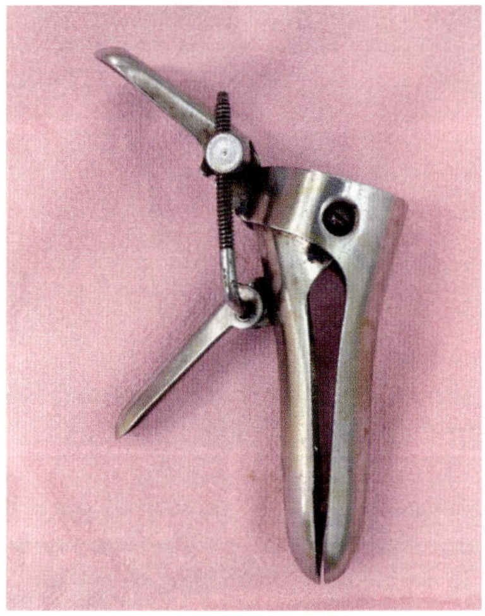

Figure 42.13 Cusco speeculum.

- It helps to break adhesions in Asherman syndrome.
- It differentiates between chronic inversion and fibroid polyp.
- In a misplaced IUCD, the uterine sound can be inserted and X-ray of the pelvis taken, and the position of IUCD in relation to the uterine sound shows if IUCD is perforated.

OTHER TYPES OF SPECULUM

- Cusco speculum (Chapter 1, see also Fig. 42.13).
- Auvard speculum (Fig. 42.14A) is a heavy retractor provided with a heavy metal ball and is self-retaining. It is employed in vaginal hysterectomy to retract the posterior vaginal wall. A channel is provided in the handle to collect the blood and drain.

The ovum forceps is a noncrushing forceps which does not have a catch or lock on its handle and is meant to grasp the products of conception. The forceps is introduced closed into the uterine cavity. It is then opened, the products of conception grasped, the instrument closed and rotated to detach the products from the uterine wall.

Fractional Curettage: It is a modification of D&C where initially, curettings are obtained from endocervical canal before dilatation of os followed by dilatation of os and curettage of endometrium. Specimen obtained from endocervical canal is separately sent for histopathology in addition to endometrial curettings. In the past, it was a commonly done procedure in a suspected case of endometrial cancer to know whether the disease has spread downwards to involve endocervix.

Endometrial Aspiration + Endocervical Curettage (EA+ECC): This procedure, being less painful has replaced fractional curettage. Dilatation of internal os is avoided, so it makes procedure pain-free and an OPD procedure. Tissue specimens from endocervix and endometrium are sent separately for histology.

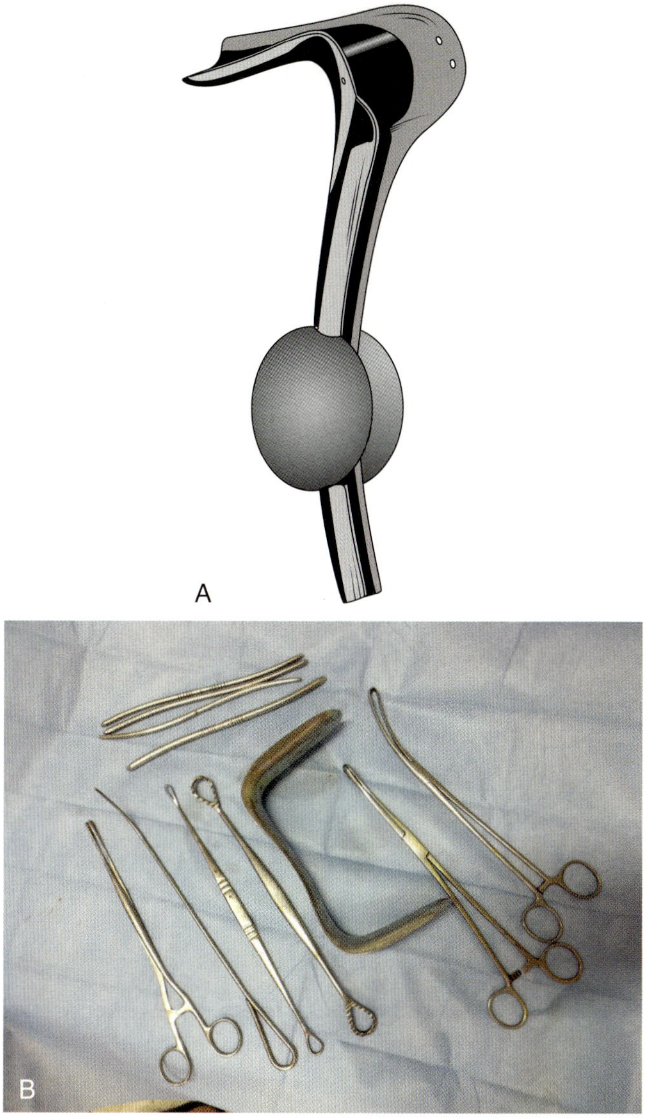

Figure 42.14 (A) Auvard speculum (B) Instruments required for D&C.

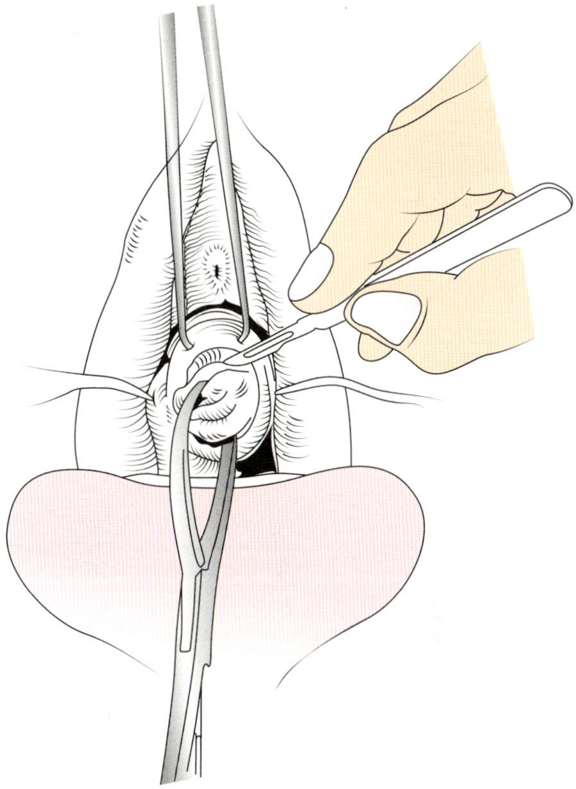

Figure 42.15 Cone Biopsy of Cervix.
⊙ Play to scan Cervical Biopsy-Conisation

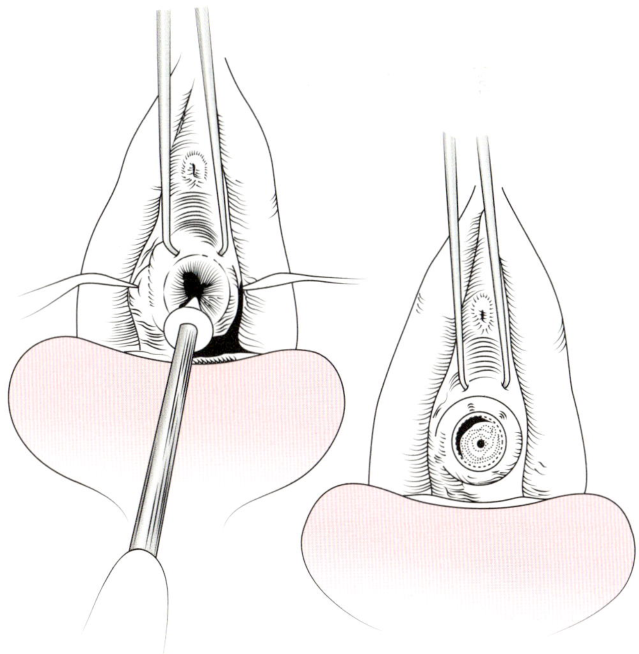

Figure 42.16 Cryotherapy of Cervical Lesion.

CONE BIOPSY OF CERVIX (CONISATION)

Cone Biopsy is a procedure in which a cone shape tissue of cervix is obtained under anaesthesia (Fig. 42.15⊙). This procedure can be used both for diagnostic and therapeutic purposes. A detailed description of the procedure has been given in Chapter 33.

CRYOTHERAPY OF CERVIX

This is a minor procedure done in OPD to treat benign and pre malignant lesion of cervix. In this procedure a cone shape probe is attached to a source of CO2 gas and probe is applied to surface of cervix for a duration of 3min. Under the effect of cryo probe, the underline tissue undergoes freezing subsequently, this tissue slowly heels replacing the unhealthy tissue. This procedure is commonly used in the treatment of cervical erosion (Fig. 42.16).

- Preoperative workup
- Purposc of prcopcrative workup

MAJOR PROCEDURES IN GYNAECOLOGY

Hysterectomy or removal of the uterus is a fairly common gynaecological operation done for a variety of conditions such as fibroid uterus, AUB, adenomyosis and gynaecological malignancies.

Removal of the body of the uterus with cervix is called *total hysterectomy*, if only body of the uterus is removed and cervix is retained it is called *subtotal hysterectomy* (supracervical hysterectomy). Removal of the uterus with cervix and both tubes and ovaries is called *total abdominal hysterectomy with bilateral salpingo-oophorectomy* (TAH with B/L SO). In cases of malignancies where besides removal of the uterus, cervix, tubes and ovaries, other structures such as upper vagina, parametrial tissue and lymph nodes from pelvis and para-aortic area are removed are labelled as *Radical Hysterectomy.*

Routes of hysterectomy: Depending on the expertise of surgeon, size of uterus, underlying pathology, removal of the uterus can be carried by open abdominal surgery or by laparoscopic approach or by vaginal route.

Preoperative workup and preparation for major gynaecological surgery.

PREOPERATIVE INVESTIGATIONS

Before the submission of the patient to any major gynaecological surgery, it is necessary to evaluate her fitness for it. The preoperative investigations include the following:

- *Complete blood count.* This includes haemoglobin assessment and total and differential leucocyte count.
- *Urinalysis.* This includes routine and microscopy urinalysis. Culture examination is requisitioned, if microscopy reveals significant number of pus cells (more than 5) or history of urinary tract infection (UTI), especially in women with cystocele, urinary complaints and fistula.
- Fasting and postprandial blood sugar estimations.
- *Kidney function tests.* Blood urea, serum creatinine and uric acid.
- *Liver function tests.* Particularly in women with a history of jaundice and in all women undergoing cancer surgery.
- *Blood tests for VDRL,* Australia antigen and HIV-I and II.
- *Serum electrolytes.* Na, K, Cl and HCO_3.
- *Radiograph of the chest,* preoperatively or in genital cancer for metastasis.
- *ECG and stress test* whenever indicated.
- *Intravenous pyelography (IVP)* in case of cancer cervix and urinary fistulae.
- *Blood group and Rh factor.*
- *Bleeding time and clotting time.*

PREOPERATIVE WORKUP

PURPOSE OF PREOPERATIVE WORKUP

It is the cornerstone for successful surgical outcome.

- To make the correct diagnosis.
- To decide on the need for surgery and its correct selection.
- Investigations to:
    - confirm the diagnosis.
    - fitness for anaesthesia and surgery.

Identify the risk factors, any abnormal condition and rectify this before undertaking surgery.

CORRECT DIAGNOSIS

Detailed history and clinical examination can lead to correct diagnosis in most cases. History includes the presenting symptoms, drugs taken, any allergy and previous blood transfusion and surgery.

CLINICAL EXAMINATION

Apart from abdominal, speculum and bimanual examination, general examination rules out hitherto undetected anaemia, thyroid enlargement, breast disease and cardiovascular examination besides blood pressure. Pap smear is taken as required.

INVESTIGATIONS

These include the following:

- Confirmation of clinical diagnosis by ultrasound, CT and MRI.
- To assess the extent of the disease, any anatomical distortion of bladder, ureter by the pelvic tumour and malignancy.
- Staging and feasibility of surgery. In case of uterine fibroids, the number, size and location of fibroids decide the type of surgery appropriate to the case.
- Decide on the type and route of surgery.

FITNESS FOR SURGERY

It is necessary to ensure that the woman is fit for surgery, by performing the following investigations:

- BP check-up.
- Hb% white cell count, differential count, blood group-Rh.
- Routine urine examination for pus cells, sugar and protein.
- Kidney function tests.
- Liver function tests in cancer surgery and in previous liver disease.
- Blood sugar. In a known diabetes patient, to check on sugar control.
- X-ray of the chest, routine and for secondary malignancy.
- ECG.
- Thyroid function tests if required.

If any abnormality is detected, the woman is referred to the appropriate specialist for treatment and the operation is postponed until the woman is considered fit.

To protect the surgical staff regarding hepatitis B virus, HIV in high-risk patients. Patient test such as HBsAg, HIV should be done.

In an emergency and life-saving condition, minimal essential investigations are done, blood arranged and the risks of operation explained.

In a planned surgery, some gynaecologists prefer autotransfusion, and blood of the woman is withdrawn 2 days before surgery and preserved. Alternately, a relative donor is arranged. This avoids the risk of HIV and other sexually transmitted diseases, hepatitis B virus.

By assessing the fitness in this way, sudden cancellation and prolonged postoperative hospitalization due to complications are avoided.

DRUGS

Woman on any drug needs counselling, regarding temporary stoppage or addition of alternative drugs or a new drug. Any allergy to a particular drug should be noted. History of previous blood transfusion, the reason for transfusion and any adverse reaction is noted.

Oral contraceptive pills should be stopped 4 weeks before surgery. These can cause thromboembolism. Warfarin should be stopped and replaced by heparin with good monitoring. Aspirin is also best avoided as it can cause bleeding. Anaemia should be treated and Hb% should be at least 10 g%. Any infection should be cleared with antibiotics.

Smoking and alcohol should be stopped for a few days before surgery. Lithium and tricyclic anti-depressants should also be stopped. The drugs for hypertension and diabetes should continue. Many prefer to switch to insulin before and after the surgery. Thyroid drugs need to be continued.

THROMBOPROPHYLAXIS

Prophylactic heparin is needed in a high-risk woman for thromboembolism and it should be continued for a variable period postoperatively.

CONSENT

Proper counselling and informed consent should be obtained in writing. A girl younger than 18 years and a woman with a psychiatric problem are considered unfit to give consent and the guardian's signature is required.

PREOPERATIVE PREPARATION

- The woman should not take any food or liquid at least 12 hours before surgery.
- **Bowel preparation**. The patient is advised to take Dulcolax or other laxatives at night so that her bowels move well, and it is empty during surgery. It is important so that the bowels do not move and soil the operation table, and also intestines are not distended and obstruct the surgery. Some recommend enema early in the morning, but this is cumbersome and some enema water may be retained.

Preoperative bowel preparation is required for laparoscopic surgery and surgery for a malignant tumour. This is necessary in case bowel injury occurs during surgery.

Nowadays, the vaginal wall is cleaned just before surgery with Betadine after the bladder is catheterized. The bladder needs to remain empty throughout the surgery. If spinal or epidural anaesthesia is employed, the woman may not be able to micturate as such and bladder catheter for 24 hours postoperatively becomes necessary.

In prolapse, if infection or a decubitus ulcer is present, vaginal packing with Betadine for a few days heals the ulcer. Menopausal woman may require oestrogen vaginal cream for a few days.

Most women are now admitted early on the day of the operation, and this saves the cost. Only those at high risk or with a medical disorder get admitted one day before surgery.

Shaving the part is essential. The area for surgery is cleaned with Savlon and spirit in the operation theatre. The vagina is cleaned with Savlon or Betadine lotion. The bladder catheter keeps the bladder empty throughout the surgery. This avoids injury to the bladder.

ANAESTHESIA

It is left to the choice of the anaesthetist, and this partly depends on the condition of the woman.

ANTIBIOTICS

Today's practice is to start intravenous antibiotics intraoperatively. In caesarean section, antibiotic is administered after the delivery of the baby.

STEPS OF ABDOMINAL HYSTERECTOMY

▶ Scan to Play Total Abdominal Hysterectomy

For removal of uterus per abdomen following are necessary steps. However, a small variation in steps may occur depending on the underlying disease, size of uterine and practice of surgeon.

1. Indwelling catheter for drainage of urine during procedure.
2. Antiseptic preparation of area of operation.
3. Choice of anaesthesia: It is at the discretion of anaesthetist.
4. Abdominal wall incision: Both a transverse suprapubic incision and a vertical midline incision can be used depending on the underlying disease, size of the uterus and previous laparotomy scar.
5. Inspection and palpation of pelvic organs and exploration of remaining part of abdomen. Ascitic fluid/peritoneal washings may be obtained in case of suspected malignancies.
6. Packing away of intestines and retracting bladder with the help of retractor. This provides adequate exposure of pelvic organs facilitating surgery.
7. Decision regarding preservation of ovaries: It will depend on age of women, diagnosis and her desire to preserve uterus.
8. Clamping of round ligaments and dividing them between two clamps and suturing the lateral ends with absorbable suture.
9. Clamping, division and suturing of infundibulo pelvic ligaments in case ovaries are to be removed. In case ovaries are to be preserved, clamp is placed close to uterine fundus and ovarian ligament and the fallopian tubes are divided close to lateral wall of the uterus and stitched.
10. Opening of utero-vesical fold of peritoneum and displacing bladder away from anterior aspect of cervix.
11. Tying of uterine vessels close to lateral border of the uterus.
12. Division, tying of Mackenrodt's and Uterovesical ligaments close to lateral margin of cervix.
13. Opening of vagina at junction of cervix and vagina. After hysterectomy specimen is removed, edges of vaginal cuff are stitched.
14. Obtaining haemostasis; counting of sponges and instruments and needles.
15. Closure of abdomen in layers.

Surgical specimen should be cut open to see inside of endometrial cavity, endocervix and ret of the specimen (ovaries & fallopian tubes).

VAGINAL HYSTERECTOMY

▶ Scan to play Vaginal hysterectomy for prolapse uterus

Removal of the uterus by vaginal route is called vaginal hysterectomy. This procedure is mostly carried out for prolapse of the uterus and is called 'vaginal hysterectomy with pelvic floor repair' as in the operation simultaneously repair of anterior vaginal prolapse (cystocele, urethrocele) and posterior vaginal wall prolapse (rectocele and enterocele) is carried out. However, some gynaecologist perform vaginal hysterectomy in the absence of associated prolapse of the uterus, this procedure is labelled as 'nondescent vaginal hysterectomy'.

STEPS OF VAGINAL HYSTERECTOMY

1. Anaesthesia
2. Lithotomy position
3. Antiseptic preparation of operative area
4. Emptying bladder
5. Exposure of vaginal walls by placing Sims speculum, labial retraction suture and pulling cervix downwards by holding with a vulsellum
6. Placing a transverse incision on cervix at the lower limit of bladder
7. Separating vaginal mucosa from underlying bladder
8. Displacing bladder upwards till one reaches uterosacral fold of peritoneum and opening of peritoneum
9. Posteriorly opening of the pouch of Douglas
10. To clamp cut and ligating attachments of the uterus from below upwards (Mackenrodt's ligament, uterine vessels, fundal structures)
11. After removing the uterus, securing all the pedicles and checking haemostasis
12. Closure of vault
13. Repair of cystocele, repair of enterocele
14. Gentle packing of vagina and leaving behind Foley's catheter for a continuous drainage of urine

POSTOPERATIVE CARE

Postoperative care is important if surgical complications are to be avoided.

IMMEDIATE CARE (24 HOURS)

Vital signs such as

- Pulse, temperature, BP and respiration chart to be maintained.
- The patient needs intravenous fluid for first 24 hours. Following a minor surgery, oral fluids are allowed 4 hours after the surgery, and a soft diet is given on the day of surgery.

The average patient needs 2 L of fluid intravenously for 24 hours. This comprises 1 L of 5% glucose, 1/2 L of glucose saline and 1/2 L of Ringer's lactate to maintain electrolyte balance. If the woman vomits, extra fluid is required to make up for the loss.

- Intake–output chart should be maintained to monitor renal function as well as to decide on the amount of intravenous fluid required. Catheter for 24–48 hours prevents urinary retention.
- Antibiotics are best administered intravenously in the first 24 hours. The first dose is given during surgery. Later, oral antibiotics can be started. The choice of antibiotics depends on the surgeon, but it is prudent to administer i.v. metrogyl for the first 24 hours to combat anaerobic organisms in addition to other antibiotics.
- Analgesics are required for a day or two, and the choice depends on the need of the woman. Night sedation allows the woman to sleep well and wake up fresh. NSAID should be avoided in a woman with asthma and gastric ulcer.
- The patient should be observed for respiratory complications and pain in the legs (thrombosis).
- The abdomen is watched for distension and bowel sounds. Once the bowel sound returns, oral soft diet is started (Fig. 42.16).
- Urine culture should be obtained, if the indwelling catheter is placed for 2 days or more.
- The patient should be observed for vaginal bleeding. A slight bleeding is noted during the first few days, and this wears off gradually.
- Blood transfusion should be avoided as far as possible. If postoperative haemoglobin falls below 8 g%, iron therapy will restore it to normal. It should be noted that one unit of blood raises haemoglobin by just 1 g, with its other associated risks of blood transfusion.
- Early ambulation is practiced nowadays to avoid thromboembolism. The patient is advised to move out of bed once the intravenous fluid is stopped.
- Bowels should be moved with Dulcolax suppository or enema on the 3rd or 4th day once she is on a solid diet.
- The abdominal dressing should be changed on the third day and when the sutures are removed. Nowadays, subcuticular catgut suture for the skin does not require removal.
- The woman is normally discharged home on the 4th or 5th day of operation. The patient is advised against intercourse for 1 month.

Follow-up is done a month after the surgery to check all is well. The woman needs counselling regarding lifestyle, sexual activity and any special precaution. A woman operated for cancer needs prolonged chemotherapy and radiotherapy and should be under observation for recurrence.

Immediate Postoperative Complications are as Follows

- Haemorrhage
- Infection such as wound infection, chest infection, urinary infection
- Paralytic ileus
- Embolism
- *Burst abdomen.* Burst abdomen in gynaecological surgery is now rare with the use of Pfannenstiel incision.
- *Bowel perforation:* A rare complication which can occur in patients with extensive bowel adhesions (Fig. 42.1).
- Pelvic vein thrombosis with fever and tachycardia is less common with early ambulation and prophylactic antibiotics. CT is useful in the diagnosis of pelvic vein thrombosis. Heparin and antibiotic are needed.

Late sequelae are as follows:

- Scar site hernia
- Dyspareunia in vaginal surgery
- Abdominal adhesions causing chronic pain
- Recurrence of fibroids and endometriosis
- Recurrence of malignancy

KEY POINTS

- To make any surgery safe, preoperative and postoperative care are as important as the surgical technique.
- Preoperative care includes confirmation of the clinical diagnosis, assessment of the extent of the surgery required and making the patient fit for anaesthesia as well as surgery.
- Postoperative care looks after her nutrition, prevention of infection with appropriate and adequate antibiotics, prevents thromboembolism by early ambulation and makes this period as pain-free and comfortable as possible.
- D&C is a minor diagnostic procedure.
- Dilatation of cervix is required in a few cases.
- Endometrial study is required in AUB, secondary amenorrhoea and postmenopausal women suspected of endometrial cancer.
- Conization of the cervix is restricted to therapeutic procedure in young women with CIN III. As a diagnostic procedure, it has been replaced by colposcopic biopsy, LLETZ and LEEP.

SELF-ASSESSMENT

1. Discuss the indications of D&C.
2. What are the complications of D&C?
3. Discuss the role of conization.
4. Describe indications and steps of abdominal hysterectomy.

SUGGESTED READING

Hacker and Moore's Essentials of Obstetrics and Gynecology 2010.

43 Obesity and its Significance in Gynaecology

CHAPTER OUTLINE

Obesity is on an increase the world over. In India, the incidence is reported to be 10%–15%. Obesity affects menstrual functions, reproductive functions and other organ systems in the body with a profound effect on the incidence of PCOD, infertility, pregnancy outcome, endometrial cancers (increased) and a variety of menstrual irregularities. With an ever-increasing incidence of obesity, it looks like a major factor which will influence health of the people in the next few decades.

Obesity until recently was considered a cosmetic nuisance, personal issue and social problem, but now it is realized that it also poses a major health hazard in later years, causing morbid conditions and, at times, early death. Now considered a metabolic disorder, its prevalence has increased globally and threatens the health of the individual. Once acquired, it is difficult to get rid of, despite dietary control and exercise. It is therefore important to check the growth and weight of adolescents and adults before it creates health problems.

PREVALENCE

Increased prevalence over the previous years is because of several factors:

- *Lifestyle change:* Better social and economic environment has changed the lifestyle of people; overeating and overindulgence in wrong foods has led to obesity (fatty food)
- Lack of exercise because of heavy and prolonged hours at work, physical disability and sedentary life, causing less utilization of calories and accumulation of body fat
- Genetic
- Increased birthweight and maintenance of increasing weight through childhood and adolescence

DEFINITION

Obesity is defined in terms of body weight over height. Body mass index (BMI) is expressed as follows:

$$\text{BMI} = \frac{\text{weight(kg)}}{\text{height(m}^2\text{)}}$$

- Normal BMI is between 18 and 25.
- Below 18 is considered underweight.
- Between 25 and 29.9 is overweight.
- Between 30 and 35 is obese.
- BMI over 35 is considered morbidly obese.
- Waist-to-hip ratio should not exceed 0.8.

AETIOLOGY

Apart from the above-mentioned factors well known for gain in weight, obesity is considered a metabolic disorder originating in the fetus itself, partly contributed by mother's environment during pregnancy. Maternal conditions during pregnancy are overnutrition, glucose intolerance and diabetes, leading to macrosomic fetus. The metabolic changes in this fetus persist through childhood, adolescence and adulthood leading to overweight and obesity.

Other factors are as follows:

- *Genetic*: Family history reveals obesity.
- *Prepregnancy weight*: Overweight mothers gain more weight than normal women during pregnancy. They also retain increased weight gain postpartum, and put on some extra pounds or so following each delivery; multiparae therefore tend to be overweight compared to primis and those with lesser pregnancies.
- *Menopause*: Low metabolic rate and inactivity add to the woman's weight after the menopause.

- Overeating and eating wrong food also lead to obesity.
- Lack of exercise and sedentary lifestyle lead to an increase in the woman's weight.
- *Diseases:* Thyroid (hypothyroidism) and oedema occur because of hepatorenal disorders.
- *Drugs*: Corticosteroids over a prolonged period, androgens and oral hormonal contraceptives tend to increase the woman's weight.

PATHOPHYSIOLOGY

Bones make up 12% of the total body weight, muscles 35% and body fat 27%. The rest comes from other organs and blood and body fluid.

Of the total fat, abdominal and visceral fat (waist circumference) is linked to diseases in the adult life. Women tend to accumulate more fat over the abdomen than over the hips, as compared to men, they tend to suffer from obesity more than men.

Leptin (167–amino acid protein) is a hormone secreted by adipocytes in the fat that influences hypothalamus regarding appetite. Increased leptin increases fat accumulation. Leptin secretion is also regulated by insulin which stimulates leptin secretion. In pregnancy, some women develop insulin resistance, and hyperinsulinaemia may be responsible for excessive weight gain through fat deposition and retention of weight gain postpartum.

CLINICAL FEATURES

- *Age*: Pregnancy and menopause are linked to obesity in women.
- *Parity*: Multiparous women tend to be more overweight than less parous women.
- Family history (genetic) also leads to obesity.
- Many obese women are born overweight.

COMPLICATIONS AND SEQUELAE (Fig. 43.1)

- Obese adolescents tend to have precocious puberty which in turn reduces their height overall (see Chapter 6).
- There may be menstrual dysfunction because of hormonal and metabolic dysfunction.
- Polycystic ovarian syndrome (PCOS) is nowadays seen in young women who are overweight. They also demonstrate insulin resistance.
- Anovulatory infertility may occur because of anovulation and PCOS.
- The success of in vitro fertilization (IVF) in infertile obese women is reported to be low.
- Breast, uterine and colonic cancer are reported to be higher in obese women than in lean women.
- Stress incontinence of urine is more prevalent amongst overweight women.
- Fungal and urinary infection are more common in obese women.
- *Diseases*: Obese women tend to suffer more from the following medical problems than lean women:
  - Gall bladder stones
  - Cardiovascular disease, especially myocardial infarct
  - Stroke and osteoarthritis
  - Thromboembolism and pulmonary embolism
  - Respiratory problems such as asthma
  - Sleeping disorders

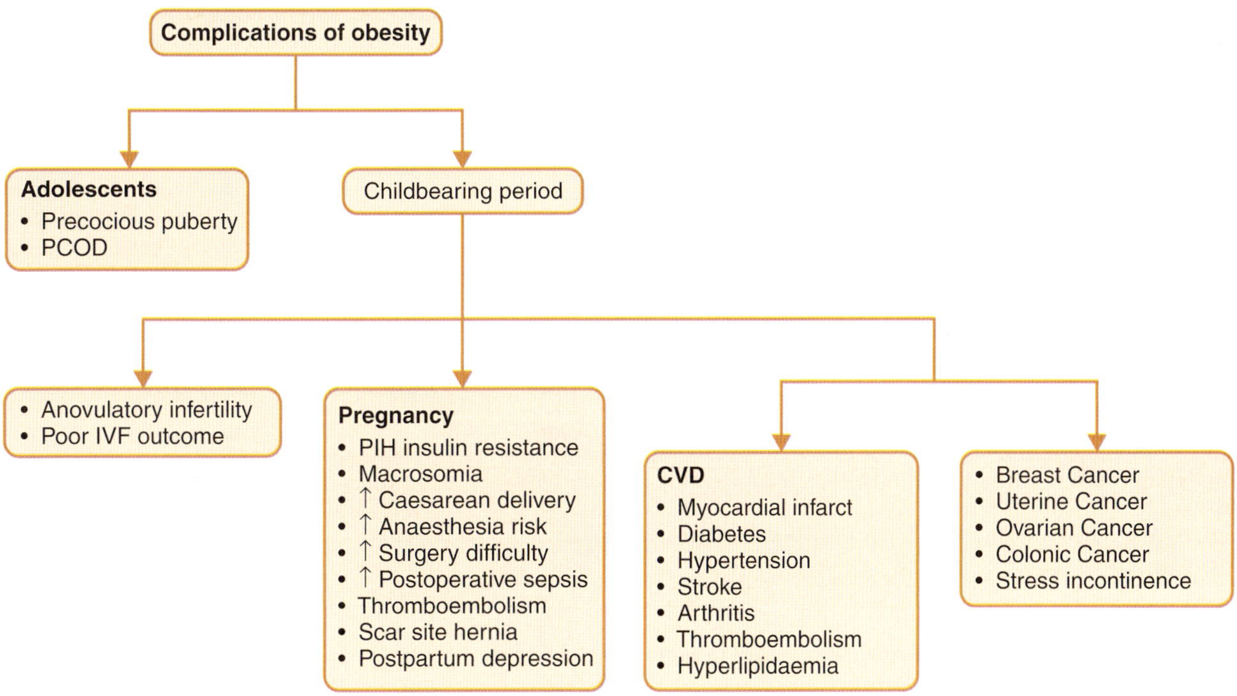

Figure 43.1 Complications of obesity.

  - Diabetes II
  - Hyperlipidaemia
- *Surgery:* It is difficult to procure a vein for intravenous drip during surgery.
  - Intubation during general anaesthesia and getting into an epidural space for spinal anaesthesia could be a problem.
  - Laparoscopic surgery is technically difficult.
  - During laparotomy, inadequate space and exposure of organs may make surgery difficult. Trauma to organs occurs more in obese women, so also bleeding during surgery.
  - Postoperative period may be complicated by infection, poor wound healing, thromboembolism and scar hernia.
- *Pregnancy*
  - Pregnancy-induced hypertension
  - Insulin resistance and gestational diabetes
  - Macrosomic baby
  - Increased incidence of caesarean section likely because of abnormal position caused by macrosomia, cephalopelvic disproportion and fetal distress
- *Postpartum complications:* Retention of weight gain, postpartum depression, thromboembolism and poor lactation. Poor lactation is seen in obese women. This, in turn, causes overweight infants through bottle feeding.
- *Contraceptives:* Hormonal contraceptives are contraindicated in obese women.
- Functional limitations because of overweight are well known.

MANAGEMENT

Management comprises:

- Prophylaxis (prevention)
- Treatment

PROPHYLAXIS

DIET

Proper balanced diet is the essential step in maintaining normal weight. A balanced diet should contain 60% carbohydrate, 20% protein and 15%–20% fat. Intake of diet with 1800–2000 cal daily is adequate, but also depends on body weight (body weight [kg] × 35).

A diet containing fibres delays absorption and lowers the glucose level.

Carbohydrates should be mainly of low glycaemic index. Animal proteins with amino acids are preferred.

EXERCISES

Yoga, meditation and regular exercises help in reducing weight. Rapid weight loss is not recommended, but 1 lb/week is safe.

Walking for half an hour daily for 5 days is sufficient to maintain weight.

PREGNANCY

- Prepregnancy weight should be normal. Overweight women should be asked to reduce weight before conception.
- Weight gain should be monitored regularly.
- Postpartum weight should be carefully monitored. Most women reduce weight and return to prepregnancy weight by the end of 3 months postpartum; otherwise, diet control and exercises are recommended.

Breastfeeding prevents obesity in infants. Obese infants tend to remain obese throughout life, exposing themselves to diabetes, hypertension, hyperlipidaemia and certain cancers.

MANAGEMENT OF OBESITY

- Diet
- Exercises
- Drugs – lipase, inhibitors
  - Orlistat
  - Rimonabant
  - Sibutramine
- Surgery – bariatric lipectomy
- Gene therapy

DRUGS

Lipase inhibitors are prescribed for obese women. These are as follows:

- Orlistat (Reshape) is an antiabsorbent of fat and 120 mg daily reduces 30% of fat absorption from intestinal tract. It also prevents absorption of fat-soluble vitamins which is a disadvantage. It also causes fatigue and depression.
- Rimonank reduces food intake.
- Sibutramine enhances safety and is thermogenic by inhibiting serotonin and noradrenaline reuptake. It acts centrally.

FETAL OBESITY

Apart from changing lifestyle, diet and exercise, the important cause of adult obesity and its sequelae is fetal obesity or what is also known as macrosomia. It is now realized that fetal macrosomia is because of a disorder in the maternal environment causes fat deposition in the newborn and infant. Metabolic disorder thus sets in and continues through adolescence and adulthood. Pregnancy adds to this metabolic disorder and increasing weight gain during pregnancy worsens the situation. Once obesity sets in, it is extremely difficult to shed it off. Various sequelae of diseases follow, impairing life and even causing early death (Table 43.1).

Prevention therefore lies in managing pregnancy, controlling weight gain and bringing back the original prepregnancy weight in the postpartum period. Controlling

Table 43.1 Classification of Disorders of Obesity

BMI	Classification
<18.5	Underweight
18.5–24.9	Normal weight
25.0–29.9	Overweight
30.0–34.9	Class I obesity
35.0–39.9	Class II obesity
>40.0	Class III obesity

preconceptional weight and avoiding obesity before pregnancy are also very important for optimal outcome for the individual and long-term health benefit.

TREATMENT

SURGERY

When medicines fail, surgery is resorted to as follows:

- Sleeve gastrectomy and gastric bypass surgery are two commonly done procedures for morbid obesity.
- Gastric Bypass surgery takes 3 hours to perform, but is a one-time procedure.
- Lipectomy may be helpful.
- Laparoscopic adjustable gastric band (Lap Band) takes half an hour to perform, but the band needs periodic adjustments, so follow-up is necessary.
- Gastrointestinal implantable electrical stimulation of nerves is being tried.
- Gene therapy may prevent obesity.

KEY POINTS

- BMI is used to rate a person as overweight or obese.
- Obesity poses many health hazards in adult life and some can be life-threatening.
- Common causes of obesity are well known and can be rectified.
- Gynaecological problems related to obesity are menstrual dysfunction, anovulatory infertility, PCOS and certain malignancies. IVF also yields poor results.
- Obstetric problems to obesity are considerable. Apart from maternal complications, fetal macrosomia is now considered a very important cause of adult obesity.
- Surgery increases morbidities in obese women in the form of infection, respiratory problems and thromboembolism.
- Medical problems in adults impair quality of life and may even cause early death.
- Prevent treatment, treatment of obesity often fails and can be frustrating.

SELF-ASSESSMENT

1. Discuss the hazards of obesity in reproductive functions.
2. Discuss the sequelae of obesity.

SUGGESTED READING

Green BB, Weiss NS, Daling JR. Risk of ovulatory infertility in relation to body weight. Fertil Steril 50(5): 721–726, 1988.

Laros, Abrams BF, Laros RK Jr. Am J Obstet Gynecol 154(3): 503–509, 1986.

Maggard MA, et al. J Am Med Assoc 300: 2286, 2008.

Rayburn WF. Clinics of North America 36(2), 2009.

WHO. Obesity. Technical report series, 894, 2000.

44 Instruments Used in Gynaecology

CHAPTER OUTLINE

A variety of instruments are used in gynaecology during clinical examination, minor and major operations. Following section describes these instruments.

INSTRUMENTS USED TO RETRACT VAGINAL WALL AND EXPOSE CERVIX

SIMS SPECULUM WITH ANTERIOR VAGINAL WALL RETRACTOR

This is the most commonly used instrument in gynaecological practices (refer chapter 42, Fig. 42.9). Its uses include:

- Exposure of cervix to obtain Pap smear or cervical biopsy
- Exposure of cervix to catch its anterior lip before minor and major operations on cervix, endocervix or endometrium

Disadvantage: Help of an assistant is needed if some procedure is to be performed.

Method of sterilization of instrument: It is done by autoclaving/boiling in water/placing in glutaraldehyde solution (Cidex) for at least 15 minutes.

CUSCO'S SELF-RETAINING SPECULUM

This bivalve speculum when introduced in vagina gives a good exposure of cervix for the purpose of OPD examination, obtaining Pap smear, obtaining cervical biopsy or removing a small cervical polyp (refer chapter 42, Fig. 42.13).

Advantage: It does not require the help of an assistant.

Disadvantage: It covers anterior and posterior vaginal walls; hence, conditions such as fistula in anterior or posterior vaginal wall can be missed.

Method of sterilization: It is done through autoclaving/heat boiling/Cidex.

INSTRUMENTS USED TO CATCH ANTERIOR LIP OF CERVIX

While performing any procedure on endocervix and endometrium, one needs to hold the anterior lip of cervix to stabilize the uterus. Some of these procedures are endometrial biopsy, endometrial aspiration for histology/cytology, endocervical biopsy, dilatation and curettage, hysteroscopy, HSG and those during laparoscopy.

Commonly used instruments for this purpose are tenaculum, vulsellum, long Allis forceps or a sponge-holding forceps in pregnancy.

TENACULUM

It has a single pair of teeth to grasp the anterior lip of cervix (Fig. 44.1). It is useful to catch the anterior lip of cervix for procedures where dilatation of cervix is not needed such as EB, EA, ECC, Copper-T insertion and HSG.

Disadvantage: If a force is used to pull on cervix, it can cut through substance of cervix.

Method of sterilization: It is done through autoclaving/heat boiling/Cidex.

To view the lecture notes scan the symbol or log in to your account on www.MedEnact.com

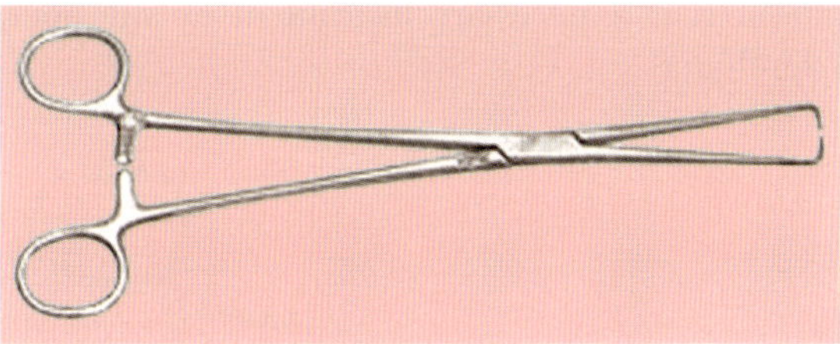

Figure 44.1 Tenaculum.

VULSELLUM

This instrument has three to four pairs of teeth at its catching end, thus giving a good grip of cervix. It is useful in procedures where dilatation of internal os needs to be carried out such as in dilation and curettage (D&C), hysteroscopy, removal of submucous polyp or fibroid or suction evacuation of pregnancy (refer chapter 42, Fig. 42.10).

Disadvantages: It may cause a small amount of pain while catching cervix. It cannot be used to catch pregnant cervix as it may cause local bleeding.

Method of sterilization: It is done through autoclaving/heat sterilization/Cidex.

LONG ALLIS FORCEPS

Long Allis forceps can also be used to catch the anterior lip of cervix but gives a poorer grip of cervix as compared to vulsellum. It may be desirable to catch the anterior lip of cervix in a pregnant state by either sponge-holding forceps or Allis forceps (refer chapter 42, Fig. 42.11).

Method of sterilization: It is done by autoclaving/heat sterilization/Cidex.

SPONGE-HOLDING FORCEPS

The anterior lip of cervix can also be held with a sponge-holding forceps especially in a pregnant state such as during McDonald stitch application or in a case of traumatic postpartum haemorrhage to explore cervix for tear (Fig. 44.2).

Method of sterilization: It is done by autoclaving/heat sterilization/Cidex.

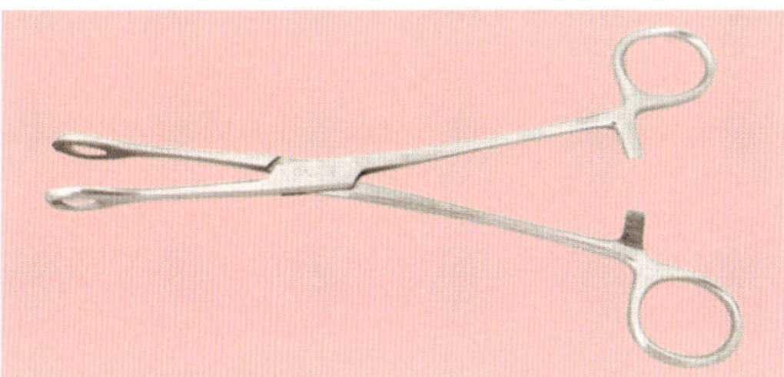

Figure 44.2 Sponge Holding Forceps.

INSTRUMENTS USED FOR DILATATION OF CERVIX

For a variety of conditions in gynaecological practice, one may have to dilate internal os of cervix to gain access to endometrial cavity. A number of metal dilators are used to dilate internal os such as Hegar dilator and Pratt dilator but slow dilatation of cervix can also be achieved by devices such as laminaria tent/Isabgol tent or by use of prostaglandin gels or tablets.

HEGAR DILATORS

This is the most commonly used metal dilator used to achieve dilatation of cervix. Dilatation of cervix is needed in a variety of gynaecological procedures such as D&C, fractional curettage, hysteroscopy and hysteroscopic procedures, for drainage of pyometra and haematometra. Dilatation of cervix is also needed for MTP and evacuation of missed abortion. Dilatation is a part of conservative operation for prolapse uterus (Manchester operation). In the management of cancer cervix by placing intrauterine source of irradiation, dilatation of os is needed.

Hegar dilator has two ends which are used for dilatation of os. Hegar dilators are available with various diameters which are numbered at the end of dilatation (refer chapter 42, Fig. 42.2).

Generally for gynaecological operations, dilatation up to number 7–8 is needed. However, for hysteroscopic procedures such as polypectomy, resection of septum and myomectomy, a greater degree of dilatation up to number 11–12 may be needed to be able to introduce resectoscope.

Complications with the use of dilators: It is a painful procedure; hence, adequate anaesthesia should be given as either general anaesthesia or local paracervical block anaesthesia.

Perforation of uterus: Introduction of Hegar dilator with force without adequate anaesthesia can cause perforation of uterus. Two common sites of perforation are just above internal os or fundus of uterus. Management of uterus requires immediate suspension of procedure, checking pulse and blood pressure, looking for signs of intraperitoneal bleeding and giving prophylactic antibiotics. Laparoscopy/laparotomy may be needed for features of intraperitoneal bleeding or sepsis.

OTHER TYPES OF DILATORS

A variety of cervical dilators are available; these include Hawkins (refer chapter 42, Fig. 42.4), Pratt, etc.

OTHER COMMONLY USED INSTRUMENTS IN VAGINAL GYNAECOLOGICAL OPERATIONS

UTERINE SOUND

This long, fine instrument is used to confirm the length of uterine cavity and its direction before insertion of Copper-T, before EA, D&C, hysteroscopy, etc. It can also be used to locate a misplaced Copper-T if strings of Copper-T are not visible on per speculum examination (refer chapter 42, Fig. 42.12).

Complication: It may lead to perforation of uterus.

BLUNT AND SHARP CURETTE

This metal instrument has blunt and sharp curette at two ends. It is used to curette endometrium in gynaecological and obstetric conditions. Generally, blunt is performed for a soft, pregnant uterus, whereas sharp end is used to curette for gynaecological conditions (refer chapter 42, Fig. 42.7).

Complications: Perforation of uterus, haemorrhage and excessive curettage give rise to adhesion formation in endometrial cavity (Asherman syndrome).

TUBAL INSUFFLATION CANNULA (RUBIN CANNULA)

It is used to introduce dye in uterine cavity during hysterosalpingography or diagnostic laparoscopy (Fig. 44.3).

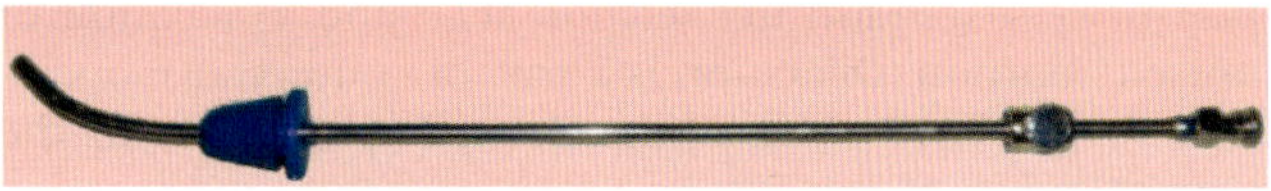

Figure 44.3 Rubin's Cannula.

INSTRUMENTS NEEDED FOR ALL GYNAECOLOGICAL OPERATIONS (ABDOMINAL OR VAGINAL SURGERIES)

SPONGE-HOLDING FORCEPS

This instrument is needed in all abdominal and vaginal operations. A gauge piece held at the tip of this forceps is used to clean operative field with antiseptic solution (Fig. 44.2).

In addition, this instrument is also used for a variety of other purposes during operations such as displacing bladder downwards away from cervix in caesarean, hysterectomy and other operations. In vaginal operation, it can be used to catch the anterior lip of cervix in a pregnant state; a polyp of cervix can be held with this instrument, twisted to be able to catch pedicle of polyp. For removal of Copper-T, threads of Copper-T are held with sponge holder and pulled downwards. While doing D&C for evacuating incomplete abortion or missed abortion, tissue visible at external os can be held with sponge holder.

ALLIS TISSUE FORCEPS

Available in various sizes, 6, 8 and 12 inches long, this instrument is used to catch edges of rectus sheath and edges of tissue being dissected. It is not used to catch vessel wall or soft structure as it will puncture them (Fig. 44.4).

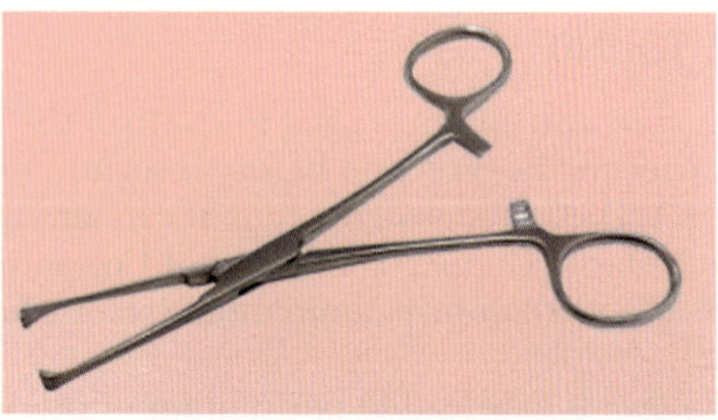

Figure 44.4 Allis Forceps.

ARTERY FORCEPS

It is available in various lengths and sizes with straight or curved ends and is used to catch bleeding points in abdominal operation. It is a necessary instrument in any operation (Fig. 44.5).

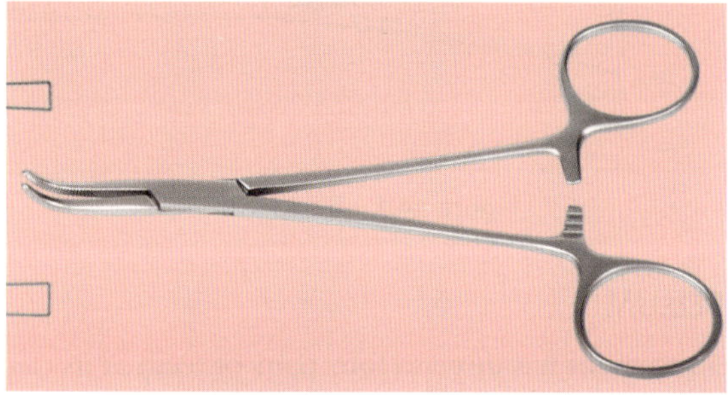

Figure 44.5 Artery Forceps.

BABCOCK FORCEPS

This necessary instrument is used for a variety of purposes. However, the most common use is to catch fallopian tube in tubectomy operation. Its ends are noncrushing, hence useful to catch other structures (Fig. 44.6).

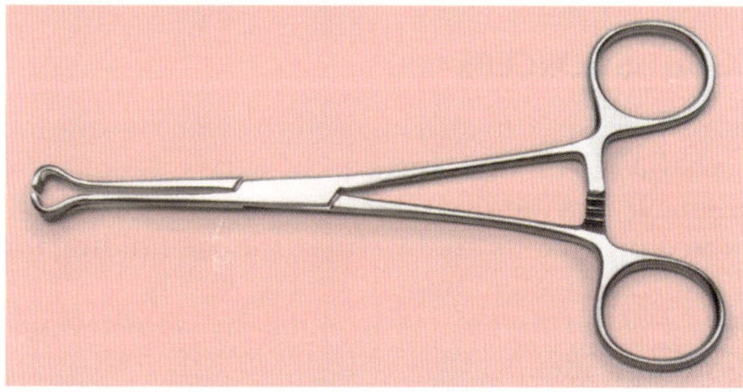

Figure 44.6 Babcock Forceps.

HYSTERECTOMY CLAMP

Available as straight or curved-tip instrument, it is extremely useful in performing abdominal and vaginal hysterectomies (Fig. 44.7).

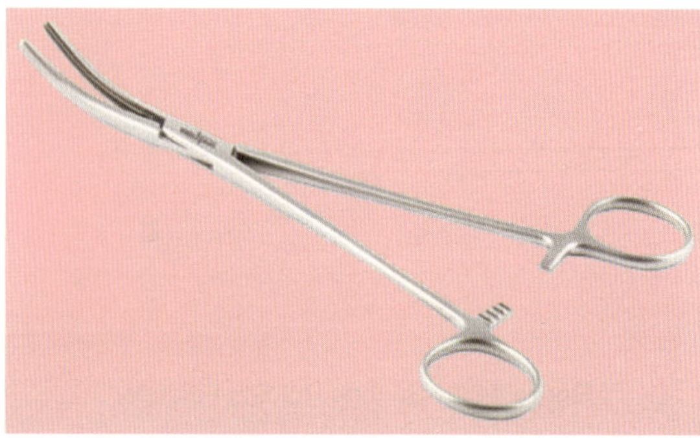

Figure 44.7 Hysterectomy Clamp.

TISSUE-CUTTING SCISSORS (METZENBAUM SCISSORS)

Available as slightly curved near tip, this instrument is used to cut rectus sheath, parietal peritoneum, tissues during hysterectomy, and surgery on fallopian tubes and ovaries (Fig. 44.8).

To avoid blunting of cutting edges, this instrument is sterilized by Cidex solution or E_2O sterilized. Autoclaving will lead to blunting of cut edges.

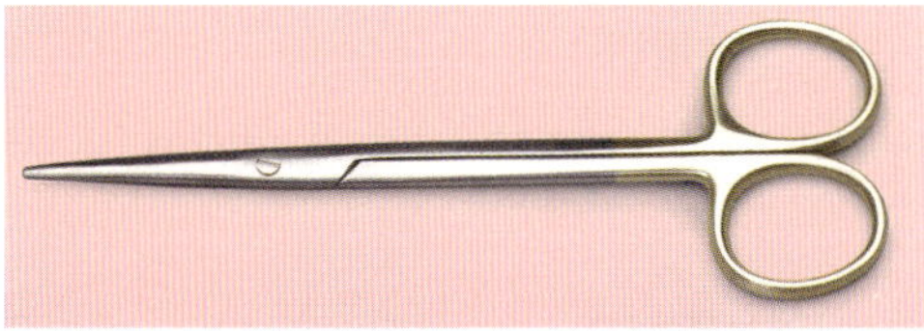

Figure 44.8 Metzenbaum Scissors.

SUTURE-CUTTING SCISSORS (MAYO SCISSOR)

Available in various sizes, this instrument is used to cut the ends of a tied suture. It is also sterilized by E_2O or Cidex solution. Autoclaving is avoided as it may result in blunting of cut edges (Fig. 44.9).

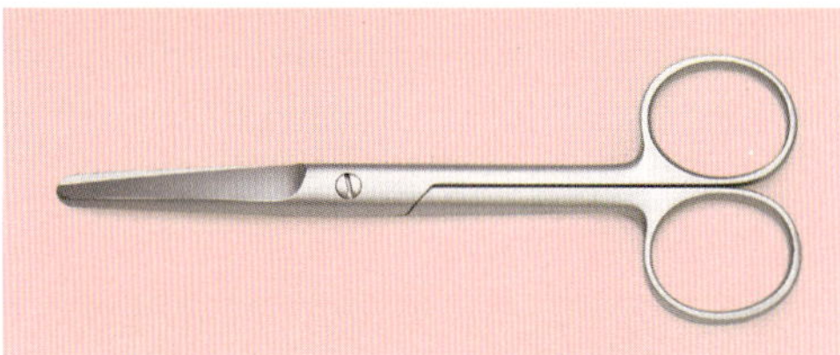

Figure 44.9 Mayo Scissors.

INSTRUMENTS USED IN SPECIALIZED PROCEDURES

MYOMECTOMY CLAMP AND MYOMA SCREWS

These are needed at times while performing myomectomy operation (refer chapter 13; Fig. 13.20 and 13.22).

TUBOPLASTY PROCEDURE INSTRUMENTS

These are fine instruments used to hold tubes while reanaesthetizing cut edges of tubes.

INSTRUMENTS IN VESICOVAGINAL FISTULA REPAIR

These curved fine instruments are used for exposure of margins of fistula, for dissection of bladder mucosa away from vaginal mucosa and for closure of fistula.

ENDOSCOPY INSTRUMENTS

These are described in the chapter 41 on Endoscopy.

INSTRUMENTS USED IN LAPAROSCOPY

Laparoscopic procedures have gained a lot of popularity in modern gynaecology. They allow early discharge from hospital with considerably less postoperative pain. However, all laparoscopic procedures require use of specially designed equipment. Most of these equipment are imported, are costly and require a very careful handling (Fig. 44.10).

SOURCE OF CO_2 GAS

It includes large or small-sized cylinders.

AUTOMATIC PNEUMOINSUFFLATOR

It indicates showing volume of gas insufflated, intraabdominal pressure and facility for automatic cut-off in case pressure becomes too high (Fig. 44.11).

ENDOVISION DISPLAY SYSTEM

It includes high-resolution TV monitor, a laparoscopic camera and a camera control unit (Fig. 44.12).

VERESS NEEDLES

Veress needles are used for insufflations of pneumoperitoneum.

TROCAR AND CANNULA

Usually a trocar with 10–11 mm diameter is used for introduction of telescope and a 5-mm trocar and cannula is used for introduction of hand instruments (Fig. 44.13).

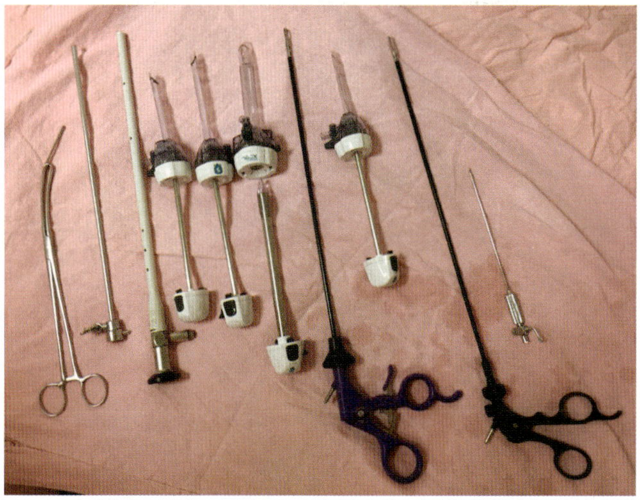

Figure 44.10 Instruments needed for diagnostic laparoscopy.

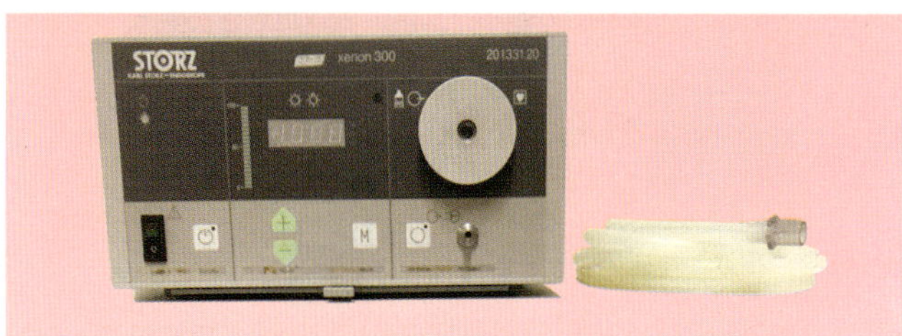

Figure 44.11 Cold light source.

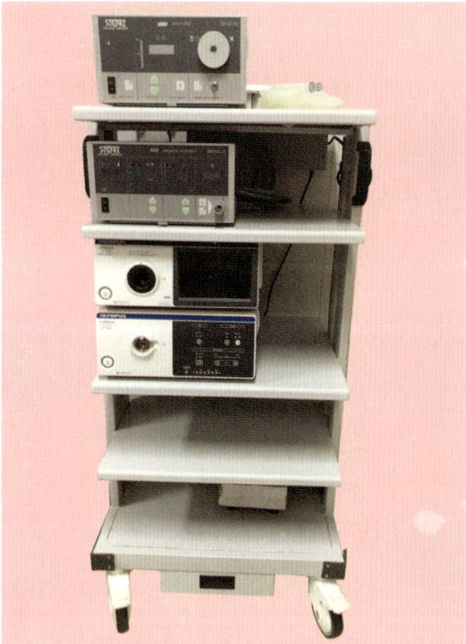

Figure 44.12A Endoscopy cart.

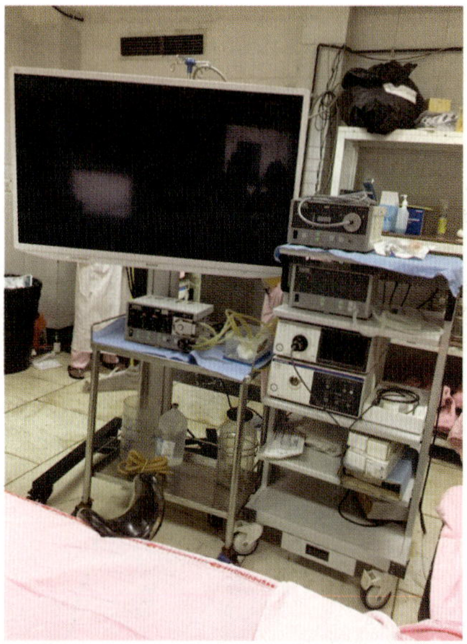

Figure 44.12B Endoscopy display system.

TELESCOPES

Telescopes of 10–11 mm diameter are used for visualization of pelvic and abdominal organs. Thinner telescopes of 4–5 mm diameter can be used for younger patients and for diagnostic procedures only.

COLD LIGHT SOURCE

For visualization of intraabdominal organs, a cold light source of xenon light is used.

HAND INSTRUMENTS

A variety of laparoscopic hand instruments are used depending on the procedure being undertaken. These include graspers, claw forceps, laparoscopic needle, laparoscopic Babcock, etc (Fig. 44.14).

VESSEL SEALING DEVICES

In advanced laparoscopic procedures such as hysterectomy, there is often a need for using Cautery source which may seal not only small size vessels but also medium size vessels. For this purpose a number of equipments are available, these include harmonic scalpel, ligasure and other similar devices as shown in Figs 44.15-44.18.

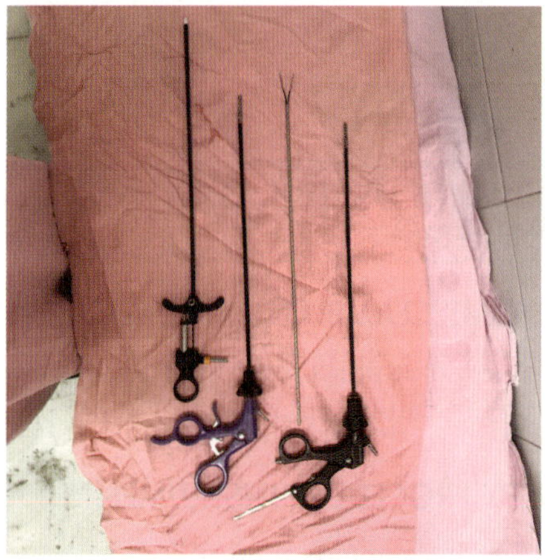

Figure 44.14 Instruments used for operative laparoscopy.

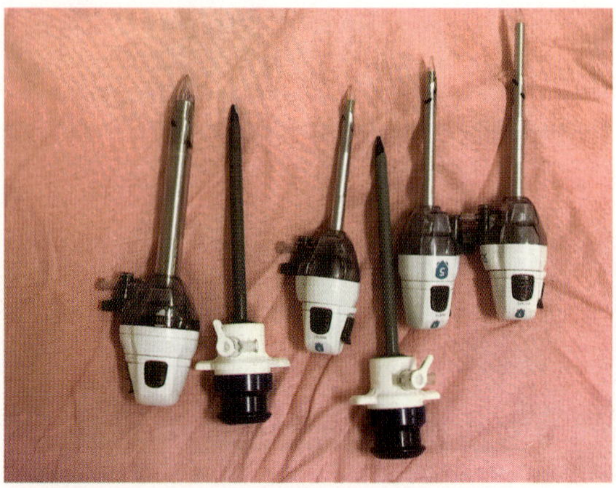

Figure 44.13 Disposable trocar and cannula.

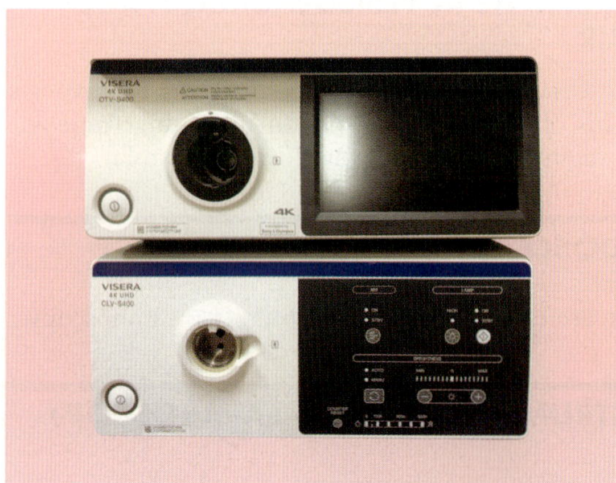

Figure 44.15 Vascular sealing device.

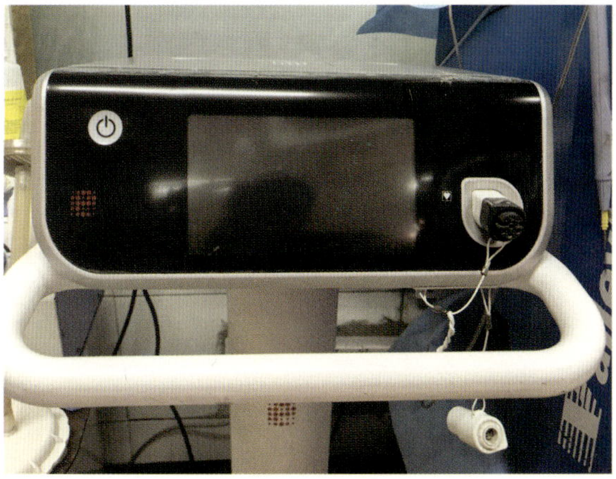

Figure 44.16 Harmonic device.

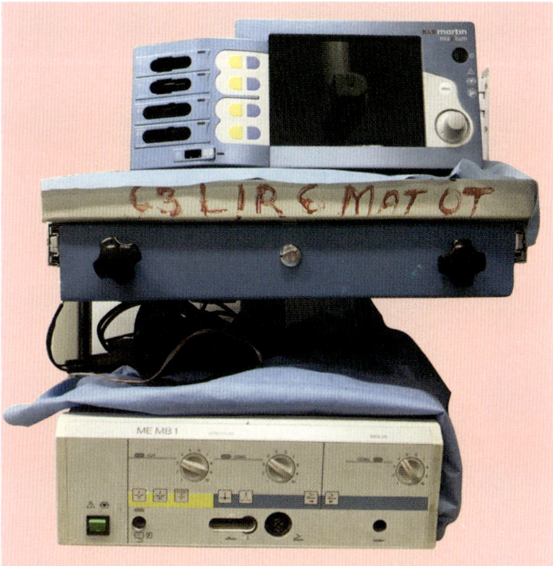

Figure 44.17 Unipolar and Bipolar Cautery.

INSTRUMENTS USED IN HYSTEROSCOPY AND HYSTEROSCOPIC OPERATIVE PROCEDURES

Close to list of equipment used in laparoscopy, a variety of equipment are used in diagnostic and operative hysteroscopy (Fig. 44.19).

TELESCOPES

These are generally 4 mm in diameter and are introduced with outer metal sheath. Mostly, the outer sheath has an inlet for introducing a distension medium. For operative hysteroscopy, an additional side channel may be available for introducing flexible instruments such as brush and biopsy forceps.

COLD LIGHT SOURCE

Some cold light sources used in laparoscopy can be used for hysteroscopy.

ENDOVISION DISPLAY SYSTEM

A system which is used for laparoscopy can also be used for hysteroscopy.

ENDOMETRIAL CAVITY DISTENSION MEDIA

Both saline and nonionic glycine are used as distension media during hysteroscopy. A check should be kept on the amount being pushed in and the amount which returns. A fluid deficit of more than 600–800 mL, especially if it is glycine solution, can lead to pulmonary oedema.

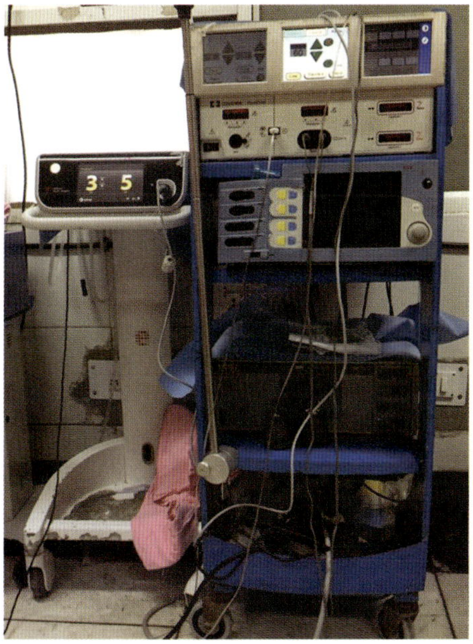

Figure 44.18 Vessel sealing device.

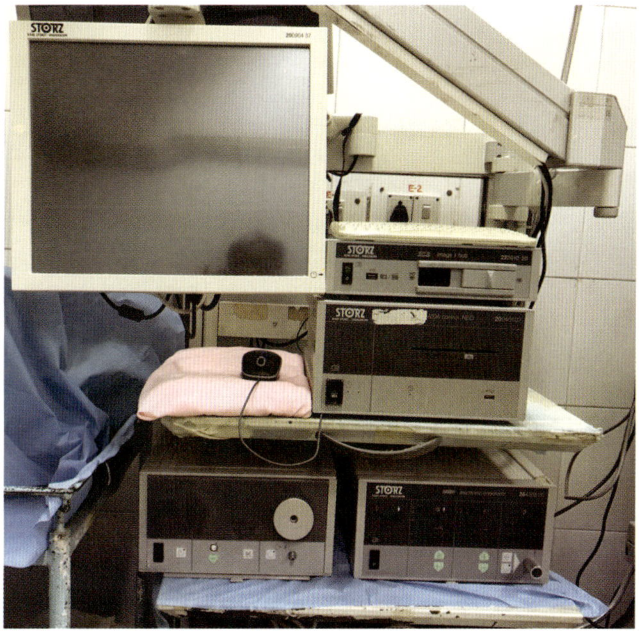

Figure 44.19 Instruments used for hysteroscopy.

AUTOMATIC FLUID INFUSION PUMP (HYSTEROMAT)

SPECIAL INSTRUMENTS FOR HYSTEROSCOPIC SURGERY

A variety of instruments are used for hysteroscopic procedures; these include Collin knife, TCRE resectoscope loupe, ball electrodes, graspers, etc.

STERILIZATION OF LAPAROSCOPIC AND HYSTEROSCOPIC EQUIPMENT

Because of risk of damage to fine optics and fine instruments, autoclaving is not preferred. There are special devices which are used to sterilize endoscopic instrument; one such device is called 'plasma'.

Index

Q

R

S

V

W

X

Y

Z